AF327169

ORTHOPAEDIC PATHOLOGY
A Synopsis With Clinical And Radiographic Correlation

GEORGE P. BOGUMILL, Ph., M.D.

Professor of Surgery (Orthopaedic)
Georgetown University
School of Medicine
Adjunct Associate Professor of
Orthopaedic Surgery
George Washington University
School of Medicine
Consultant, Orthopaedic and Hand Surgery
Walter Reed Army Medical Center
Attending Surgeon (Orthopaedic)
Veterans Administration Hospital
Washington, D.C.

HARRY A. SCHWAMM, M.D.

Chairman, Department of Pathology
The Graduate Hospital
Clinical Professor of
Orthopaedic Surgery (Pathology)
Department of Orthopaedic Surgery
Clinical Professor of Pathology
Department of Pathology
University of Pennsylvania
School of Medicine
Philadelphia, Pennsylvania

1984

W. B. Saunders Company

Philadelphia / London / Toronto / Mexico City / Rio de Janeiro / Sydney / Tokyo

W. B. Saunders Company: West Washington Square
Philadelphia, PA   19105

1 St. Anne's Road
Eastbourne, East Sussex BN21 3UN, England

1 Goldthorne Avenue
Toronto, Ontario M8Z 5T9, Canada

Apartado 26370—Cedro 512
Mexico 4, D.F., Mexico

Rua Coronel Cabrita, 8
Sao Cristovao Caixa Postal 21176
Rio de Janeiro, Brazil

9 Waltham Street
Artarmon, N.S.W. 2064, Australia

Ichibancho, Central Bldg., 22-1 Ichibancho
Chiyoda-Ku, Tokyo 102, Japan

Library of Congress Cataloging in Publication Data

Bogumill, George P.

Orthopaedic pathology.

Includes bibliographies.

1. Bones—Diseases.   2. Bones—Radiography.
  3. Orthopedia.   I. Schwamm, Harry A.   II. Title.
  [DNLM: 1. Bone and bones—Radiography.   2. Bone diseases—Pathology. WE 225 B675o]

RC930.4.B63 1984   616.7′1   83–8904

ISBN 0–7216–1169–9

Orthopaedic Pathology: A Synopsis with Clinical and Radiographic Correlation   ISBN   0-7216-1169-9

© 1984 by W. B. Saunders Company. Copyright under the Uniform Copyright Convention. Simultaneously published in Canada. All rights reserved. This book is protected by copyright. No part of it may be reproduced, stored in a retrieval system, or transmitted in any form or by any means, electronic, mechanical, photocopying, recording, or otherwise, without written permission from the publisher. Made in the United States of America. Press of W. B. Saunders Company. Library of Congress catalog card number 83-8904.

Last digit is the print number: 9   8   7   6   5   4   3   2   1

Dedication:
Lent C. Johnson, M.D.

The authors gratefully acknowledge the great debt owed to Lent C. Johnson, Chief of the Orthopaedic Pathology Branch at the Armed Forces Institute of Pathology for most of the years since the early 1940s. His concepts and philosophy form the basis of this volume. Aside from his refreshing refusal to accept the shibboleths of simply unacceptable dogma, there are the challenging definitions of the roles of the pathologist, surgeon, hospital, and Institute that remain with us long after our sojourn at the AFIP is over:

"The mission and uniqueness of the Institute is in the fashioning of its end product . . . the activity of the pathologists in supplying consultations that are reasoned explanations rather than mere diagnoses, in investigations that measure *time, place,* and *amount* of structural change, and in systematic teaching of a subspecialty as biology rather than gamuts of diagnostic criteria."*

"Pathology is the study of the *structure* of disease. Therefore we must understand the discipline of structure before we approach the structure of disease."*

"The study of structure is to biology what the study of astronomy is to physical sciences. Both are observational, involving the recording of increasingly refined details of structure and the relationship between structures. Both are nonexperimental and both are essential to the interpretation and the validation of experimental studies."*

"Disease involves no new biological mechanism. The cessation of biology is death. The essence of biology is the capacity to react. Extreme reactions, because one is no longer at ease, are considered "disease" . . . The disease from which a patient suffers is a function of his reactive state, rather than of the agent that triggers the reaction."*

"The basic principle of medicine is that disease results from disturbed function. The basic principle underlying pathology . . . is that any change of structure of necessity involves a change of function, and any alteration of function, if it persists, will eventually lead to a change in structure."*

"Perceiving all the ramifications of a disease in its cellular, focused and abscopal aspects involves:

a. assessment of changes in individual *cell*

b. exploration of the variations from one part to another of the *field* that represents the area of disease

c. search for alterations (at a distance from the site of disease) that indicate its *constitutional* reverberations."*

---

*Johnson, L. C.: Internal memo, AFIP, and repeated admonitions, 1970 to present.

"Measuring the impact of disease involves:

a. *time:* the relation of duration to anatomic changes and the sequences or stages of disease
b. *place:* the relation of zones of anatomic changes to the intensity of disease
c. *amount:* the quantitation of the various kinds of anatomic changes; at different stages and in different zones."*

This volume is our modest effort to use the principles of morphologic analysis as taught by Dr. Johnson. It is our intent to demonstrate that morphologic analysis provides data to indicate what has been, what is, and what may be expected. It is evidence to unravel a dynamic process, much as the anthropologist uses the single fragment of fossilized bone to reconstruct not only the physiognomy of the individual but also his niche in the dynamic evolutionary process. If the effort is successful, it is a tribute to Lent Johnson.

GEORGE P. BOGUMILL
HARRY A. SCHWAMM

---

*Johnson, L. C.: Internal memo, AFIP, and repeated admonitions, 1970 to present.

Preface

The analysis of orthopaedic disease requires marriage of the radiograph with the microscope. The orthopaedic surgeon will always interpret his own films and, indeed, argue at length with his radiologic colleagues. He should not shy away from the pathologist but rather strive to gain equal confidence with the images of the microscope. The pathologist, in turn, should venture into the realm of the view boxes, understand the significance of radiographic appearance, and not stake his whole reputation (and the patient's fate!) on the microscopic analysis of scattered tissue fragments, whose precise site of origin is not always clear. After all, the radiograph is simply a representation of the gross anatomy. This book therefore attempts to document the microscopic changes that lead to changes in radiographic appearance. *Understanding* the change, rather than simply labeling it, is the key to successful therapy.

We have deliberately emphasized morphology at the expense of basic physiologic and biochemical concepts in an effort to confine this book to a study of structural alterations. Because of the importance of early development and growth of the skeleton as the basis for understanding of disease processes, we have stressed skeletal embryology. The difficulties of diagnosis have prompted the inclusion of a final chapter in which apparently similar entities are discussed from a differential diagnostic viewpoint. An inclusive text of moderate proportions such as this one is of necessity brief, confined to the salient features and limited in scope. The profuse illustrations are intended to form a separate sequential entity of their own, expanding upon as well as visualizing material from the sparse text.

The Orthopaedic Pathology Branch of the Armed Forces Institute of Pathology, under the leadership of Lent C. Johnson, M.D., has played a significant role in the education of orthopaedic surgeons, pathologists, and radiologists since the early 1940s. Numerous courses have been conducted for the study of orthopaedic pathology. Teaching sets have been developed, and this book is an extension of the material from the study sets at the Institute, prompted by the numerous requests for a source to use after completion of the AFIP course. We have added extensive case material from our own experience.

The cooperative efforts of physicians from many federal and civilian institutions provided much of the initial study material. Many physicians participated in the preparation of study sets and the direction of courses that ultimately led to this book. A partial list includes Roger Terry, Jack D. Hansen, John R. Archdeacon, James J. Schubert, Byron A. Genner, III, Morris A. Schultz, David F. Henges, Robert G. Kindred, H. Todd Stradford, Robert Brown, Harold R. Noer, Charles E. Nye, Barton K. Slemmons, Alfred O. Heldobler, George E. Omer, Robert E. Cranley, Jr., Claude A. Leukens, Jr., Monroe I. Levine, James J. Hamilton, William L. Thompson, Elios G. Theros, Richard K. Cavanaugh, Robert M. Allman, and John E. Madewell from the Armed Forces and James W. Milgram. Doctors Donald E. Sweet and Bruce D. Ragsdale of the Institute have continued in the tradition of open-door willingness to consult in depth on any problem and have provided photos of recent cases.

This book could not have been written without the arduous work of our secretarial staff, in particular Nancy Park, who performed miracles through her expertise with word processing equipment and patiently labored through endless text revisions while two geographically separated, somewhat stubborn coauthors went through the penultimate revision of the revision. Linda Wassman and Mara Weitzman assisted in the revisions and corrections of the manuscript. Gary Pfaff labored to produce all the original photographic material in this text. The medical illustration section of the Armed Forces Institute of Pathology processed many of the gross specimens, radiographs, and histologic material, ultimately incorporated into the text. To all our colleagues, associates, and friends who contributed to this text, our heartfelt thanks. To our wives, Bonnie and Ruth, our gratitude for their patience and forbearance during our preoccupation with this project.

Finally, we salute those who by their courage and example spur us on to achieve our goal.

GEORGE P. BOGUMILL
HARRY A. SCHWAMM

Contents

1

NORMAL DEVELOPMENT AND GROWTH

The development of the musculoskeletal system follows a pattern of sequential formation, maturation, and removal of mesenchymal tissue. Cartilage is formed, only to be removed and replaced by bone. Bone itself is removed and replaced by more mature bone. The process is continuous throughout life; we never cease to "grow." The adult skeletal system undergoes formation and removal in response to increasing or decreasing mechanical demands. Bone is viable tissue; therefore, inactivity will result in loss of bone; exercise increases not only muscle mass but also the mass and quality of bone. The remodeling processes of the fetus are adapted and persist throughout the life of the individual.

LIMB BUD DEVELOPMENT

A limb bud is first seen on the 4-week embryo as a rounded prominence on the lateral body wall (Fig. 1–1). During the next 10 to 14 days, the limb bud rapidly elongates. The end of each bud becomes shaped like a mitten, with longitudinal ridges indicating the site of future metacarpals. Small projections on the rim of the "mitten" become digits. Lower limb development begins approximately 1 week later than upper limb development (Fig. 1–2), and this craniocaudal lag persists throughout gestation. By the end of the seventh week, rapid differentiation has resulted in well-defined fingers and toes.

Because early limb buds develop from the unsegmented mesoderm (somatopleure) of the lateral body wall, they are unrelated to somite formation. Each bud consists of an ectodermal covering and a central condensation of mesoderm. The apical ridge ectoderm is an essential antecedent to the development of additional mesenchymal structures. Poisoning of the epithelium (e.g., with thalidomide, phenytoin, radiation) interrupts epithelial development, and, consequently, further mesenchymal (i.e., skeletal) development is altered or even arrested.

Differentiation of the limb structures proceeds in a proximal to distal sequence. Thus, the shoulder girdle, arm, elbow, forearm, wrist, and hand differentiate and

1

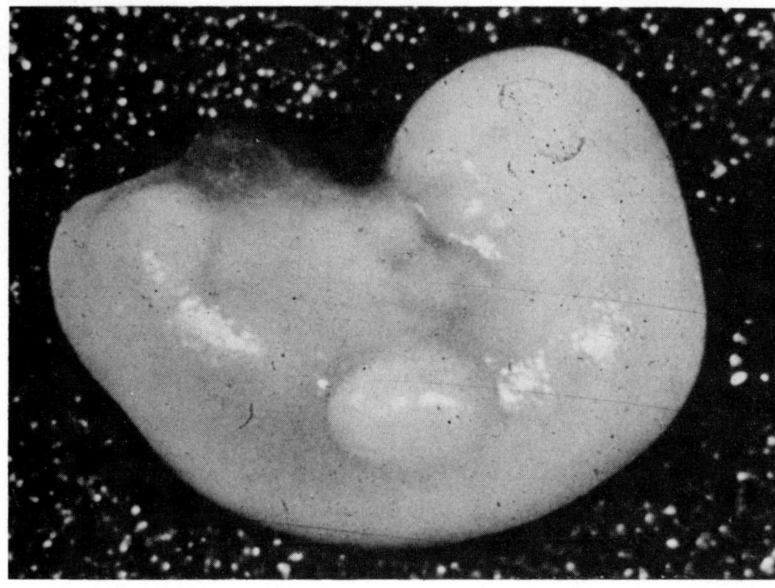

Figure 1–1. Fetus, approximately 4 weeks' gestation. Each limb bud is visible as a rounded eminence on the lateral body wall.

develop sequentially and not simultaneously. Rapid reproduction of mesenchymal cells results in a condensation of cellular material within the core of the limb bud. Mesenchymal cells are totipotential. Within certain limits, they are able to modulate into any of the skeletal structures of the field in which they are placed. The condensed cells in the center of the limb bud form the cartilage, whereas similar mesenchymal cells near the surface of the limb bud modulate to form skeletal musculature, tendon, periosteum, blood vessels, and fat (Fig. 1–3). At any age and under appropriate circumstances (e.g., trauma) blastema formation, or reversion to mesenchymal status, occurs, and cells regain their ability to transform and modulate into the differentiated structures of the musculoskeletal system. Nerves are the only structures present in the fully mature limb that do not develop in situ. They extend outward from the central nervous system into the base of the limb bud and attach themselves to developing muscles and other structures. Since the limb buds develop in the lower cervical and lumbar regions, nerve plexuses that supply the limbs originate in the cervical and lumbosacral regions of the spinal cord.

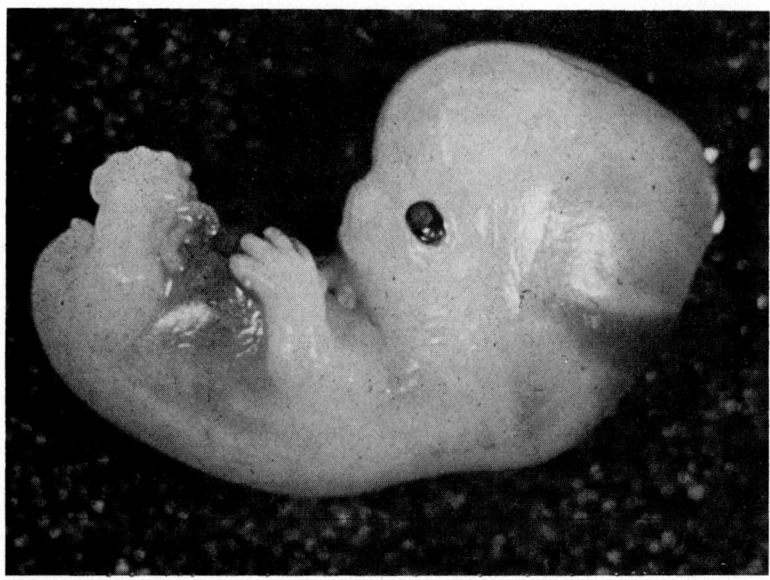

Figure 1–2. Fetus, approximately 6 to 7 weeks' gestation. Limb bud development exhibits craniocaudal lag. Identifiable digits are present on the upper extremity, but incomplete development with ridges on a "mitten" is present in the lower extremity.

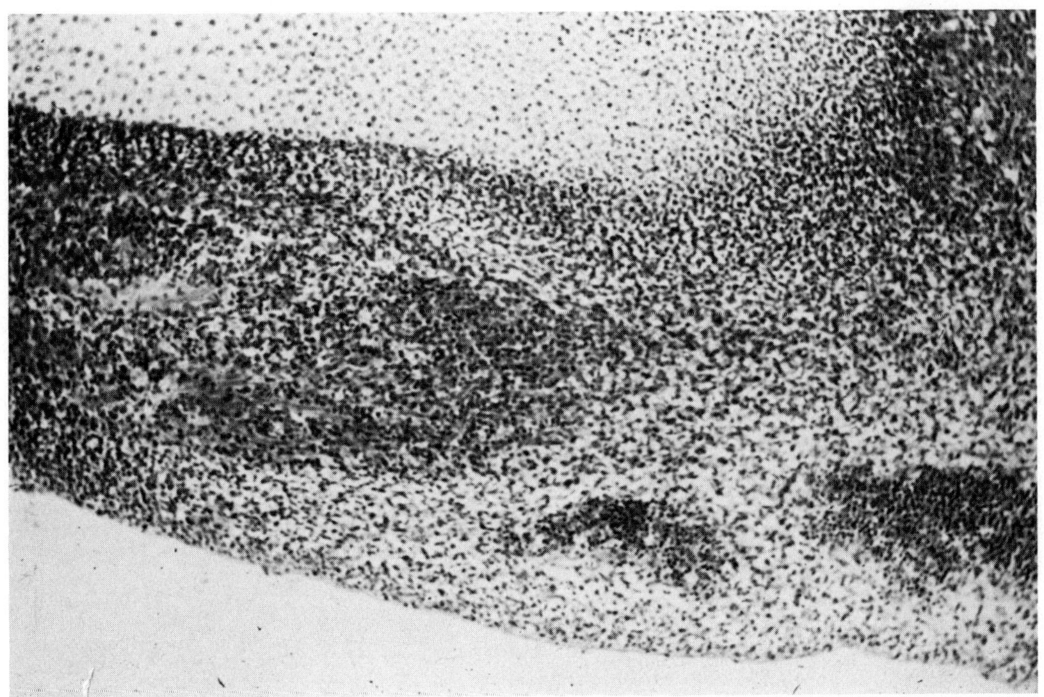

Figure 1–3. Histologic study of fetus, approximately 4 weeks' gestation. Undifferentiated mesenchymal tissue within the limb bud, with early central condensation forming "anlage" of musculoskeletal structures.

BONE FORMATION

In the sixth week of embryonic development, cells in the core of the limb bud secrete a matrix about themselves and form the cartilage model of future osseous structures. By the end of the embryonic period (8 weeks), most of the skeleton is cartilaginous (Fig. 1–4).

The cartilage model represents only one form of bone formation, the "endochondral" type. All bones in which there is no specific cartilage model, but instead a direct transition from fibrous stroma to bone, form by "intramembranous" ossification. Because cartilage as well as the fibrous mesenchymal tissue must be removed to make room for bone, more appropriate terms are "collagen model bone" for intramembranous ossification and "cartilage model bone" for endochondral ossification. In actuality, bone is formed by a combination of the two processes. The distal portion of the distal phalanx of all digits is formed by direct transition from primitive connective tissue (collagen model), but the shaft is preformed in cartilage (cartilage model) (see Fig. 9–141A). The skull vertex, clavicle, mandible, and other facial bones form primarily from the mesenchymal matrix (collagen model). The clavicle and mandible acquire cartilage growth centers at their ends to provide for longitudinal growth (Fig. 1–14). The progressive thickening of the diaphyseal shafts of all long bones, which contributes a majority of bone mass to any given long bone, is a result of appositional bone growth from the outer periosteum (i.e., collagen model bone). Thus, bone is formed through a combination of both processes, and "collagen model" (intramembranous) and "cartilage model" (endochondral) bone formation refers only to the initial model, not the entire process.

Regardless of prior model, all bones in the body are produced by osteoblasts. Osteoblasts synthesize and extrude collagen fibrils. Intramolecular cross-linkage is required prior to mineralization. During this "maturation," unmineralized osteoid can be identified and the rate of osteoid formation can be established by tetracycline

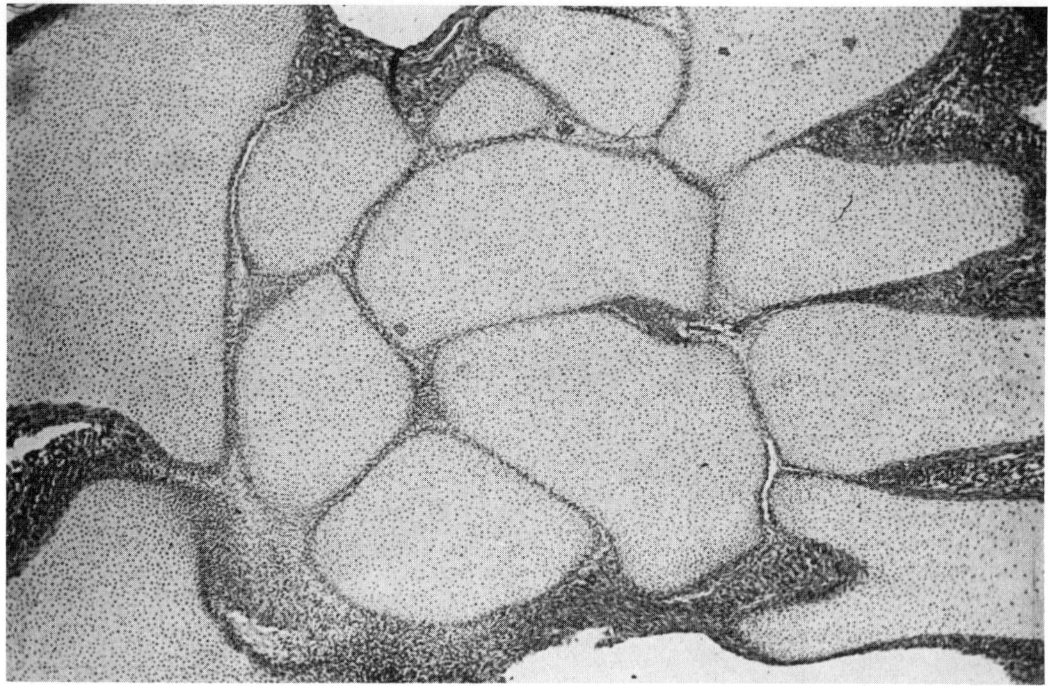

Figure 1–4. Histologic study of fetus, approximately 3 months' gestation. Chondrification of mesenchymal model tissue will form the more mature cartilage and joint structures. Secretion of matrix by the mesenchymal cells has resulted in bars of cartilage separated by noncartilaginous interzones.

labeling. The precise mechanism of calcification is a matter of controversy. It may be spontaneous ion precipitation, creation or unmasking of nucleating sites, or removal of substances, such as proteoglycans, that prevent mineral formation. Possibly all three mechanisms play a role (Teitelbaum and Bullough, 1979).

Once the bones are formed, there is no identifiable difference in those from various body regions, and there is no structural difference between endochondral and intramembranous bone (see discussion of bone structure, p. 37).

THE PRIMARY OSSIFICATION CENTER

The initial formation of bone consists of a sleeve surrounding the central portion of the cartilage model. This "sleeve," "collar," or "ring of Ranvier" is formed by direct transition from the mesenchymal connective tissue (periosteum) surrounding the cartilage model (Fig. 1–5). As the cartilage skeleton enlarges, distinct zones are established. The cells in the central portions proliferate, secrete matrix, hypertrophy, absorb water, and die. The secreted matrix left behind is dehydrated, becomes calcified, and provides the lattice framework on which bone formation occurs.

Dead cartilaginous cells induce vascular buds to grow in from the periosteum, and possibly vessels enter cartilage prior to the death of the cell. Whatever the process, the end result is the same: vascular invasion of the skeletal anlage. Blood vessels are accompanied by undifferentiated mesenchymal cells capable of forming the differentiated structures of the skeleton, including osteoblasts, osteoclasts, fat cells, vessels, and marrow elements. Cellular debris is removed, and osteoid is formed and deposited on the remaining calcified cartilage. The combination of sleeve bone, calcified cartilage matrix and bone is known as the "primary ossification center" (Figs. 1–6 to 1–8). Once the central portion of the cartilage model has been replaced by the primary

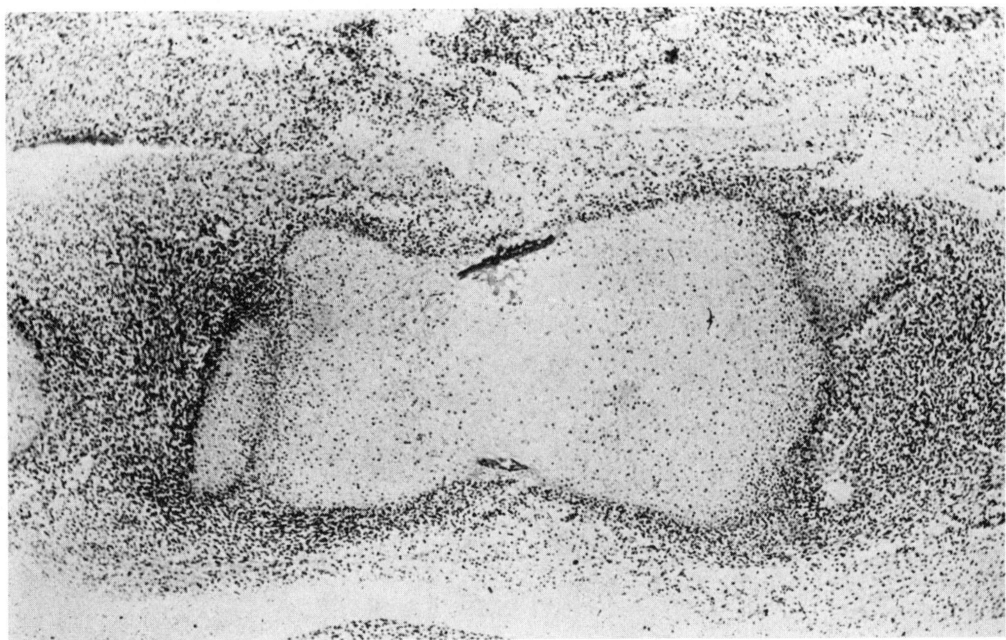

Figure 1–5. Histologic study of fetus, approximately 8 weeks' gestation. Earliest ossification is depicted here. A sleeve, or collar, of bone is present on the outer surface of the cartilage model.

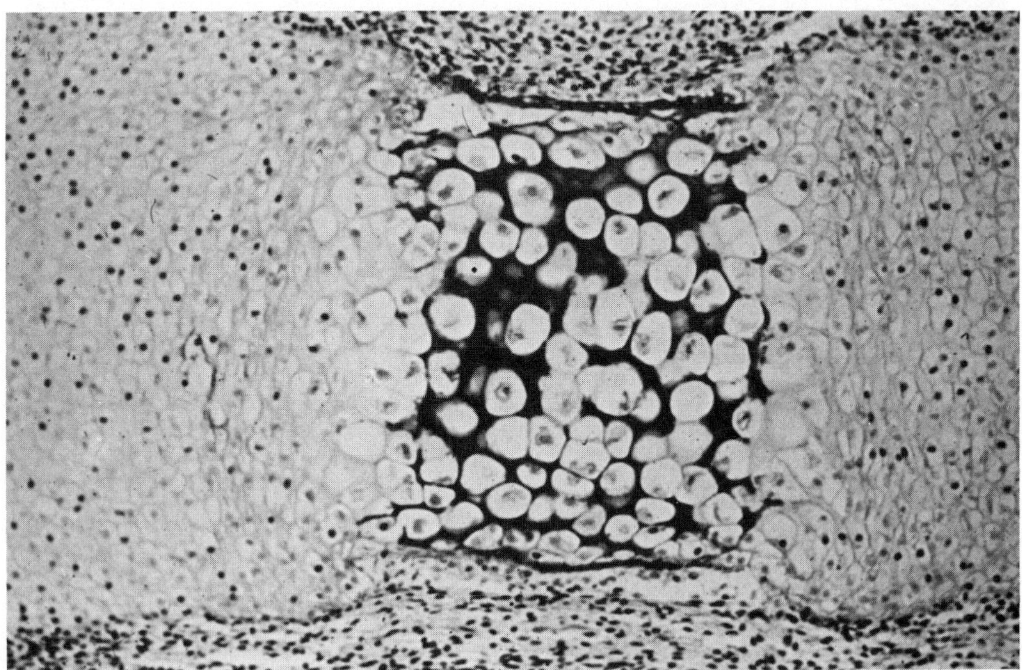

Figure 1–6. Histologic study of fetus, approximately 10 weeks' gestation. The central cartilage cells have hypertrophied, and many are undergoing necrosis. The intercellular matrix is calcified, and vascular invasion is beginning at the periphery. A thin sleeve of bone is present at the periphery of the cartilage. This combination of calcified cartilage core and sleeve bone collar constitutes the primary ossification center.

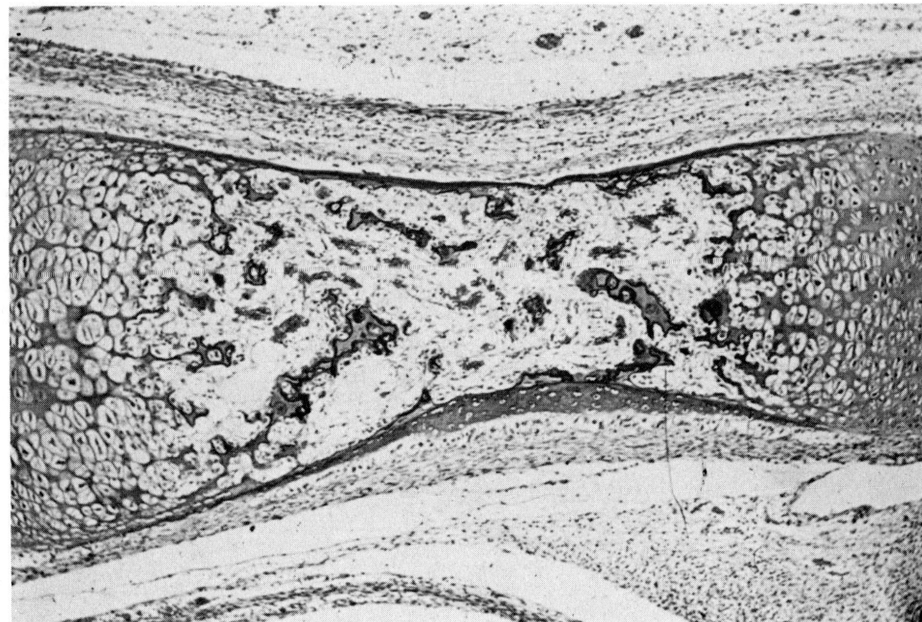

Figure 1–7. Primary ossification center of fetus, approximately 14 weeks' gestation. The cartilage cells have been removed almost entirely from the center, leaving remnants of acellular cartilage matrix. Bone deposits on the cartilage remnants will form primary trabeculae. Note that the primary sleeve, or collar, of bone has extended along both margins and is located adjacent to the hypertrophied cartilage at each epiphyseal end.

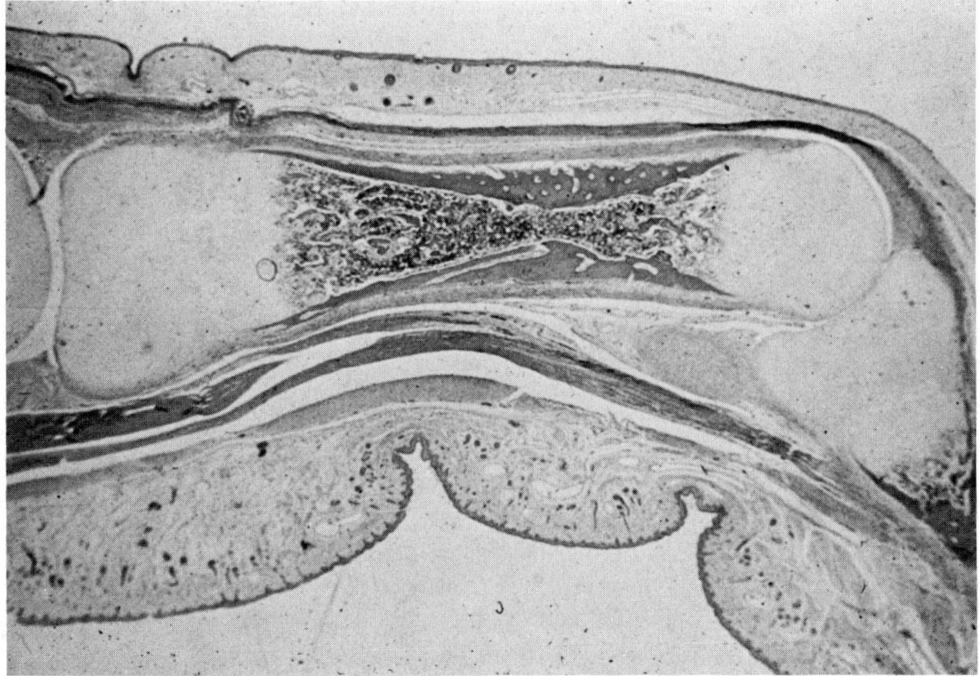

Figure 1–8. Primary ossification center, near term. There is complete replacement of cartilage in the diaphyseal portion of the cartilage model. The remaining cartilage is confined to both epiphyseal ends of the model. Note the increasing thickness of the cortical portion of bone, which is a result of conversion of periosteum to bone. A light-staining cambium layer is identifiable. The narrowest portion of the shaft is the site of initial vascular invasion and remains identifiable throughout life in many bones, especially in hands and feet. The eccentric position of this narrowed area indicates the disproportionate contribution to growth in length from each epiphysis.

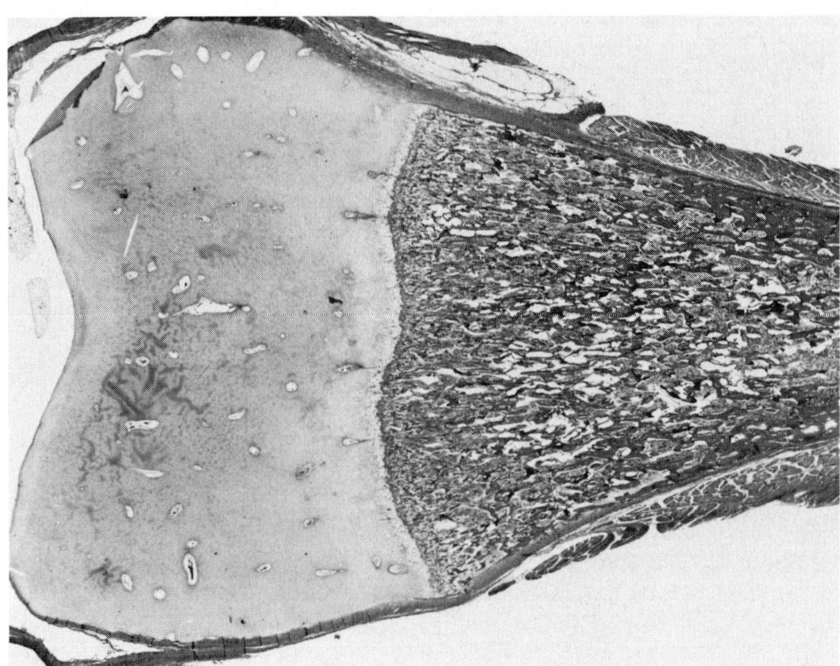

Figure 1–9. Histologic study of fetus, approximately 30 weeks' gestation. There is a fully developed primary ossification center, but as yet there is no evidence of ossification in the cartilaginous epiphysis.

Figure 1–10. Histologic study of fetus, 30 weeks' gestation, exhibiting numerous cartilage canals. These canals contain arterioles and venules with no associated capillary network.

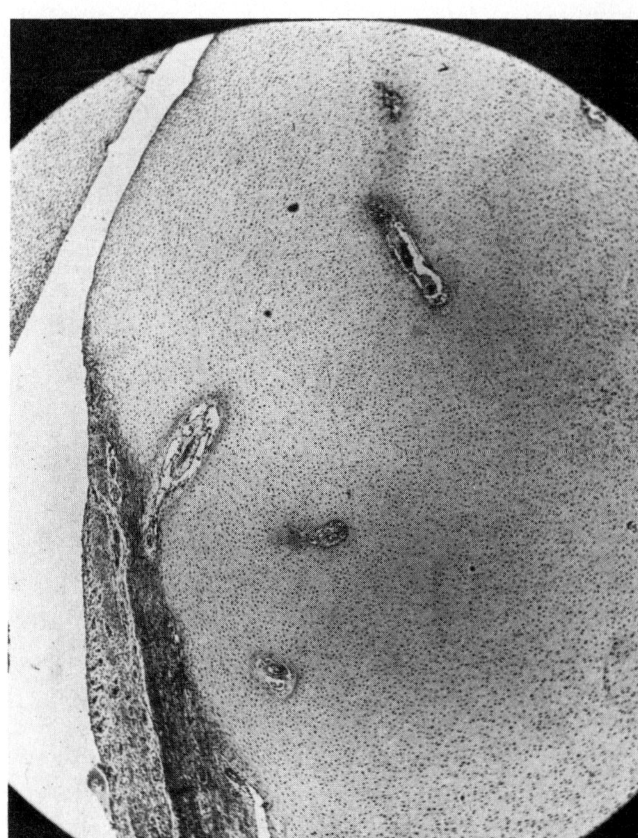

ossification center, the process progresses towards each end of the cartilage model. By birth, most of the long bones have been ossified through a major portion of their length.

SECONDARY OSSIFICATION CENTER

The development of the primary ossification center results in a shaft of bone with a cartilaginous cap at either end. As this epiphyseal cartilage mass increases in size it incorporates adjacent vessels, forming cartilage canals in the midst of the cartilage ball, but there is no associated capillary network (Figs. 1–9 to 1–11). At different times for each bone, epiphyseal maturation of cartilage occurs, similar to the maturation and transition noted in the primary ossification center. Secretion of matrix, hypertrophy, and death of cartilage cells is followed by vascular invasion and removal of the dead cellular material. Invasion of the cartilage matrix originates from vessels at the periphery as well as from vessels located within the cartilage canals. This secondary ossification center continues to enlarge until it is surrounded by a thin rim of articular cartilage at the surface and a thin strip of cartilage separating the epiphysis from the metaphysis. This layer of cartilage becomes the growth plate (epiphyseal plate, physis) (Figs. 1–9 to 1–13).

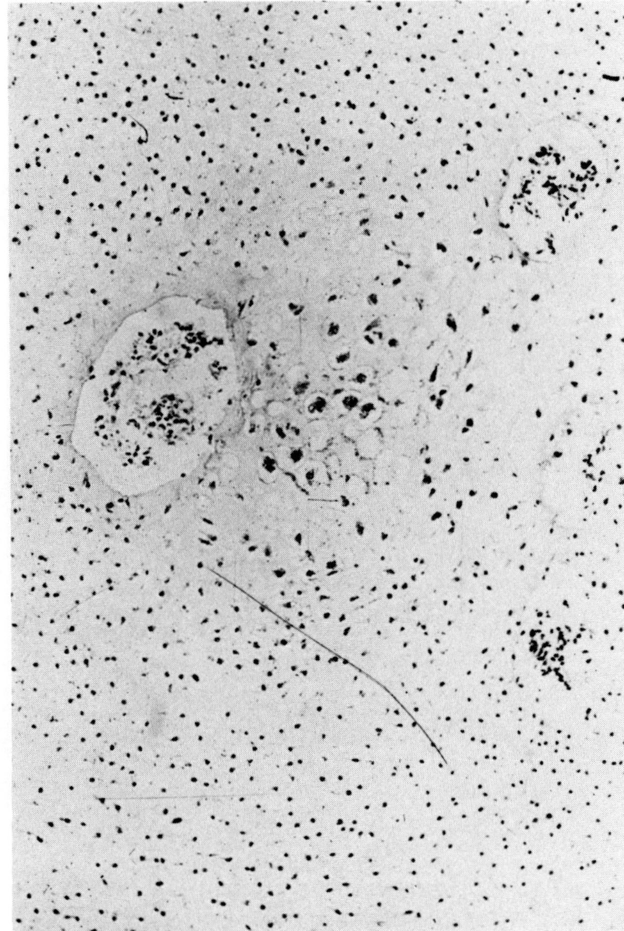

Figure 1–11. Higher magnification of early secondary ossification center. Hypertrophy of epiphyseal cartilage cells between three cartilage canals is evident.

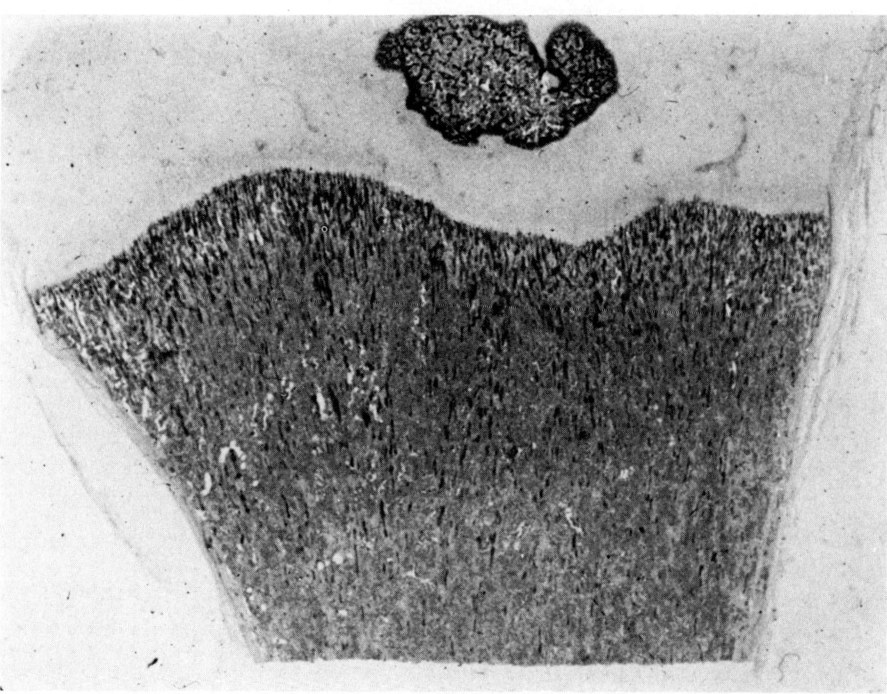

Figure 1–12. Early secondary ossification center of mature fetus. The formation of the secondary ossification centers in the lower tibia and upper femur coincide with fetal maturity. The secondary center does not begin in the center of the epiphysis, but nearer the growth plate. Expansion, therefore, is eccentric.

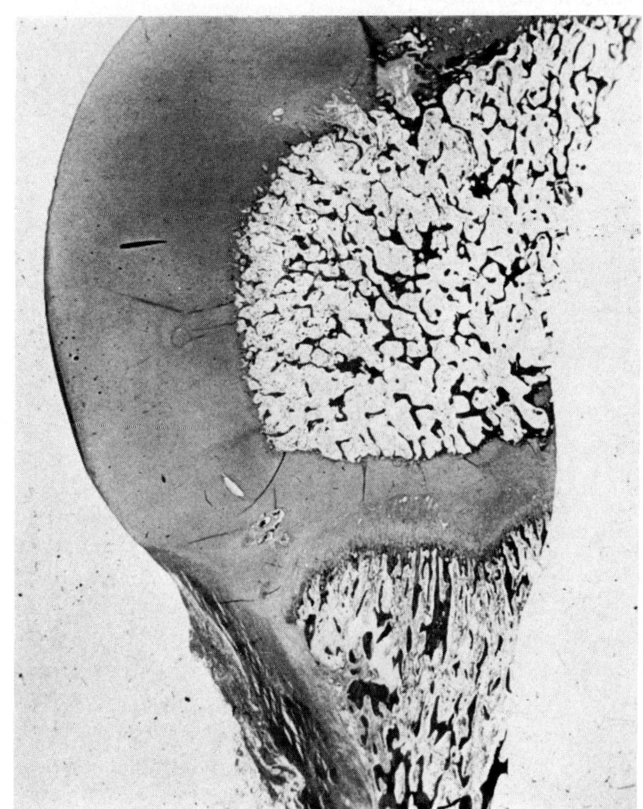

Figure 1–13. Histologic study of adolescent. Note the expansion of the secondary ossification center by conversion of the remaining epiphyseal cartilage model to bone. The histologic changes of cartilage maturation, removal, and replacement by bone are evident at the rim of this secondary center, especially where it expands towards the articular surface.

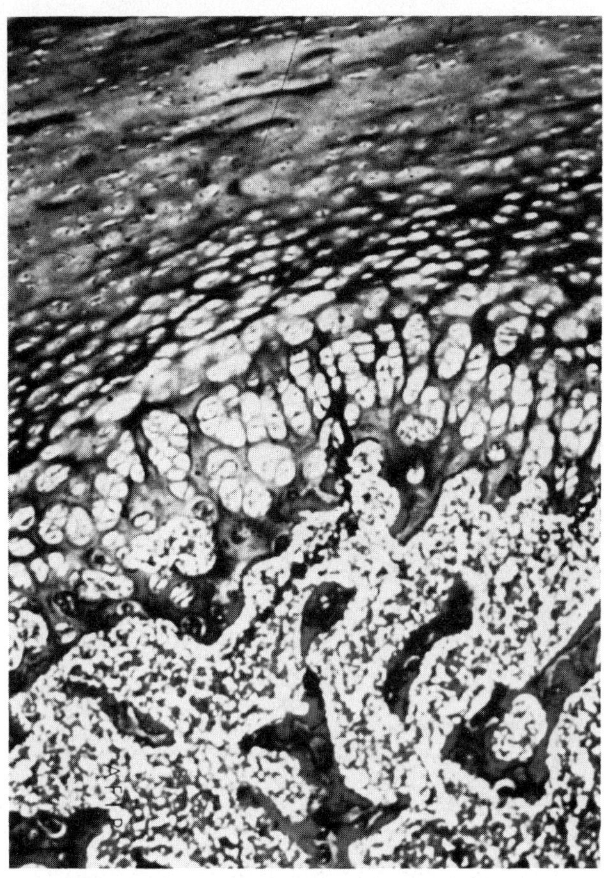

Figure 1–14. Clavicle. The articular surface (top) also provides transition of cartilage to bone. Note the horizontally layered articular cartilage elements near the surface, columnization of the deeper layers of the cartilage, and transformation of cartilage to bone similar to that seen in a growth plate.

GROWTH PLATE (PHYSIS)

The narrow rim of cartilage that remains between the primary and secondary ossification centers exhibits orderly transition of cartilage to bone and is responsible for growth in length. The entire activity can be divided into a zone of resting cartilage; zones of proliferating, hypertrophied, and secretory cartilage; and a zone of provisional calcification. In general, cartilage can expand either by cell multiplication or by production of matrix, but once the matrix becomes mineralized, cells within the matrix can no longer expand. At that point, enlargement is possible only by apposition to the surface, but not by interstitial cell duplication. The growth plate exhibits orderly interstitial *cellular* growth, both by cell multiplication within the growth plate and by cell additions from the encircling perichondrial ring.

The most proximal zone is the resting zone, in which sparse cartilage cells are embedded in a cartilaginous matrix. Here, isolated cartilage cells are undergoing necrosis. It is conceivable that the death of these cartilage cells stimulates the remaining cartilage cells to undergo mitotic division and proliferate. At the same time, the cartilage cells secrete matrix. This matrix will form the "territorial cartilage" as opposed to the "cellular cartilage" of the reproducing cell. The territorial cartilaginous matrix contains copious quantities of water. As the process continues, water is imbibed (i.e., transferred from the territorial cartilage into the cell). This activity causes massive enlargement (hypertrophy) of the cell while dehydrating the adjacent territorial cartilage. The increased size of the cartilage cell is a result of hydraulic enlargement of the lacunar space and serves to lift the epiphyseal cartilage and bone away from the growth plate. At the same time, the dehydrated territorial cartilage matrix calcifies. Dehydration is characterized by fibrillary change, easily demonstrated in the territorial cartilage between the rows of hypertrophied cartilage cells (Figs. 1–16 to 1–24).

Cartilage cells thus imbibe water, increase their size and therefore the length of the bone, and then die. Vascular buds from the metaphysis invade the dead cellular debris, and cellular elements remove it, leaving only the calcified cartilage bars projecting into the metaphysis like docks into a lake (Figs. 1–21 to 1–24). The bars form the latticework for bone formation, prevent collapse during the death of the hypertrophied cartilage cell, and provide the firm unyielding base on which growth takes place. Osteoblasts, emerging from the vascular bud, form primitive bone that develops on the cartilage-bar framework. The combination of calcified cartilage bars with primitive bone on the surface constitutes the primary trabeculae. "Growth" is a function of the normal cartilage cell: The cell replicates and increases the size of the lacunar space. Failure of the cartilage cell to develop results in arrested growth (see Achondroplasia, Chap. 2). Osteoid formation adds strength and resilience to the skeletal structure, but it is not responsible for growth. The patient with improper osteoid formation does not suffer from short stature (see Osteogenesis Imperfecta Tarda, Chap. 2).

The picture of growth-plate development and function as viewed in a longitudinal fashion is the usual classic presentation (Fig. 1–25). Studying the growth plate in horizontal sections provides a three-dimensional perspective and adds to our comprehension of the sequential processes involved.

In the resting zone, isolated cells per lacuna are widely interspersed between large areas of acellular matrix (Fig. 1–26). Nearer the metaphysis, lacunae contain two or more cells (Fig. 1–27). The cellular expansion begins to crowd the intervening matrix (Fig. 1–28). Not all the original resting cells proliferate, and empty lacunae

Text continued on page 17

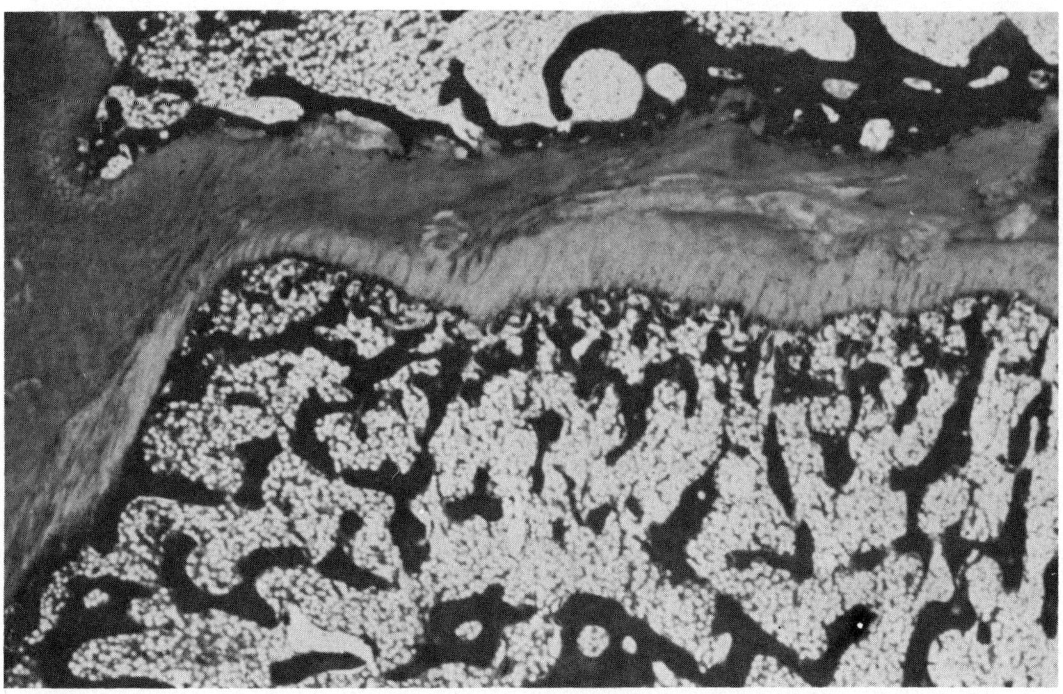

Figure 1–15. Growth plate, Masson stain. Note the light staining of the lower portion of the growth plate, indicating higher water content.

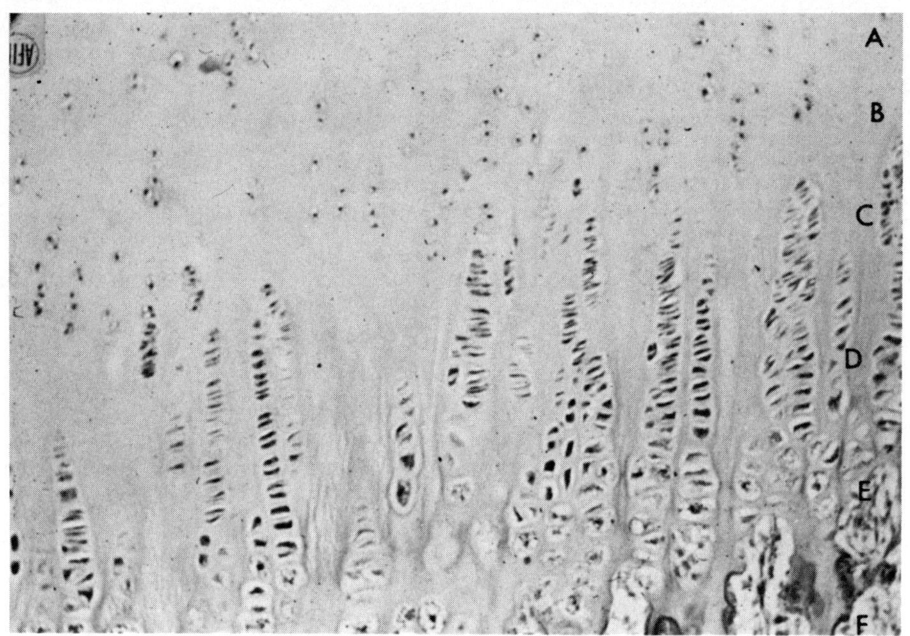

Figure 1–16. Growth plate. Low-power view showing entire plate. At *A*, resting zone has isolated cartilage cells in the upper portion together with empty lacunae. At *B*, cell reproduction produces cloning of cells that "stack-up" longitudinally. Successive generations occupy more space than each single progenitor cell and thus increase the length of the cartilage model. Secretion of new matrix at *C* is followed by dehydration with accompanying fibrillation of the territorial cartilage matrix between the "dinner plates" at *D*. Hypertrophy of cartilage cells at *E* is due to imbibition of water. Calcification of matrix is followed by vascular invasion at *F*.

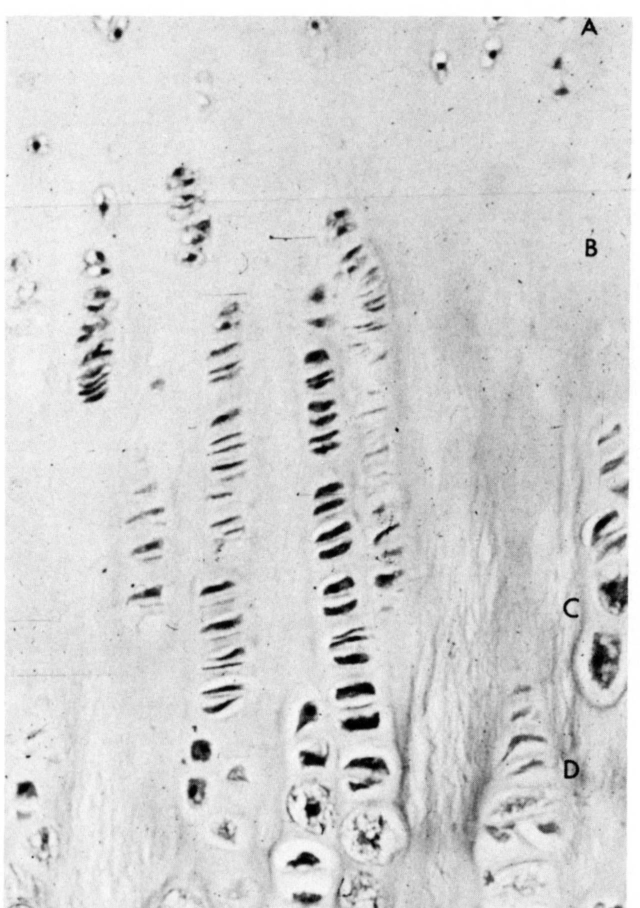

Figure 1–17. Slightly higher magnification illustrating resting zone *A*, proliferation zone *B*, hypertrophic zone *C*, and zone of provisional calcification *D*.

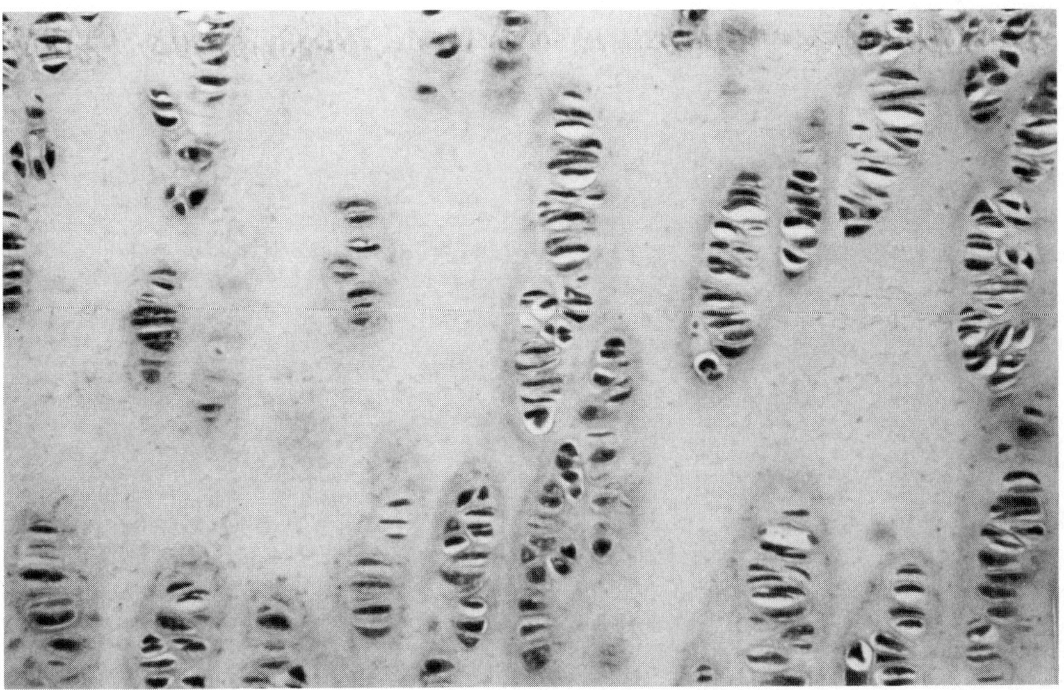

Figure 1–18. Growth plate, zone of proliferation. Cloning of cartilage cells produces stacked "dinner plates." Note darker staining and newly secreted matrix around each of the clones, which is distinct from the older, acellular territorial cartilage destined to become the calcified central cores of primary trabeculae.

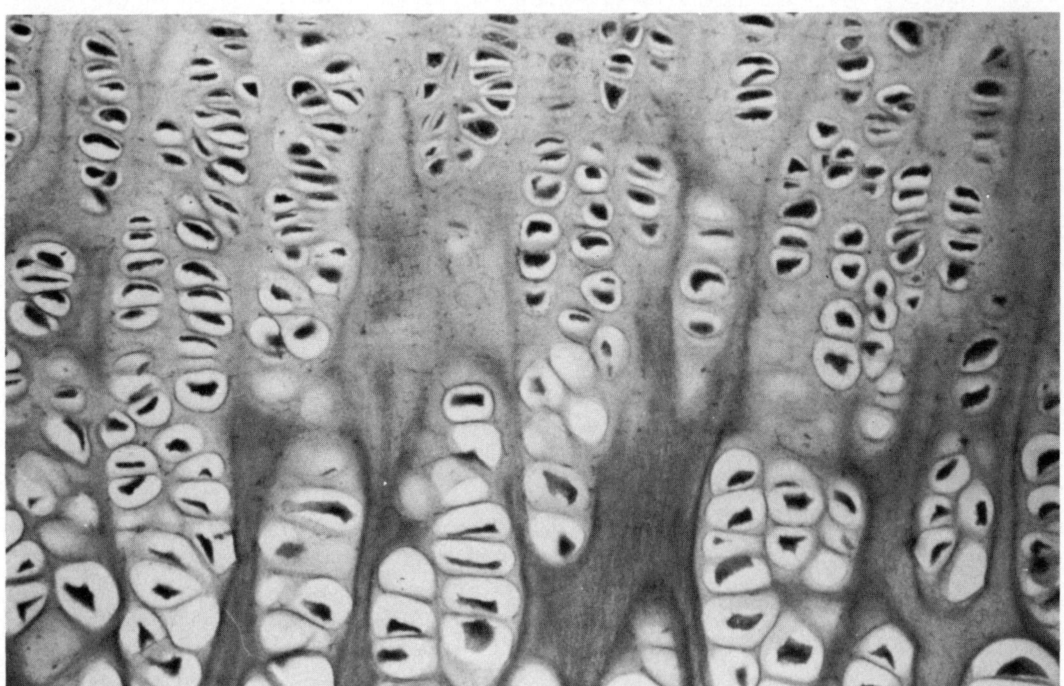

Figure 1–19. Growth plate, zone of proliferation merging with zone of hypertrophy. Note swelling of cartilage cells and much-darker-staining fibrillary territorial cartilage matrix. Removal of water by the cells leaves longitudinally oriented collagen bundles that become calcified and provide the lattice for later bone deposition.

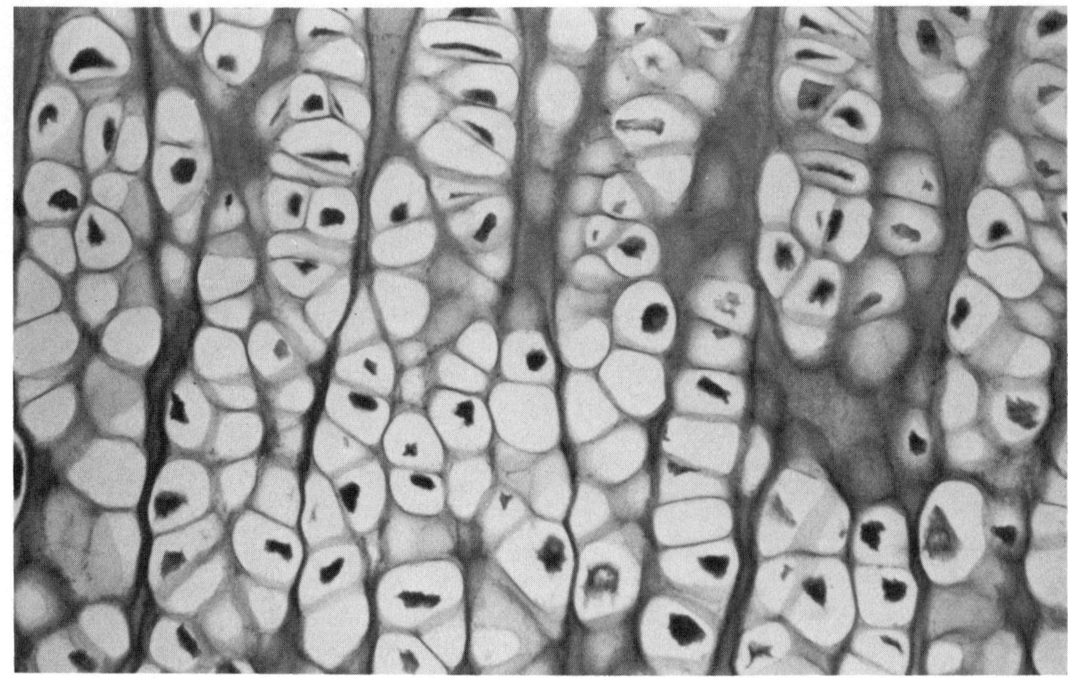

Figure 1–20. Growth plate, zone of hypertrophy. Cartilage cells are swollen, enlarged with loss of nuclei. The matrix is condensed, forming thin bars oriented in the long axis of the bone.

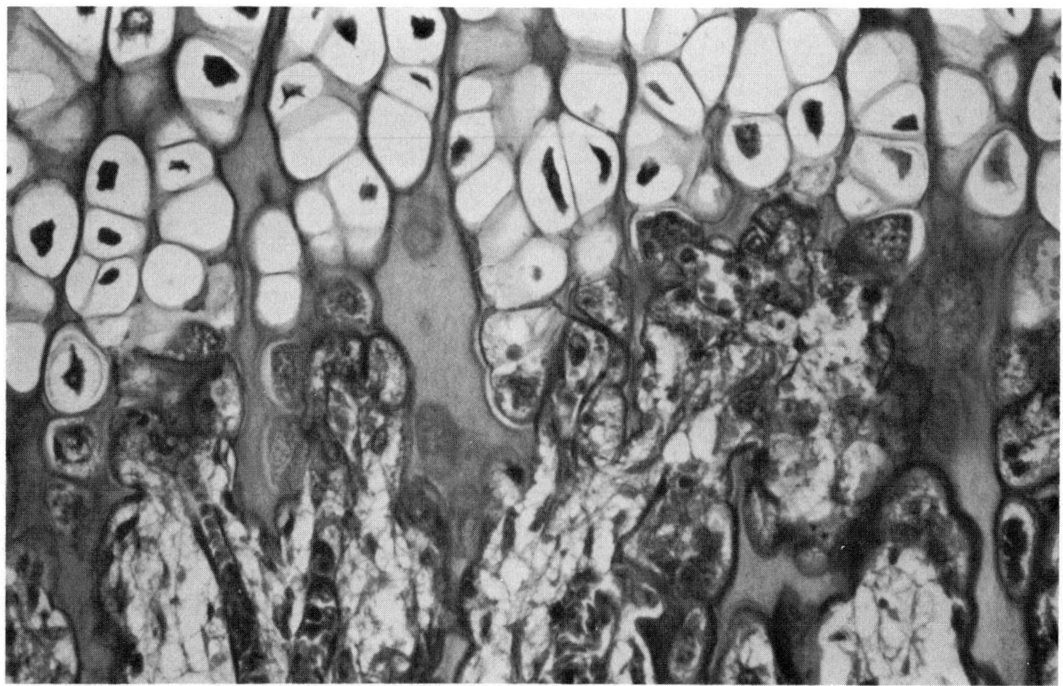

Figure 1–21. Growth plate, zone of hypertrophy merging with zone of provisional calcification. Nuclei have disappeared from many lacunae. Horizontal septa between lacunar spaces are eroded by cellular elements (chondroclasts) originating in the vascular fountain from the metaphyseal side of the growth plate. The longitudinally oriented, calcified cartilage bars remain as the "scaffolding" on which the bone will be deposited.

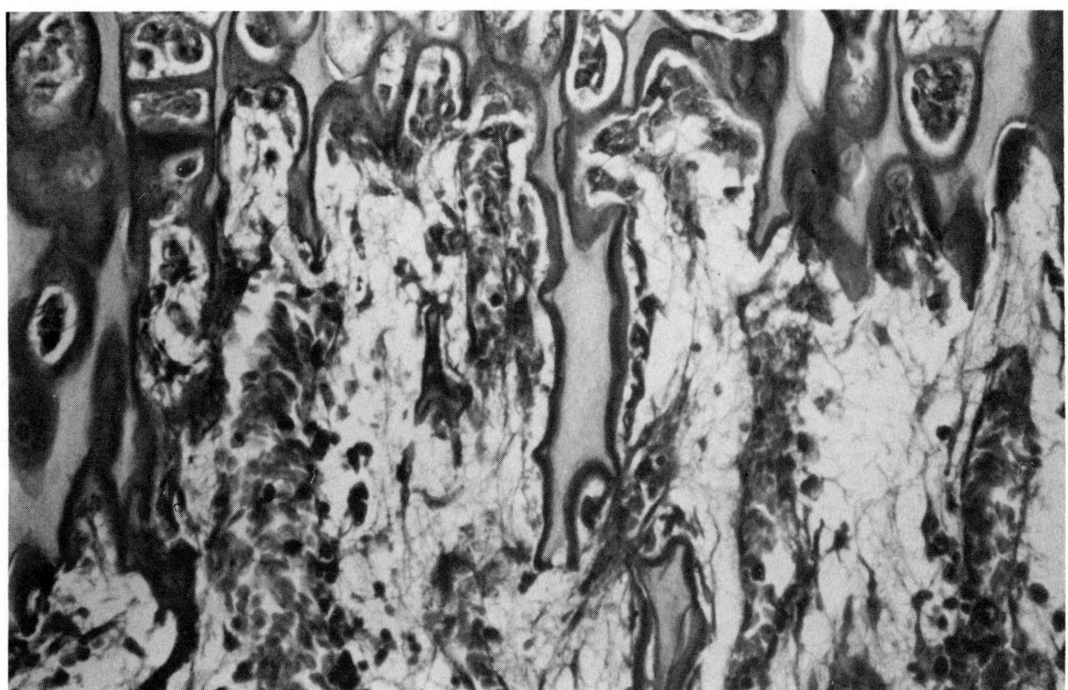

Figure 1–22. Growth plate. Calcified cartilage bars remaining after removal of dead cartilage cells form the "scaffold" on which osteoblasts deposit osteoid. The presence of darker-staining cellular bone surrounding a lighter-staining acellular cartilage matrix core constitutes a "primary trabecula."

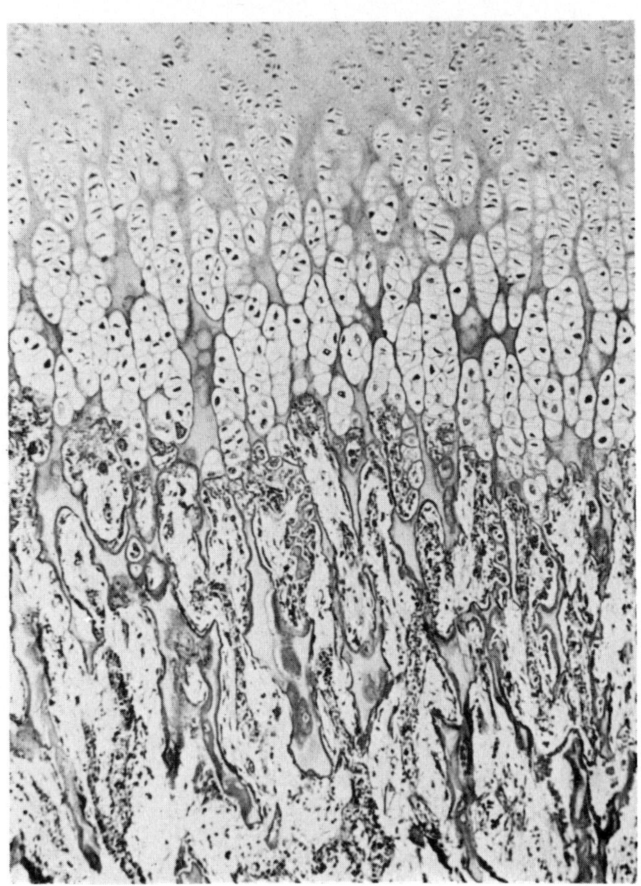

Figure 1–23. Active growth plate, lower end of femur of newborn. Hypertrophic cartilage, dead cartilage cells, vascular buds, zone of provisional calcification, and deposition of newly formed osteoid on remaining calcified cartilage matrix are evident. Note the undulating configuration of the advancing edge of vascular invasion ("hills and valleys").

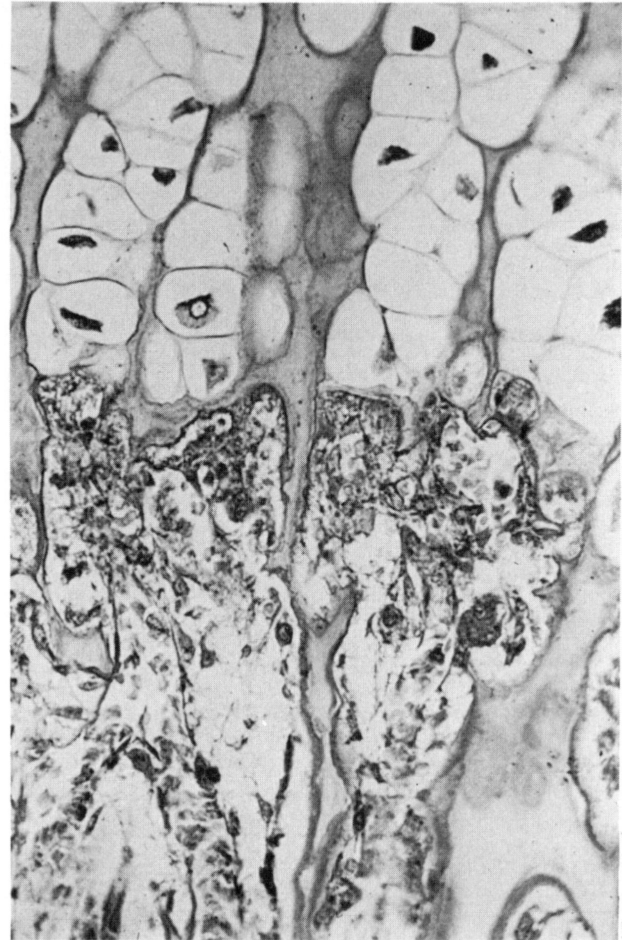

Figure 1–24. Higher magnification of growth plate shown in Figure 1–23. The vascular buds entering the area of hypertrophied cartilage are illustrated. Chondroclasts serially remove intercellular septa opening and emptying the lacunae of cellular debris. Osteoid deposits on the remaining calcified cartilage matrix bars. The combination of calcified matrix core with osteoid on its surface constitutes primary trabeculae.

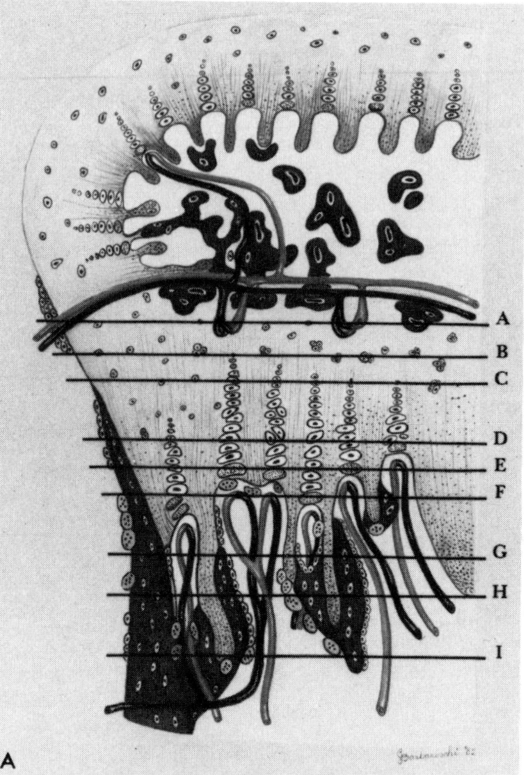

Figure 1–25. Schematic diagrams of growth plate. Levels *A* to *I* correspond to cross sections of the growth plate illustrated in Figures 1–26 to 1–34. The cross-sectional view helps place events at the growth plate in three-dimensional perspective.

Illustration continued on opposite page

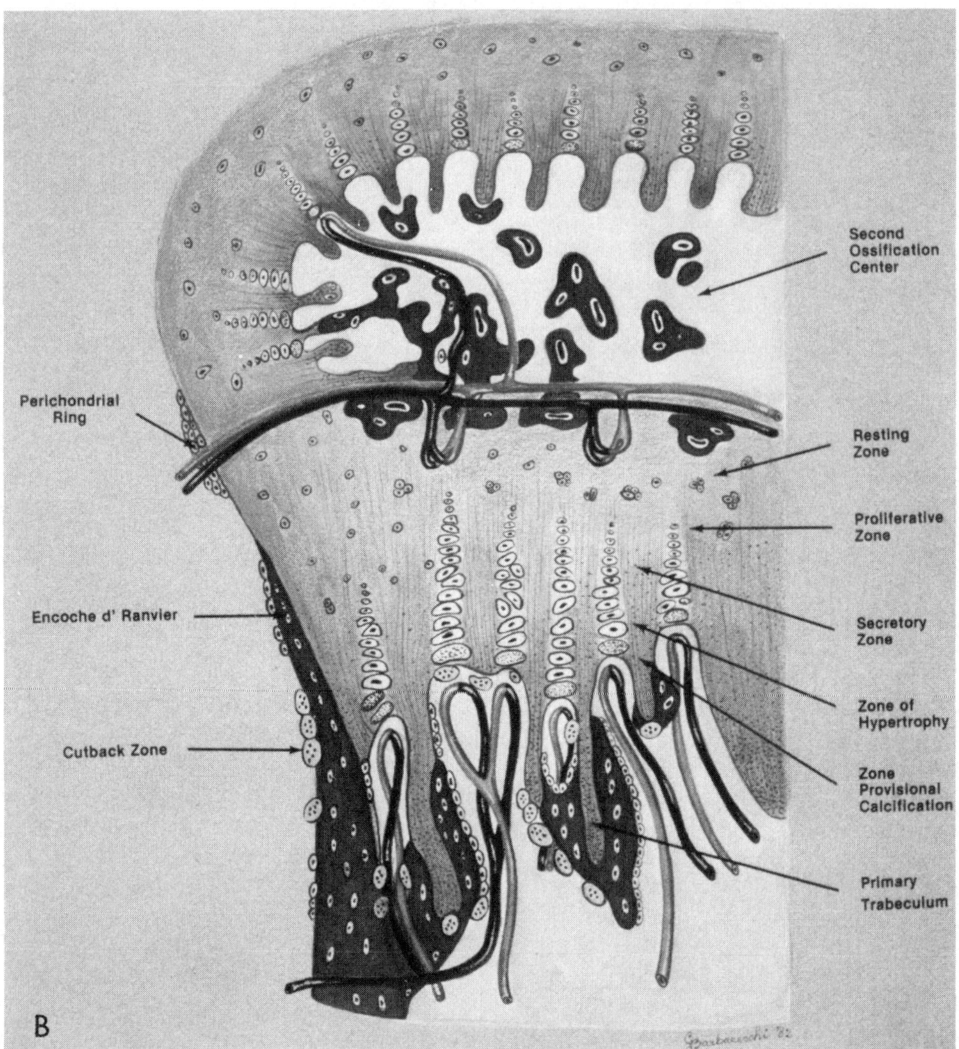

Figure 1–25 *Continued.*

and "ghosts" indicate cellular death (Fig. 1–26). A horizontal section through the secretory zone shows new matrix around each of the cartilage-cell clones (Fig. 1–28). This new matrix is distinct from the calcified cartilage matrix that remains as a "scaffold" for bone production when the cartilage cells are removed. Continued cell reproduction in the clones and alignment in columns occupy greater space; this interstitial cell growth results in elongation of the physis.

Cells in the zone of hypertrophy enlarge by imbibing fluid from the adjacent acellular territorial cartilage (Fig. 1–29). As the fluid is removed from this matrix, the intervening territorial cartilage contains visible strands of fibrillary collagen between the cells. The dehydration is associated with calcification.

As hypertrophied cartilage cells die, vascular buds enter from the metaphysis (Figs. 1–30 and 1–31). This process is not uniform across the entire hypertrophied zone. On any given transverse section, there are portions from which the cartilage cells have already been removed and in which new blood vessels are present, but there are also other adjacent portions that still contain hypertrophied cells. The purpose of this hill-and-valley effect is to lend stability to the growth plate and prevent lateral slippage.

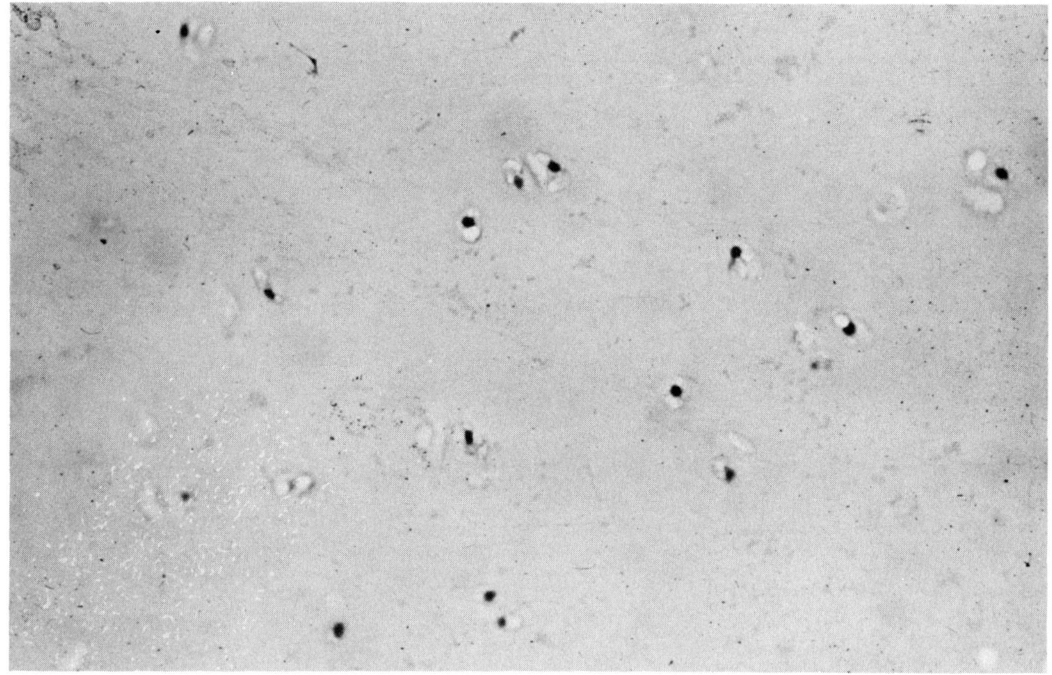

Figure 1–26. View of level *A* of Figure 1–25, resting zone. Isolated cartilage cells are associated with empty lacunae and large amounts of intercellular matrix.

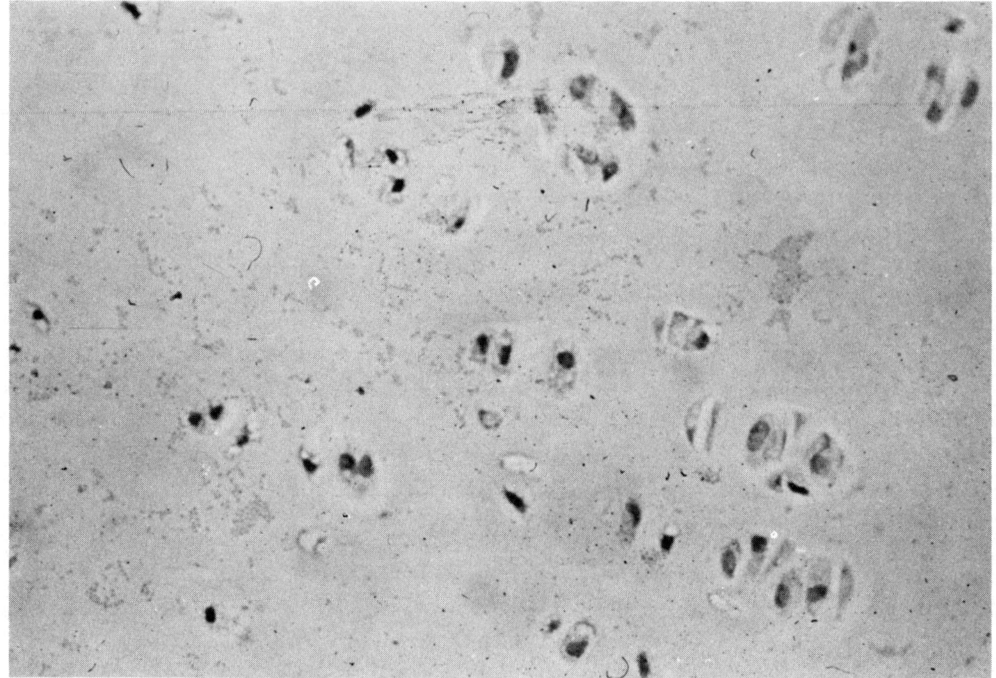

Figure 1–27. View of level *B* of Figure 1–25, resting zone–proliferative zone. Note cloning of cartilage cells.

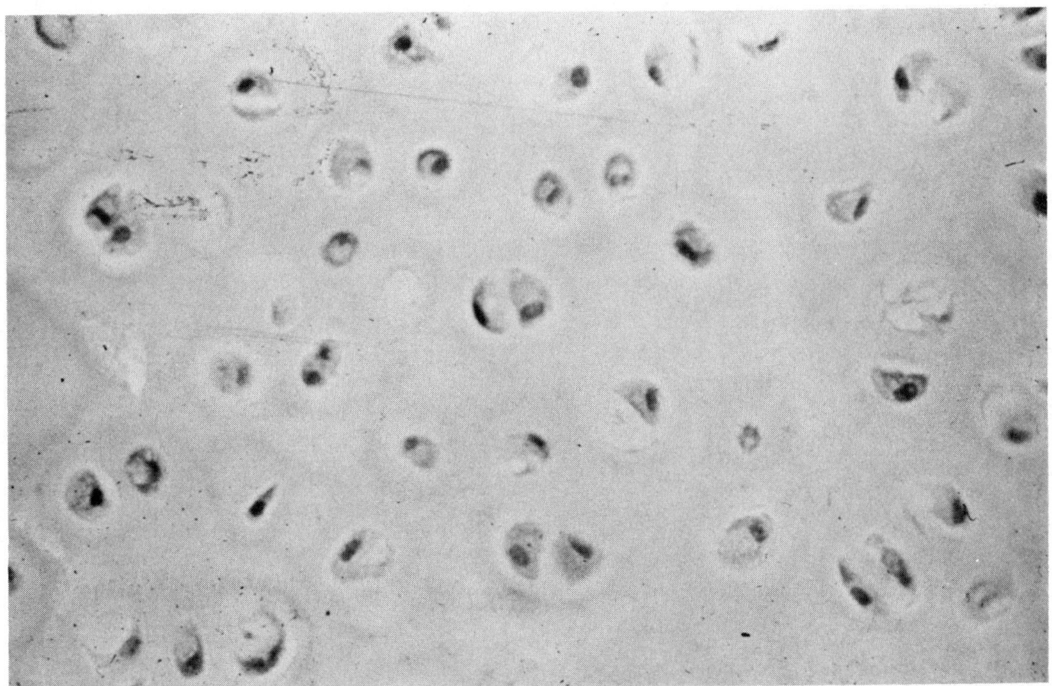

Figure 1–28. View of level *C* of Figure 1–25, proliferative zone. Note the cloning of cartilage cells with a halo of new matrix about the clones. The intervening older territorial cartilage matrix is compressed by the combination of new cells and matrix.

As soon as the vascular bud invades from the metaphysis, osteoclasts remove some of the walls between the columns of hypertrophied cells. Osteoblasts appear and deposit bone in globules on the calcified cartilage wall (Fig. 1–32). This is a continuous process that results in removal of more calcified cartilage and deposition of more bone (Figs. 1–33 and 1–34). What appeared on longitudinal section as bars of calcified cartilage projecting into the metaphysis are in reality the interconnecting components of a meshwork of calcified cartilage with bony deposition. The primitive marrow with its marked vascularity is contained in fairly rigid spaces. The vascular spaces contain numerous sinusoidal vessels with sluggish vascular flow. The flow accelerates nearer the diaphysis with smaller and smaller vessels, deposition of primitive marrow elements, and larger marrow spaces. Blood-flow characteristics are important in numerous diseases of bone (see Chapter 5).

Three-dimensional analysis emphasizes that all the primary trabeculae are interconnected. Remodeling with its constant removal and replacement of bony walls and enlargements of marrow spaces results in thickening and lends stability to the bone.

The growth plate represents rapid transformation of cartilage to bone, but this transformation occurs at all cartilage-bone interfaces, albeit at a slower rate. The secondary ossification center enlarges by transforming the entire ring of epiphyseal cartilage to bone; zones of proliferation, secretion, hypertrophy, and provisional calcification can be identified as in the physis. Bones formed without a secondary ossification center adapt by converting articular cartilage to bone and thus adding to the length of the structure (Fig. 1–14). Even the adult, under appropriate mechanical, metabolic, or endocrine stimuli, will slowly convert articular cartilage to bone (acromegaly).

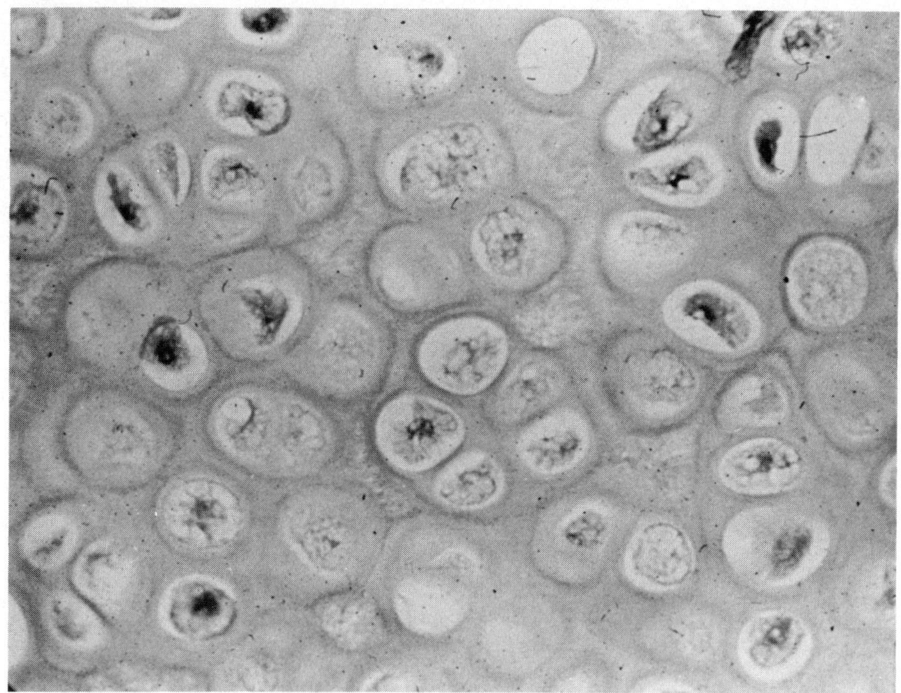

Figure 1–29. View of level *D* of Figure 1–25, hypertrophic zone. Cell multiplication, secretion of new matrix, and swelling of cartilage cells take up space by encroaching on the territorial cartilage between the cell columns. Note fibrillary changes in the territorial cartilage, as well as beginning necrosis of cells.

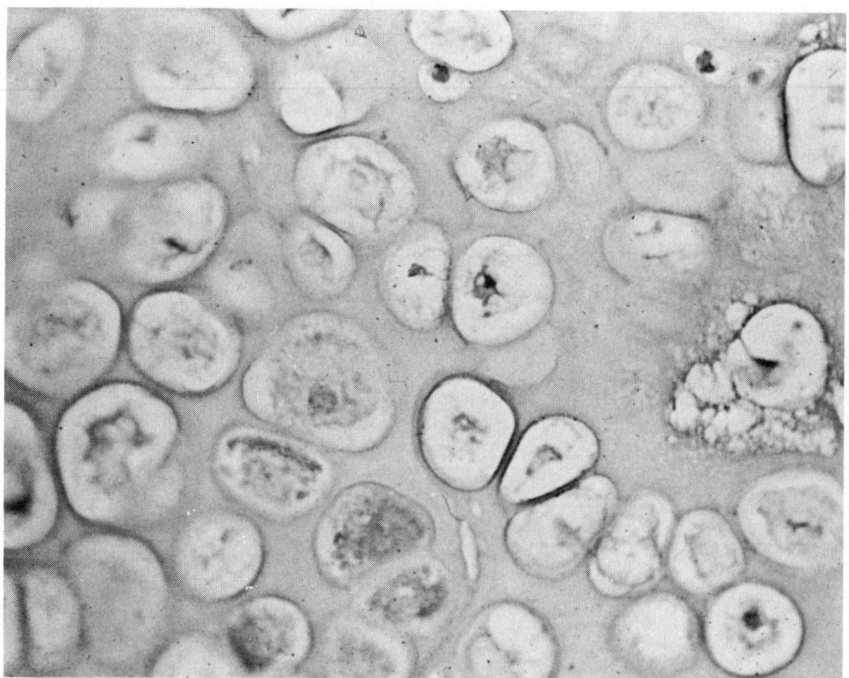

Figure 1–30. View of level *E* of Figure 1–25, hypertrophic zone. Almost all cartilage cells are dead, showing nuclear pyknosis and disintegration.

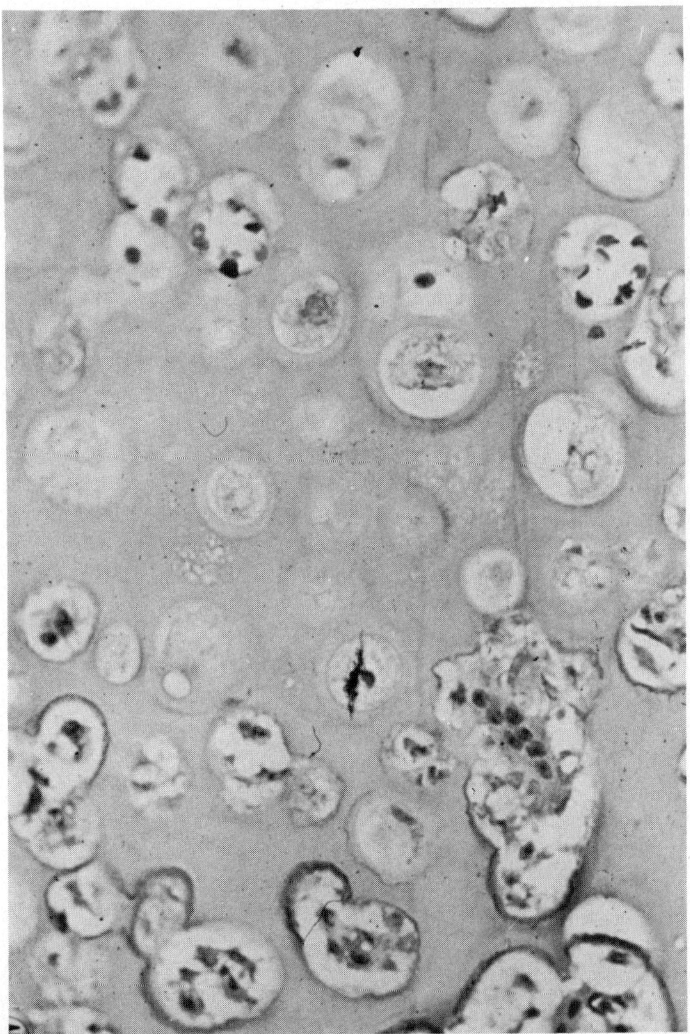

Figure 1–31. View of level *F* of Figure 1–25, zone of provisional calcification. Beginning vascular invasion is evident in some of the lacunae. Chondroclasts appear with the vascular granulation and remove cartilage cell debris. Septa between lacunae are removed resulting in enlargement of the primitive medullary cavity. Osteoblasts and osteoclasts are present in the larger spaces, and osteoid formation is on the latticework of the calcified cartilage at the lower edge of the photograph.

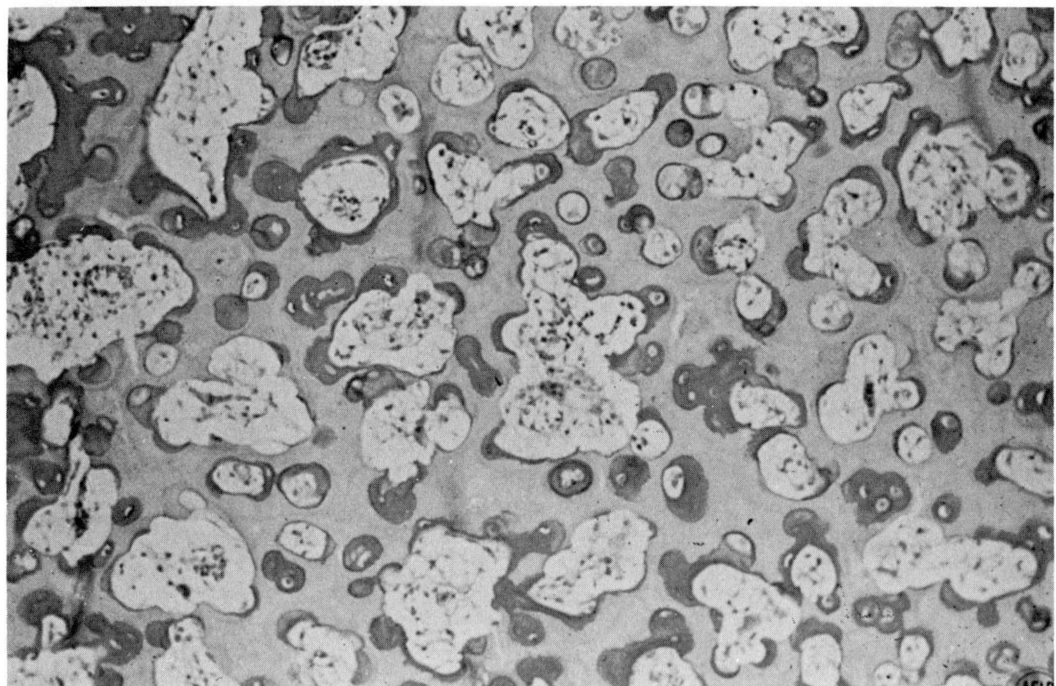

Figure 1–32. View of level *G* of Figure 1–25, zone of provisional ossification. Large areas of territorial cartilage persist. Many lacunar walls are being removed by osteoclasts to make larger marrow spaces. Osteoblasts have deposited small globules of bone in empty spaces left by cartilage cell removal. The process of vascular invasion is not uniform across the width of the growth plate, thus producing areas resembling hills and valleys (see Fig. 1–17). This provides lateral stability to the growth plate.

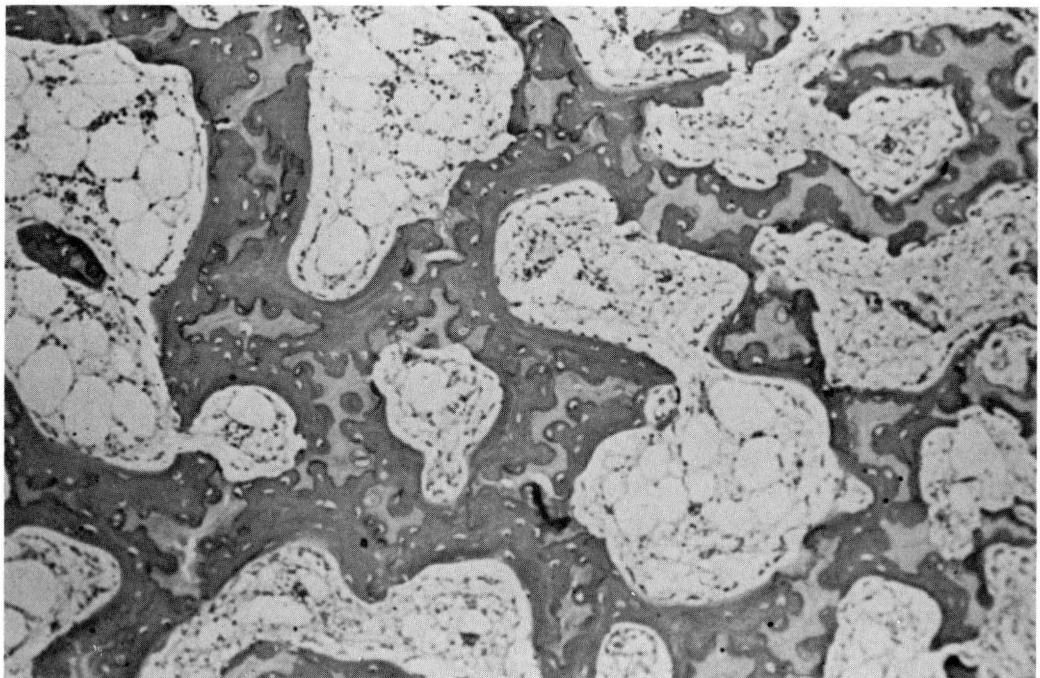

Figure 1–33. View of level *H* of Figure 1–25, metaphysis. Note the progressive enlargement of marrow spaces with deposition of increasing amounts of bone on the cartilage scaffold. Hill-and-valley effect is evident, with greatest number of cartilage cores in the lower right corner. There are numerous small vessels in the marrow spaces with a loose intervascular stroma.

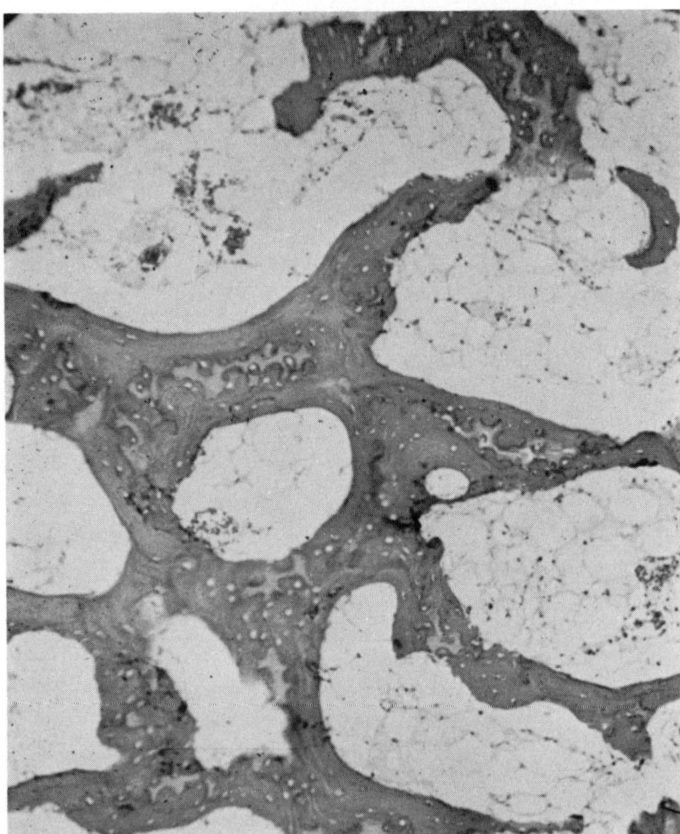

Figure 1–34. View of level *I* of Figure 1–25. Metaphysis with primary trabeculae and early marrow elements is shown here. Continued remodeling results in removal of cartilage cores of primary trabeculae and increasing amounts of bone in fewer trabeculae. Vessels are larger, and early marrow cells appear.

METAPHYSEAL REMODELING

Without the presence of a broad, firm base, growth could not occur; however, such a base does not provide the strength and resilience required in mature bone; "tubular steel" is required. The primary trabecular meshwork must be removed and replaced by structures able to withstand the stresses of muscular pull and weight. It is therefore no surprise that primary trabeculae are removed almost as quickly as they are formed. Successive layers of osteoclasts allow alternate trabeculae to mature and ultimately eliminate 90 per cent of the original trabeculae, allowing only 10 per cent to mature to their full thickness. These thickened primary trabeculae, characterized by their central core of cartilage, are found in the metaphyses and diaphyses of the growing child (Fig. 1–35).

As the diaphysis elongates, new sleeve bone continues to develop adjacent to the growth plate and remains at the level of the hypertrophied cartilage. This sleeve-bone extension, the ring of Ranvier, ensures correct directional growth of cartilage. The hypertrophied cartilage cells are directed downward toward the growth plate (Fig. 1–36).

The diameter of the growth plate is much wider than that of the diaphysis. Remodeling of the metaphysis is necessary to accomplish the essential reduction in diameter. "Funnelization" is accomplished by extensive osteoclastic activity and removal of the outer circumference of bone until the narrow diaphyseal diameter is established (Figs. 1–37 and 1–38). At the same time, in order to maintain the structural integrity of bone, fierce osteoblastic activity must take place on the inner surface to strengthen the cortical rim. Both activities occur simultaneously and involve zones of osteoclastic resorption and osteoblastic refill (Fig. 1–39).

Text continued on page 28

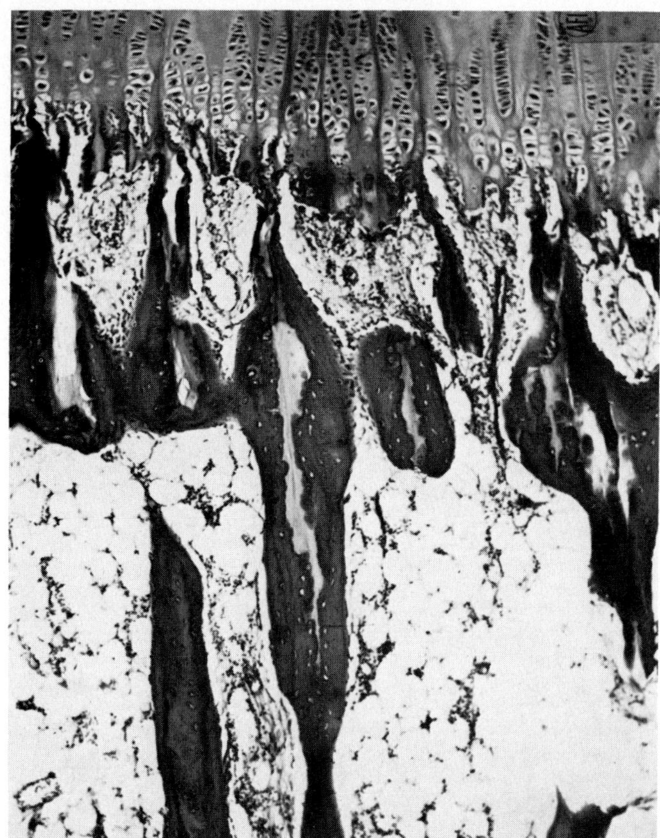

Figure 1–35. Metaphysis. This histologic study of primary trabeculae exhibits reduction in the number of trabeculae, thickening in the remaining trabeculae, and only isolated cartilage cores in the center of the trabecular network. Further remodeling has resulted in more bone in fewer trabeculae and decreasing residual cartilage. The larger marrow spaces contain fewer but larger vessels, fat, and early hematopoietic cells. All trabeculae are connected to each other (and to the cortex) and form a honeycomb of marrow spaces surrounded by rigid walls.

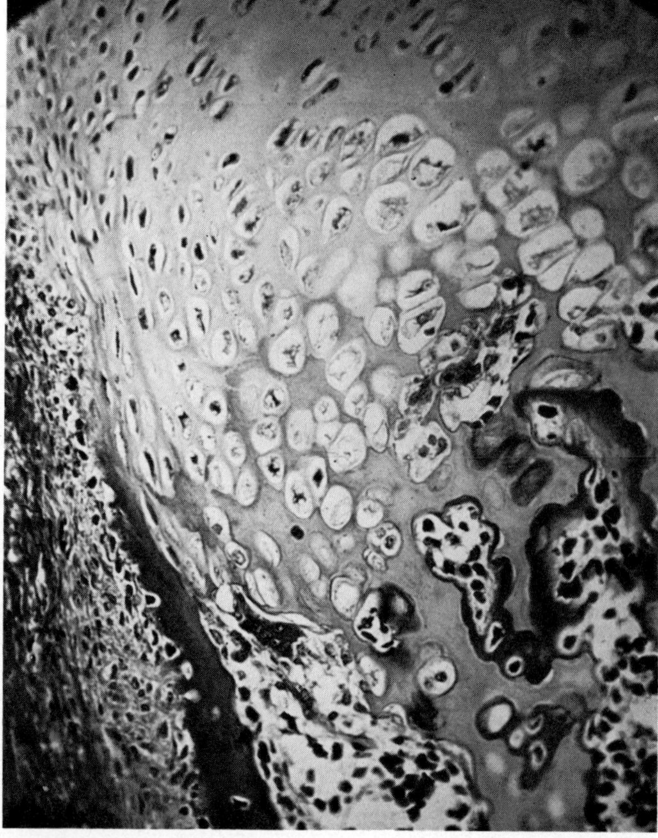

Figure 1–36. Higher magnification of sleeve bone exhibiting osteoblastic seam, osteoid, and bone formation extending above the level of cartilage hypertrophy.

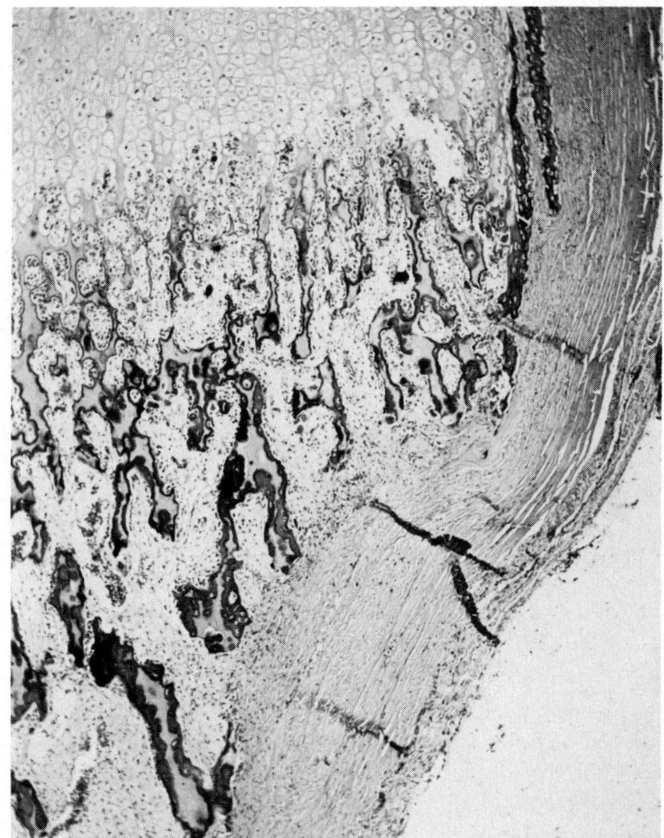

Figure 1–37. Metaphyseal remodeling. Cutback zone with extensive osteoclastic activity on the lateral surface to narrow the metaphysis from the width imposed by the growth plate is shown here. Successive waves of sleeve bone formed at the lateral margin of the growth plate ensure metaphyseal direction of the proliferating cartilage.

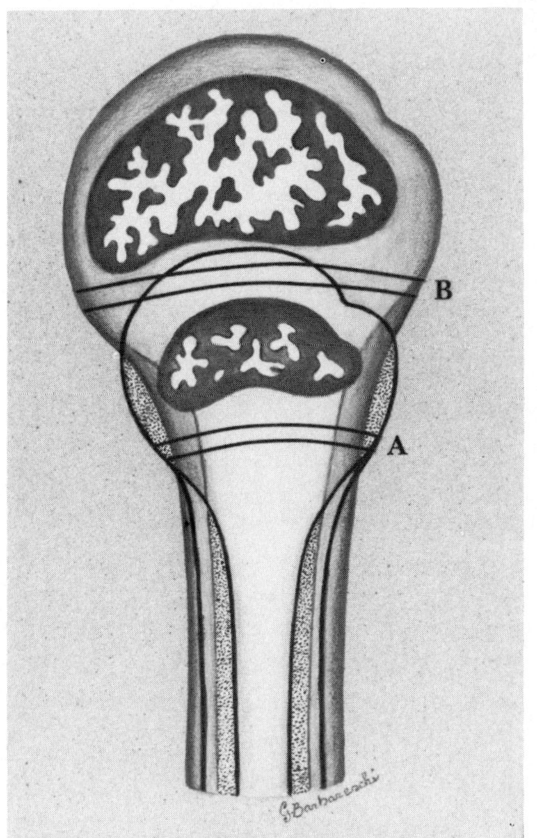

Figure 1–38. Schematic diagram of metaphyseal remodeling (funnelization). Stippled area indicates bone to be removed by osteoclasts to transform the bone from the shape and size indicated in A to that in B.

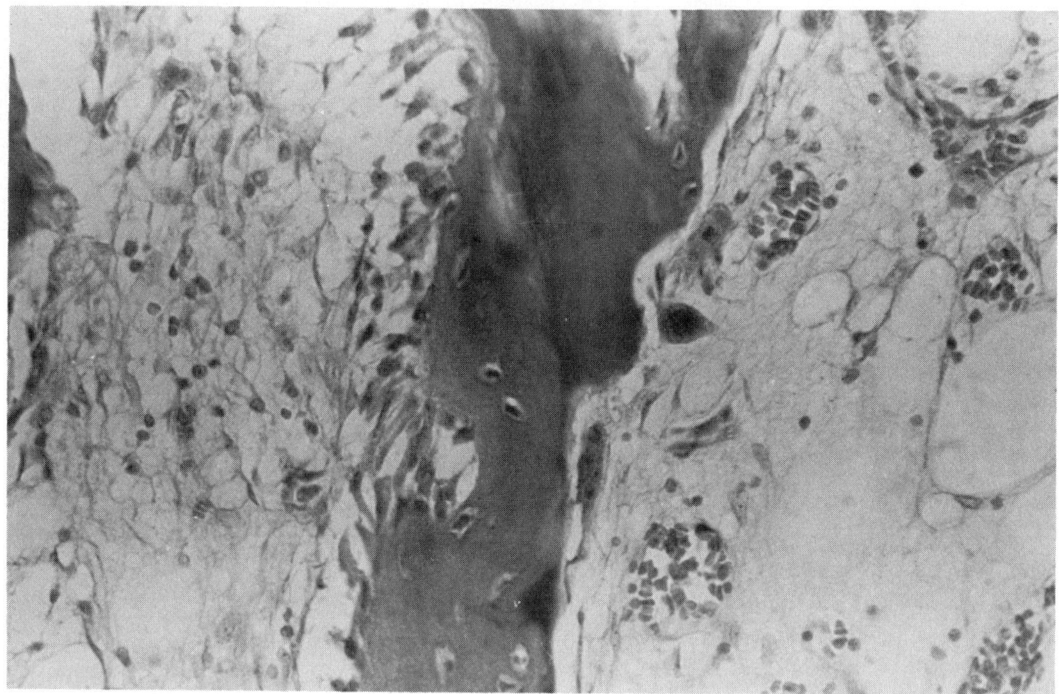

Figure 1–39. Higher magnification of metaphysis near cutback zone. Osteoclastic activity on the outer (right) side, of the trabecula, accompanied by intense osteoblastic activity on the inner (left) side, with the skewed growth occurring in response to mechanical (muscular) stresses.

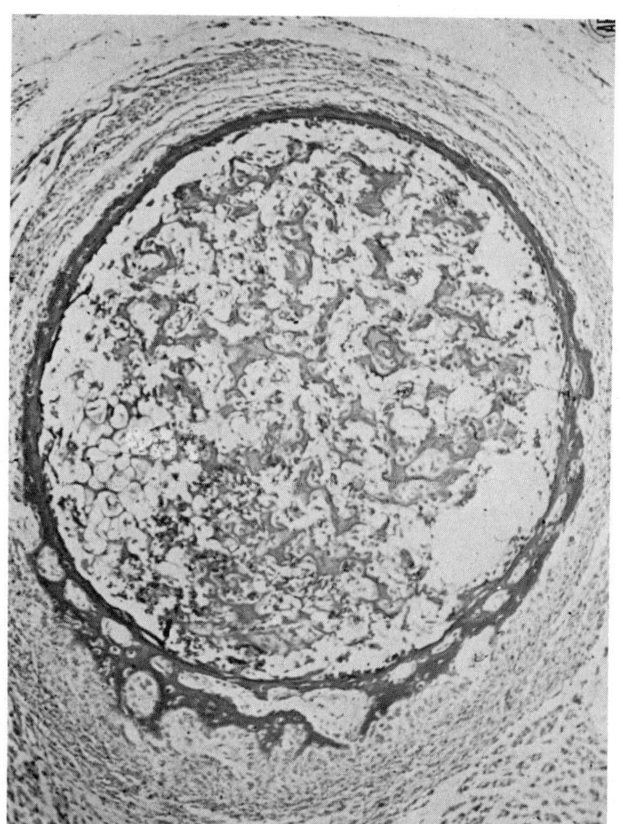

Figure 1–40. Cross section of bone just beneath the growth plate in a fetus. Note cartilage cells and primary trabeculae in the medullary cavity. The periosteum can be divided into an outer fibrous and lighter staining inner cambium layer with new bone formation producing successive layers outside the primitive cortical shell of sleeve bone.

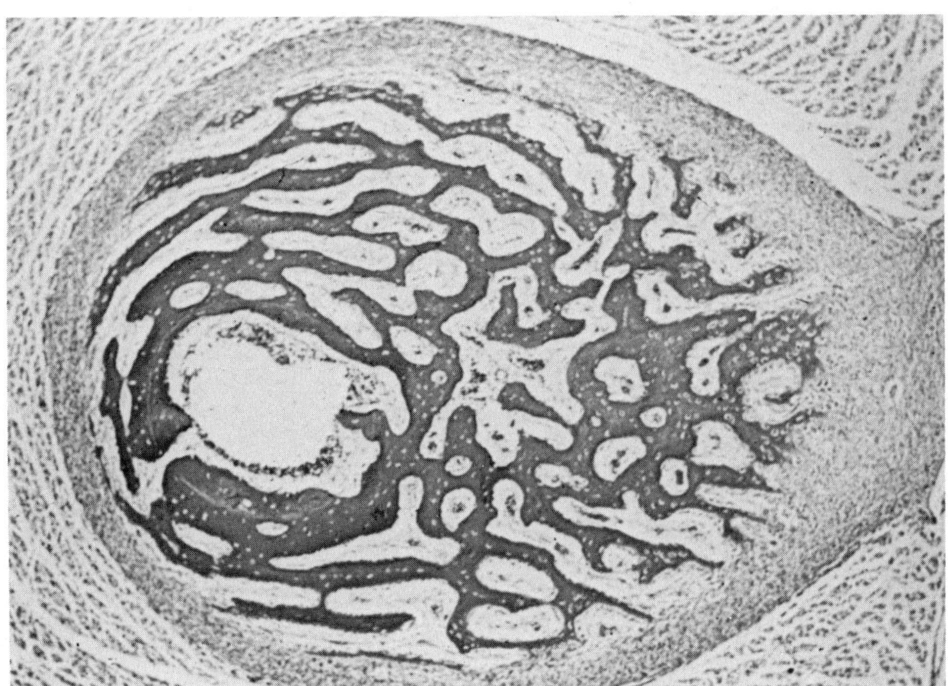

Figure 1–41. Streamers of bone extending centrifugally from the original cortex in a fetus. Note the prominent periosteum with inner cambium layer. Also note the skewed growth toward the right side of the photograph. These rapidly produced streamers of bone have a loosely woven collagen pattern and many cells per unit volume.

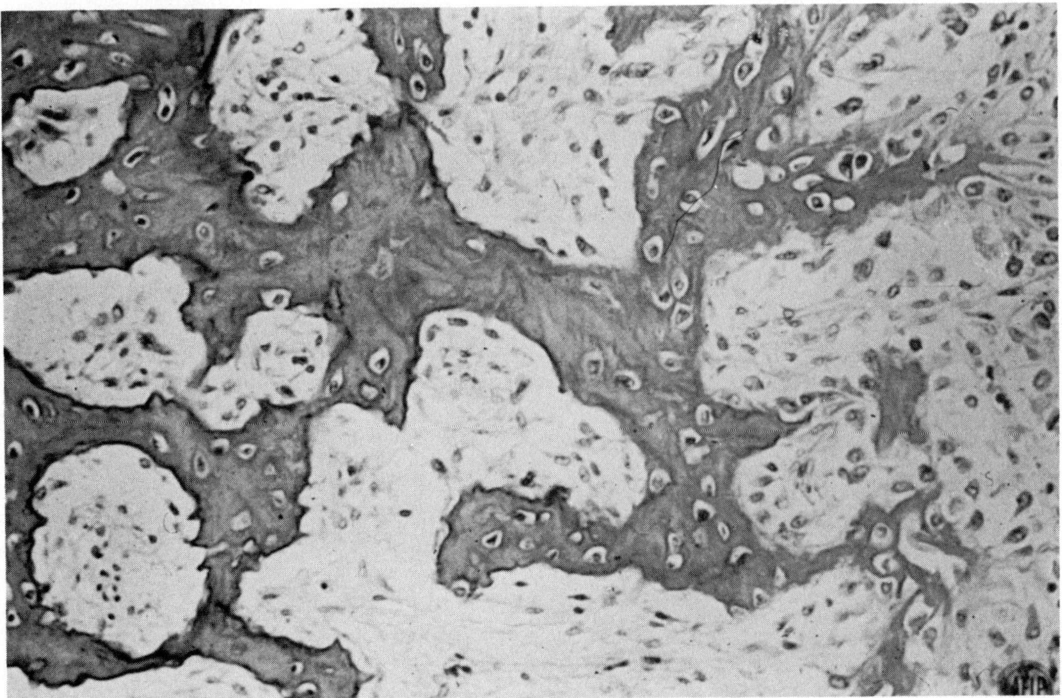

Figure 1–42. Collagen model bone (intramembranous ossification). Cells in the cambium layer proliferate and modulate to osteoblasts that deposit collagenous matrix (osteoid) around themselves. As the matrix mineralizes, some of the osteoblasts become incorporated and modulate to osteocytes (right of photograph). This type of rapid bone formation is seen in many conditions, including fracture callus and Codman's triangle.

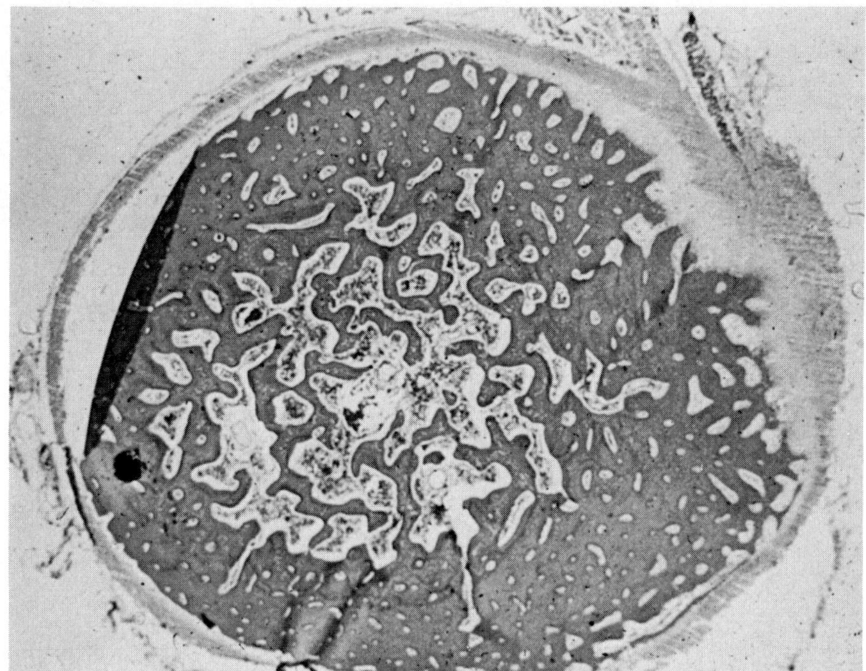

Figure 1–43. Streamer and inlay bone in a fetus. The space between the rapidly deposited streamers has been filled by slowly deposited new bone, adding to the overall thickness of the cortex. Most of the primary trabeculae have been removed from the marrow.

CORTICAL DEVELOPMENT

The growth process at the epiphyseal plate is responsible for increase in length; however, if this were the only type of growth that occurred in bones, we would all be walking on long, thin pencil-like structures. The major mass of bone in the adult is produced by lateral growth from the shaft of the bone in the subperiosteal area of the diaphysis.

After the initial sleeve bone is laid down, the periosteum becomes thickened and can be differentiated into an outer and inner (cambium) layer. Perpendicular spicules of bone are laid down, replacing the periosteal tissue (collagen-model bone). In the early phase, thin streamers of bone are formed and radiate outward (Figs. 1–40 to 1–43). In this immature bone, the collagen fibers are not arranged in symmetric bundles, but rather in the criss-cross pattern similar to that seen in fabric. Depending on the rate of production and the similarity to the type of fiber, it may be termed "burlap," "woven," or "linen" bone. The coarser the fiber structure, the more rapid the production. Lamellar bone and osteonal bone represent slower deposition in which the fiber structure is organized in concentric layers. The structural pattern of the collagen fiber is apparent only under polarized light (Figs. 1–44 and 1–45).

As growth in diameter slows, osteoblasts appear, align themselves on the surface of the streamers of bone, and slowly deposit lamellar bone as an inlay into the spaces between the streamers. This inlay bone will polarize better because collagen fibers are aligned parallel to each other. Filling of the space between osteophytic streamers results in the formation of a solid cortex.

Once the cortical surface is formed, layer after layer of bone is deposited on this surface, forming outer circumferential lamellae (Fig. 1–46). The marrow cavity is progressively enlarged, and all original primary trabeculae are removed.

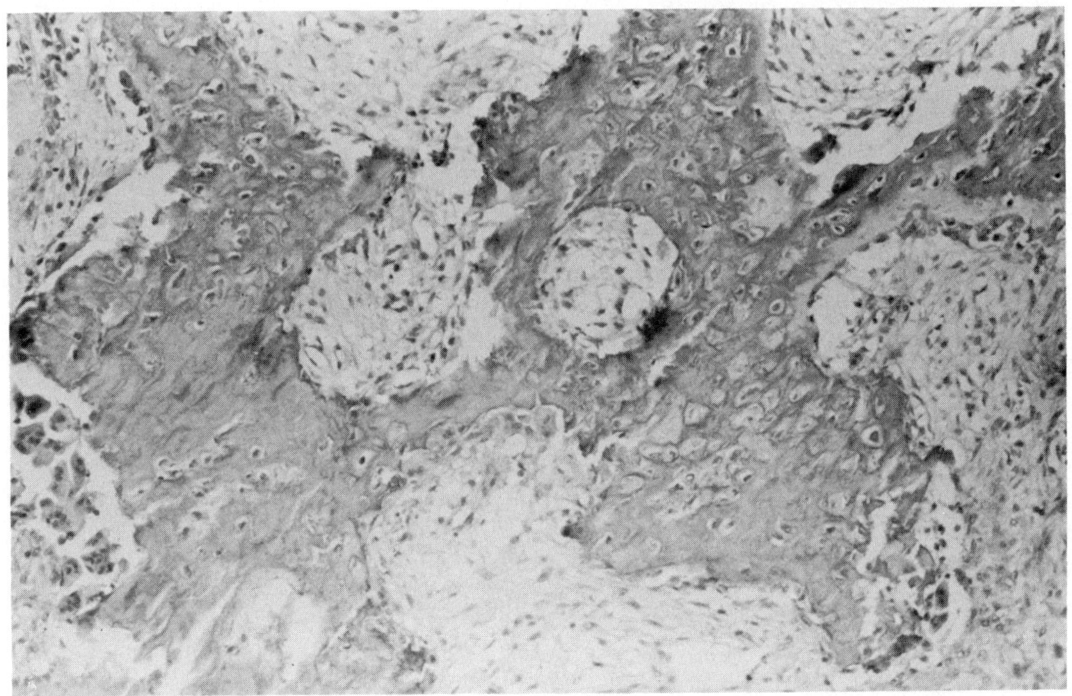

Figure 1–44. Immature bone (early callus). Note the large number of osteoblasts and osteocytes.

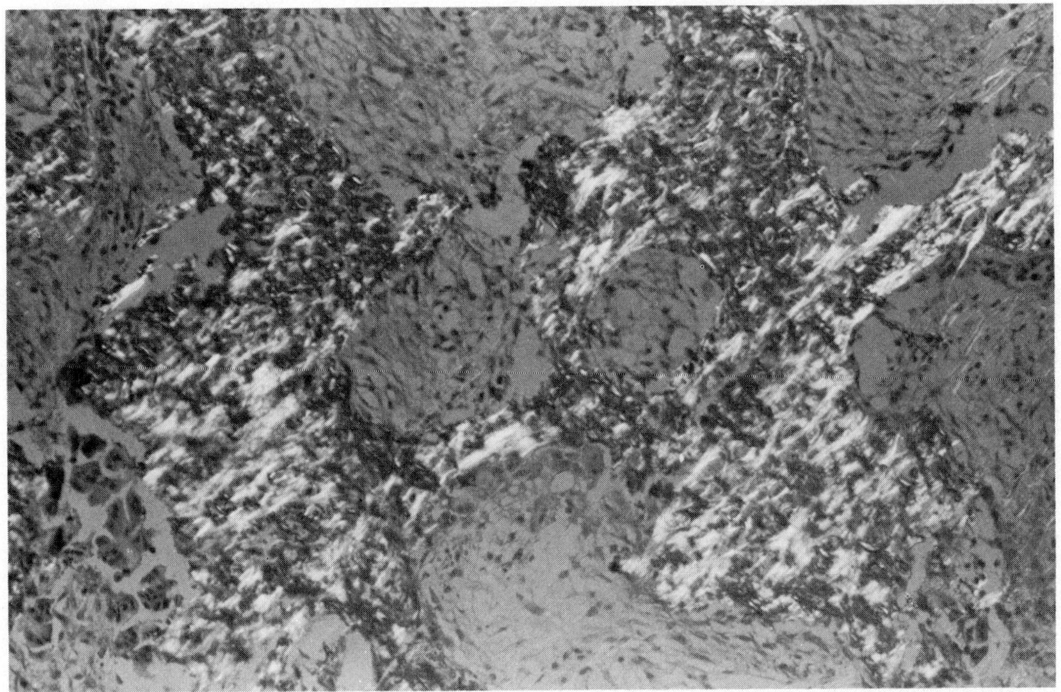

Figure 1–45. Fragment depicted in Figure 1–44, here shown under polarized light. The woven pattern of immature bone is clearly identifiable.

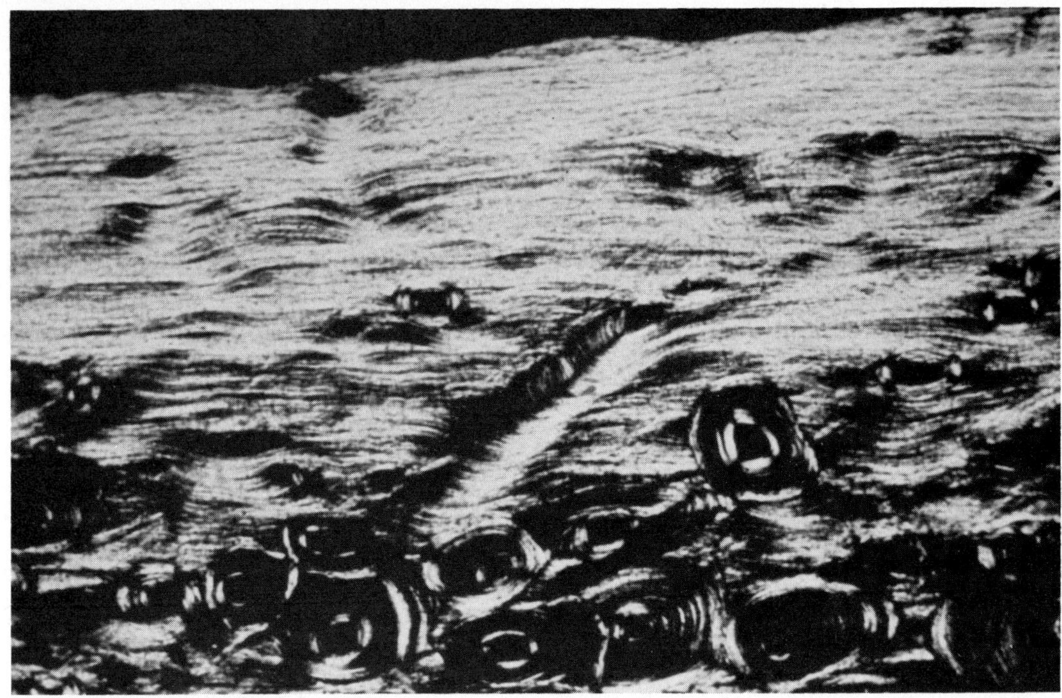

Figure 1–46. Section of outer cortex viewed under polarized light. Outer circumferential lamellae consist of concentric layers of bone on the periphery of the cortical shaft. Some osteons are evident in the lower portion of the photograph. The polarized light is absorbed by fibers at right angles to the light and transmitted by fibers parallel to the light rays (birefringence). Orientation of fiber structure indicates greater maturity and is reflected by greater birefringence.

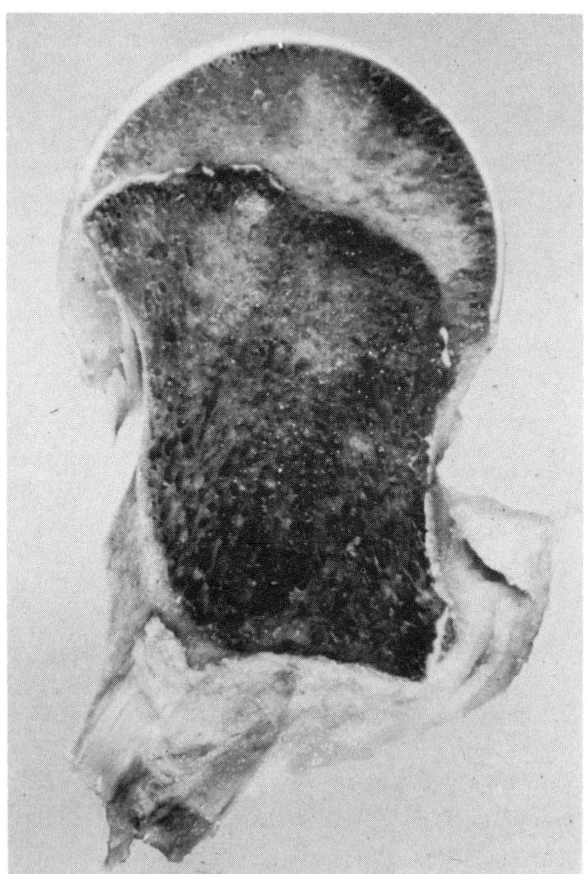

Figure 1–47. A gross specimen of the head of the femur from a 16-year-old patient exhibits partial growth-plate closure. Cartilage is visible near the periphery of the remaining growth plate.

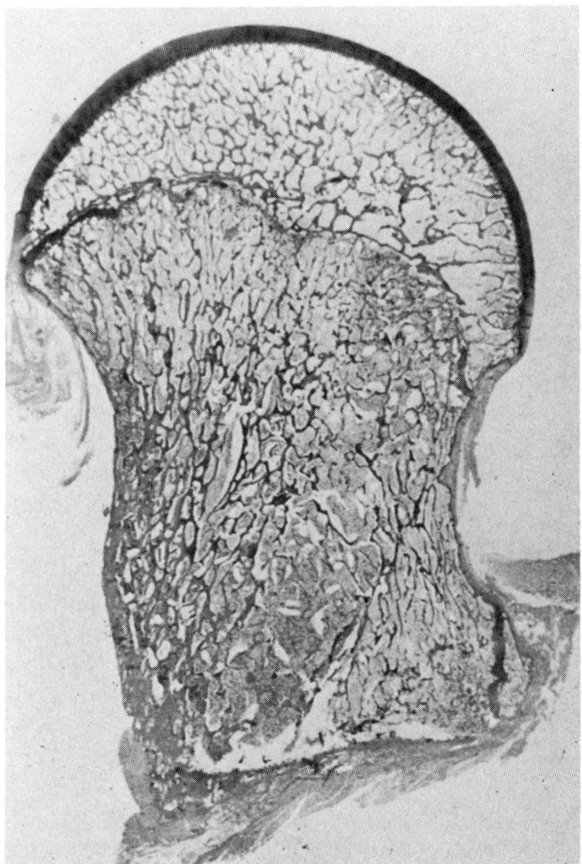

Figure 1–48. Macrosection of the femur shown in Figure 1–47 exhibiting the trabecular meshwork of the epiphysis and metaphysis with focal cartilage remnants of the growth plate. Note the lack of trabecular continuity across the growth-plate scar. Intense remodeling is necessary to realign these trabeculae. Much of this has already been done at the greater trochanteric growth plate.

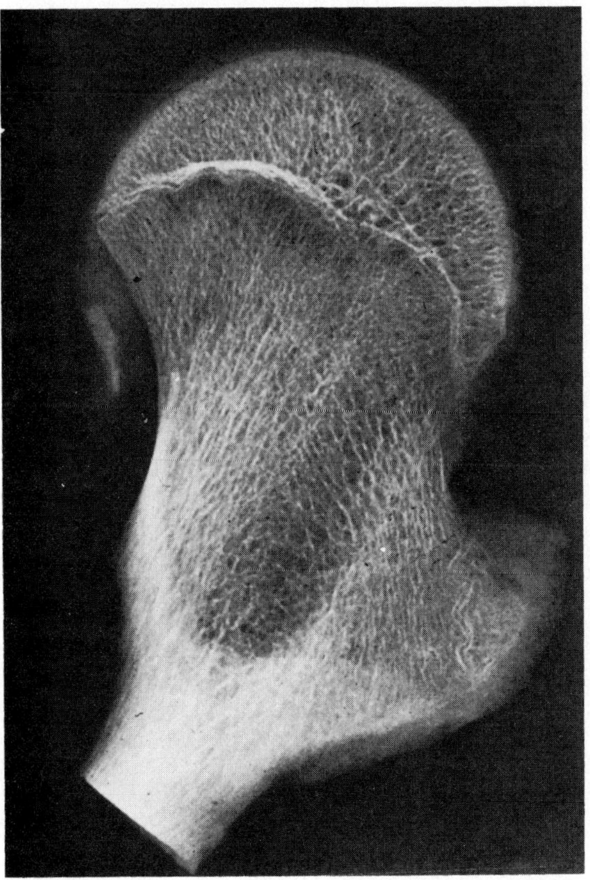

Figure 1–49. Specimen radiograph of the femur shown in Figures 1–47 and 1–48 illustrating lines of stress. A separate meshwork exists in the epiphysis and metaphysis.

INTERNAL REMODELING

At a fairly constant age for each bone, cellular replication of growth-plate cartilage ceases and the remaining cartilage is completely converted to bone. The growth plate "fuses." The trabecular meshwork of the epiphysis is united with the meshwork of the metaphysis, but extensive remodeling is required for realignment of all trabeculae into functional lines of stress (Figs. 1–47 to 1–51). The vascular network of the growth plate persists and can be reactivated under appropriate circumstances (see discussion of fracture, p. 72, and Figs. 3–4 and 3–5).

As the organism grows and becomes active, bones become subject to muscular stresses during walking, running, standing, and other physical activity. Bone must adapt to these changing mechanical demands, and there is a need for remodeling of the skeleton that continues throughout life (Fig. 1–52).

Before new structures can be formed, existing bone must be removed. In cortical areas, a "cutting cone" of osteoclasts appears and progresses along the course of a vessel, producing a resorption cavity (Fig. 1–53). Following behind this cutting cone, osteoblasts align themselves on the wall of the formed cavity and secrete a "cement" or "reversal" line of proteoglycans (Fig. 1–54). Successive relays of osteoblasts produce layers of bone, filling this space from outside in, leaving a small central canal that contains the vessel (haversian canal). A few of the osteoblasts encase in spaces within the bone and become osteocytes. This osteonal system is the basic structural unit of mature bone (Figs. 1–55 to 1–58).

Text continued on page 37

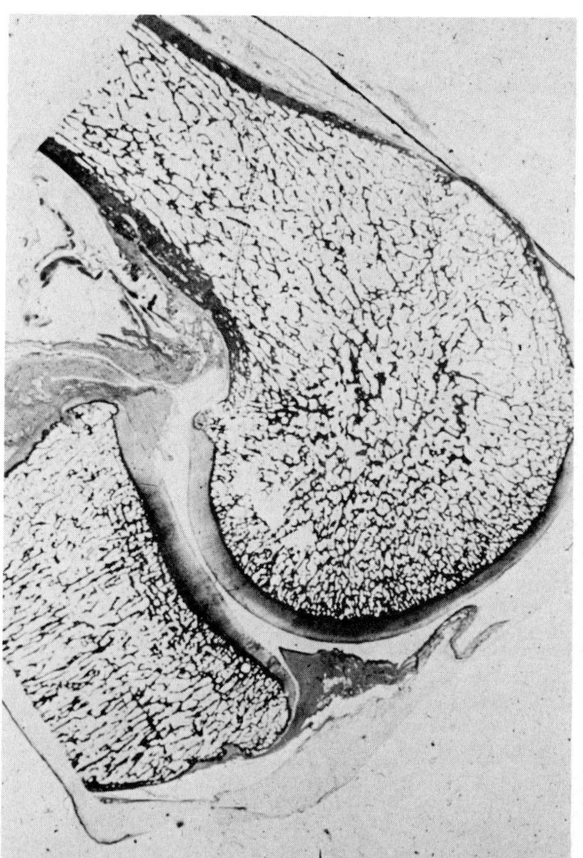

Figure 1–50. Macrosection of adult knee joint illustrating the realignment and fusion of the epiphyseal and metaphyseal trabeculae into one functional unit.

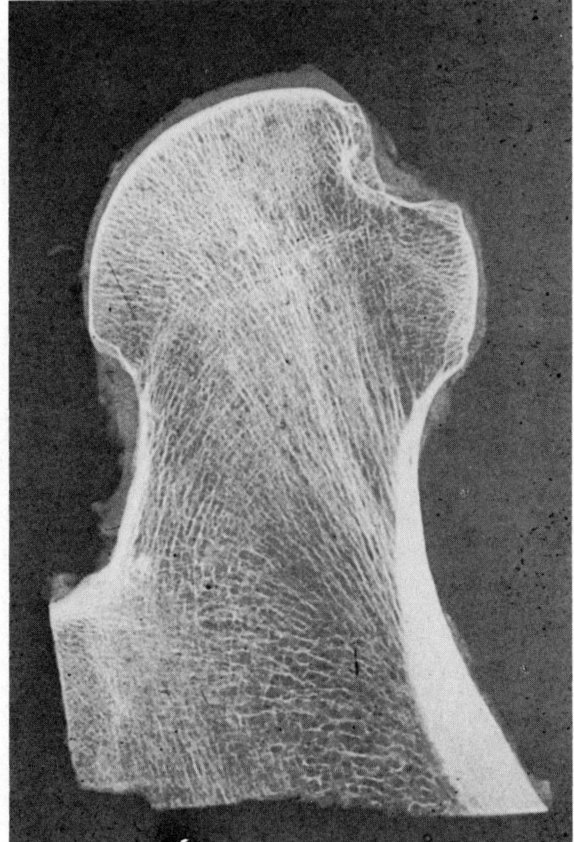

Figure 1–51. Specimen radiograph of mature femur from a young adult showing fusion of epiphyseal and metaphyseal trabecular meshwork into a single functional unit. Compare with Figure 1–49. Extensive remodeling is required to restructure the trabeculae in lines of stress. A bony "scar" persists for years in most bones and marks the site of the earlier growth plate. The metaphyseal vascular bed also persists for years in relation to this scar and can be reactivated by trauma or neoplasm.

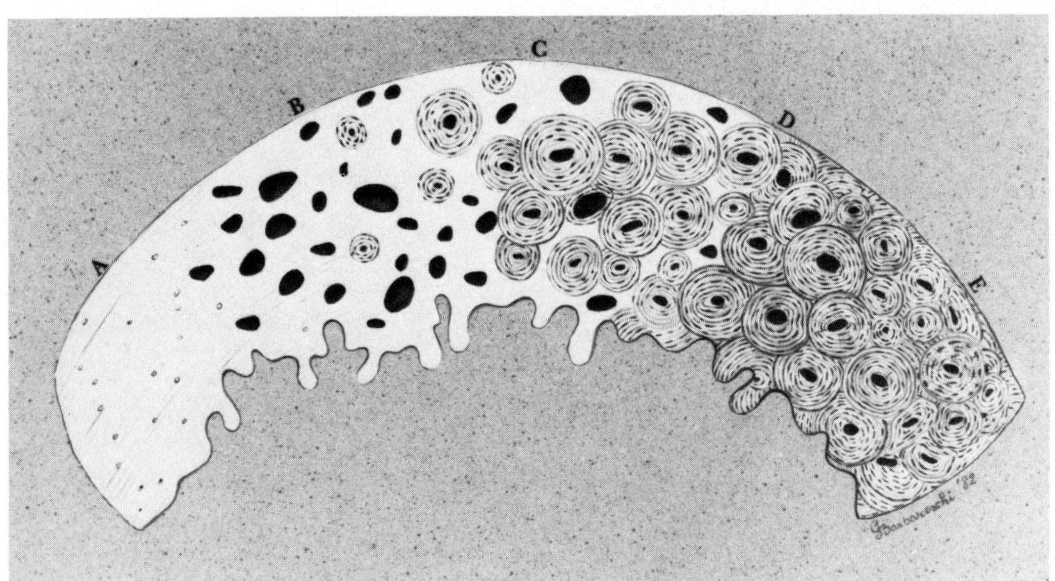

Figure 1–52. Schematic diagram of remodeling from lamellar *(A)* to osteonal bone. The initial step in any remodeling process is activation of osteoclasts with removal of existing bone along blood vessel tracks, resulting in numerous resorption cavities *(B)*. These fill with new bone to produce osteons *(C)*. Further waves of resorption *(D)* and refill result in numerous osteons and fragments *(E)*.

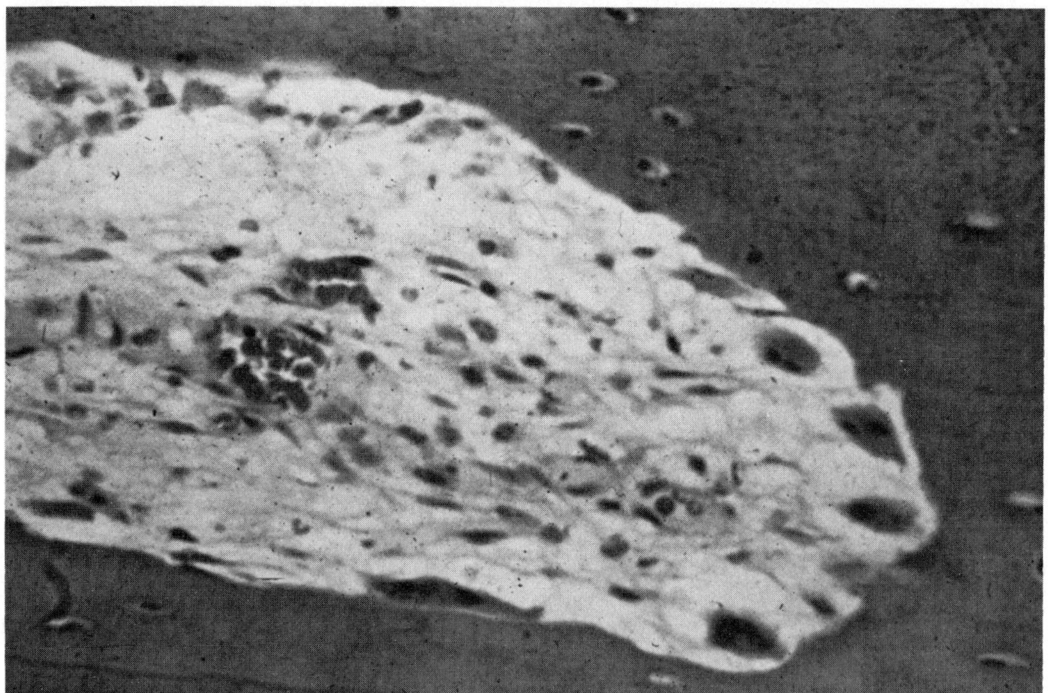

Figure 1–53. "Cutting cone." Successive relays of osteoclasts on the right resorb a tunnel of bone, making it longer and wider with each relay. Behind the cutting cone is a "filling cone" of successive relays of osteoblasts secreting osteoid. Resorption is facilitated by high-speed flow of well-oxygenated blood in small vessels, whereas refill is accompanied by dilated sinusoidal vessels with sluggish flow and low oxygen content.

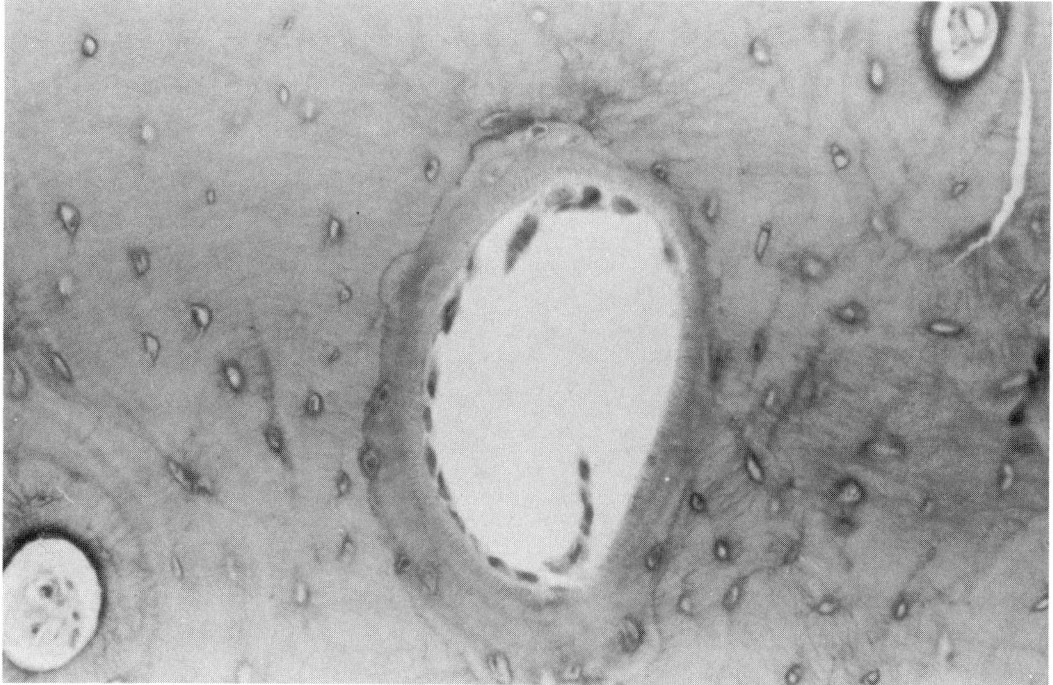

Figure 1–54. Transverse section through cutting cone distal to site of osteoclastic resorption. The osteoblasts have secreted a proteoglycan reversal line, and concentric layers of osteoid matrix are being laid down by the osteoblasts. Osteons are thus cut from inside out and filled from outside in.

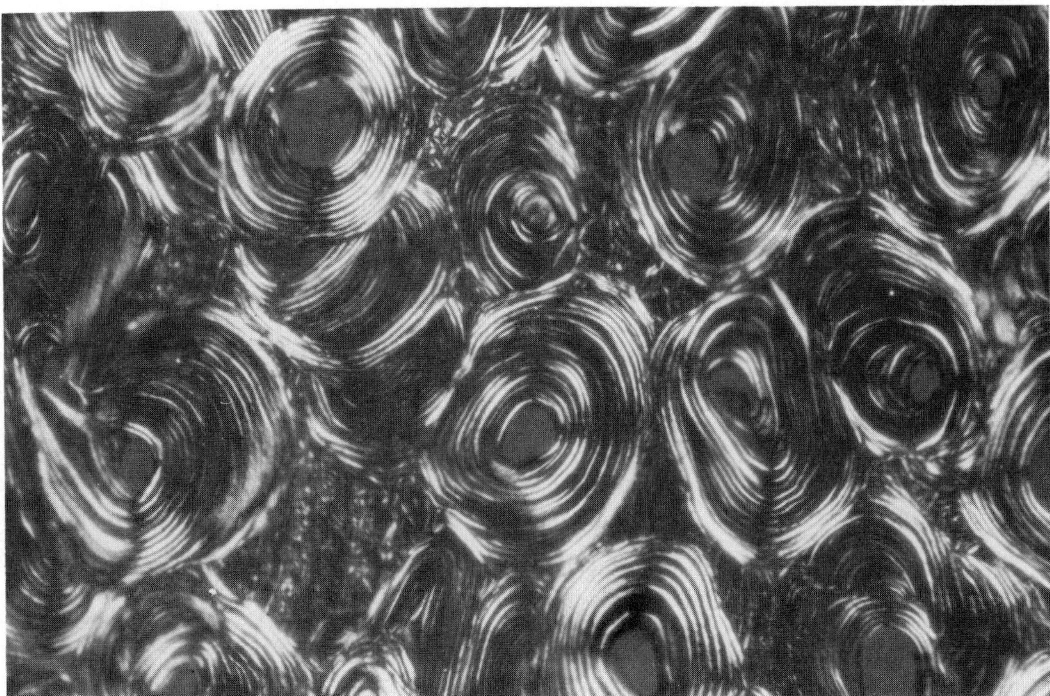

Figure 1–55. Osteons exhibiting circular collagen pattern under polarized light. The central dark space is a haversian canal that contains blood vessels. Small fragments of nonosteonal bone remain. There have been several waves of osteonal remodeling with creation of secondary osteons.

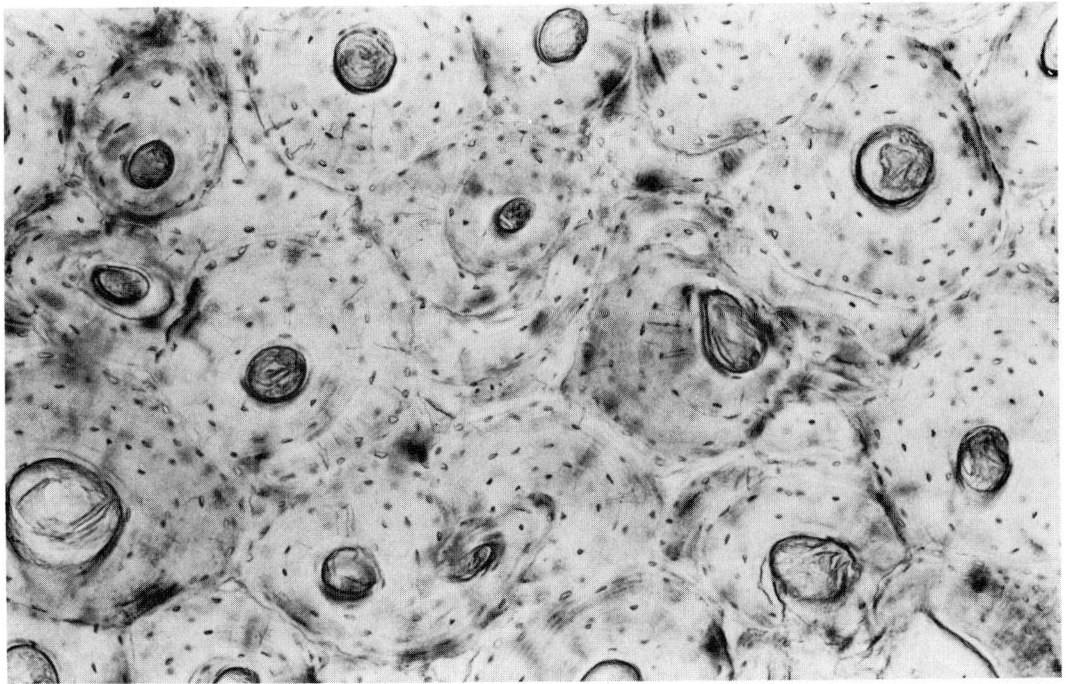

Figure 1–56. Mature bone; osteonal structure as seen in undecalcified material. Numerous interstitial fragments (osteonal fragments without an associated haversian canal) are readily observed.

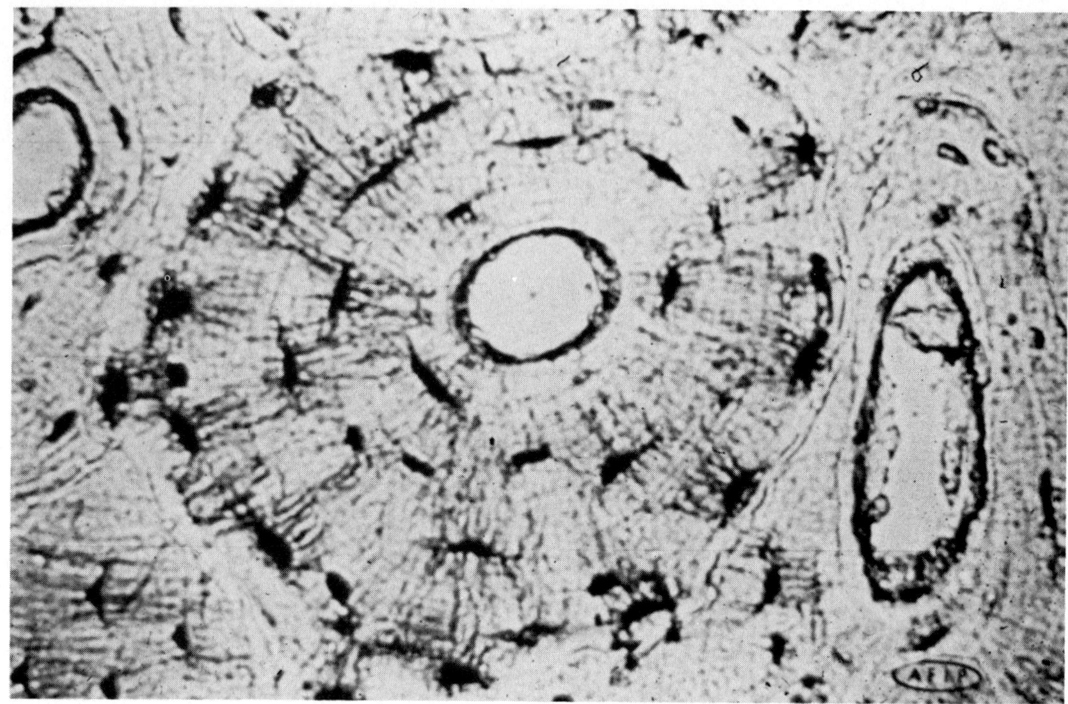

Figure 1–57. Mature bone; reticulin stain. The osteon exhibits a central haversian canal, numerous canaliculi radiating outward from the haversian canal, and osteocytes encased in their lacunae. The canalicular and lacunar system serves to transmit nutrients throughout the osteonal system.

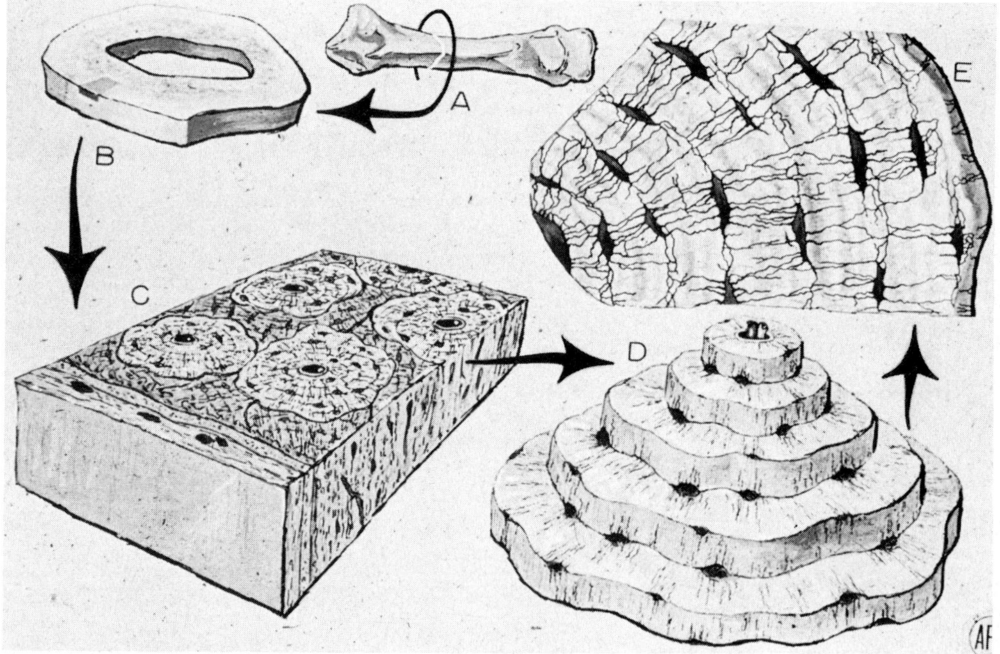

Figure 1–58. Schematic drawing of the osteon and its relationship to bone as a whole. *A,* Whole bone. *B,* Bone with cortical slice removed. *C,* Segment of outer rim of cortex with outer circumferential lamellae and four osteons. *D,* Three-dimensional diagram of osteon illustrating positioning of osteocyte lacunae between layers of osteonal bone and their connections with other osteocytes by cell processes within canaliculae. *E,* Single osteon showing connection from central canal to reversal (cement) line, marking outer limit of osteonal unit.

BONE STRUCTURE

Each osteon consists of a central haversian canal surrounded by concentric layers of bone and defined at its periphery by the reversal line (Fig. 1–56). Lacunae are spaces between the concentric layers of bone that contain the cell body of the osteocyte (Fig. 1–57). Osteoblasts normally interconnect by cell processes; when they become osteocytes, the processes retain the cell-to-cell connections via canaliculi (Figs. 1–57 and 1–58). Each haversian unit, or osteon, is thus a single metabolic unit nourished by the vessel in the central canal.

As the concentric rings of the osteon are formed, the osteoid deposited is mineralized very rapidly to approximately 70 per cent of its capacity. The remaining 20 to 30 per cent of the mineral deposits at a much slower rate.

Primary osteons are usually well developed at the time of growth cessation. During adult life, stresses will continue to vary, and replacement of existing osteonal structure will continue. The process remains the same. A cutting cone is established, bone is removed, and a new osteon is formed. Whether osteoclasts are the only cells capable of removing bone or whether other mechanisms for bone removal exist remains a point of contention (Jaffe, 1972; Koeffler et al., 1978), but in our experience, osteoclasts are always demonstrable.

Each osteon has a finite life span. It will vary from 2 to 3 years in a very young child and up to 15 years in an adult. During remodeling, as the cutting cone removes bone, it may cross osteonal boundaries and remove portions of several adjacent osteons (Fig. 1–56). When this cavity is refilled, portions of the initial osteon may remain. After several waves of such activity, small interstitial fragments that are not

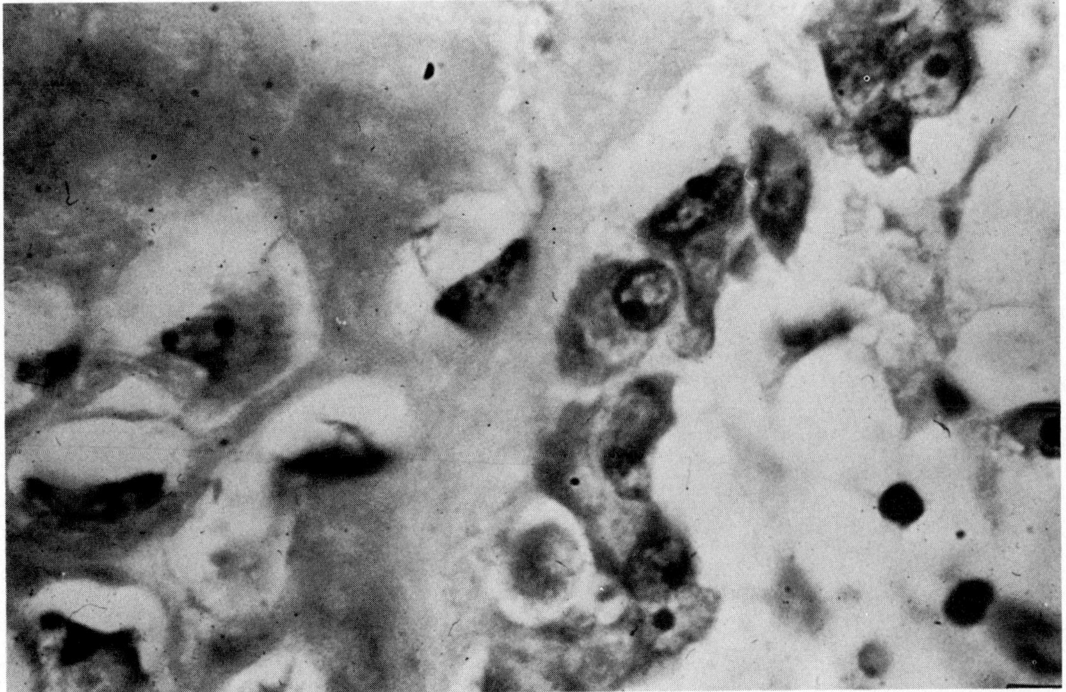

Figure 1–59. Osteoblasts secreting osteoid matrix. The light-staining matrix is deposited on the surface of existing bone. Some of the osteoblasts become encased in the osteoid matrix and modulate to become osteocytes (evident on the left). New relays of osteoblasts appear on the right. The large nucleus with prominent nucleolus, bluish-staining cytoplasm due to numerous ribosomes, and large demilune (Golgi apparatus) are characteristic of cells actively producing protein (osteoid).

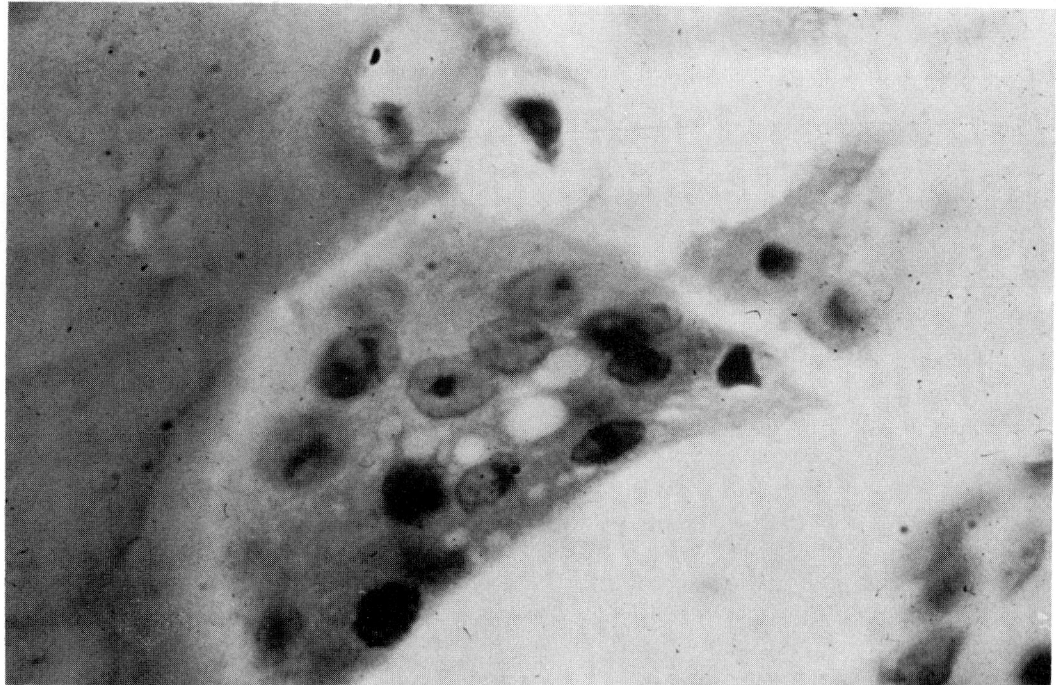

Figure 1–60. Osteoclasts removing bone. The multinucleated osteoclast contains many mitochondria and proteolytic enzymes. The pale area adjacent to the bone is due to large numbers of villi and infolding of cell membrane typical of resorption surfaces. Digestive vacuoles are evident in the cytoplasm. Action by the osteoclast is rapid. Occasionally the osteoclast will have disappeared, leaving the empty space behind. These spaces are called "Howship's lacunae."

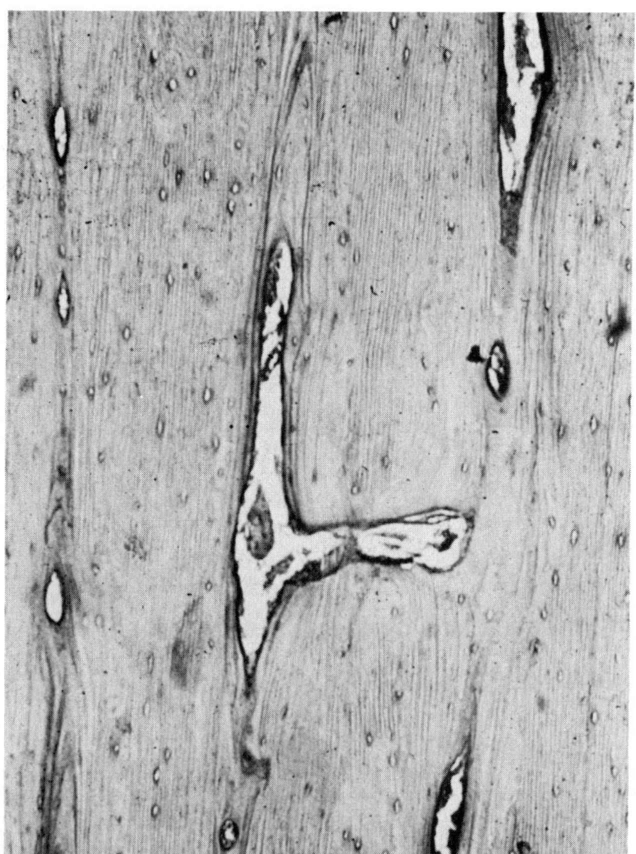

Figure 1–61. Volkmann canal, connecting one haversian system with another. The canal is perpendicular to the haversian system but does not have an osteonal system of its own.

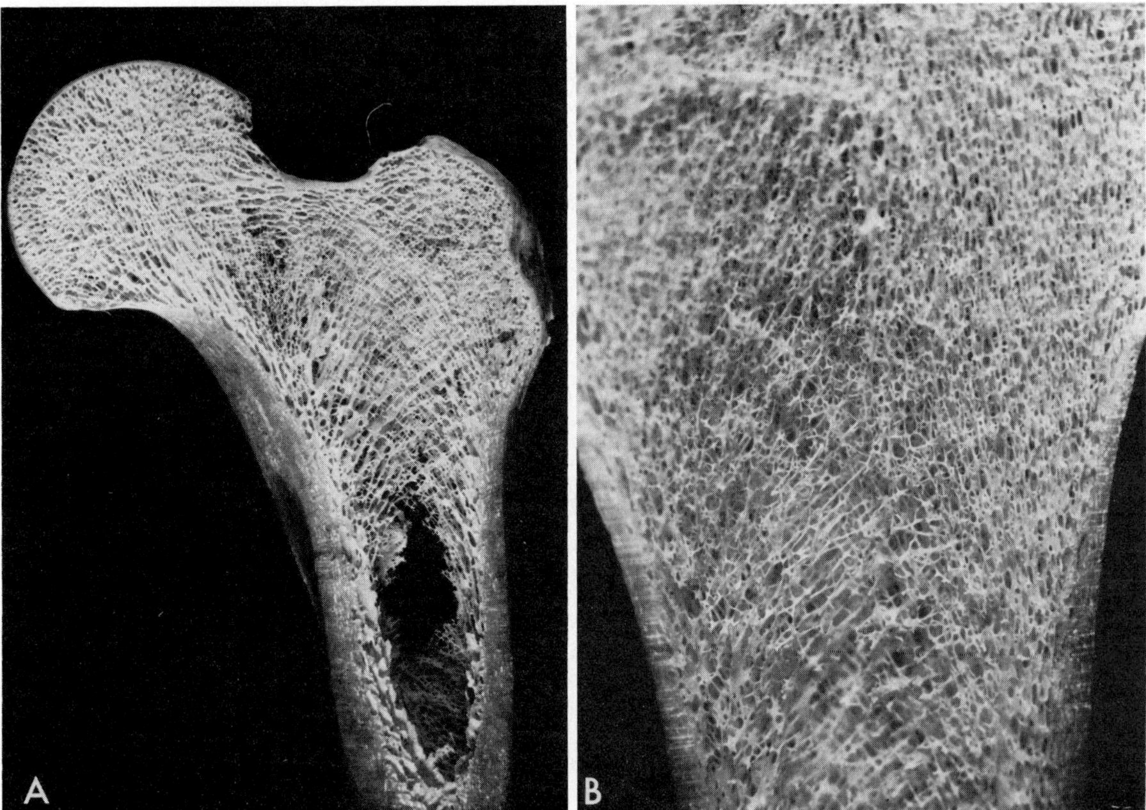

Figure 1–62. Gross specimen of femur illustrating cortical and trabecular bone. Note the fine trabecular meshwork in the spongiosa. The thin trabeculae are characteristic findings in a younger individual.

connected to any haversian system are evident. After many waves of remodeling activity, the number of interstitial fragments increases. The age of a bone can be approximated by the number of osteonal interstitial fragments as well as the number of rings within the osteon. Younger individuals have more osteonal rings and fewer interstitial fragments. Haversian canals are generally oriented longitudinally along the cortex of the bone. They are connected by transversely situated Volkmann's canals (Fig. 1–61).

The blood supply to the bone consists of two independent networks that anastomose with each other. Blood vessels enter the medullary cavity via the nutrient canal, located in the diaphysis of the long bone. Additional vessels enter the metaphyseal and epiphyseal portion of the bone. A single trunk supplies vessels to the epiphysis and metaphysis of both bones in a joint complex. Vascular alterations will therefore affect these structures equally on both sides of the joint, even if the stimulus for the vascular reaction is located in only one bone. (See Fracture, Chapter 3; Tuberculosis, Chapter 4; Sudeck's Atrophy, Chapter 5; and Rheumatoid Arthritis, Chapter 7.)

Within the cortex, the branches of the nutrient vessel split and branch to supply the entire spongiosa. In the growing child with an open growth plate, these vessels form the arcades underneath the hypertrophied cartilage. Branches of the nutrient artery supply the cortex of the bone from the endosteal surface, where they anastomose with numerous branches that supply the periosteum. The periosteum is also supplied with lymph vessels as well as numerous nerves. Periosteum is thus extremely sensitive to pain, but there are no identifiable nerve structures within the medullary cavity. Sympathetic trunks to major vessels terminate when the vessel enters the medullary cavity.

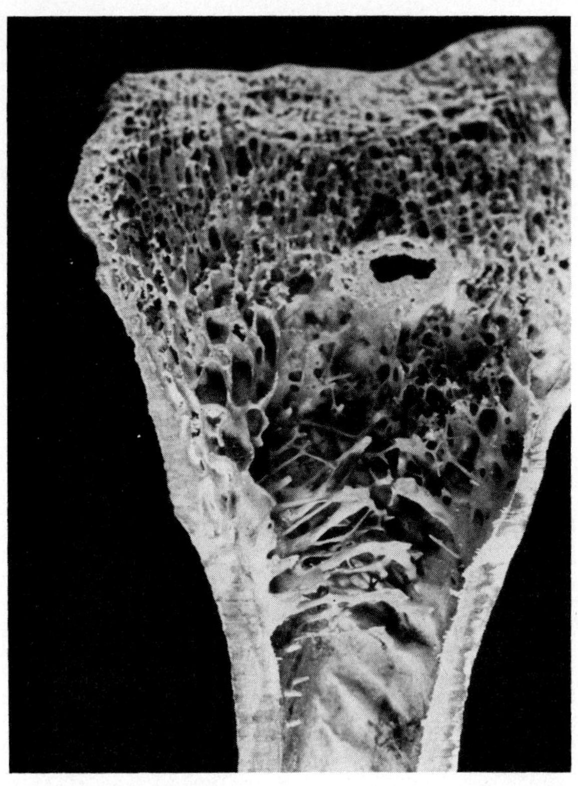

Figure 1–63. Gross specimen of cortical and medullary bone in an older individual, exhibiting the relatively coarse trabeculae in the spongiosa. As individuals age, the cortex widens, medullary trabeculae are reduced in number but become thicker and more prominent.

SUMMARY

Bone may be premodeled in cartilage or in collagen. For most of the bones of the human skeleton, mesenchymal condensation results in a primitive cartilaginous skeleton. Cartilage cells proliferate, secrete matrix that becomes calcified, imbibe water to hypertrophy, and then die. Dead cartilage induces blood vessel invasion, and bone formation follows on the surface of the remaining calcified matrix. This first visible bone formation is termed the "primary ossification center." As it enlarges, bone and marrow gradually replace the center of the previously formed cartilaginous structure. In long bones, secondary ossification centers form in the epiphyseal areas, resulting in a layer of cartilage between the primary and secondary ossification center. This layer of cartilage is the epiphyseal growth plate and continues to proliferate, secrete matrix, hypertrophy, and convert to bone throughout the growth phase of the individual's life span. "Growth" occurs during the hypertrophy of the cartilage cell; it is the result of cell multiplication and hydraulic lifting of the epiphyseal cartilage over the underlying bone platform. Primary trabeculae of bone are those that are formed on the surface of the calcified cartilage matrix framework. Trabeculae are constantly being remodeled through the action of osteoclasts and osteoblasts. In normal adult bone, no primary trabeculae remain.

Increasing thickness of bone is required by the growing individual to cope with muscular stress and activity. Periosteal proliferation results in lateral growth through direct conversion of the connective tissue cambium layer to bone. Streamer bone is formed beneath the periosteum, followed by inlay bone, which fills the space between the streamers, then by addition of circumferential lamellar bone, and next by successive generations of osteon formation. Osteons are the structural units of adult bone. Bone growth is a continuous process that never completely ceases, and it responds to periods of activity or rest by increasing or decreasing bone thickness. The epiphyseal growth plate, however, disappears at a fairly constant age through fusion of the primary and secondary ossification centers. Some conversion of cartilage to bone (i.e., "growth") occurs at the articular end of the bone throughout life.

CITED REFERENCES

Jaffe, H. L.: Metabolic, Degenerative and Inflammatory Diseases of Bones and Joints. Philadelphia, Lea and Febiger, 1972, p. 73.
Koeffler, H. P., Mundy, G. R., Golde, D. W., and Cline, M. J.: Production of bone resorbing activity in poorly differentiated monocytic malignancy. Cancer 41:2438, 1978.

GENERAL REFERENCES

Aegerter, E., and Kirkpatrick, J. A., Jr.: Orthopedic Diseases. 4th ed. Philadelphia, W. B. Saunders Company, 1975.
Jaffe, H. L.: Metabolic, Degenerative and Inflammatory Diseases of Bones and Joints. Philadelphia, Lea and Febiger, 1972.
Johnson, L. C.: Morphologic analysis in pathology: the kinetics of disease and general biology of bone. *In* Frost, H. M.: Bone Biodynamics. Boston, Little, Brown and Co., 1964.
Johnson, L. C.: Birth defects. Original Article Series II, No. 1. National Foundation March of Dimes, April, 1966.
Lichtenstein, L.: Diseases of Bone and Joints. St. Louis, C. V. Mosby Co., 1970.
O'Rahilly, R., and Gardner, E.: The embryology of bone and bones. *In* Ackerman, L. V., Spjut, H. J., and Abell, M. R. (Eds.): Baltimore, Williams and Wilkins Co., 1976, pp. 1–15.
Teitelbaum, S. L., and Bullough, P. G.: The pathophysiology of bone and joint disease. Am. J. Pathol. 96:283, 301, 1979.

SKELETAL SYSTEM
NORMAL GROWTH AND DEVELOPMENT: GLOSSARY

Terms	Definition	Illustration
Bone formation		
Cartilage model bone; endochrondral bone formation	Bone preformed in cartilage	Fig. 1–4
Collagen model bone; intramembranous bone formation	Bone formed directly in connective tissue, without pre-existing cartilage model.	
Bone types		
Compact	Cortex	Figs. 1–62 and 1–63
Cancellous	Trabeculae, spongiosa	
Growth plate		
Resting	Layers of cartilage leading to formation of bone	Figs. 1–16 to 1–34
Proliferating		
Secretory		
Hypertrophic		
Provisional calcification		
Ossification centers		
Primary	Central; diaphyseal precedes formation of secondary ossification center in epiphysis	Figs. 1–7 and 1–8
Secondary	Epiphysis; appear and fuse at uniform age and can be used to evaluate fetal maturity	Figs. 1–12 and 1–13
Terms		
Osteoblasts	Form bone; encase within matrix to become osteocytes in lacunae; lacunae are connected by canaliculi and contain cell processes of the osteocytes	Fig. 1–59
Osteoclasts	Remove bone; Howship's lacunae remain after removal	Fig. 1–60
Haversian canals	Central canals of osteons; contain blood vessels	Fig. 1–57
Volkmann's canals	Connect one Haversian system to another	Fig. 1–61
Cutting cone	Relay of osteoclasts for removal of bone prior to remodeling	Fig. 1–53
Filling cone	Osteoblastic activity to restructure cortical bone into osteons after osteoclastic resorption	Fig. 1–54
Cambium layer	Prominent periosteal layer seen during growth phase on the lateral surface of bone	Figs. 1–40 and 1–41
Collagen patterns (under polarized light)		
Woven bone A. Coarse: "burlap" (rapid) B. Fine "linen" (slower)	Appearance of collagen pattern in bone; structure depends on rate of formation	Figs. 1–45 and 3–32
Lamellar bone A. Outer circumferential lamellae	Without osteons; parallel bands of collagen	Fig. 1–46
B. Osteonal lamellae	Basic structural unit of mature bone with central Haversian canal surrounded by concentric lamellae	Fig. 1–55

2

CONGENITAL DYSPLASIAS

The identified skeletal dysplasias comprise more than eighty distinct conditions with variable expression that can be distinguished on the basis of morphologic and radiographic findings. Detailed analysis of these abnormalities is beyond the scope of this book; the reader is therefore referred to the classic monograph by Rubin and the more recent review by Sillence and coworkers. Achondroplasia represents failure of cartilage formation, osteogenesis imperfecta represents abnormal bone formation, and osteopetrosis represents faulty bone remodeling; variations of these basic defects account for the vast majority of the remaining numerous but rare dysplasias. The morphologic findings of the three fundamental defects are summarized below.

ACHONDROPLASIA

Achondroplasia is a congenital hereditary disturbance of the growth plate characterized by failure of cartilage maturation. Bone formation is normal, as is collagen fiber formation. All bones preformed in cartilage are thus affected; in contrast, the dome of the skull is normal because it is formed directly from collagen without a cartilage model. In the most severe form of this disorder, the chest cavity fails to expand sufficiently for survival, and an affected child dies in utero. The more classic achondroplastic dwarf is a familiar sight, with short legs, more or less normal torso, and lordotic deformity of the spine. The lordosis is due to the deranged growth centers in the body and lateral masses of the vertebral column.

The histologic manifestations of achondroplasia are seen at the growth plate. Although there is some cartilage maturation, it is severely inhibited and inconsistent with the normal length of the hypertrophied cartilage columns (Figs. 2–1 and 2–2). When evaluating a growth plate for evidence of retarded development, one must always compare it with the corresponding growth plate of a normal individual at the same chronologic age (Figs. 2–3 to 2–14).

Text continued on page 51

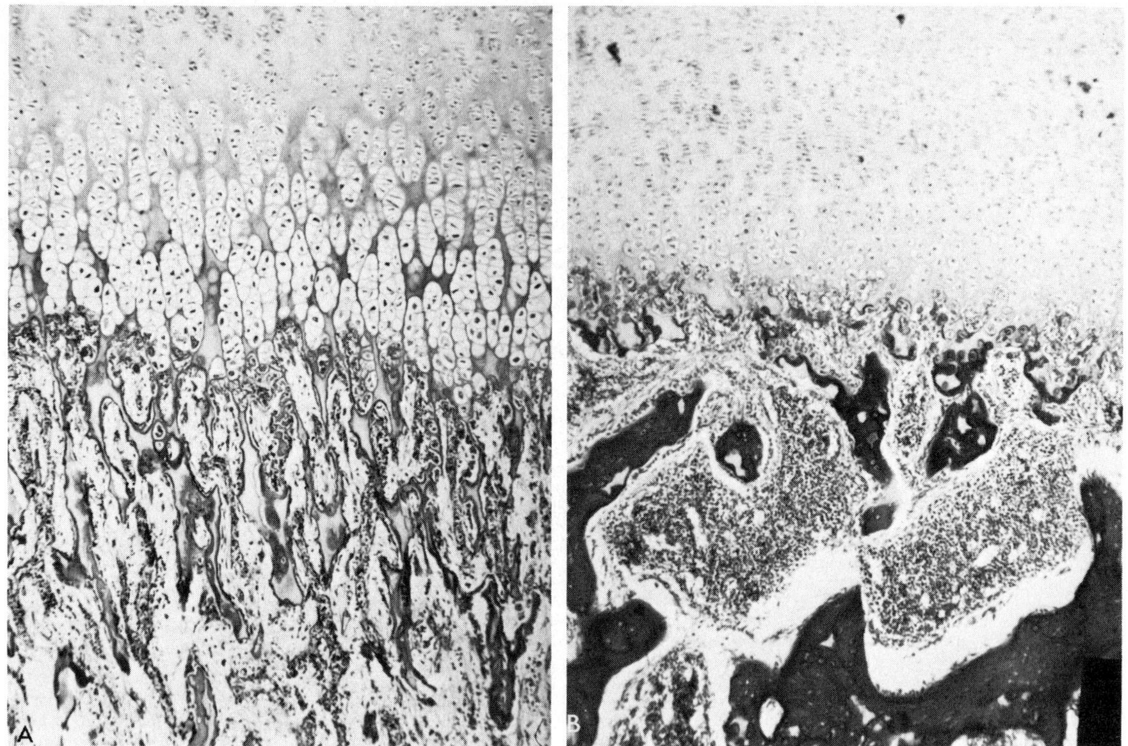

Figure 2–1. Histologic study of growth plate of lower end of femur in normal 1-year-old patient *(A)* compared with section from achondroplastic dwarf *(B)*. Note the fairly long columns of hypertrophied cartilage and bone formation on the slender cartilaginous matrix bars in the normal section. The section from the achondroplastic dwarf has little normal hypertrophied zone, no discernible columnization, and haphazard bone formation on those isolated fragments of cartilage that are developed.

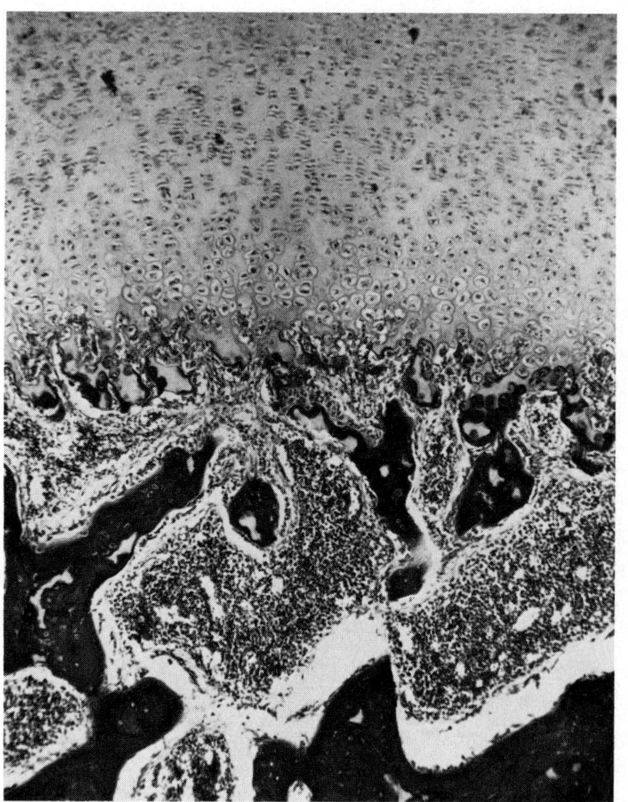

Figure 2–2. Histologic appearance of growth plate exhibiting lack of cartilage maturation. Failure to produce normal cartilage scaffold causes abnormal activity at the cartilage-bone interface, even though bone production itself is normal. Growth plates must be compared with similar growth plates in normal children at same chronologic age.

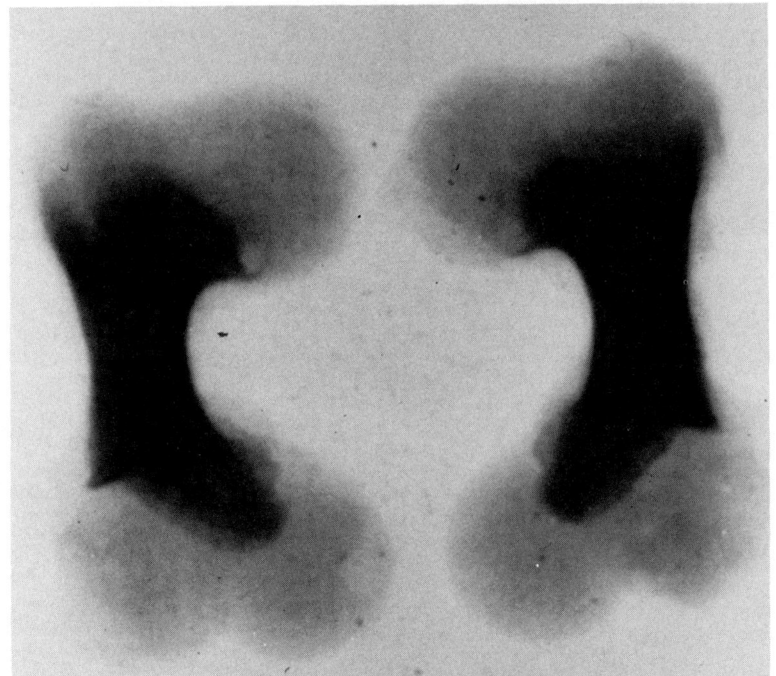

Figure 2–3. Specimen radiograph of achondroplastic femurs. Failure of normal conversion of cartilage to bone results in short, broad bones with enlarged bulbous cartilage ends.

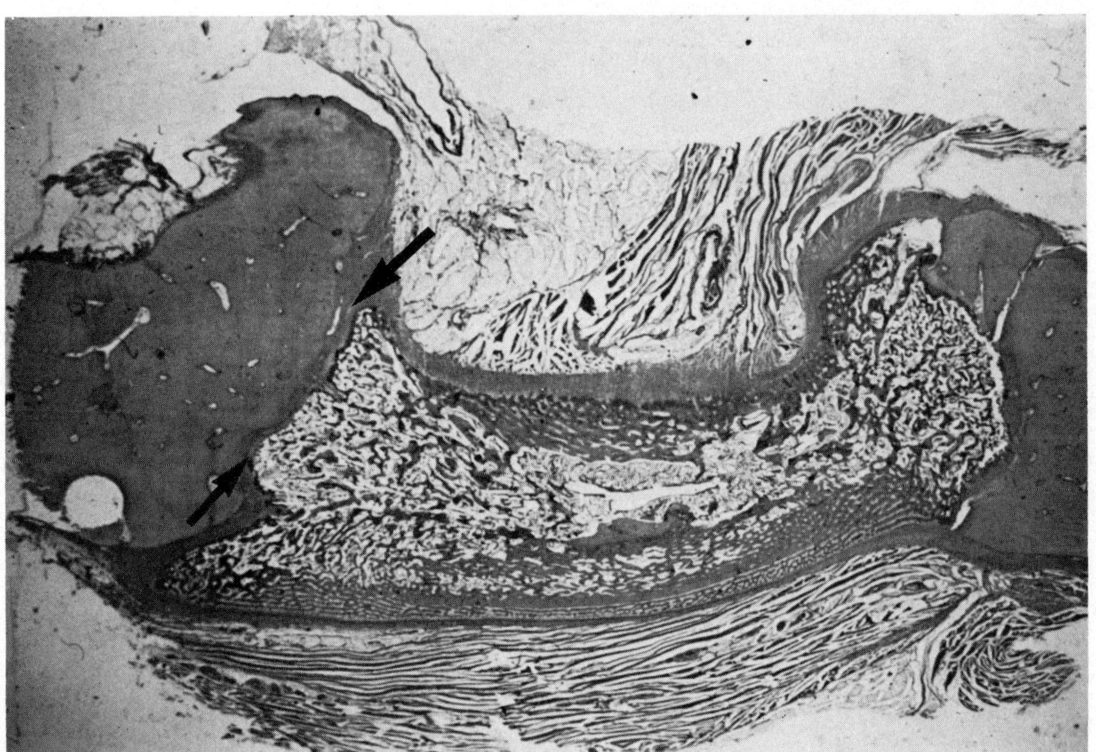

Figure 2–4. Macrosection of achondroplastic bone. Lack of cartilage maturation results in markedly decreased length of long bones. There is also decreased width of the growth plate despite overall increase in diameter of the cartilage epiphysis. Normal periosteal bone growth with narrowed growth plate is seen with infolding and apposition of periosteum and perichondrium at level of perichondrial ring (arrows).

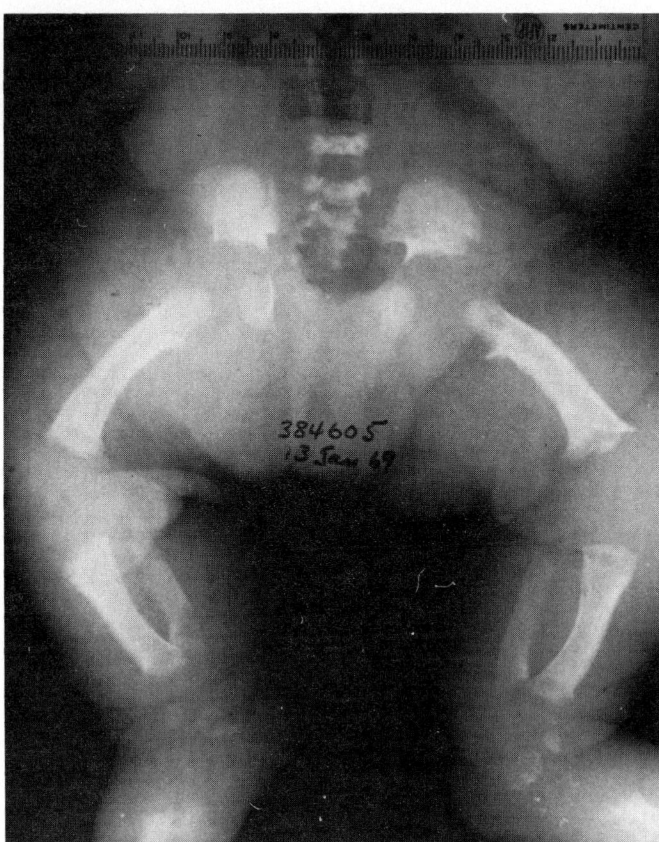

Figure 2–5. Radiographic appearance of lower limbs in a patient with achondroplasia. Note the narrow sciatic notch and flat broad acetabulum due to inadequate growth of "Y" cartilage in acetabulum. Shortened, thick femurs, tibias, and fibulas are bowed. Bone density is normal. Epiphyses do not yet exhibit secondary ossification centers.

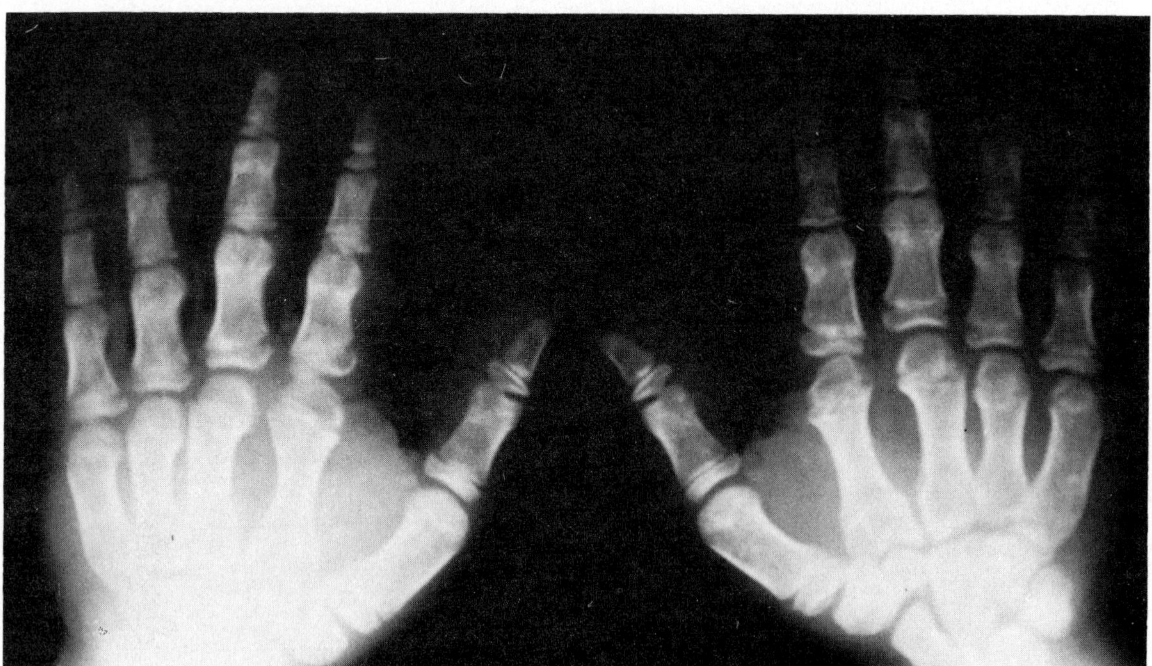

Figure 2–6. Radiograph of hands of achondroplastic child. Deformities are accentuated where growth normally is greatest (distal femurs, proximal tibias, etc.) or where multiple growth plates are present in a small area. Short, stubby fingers are characteristic of achondroplasia.

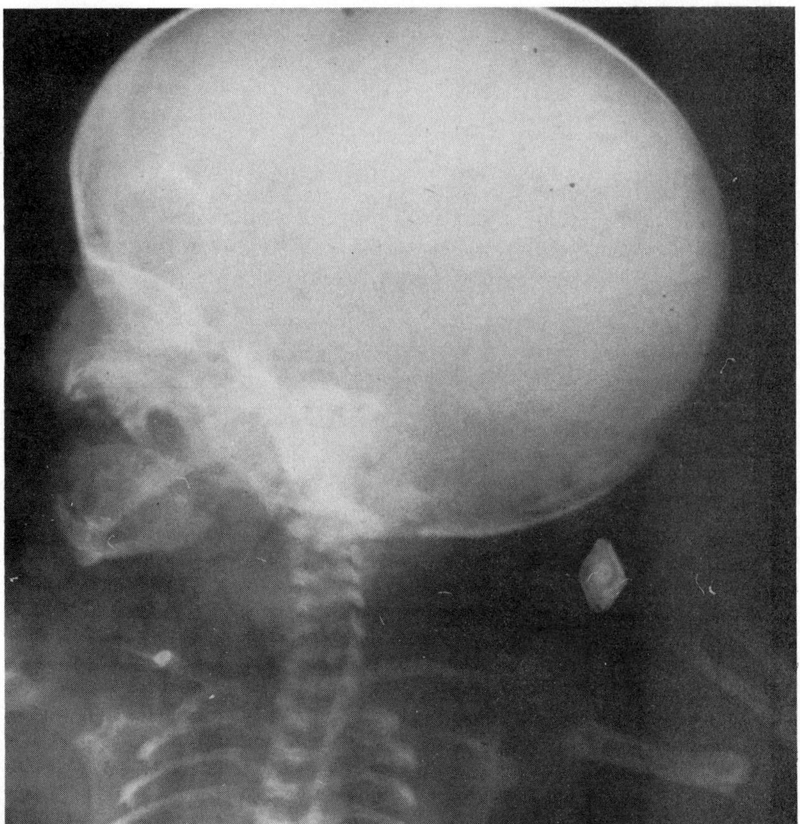

Figure 2–7. Lateral skull radiograph of patient with achondroplasia exhibiting abnormal skull formation. Bones of cranial vault are formed from collagen model and are not affected by the chondrodystrophic process. The bones of the basicranium are cartilage model and are shortened relative to the vault, causing frontal bossing and appearance of hydrocephalus.

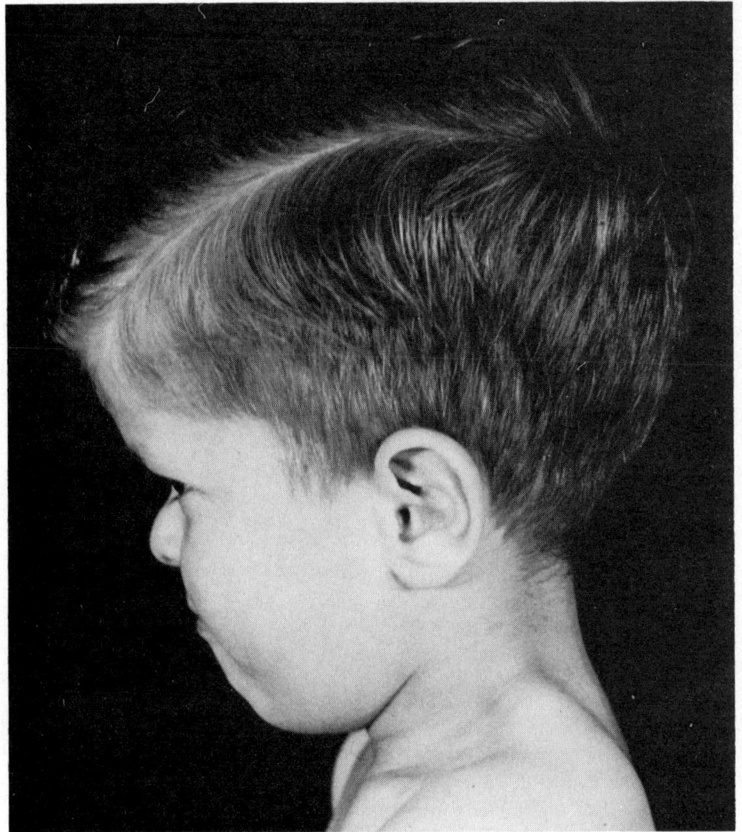

Figure 2–8. Inadequate growth of base of skull and of mandible causes characteristic frontal prominence, depressed nasal bridge, shortened jaw, and disproportion between face and cranial vault. Appearance of hydrocephalus is deceptive, since many children with these findings are very bright.

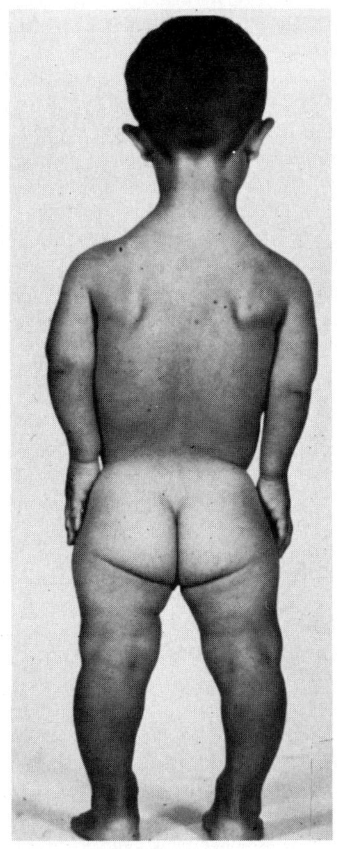
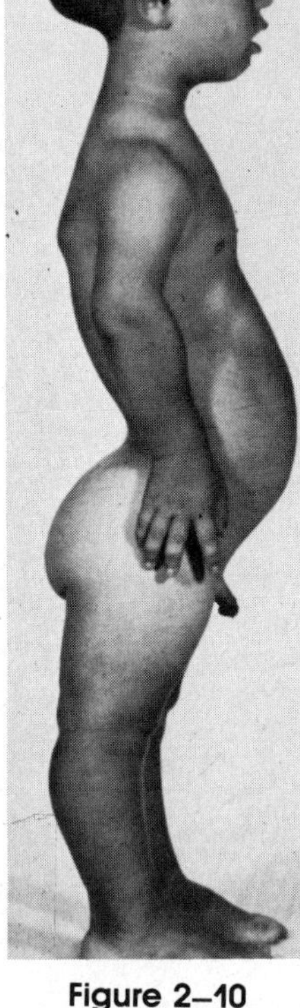

Figure 2–9. Photograph of achondroplastic dwarf showing distorted growth of long bones. The proximal limb segments are proportionately shorter than the distal, with the hands reaching only to the hip region. The legs are bowed, and the scapulae and pelvis are smaller than normal. Scoliosis is uncommon.

Figure 2–10. Child with achondroplasia. Note marked lumbar lordosis with prominent buttocks due to pelvic tilt. The lordosis is due in part to differential growth of vertebral body versus posterior elements.

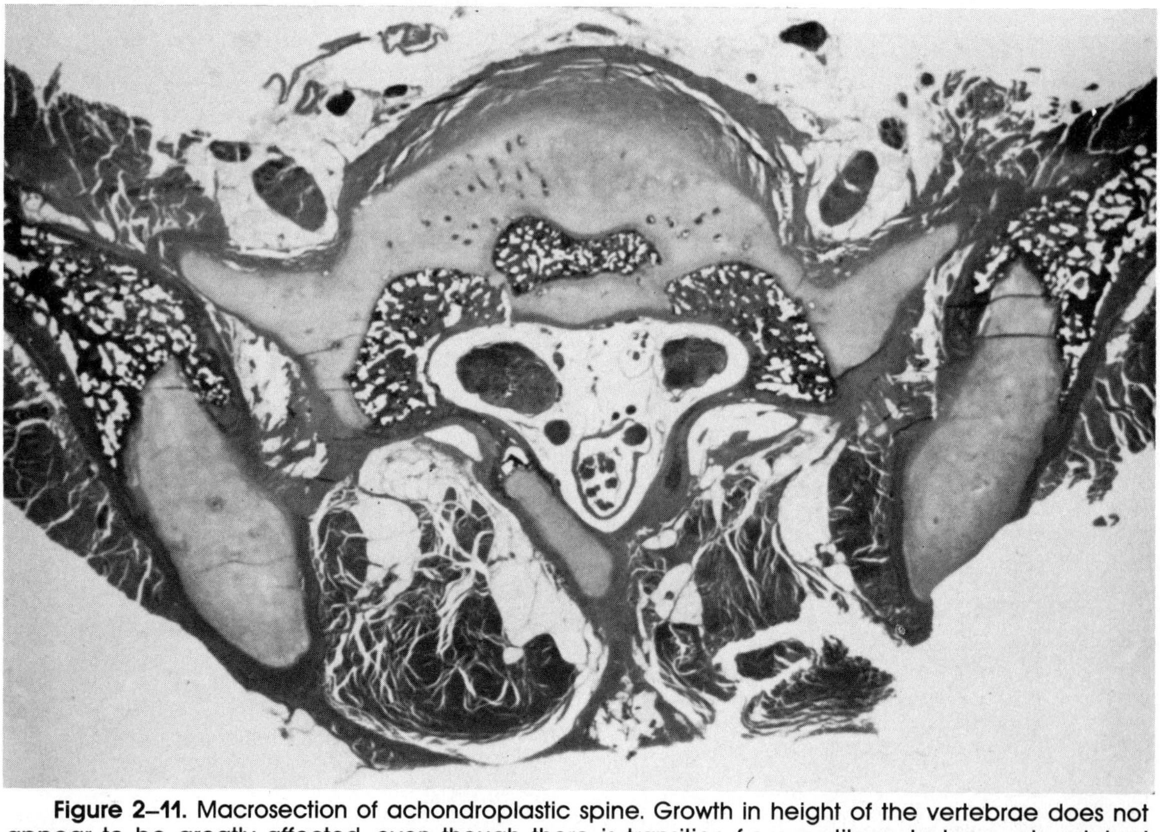

Figure 2–11. Macrosection of achondroplastic spine. Growth in height of the vertebrae does not appear to be greatly affected, even though there is transition from cartilage to bone at vertebral end-plates.

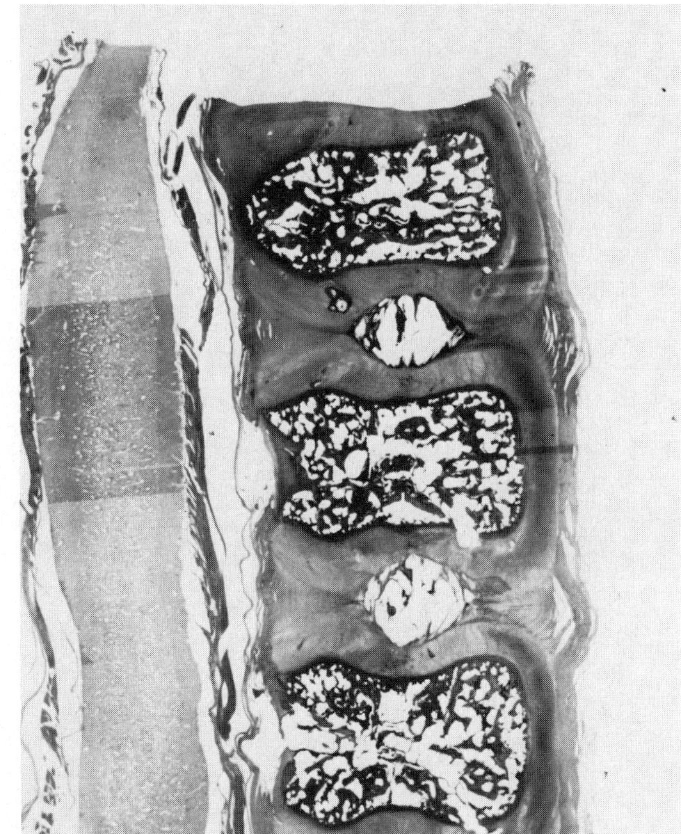

Figure 2–12. Macrosection of achondroplastic vertebrae. Growth of primary ossification centers in body and lateral masses is severely affected, causing shortened pedicles and laminae with narrowed intervertebral foramina.

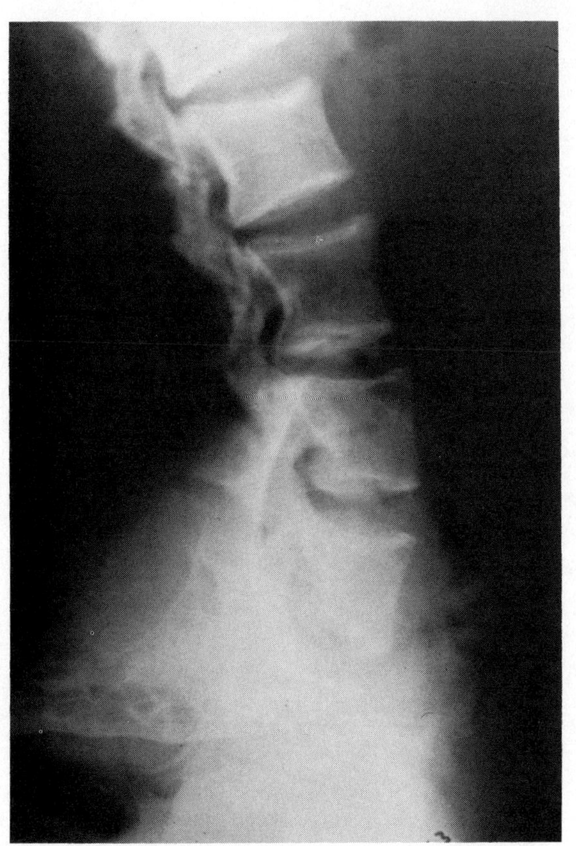

Figure 2–13. Lateral radiograph of lumbosacral spine and pelvis. Abnormal vertebral growth posteriorly results in short pedicles and markedly narrowed intervertebral foramina. The accentuated lumbar lordosis and pelvic tilt cause prominent buttocks and waddling gait. Note horizontal sacrum. Lumbar disc disease with nerve compression is very common in achondroplastic adults.

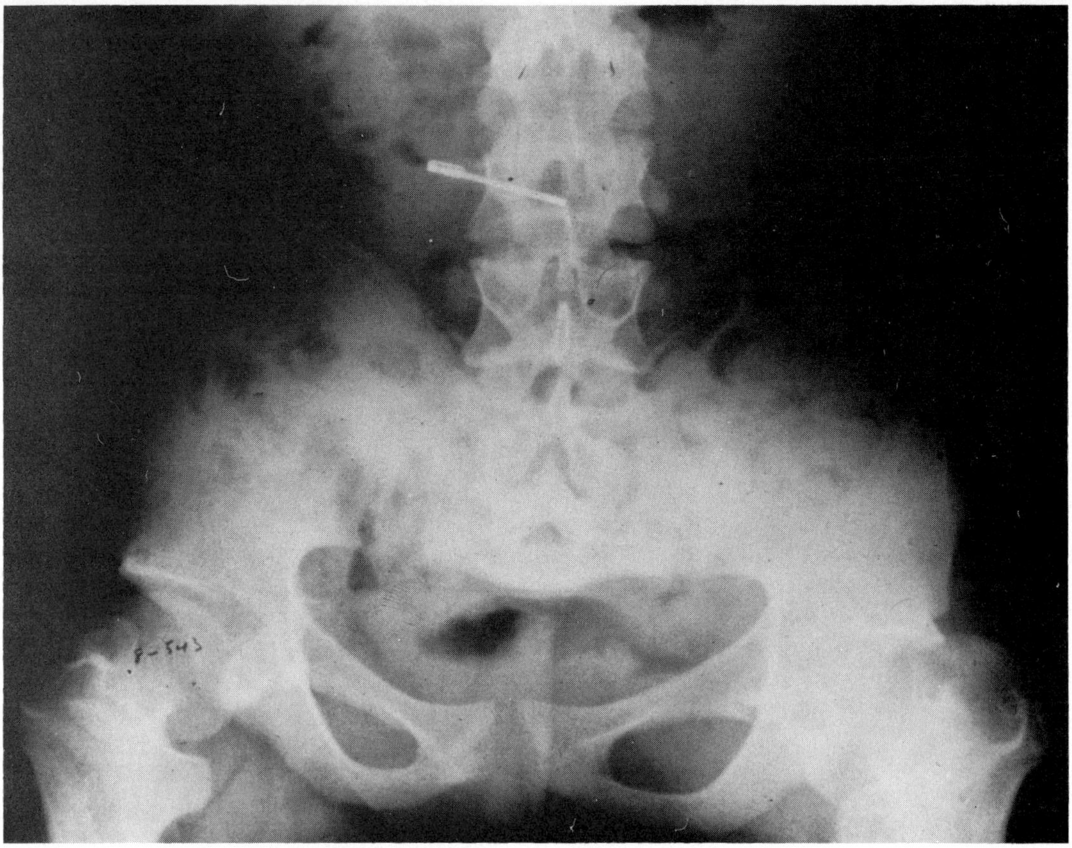

Figure 2–14. Anteroposterior radiograph of lumbosacral spine and pelvis. Vertebral body growth abnormalities are seen in decreasing interpedicular distances from L-1 to L-5. Marked lumbar lordosis and pelvic tilt are evident in the appearance of fifth lumbar vertebra, seen "on end" with the vertebral canal clearly visualized.

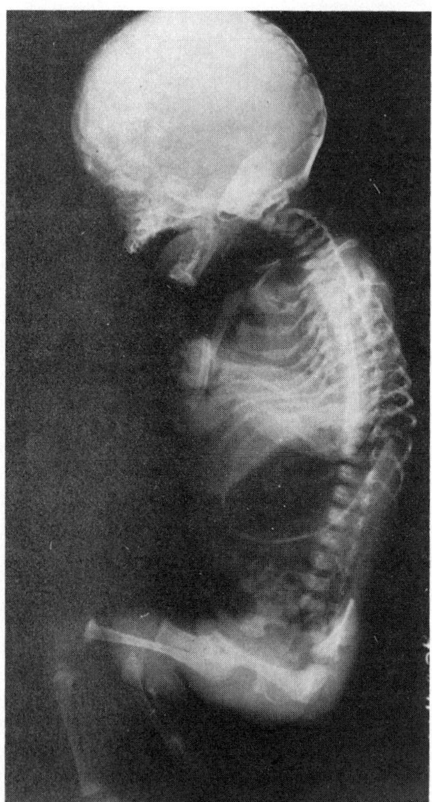

Figure 2–15. Radiograph of stillborn infant with osteogenesis imperfecta. Note multiple fractures of ribs, femurs, and other bones. All bones are severely osteopenic.

OSTEOGENESIS IMPERFECTA

Osteogenesis imperfecta comprises a group of generalized hereditary defects in which fibroblasts, chondroblasts, and osteoblasts are unable to produce normal collagen (Sykes et al., 1977). Although osteoblasts are present, the defective collagen results in poor osteoíd that is not easily mineralized and is subject to bowing and fracture. Collagen synthesis is affected throughout; the patient therefore has multiple defects, including the characteristic blue sclerae (Teitelbaum and Bullough, 1979).

Radiographically, the bone that is formed is severely osteoporotic, and it is subject to numerous fractures. In the majority of fractures, callus formation results in healing with development of similar immature osteoporotic bone. Occasional fractures are characterized by exuberant callus formation, disproportionate with the actual fracture. Despite the extensive callus, the bone remains osteoporotic and of poor quality.

Histologically, the bone is characterized by a primitive collagen pattern, reminiscent of "burlap," or "woven," bone (Figs. 2–15 to 2–35). Lamellar bone or osteon formation is scanty and occurs in the less severely involved disease states (tarda) (Fig. 2–36).

Text continued on page 63

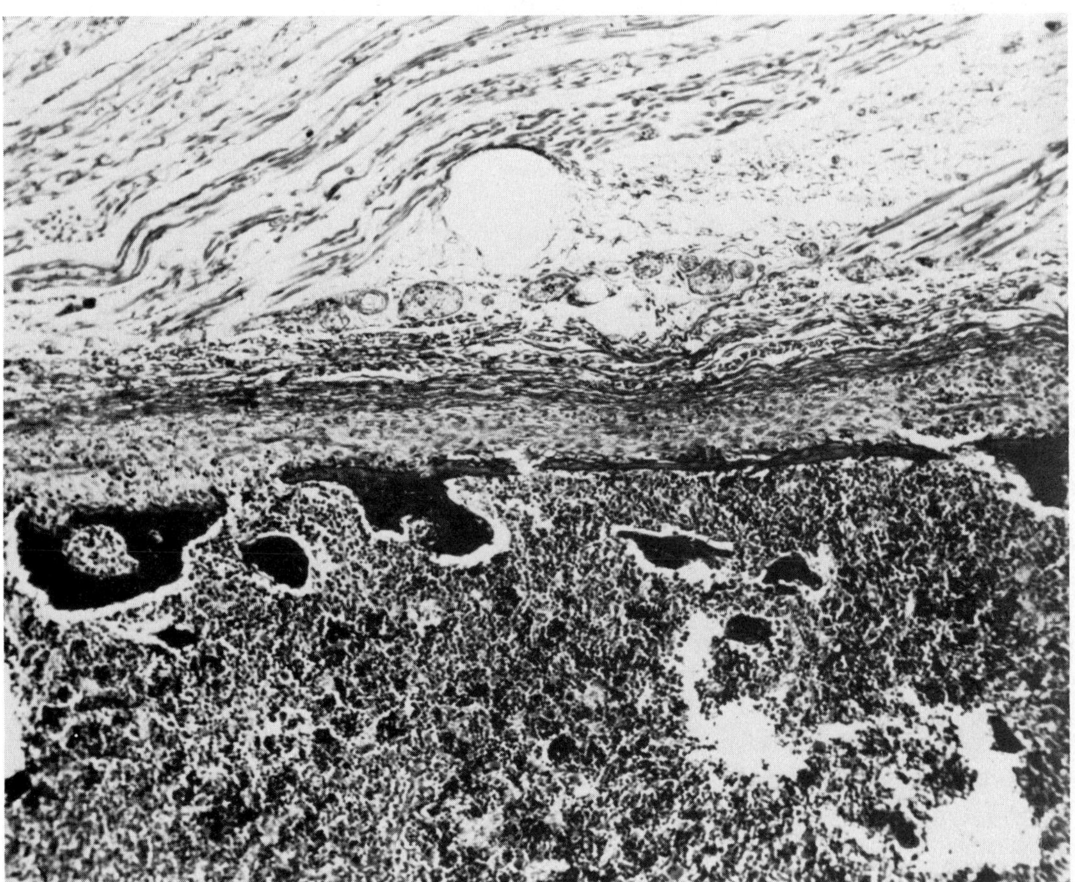

Figure 2–16. Longitudinal section of severely involved long bone with only minute amount of woven bone evident beneath the periosteum. There are no trabeculae seen in the medullary cavity.

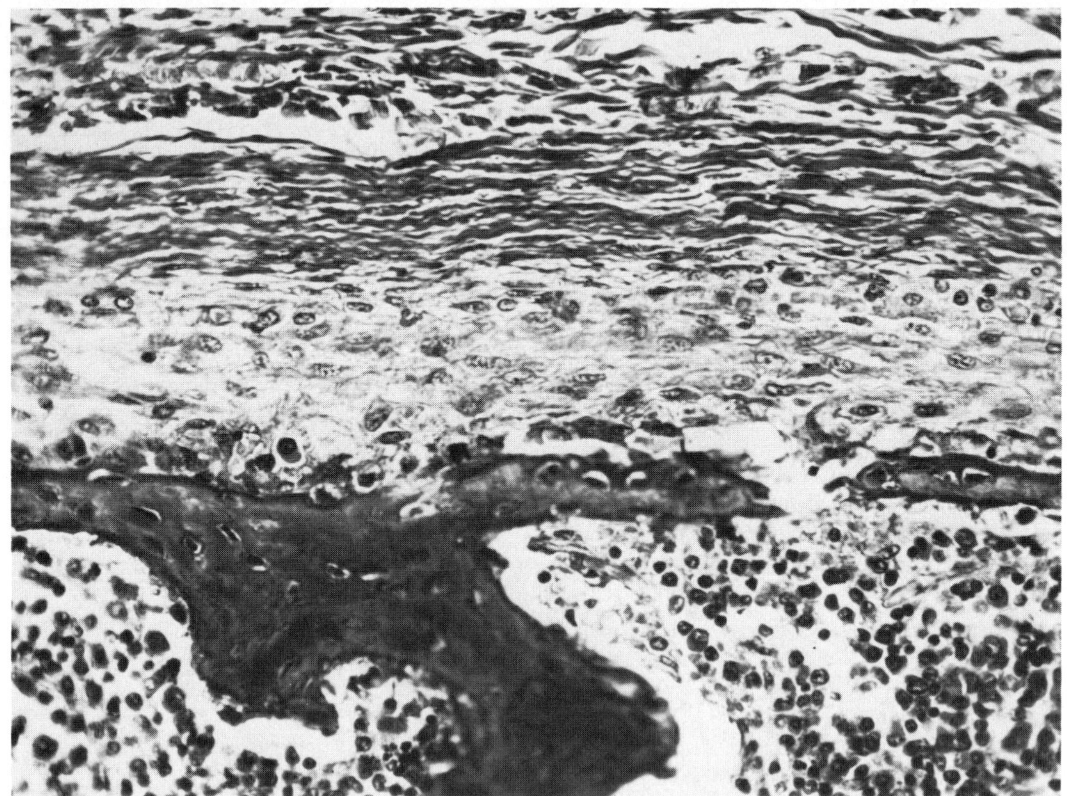

Figure 2–17. High-power view of cortex. A prominent periosteal membrane is present with a cellular cambium layer. Many osteoblasts are evident, but their product is scanty and primitive.

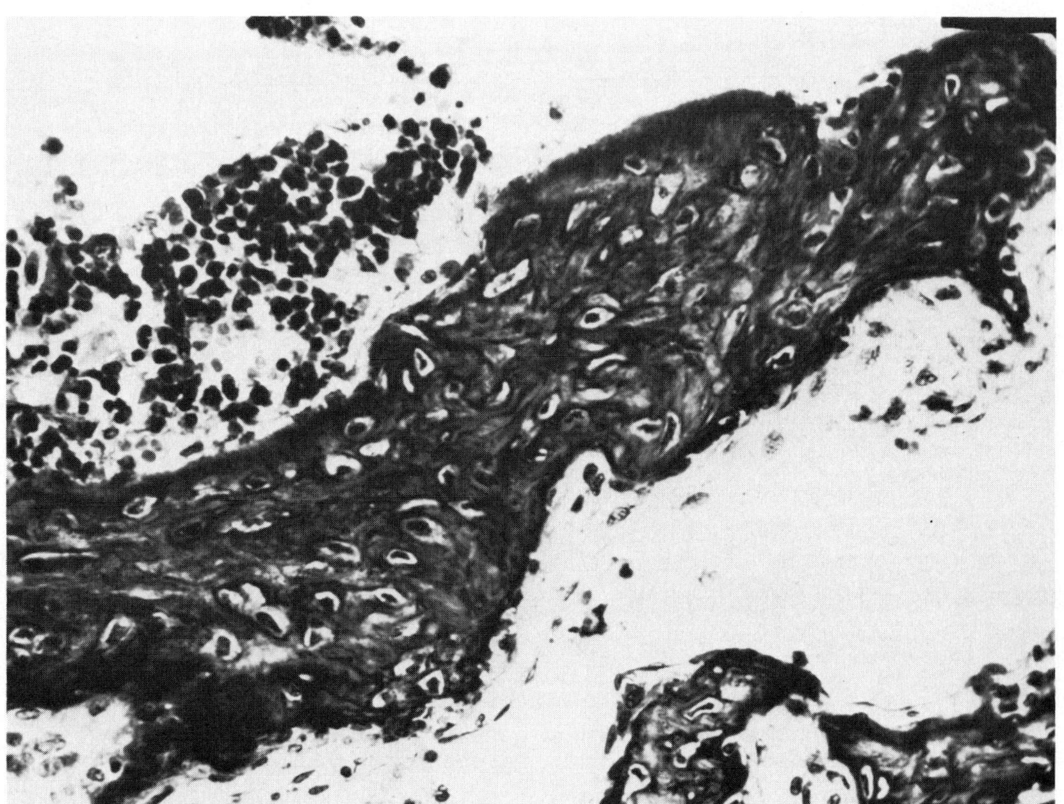

Figure 2–18. Intramedullary trabeculae of bone exhibiting primitive woven pattern with numerous cells per unit volume. Woven bone is normal in the early stages of bone formation but is progressively replaced by lamellar bone during normal development. In osteogenesis imperfecta, bone structure does not progress beyond this primitive woven bone.

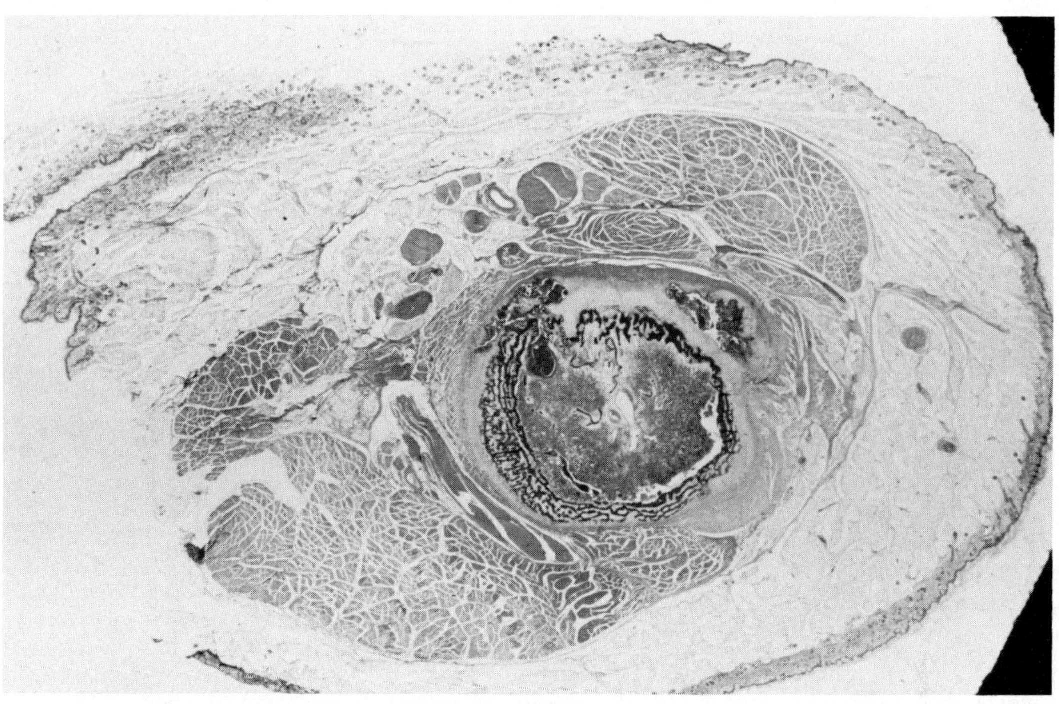

Figure 2–19. Cross section of humerus exhibiting several layers of primitive woven bone but no lamellar bone formation.

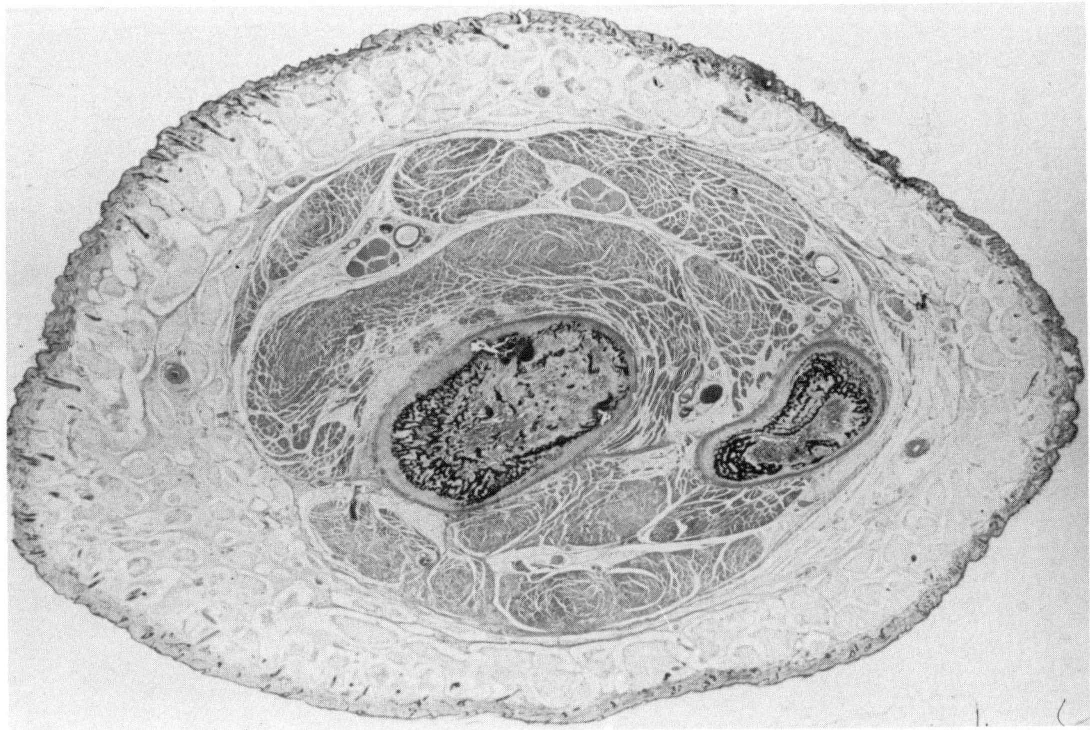

Figure 2–20. Cross section of forearm exhibiting type of bone similar to that seen in Figure 2–19. There is some attempt at normal skew of growth, as evidenced by increased bone production on one side of each bone.

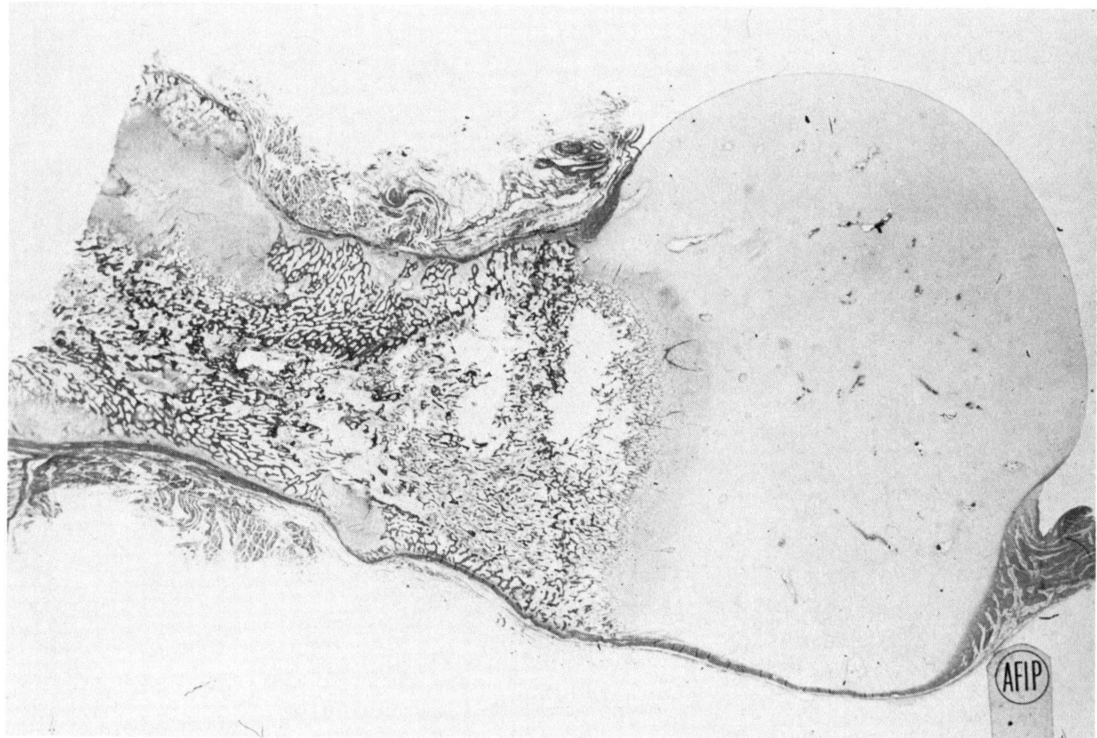

Figure 2–21. Macrosection of upper humerus. The cartilage appears normal, although the bone is severely involved. Very few bone trabeculae are evident in the upper metaphysis near the growth plate. A number of fractures are present. They are characterized by the presence of cartilage in the cortical area of the bone shaft.

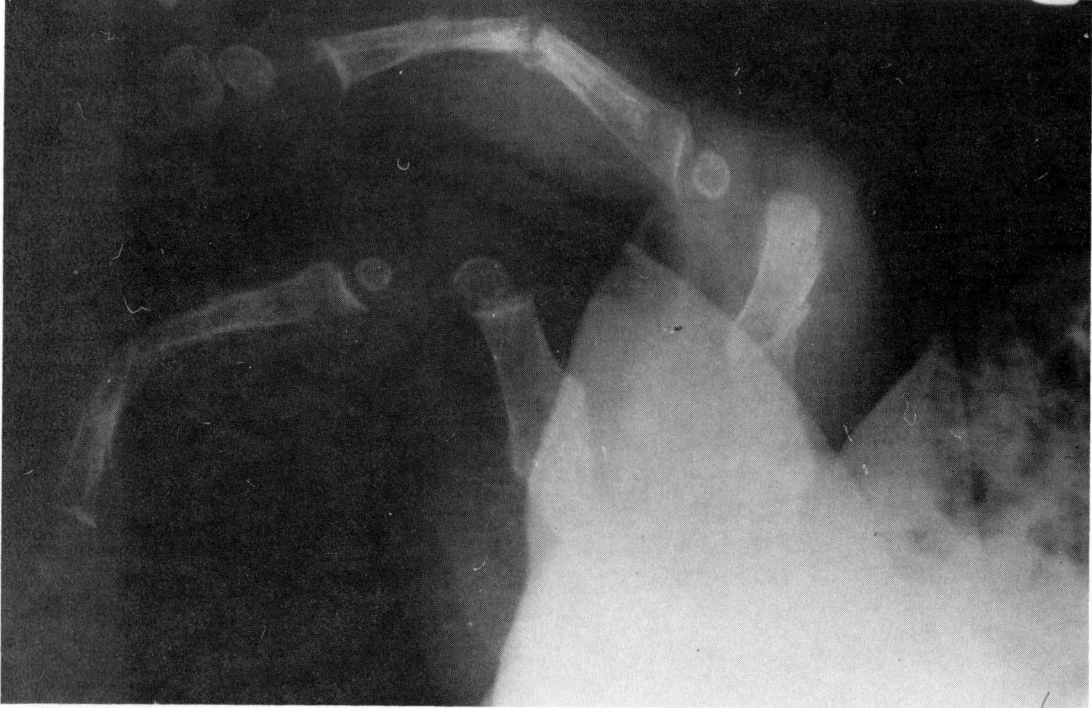

Figure 2–22. Characteristic clinical picture of osteogenesis imperfecta, with numerous fractures at different stages of healing. This is not to be confused with the battered-child syndrome.

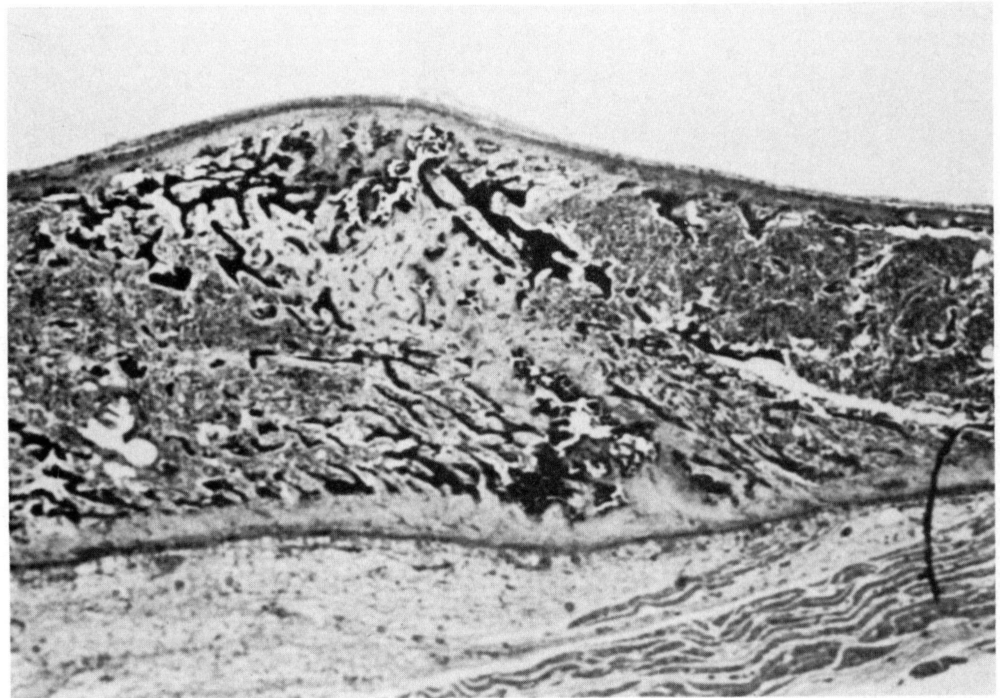

Figure 2–23. Histologic study of healed fracture. Fractures occur with minimal trauma, are painful, and, because there is not much soft tissue damage, heal in the usual time with minimal or normal amount of callus. Callus is composed of the same primitive woven bone that the patient has elsewhere and does not progress beyond that stage into more mature structure.

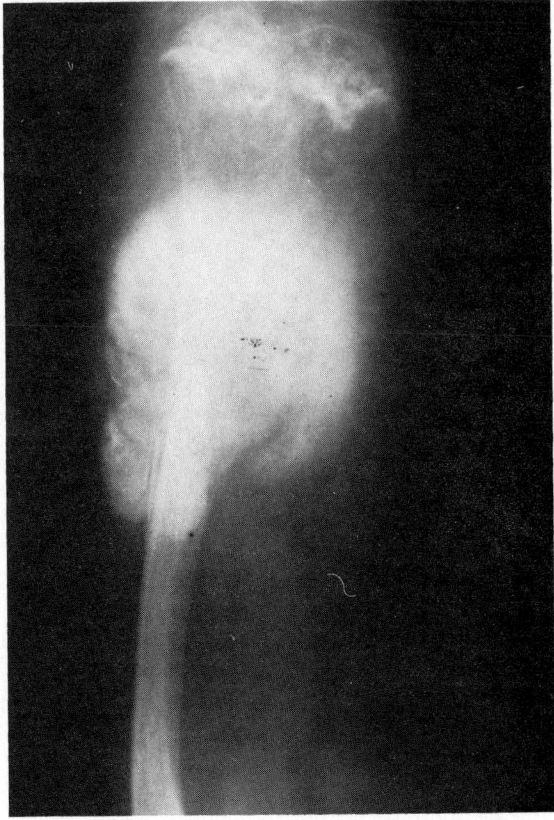

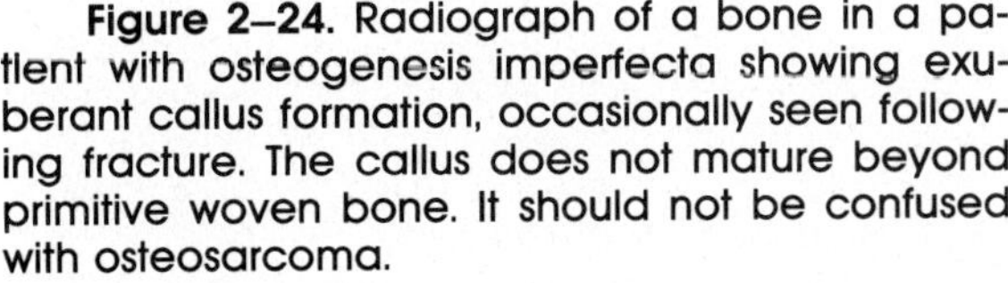

Figure 2–24. Radiograph of a bone in a patient with osteogenesis imperfecta showing exuberant callus formation, occasionally seen following fracture. The callus does not mature beyond primitive woven bone. It should not be confused with osteosarcoma.

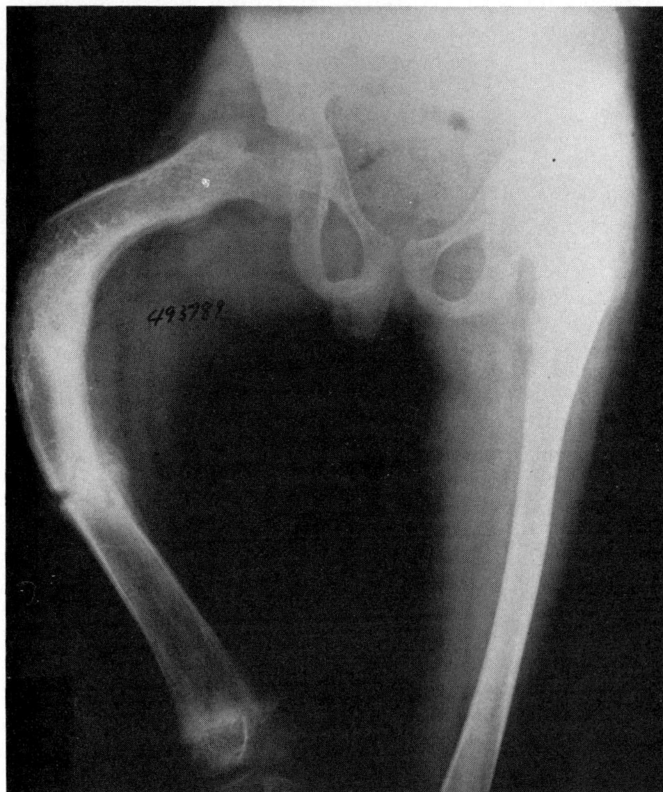

Figure 2–25. Bowed femur. After repeated fractures, bowing is common owing to the angulation during the healing process. These bones are brittle rather than soft or pliable.

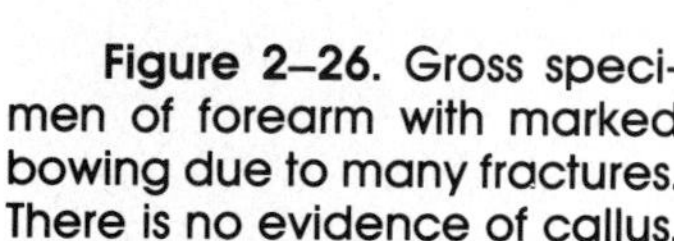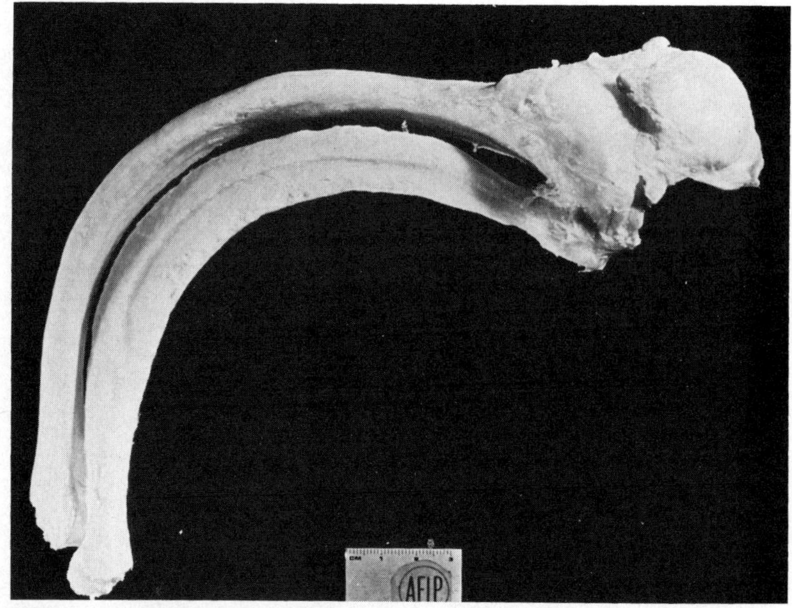

Figure 2–26. Gross specimen of forearm with marked bowing due to many fractures. There is no evidence of callus.

Figure 2–27. Growth plate of osteogenesis imperfecta. Since all bones are involved there is a severe effect at the growth plate. Cartilage production and maturation is essentially normal but scanty bone is formed on the cartilaginous scaffold and few primary trabeculae are formed.

Figure 2–28. Radiograph of lower limbs in osteogenesis imperfecta showing marked bowing. Irregular calcification in the epiphysis is evidence of severe derangement of growth. This will affect all subsequent stages of development at the growth plate.

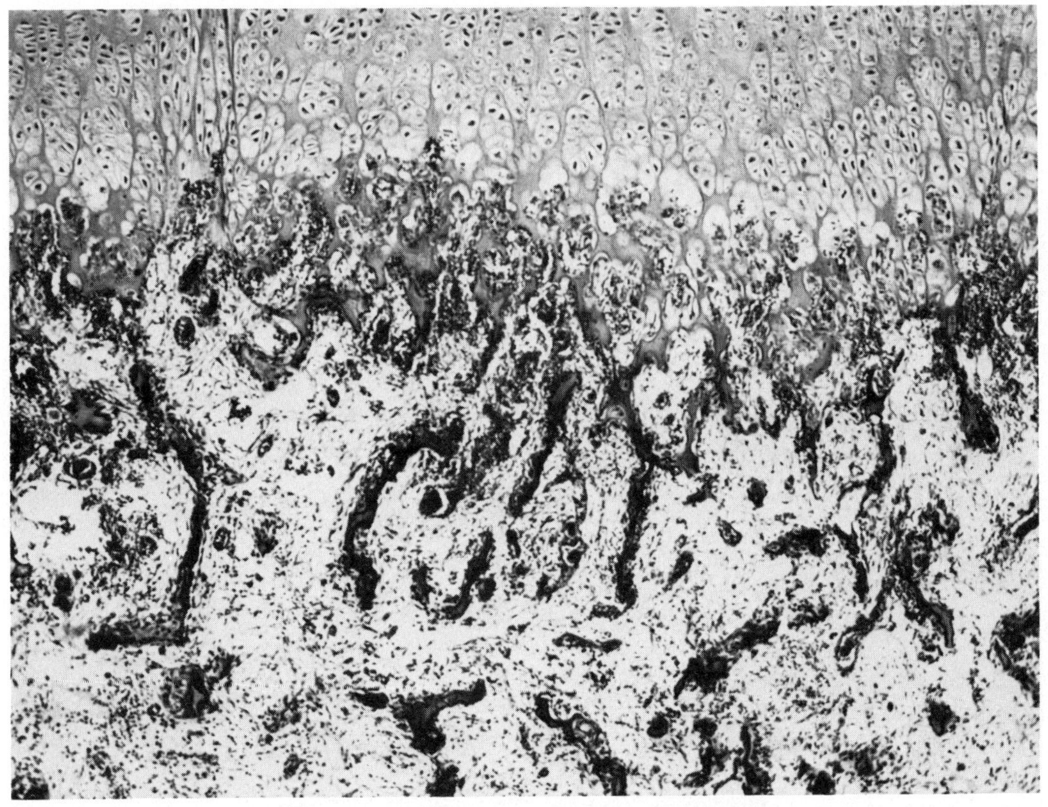

Figure 2–27. *See legend on opposite page.*

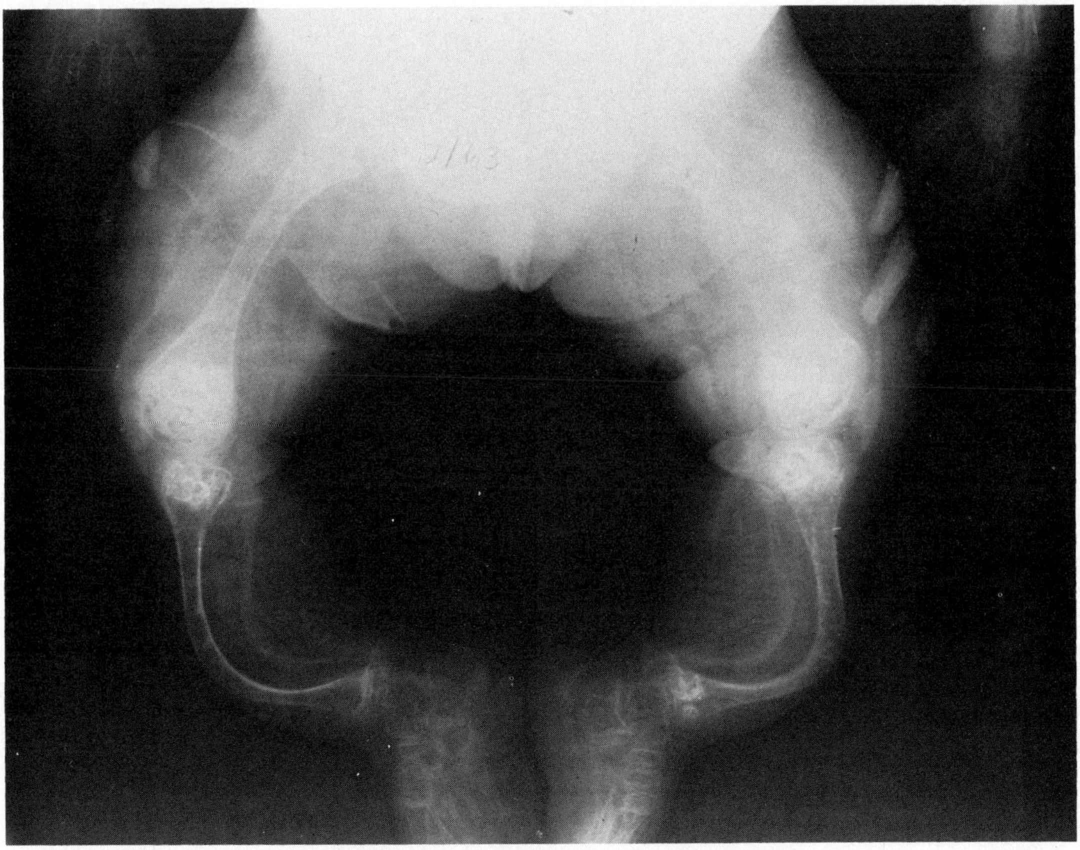

Figure 2–28. *See legend on opposite page.*

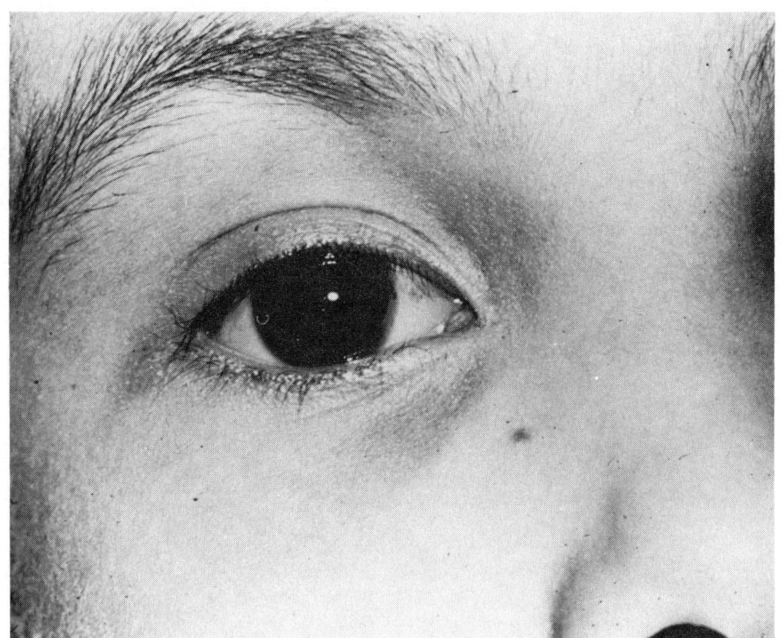

Figure 2–29. General defect in fibrous tissue production is also present in many cases of osteogenesis imperfecta. This collagen defect is characterized by blue sclerae, retinal pigment showing through thinned fibrous sclerae.

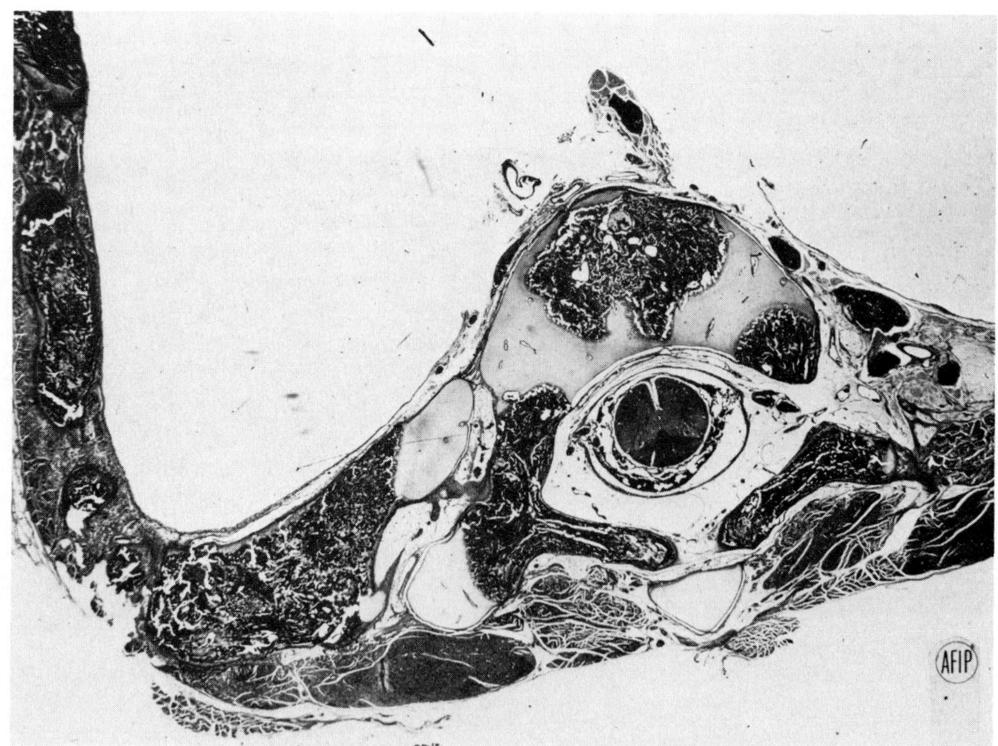

Figure 2–30. Macrosection of bone in a patient with osteogenesis imperfecta. The cartilage model is normal but bone production is abnormal. Note rib deformity from fractures.

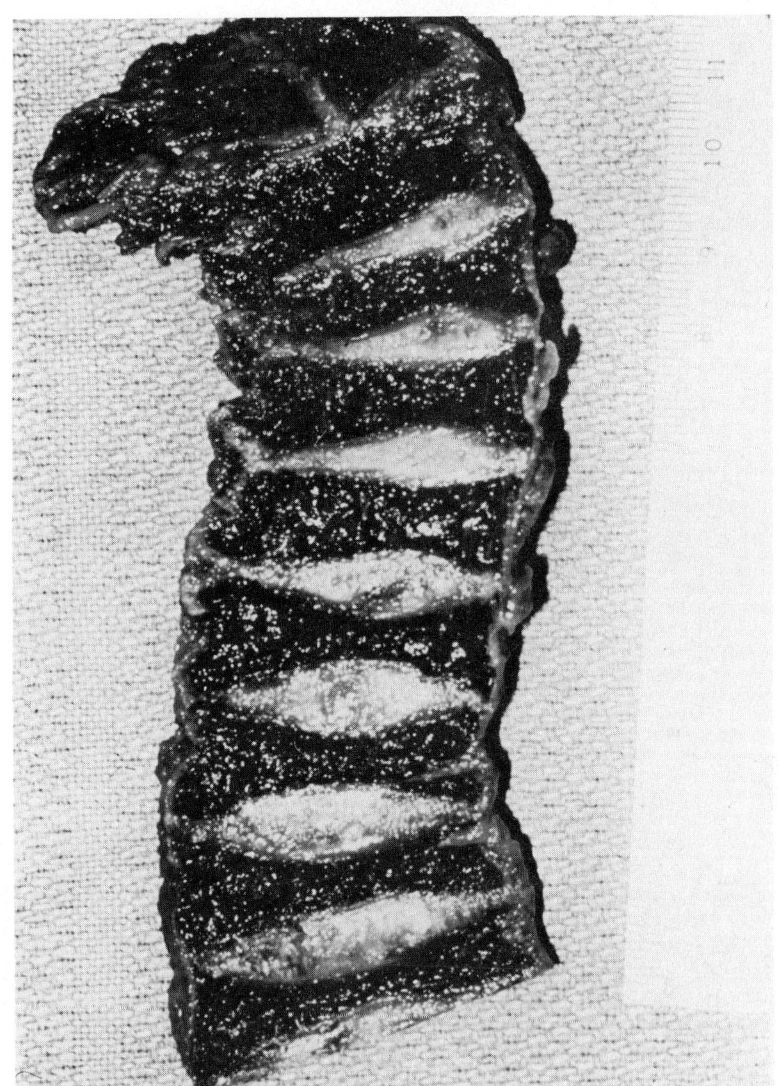

Figure 2–31. Gross specimen of spine. Expansile pressure of intervertebral discs associated with multiple microfractures causes "codfish vertebrae" with biconcave shape.

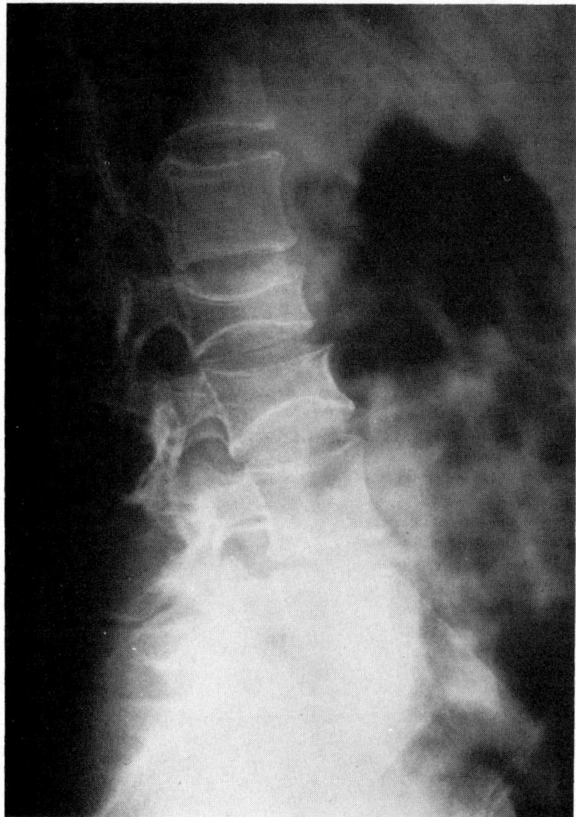

Figure 2–32. A lateral radiograph of the lumbar spine exhibiting "codfish vertebrae" and severe osteopenia.

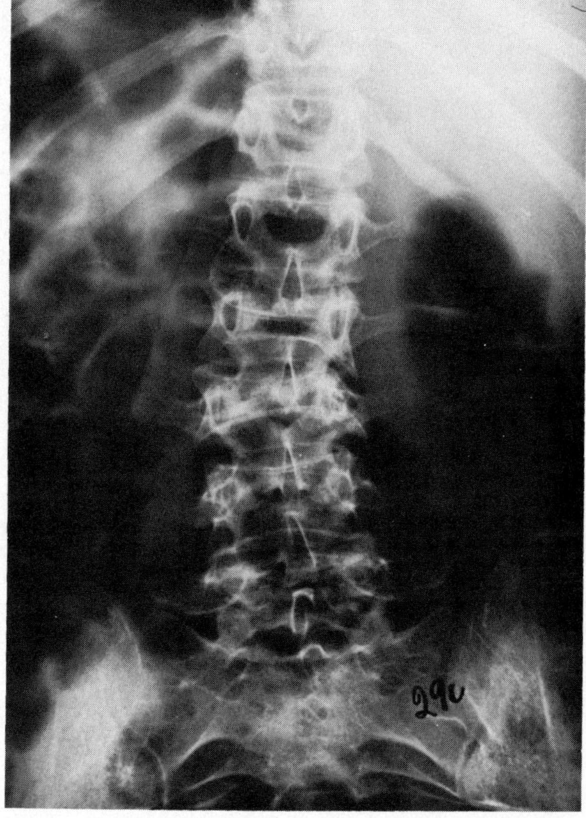

Figure 2–33. Anteroposterior radiograph of lumbosacral spine. Fractures have led to decrease in height of the vertebral bodies associated with increased width. Scoliosis is common following multiple fractures.

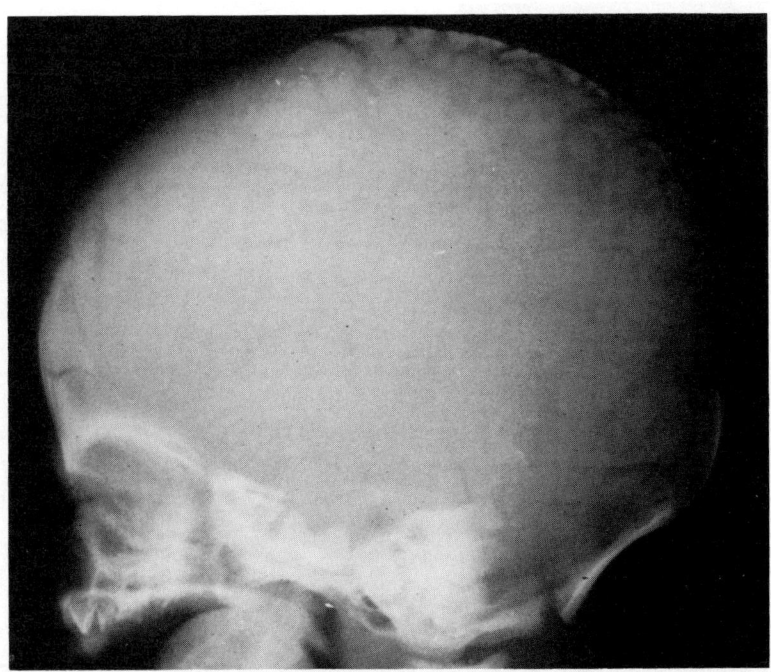

Figure 2–34. Lateral radiograph of skull. The collagen model bone of the cranial vault is severely affected, as are the bones of the face and basal portion of the skull. Dentition is usually poor because the enamel organ is equally affected. Numerous wormian bones are present in the calvarium.

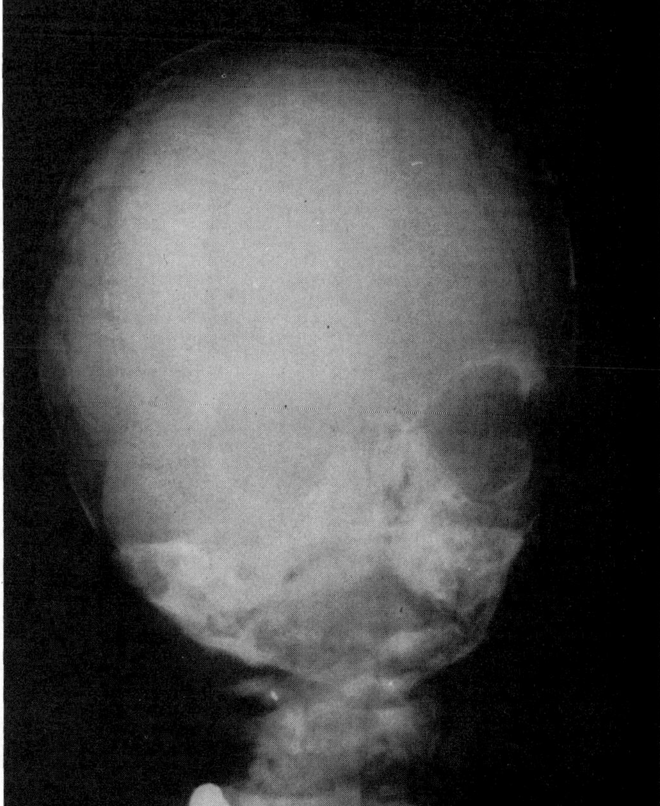

Figure 2–35. Anteroposterior radiograph of skull. The egg-shell–thin calvarium will "crackle" with palpation. The poor bone present in the mandible associated with abnormal dentition results in early loss of multiple teeth.

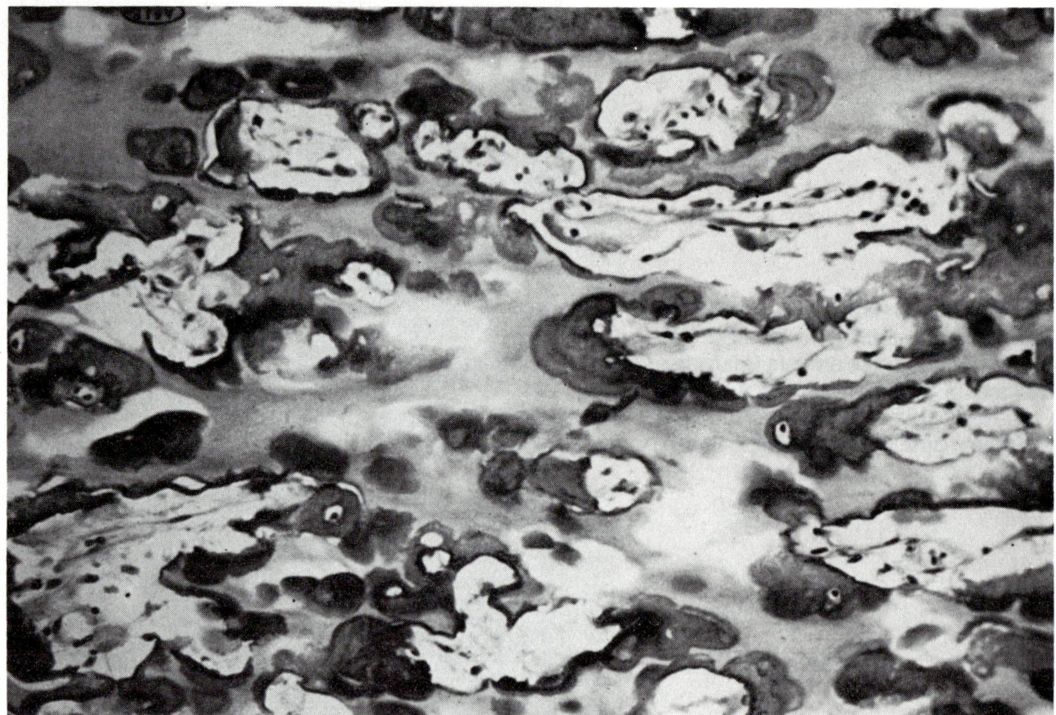

Figure 2–43. Higher magnification of patient with osteopetrosis exhibiting maintenance of primary trabeculae with bone formation onto the cartilage scaffold and extremely limited marrow space formation. Extramedullary hematopoiesis becomes necessary for survival.

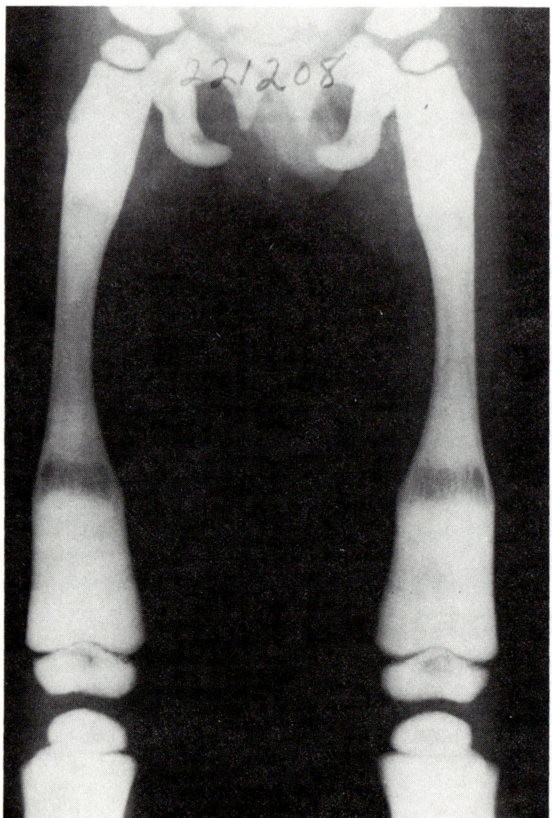

Figure 2–44. Radiographic manifestations of osteopetrosis, with characteristic dense sclerotic bone. Lack of metaphyseal remodeling in the cutback zone of the metaphysis produces the so-called "Erlenmeyer flask" deformity. Focal areas of normal density and shape occur at times when the process is inactive.

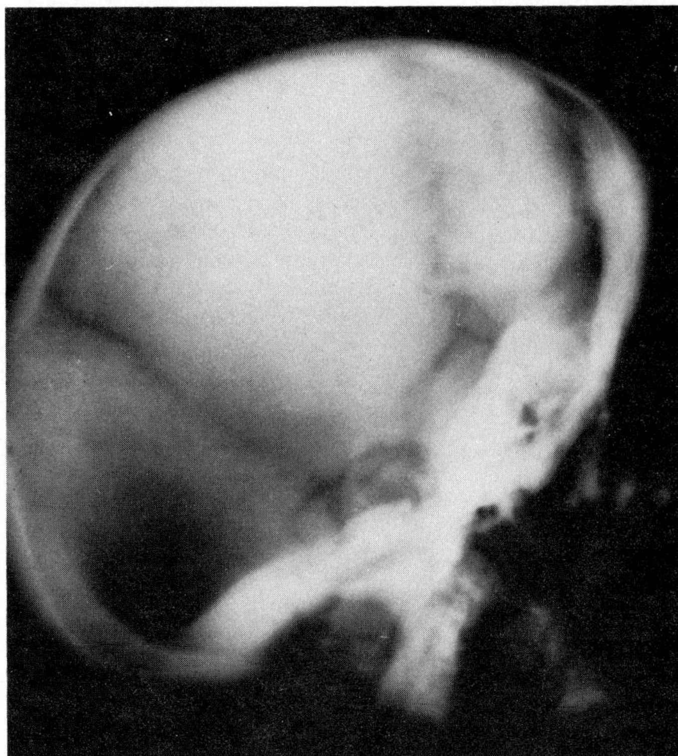

Figure 2–45. Dense skull of patient with osteopetrosis. Note the thickening of the base of the skull and the poor dentition. The cranial vault also exhibits increased density, even though it is not preformed in cartilage. It indicates a generalized defect in the remodeling process.

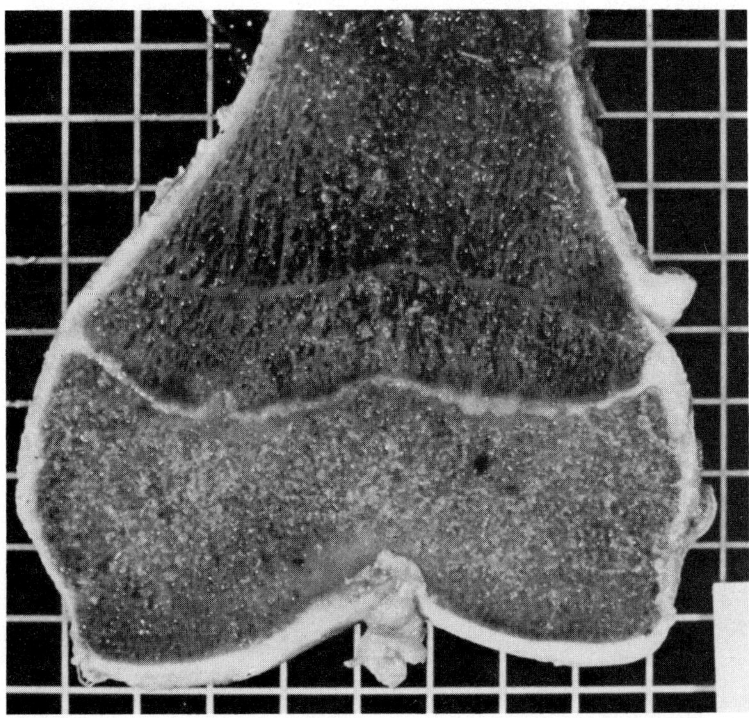

Figure 2–46. Growth-arrest line, lower end of femur. Note the horizontal condensation of the bone on the metaphyseal side of the epiphyseal growth plate. These growth-arrest lines indicate osteoclastic failure of limited duration and may be secondary to periods of malnutrition, disease, or other episodes of limited duration. The mechanism is similar to that in osteopetrosis.

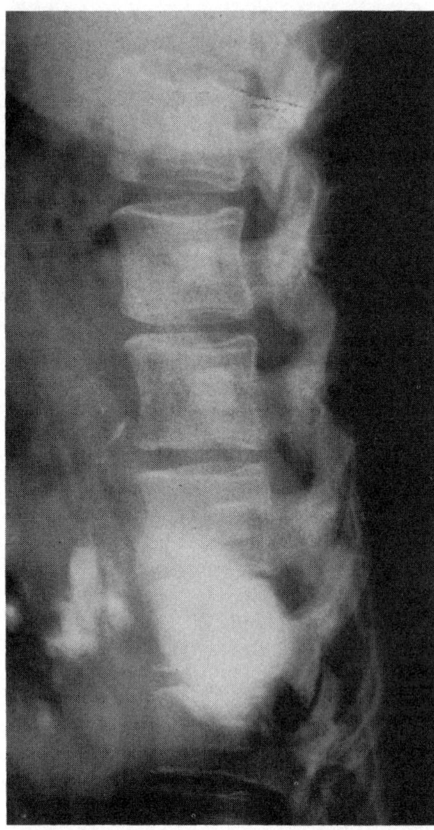

Figure 2–47. Thorotrast toxicity. Radiographic manifestation of "bone within bone" in patient who received thorotrast for gallbladder visualization. Thorotrast caused limited osteoclastic failure. Sarcoma has been associated with the deposition of the radioactive material in bone (Harrist et al., 1979).

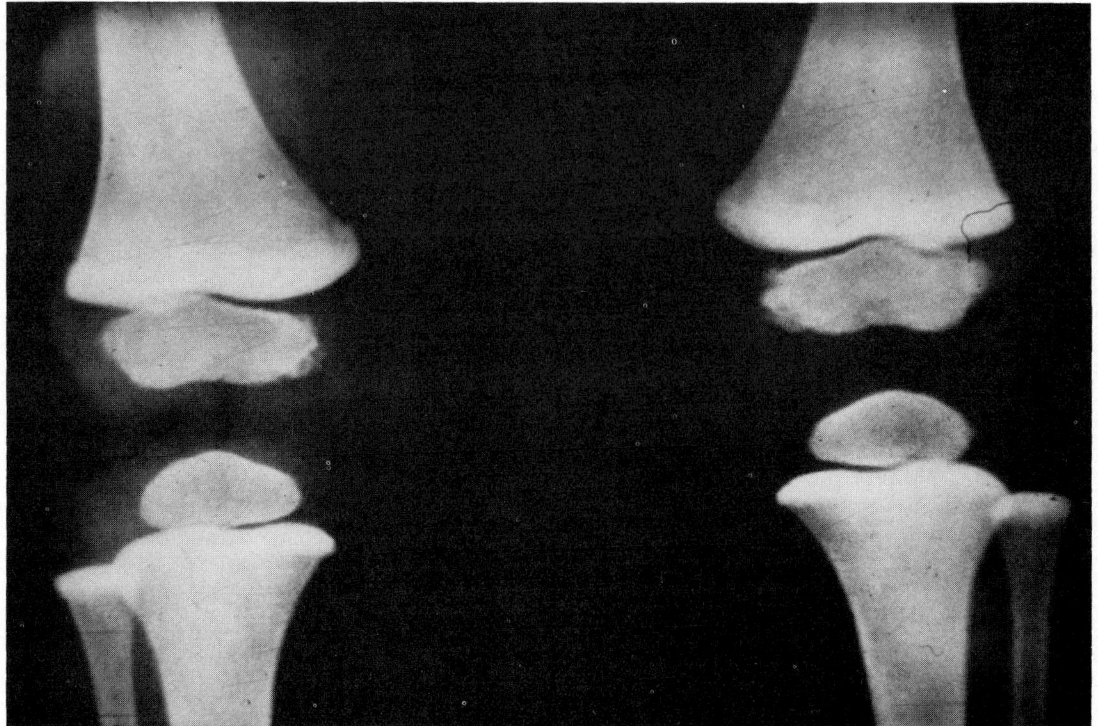

Figure 2–48. Radiographic manifestation of lead toxicity. Lead causes osteoclastic failure, with resultant remodeling failure. The dense bone is an expression of the osteoclastic malfunction.

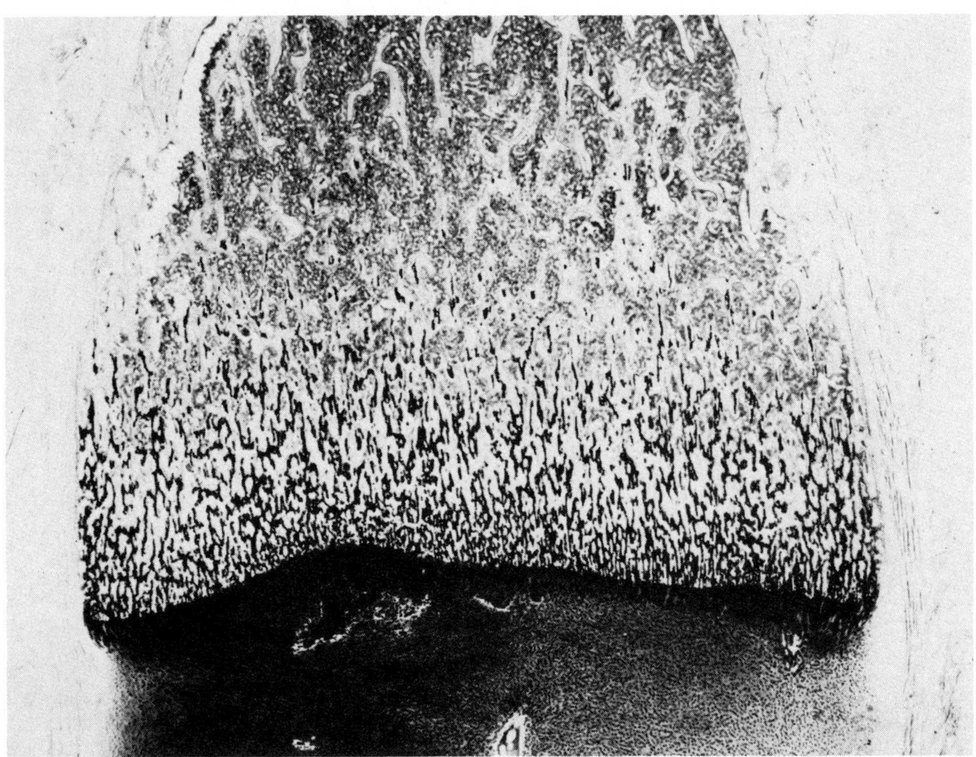

Figure 2–49. Macrospecimen of "lead line" indicating persistence of trabeculae and dense bone formation with osteoclastic failure in the immediate subepiphyseal portion of growth plate. Note the absence of funnelization, similar to what is seen in osteopetrosis.

CITED REFERENCES

Case Records of the Massachusetts General Hospital (Case 37–1982). N. Engl. J. Med. *307*:735, 1982.

Coccia, P., Krivit, W., Cervenka, J., Clawson, C., Kersey, J. H., Kim, T. H., Nesbit, M. E., Ramsay, N. K. C., Warkentin, P. I., Teitelbaum, S. L., Kahn, A. J., and Brown, D. M.: Successful bone-marrow transplantation for infantile malignant osteopetrosis. N. Engl. J. Med. *302*:701, 1980.

Harrist, T. J., Schiller, A. L., Trelstad, R. L., Mankin, H. J., and Mays, C. W.: Thorotrast-associated sarcoma of bone. A case report and review of the literature. Cancer 44:2049, 1979.

Milgram, J. W., and Jasty, M.: Osteopetrosis, a morphologic study of twenty-one cases. J. Bone Joint Surg., *64A*:912, 1982.

Sykes, B., Francis, M. J. O., and Smith, R.: Altered relation of two collagen types in osteogenesis imperfecta. N. Engl. J. Med. *296*:1200, 1977.

Teitelbaum, S. L., and Bullough, P. G.: The pathophysiology of bone and joint disease. Am. J. Pathol. *96*:283, 1979.

GENERAL REFERENCES

Rubin, P.: Dynamic Classification of Bone Dysplasias. Chicago, Year Book Medical Publishers, Inc., 1964.

Sillence, D. O., Horton, W. A., and Rimoin, D. L.: Morphologic studies in the skeletal dysplasias. A review. Am. J. Pathol. *96*:811, 1979.

3 *TRAUMA*

FRACTURE

In response to trauma or other injury, the musculoskeletal system attempts to re-establish functional and anatomic integrity. Repair requires reversion to basic mesenchymal tissue (blastema) with subsequent wound closure and scar formation. The scar tissue of bone is bone; thus, recapitulation of many of the steps of normal bone development and growth is necessary for healing.

Fracture healing consists of three separate healing phases that can be individually identifed:

1. *Circulatory*, which leads to the closure of the wound and the formation of the primary callus.

2. *Metabolic*, during which the primary callus is reinforced and strengthened, leading to clinical union.

3. *Mechanical*, during which the united bone is remodeled and adapted to lines of stress.

The interaction of these processes and the speed of healing depends on many factors, including age, general health, nutrition, and degree of activity.

CIRCULATORY PHASE

The circulatory phase is conveniently subdivided into three distinct components: (1) cellular, (2) vascular, and (3) primary callus, each approximately 10 days in duration.

Cellular Phase

Trauma sufficient to cause fracture in bone also damages the overlying muscle, tendon, periosteum, numerous blood vessels, and marrow tissue, resulting in hematoma formation. The injured cells as well as the hematoma incite a cellular inflammatory response, particularly prominent during the first 5 days of the fracture. Surviving cells in the area of injury and new cells brought in by the granulation tissue create a blastema of undifferentiated mesenchymal cells. This granulation tissue invades and replaces the hematoma. These cells are ultimately capable of modulating into the mature components of callus (Figs. 3–1 and 3–2).

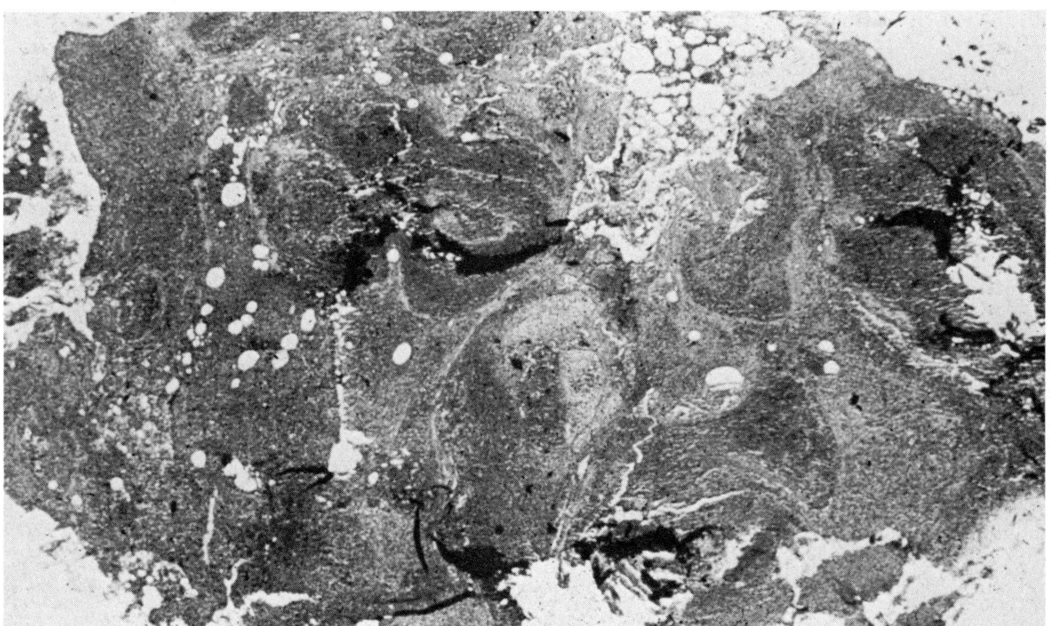

Figure 3–1. Fracture callus, 3 days old. Hematoma plus damaged periosseous tissue. There is no identifiable osseous differentiation.

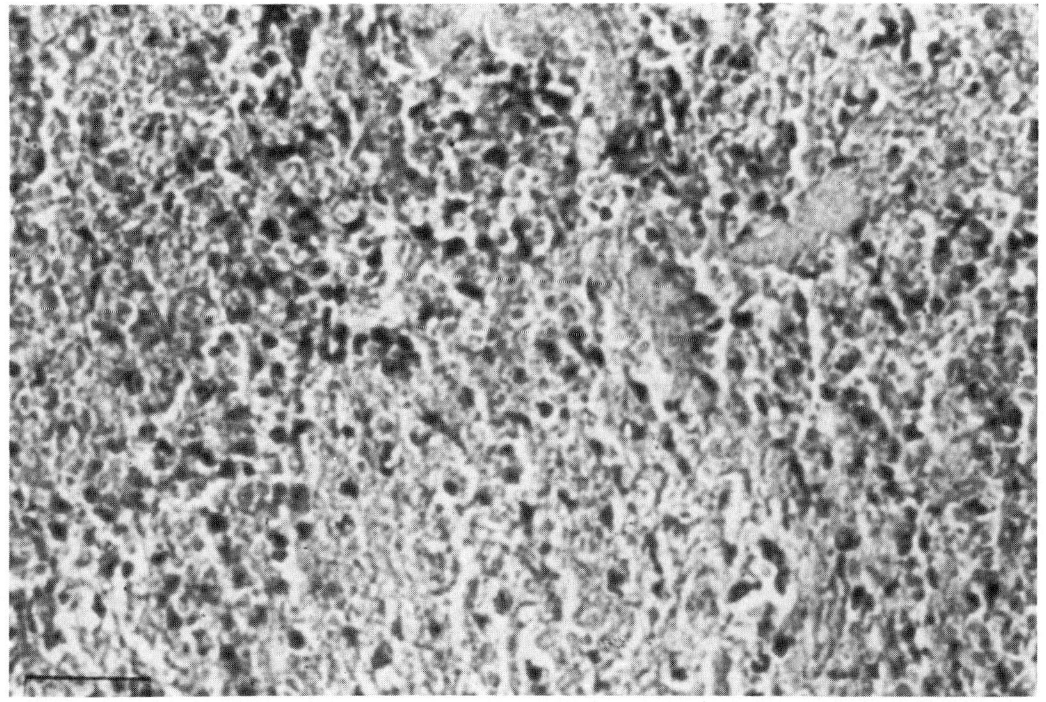

Figure 3–2. Callus, 3 days old, with no identifiable differentiation into bone. There are "blastema" cells with extensive hemorrhage undergoing partial organization.

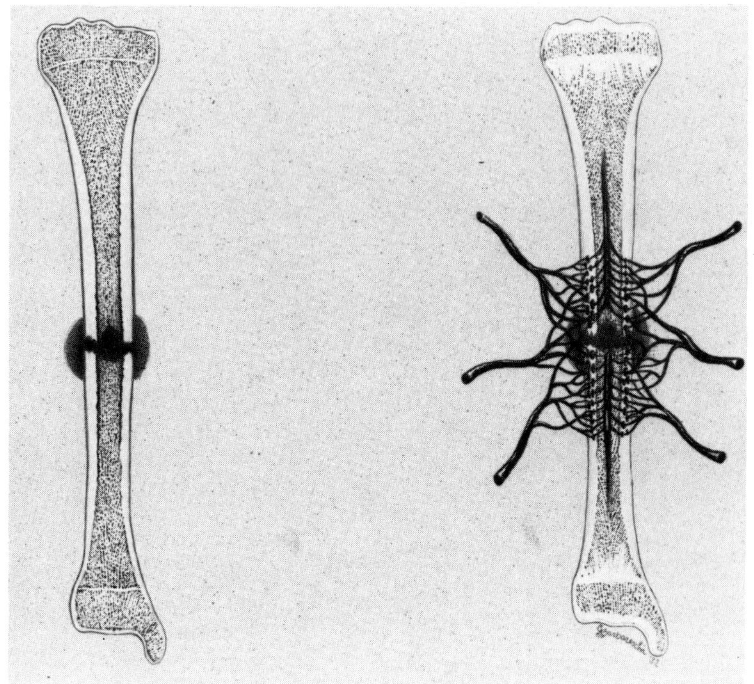

Figure 3–3. Schematic diagram of vascular meshwork created during fracture healing. Fracture hematoma (left) induces cellular and vascular changes with creation of vascular "spindle" (right). The active hyperemic, high-speed, well-oxygenated flow on the periphery results in resorption of cortex, whereas the sinusoidal, slower-speed, lower-oxygenated flow centrally favors osteoblastic activity, enhancing callus formation. Activation of vascular beds in an entire limb occurs reflexively and results in resorption bands at ends of bones.

Vascular Phase

The cellular phase is promptly followed by the vascular phase. A specialized circulatory network develops about the fracture (Fig. 3–3). It consists of dilated tributaries of major vessels that form around the periphery of the injured area and a central swamp-like area of wide-open capillaries, resulting in formation of a vascular spindle. Following injury, the blood flow of the entire limb is augmented, with active hyperemia at the edges of the injured area. The vigorous blood flow in the arteries and arterioles is slowed when it reaches the vascular "swamp," and passive hyperemia or congestion occurs. This passive hyperemia establishes the milieu for the active secretion of osteoid matrix by the mesenchymal cells that have migrated into the area.

The active hyperemia on the periphery of the vascular spindle with its high-speed, well-oxygenated blood flow induces osteoclastic activity in the cortex surrounding the fracture, easily demonstrable on sequential radiographs. It also activates the vascular bed of the old growth plate and subchondral plate, producing radiographically identifiable subchondral and submetaphyseal resorption bands (Figs. 3–4 and 3–5). Augmented circulation to the entire limb also produces hypertrichosis due to stimulation of hair follicles and tanning of the skin due to stimulation of the melanocytes.

Trauma in the muscle and stripping of the periosteum add to the initial fracture hematoma. Periosteal cells adjacent to the fracture become activated, reproduce, and secrete a matrix about themselves, in effect "elevating" the periosteum. Simultaneously, changes take place in the injured muscle tissue outside the periosteum, with granulation tissue replacing muscle cells. These cells will give rise to mature callus (Figs. 3–6 to 3–10). As the process continues, a new periosteum will be formed at the line of demarcation between the normal muscle and callus (Fig. 3–8). This makes moot the argument of whether to put plates beneath or outside the injured periosteum, since the eventually healed periosteum is a newly formed structure. Periosteum is not "elevated"; the old is destroyed, and a new membrane is formed. "Elevated" periosteal callus, when mineralized, will produce a Codman's triangle on radiographs.

Text continued on page 77

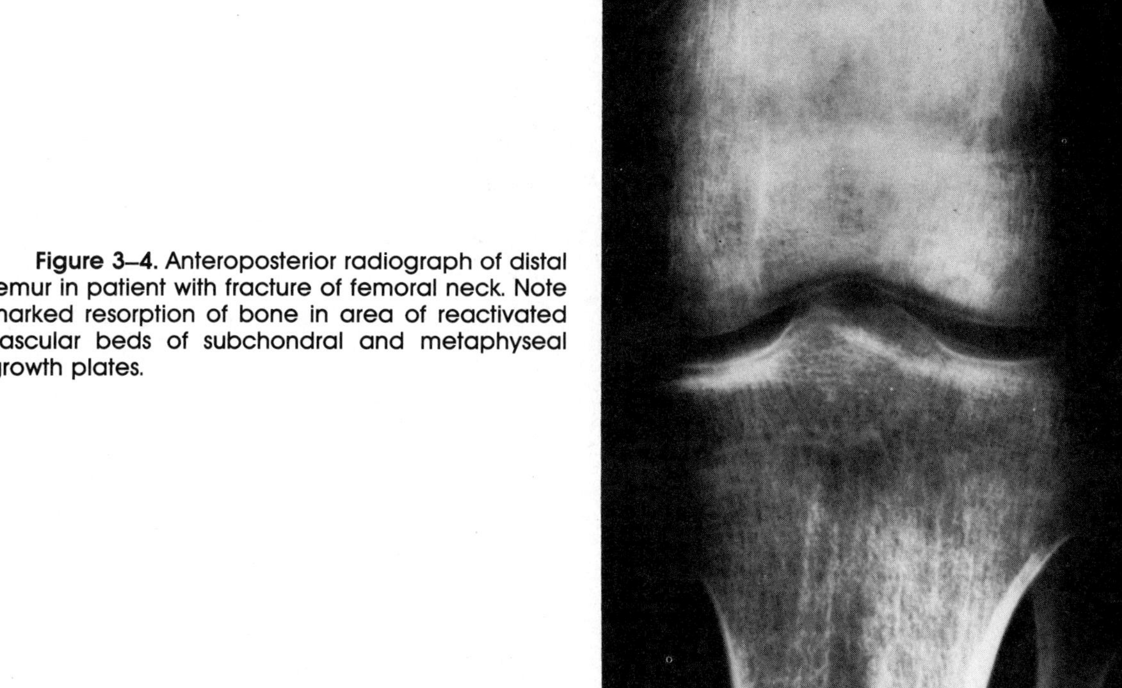

Figure 3–4. Anteroposterior radiograph of distal femur in patient with fracture of femoral neck. Note marked resorption of bone in area of reactivated vascular beds of subchondral and metaphyseal growth plates.

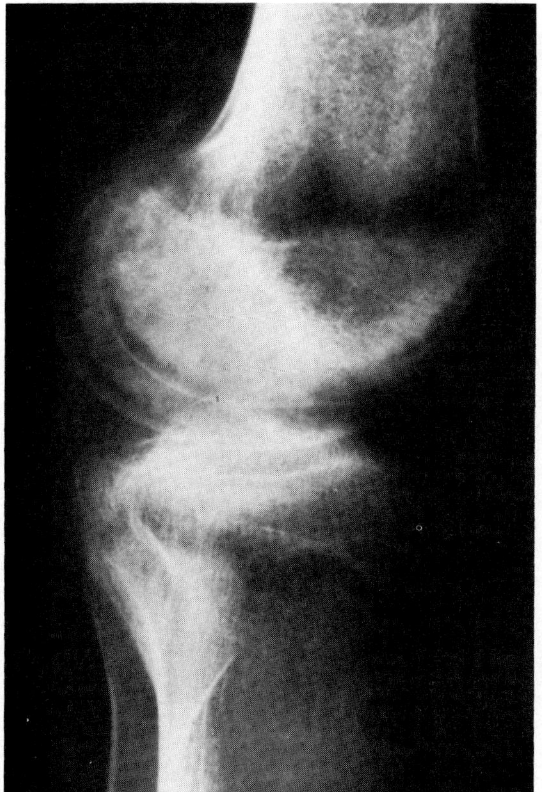

Figure 3–5. Lateral radiograph of same leg seen in Figure 3–4. Knee pain was severe whenever patient tried to put weight on these porotic bones.

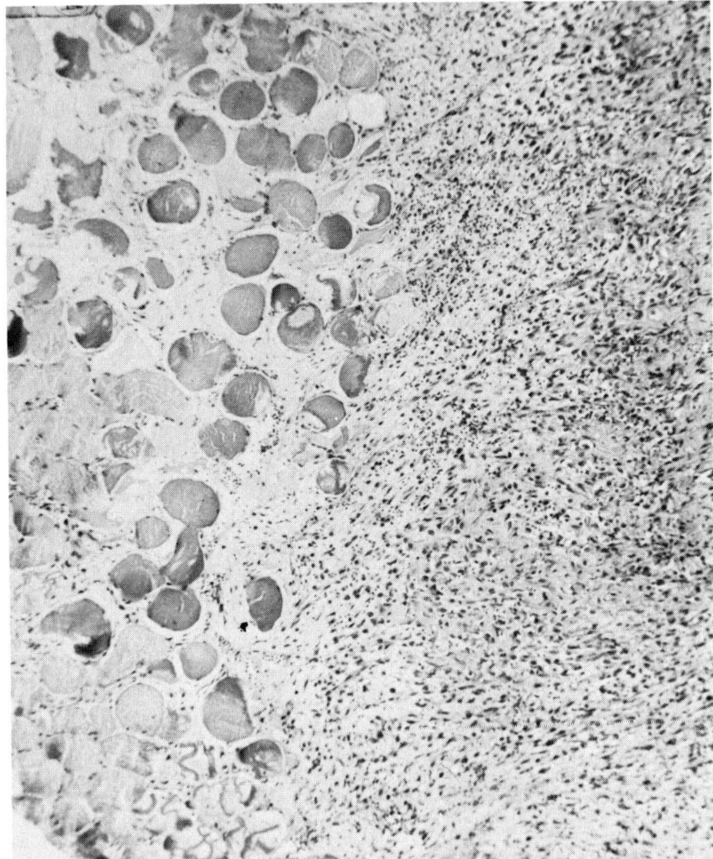

Figure 3–6. Margin of fracture hematoma and reactive periosteal change adjacent to muscle fibers undergoing breakdown and replacement. This same process is seen in myositis ossificans and results in heterotopic ossification as part of the fracture callus.

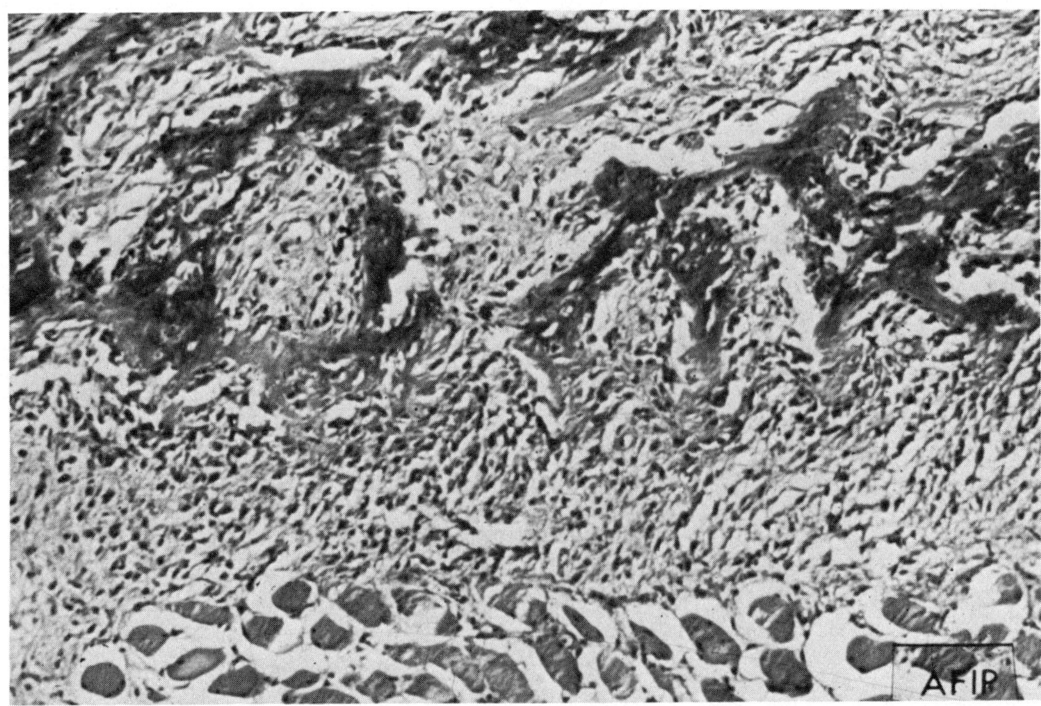

Figure 3–7. Edge of callus, approximately 3 weeks old, with sharp demarcation from surrounding striated musculature.

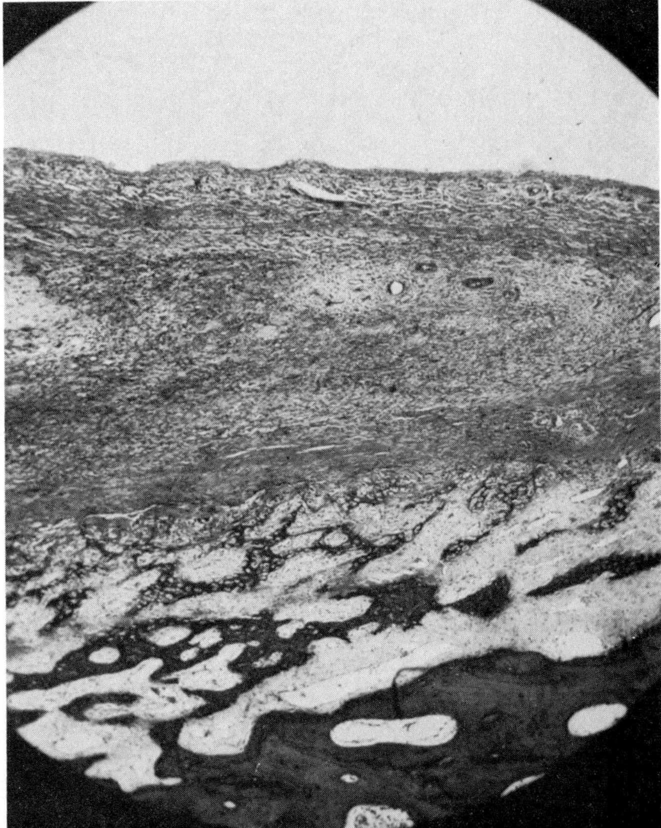

Figure 3–8. Further maturation of periosteal change with elevation, bone production, and formation of new, thickened periosteum from modulation of muscle tissue. This slide shows a region of a Codman triangle and would present the same appearance, regardless of whether the inciting cause was trauma, inflammation, or neoplasm.

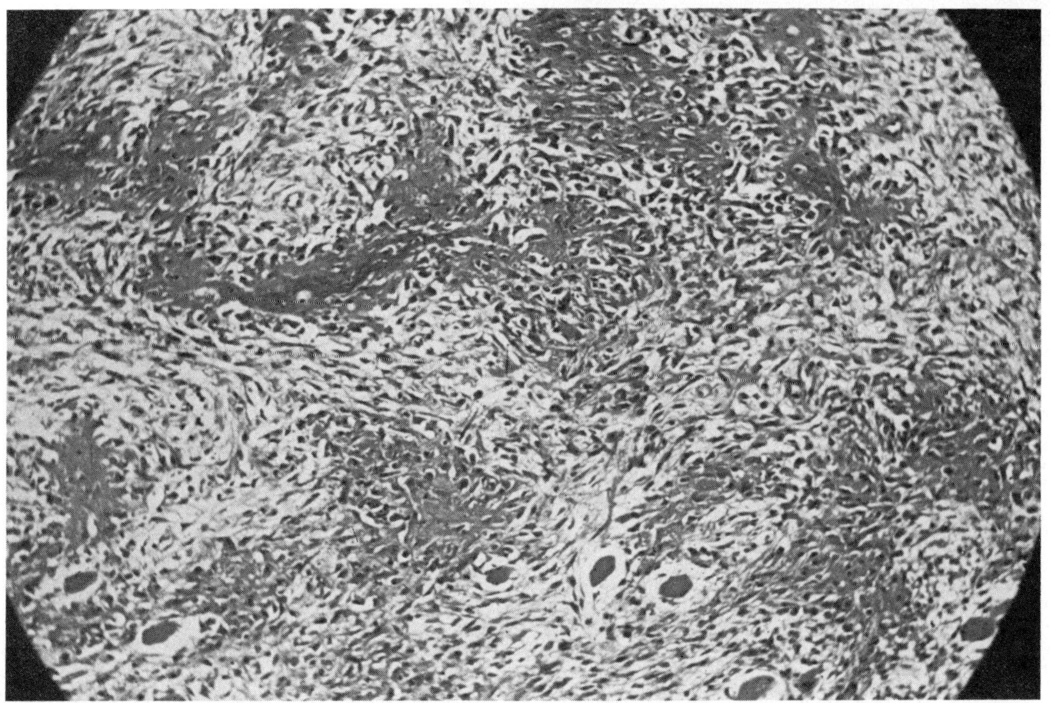

Figure 3–9. Callus, 10 days old. Earliest differentiation into recognizable osteoid. The amount is not enough to be visible on a radiograph. Note the incorporation of isolated muscle fibers into the callus.

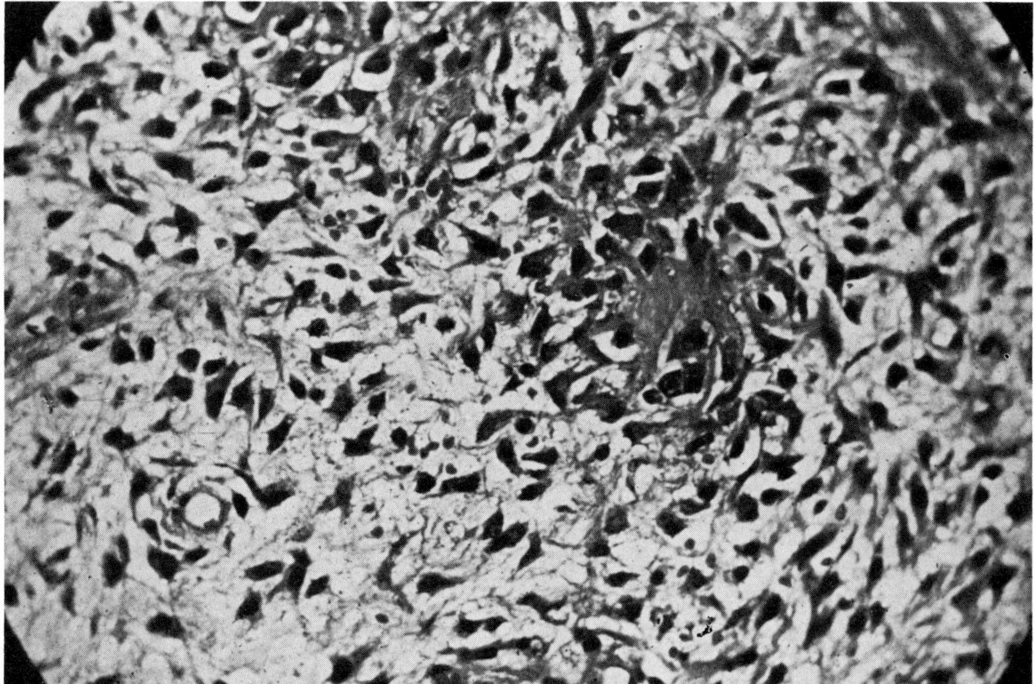

Figure 3–10. Callus, approximately 10 days old, with formation of primitive osteoid. Cellularity and pleomorphism, if considered out of the context of the entire clinical picture, could be confused with neoplasm by an inexperienced observer, a danger that is possible when a pathologic fracture is biopsied 2 to 3 weeks after fracture.

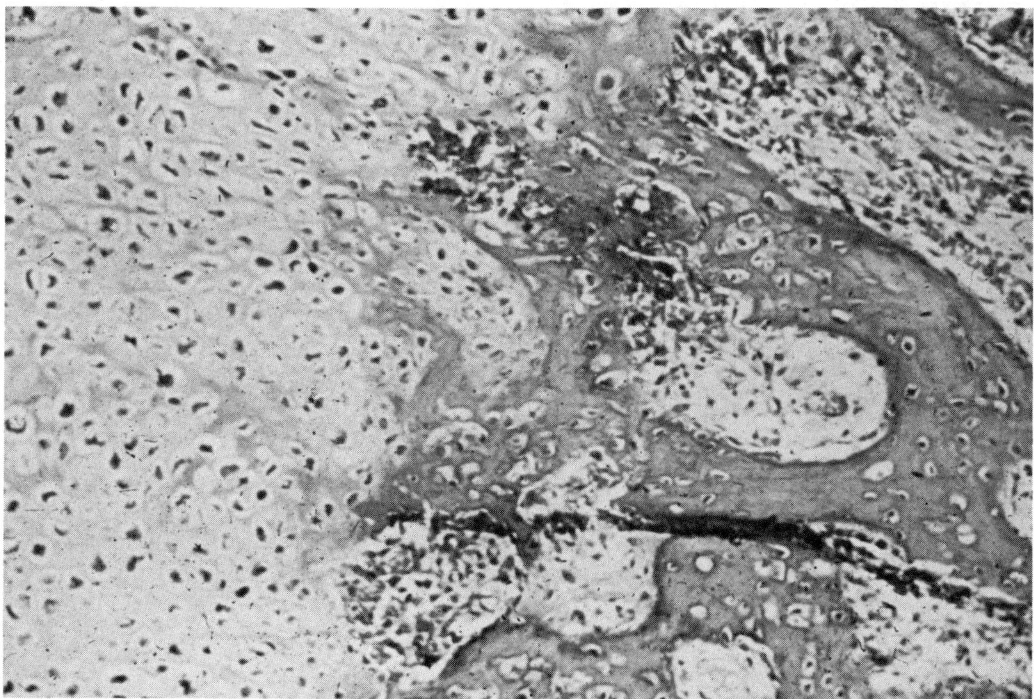

Figure 3–11. Callus, approximately 3 weeks old, with prominent cartilage component. The cartilage converts to bone whenever vascularity is sufficient for the conversion, or when motion is minimized.

Phase of Primary Callus

Once the vascular phase is well established, more and more "raw material" becomes available. Cellular elements arise from injured bone, connective tissue, marrow, and muscle to form undifferentiated mesenchymal cells. Whether these cells are modulated rhabdomyoblasts, fibroblasts, or osteoblasts or are new cells arising out of the necrotic tissue has not been resolved; nevertheless, muscle, connective tissue, and bone marrow are all essential in producing a blastema that accounts for approximately 70 per cent of the callus in a femur-shaft fracture. High-speed deposition of osteoid occurs in the form of coarsely woven bone, deposited in a more or less haphazard fashion in the area of the fracture. This osteoid becomes mineralized. Earliest radiographic visualization occurs after 14 days. Depending on the degree of motion and vascularization, cartilage is formed within the callus at the same time (Fig. 3–11).

The development of this primitive material in the blastemal zone represents the formation of the primary callus. The first stage of fracture healing can be summarized as (1) necrosis, hematoma—approximately 10 days; (2) vascular spindle formation—approximately 10 days; and (3) primary callus.

METABOLIC PHASE

The second stage of fracture healing is characterized by more orderly secretion of callus and the removal and replacement of coarsely woven osteoid by a more mature form of bone. The process is one of remodeling, mimicking the generalized remodeling processes that occur during normal growth and development (Fig. 3–12). The callus

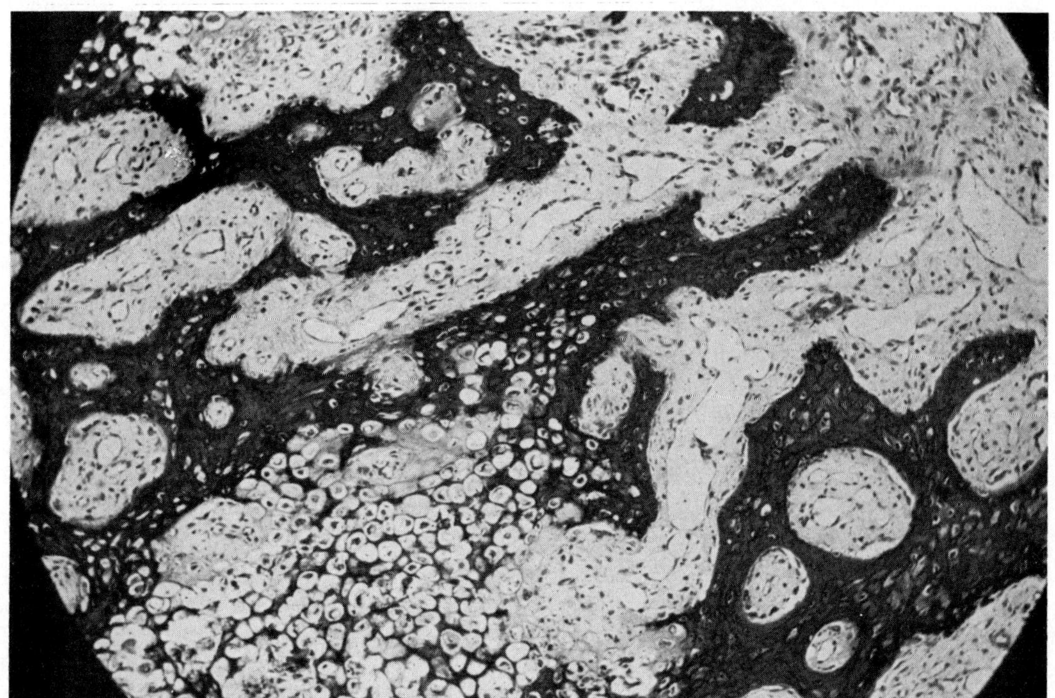

Figure 3–12. Callus, approximately 3 weeks old, with primitive bone trabeculae and masses of cartilage with endochondral ossification. It is frequently difficult to define the distinct junction of cartilage and bone, as many cells show characteristics of both, forming what is known as "chondro-osseous bone."

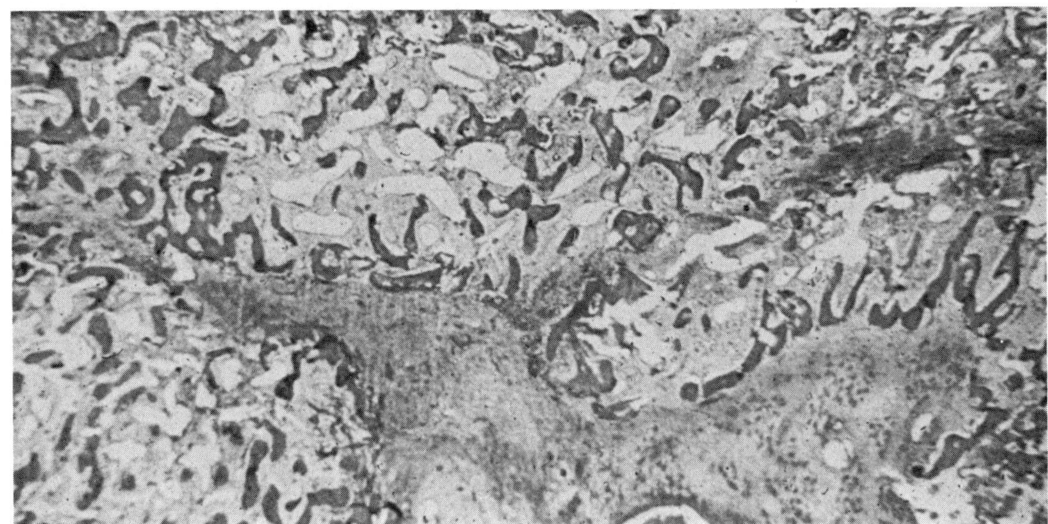

Figure 3–13. Callus, 4 weeks old. Note numerous sinusoidal vessels adjacent to trabeculae of bone, which create a swamp-like appearance.

can be divided into separate entities, separated more by nomenclature than function, but nevertheless identifiable as sealing, buttressing, bridging, and uniting callus (Fig. 3–14). Buttressing callus is adjacent to the outer surface of the cortex and is formed by periosteum as well as the surrounding skeletal musculature. Sealing callus fills the medullary cavity and arises from the marrow to "seal" it from the fracture site. Bridging callus unites the gap between the two buttress ends, and uniting callus joins the cortical portions of the fractured bone. Clinical union is achieved when the callus is sufficiently developed to allow weight-bearing or similar stress.

MECHANICAL PHASE

The mechanical phase involves realignment and remodeling of bone and callus along lines of stress. Extra bone is deposited in stress lines and removed in areas in which stress is not applied (Wolff's law). The final stage of fracture healing is restoration of the medullary cavity and bone marrow.

The sequence of events in the healing of a fracture described previously have definite practical consequences in the management of the patient:

1. Although a hematoma is not essential to the healing of a fracture, the hematoma plays a role in inducing granulation tissue response. The greater the response, the more cellular the granulation tissue and the better the ultimate callus. Therefore, the less disturbance of the hematoma the better.

2. Large necrotic bone fragments will have to be removed by phagocytic processes and may impede callus formation. Sequestered bone fragments may require removal to help the healing process. Injury induces increased vascularity, which promotes callus. Injured soft tissue should therefore be left alone. Muscle contributes extensively to formation of callus and is richly vascularized, and it should be minimally disturbed despite injury. Poor fracture healing usually occurs in bones with little or no adjacent musculature.

3. Clinical healing will precede anatomic reconstitution. Extensive remodeling will proceed for years after the fracture; therefore, realignment of fracture fragments should emphasize maintained viable bone and all fragments within the field of the

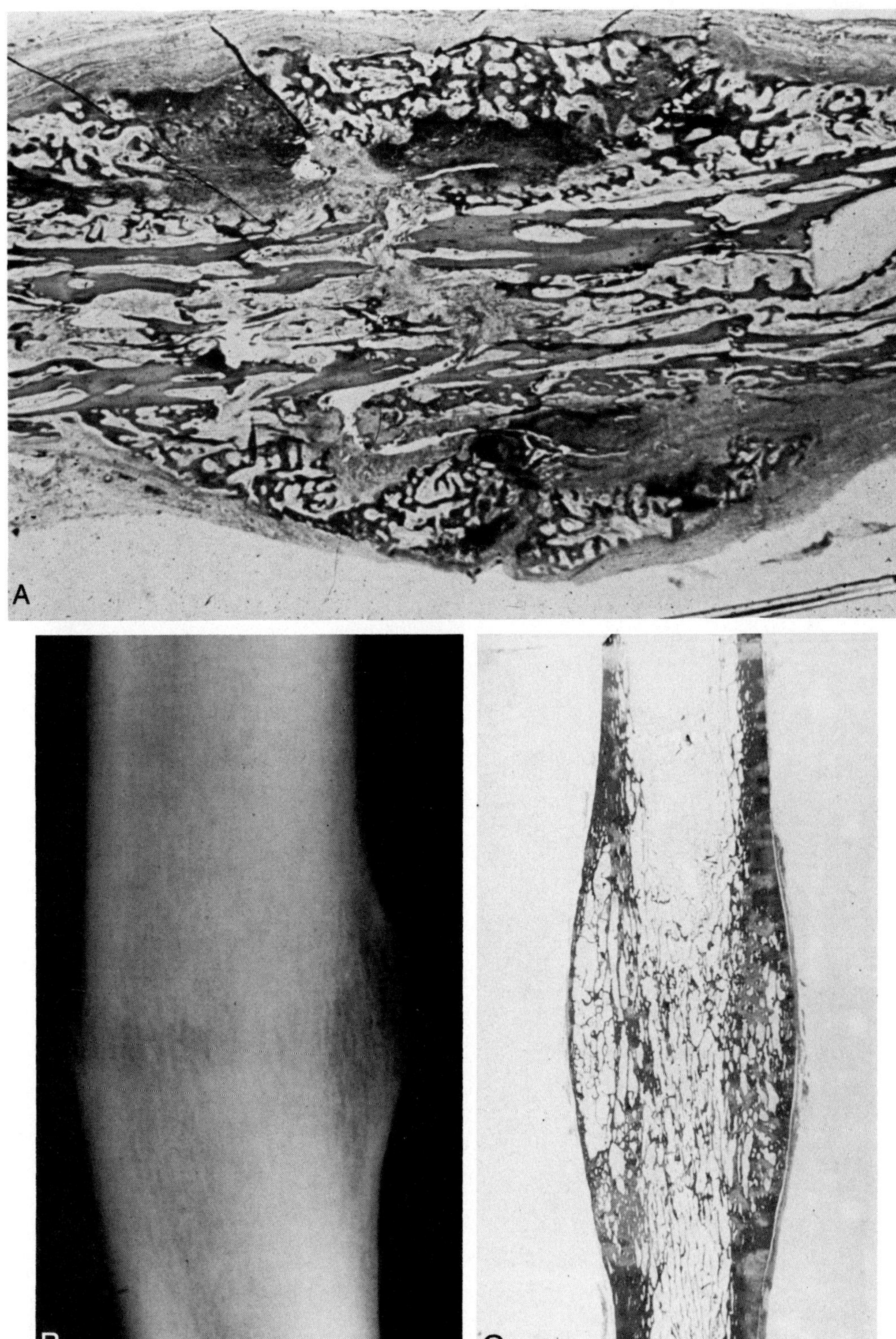

Figure 3–14. *A,* Histologic study of healing fracture, with sealing, buttress, uniting, and bridging callus and reconstitution of marrow cavity. *B,* Radiographic appearance of another healing fracture, late stage, with reconstitution of marrow cavity and remodeling. *C,* Histologic appearance of healing fracture in *B* showing almost complete restoration of normal structures.

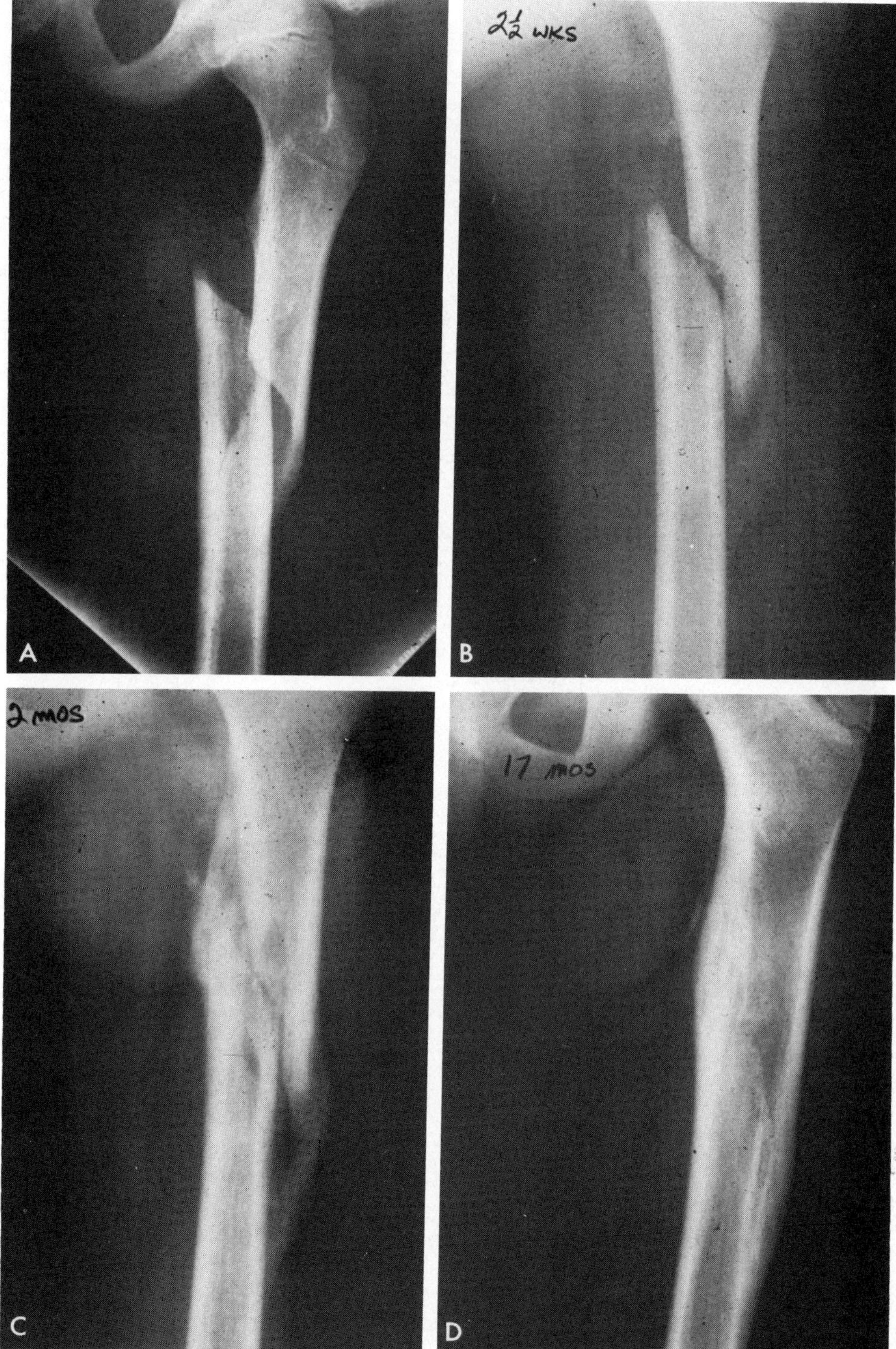

Figure 3–15. Sequence of events in spiral fracture of femur. Notice the sharp delineation of fracture fragments at the time of the acute episode *(A)*. At 2½ weeks *(B)*, the margins are indistinct, early callus is visible, and there is definite loss of density of the cortex. At 2 months *(C)*, the callus is sharply delineated against the surrounding tissue, the callus density is markedly increased, and there is significant resorption of the residual cortical remnants. At this point, the patient is clinically healed and resumes normal activity. At 17 months *(D)*, the full extent of the remodeling process can be recognized. Although completely normal anatomic reconstitution cannot be achieved, remodeling persists for many years.

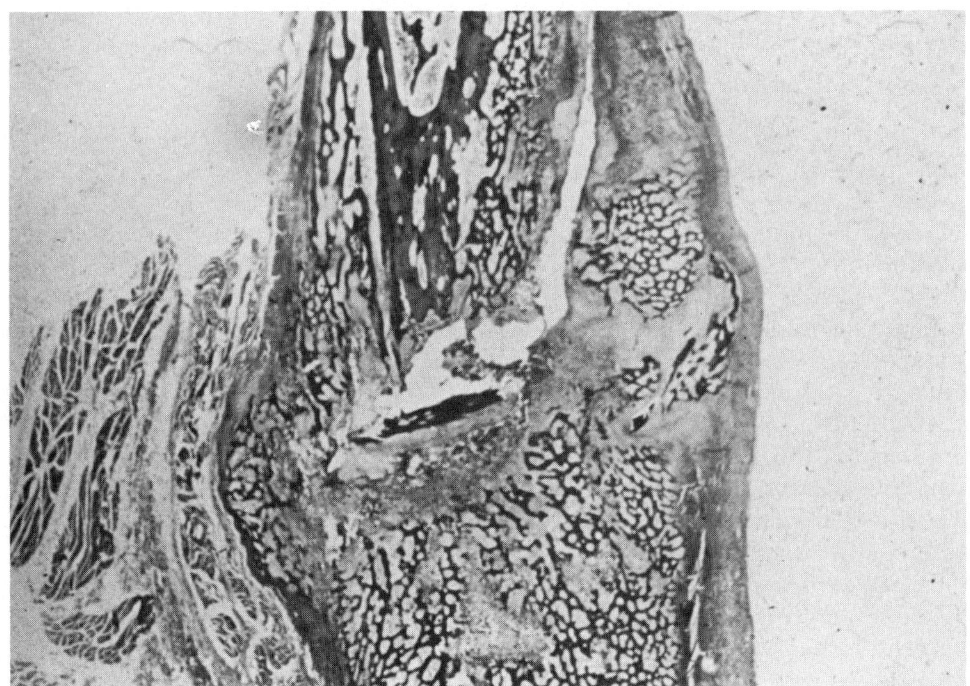

Figure 3–16. Fracture callus with small sequestered fragment in midst of callus.

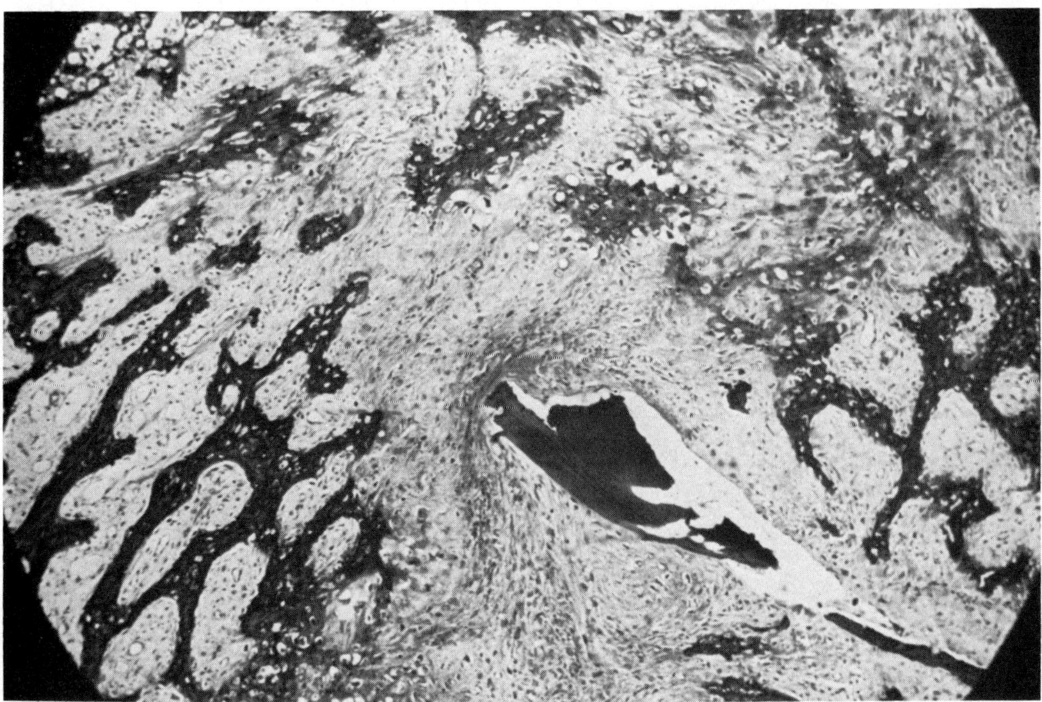

Figure 3–17. High-power view of sequestered fragment in midst of callus. A small fragment of this nature will not significantly interfere with callus formation and will probably be subject to complete resorption within a short period of time. Note the increased density of the sequestered fragment as compared with that of the new osteoid being laid down in the callus.

vascular spindle. Anatomic reconstitution will usually occur as a consequence of extensive remodeling and does not require exact replacement of fracture fragments (Fig. 3–15).

COMPLICATIONS

Fibrous Union. Bones with relatively poor blood supply and little or no associated muscle tissue (lower end of tibia, carpal navicular) have difficulty establishing the normal vascular spindle when fractured. The resultant poor blood supply tends to propagate primitive scar tissue rather than bony callus (Fig. 3–18). The bridge between the two fractured bone fragments is consequently filled by relatively avascular fibrous connective tissue rather than bone or cartilaginous elements. The only method of converting the ineffective fibrous connective process into bona fide bone is to keep stimulating the fracture site until sufficient vascularity is established. As a general principle, measured and repetitive "pounding" of the fracture is essential. Carefully selected electrical stimulation has caused dramatic improvement in the effort to induce bony callus formation from fibrous union (Brighton et al., 1981).

Pseudarthrosis. If the fracture is not adequately immobilized, motion between the fractured bony ends persists, and small vessels that grow into the fracture site are constantly sheared. The callus is thus poorly vascularized and tends to produce cartilage instead of bone (Figs. 3–19 to 3–24). Continued motion results in myxoid degeneration and liquefaction of the cartilage, with the formation of a pseudo–joint space. The pseudarthrosis, once established, can be healed only by refracture, removal of the cartilaginous component, and the re-establishment of a vascular spindle with new callus formation.

Text continued on page 87

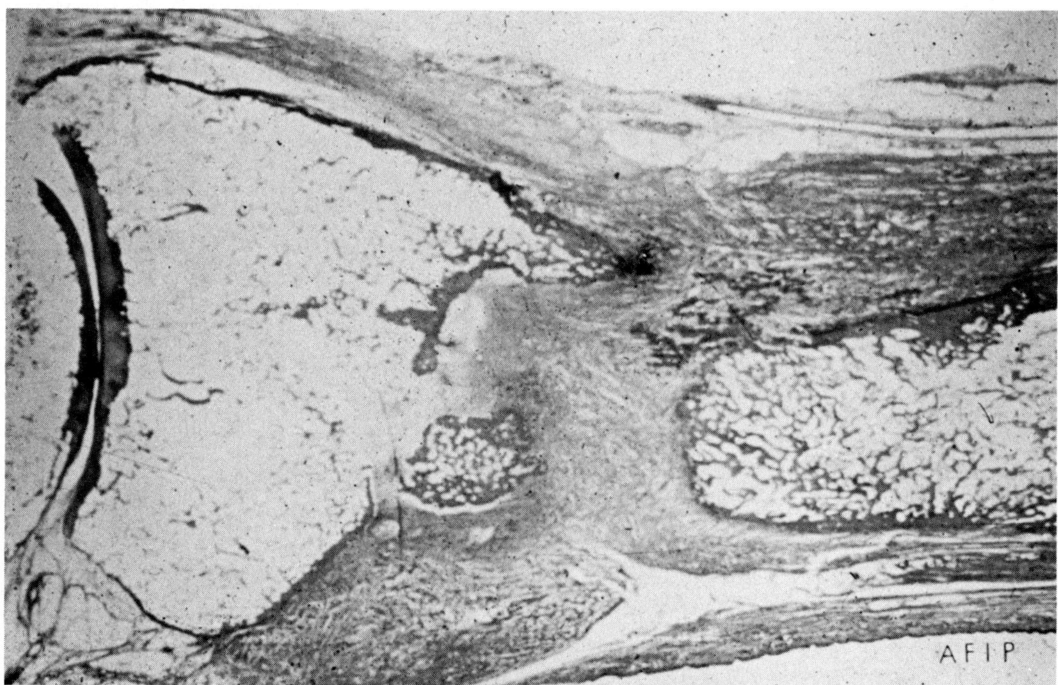

Figure 3–18. Fibrous union, with extensive fibrotic tissue, some poorly formed osteoid in the midst of the fibrous connective tissue, and marked osteoporosis.

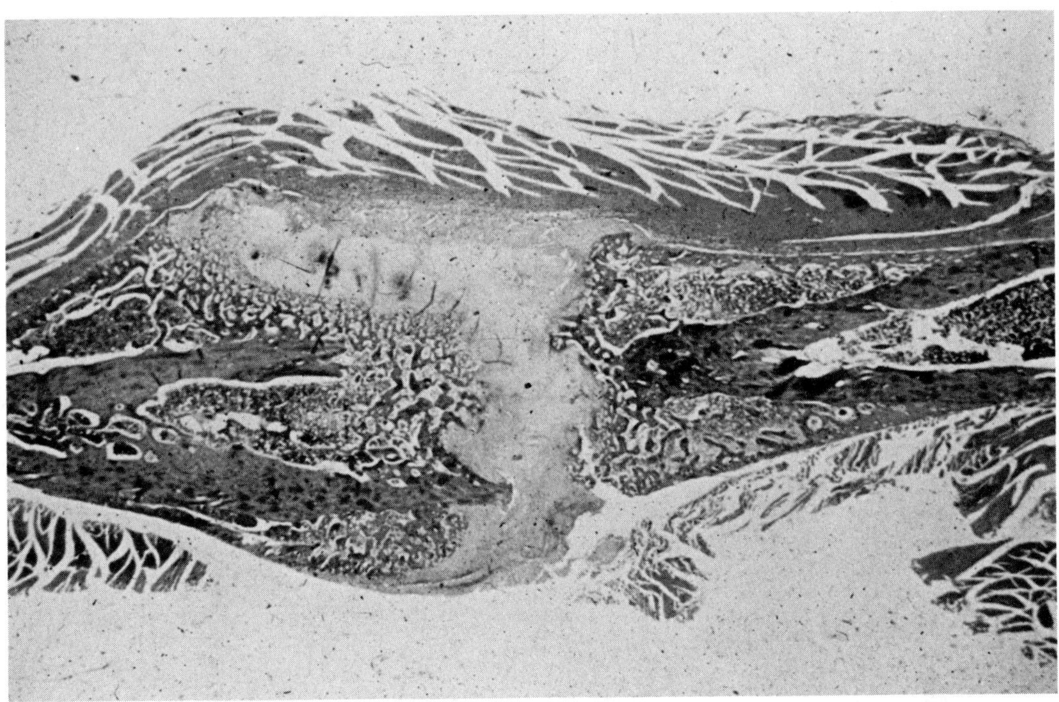

Figure 3–19. Delayed union, with formation of cartilage across the fracture gap. If motion persists, a true pseudarthrosis may result.

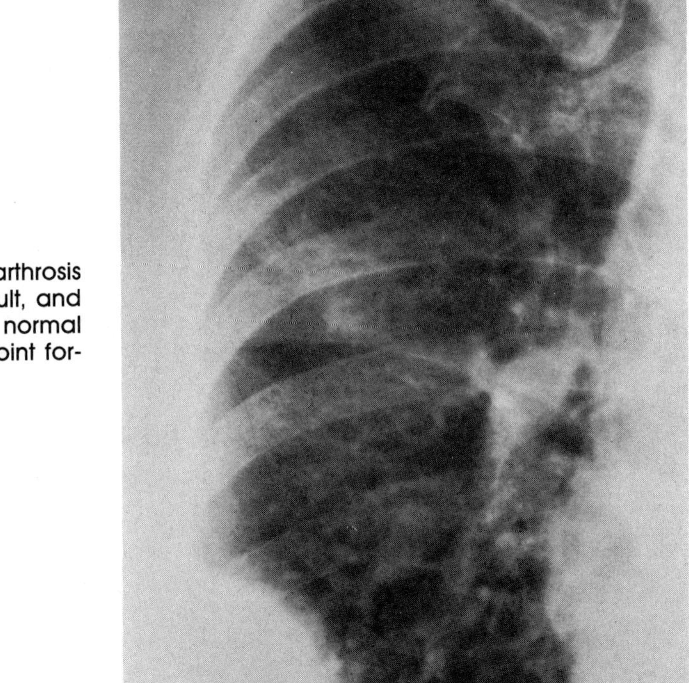

Figure 3–20. Radiograph of pseudarthrosis of rib. Immobilization of the rib is difficult, and the continuous shear of vessels prevents normal callus formation. The fracture site and joint formation are easily identified.

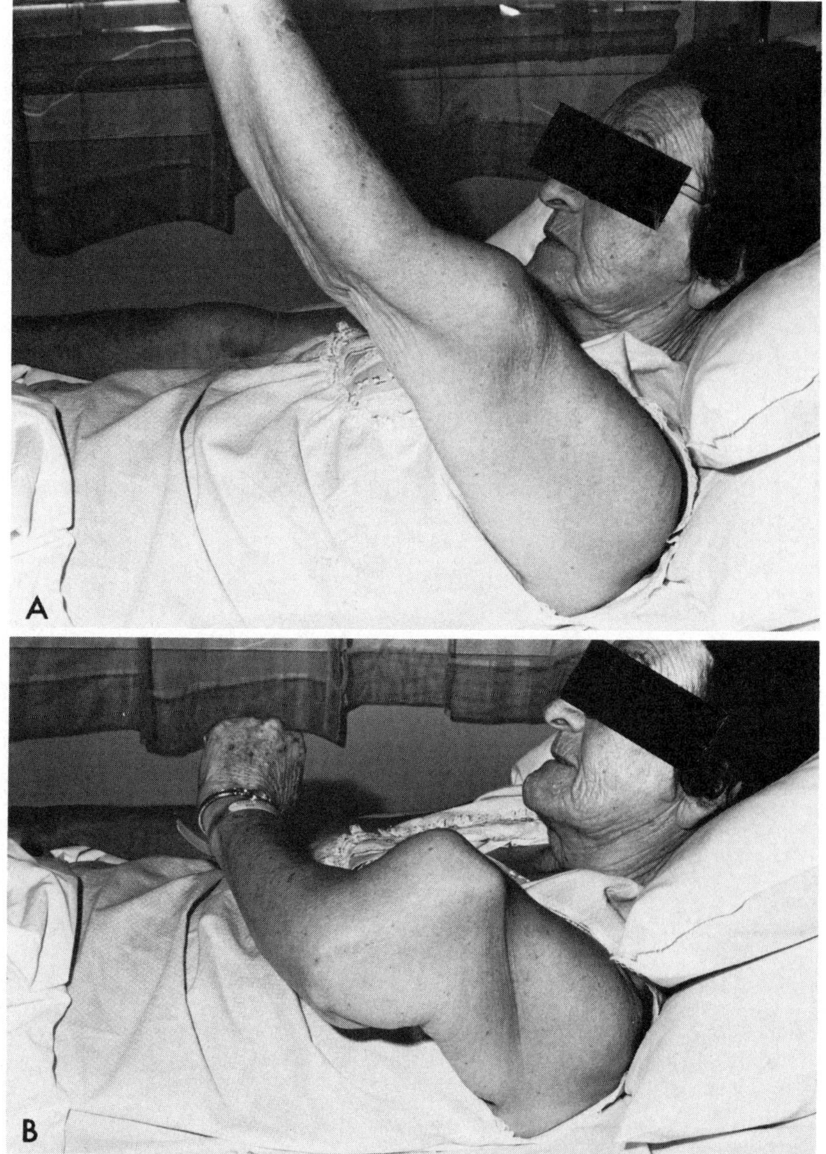

Figure 3–21. Pseudarthrosis. Extension *(A)* and flexion *(B)* photographs of 76-year-old woman with painless pseudarthrosis of the humerus, 25 years' duration.

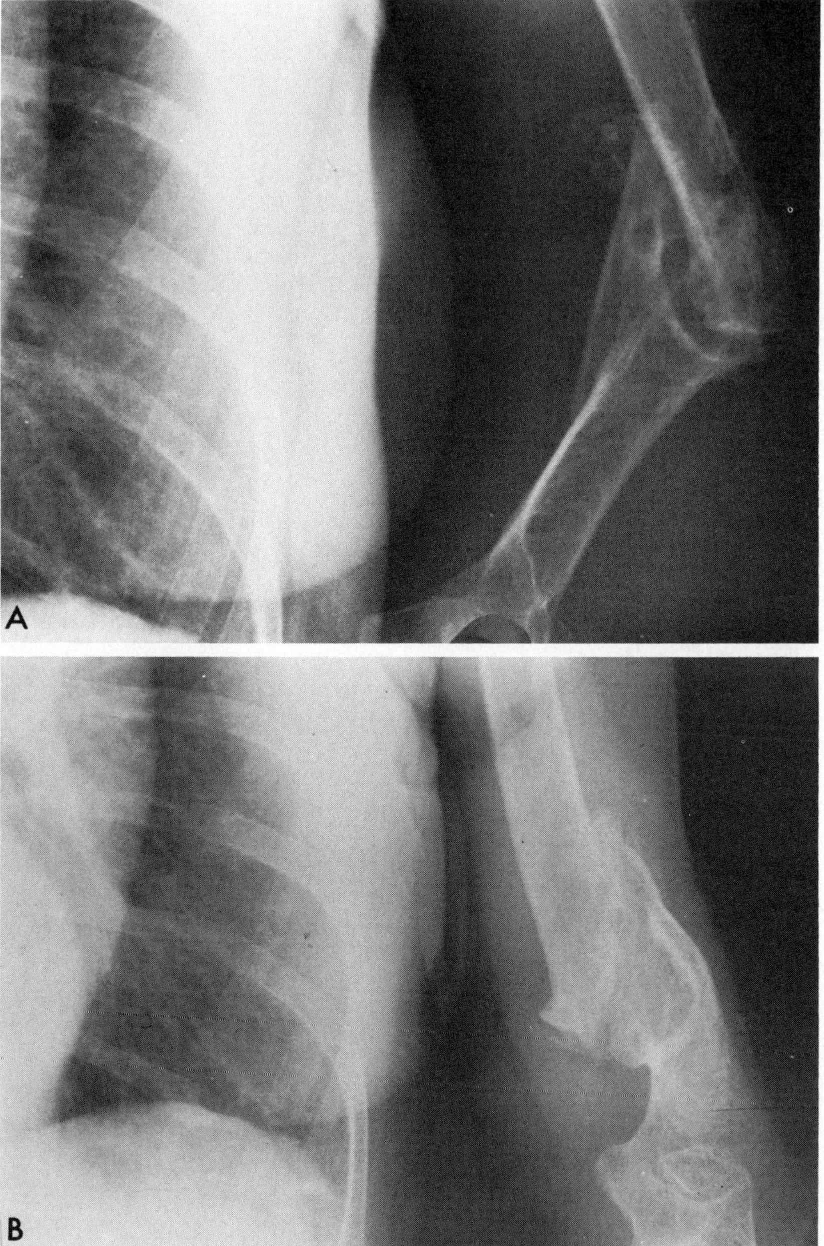

Figure 3–22. Radiographs of patient shown in Figure 3–21 exhibiting deformity of fracture ends with clear-cut space between fragments. There is more motion at the site of the pseudarthrosis than at the elbow joint.

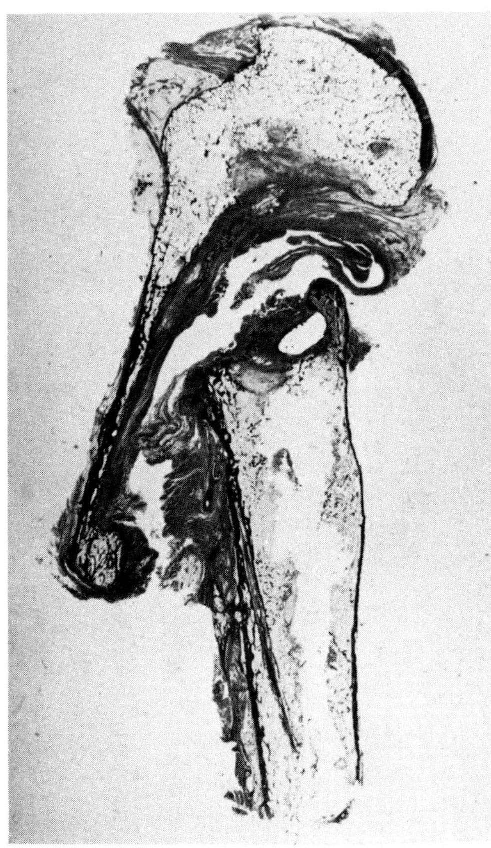

Figure 3–23. Macrosection of pseudarthrosis of distal femur. All attempts at fracture healing have ceased. The bone surfaces are capped with fibrous tissue, and the clear space represents the false joint. Note the marked osteoporosis secondary to disuse. The patient is not able to use the limb normally.

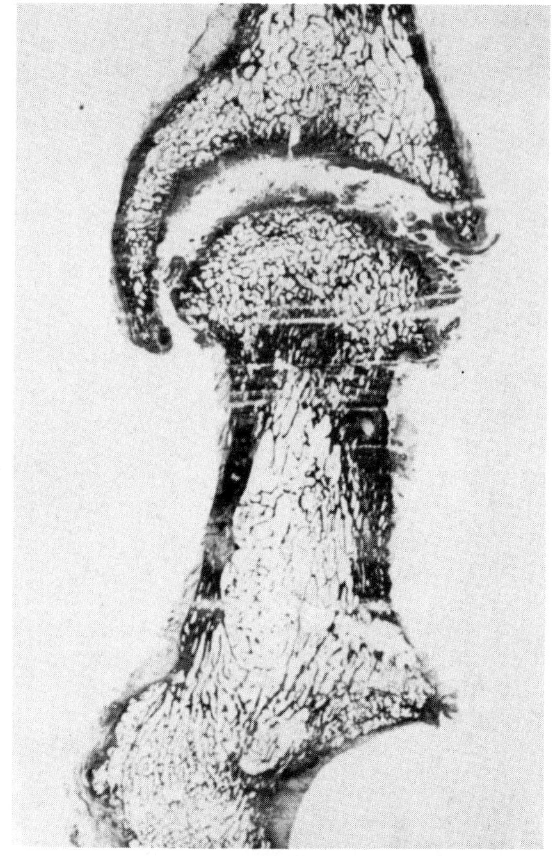

Figure 3–24. Macrosection of ulna with pseudarthrosis of long duration. The remodeling process has resulted in the formation of a rudimentary ball-and-socket configuration seen in such cases of long-standing pseudarthrosis.

STRESS FRACTURE

Accentuation or lag in any of the phases of normal growth and development will result in predictable morphologic alterations that, in turn, will produce a characteristic clinical syndrome. Stress fracture is a classic example produced by unusual demands for remodeling (i.e., unusual stress).

Basic to understanding of the stress fracture is analysis of the speed of osteoclastic and osteoblastic activity. Under appropriate stimuli, osteoclasts can resorb bone within hours, presenting visible macroscopic evidence of bone resorption within 1 or 2 days. This can be observed in an acute fracture or in hyperparathyroidism. Osteoblastic activity is slower. A minimum of 10 to 15 days is required before any visible bone can be seen following periosteal elevation or fracture. It has been calculated that the activity of one osteoclast equals the activity of 150 osteoblasts over a single unit of time (Johnson, 1964). With this relationship in mind, one should remember that the stimulus for remodeling is initiated by muscular stress; osteoclastic activity is required for the resorption of existing structures, followed by the osteoblastic refill to meet the demands of the additional stress. The remodeling process occurs in all bones and at all times during life (see Figs. 1–53 and 1–54).

Individuals subject to stress fractures have typical histories. Enthusiastic joggers and tennis players are the latest groups to join the ranks, and even well-conditioned professional and amateur athletes are often plagued by recurrent stress fractures

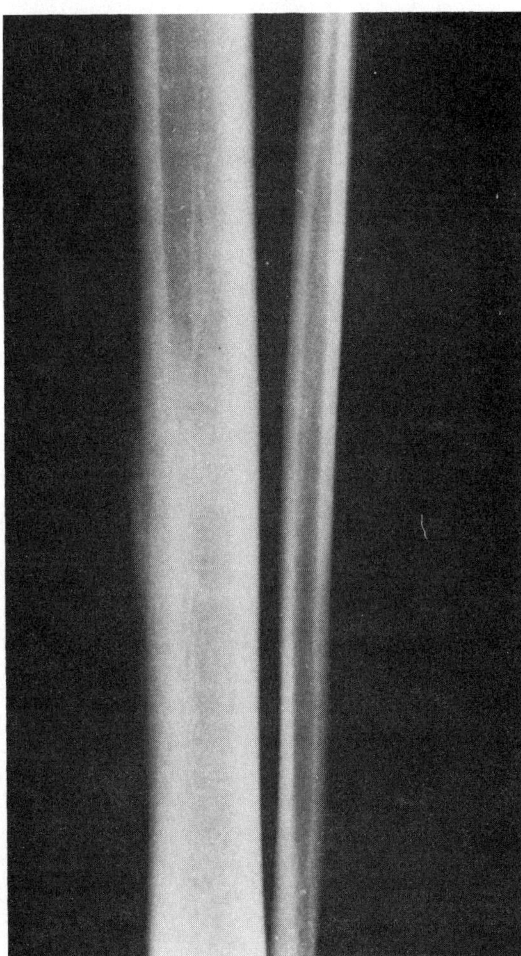

Figure 3–25. Clinical film of a military recruit who complained of pain during basic training. Radiographically, the cutting cones are made visible by decreased cortical density; there is a limited periosteal reaction.

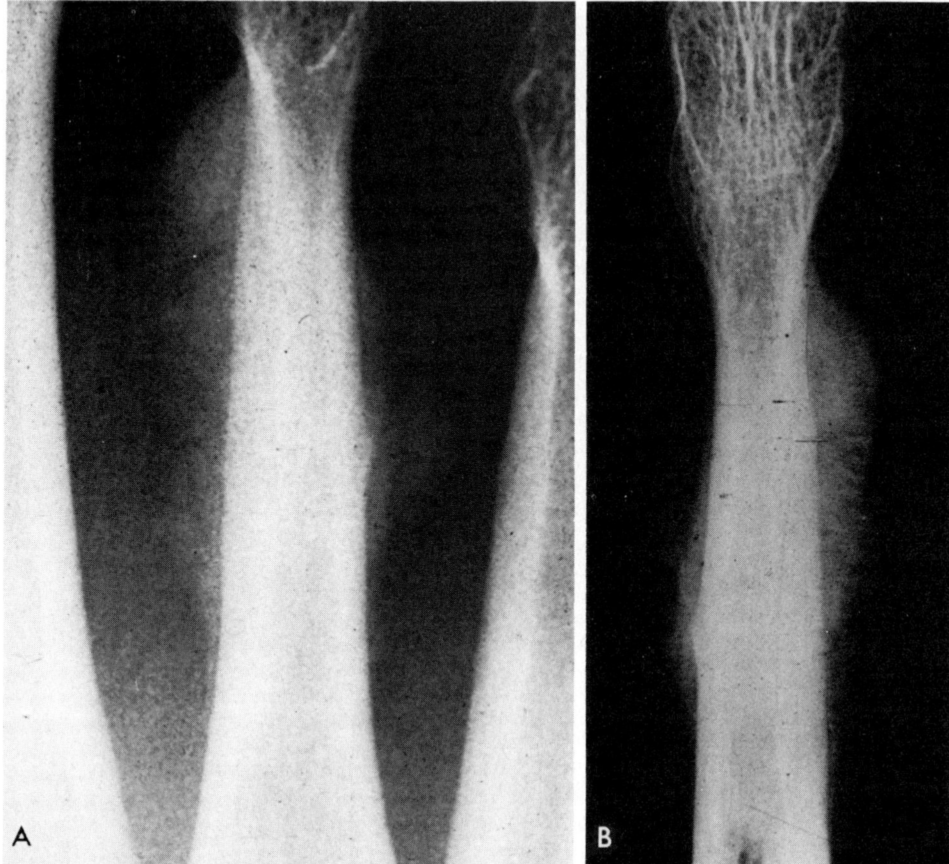

Figure 3–26. Clinical *(A)* and specimen radiographs *(B)* of stress fracture of the second metatarsal in a 34-year-old woman that occurred after strenous physical activity (tennis).

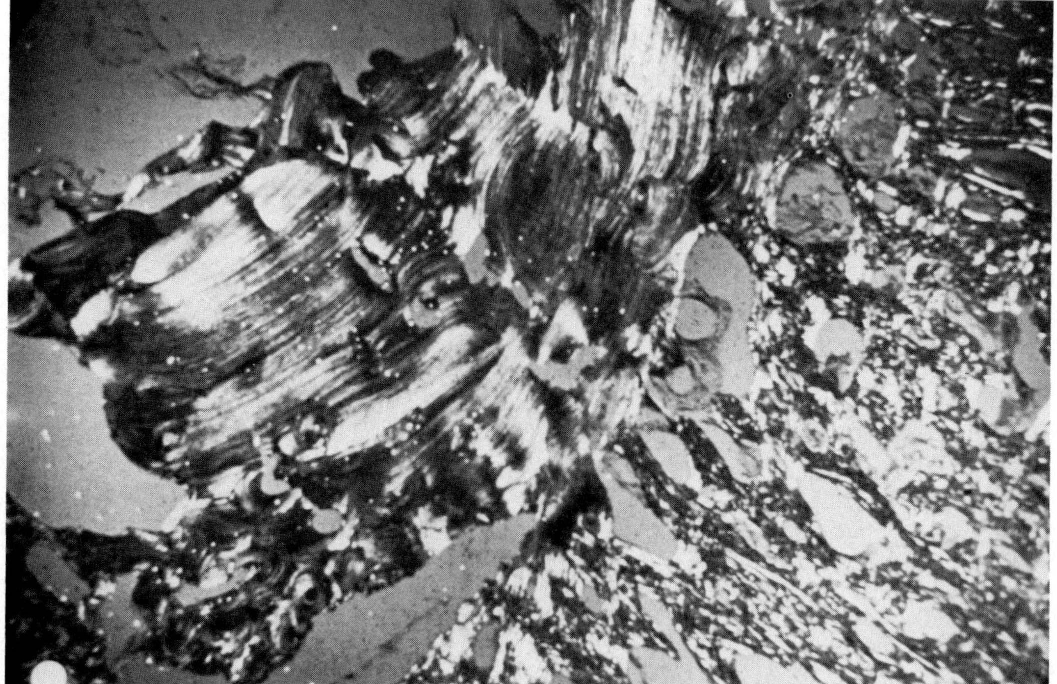

Figure 3–27. Cross section of bone exhibiting circumferential lamella without significant osteonization.

(Pavlov et al., 1982; Torg et al., 1982). Stress fractures are traditionally recognized in military medical practice, usually during basic training. A young adult who has been relatively inactive is likely to develop pain in the lower extremity during the rigors of physical activity of the training camp. Localized pain and tenderness will probably persist, and examination may indicate some local heat. Radiographic examination during the early stages may be negative. The most common location of stress fracture in the military recruit is the proximal posterior medial aspect of the tibia.

Histologic examination of the bone, biopsied in this early stage, shows a large number of longitudinally oriented resorption cavities created by cutting cones of osteoclasts (Figs. 3–27 to 3–30). Examination under polarized light shows that the cortex consists primarily of circumferential lamellar bone and that osteonization has lagged behind normal development for this age and location (Fig. 3–27). The process of accelerated resorption may continue for a number of weeks, and the weakened bone structure is the cause of pain as well as the stimulus for initiating osteoblastic refill.

The first radiographic manifestation is a periosteal reaction after approximately 2 to 3 weeks. New bone formation may also occur on the endosteal surface (Fig. 3–30). Periosteal and endosteal reaction is a scaffolding device to maintain the integrity of the anatomic structure while the cortex is being remodeled. Any weakening of the cortex, be it by accelerated cutting cone activity due to remodeling as in stress fracture, active hyperemia accompanying inflammation, or permeative destruction due to tumor, will give rise to a periosteal reaction that will persist until osteoblasts can completely repair and remodel the weakened cortex so that it can respond to the increased demands. Excessive osteoclastic resorption weakens the cortex, and significant time is required before the osteoblastic refill can cope with the demands placed on the bone. If the stresses are continued despite the pain and periosteal reaction, outright fracture may result.

Stated briefly, the events in stress fracture are the appearance of osteoporosis from the accelerated resorption of circumferential lamellae, periosteal and endosteal

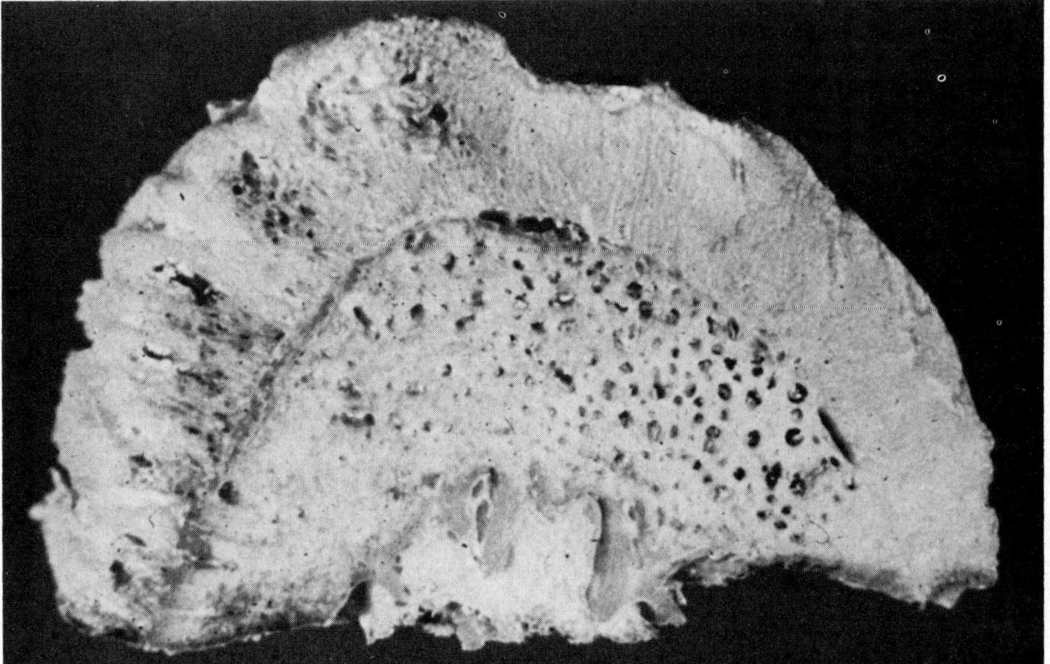

Figure 3–28. Gross specimen of stress fracture exhibiting numerous resorption cavities caused by relays of osteoclasts forming cutting cones prior to osteoblastic refill and osteonization. See Figure 3–29 for corresponding macrospecimen.

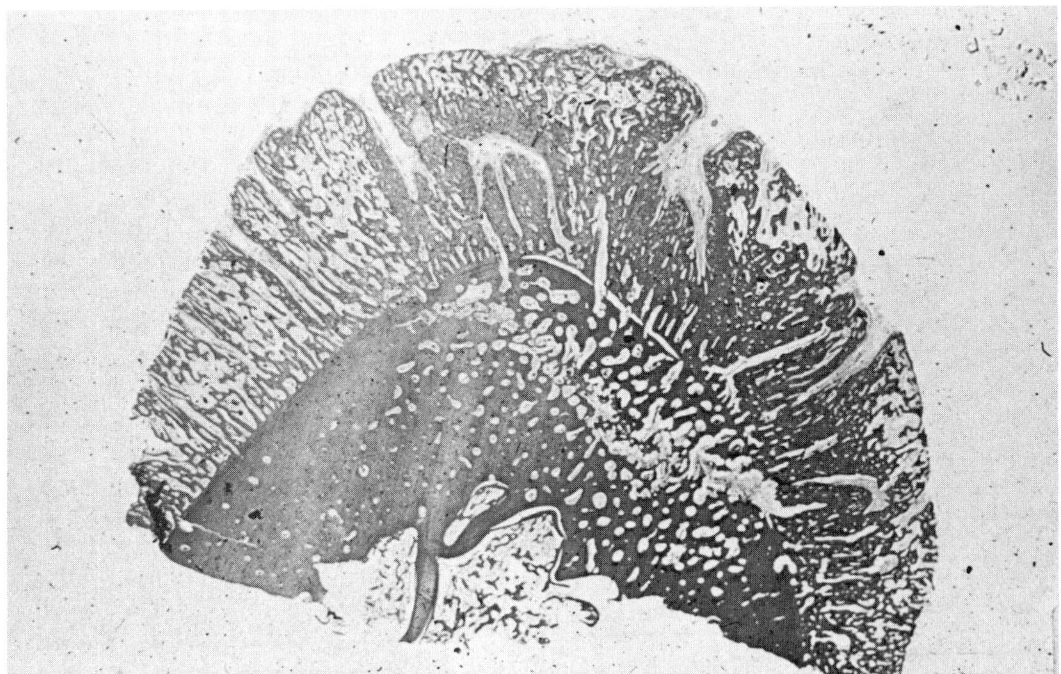

Figure 3–29. Macrospecimen of stress fracture depicted in Figure 3–28 exhibiting cutting cones, extensive resorption cavities, and periosteal reaction that has begun to solidify.

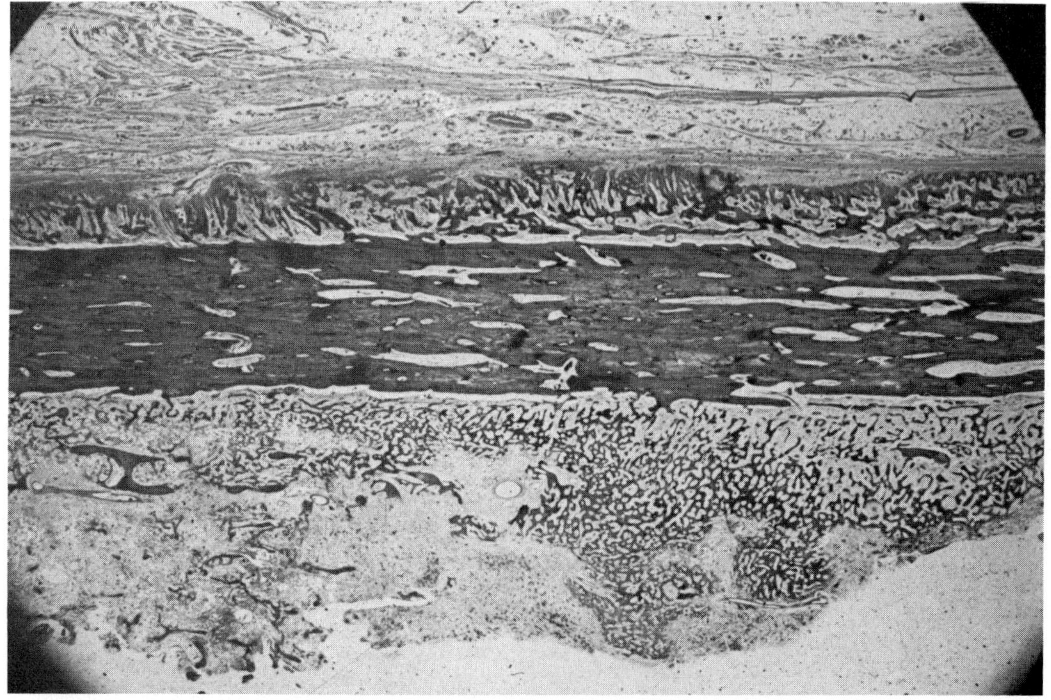

Figure 3–30. Macrospecimen, longitudinal view, exhibiting cutting cones and periosteal reaction as well as endosteal reaction.

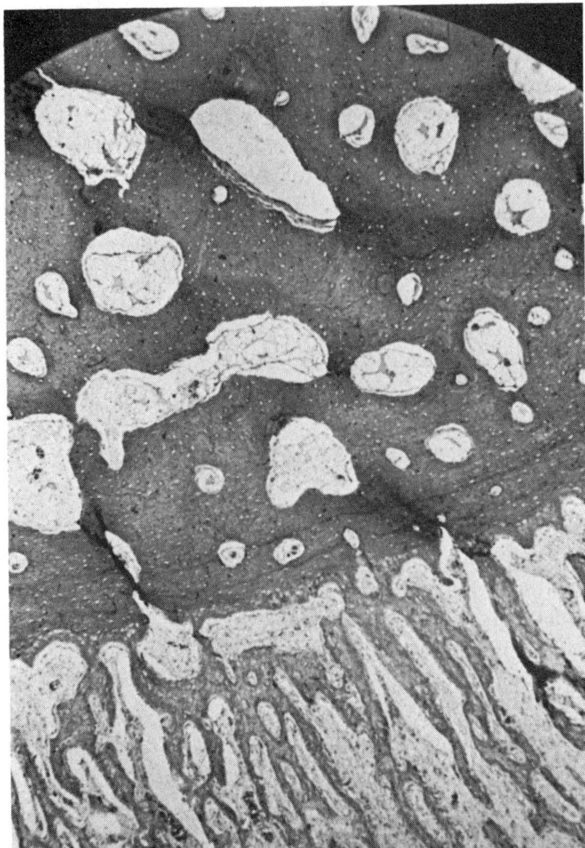

Figure 3–31. Cross section of specimen exhibiting a stress fracture with periosteal reaction and numerous cutting cones resulting in extensive resorption of cortical bone.

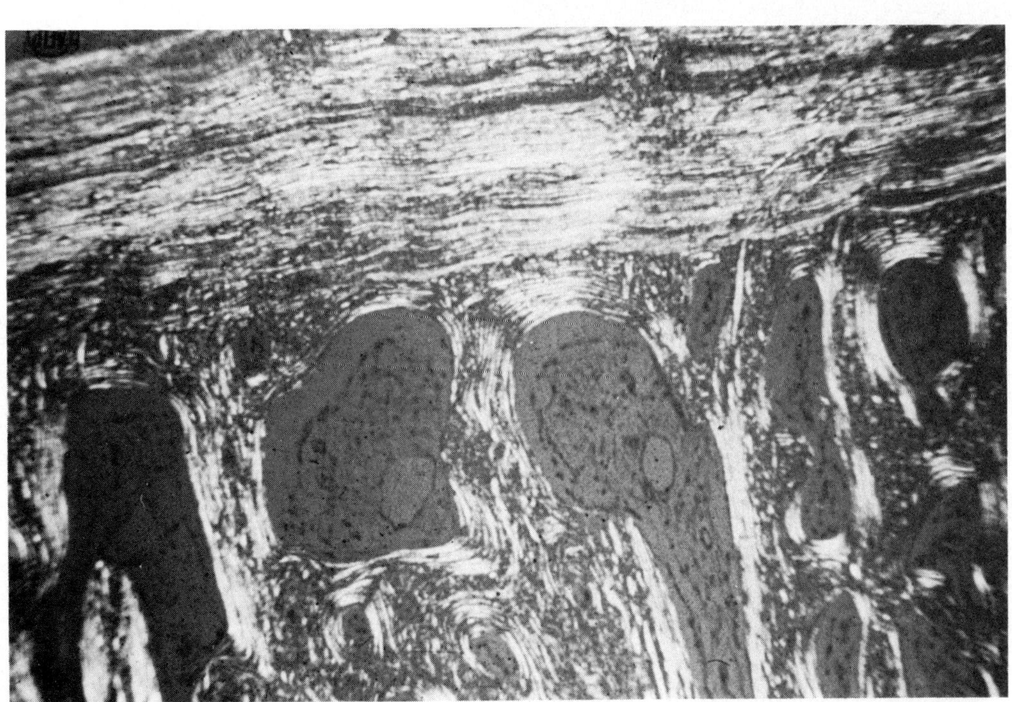

Figure 3–32. Fragments of bone from a stress fracture shown under polarized light exhibiting circumferential lamellar pattern and periosteal streamer bone. The relatively recently formed periosteal streamer bone has a "linen"-weave appearance under polarized light, as opposed to the "burlap"-weave appearance of younger bone (see Fig. 1–45).

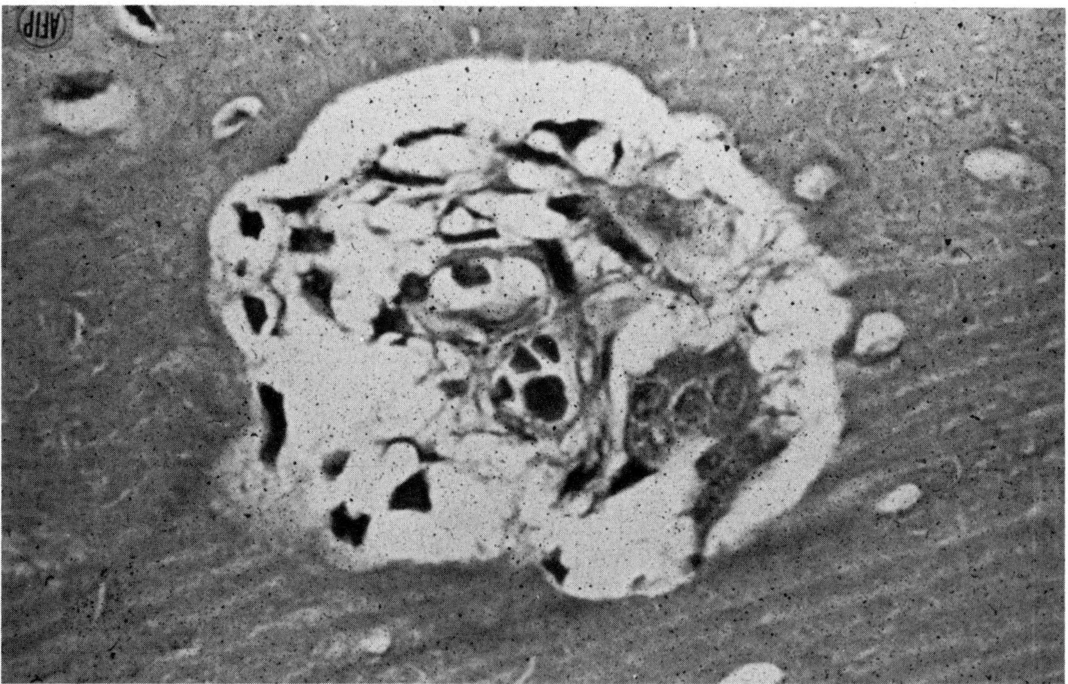

Figure 3–33. Histologic section exhibiting cutting cones with osteoclasts removing bone. Osteoblasts are visible on the left, preparing to deposit bone to produce an osteon (see Figs. 1–53 and 1–54).

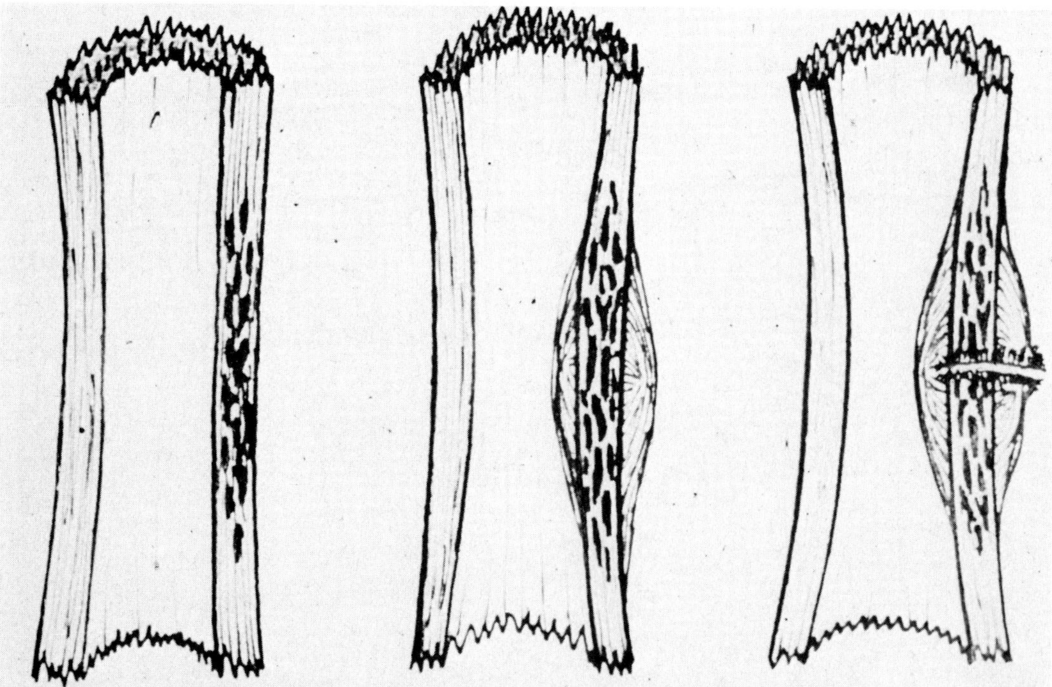

Figure 3–34. Schematic diagram of sequence of events leading to stress reaction and stress fracture. Increased stress results in the formation of numerous cutting cones and resorption of cortical bone, leading to weakened structure (left). Periosteal reaction occurs on the surface, and endosteal new bone is present as well (center). The periosteal reaction is the normal reaction of bone to weakened cortex, regardless of cause. If the stress continues, the weakened cortex may fracture (right) (Johnson, 1964).

reinforcement of this area, and, finally, outright fracture. The last event may never occur if effective treatment is begun early enough. Appropriate treatment is to diminish but not totally cease the activity. The goal is to provide continued mechanical stimulation for the area to remodel and heal, but not so much that the healing process is overwhelmed. Hence, joggers with stress fracture should not be placed at bed rest, but they should walk instead of run.

CORTICAL DESMOID (PERIOSTEAL DESMOID*; CORTICAL IRREGULARITY SYNDROME†)

Cortical desmoid is characteristically seen in the lower end of the femur. It arises as a result of osteoblastic failure to maintain remodeling activity during a combination of unusual growth spurts as well as muscular activity. Under normal circumstances, metaphyseal bone must be remodeled to assume the thinner diaphyseal diameter. Maximum reduction occurs in the lower end of the femur, where the epiphyseal diameter is twice that of the diaphysis.

The lower margin of the linea aspera serves as the site of insertion of the tendon of the adductor magnus and is a location in which there is maximum remodeling with reduction in overall diameter of bone. Teenagers often undergo spurts of growth, and if this experience is coupled with unusual muscular activity involving the adductors (athletes, cheerleaders, etc.), normal osteoclastic resorption and reinforce-

---

*Kimmelstiel and Rapp, 1951.
†Mirra, 1980.

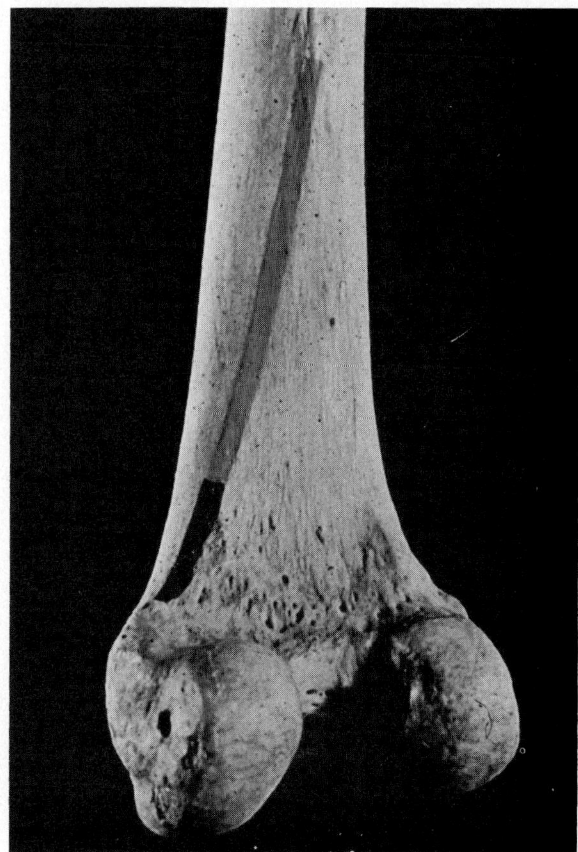

Figure 3–35. Anatomic model of lower femur illustrating the location of the linea aspera (insertion of adductor magnus muscle).

ment of the cortex may be accentuated by added demands of osteonization. At times the osteoblastic lag is pronounced, and instead of new cortical osteonal bone being formed, primitive fibrous connective tissue is deposited (scar tissue), to be replaced by bone later. The site of this connective tissue defect is always on the medial aspect of the lower end of the femur and consists of a sharply circumscribed external defect on the outer cortical rim (Figs. 3–37 and 3–38). Bilaterality is common. Although the defect is most commonly identified in the lower end of the femur, isolated instances of its appearance in other bones have been noted. The defect is by no means uncommon and is seen quite often in radiologic practice.

During its initial stage, the fibrous fill-in may be quite cellular and therefore worrisome (Fig. 3–39). As the lesion is allowed to mature, the cellular material becomes more heavily collagenized, and biopsies of the lesion at this stage reveal heavily collagenized connective tissue, findings reminiscent of the characteristics of extra-abdominal desmoid (Figs. 3–40 and 3–41). There is, however, no kinship to the fibromatosis encountered in skeletal musculature; if left alone the lesion will ultimately heal, with the formation of normal bone replacing the fibrous tissue (Fig. 3–42). Occasionally, the cortical desmoid will be complicated by microavulsion fractures with the formation of periosteal callus (Figs. 3–43 to 3–50).

One may establish the correct diagnosis by observing the characteristic age and activity of the individual involved, the common bilaterality of the disease process, the cortical excavation under appropriate radiographic positioning (external rotation views), the location of the lesion at the site of a muscle insertion, and, if the lesion is biopsied, its innocuous histologic appearance. The majority of these lesions do not require biopsy.

Text continued on page 103

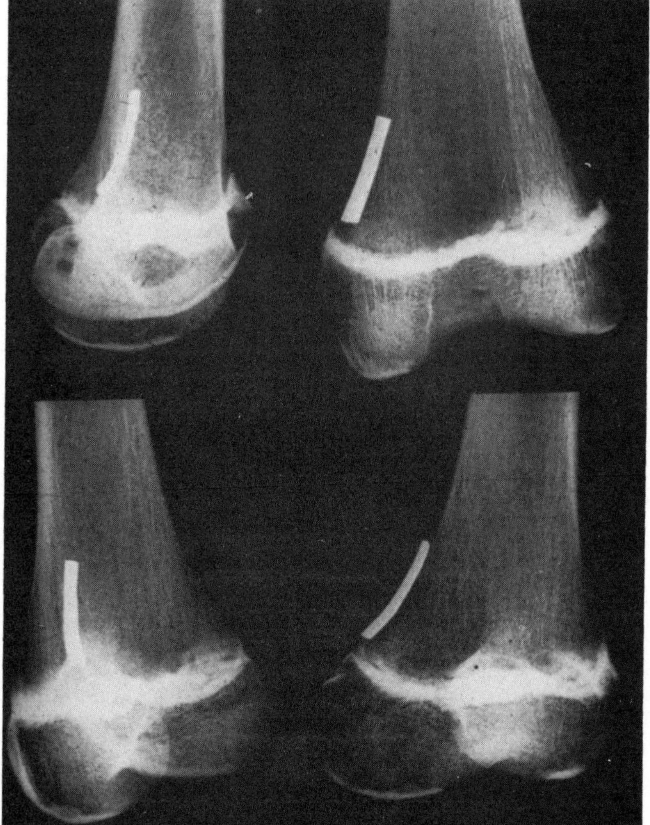

Figure 3–36. Radiographic projection of linea aspera in anteroposterior, lateral, and oblique projections of femur. In the straight anteroposterior and lateral projections, the linea aspera is not seen in profile at the edge of the radiographs; rather, it is obscured by overlying bone. (Courtesy of B. Genner, M.D.)

Figure 3–37. Characteristic radiographic appearance of a cortical desmoid. Notice the scalloped margin, characterized by dense sclerotic bone on the inner surface, absence of cortical margin, and a sharply circumscribed defect. Small avulsed sequestered fragments of bone may be seen radiographically (see Figs. 3–43 to 3–50).

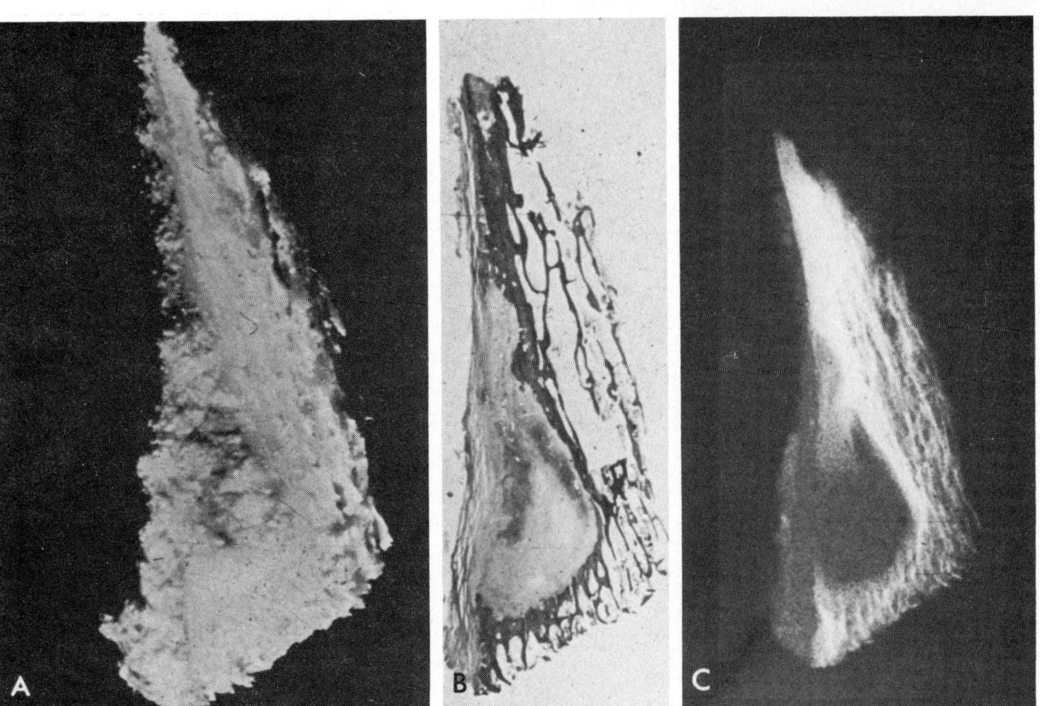

Figure 3–38. Gross specimen *(A)* macrosection *(B)* and specimen radiograph *(C)* of defect exhibiting a punched-out, sharply circumscribed, fibro-osseous defect on the surface of bone.

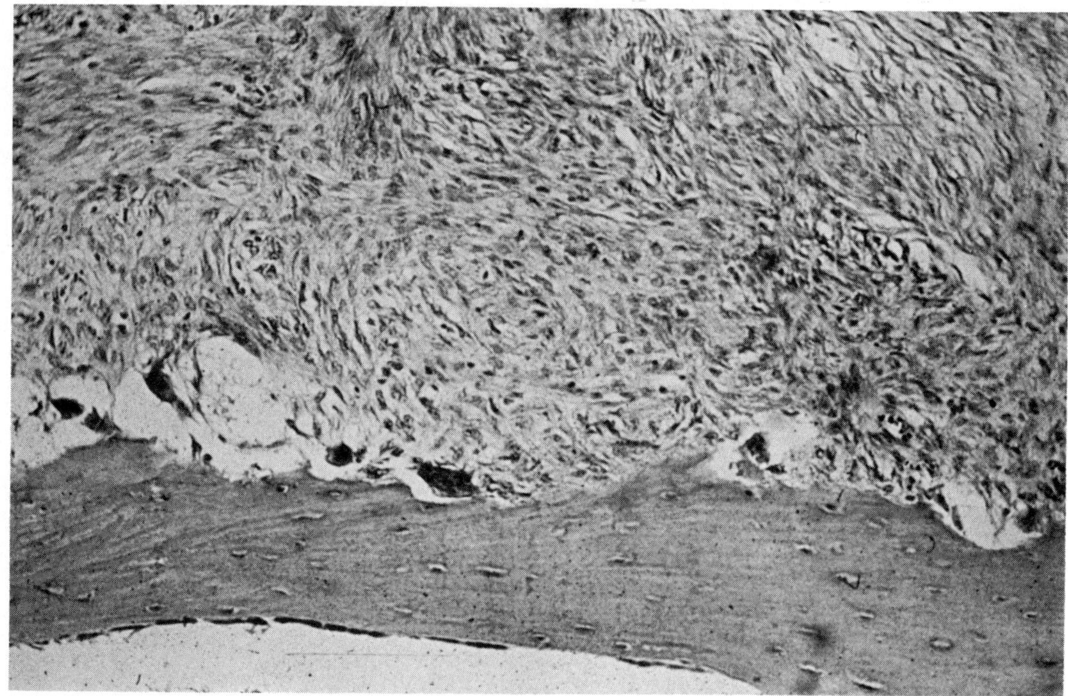

Figure 3–39. Replacement of bone by somewhat more cellular connective tissue, indicating an earlier stage of the lesion. Notice the numerous osteoclasts on the outer surface and the numerous osteoblasts on the inner surface of the cortex.

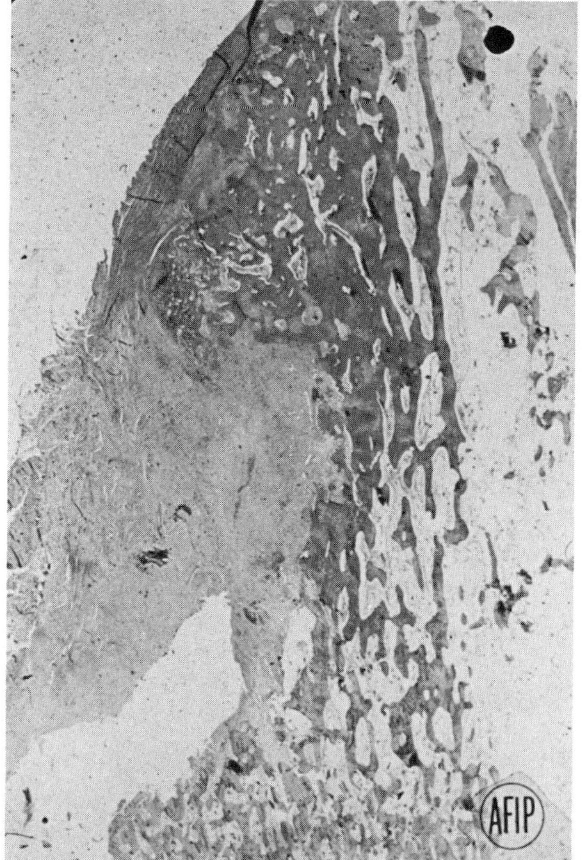

Figure 3–40. Histologic specimen exhibiting fibrous connective tissue replacing cortex and trabeculae of bone.

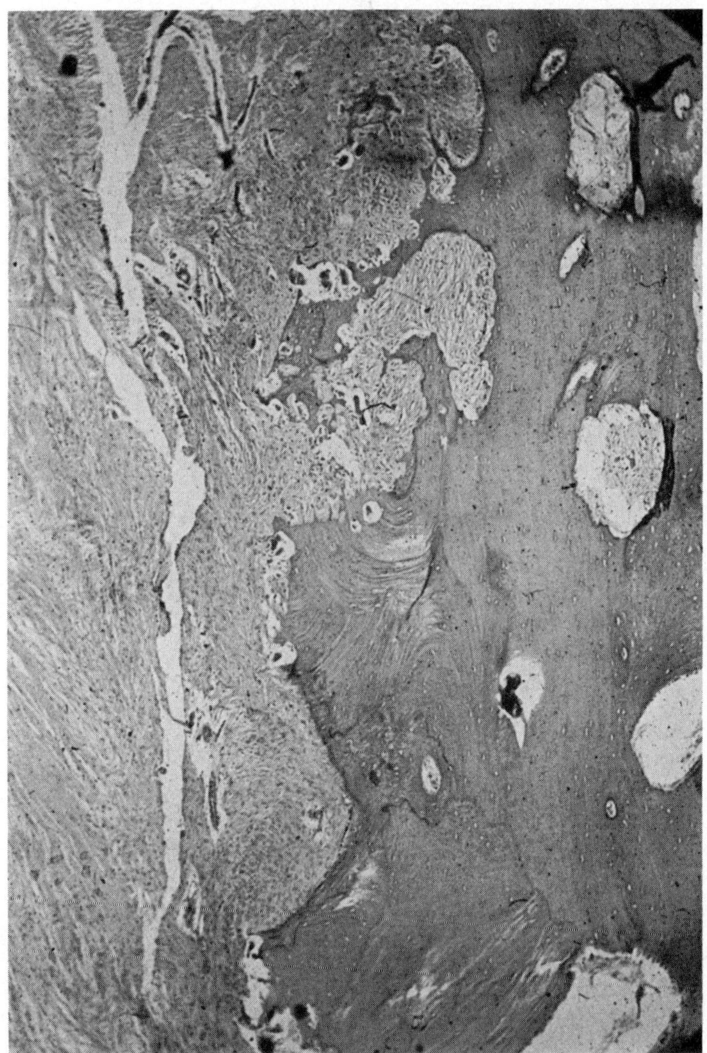

Figure 3–41. Higher magnification of the interface between cortex and lesion exhibiting irregular resorption in addition to replacement by relatively acellular fibrous connective tissue.

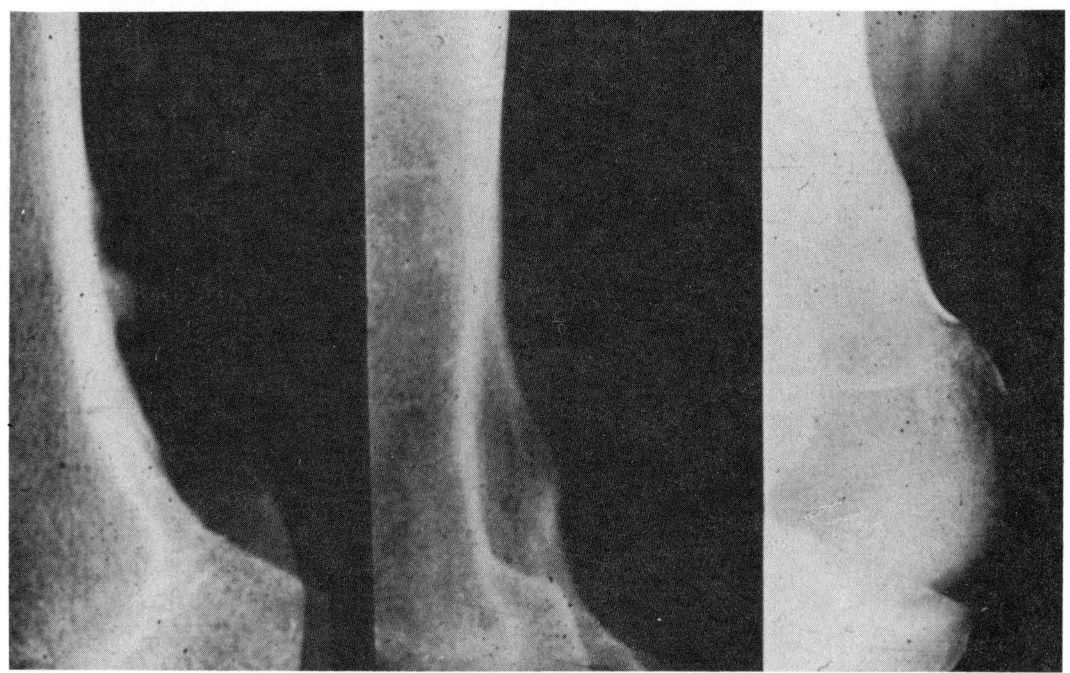

Figure 3–42. *See legend on opposite page.*

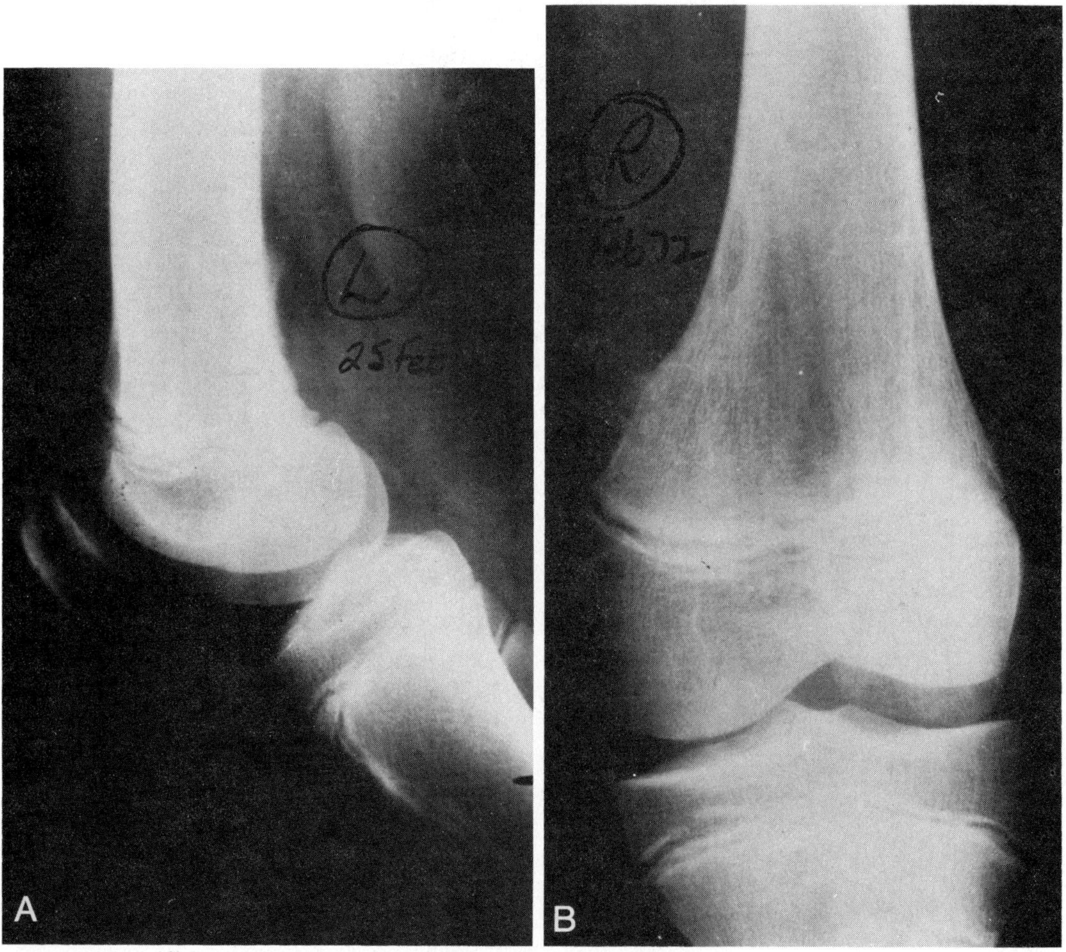

Figure 3–43. *See legend on opposite page.*

Figure 3–44. Anteroposterior radiograph of distal femur. The lesion appears in typical location as a punched-out area in bone surrounded by sclerotic rim. It is clearly visible because it represents loss of cortical rather than cancellous bone. The repair process accentuates the margin.

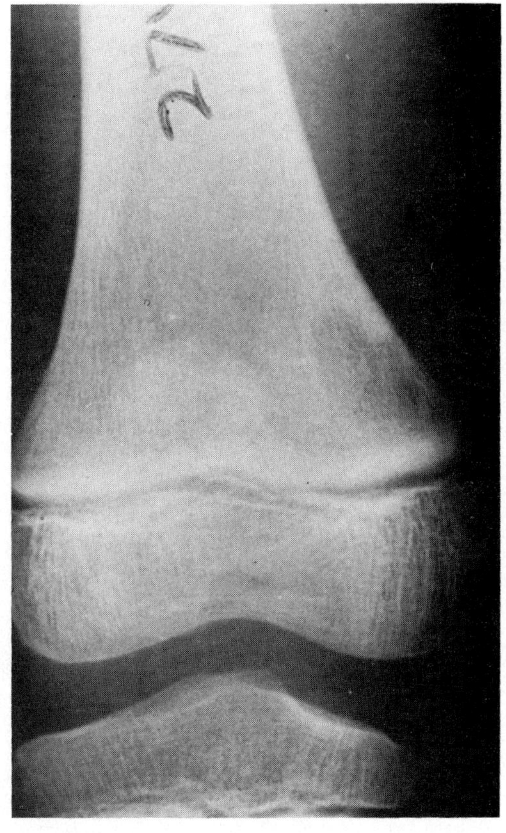

Figure 3–42. Radiographic appearance of healed cortical desmoid. When the stress leading to the defect is removed, bone will ultimately fill in, leaving only a slight protuberance that will eventually be remodeled into the normal contour of the femur.

Figure 3–43. Lateral *(A)* and anteroposterior *(B)* radiographs of cortical desmoid with periosteal reaction and early callus, characteristic of cortical desmoid in young teenagers. Note that the lesion is bilateral, a frequent presentation.

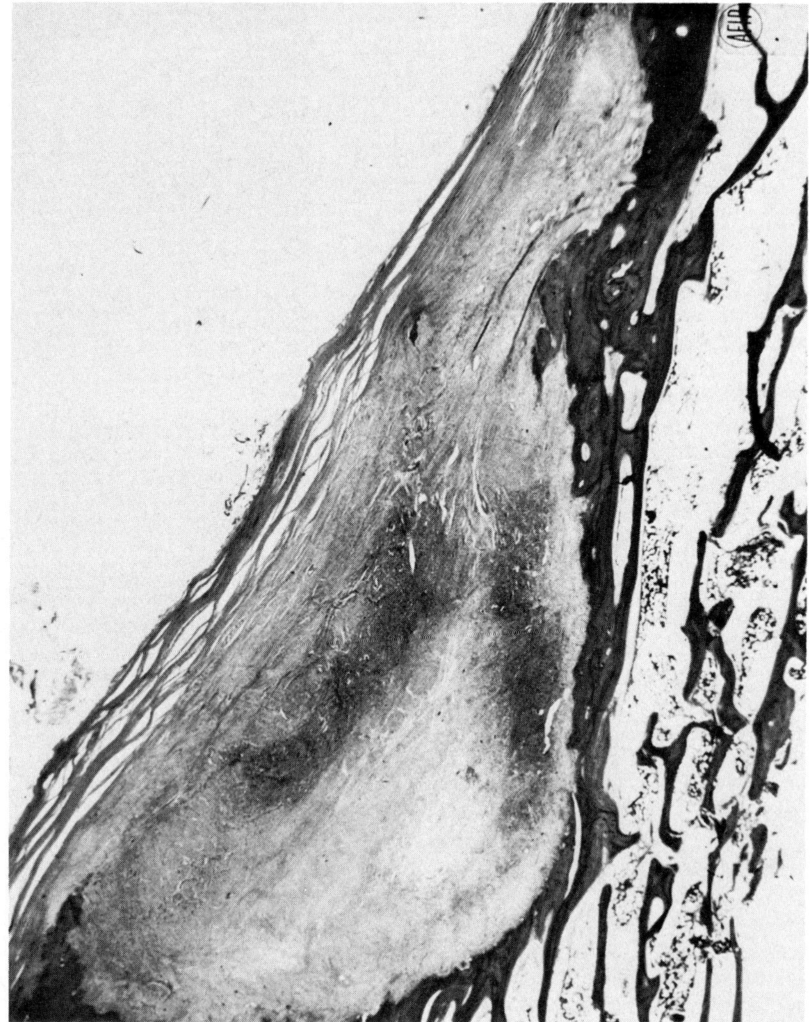

Figure 3–45. Macrosection of fibrous defect in the cortex. Bony reinforcement in the depth of the lesion indicates long duration.

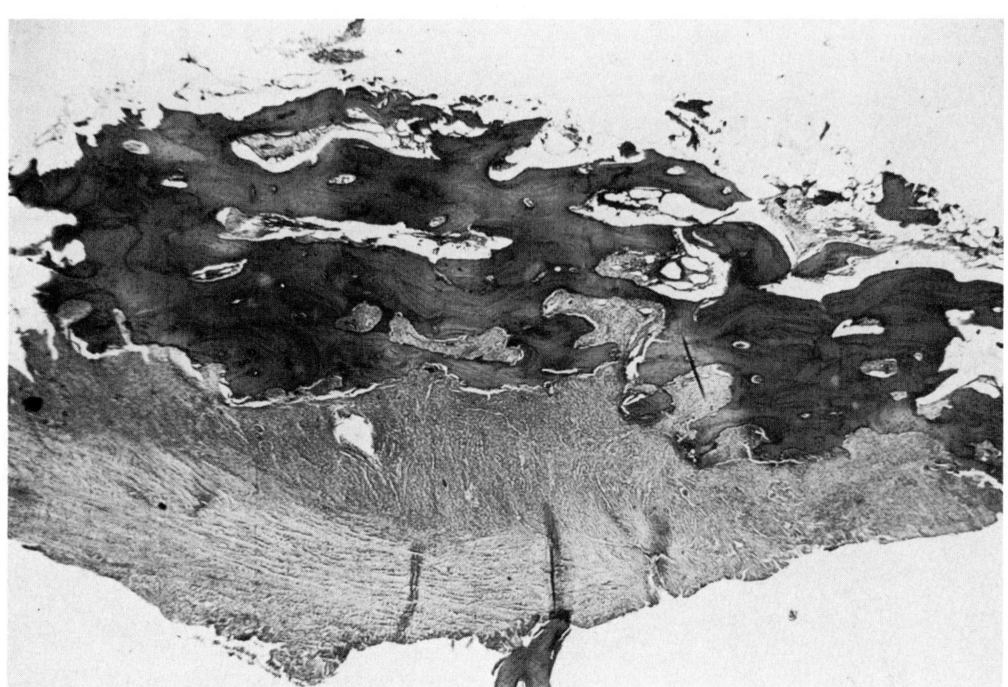

Figure 3–46. Section of cortical desmoid. Dense collagenized lesion with little cellular activity. Note large resorption cavities in the underlying cortex, indicating remodeling activity.

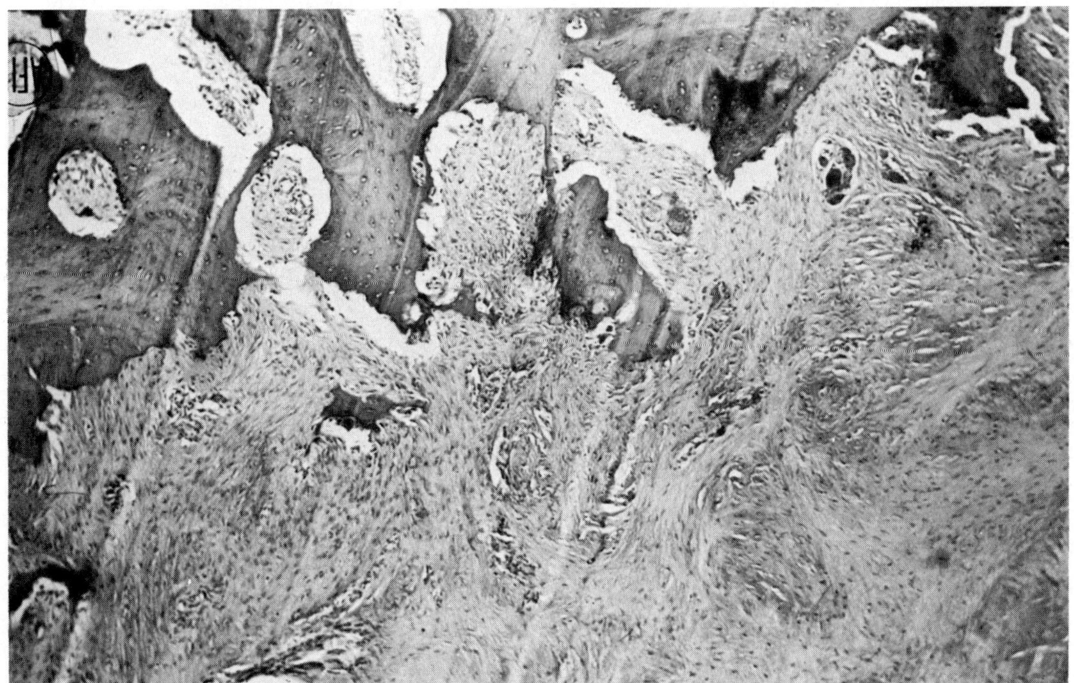

Figure 3–47. Cortical desmoid. Higher magnification of area with poor cellularity and extensive collagenization.

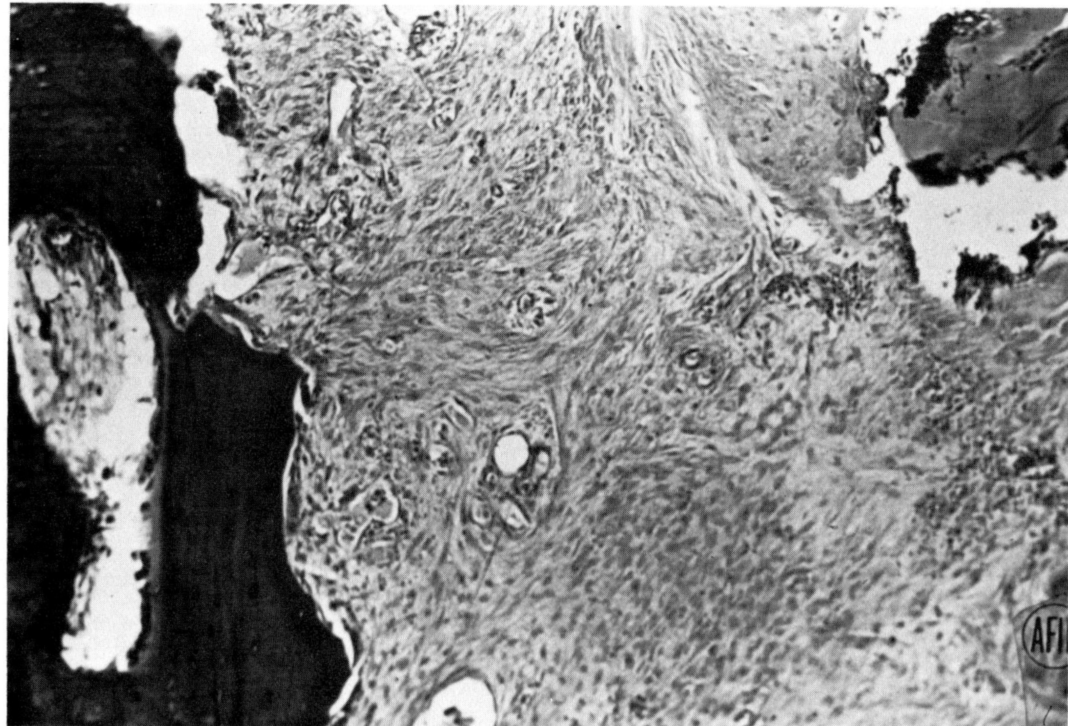

Figure 3–48. Cortical desmoid. A more cellular lesion suggesting more recent onset. The lesion may be confused with sarcoma by an observer who is unfamiliar with cortical desmoid.

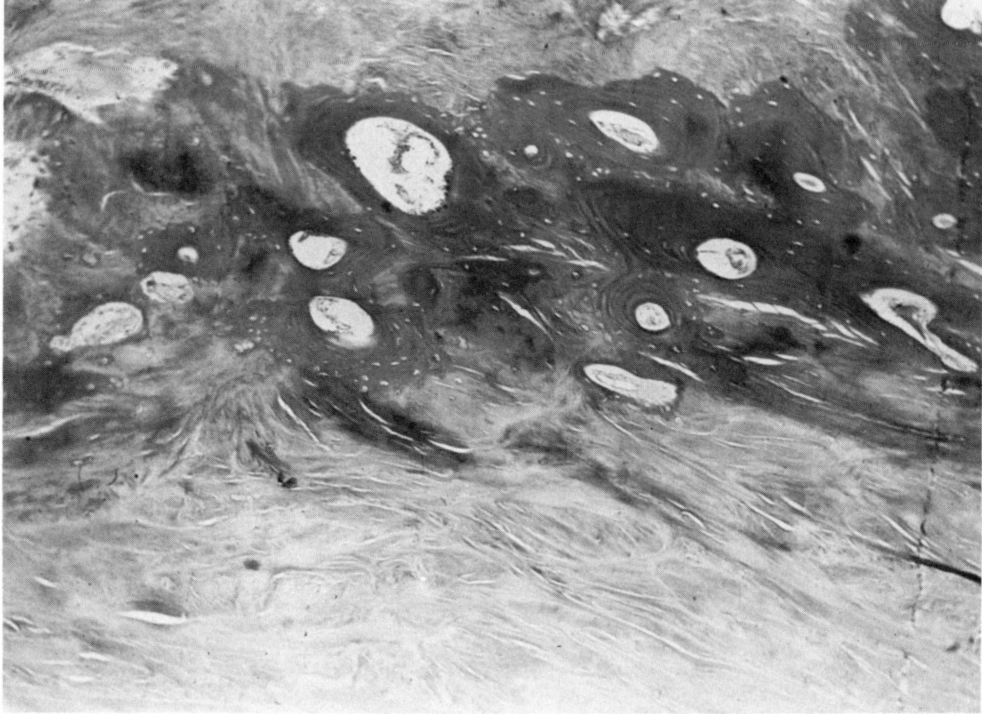

Figure 3–49. Cortical desmoid. An older lesion may be completely acellular and quiescent. The diminished activity is probably related to the long-term persistence of the radiographic defect.

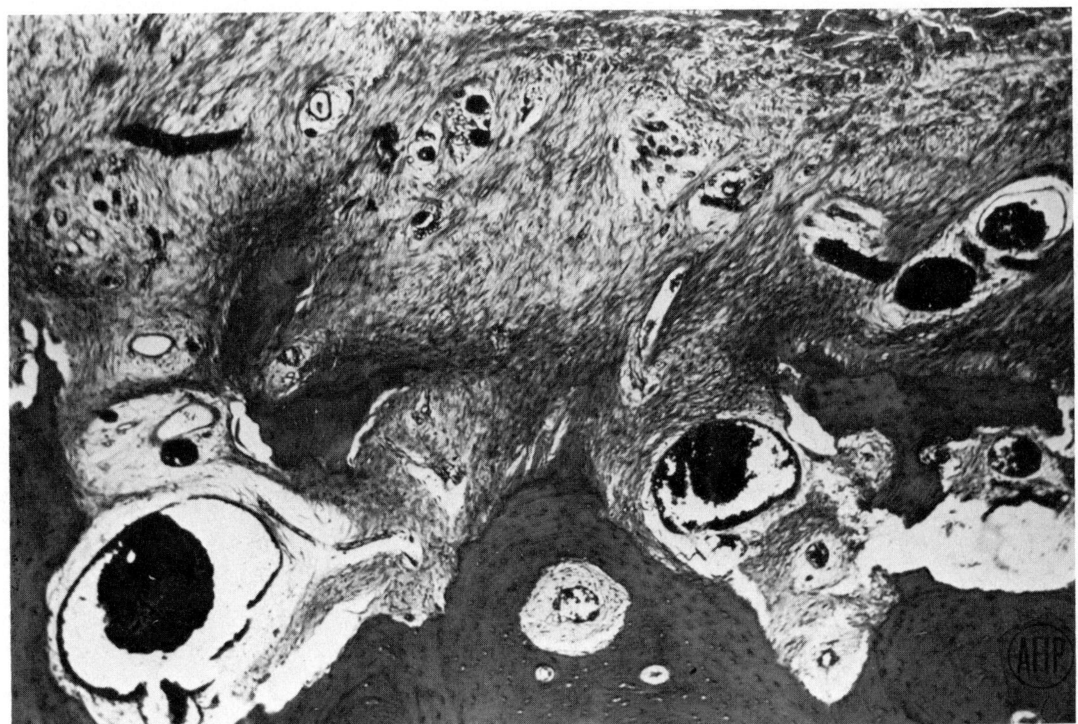

Figure 3–50. Cortical desmoid. Occasional lesions exhibit unusual cellularity. Numerous vessels are present, there is extensive resorption of cortex, and there is a greater periosteal reaction.

MYOSITIS OSSIFICANS

"Myositis ossificans" is a generic term for a class of lesions characterized by metaplasia of soft tissue to bone. The process occurs most often in muscle (Figs. 3–51 and 3–52) but may also occur in fascia, tendon, joint capsule (Fig. 3–53), and occasionally in fatty tissue. The process can be divided into three stages. The first stage, lasting 4 to 6 weeks, is known as the "pseudosarcoma stage" because it is the period of massive necrosis, degeneration, early regeneration, and marked cellular proliferation with immature structures, findings reminiscent of those seen in sarcoma. The second stage, approximately 6 weeks in duration, is a period of differentiation. The third stage, which lasts a number of months, is a period of maturation.

PSEUDOSARCOMA

The sequence of events begins with a traumatic incident in which tissue is crushed or torn. Blunt trauma is common. The precise stimulus that causes metaplastic formation of bone instead of normal repair and scar formation is unknown. With the crush of muscle, there is extensive damage and cell death. Holes appear in the sarcolemmal sheath, and fluid accumulates. The sarcolemmal nuclei proliferate, the sarcolemma disappears, and the fluid diffuses into the tissues. Phagocytes invade and remove the fibers, enlarging the holes. The capillary bed dilates, as in a fracture, producing the clinical symptoms of heat, swelling, and tenderness ("charley horse"). Since the damage is greatest in the center of the traumatized area, these tissues may totally liquefy or be replaced by sheets of nonspecific cells. The breakdown of cellular

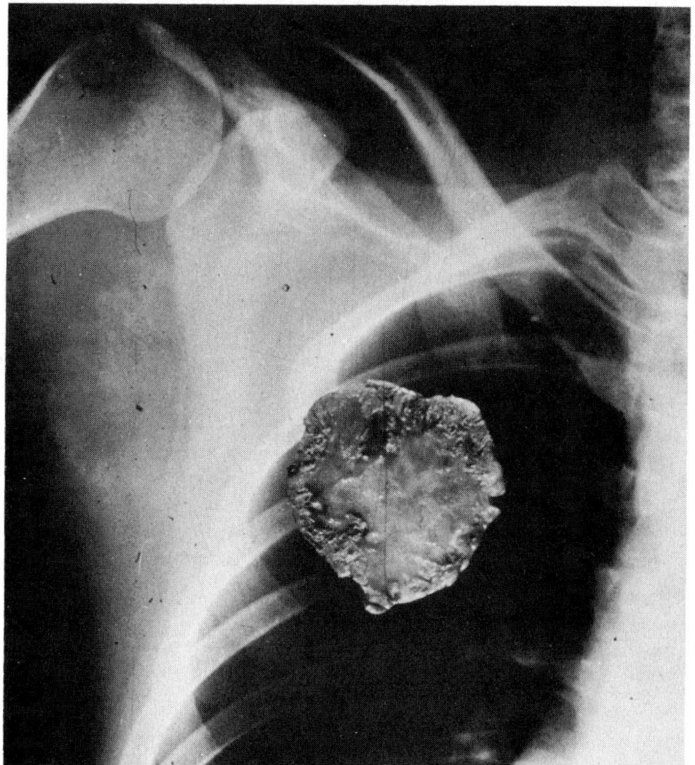

Figure 3–51. Myositis ossificans occurring on the medial surface of the scapula. The patient, a particularly strong individual, lifted a car with his shoulder instead of using a jack. The lesion appeared approximately 3 weeks after the traumatic episode.

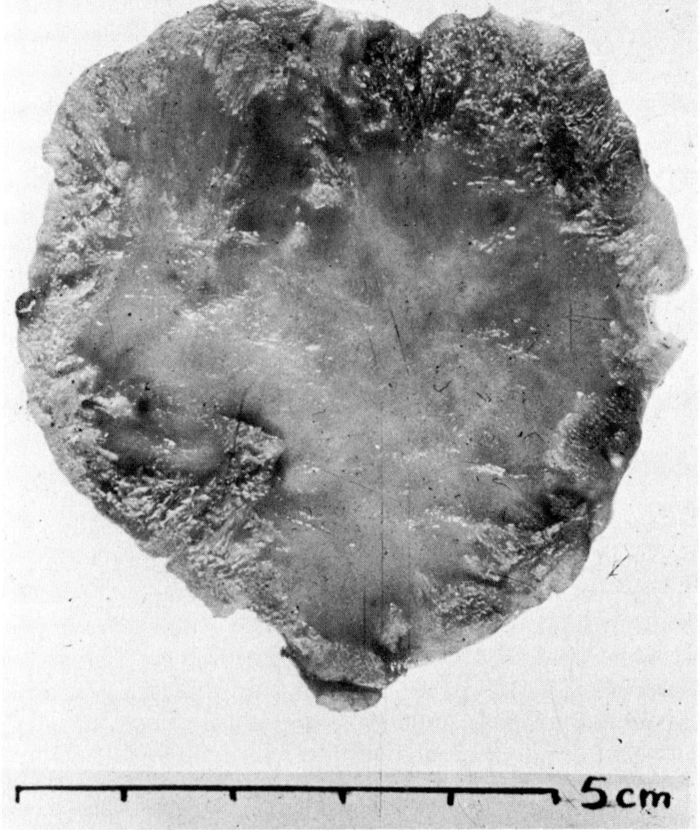

Figure 3–52. The peripheral maturation of the lesion shown in Figure 3–51 is easily seen in this specimen photograph.

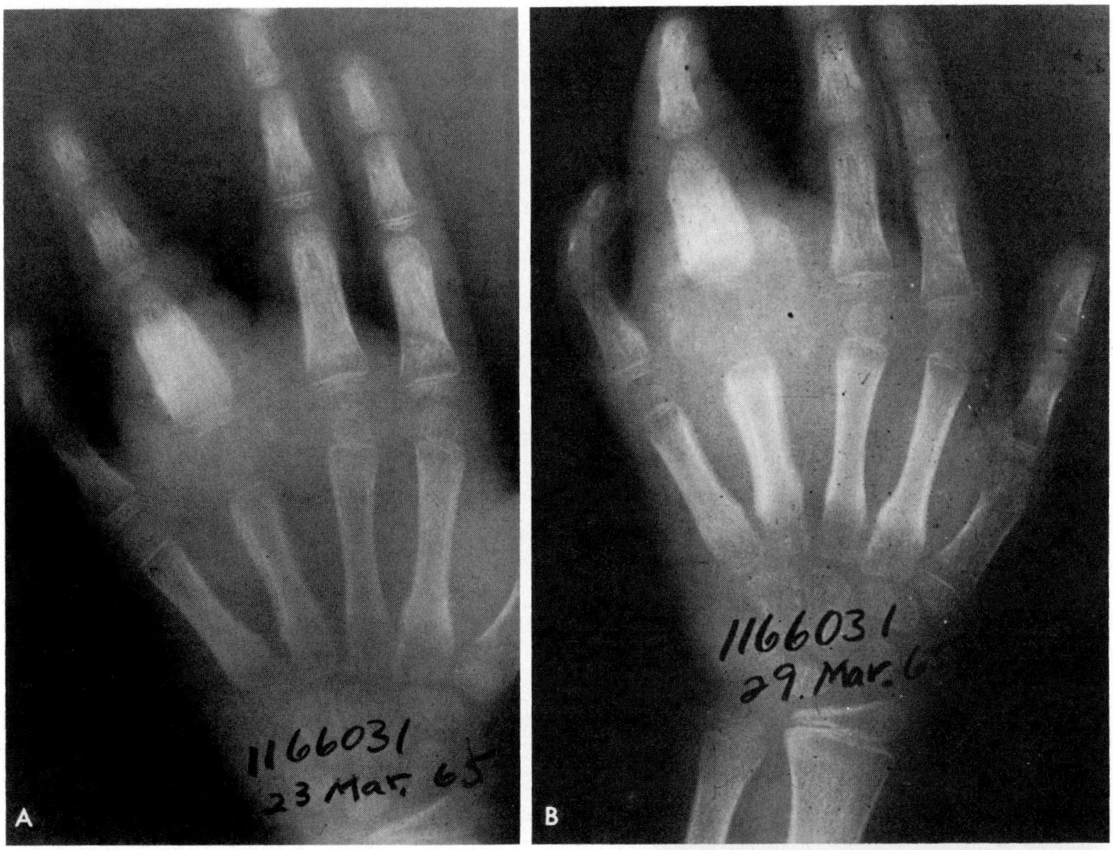

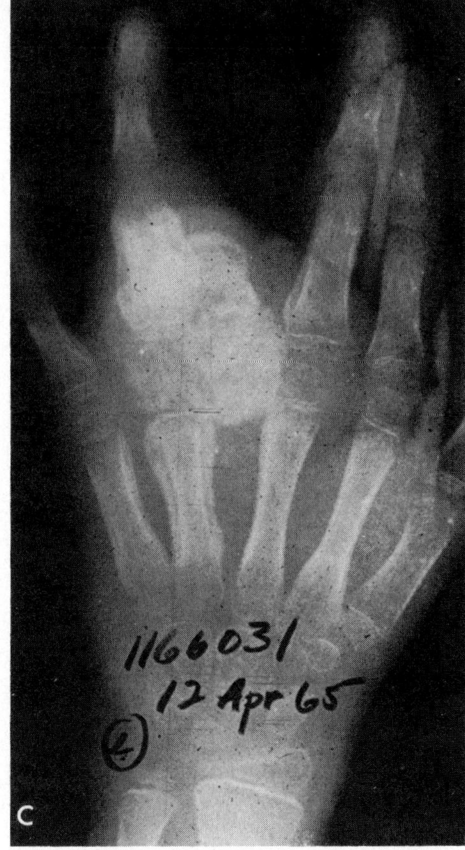

Figure 3–53. Radiographs of the hand illustrating sequence in the formation of myositis ossificans. At the end of 3 weeks, the peripheral maturation is clearly identifiable radiographically. The speed of the reaction is diagnostic, eliminating the possibility of neoplasm.

material in the traumatized area induces a transient inflammatory infiltrate ("myositis"). Unless further trauma is added by injudicious massage, excessive stretching, surgery, or other activity, the stage of degeneration lasts approximately 15 days. It is followed by a phase of activity with extensive proliferation of all mesenchymal cell types. Identifiable osteoid formation is minimal at this stage. A biopsy during this 2- to 4-week period can lead to erroneous diagnosis of neoplasia. It is a period of indecision for the clinician, radiologist, and pathologist. The clinical history of blunt trauma at the appropriate time is essential to reaching a proper diagnosis.

During the initial 6-7 week period, the lesion has identifiable zones only if excised in its entirety. The center of the lesion is necrotic, surrounded by zones with less tissue damage.

DIFFERENTIATION

During the second and third months following injury, the mesenchymal cells differentiate into fibroblasts, osteoblasts, chondroblasts, and so forth. Giant cells are numerous and remove the necrotic debris. Fibrous tissue formation and some primitive osteoid deposition occur. Blood supply to the center of the lesion is precarious. Most of the necrotic cells undergo liquefactive necrosis and resorption, which may leave a cyst filled with fluid, or the area may fill with sheets of nonspecific cells. Near the periphery of the lesion, where the damage is least, repair is more prompt and complete, leading to mineralization. The matrix will proceed to ossification with the best developed, mature trabecular bone at the periphery and progressively less differentiated zones in the central portion. The characteristic zoning of the myositis ossificans, with the *most* mature tissue at the periphery, distinguishes it from neoplasms of bone in which the *best* differentiated portions are in the center of the lesion and the *least* differentiated are at the periphery (Figs. 3–54 to 3–60).

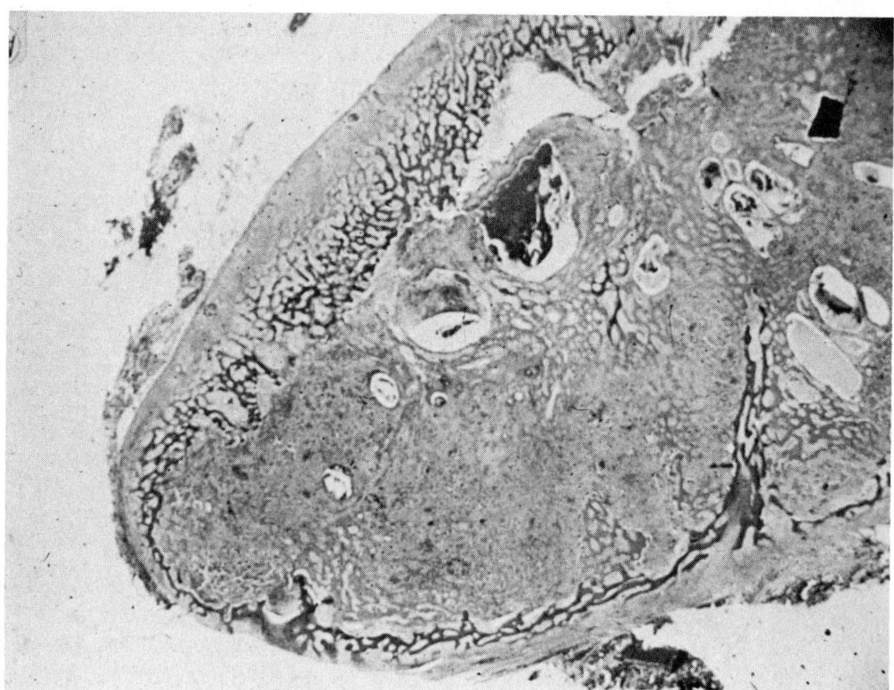

Figure 3–54. Section from a patient with myositis ossificans of the hand exhibiting a pattern of peripheral maturation and central immaturity with cyst formation from more extensive tissue damage.

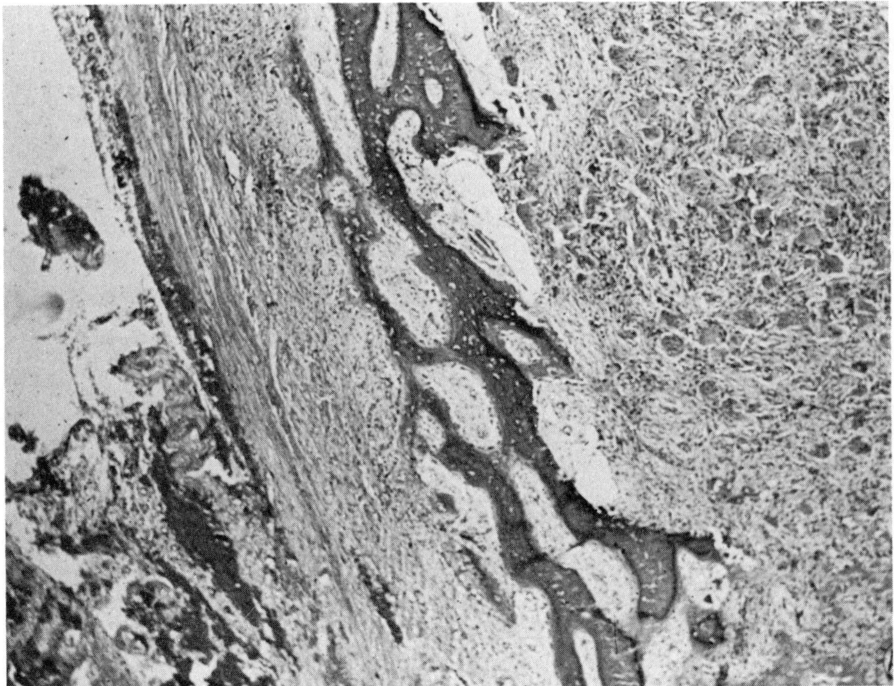

Figure 3–55. Outer rim of myositis ossificans exhibiting well-differentiated bony trabeculae covered by a "periosteum" exactly as seen in fracture callus.

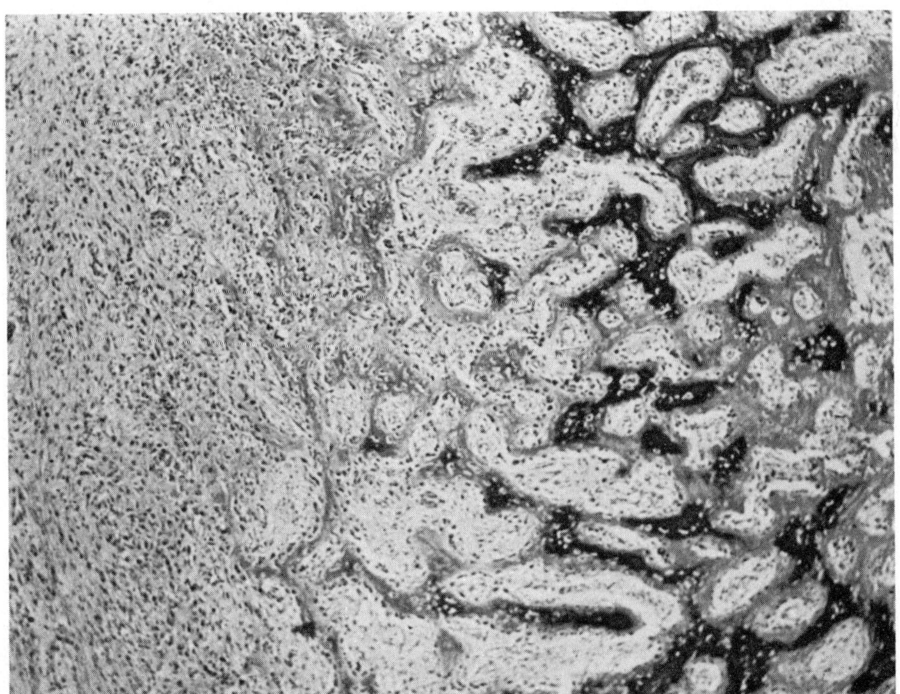

Figure 3–56. Well-differentiated trabeculae of the bone giving way to more undifferentiated tissue in the center of the lesion. Notice the decreased cellularity and sinusoidal structures accompanying the well-differentiated trabeculae at the periphery.

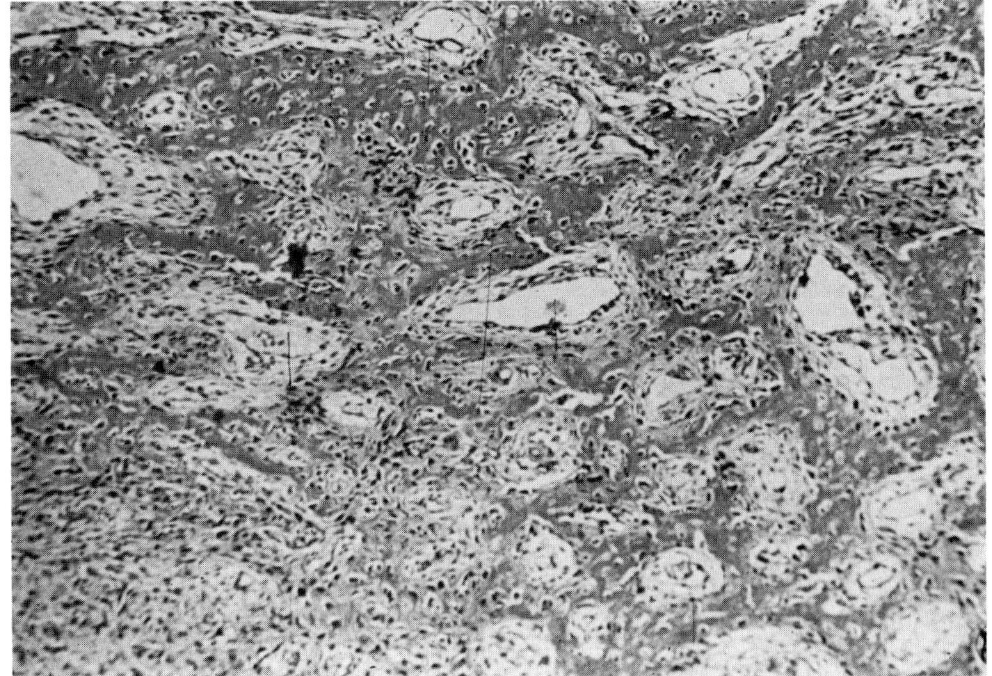

Figure 3–57. Poorly differentiated trabeculae of bone accompanied by relatively undifferentiated connective tissue from the central portion of a myositis ossificans.

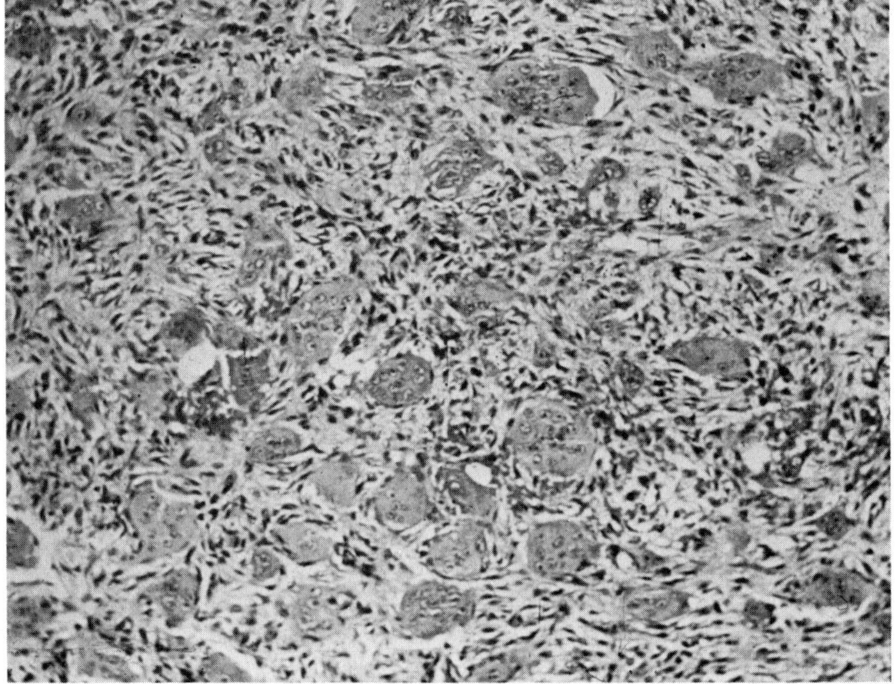

Figure 3–58. Foci of well-differentiated osteoclasts in the center of a myositis ossificans.

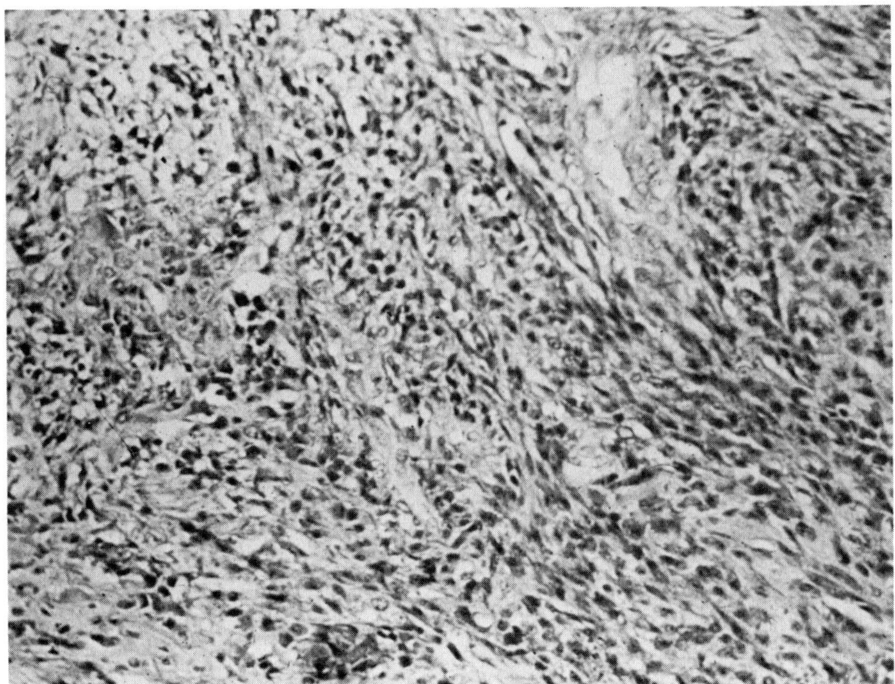

Figure 3–59. Poorly differentiated connective tissue from the center of a myositis ossificans. A small biopsy from an early lesion can be confused with a malignant process. As always, but especially in lesions of bone, careful history, correlation with radiographs, and appropriate sampling of the lesion are essential to proper diagnosis.

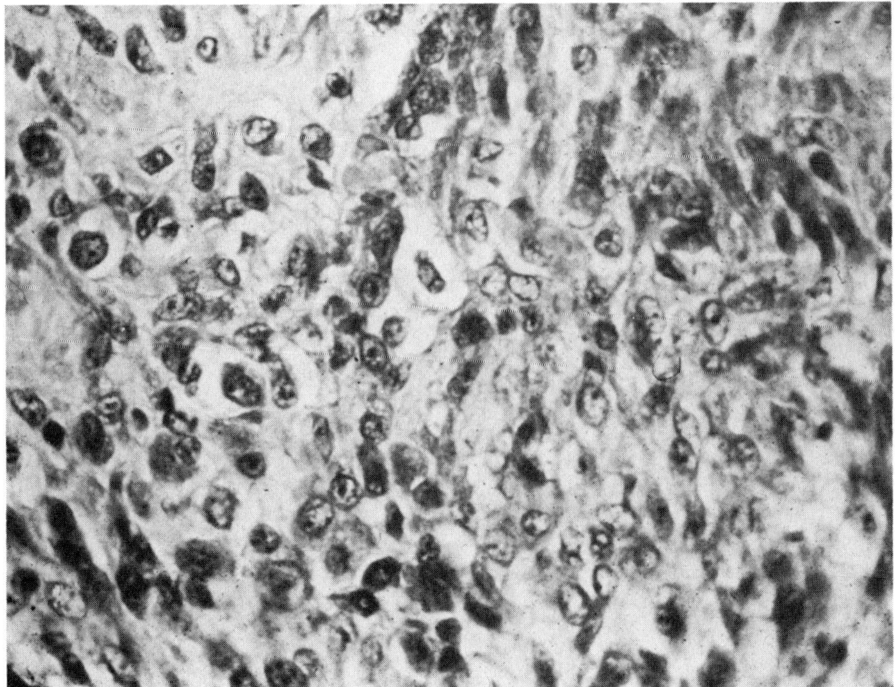

Figure 3–60. Extremely poorly differentiated connective tissue from the center of a myositis ossificans. Such foci are difficult to differentiate from a neoplastic process without a proper history, radiologic correlation, and awareness of the biopsy site.

MATURATION

As the lesion matures, it shrinks in size and the periphery becomes heavier and more developed, as is the case with fracture callus. It develops a "periosteum" that separates it from the surrounding tissue, although muscle fibers are frequently attached to the peripheral portion. The inner central area may become entirely cystic, showing removal of liquefied debris, or may become demarcated as in an infarct and never become replaced. Eventually, the activity subsides and the lesion becomes stable. Once the periosteum develops, it is easier to remove the lesion surgically. Surgical removal of immature lesions is contraindicated because of the high incidence of recurrence, often with involvement of a larger area than that included in the original lesion.

The pattern around the spine is confusing because of the bony projections, tendons, tissue planes, and so forth. Myositis ossificans is misdiagnosed as atypical osteochondroma, aneurysmal bone cyst, and even sarcoma.

The pathologist and clinician have difficulty with the lesion during its earliest stages. Regardless of the undifferentiated nature of the cellular material in the center of the lesion, the peripheral maturation, zoning, and mature bone formation serve to distinguish it from neoplastic processes.

CITED REFERENCES

Brighton, C. T., Black, J., Friedenberg, Z. B., Esterhai, J. L., Day, L. J., and Connolly, J. F.: A multicenter study of the treatment of nonunion with constant direct current. J. Bone Joint Surg. *63A*:2, 1981.

Johnson, L. C.: Morphologic analysis in pathology: the kinetics of disease and general biology of bone. *In* Frost, H. M.: Bone Biodynamics. Boston, Little, Brown and Co., 1964.

Kimmelstiel, P., and Rapp, I.: Cortical defect due to periosteal desmoids. Bull. Hosp. Joint Dis. *12*:286, 1951.

Mirra, J. M.: Bone Tumors, Diagnosis and Treatment. Philadelphia, J. B. Lippincott Company, 1980, pp. 564–566.

Pavlov, H., Nelson, T. L., Warren, R. F., Torg, J. S., and Burstein, A. H.: Stress fractures of the pubic ramus. J. Bone Joint Surg. *64A*:1020, 1982.

Torg, J. S., Pavlov, H., Cooley, L. H., Bryant, M. H., Arnoczky, S. P., Bergfeld, J., and Hunter, L. Y.: Stress fractures of the tarsal navicular. A retrospective review of twenty-one cases. J. Bone Joint Surg. *64A*:700, 1982.

GENERAL REFERENCES

Aergerter, E., and Kirkpatrick, J. A., Jr.: Orthopedic Diseases. 4th ed. Philadelphia, W. B. Saunders Co., 1975.

Heppenstall, R. B.: Fracture Treatment and Healing. Philadelphia, W. B. Saunders Co., 1980.

Jowsey, J.: Metabolic Diseases of Bone. Philadelphia, W. B. Saunders Co., 1977.

4

INFLAMMATION

OSTEOMYELITIS

Inflammation is the protective response that occurs whenever cells or tissues are injured by biological, chemical, or physical agents. It is similar in all mammals and involves a combination of cellular and circulatory reactions, both generalized and local. The purpose of the inflammatory response is to destroy, dilute, or divert the injurious agent and repair the damaged tissue.

The damaged cells or tissues release humoral substances to initiate the inflammatory response. Vascular changes occur and signal a complex, integrated sequence of events. Vasodilation occurs. This increases the rate of blood flow through the arterioles, capillaries, and venules. Capillary permeability is increased with transudation of fluid and plasma proteins into the tissue spaces, producing edema and increased hydrostatic pressure. Capillary dilatation occurs, producing slowing and turbulence of the blood flow. Within the capillaries, red cells aggregate in the axial portion of the stream while white cells orient themselves laterally and stick to the capillary membrane ("pavementing"). Stasis due to the large number of dilated capillaries can lead to complete stagnation with cessation of flow in many vessels or in an entire area.

Cells gradually concentrate in this protein-rich fluid and produce an exudate. White blood cells stick to the vessel walls then creep through the capillary membrane by ameboid movement. Initially, the polymorphonuclear leukocytes constitute most of the white-cell population. They are replaced by mononuclear cells arising from the blood stream, from vessel walls, and possibly from the damaged tissue. The ultimate presence of lymphocytes and plasma cells signifies a more chronic situation and is associated with antibody formation.

The classic clinical signs of inflammation are rubor (redness), calor (heat), tumor (swelling), dolor (pain), and functio laesa (loss of function). The classic signs of inflammation are actually due to vascular changes, including the inhibition of local vasoconstriction; dilatation of arterioles, capillaries, and venules; transudation of fluid; and exudation of cellular debris.

The inflammation can be classified according to (1) duration (acute, subacute, or chronic); (2) the predominant exudate (hemorrhagic, pyogenic, suppurative, or non-suppurative); (3) the location (bone, periosteum, epiphysis, etc.); and (4) etiology (biologic organism, i.e., *Staphylococcus aureus;* radiation, etc.). The inflammatory response in bone is basically similar to that in other tissue. However, there are factors peculiar to bone that alter the course of the inflammatory process.

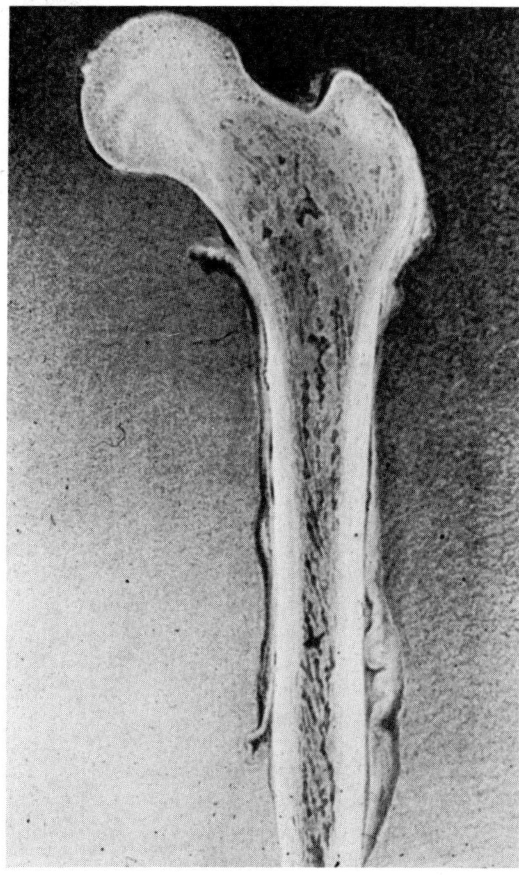

Figure 4–1. Artist's rendition of untreated osteomyelitis, Civil War era. A purulent exudate has filled the medullary cavity of the bone and has penetrated between the cortex and periosteum, elevating the periosteum into irregular folds. Sequestration of the entire cortex will follow.

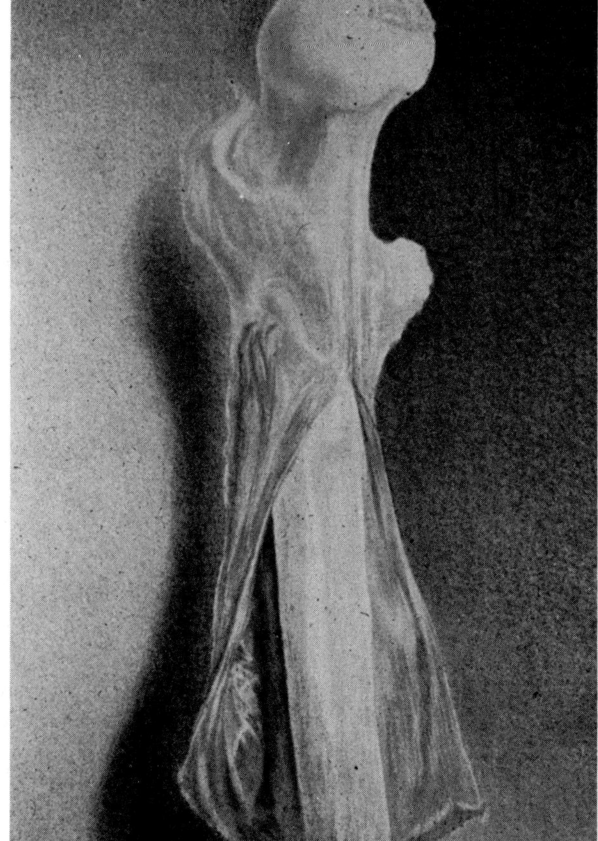

Figure 4–2. Artist's rendition of untreated osteomyelitis, Civil War era. Separation of the periosteum secondary to pyogenic infiltrate penetrating between cortex and periosteum.

Inflammation in bone, as elsewhere, begins by an insult to the tissue followed by the vascular and cellular response. The process is modified by the rigid wall of the bony cortex and by the baffle system created by the cancellous bone. Increased pressure cannot be dissipated into the soft tissue; there is no "tumor."

As a result of increased intramedullary pressure, there is compression of the capillaries and sinusoids in the marrow cavity. This produces infarction of marrow fat, hematopoietic tissue, and bone. At the margin of the area of infarction, there is active hyperemia, just as in any other soft tissue infarct. Increased hyperemia is accompanied by osteoclastic activity, which results in removal of bone and localized osteoporosis. The inflammatory exudate will form at the margin of the infarct.

The inflammatory process penetrates through the cortex into the subperiosteal area via Volkmann's and perforating canals. In infants and other children the periosteum has very few Sharpey's fibers, and it is readily stripped from the bone surface by the increased pressure in the subperiosteal space. This results in disruption of the periosteal contribution to the blood supply of the cortex. Inasmuch as the medullary cavity is already infarcted, the subperiosteal infiltration, stripping, and removal of blood supply will result in infarction of the cortex (Figs. 4–1 to 4–3).

These cortical infarcts result in the formation of the classic sequestrum. Small sequestra can be removed by osteoclasts when vascularization is restored. However, large sequestra cannot be removed by osteoclasts. Reactive bone, the involucrum, will be formed by the periosteum surrounding the sequestered bone. The sequestrum or any other piece of infarcted bone will retain its original radiographic density until revascularization occurs and osteoclastic activity can begin. Because the infarcted sequestrum is composed of osteonal bone it will retain the original radiographic density; the involucrum is composed of more rapidly formed woven bone and is therefore less dense radiographically; there is thus a radiographic contrast between dense infarcted sequestrum and less dense viable imvolucrum (Fig. 4–4).

Radiographically, the earliest changes do not appear for 10 to 14 days after the onset of symptoms, long after infarction of large sections of bone may have occurred. Initial changes consist of localized bone removal, osteoporosis, a spotty or permeative destructive pattern within the medullary cavity, and occasionally the first attempts at periosteal repair (Figs. 4–6 to 4–8). Radioisotopic scanning with gallium or technetium will be positive before radiographic changes occur (Waldvogel and Vasey, 1980).

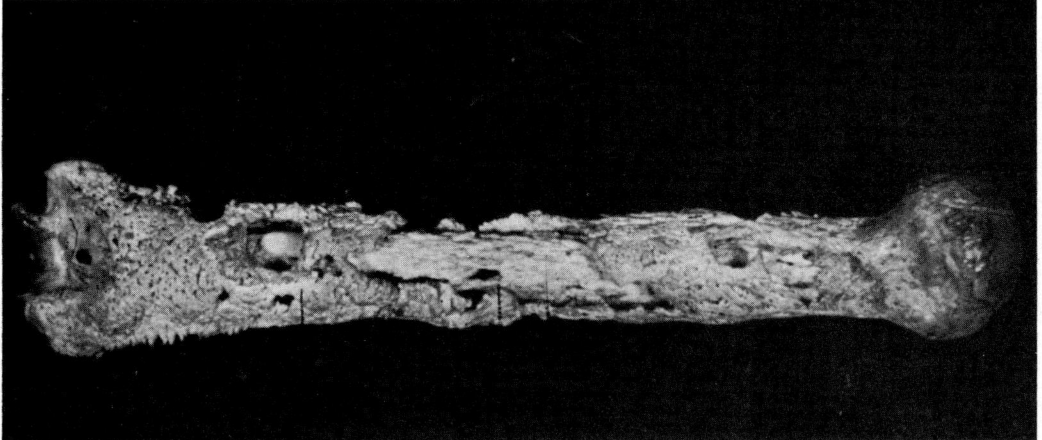

Figure 4–3. Amputation specimen of right humerus showing untreated osteomyelitis, Civil War era. The specimen was obtained 1½ years after injury. Amputation was performed at the shoulder joint after contusion by a conoidal ball. The entire shaft is necrotic and surrounded by a partial involucrum. The patient was wounded at Kane's River, LA, April 27, 1864; amputation was performed Nov. 10, 1865. The sequestered cortex is readily visible, surrounded by periosteal reaction (involucrum). The openings in the sequestra and involucra are termed "cloacae."

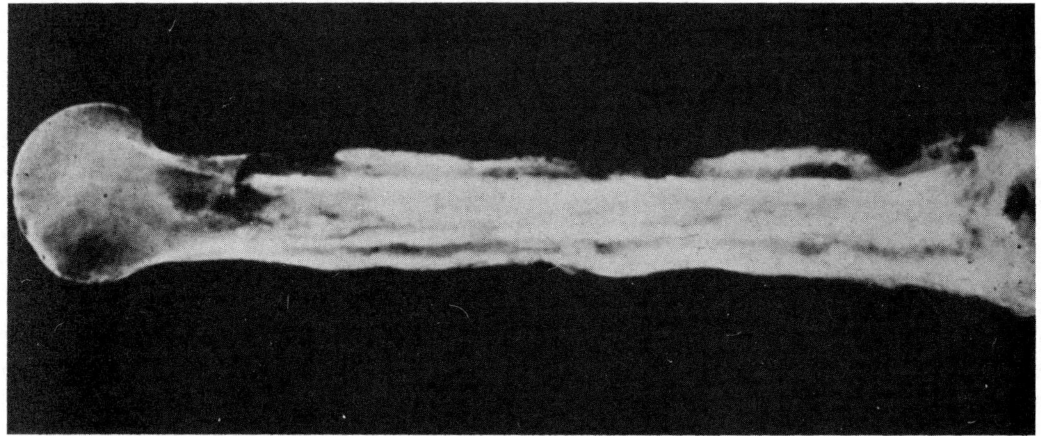

Figure 4–4. Specimen radiograph exhibiting sequestra (original dense cortex), involucrum (bone encircling sequestra), and several gaps in the involucrum (cloaca).

Histologically, acute osteomyelitis will exhibit the features usually associated with acute inflammation. There will be a loss of the normal hematopoietic marrow and fat. The leukocytic infiltrate will vary with the type of inflammation, but polymorphonuclear leukocytes are usually found (Figs. 4–12 to 4–17). A fibrous wall will be created to sequester the infarcted area or the abscess cavity. An inflammatory infiltrate of chronic nature will surround the infarcted area after it has been demarcated. The cavity may retain viable organisms for years.

Text continued on page 122

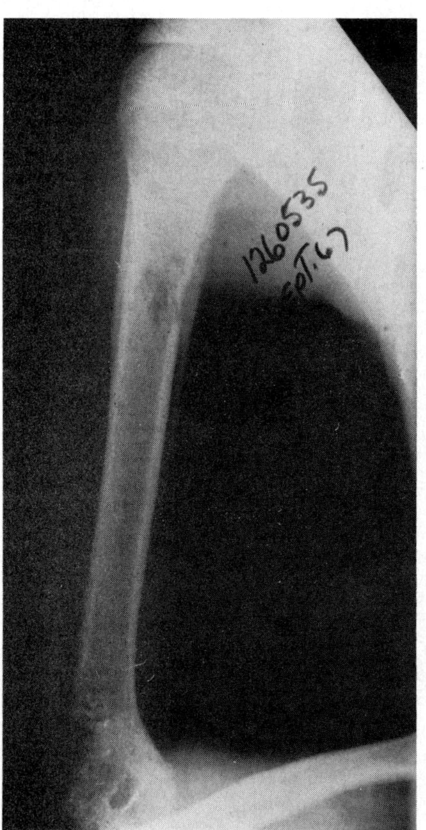

Figure 4–5. Radiograph of chronic osteomyelitis of humerus exhibiting a medially located cortical sequestrum, periosteal involucrum, and cloacae. Note the relative densities of the cortical sequestrum and periosteal involucrum.

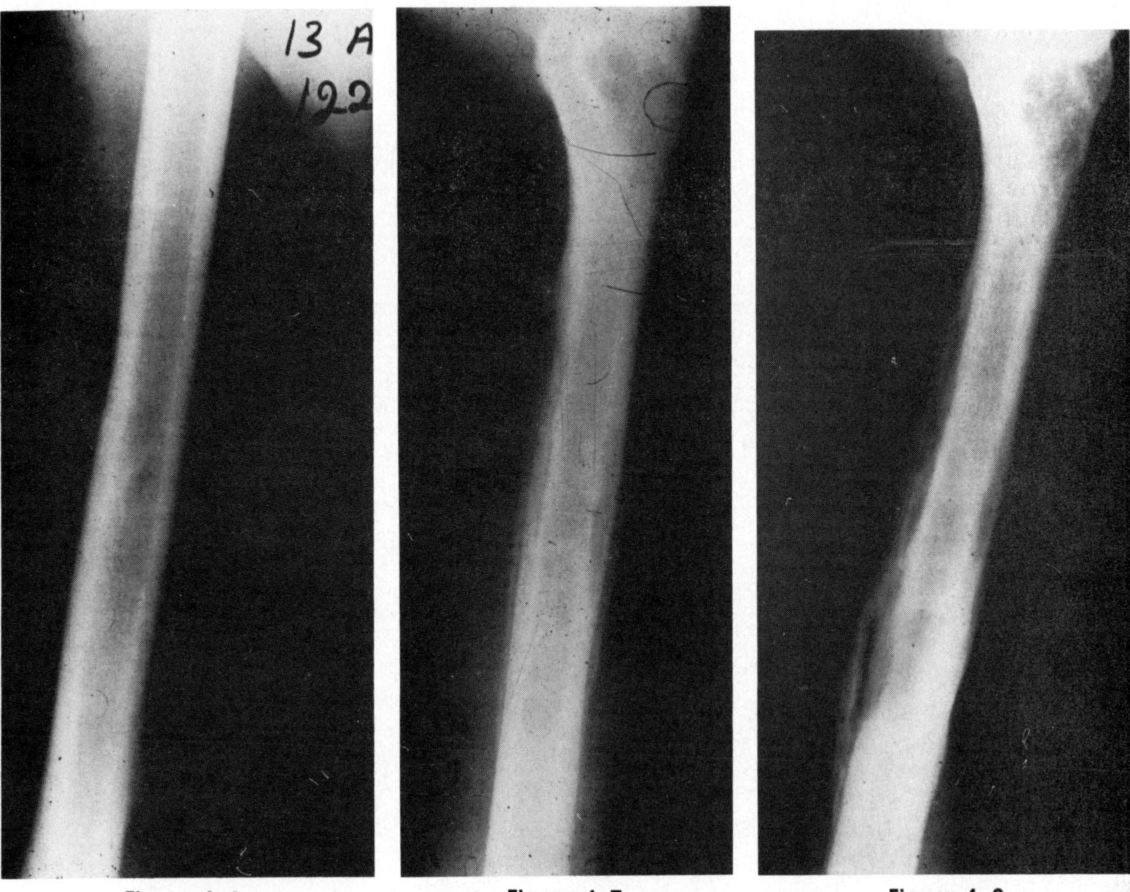

Figure 4–6   Figure 4–7   Figure 4–8

Figure 4–6. Radiograph of humerus showing osteomyelitis at time of earliest presentation. There is permeative destruction, but no evidence of periosteal reaction, and the limits of the lesion are undefinable. The early lesion of osteomyelitis is difficult to differentiate from a malignant neoplasm.

Figure 4–7. Same humerus as that illustrated in Figure 4–6, approximately 4 weeks later. There is more extensive destruction of cortex on both sides and an early but readily defined periosteal reaction. Even at this stage, the apparent rapidly progressive destructive lesion would be difficult to differentiate from a rapidly progressive malignant neoplasm.

Figure 4–8. Same humerus as that shown in Figures 4–6 and 4–7, 4 months after initial radiograph. The lesion exhibits more sharply defined geographic destruction of medullary cavity as well as cortex. The periosteal reaction has begun to fill in (inlay bone), and there appears to be no recent periosteal reaction. These radiographic features support the diagnosis of a benign reactive inflammatory process rather than a neoplasm.

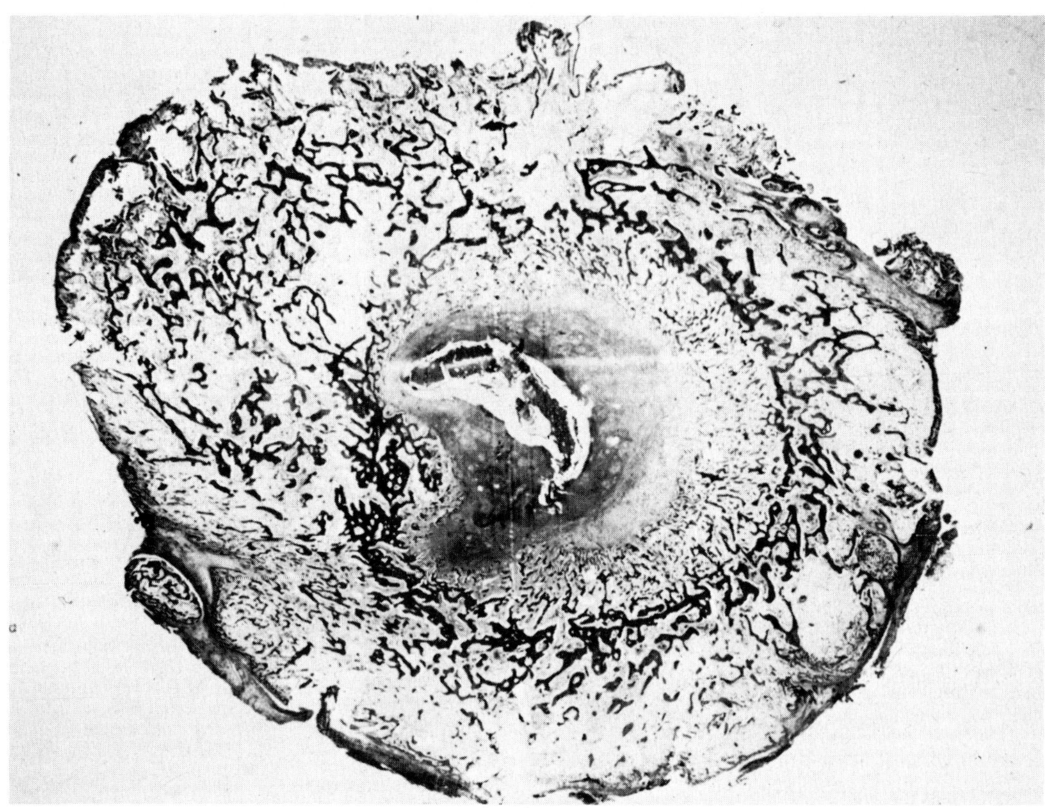

Figure 4–9. Cross section of the infected bone exhibiting centrally located sequestrum surrounded by involucrum and cloaca. Notice successive waves of periosteal reaction.

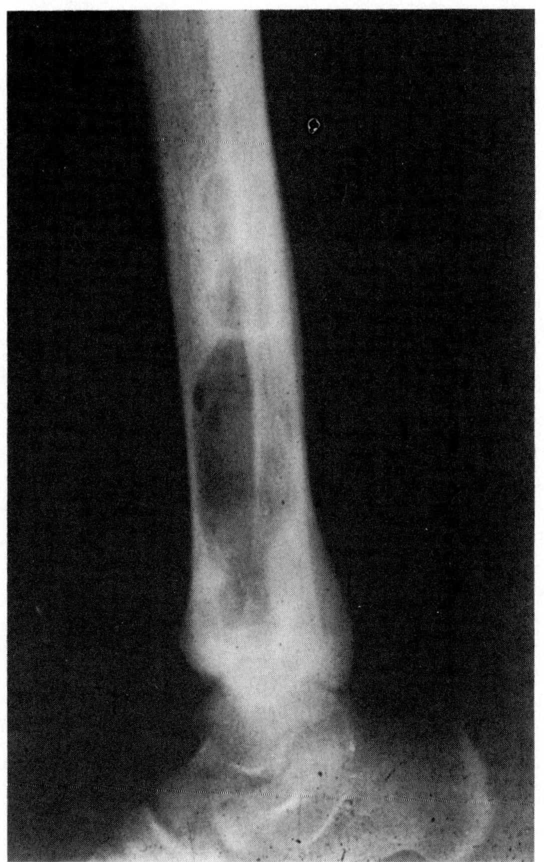

Figure 4–10. Radiograph of sharply circumscribed osteomyelitis in lower tibia with sclerotic margin.

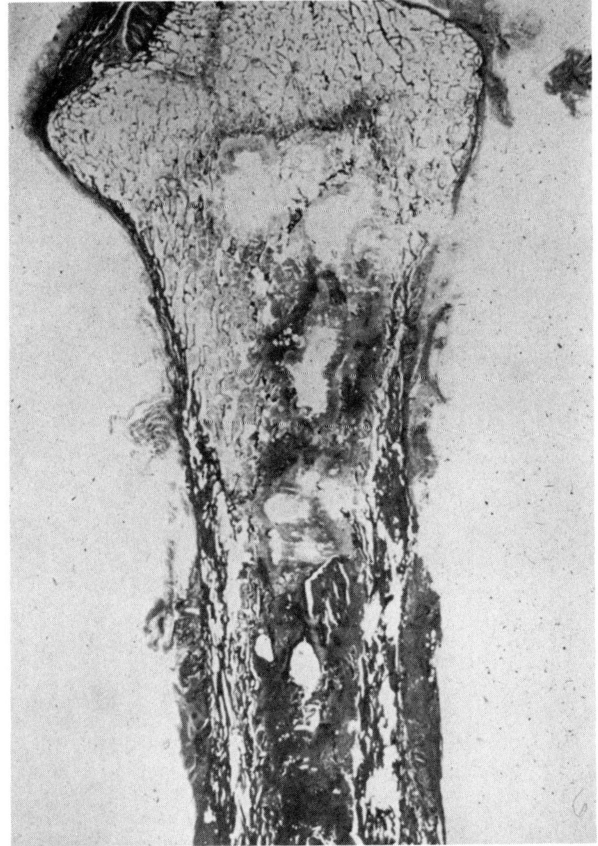

Figure 4–11. Macrospecimen exhibiting irregularly shaped central abscess cavities with some sclerosis at margin, inflammatory exudate, cortical resorption, and periosteal new bone formation.

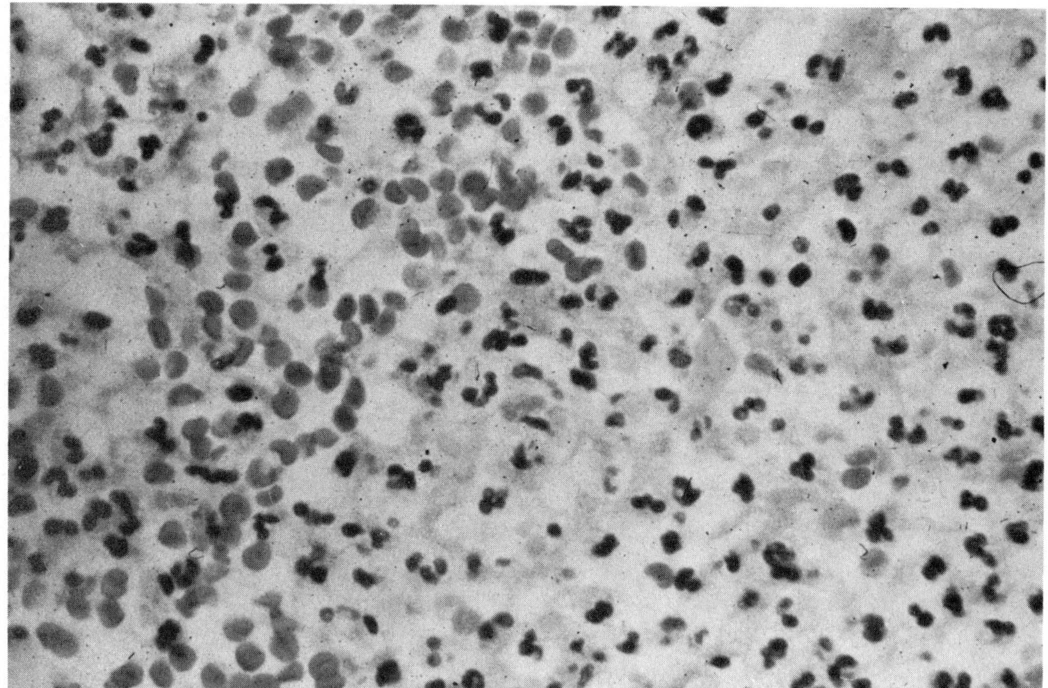

Figure 4–12. Acute inflammatory infiltrate with granulocytes and red cells.

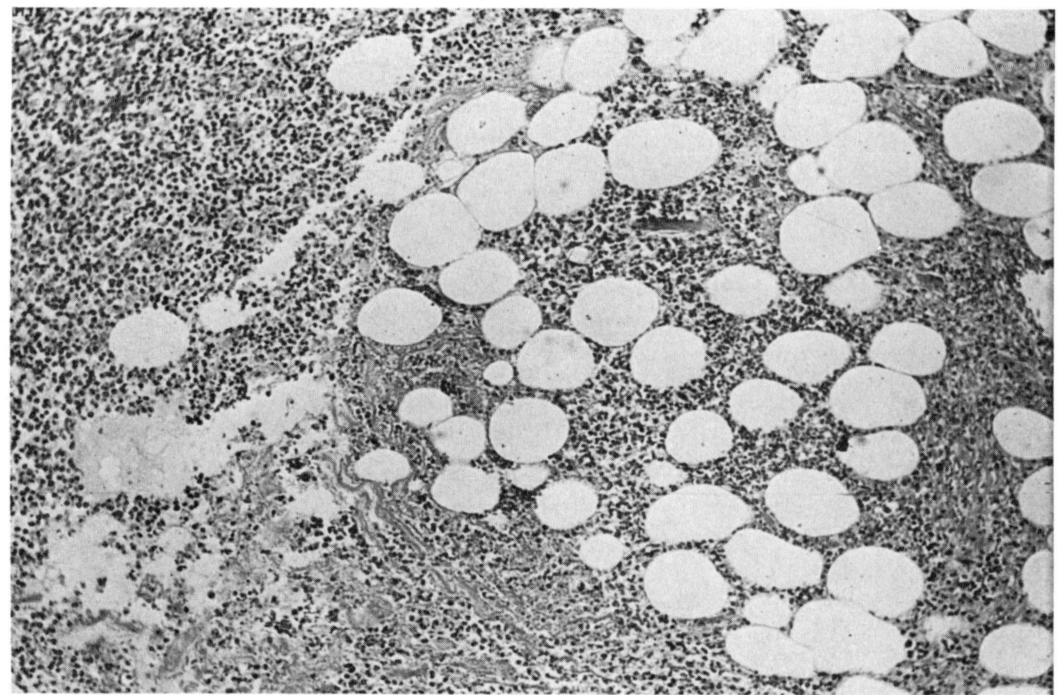

Figure 4–13. Fat necrosis in response to osteomyelitis. Normal fatty and hematopoietic elements on the right side are being infiltrated by inflammatory exudate from the left. Liquefaction of fat on the left is seen as amorphous liquid debris. Hematopoietic elements also undergo infarction and liquefactive necrosis.

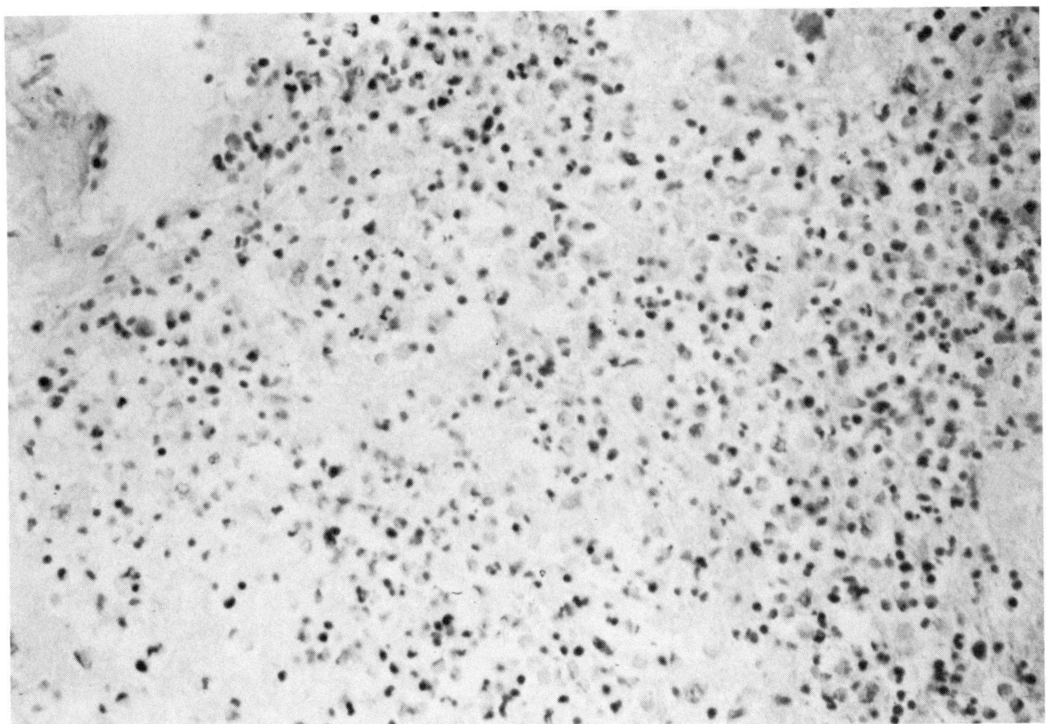

Figure 4–14. Chronic inflammatory exudate with lymphocytes, plasma cells, mononuclear macrophages, and protein-rich fluid.

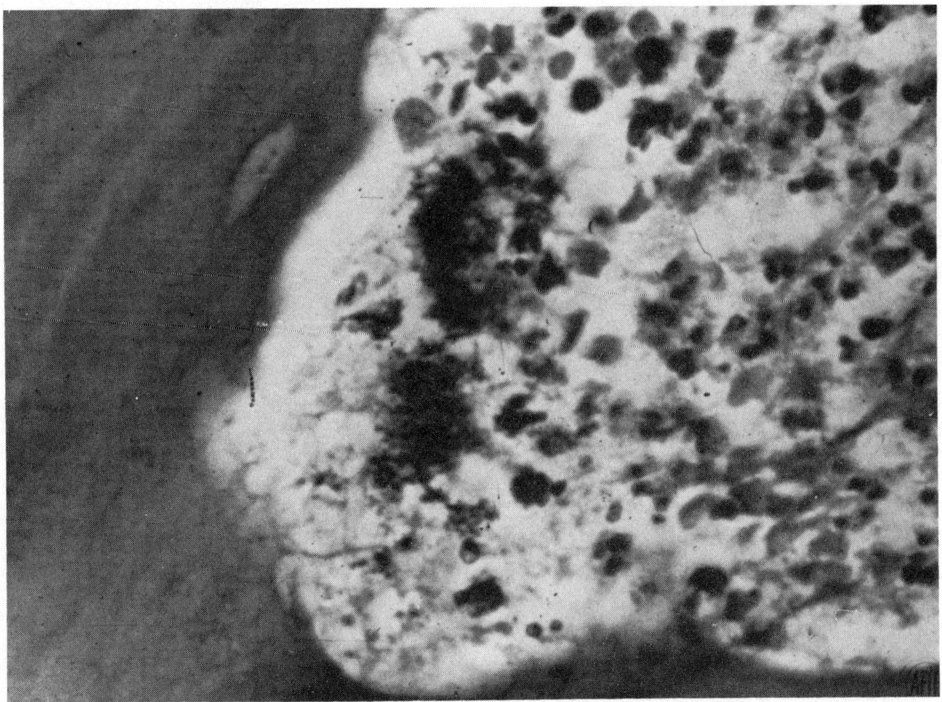

Figure 4–15. Clumps of bacteria within bone accompanied by a granulocytic infiltrate.

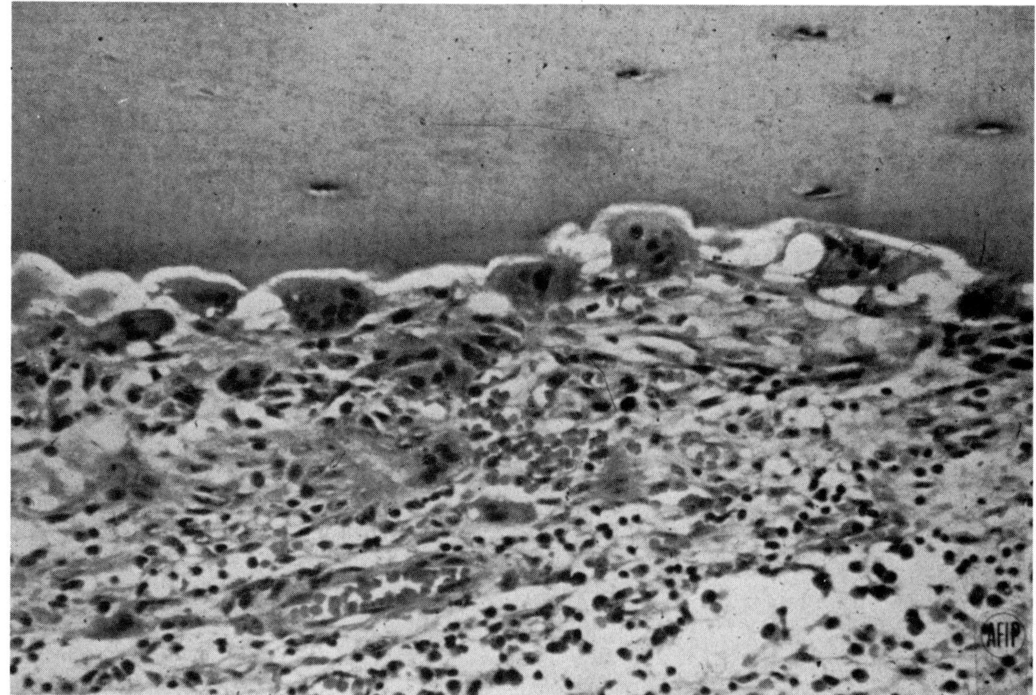

Figure 4–16. Osteoclastic resorption of bone in response to inflammation. The extensive lytic destruction of bone accompanying the osteomyelitis is a result of the stimulation of osteoclasts, and a row of such cells is illustrated removing bone adjacent to the inflammatory infiltrate.

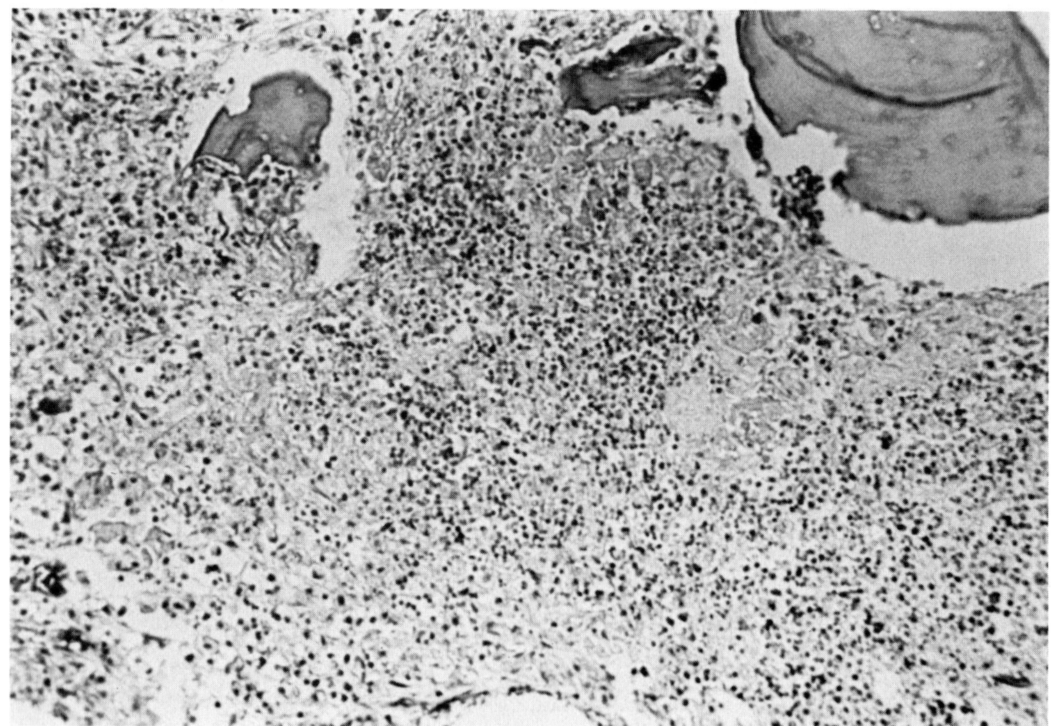

Figure 4–17. Chronic inflammatory exudate and microsequestra of trabecular bone.

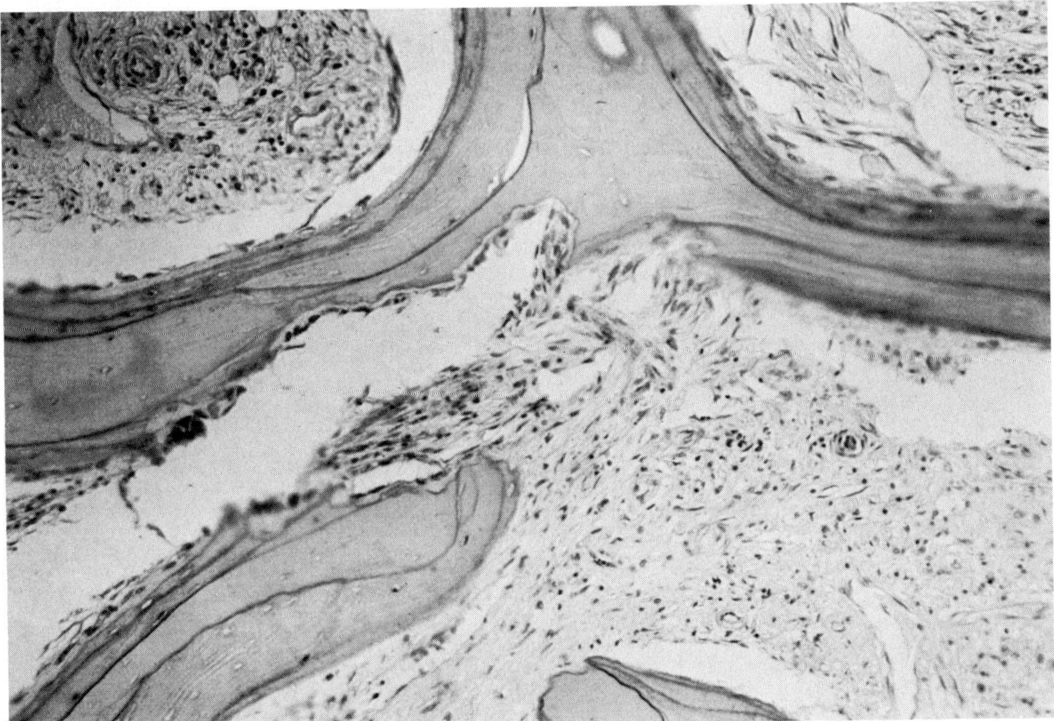

Figure 4–18. Sequestered fragment of bone in the midst of the inflammatory infiltrate. The normal marrow has been replaced by an inflammatory exudate rich in cells; the bone fragment is infarcted. Note empty lacunar spaces as well as the widened lacunar spaces. These widened spaces support the concept of osteoclastic activity by osteocytes under appropriate circumstances.

Figure 4–19. Healing osteomyelitis. Granulation tissue replaces exudate, portions of sequestrum are removed by osteoclasts, and other portions are enclosed in a "cocoon" of viable bone without waiting for removal.

The goals of therapy should be to reduce the intraosseous pressure and to prevent infarction. In principle, this is accomplished by establishing drainage and applying specific therapy against the etiologic agent. Antibiotics have limited effectiveness against bacteria harbored in either abscess cavity or infarcted tissue, and despite vigorous antibiotic therapy, recurrent infections, particularly with *Staphylococcus aureus*, are extremely common.

The scar tissue of bone is bone. Ultimately, as an osteomyelitis heals, the fibrous connective tissue is replaced by dense bone. This bone produces a mosaic pattern that may be similar to that seen in Paget's disease. The disease process may be chronic from the beginning, with sharply localized reaction to the inflammatory stimulus and without the usual abscess formation. In such instances, the only findings consist of densely scarred bone, with few clinical symptoms. The condition has been termed "chronic sclerosing osteomyelitis of Garré" (Fig. 4–22).

Osteomyelitis may also be sharply limited to one site with the formation of an abscess surrounded by sclerotic bone. The resultant Brodie's abscess may be present for extensive periods before being discovered but it usually produces pain. It must be differentiated from an osteoid osteoma; Brodie's abscess is usually larger. Brodie's abscess is usually seen in cancellous bone, and the sclerotic rim represents reinforcement of pre-existing trabeculae. The cavity contains necrotic debris, and organisms can be cultured. Granulocytes are usually present (Figs. 4–24 to 4–26). The osteoid osteoma, however, is less than 1.0 cm in diameter and contains osteoid resembling neoplastic material. The cavity is invariably sterile.

Cystic osteomyelitis is a recent addition to the spectrum of inflammatory manifestations of bone, and it probably represents an inflammatory process that aborted early, possibly through inhibition of the infectious agent by partial inadequate antibiotic therapy. The lesion manifests as a cystic cavity, usually an incidental

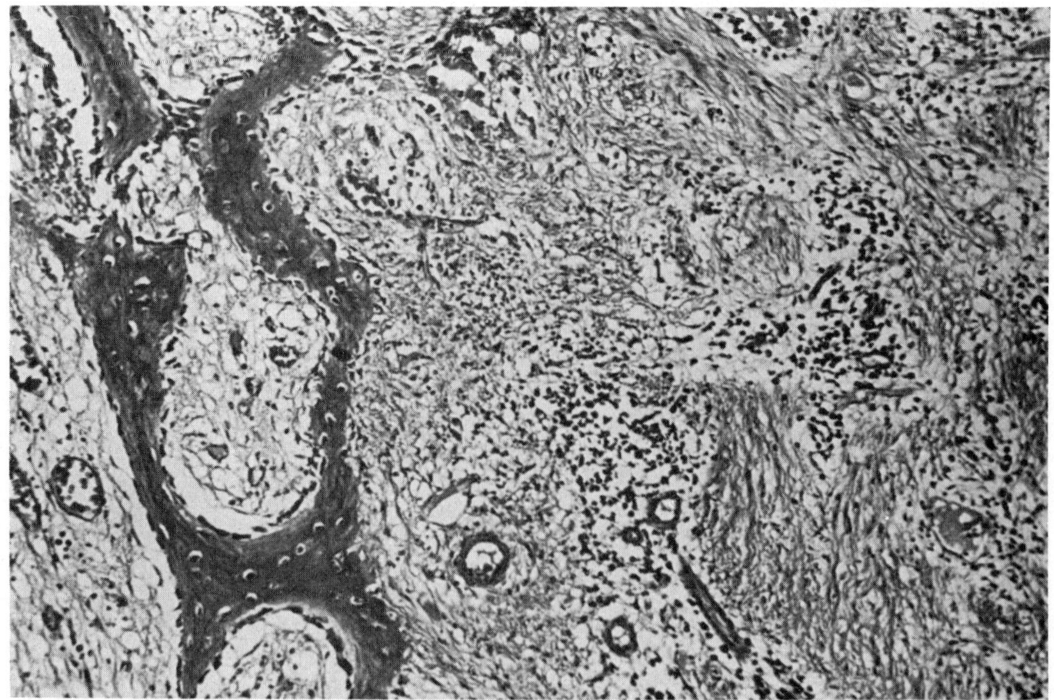

Figure 4–20. Chronic inflammatory response with fibrous scar tissue replacing exudate and bone developing at periphery of osteomyelitic focus. Fibrous abscess wall is being replaced by a bony wall.

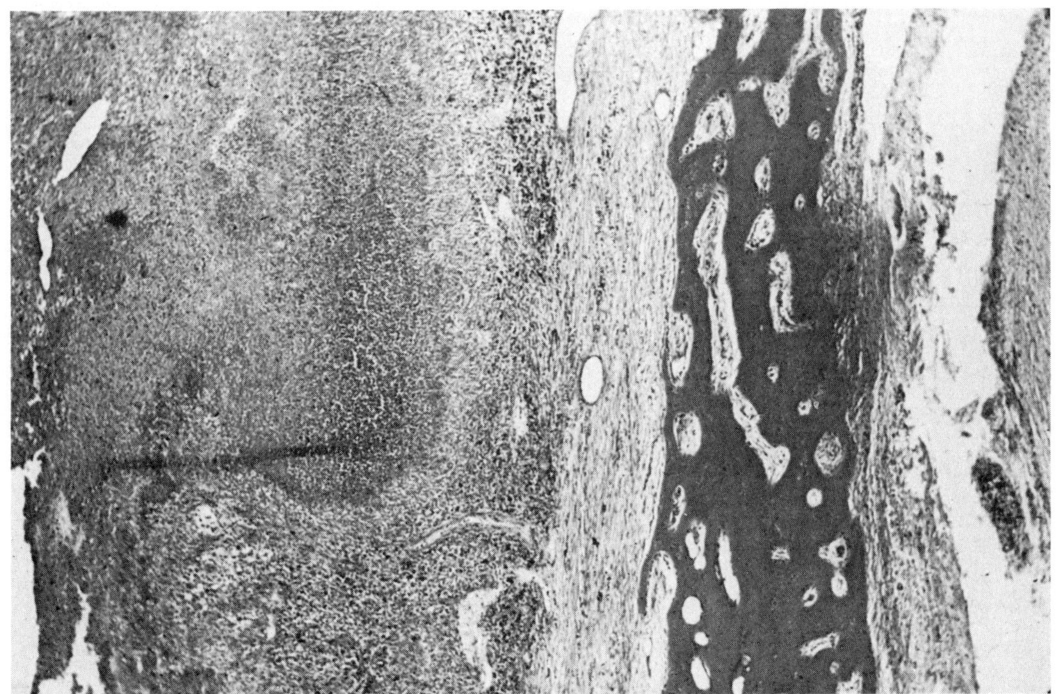

Figure 4–21. Abscess being walled off by reactive sclerotic bone at margin. This is visible radiographically as a sclerotic border around a central lytic lesion.

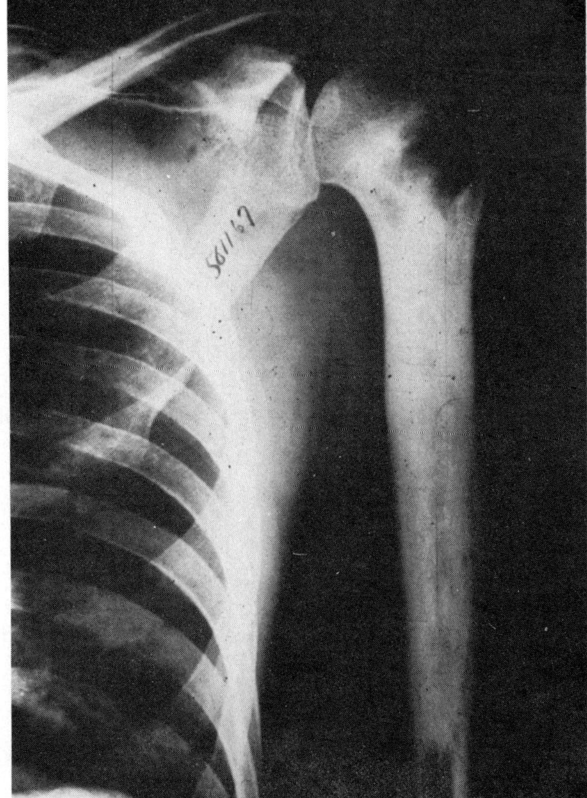

Figure 4–22. Radiograph of sclerosing osteomyelitis of Garré. The lesion simply exhibits sclerosing bone in response to the inflammatory stimulus, rather than the typical abscess. Usually, the stimulus is of lower intensity and promotes more reaction than destruction.

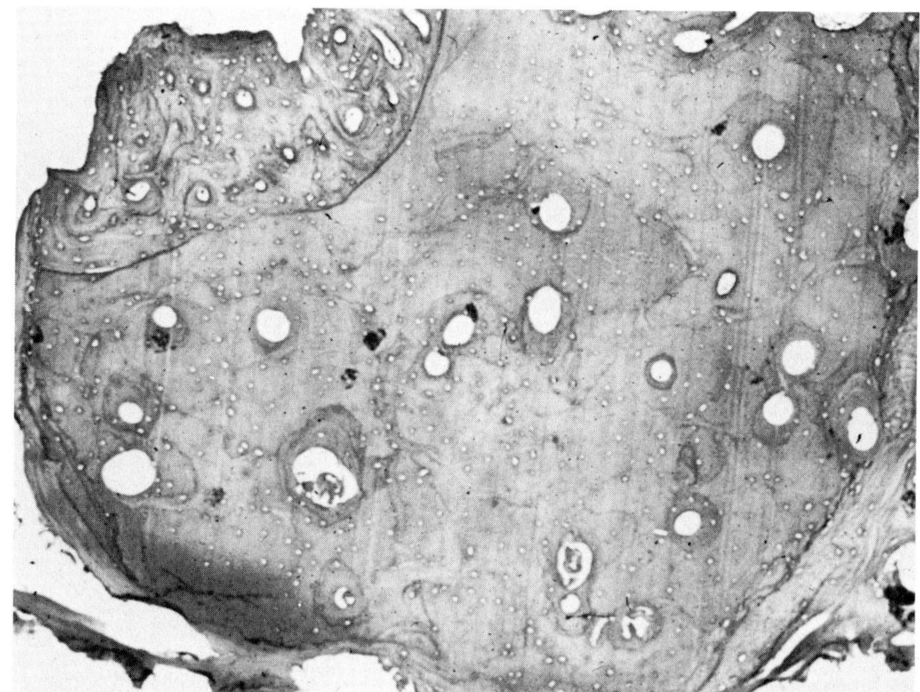

Figure 4–23. Histologic macrosection through area of sclerosing osteomyelitis exhibiting normal bone formation.

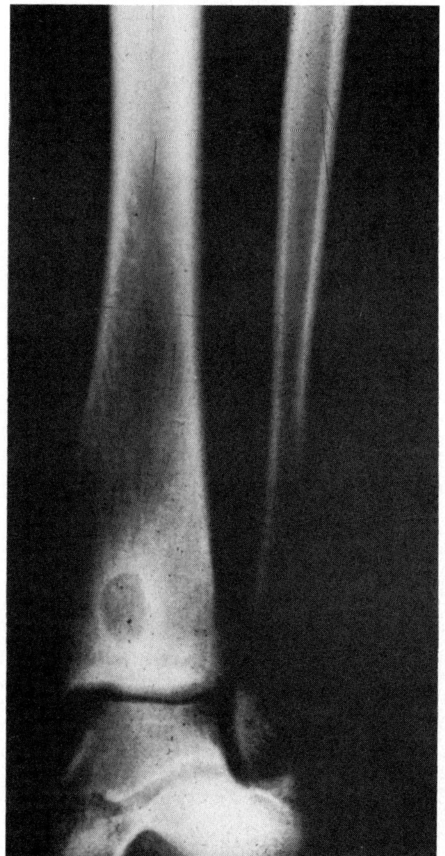

Figure 4–24. Radiograph of Brodie's abscess. The lesion is sharply circumscribed by a sclerotic rim.

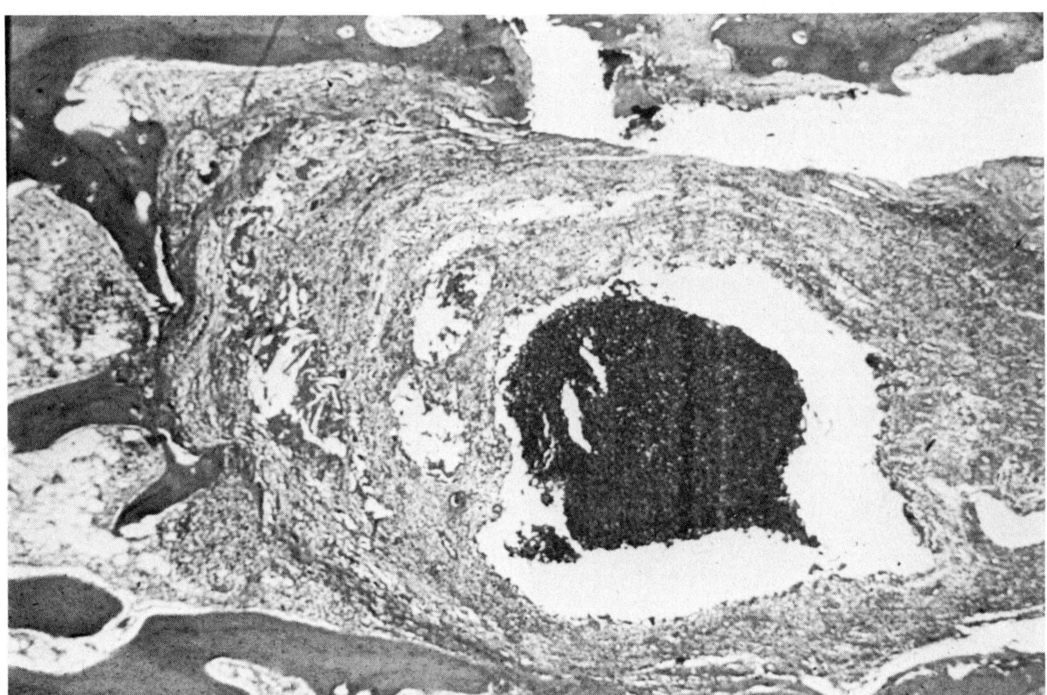

Figure 4–25. Histologic study of Brodie's abscess exhibiting sclerotic rim of bone. There is appositional new bone formation on existing lamellar bone, and the center of the cavity contains an inflammatory infiltrate.

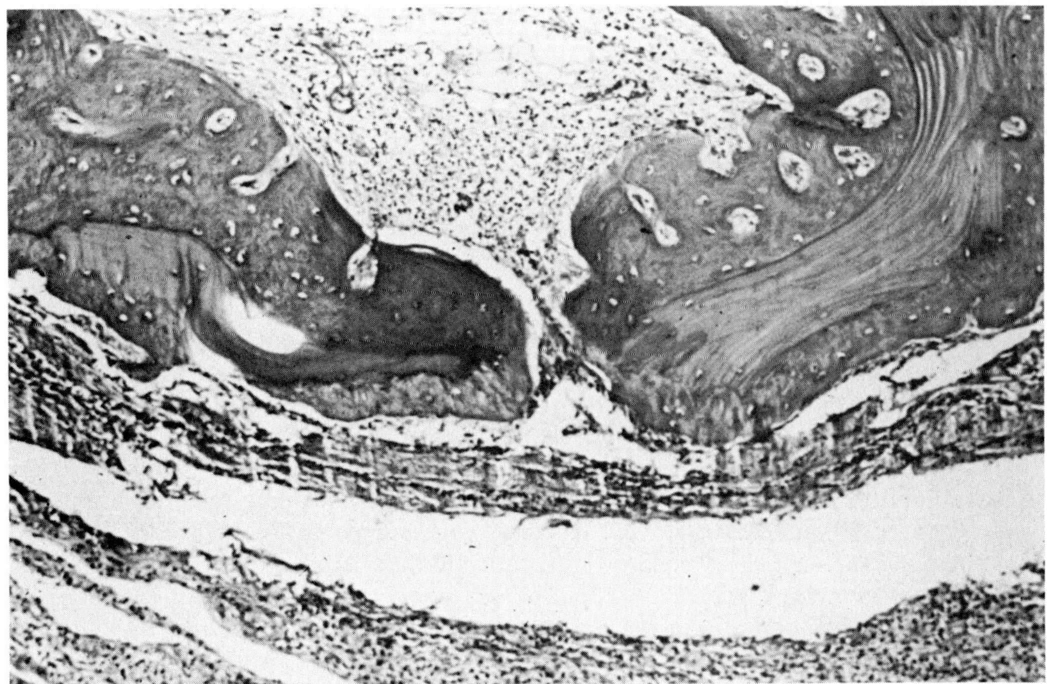

Figure 4–26. Histologic study of Brodie's abscess showing centrally located necrotic debris surrounded by connective tissue and granulocytic infiltrate, which are in turn surrounded by sclerotic bone.

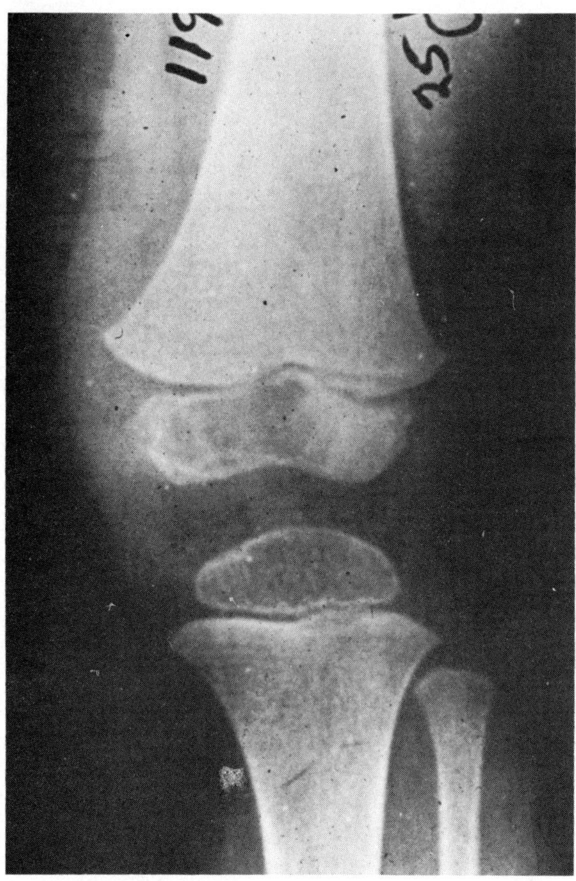

Figure 4–27. Radiograph of cystic osteo-myelitis. The lesion is sharply circumscribed and lytic, and usually contains clear fluid. It differs from the unicameral bone cyst by location as well as the sparse but readily identifiable granulocytes found within the cavity. It is postulated that this type of lesion represents an aborted osteomyelitis.

finding. Biopsy reveals a fluid-filled cavity, and only the occasional granulocyte serves to differentiate the lesion from the common unicameral bone cyst. As opposed to the unicameral bone cyst, however, cystic osteomyelitis occurs at various sites, often within the epiphysis (Fig. 4–27).

SALMONELLA OSTEOMYELITIS

Osteomyelitis usually begins as a result of hematogenous spread of organisms commonly present in children. Osteomyelitis is most often produced by *Staphylococcus* and only occasionally by *Streptococcus, Hemophilus,* or other organisms (Waldvogel and Vasey, 1980). Unusual organisms are less common causes (Case Records of the Massachusetts General Hospital, 1971). Most, but by no means all, cases of osteomyelitis in which *Salmonella* is the etiologic agent have been reported in black children with hemoglobinopathy. The exact mechanism is not clear. Sickling produces sludging or thrombosis of marrow sinusoids with actual infarction. For some unknown reason, salmonellae have a predilection for bone marrow in these individuals. The so-called "hand-foot syndrome" consists of infarcts of small bones of the hands and feet followed by osteomyelitis with *Salmonella* as the inciting organism (Fig. 4–28).

Some salmonellae inhibit systemic granulocytic response, producing leukopenia combined with a pronounced plasma-cell and lymphocyte response. The resulting plasma-cell osteomyelitis should not be confused with multiple myeloma.

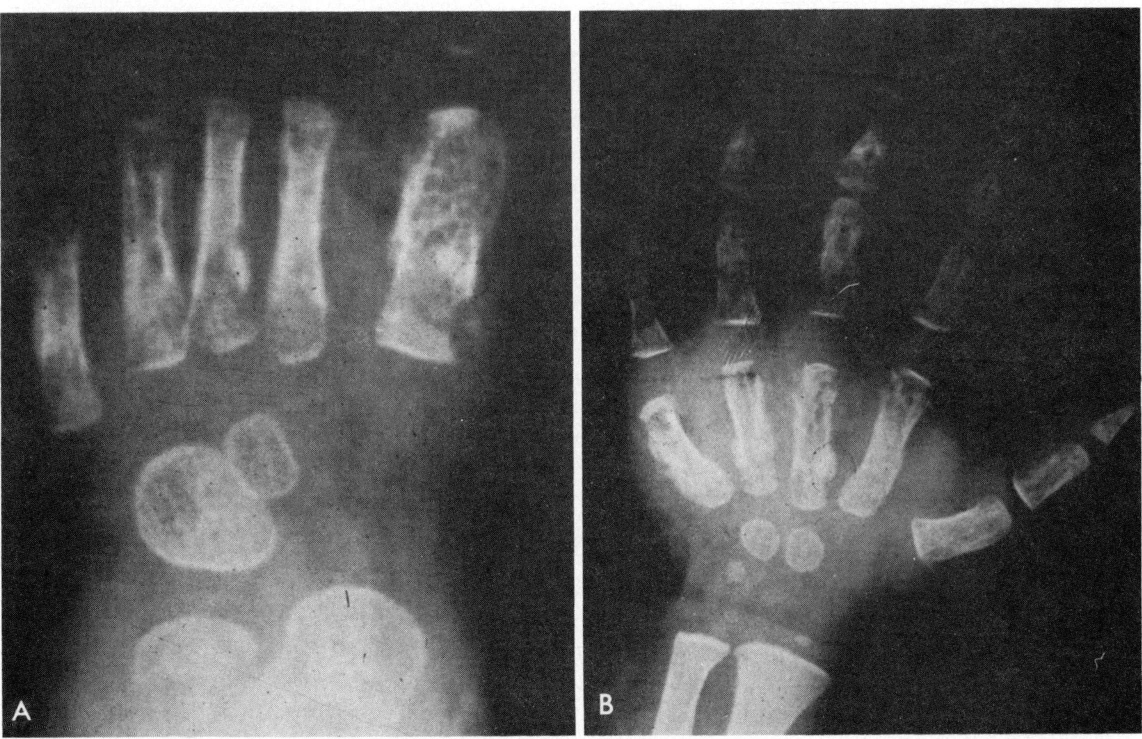

Figure 4–28. Radiographs illustrating hand-foot syndrome, exhibiting numerous areas of circumscribed lytic destruction and reactive bone formation in the small bones of the hands and feet.

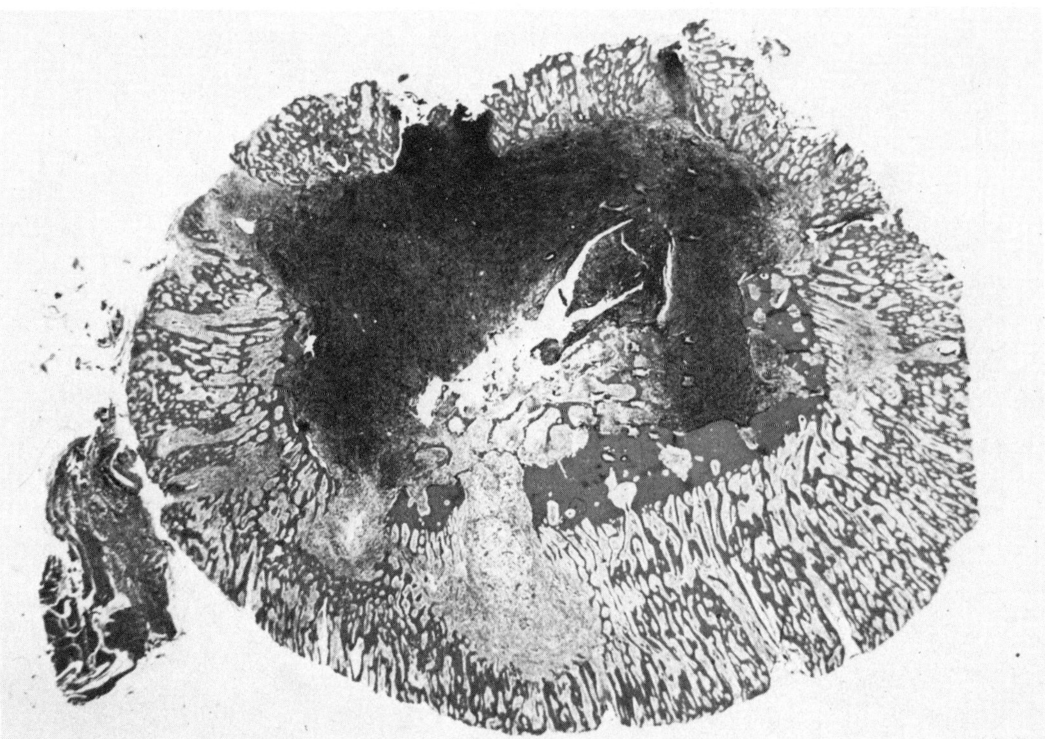

Figure 4–29. Macrosection showing congenital syphilis. Notice the major destruction of the cortex, the extensive periosteal reaction, and the replacement of cortex by extensive gumma formation. There is also an inflammatory process replacing portions of the periosteal new bone formation.

SYPHILIS

The incidence of syphilis has decreased steadily since the early twentieth century, and the disease no longer poses the public health hazard of previous times. The use of penicillin usually results in early arrest of the process, so the tertiary manifestations in bone are rarely encountered. The term "great masquerader," used because of the great variety of manifestations in multiple systems, is no longer applicable to this disease.

The causative organism of syphilis is *Treponema pallidum*. It is characterized by regularity and closeness of corkscrew-like spirals. The organism is found in early lesions but is rarely seen in late lesions, except tabes dorsalis. The basic lesion of syphilis is an angiitis of vasa vasorum, or small arterioles. The endarteritis produces necrosis of the vessel wall, with subsequent infarction of the tissue supplied by the vessel. The result is a gumma, which consists of areas of coagulation necrosis surrounded by an infiltrate of plasma cells and leukocytes (Fig. 4–30). The plasma cells are specifically located in the area adjacent to small arterial vessels (Figs. 4–31 and 4–32).

Congenital syphilis is due to spirochetemia in the mother. It results in intrauterine infection during the fifth or sixth month of pregnancy. The spirochete lodges beneath the fetal growth plates and produces a metaphysitis in which the normal vascular fountain underneath the cartilage is replaced by a syphilitic granulation. This granulation tissue interferes with bone formation and remodeling so that the bone in the zone of primary trabeculae is decreased or absent. It results in a lucent line on radiographs and weakness of bone with resultant lateral slippage through the metaphyseal zone of improper bone formation (Figs. 4–33 to 4–36).

Text continued on page 134

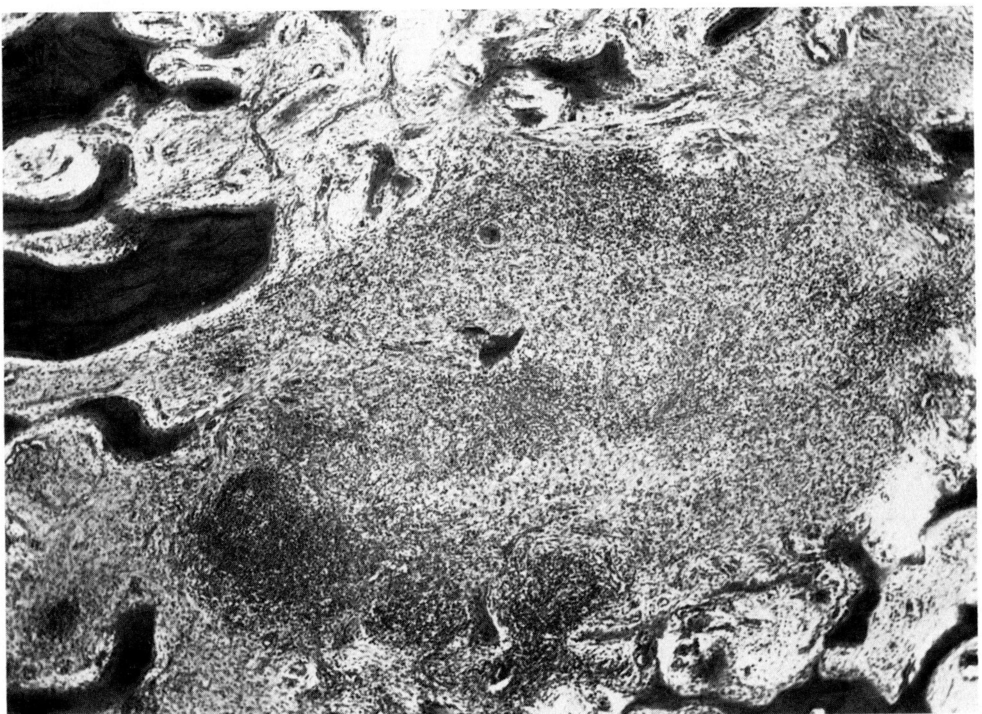

Figure 4–30. Gumma formation within the area of periostitis. The gumma is an inflammatory focus, sharply circumscribed, usually with coagulation necrosis secondary to infarction of tissue. The gumma is caused by both perivascular inflammation and vasculitis.

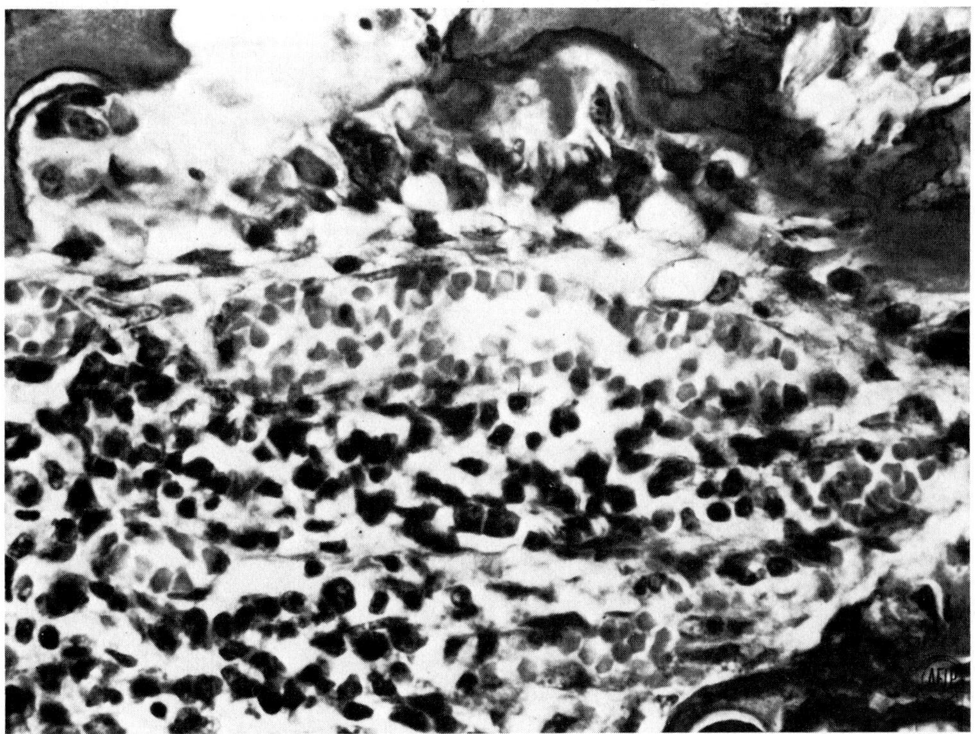

Figure 4–31. Perivascular plasma cell infiltrate, characteristic of syphilitic periostitis.

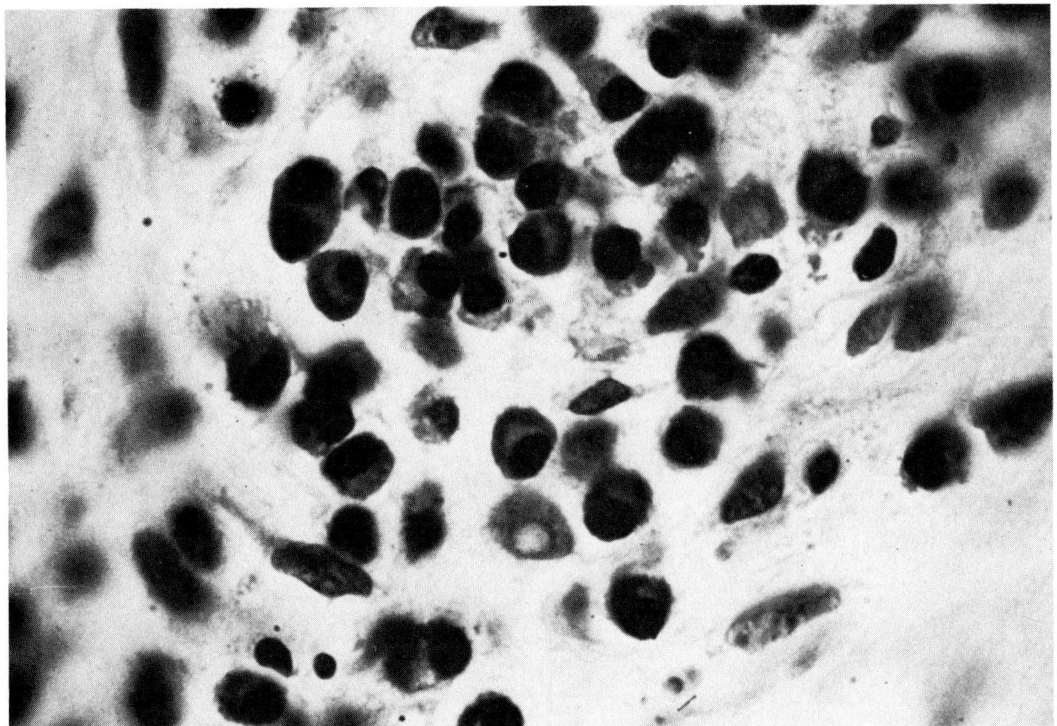

Figure 4–32. Higher magnification of plasma cells composing the inflammatory infiltrate.

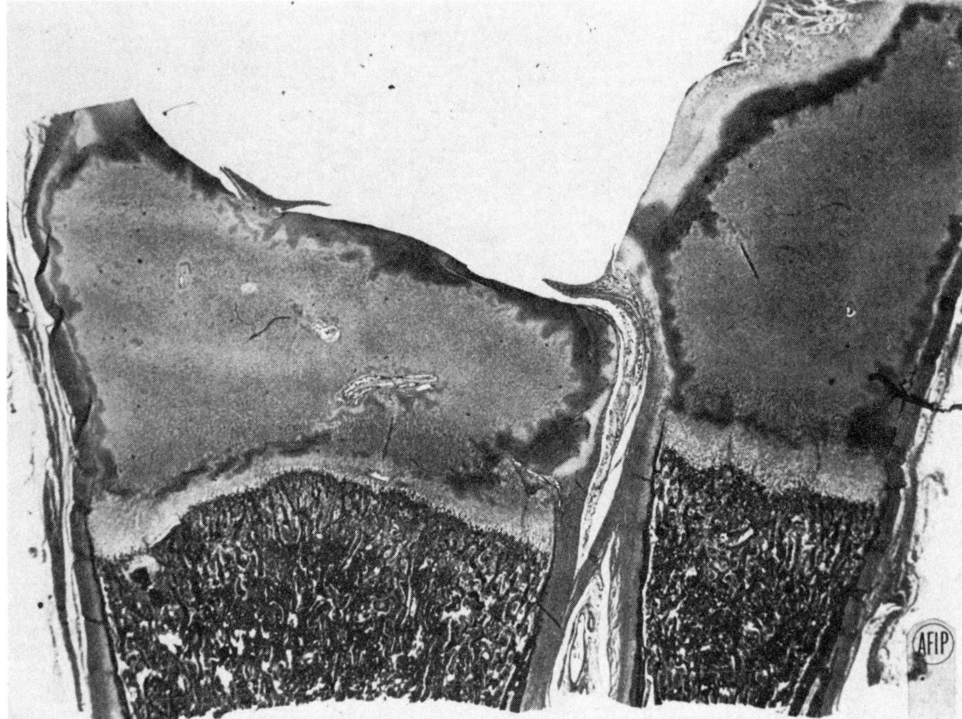

Figure 4–33. Congenital syphilis with granulation tissue at the site of new bone formation in the metaphysis. The vascular spindle that invades the cartilage columns is usually involved in the inflammatory process, leading to interference with normal cartilage removal and primary trabeculae formation.

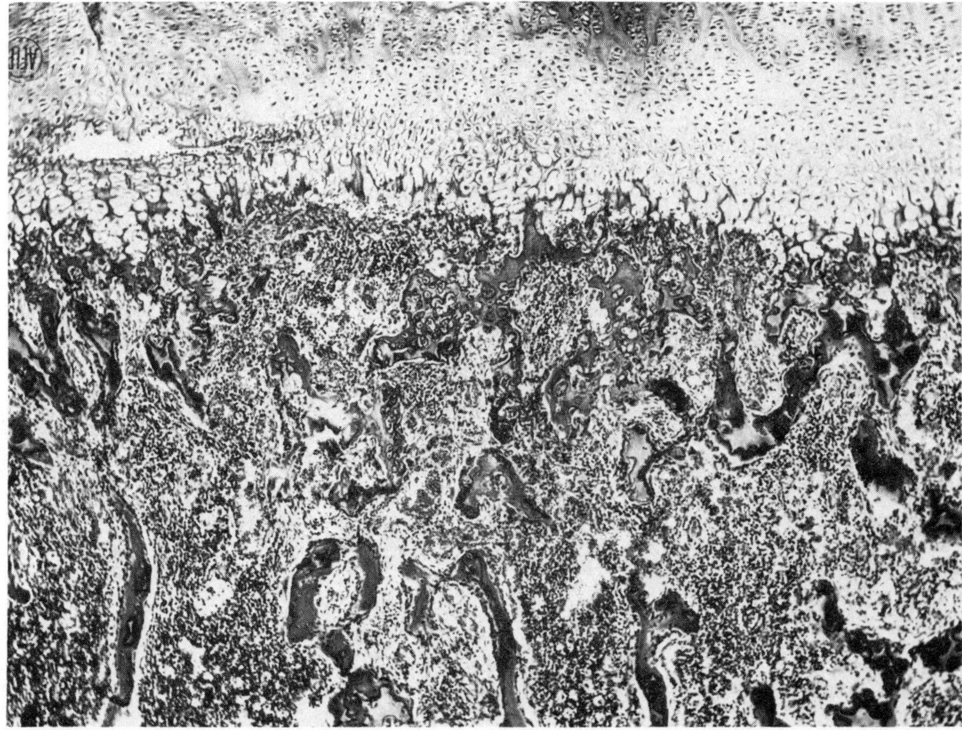

Figure 4–34. Syphilitic metaphysitis. Higher magnification of syphilitic inflammation at the growth plate. Notice normal cartilage with disruption of osteoid formation. Infected granulation tissue has replaced the normal vascular bed in the metaphysis.

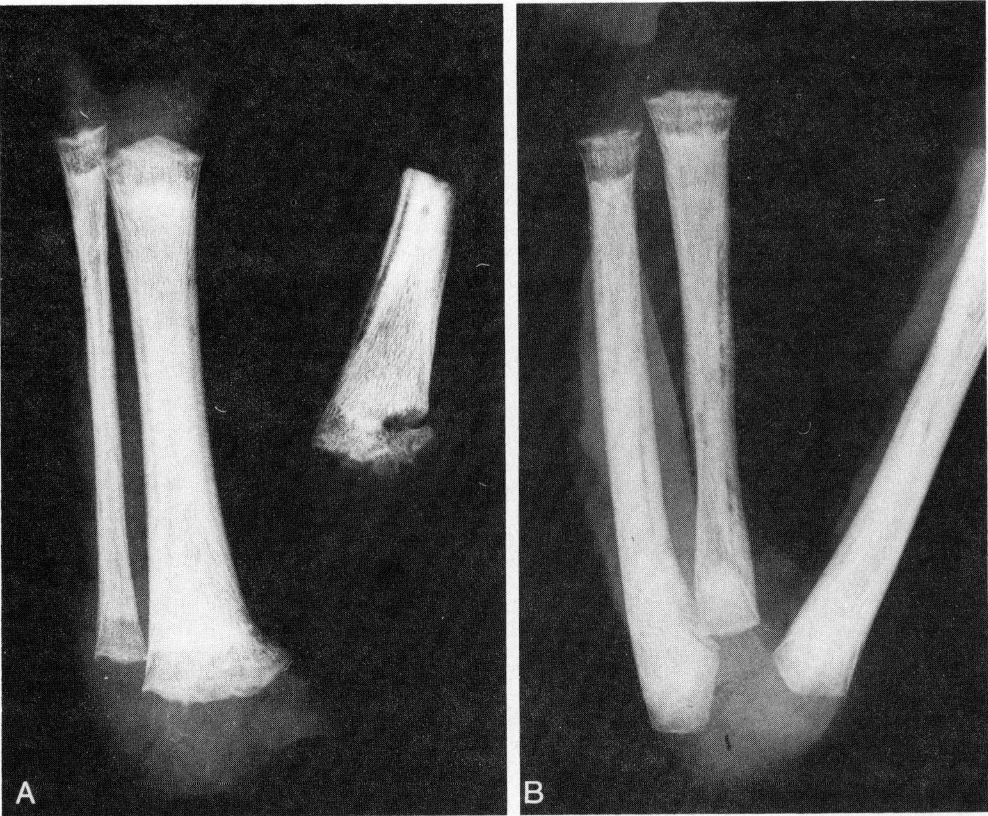

Figure 4–35. Specimen radiographs of lower *(A)* and upper *(B)* limbs of a patient with congenital syphilis. Notice the failure of metaphyseal bone to form, the irregularity of the epiphyseal growth plate with persistence of bands of calcified cartilage suggesting intermittent activity, and the periosteal new bone formation.

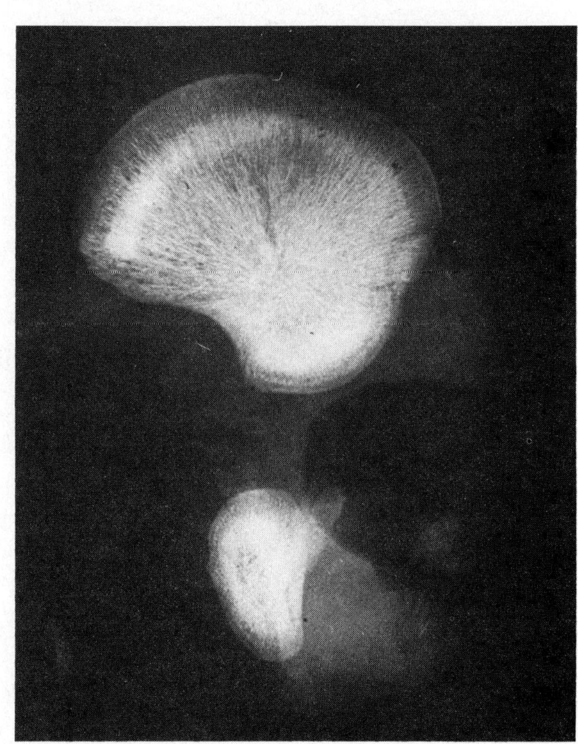

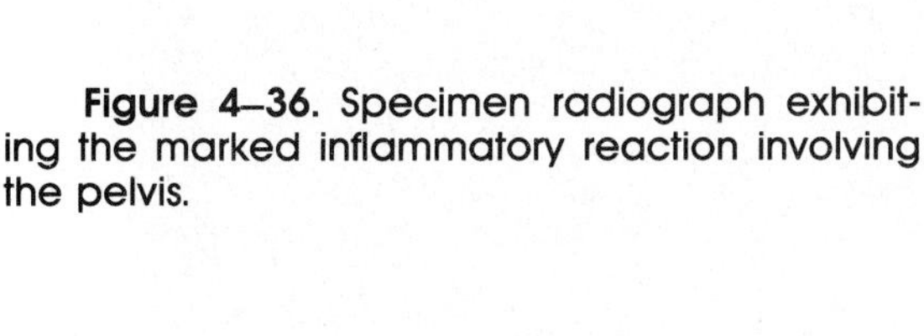

Figure 4–36. Specimen radiograph exhibiting the marked inflammatory reaction involving the pelvis.

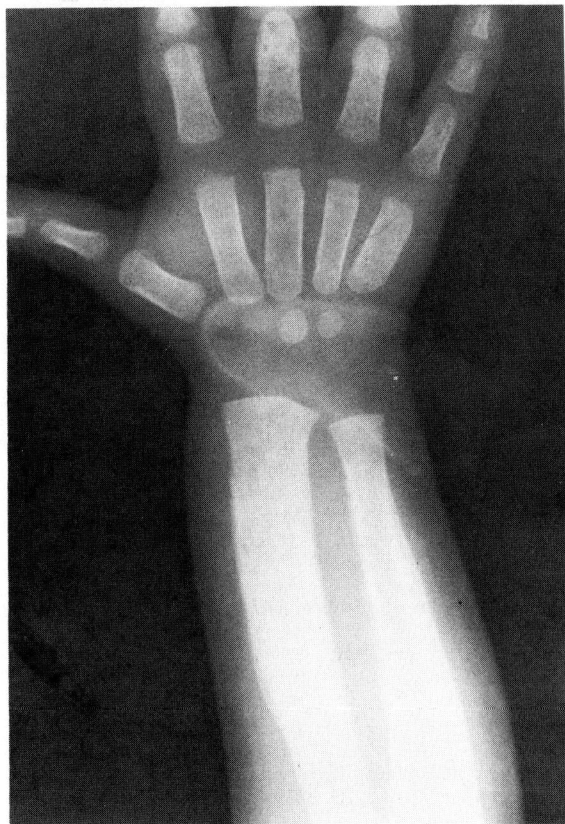

Figure 4–37. Radiograph of the hand and forearm of a somewhat older child with congenital syphilis exhibiting marked widening of both ulna and radius with fill-in. The widened diaphysis is characteristic of syphilitic periostitis and osteomyelitis. Since the process is self-limiting in the metaphysis, remodeling with growth quickly eliminates the metaphyseal stigmata of the disease in the patient.

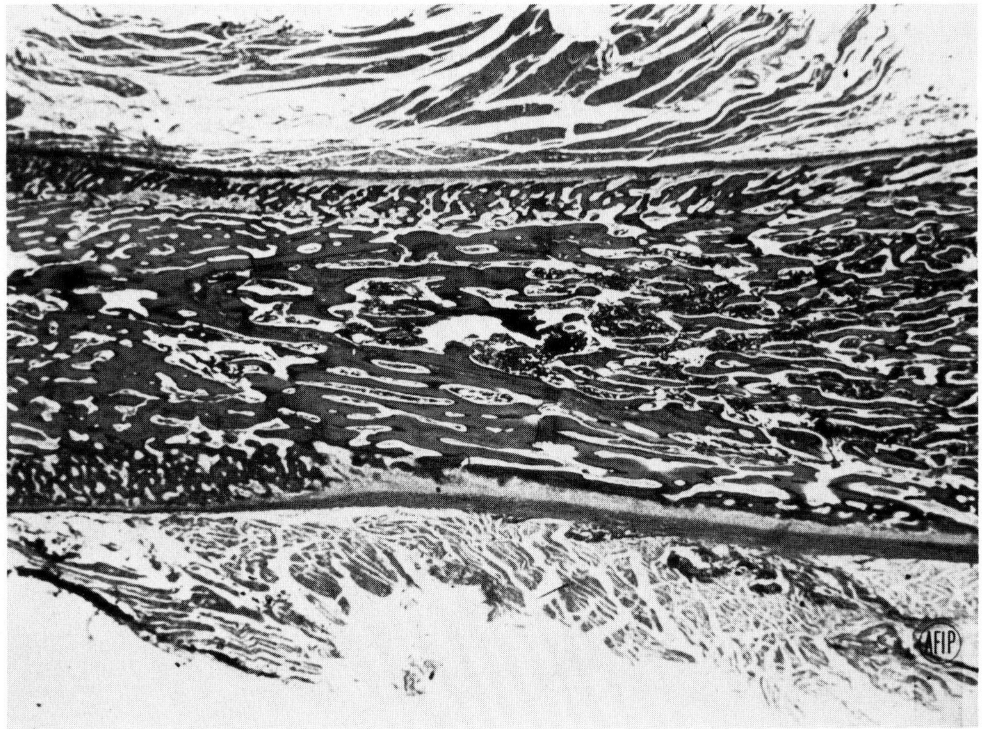

Figure 4–38. Longitudinal section through the bone of a patient with syphilis. Periostitis and osteomyelitis are present.

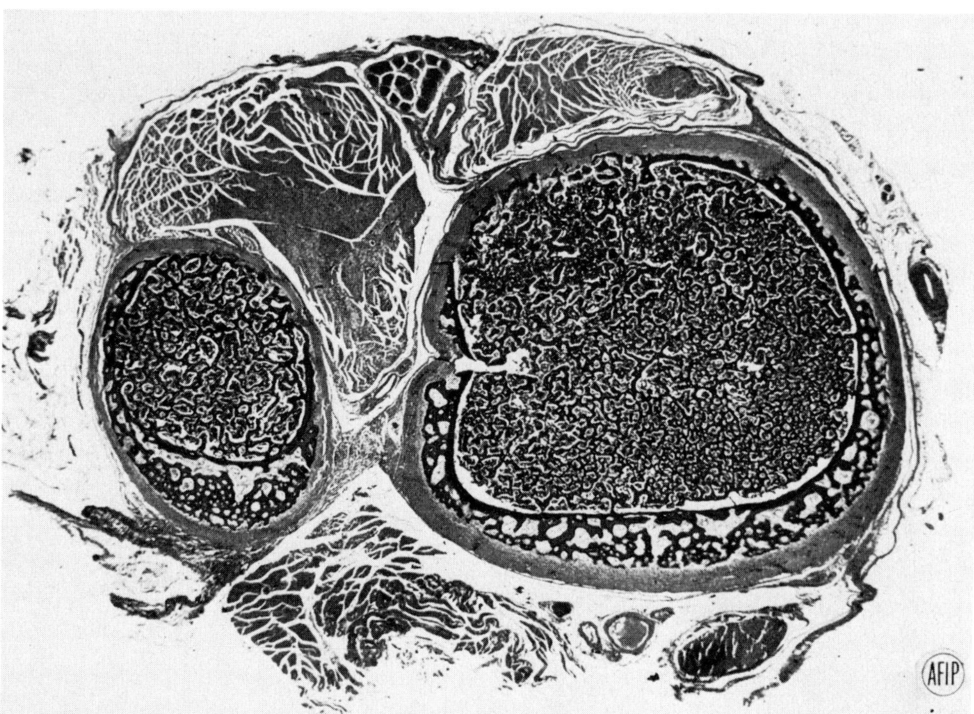

Figure 4–39. Cross section of a specimen similar to the one shown in Figure 4–38 demonstrating extensive periostitis of the tibia and fibula.

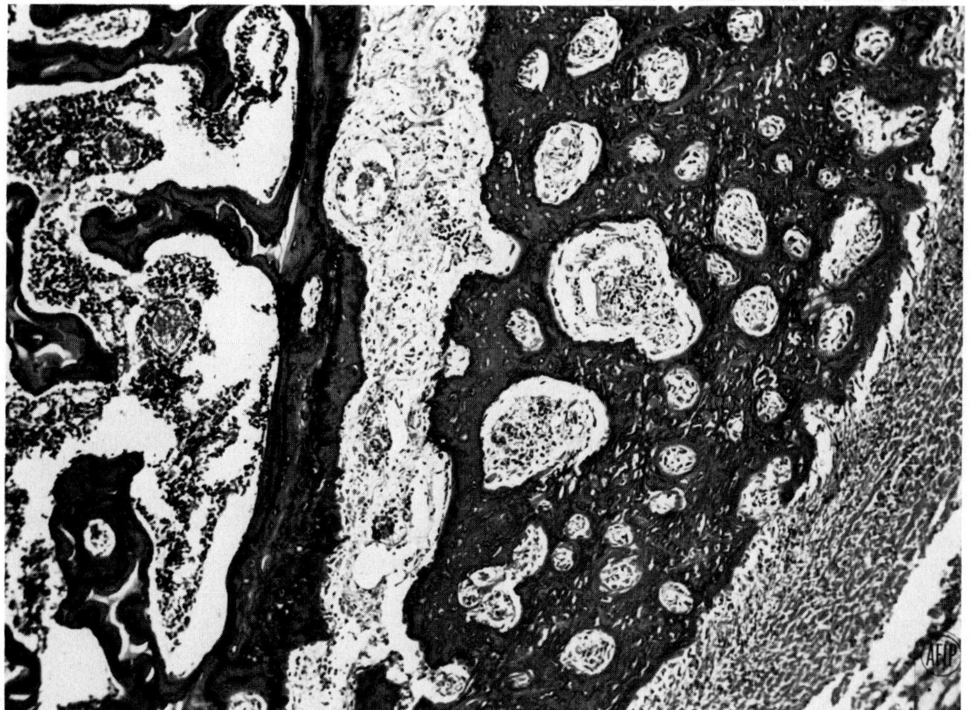

Figure 4–40. Higher-power view of periostitis with granulation tissue and periosteal new bone formation in syphilitic inflammation. Inflammatory cells are present in the medullary cavity as well as in the spaces of periosteal new bone.

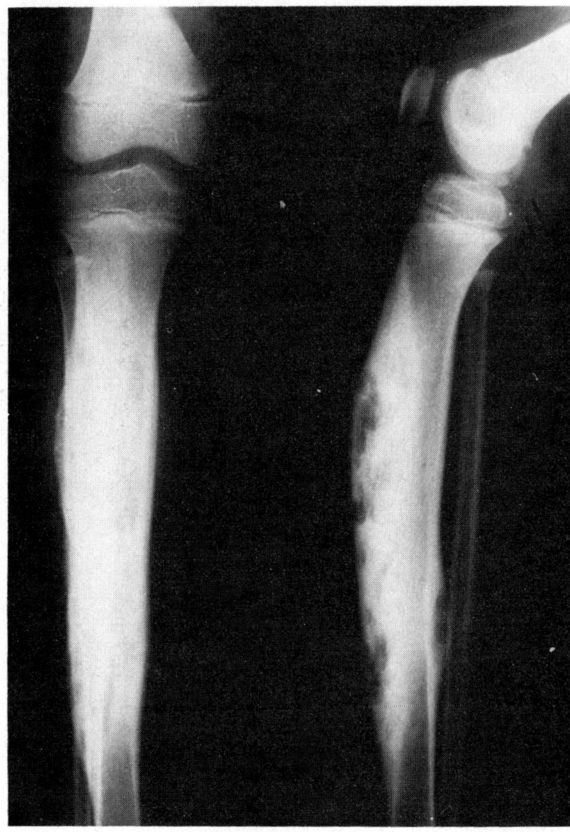

Figure 4–41. Syphilitic periostitis in a somewhat older individual. Notice the marked thickening of the bone leading to "saber shin" formation. The lytic areas represent multiple gummas.

Inasmuch as cartilage of the growth plate is avascular, the formation and maturation of cartilage are not affected by the spirochete. However, the removal of the dead cartilage cellular debris depends on the formation of normal vessels. In their absence cartilage is not removed; the remaining calcified cartilage bars persist longer owing to failure of osteoblast formation. Syphilis is thus morphologically similar to scurvy.

If the patient survives intrauterine or postnatal infection, the spirochetes tend to disappear spontaneously from the bone, and the defects at the growth plate and periosteum tend to remodel into normal bone.

In congenital as well as acquired syphilis, the periosteum is characteristically involved (Figs. 4–37 to 4–40). The inflammatory process consists of plasma-cell infiltration, fibrosis, osteoblastic activity, and fill-in. The entire shaft of bone may thicken, resulting in characteristic "saber shins" (Fig. 4–41). Hyperostosis frequently occurs at the external end of the clavicle as well as in the skull bones, particularly in the frontal and parietal regions.

Charcot's joint is a nonspecific reaction to lack of normal neurovascular stimuli and is not specific for syphilis (see Charcot's Arthropathy, Chapter 5).

GRANULOMATOUS DISEASE

A granuloma is a specific anatomic entity. It demonstrates an organoid structure that can be grossly visible as a granule, nodule, or tubercle. Histologically, the granuloma consists of a centrally located area of caseation necrosis without identifiable form or shape. This area is surrounded by a large number of epithelioid histiocytes, cells with large, clear, distinct nuclei and large quantities of cytoplasm that are capable of phagocytosis. Occasionally, multinucleated histiocytic aggregates may be seen; these are the giant cells, and specific designations, such as Langhans' or foreign-body giant cells, refer to their morphologic appearance. The function of all histiocytic giant cells is the same: phagocytosis of material.

The histiocytes, or giant cells, occupy the central position in the granuloma and surround the area of caseation. Not all granulomas are caseating; the granulomas of sarcoidosis are characteristically noncaseating. The center of the lesion is then occupied by histiocytes, or giant cells, exclusively. The histiocytes are surrounded by a rim of fibrous proliferation and lymphocytic aggregates. The caseating area may retain the offending organisms for many years; it may calcify and even ossify.

TUBERCULOSIS

Upon entry into the host tissue, the tubercle bacillus elicits an acute inflammatory response. Numerous polymorphonuclear leukocytes surround it, and the organism is phagocytosed. At this stage, the initial infection is indistinguishable from any other bacterial infection and may present with the picture of typical bacterial pneumonitis. The tubercle bacillus, engulfed within the polymorphonuclear leukocyte, continues to thrive and reproduce, and the granulocyte ultimately dies and disgorges a large number of new tubercle bacilli. As part of the response towards this inflammatory process, numerous histiocytes surround the necrotic granulocytes and form aggregates of multinucleated histiocytes (Langhans' giant cells). At some point, the proliferation of histiocytes and multinucleated giant cells results in arrest of the inflammatory

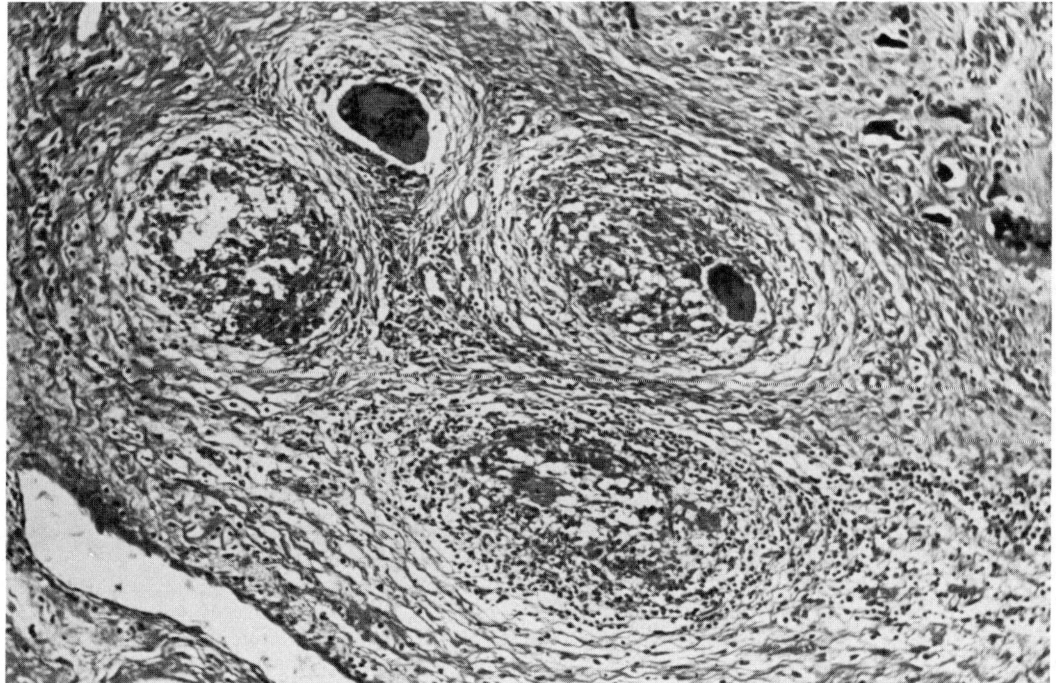

Figure 4–42. Numerous granulomas in tuberculous synovium. The granuloma is a sharply circumscribed anatomic process consisting of a central area of histiocytes and Langhans' giant cells, which is surrounded in turn by fibrous connective tissue and lymphocytes. This picture of tuberculous granulomatous disease with little caseation is characteristic of the process in the synovium.

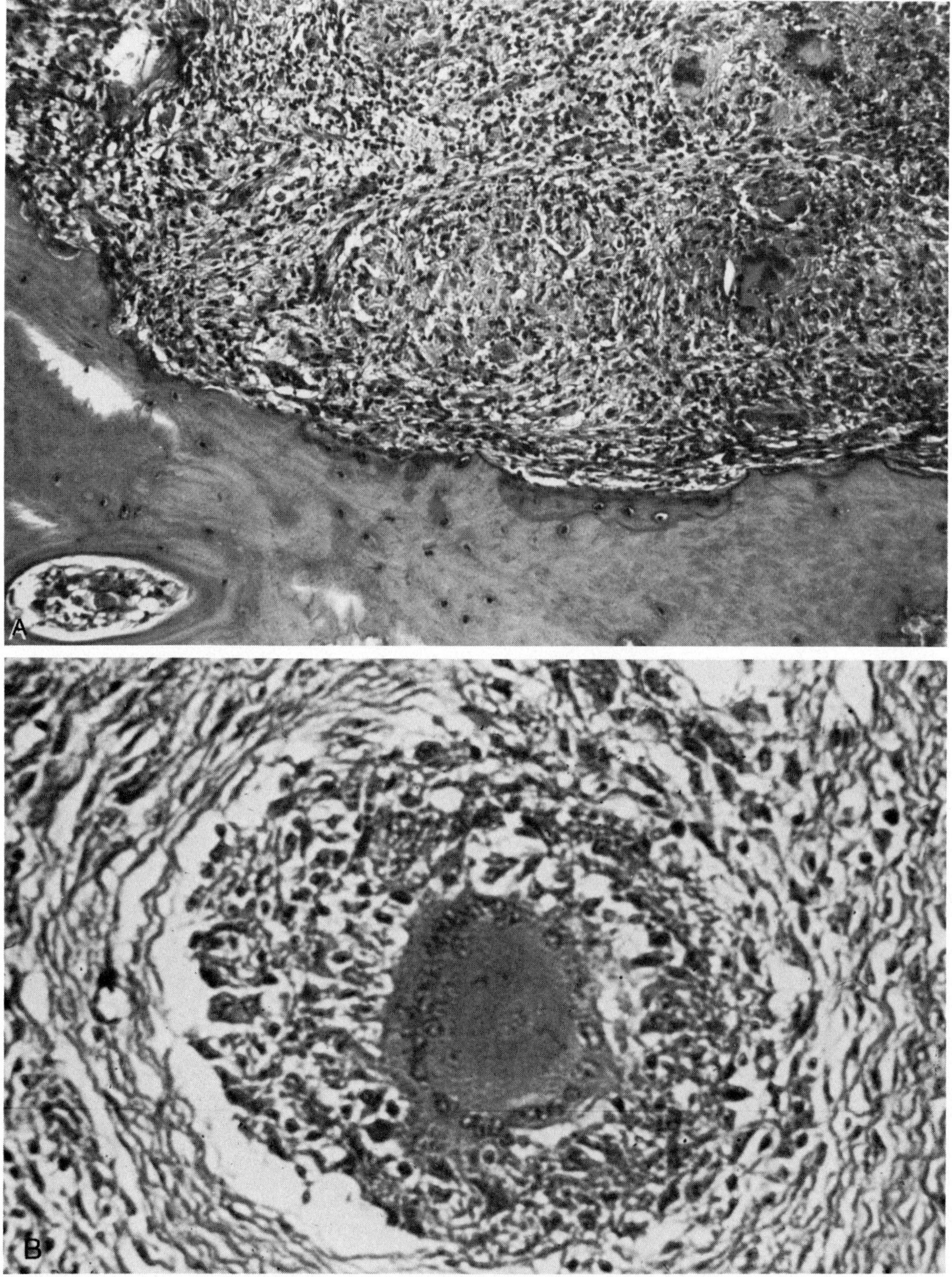

Figure 4–43. A characteristic tuberculous granuloma, with a Langhans' giant cell, surrounded by fibrous connective tissue. Note the circular and semicircular arrangement of the nuclei.

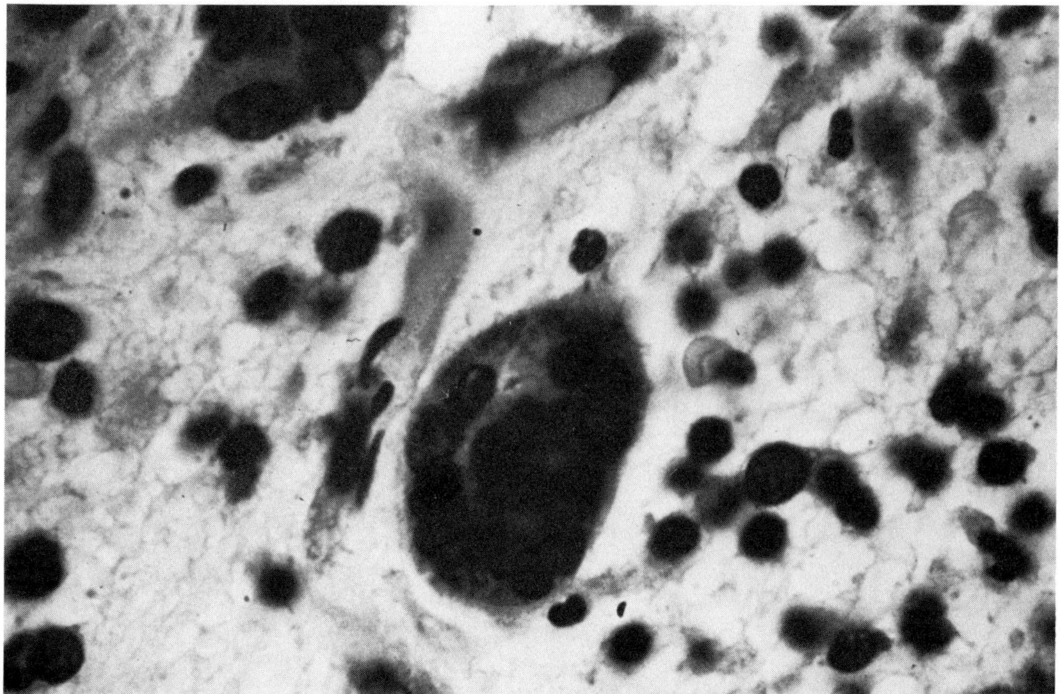

Figure 4–44. Foreign body giant cell with centrally condensed nuclei and relatively little cytoplasm.

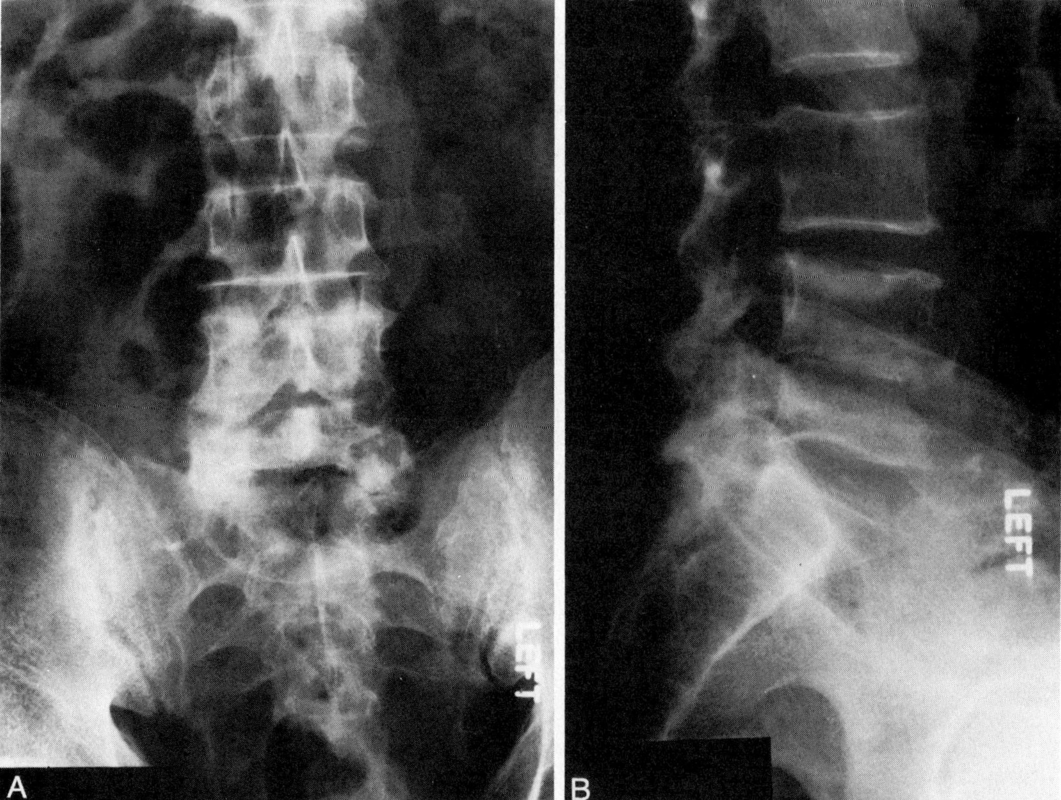

Figure 4–45. Anteroposterior *(A)* and lateral *(B)* radiographs of a tuberculous spondylitis. A large irregular lytic defect is present in the anterior portion of the vertebral body of L4 and involves the intervertebral disc and proximal half of L5. Tomograms may serve to delineate the process more precisely.

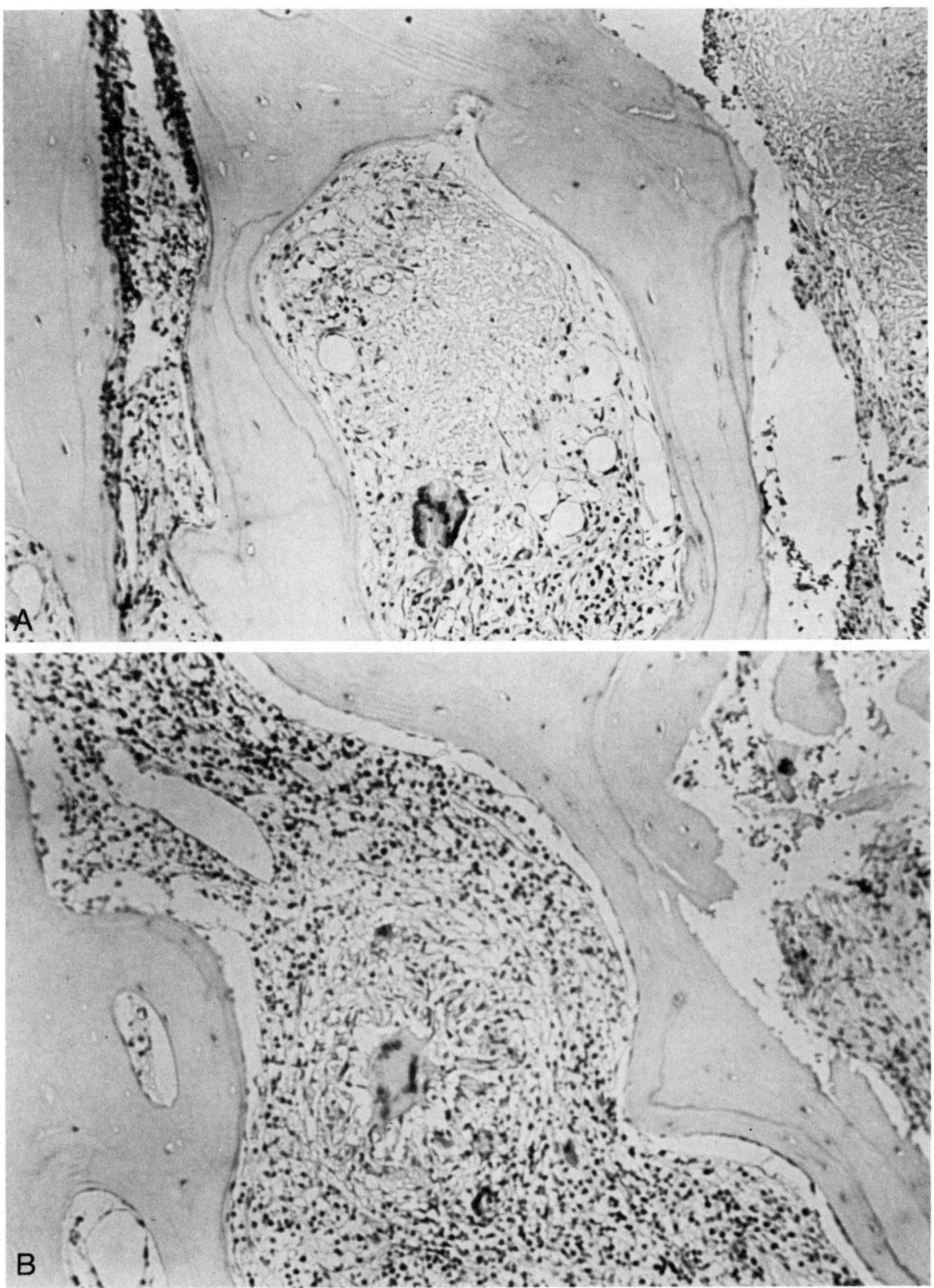

Figure 4–46. Histologic appearance of the lesion demonstrated in Figure 4–45. The lesion is composed of a granulomatous disease process in which numerous tubercle bacilli were demonstrated. The caseation is well demonstrated in *A*.

process, and the characteristic granuloma is formed, consisting of necrotic debris from dead granulocytes in the center of the lesion, which is surrounded by a wall of histiocytes and Langhans' giant cells with fibrous tissue at the periphery (Figs. 4–42, 4–43, 4–46). In humans, pulmonary tuberculosis is the necessary prerequisite to any other form of the disease. Hematogenous spread is necessary for distant tuberculosis to develop.

The tubercle bacillus is a nonmotile organism that prefers areas of high oxygen content. It will usually lodge in the synovium and possibly in associated epiphyseal or metaphyseal portion of the bone. The infected synovium becomes enlarged and occupies all the recesses of a joint, very much as pannus in rheumatoid arthritis. The interference with the free surface of the articular cartilage affects its nutrition and ultimately leads to destruction of cartilage and osteoarthritis (Figs. 4–47 and 4–51).

Tubercles often form in the subchondral marrow space and destroy the trabecular bone that provides support to the joint. This, combined with cartilage destruction from the surface, may result in a sequestrum of variable size formed by the residual articular cartilage, subchondral bone, and sequestered trabecular bone. The process may involve both surfaces of the joint, with sequestration of bone on both sides of the joint surface, leading to the characteristic "kissing sequestrum." The increased

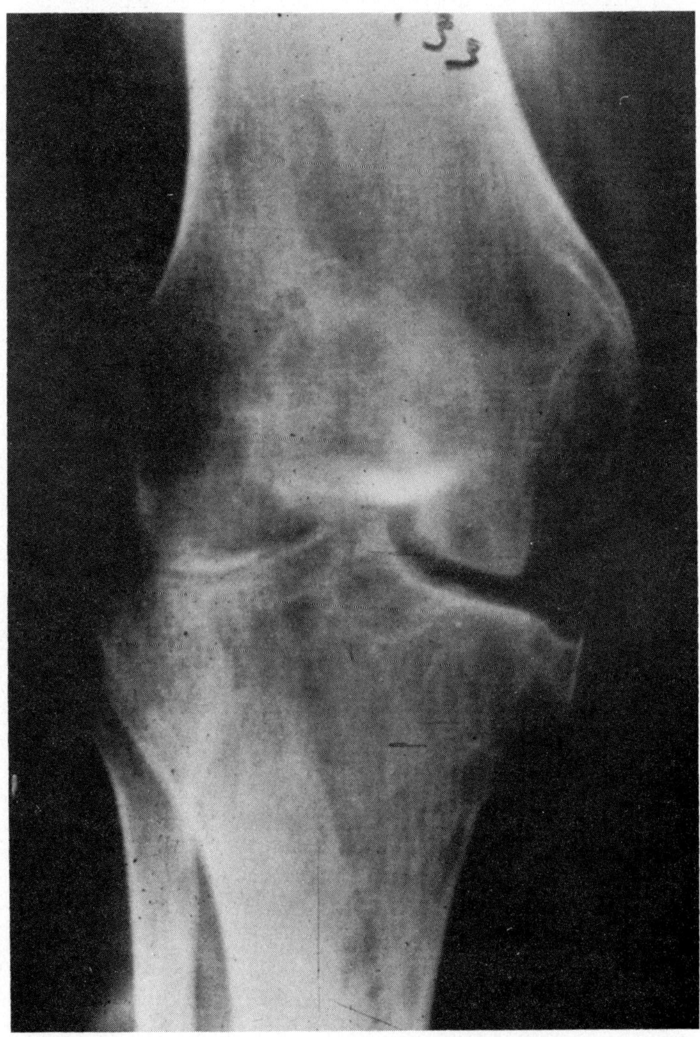

Figure 4–47. Radiograph of patient with tuberculosis exhibiting marked osteoporosis of both femur and tibia. The joint space is narrowed, and there is erosion of the margins of the articular surfaces. The osteoporosis is disproportionate with the amount of actual bone destruction. Destruction of the joint starts at the lateral margin secondary to tuberculous pannus formation. The weight-bearing areas of the joint are the last to be involved.

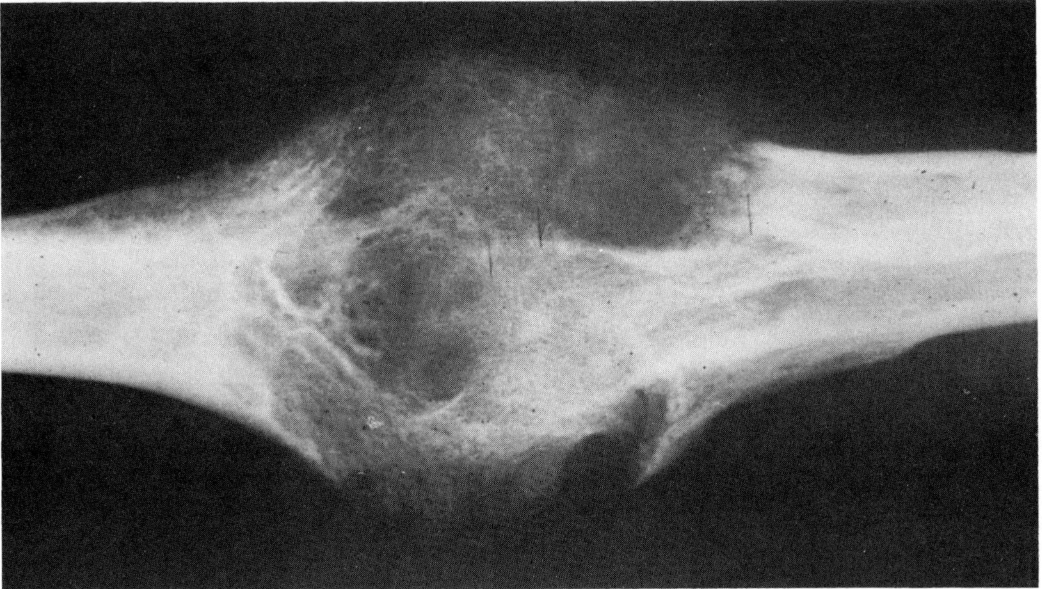

Figure 4–48. Radiograph of patient with advanced tuberculosis of the elbow joint exhibiting marked destruction of joint surfaces.

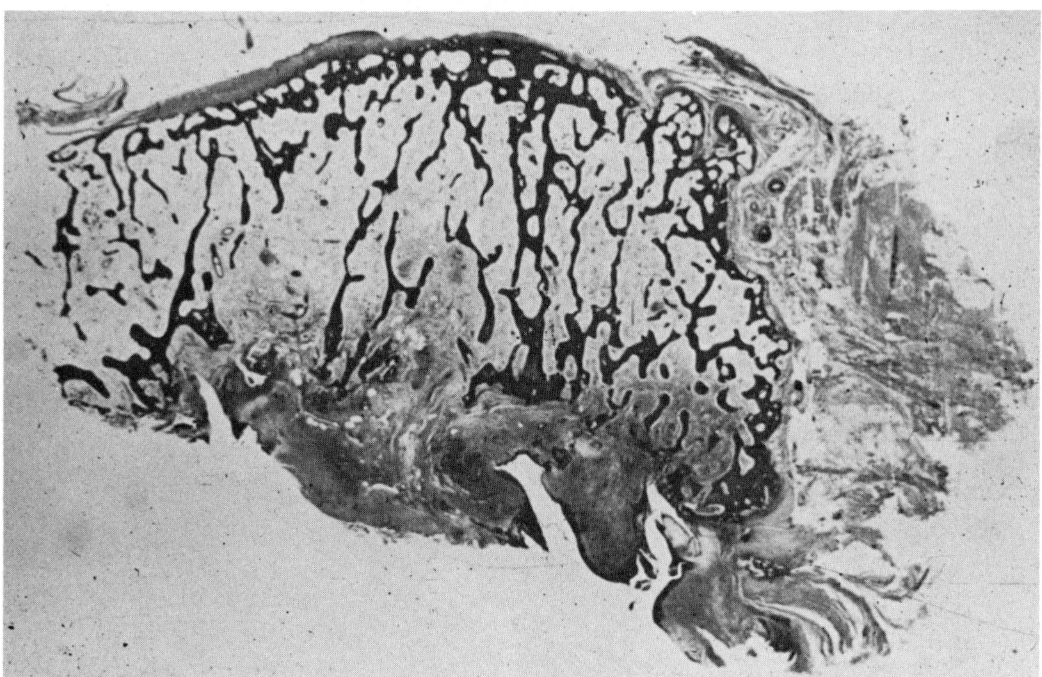

Figure 4–49. Macrosection from a patient with tuberculosis. Extensive granulation tissue and granulomatous processes are present in the synovial tissue and extend into the adjacent bone. The active hyperemia induced by the infection has stimulated the articular surface to grow and has produced a picture of progressive remodeling (see Chapter 6).

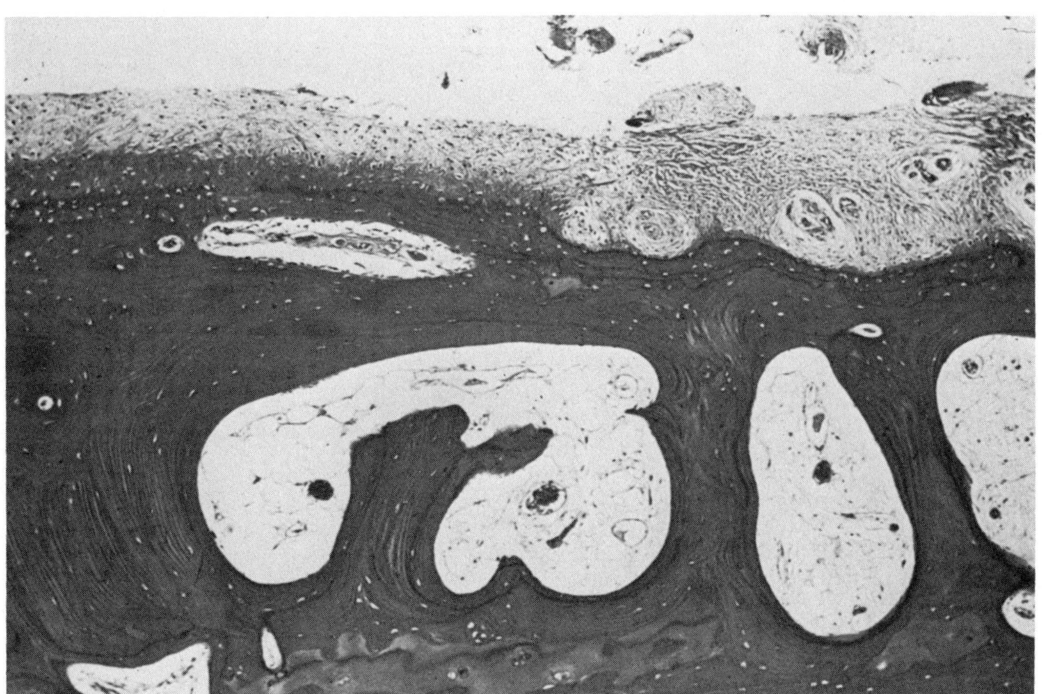

Figure 4–50. Pannus formation from tuberculosis synovitis has replaced the articular cartilage. Note the remnants of the articular cartilage at the base of the photograph, which indicate rapid forward remodeling in response to the increased vascularity of the inflammatory process (see Chapter 6).

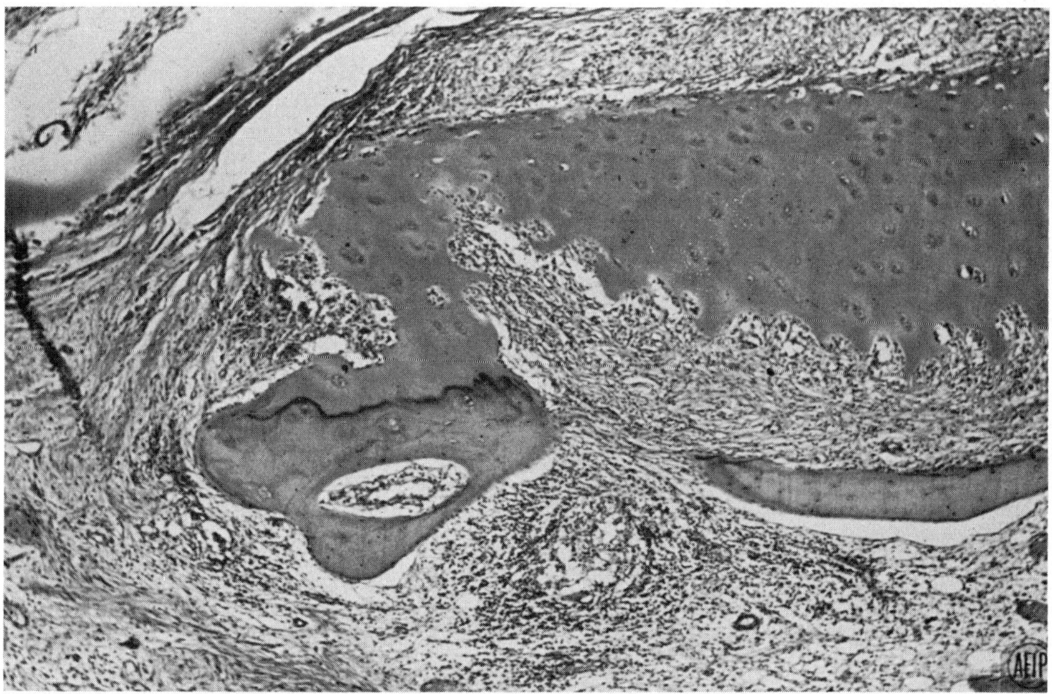

Figure 4–51. Replacement of articular cartilage and subchondral bone by the tuberculous granulomatous process has created a sequestrum of the joint cartilage and its subchondral bone.

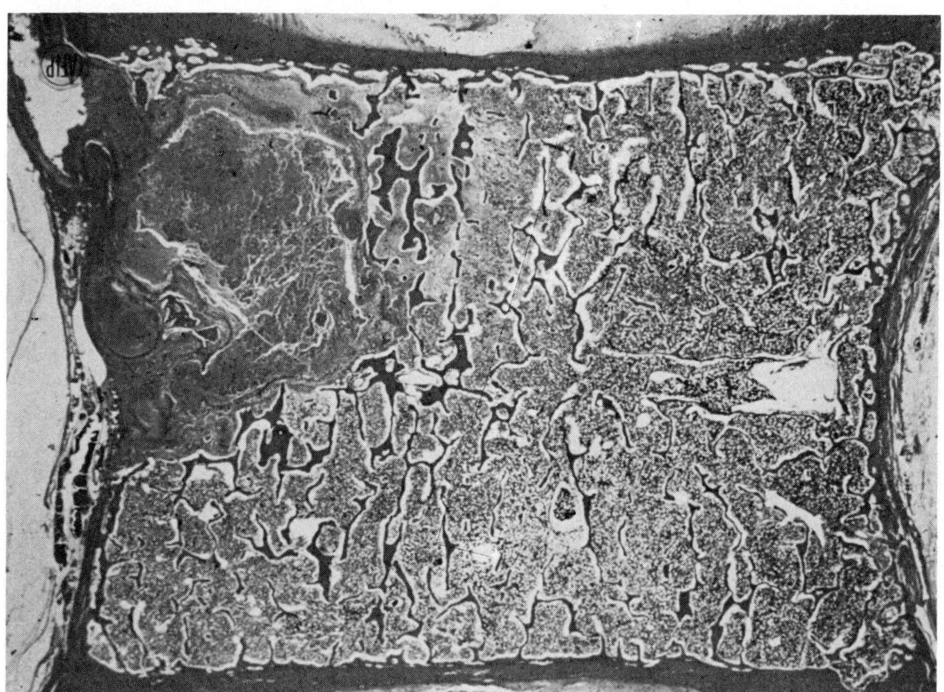

Figure 4–52. Macrosection of granulomatous disease in a vertebral body. There is replacement of bone by granulation tissue with the formation of numerous tubercles. Ultimately, this fragment of bone will collapse.

vascularity of the low-grade tuberculous inflammatory process produces osteoporosis, usually disproportionate with the degree of infection (Edeiken, 1976).

Gradual destruction of the joint surface starts at the lateral margin by pannus formation from the infected synovium. This contrasts with suppurative arthritis, in which rapid destruction by proteolytic enzymes from leukocytes destroy cartilage in the central weight-bearing portions of the joint rather than at the margin.

A very common location for skeletal tuberculosis is the spine. Deformity and crippling may be severe owing to extensive destruction of many vertebrae (Pott's disease). The disease process does not confine itself to the vertebral body but rather extends by contiguity into adjacent discs and the spinal canal, ultimately forming a draining sinus to the surface of the skin. It is frequently characterized by paraplegia and pronounced spinal deformities. Surgical intervention is still advised to prevent these complications, despite the availability of effective antituberculous chemotherapy (Figs. 4–52 and 4–53).

OTHER GRANULOMATOUS DISEASES

Sarcoidosis is a noncaseating granulomatous process presenting as small foci preferentially located in the small bones of the hand. Sarcoidosis, unlike tuberculosis,

---

Figure 4–54. The noncaseating granulomatous process of sarcoidosis tends to involve the peripheral bones, particularly the small bones of the hands and feet. Multiple punched-out lesions are present within the phalanges. These are rarely biopsied, but when they are, noncaseating granulomas are found.

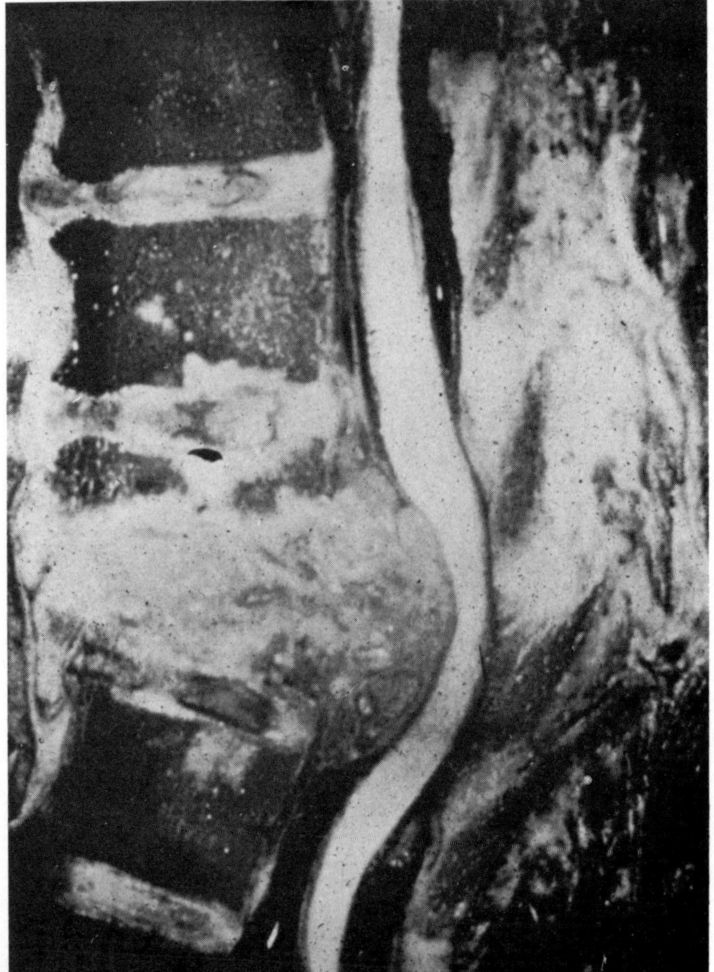

Figure 4–53. Gross specimen of Pott's disease, with tuberculous destruction of the vertebral body and extension into adjacent soft tissue resulting in compression of the spinal cord. (From Syllabus: Revised Clinical Slide Collection on Rheumatic Diseases. Atlanta, Arthritis Foundation, National Office, 1981.)

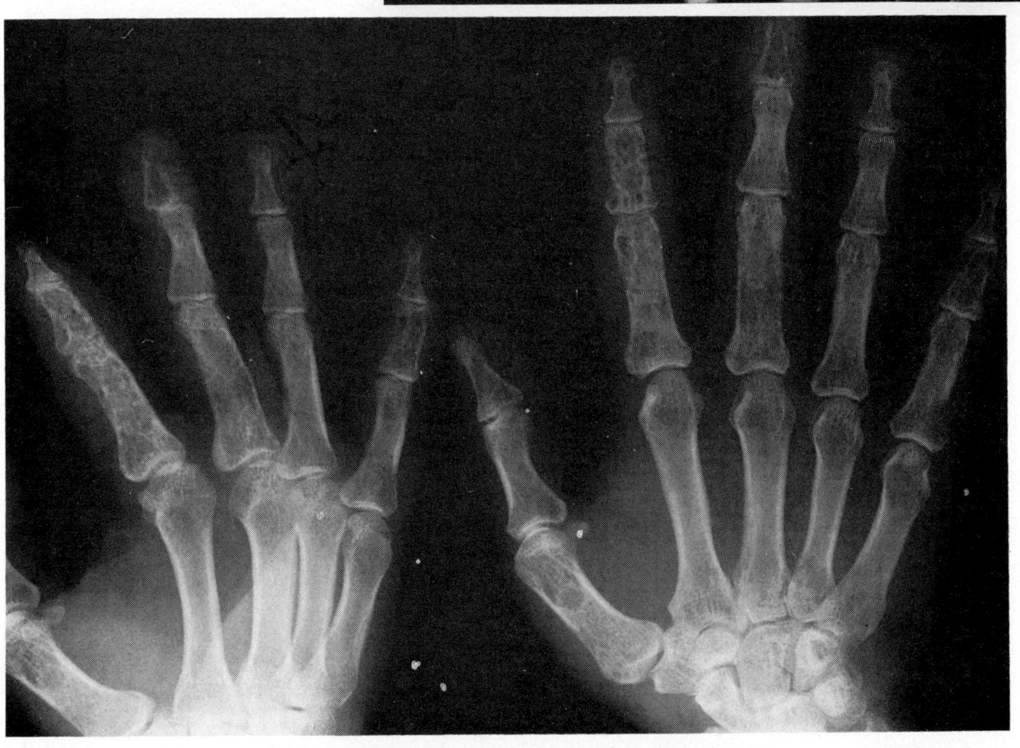

Figure 4–54. *See legend on opposite page.*

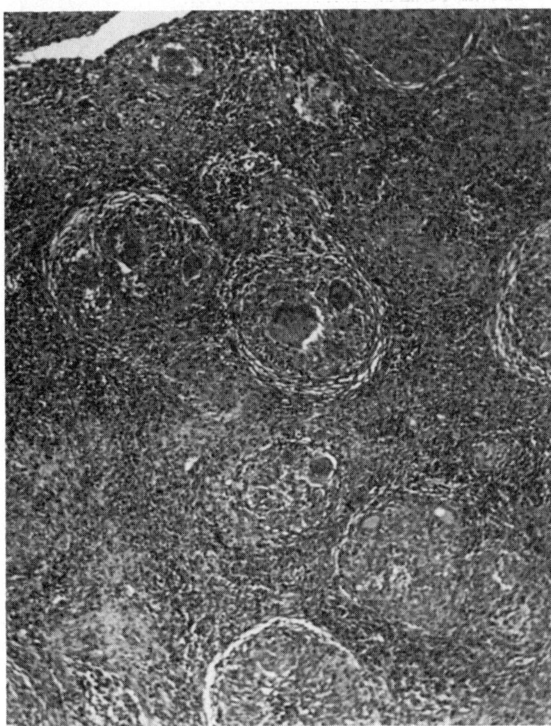

Figure 4–55. Numerous noncaseating granulomas, characteristic of sarcoidosis. Langhans' giant cells are detectable. Each of the nodules is surrounded by fibrous connective tissue septa.

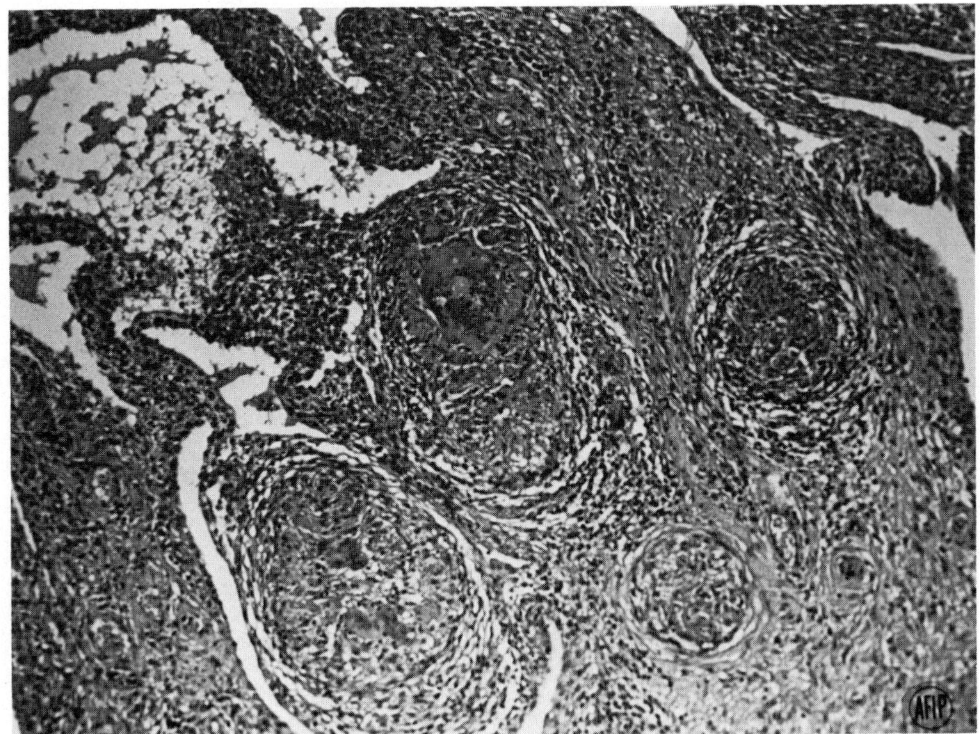

Figure 4–56. Sarcoidosis, with characteristic noncaseating granulomas.

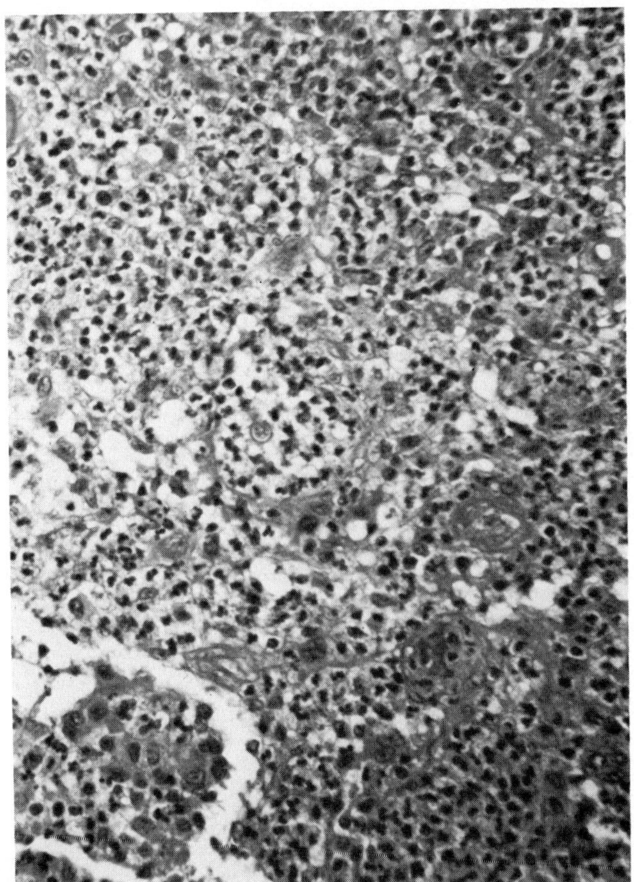

Figure 4–57. Coccidioidomycosis. Granulomatous process with numerous histiocytes and Langhans' giant cells, but also numerous polymorphonuclear leukocytes are shown. The organism is present in the center of the illustration. This large organism cannot be phagocytosed by the polymorphonuclear leukocytes. The presence of a granulomatous process with numerous granulocytes is characteristic of coccidioidomycosis.

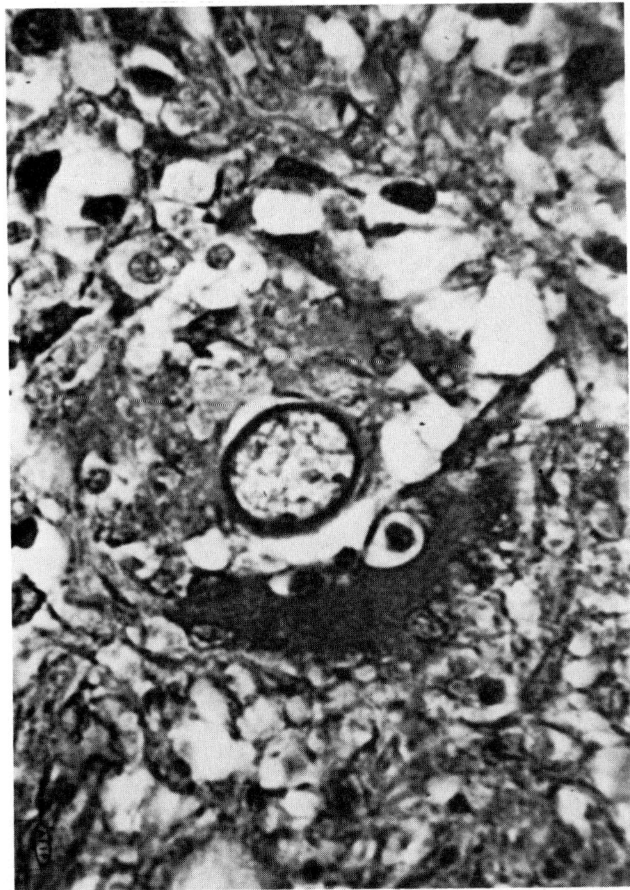

Figure 4–58. Coccidioidomycosis. Coccidioidal organism surrounded by Langhans' giant cell and histiocytes.

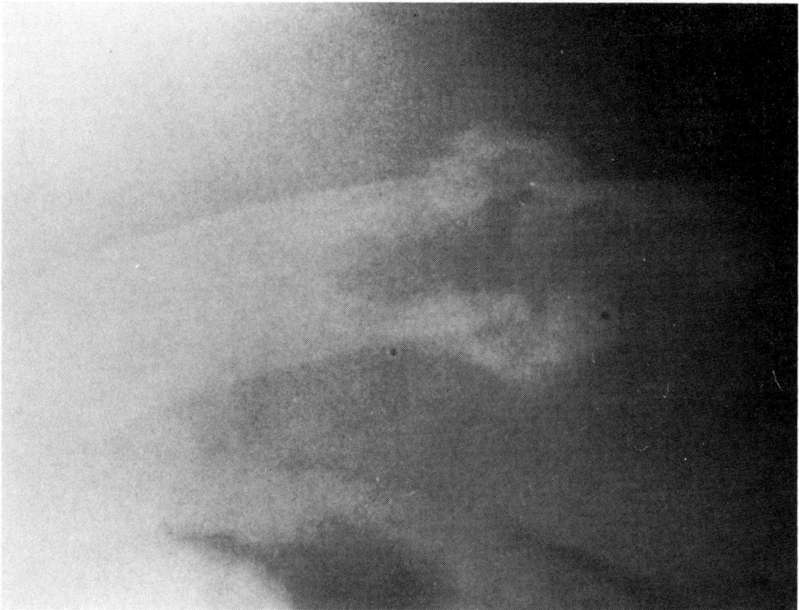

Figure 4–59. Coccioidioidomycosis. Pathologic fracture of rib with callus formation.

is not commonly associated with destruction of large foci of bone. The granulomatous process, when biopsied, exhibits a characteristic noncaseating granuloma (Figs. 4–54 to 4–56).

Fungal diseases such as coccidioidomycosis, histoplasmosis, blastomycosis, and others are capable of producing granulomatous processes in bone, just as tuberculosis. Most of these fungal diseases represent hematogenous spread from a primary pulmonary focus. The granulomatous process is identical with that of tuberculosis, and only the identification of the organism by special stains and cultures establishes definite etiology (Putschar, 1976) (Figs. 4–57 to 4–60).

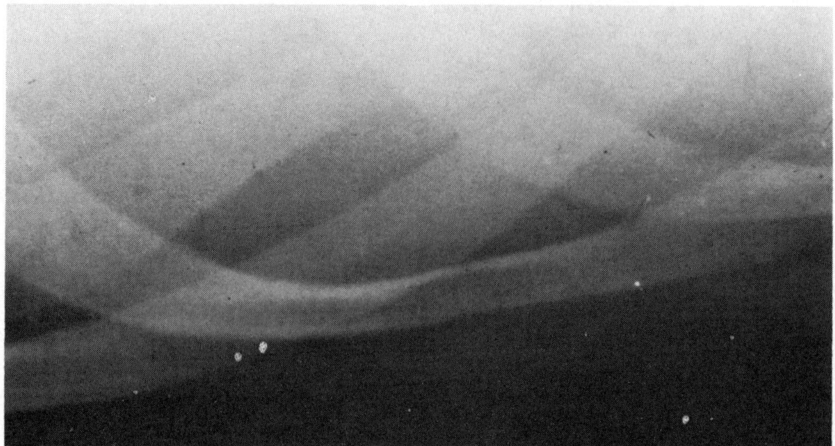

Figure 4–60. Coccidioidomycosis. Sharply circumscribed lytic defect in rib of patient with multiple skeletal lesions exhibiting granulomatous disease process. The organism was easily visualized and cultured.

INFANTILE CORTICAL HYPEROSTOSIS (CAFFEY'S DISEASE)

Infantile cortical hyperostosis (Caffey's disease) is a process of marked severe periostitis with reactive bone formation. In spite of the massive periosteal reaction with resorption of the immediate underlying cortex, the affected cortex and marrow cavity show far less inflammatory response than is usually seen in infectious disease processes of bone. The process jumps from one bone to another, with eventual spontaneous remission. The clinical course may include fever, leukocytosis, local edema, tenderness, and redness of the overlying skin. No specific etiology is known, but it is noteworthy that only bones ossified in the early stages of fetal development are involved in the process (Cremin, 1979).

The periosteal new bone formation is the most dramatic presentation of the patient with Caffey's disease (Figs. 4–61 to 4–66). The differential diagnosis of Caffey's disease must include congenital syphilis, any malignant process of the medullary cavity, osteomyelitis, trauma, and, rarely, vitamin-A poisoning. Caffey's disease

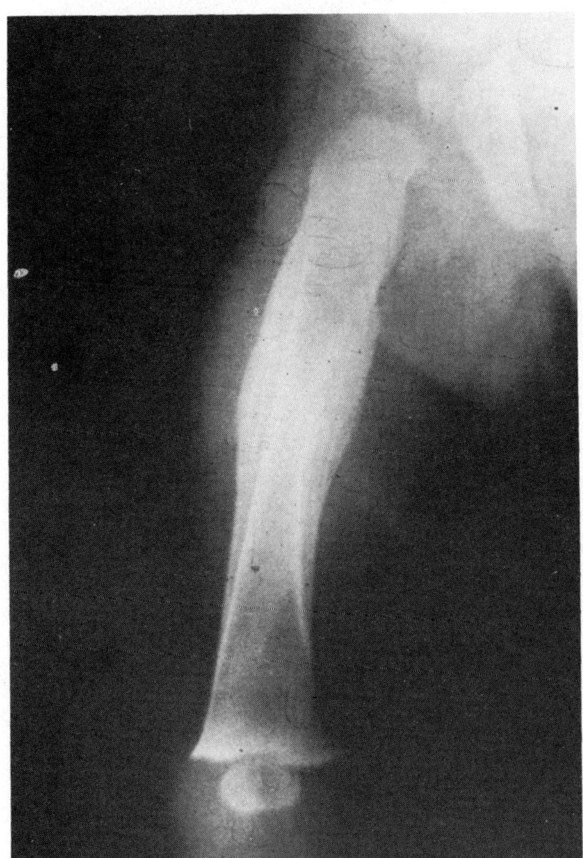

Figure 4–61

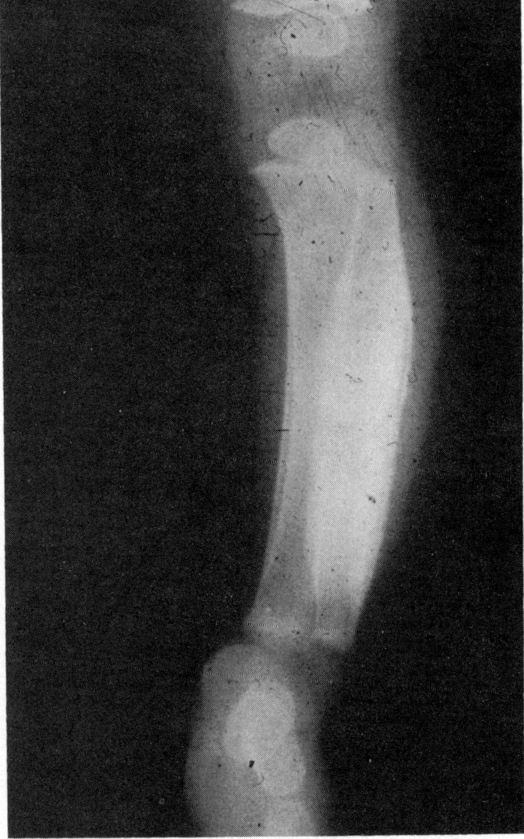

Figure 4–62

Figure 4–61. Symmetric periosteal reaction of femur in 6-month-old infant suffering from infantile cortical hyperostosis. Diaphyseal location with no intramedullary reaction is characteristic of Caffey's disease.

Figure 4–62. Periosteal reaction of tibia exhibiting symmetric periosteal elevation, predominantly diaphyseal, without identifiable endosteal lesion.

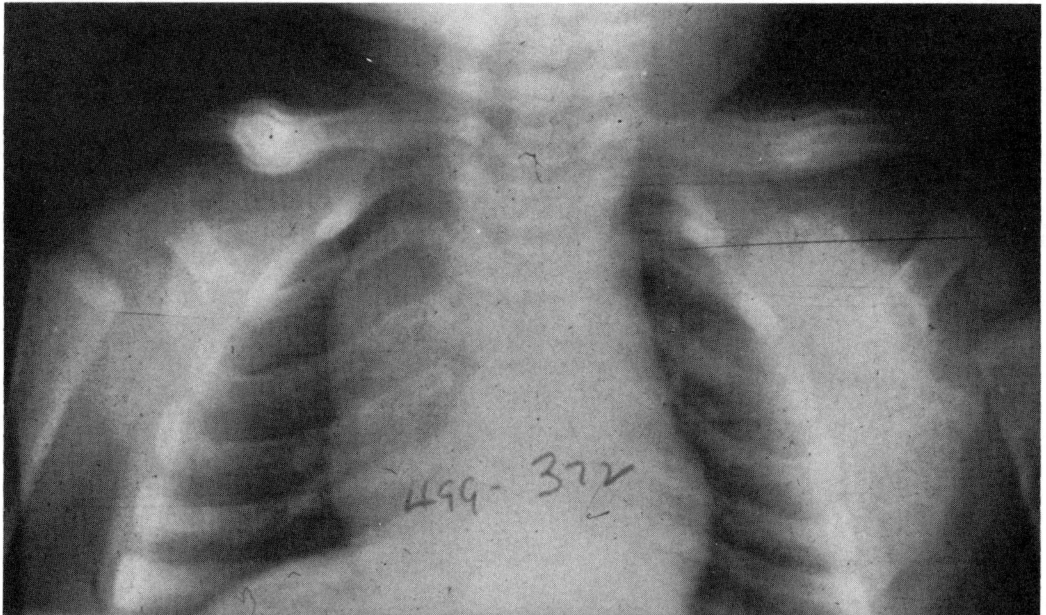

Figure 4–63. Periosteal reaction of clavicle with symmetric elevation but no identifiable endosteal lesion. The jaw is commonly involved with other bones.

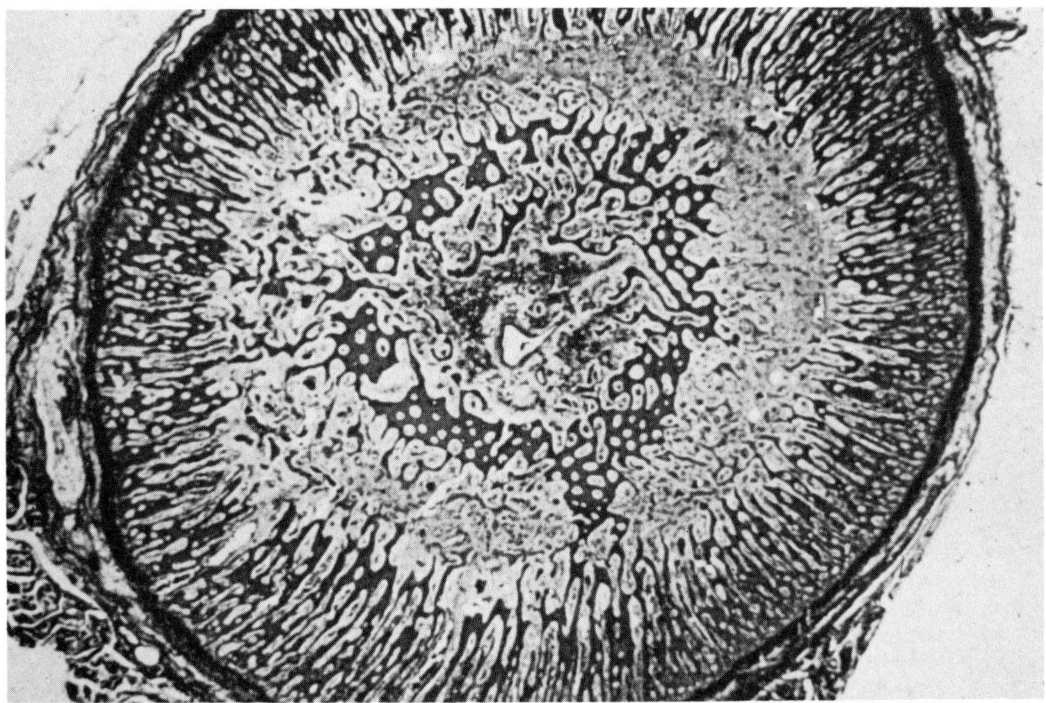

Figure 4–64. Macrospecimen from patient with Caffey's disease exhibiting an extensive periosteal reaction associated with extensive resorption of pre-existing cortex. There is no identifiable inflammatory or vascular process, and the etiology of the disease remains unknown.

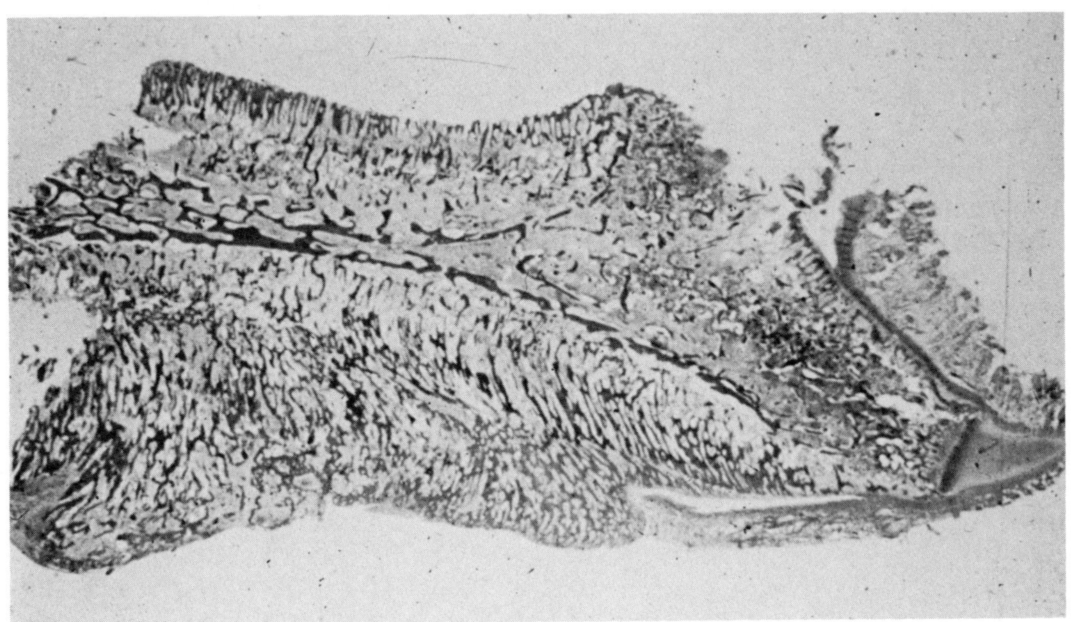

Figure 4–65. Macrospecimen of scapula with extensive resorption of cortex and periosteal reaction. The patient was biopsied for suspected osteosarcoma.

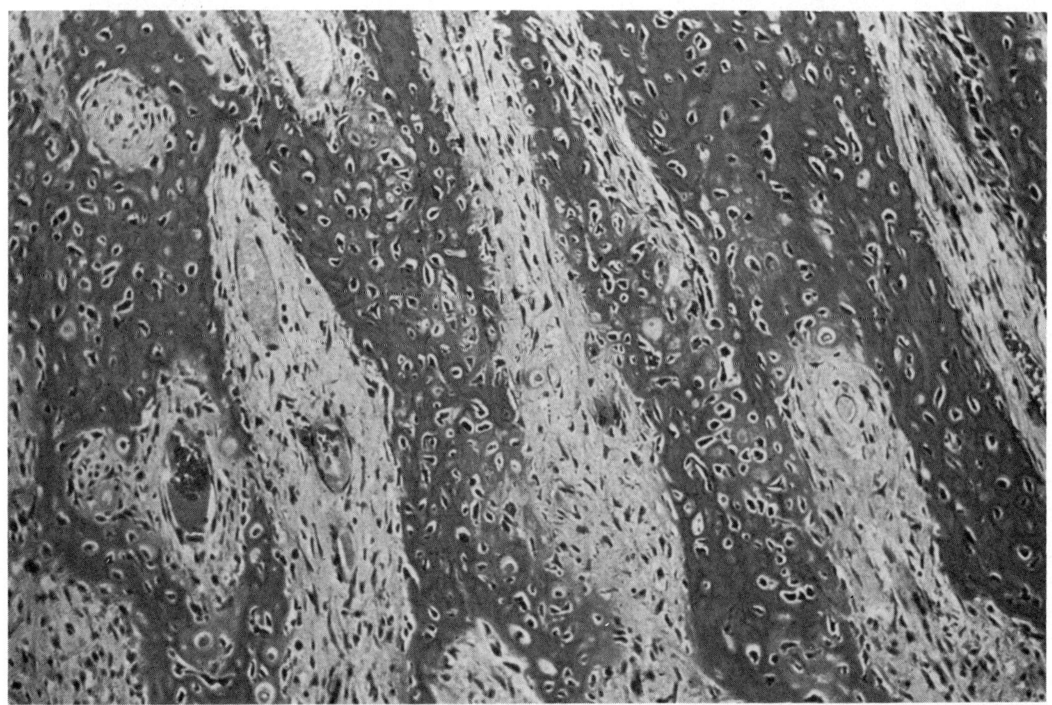

Figure 4–66. Periosteal reaction in Caffey's disease. Highly cellular streamer bone demonstrates no evidence of a pre-existing abnormality.

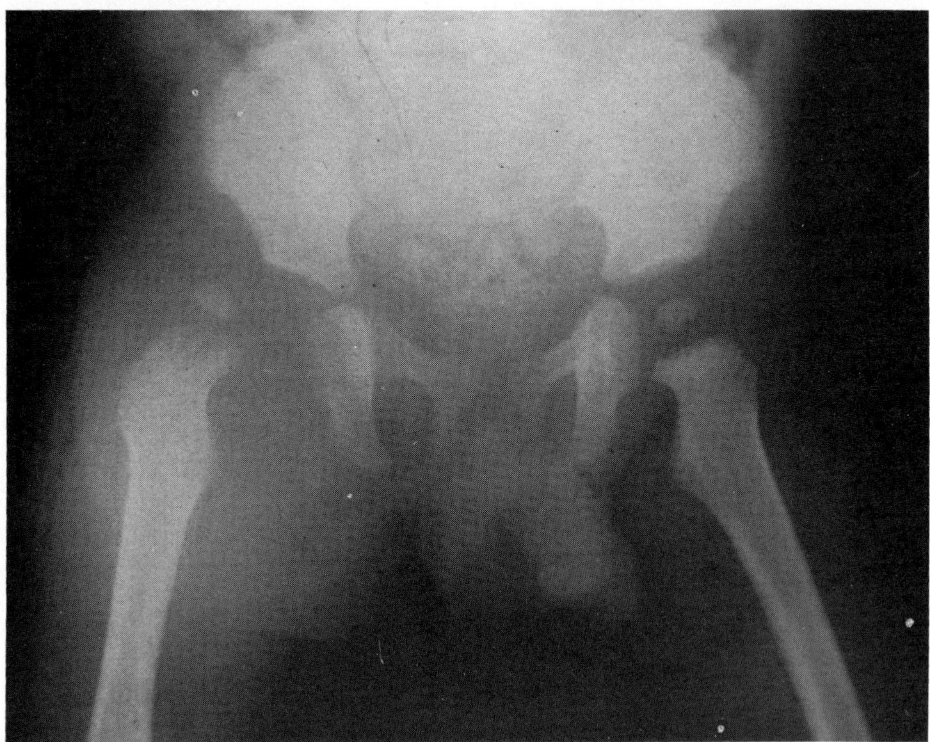

Figure 4–67. Radiograph of the pelvis of a 10-month-old male with a septic hip on the right. The femoral head is displaced from the acetabulum, and there is marked soft tissue swelling in the proximal thigh. There is a small erosion in the metaphysis of the proximal femur.

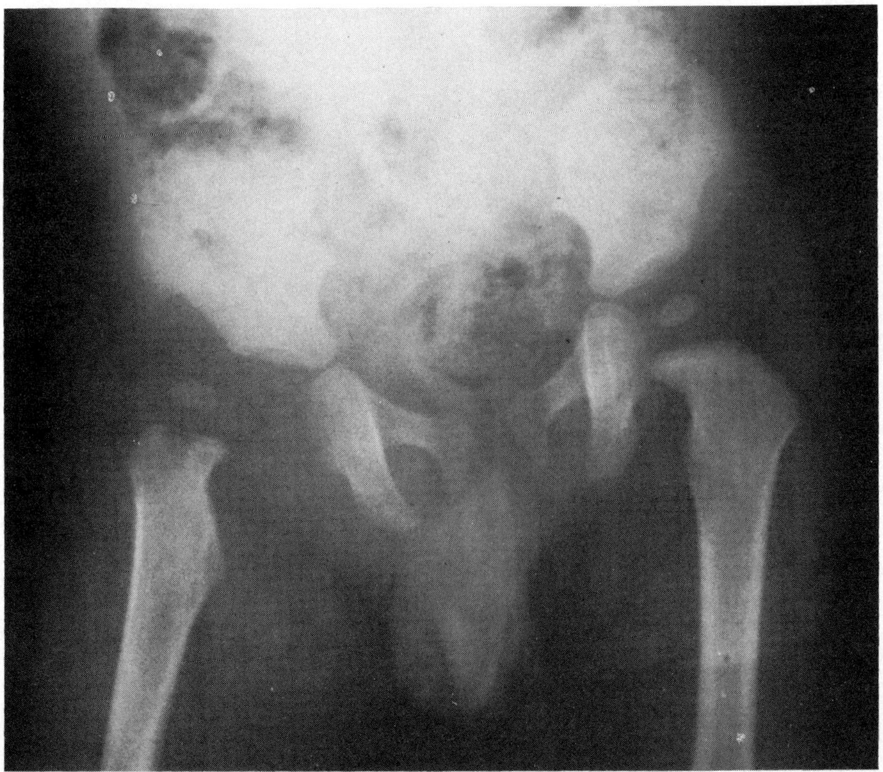

Figure 4–68. Radiograph of the case illustrated in Figure 4–67, 1 week later. The soft tissue swelling has diminished markedly. The hip is still dislocated, and the ossification center for the femoral head appears more radiolucent.

usually appears before the age of 6 months and may continue in waves of activity until age 2 years. Biopsy, when necessary, will differentiate the pure reactive process of Caffey's disease from other processes with their characteristic findings.

SUPPURATIVE ARTHRITIS

Bacterial infections of joints cause profound local destruction of cartilage and bone. Organisms most often enter the joint by direct implantation from trauma or surgery, less often by spread from an adjacent metaphyseal focus of osteomyelitis.

Accumulation of the cells and fluid of purulent exudate causes capsular distention and stretching of ligaments. The capsular distention can interfere with normal cartilage nutrition and result in death of large numbers of chondrocytes. Distention, when combined with destruction of cartilage and bone, can result in dislocation. This is especially true in the hip of the newborn. The femoral head is almost entirely cartilage, and the joint lies directly beneath the femoral artery and vein. Repeated attempts to draw blood from the femoral vein can result in direct inoculation of the joint with subsequent death of the femoral head and dislocation of the hip (Figs. 4–67 to 4–70). Subluxation or dislocation can also occur in the adult from major destruction of bone and periarticular support structures (Figs. 4–71 to 4–73).

As acute inflammatory cells and cartilage cells disintegrate, they release proteolytic enzymes from their cytoplasm, and progressive destruction of the articular

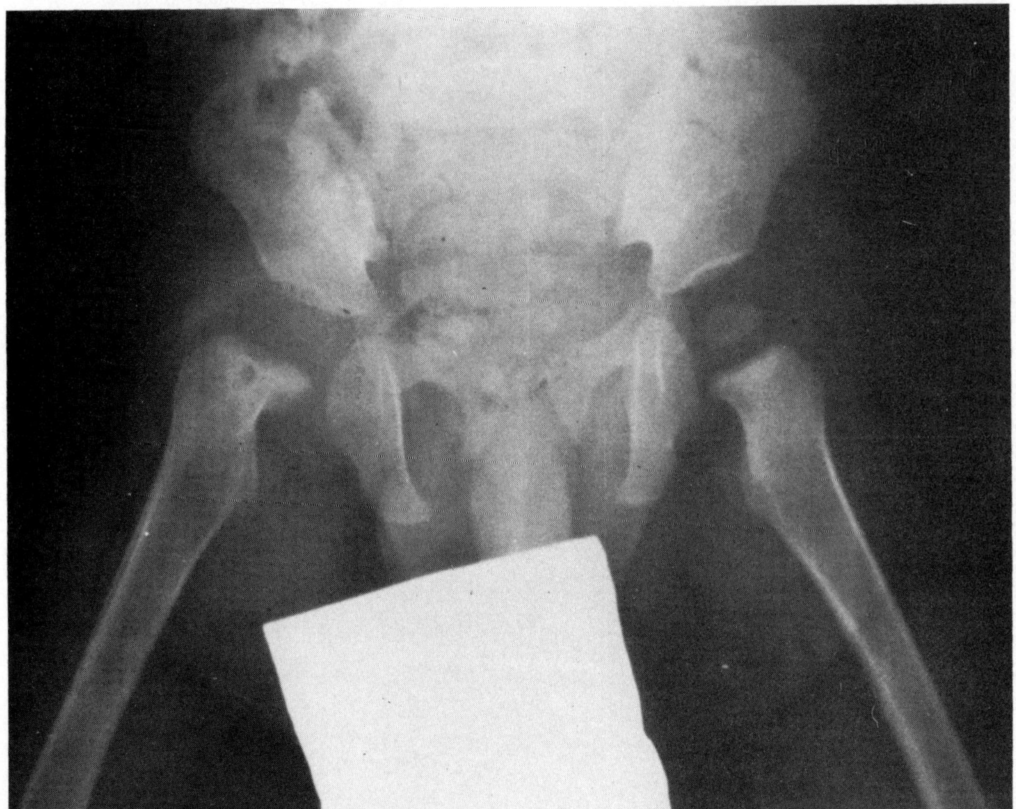

Figure 4–69. The proximal femur of the patient in Figures 4–67 and 4–68 has been repositioned in proximity to the acetabulum. The ossific nucleus for the femoral head is absent. There are changes of lucency and sclerosis in the proximal femoral metaphysis, with widening and alteration of shape.

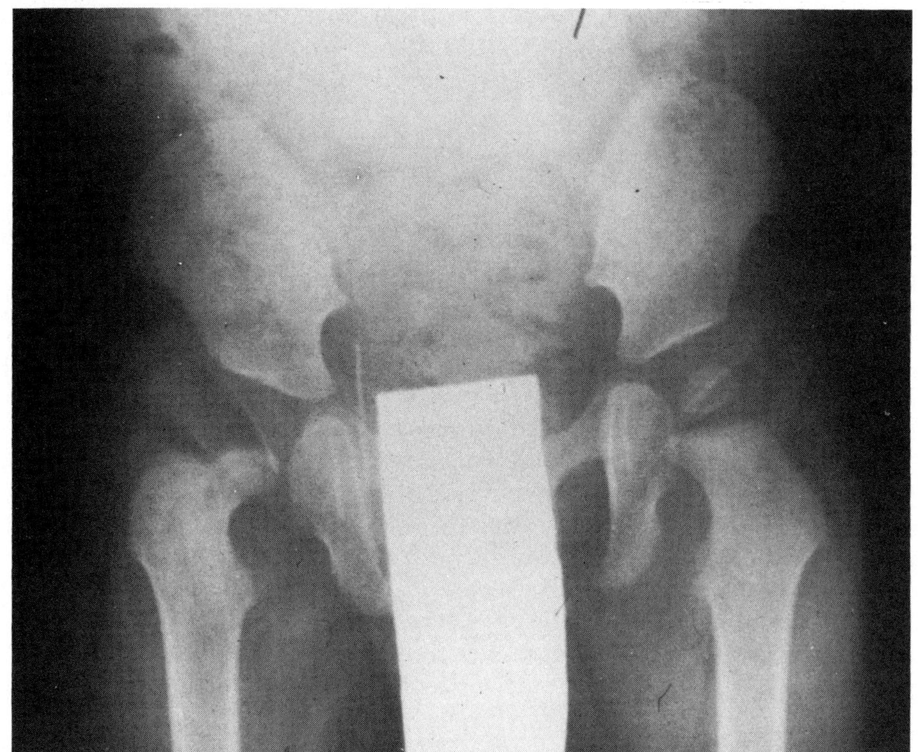

Figure 4–70. *See legend on opposite page.*

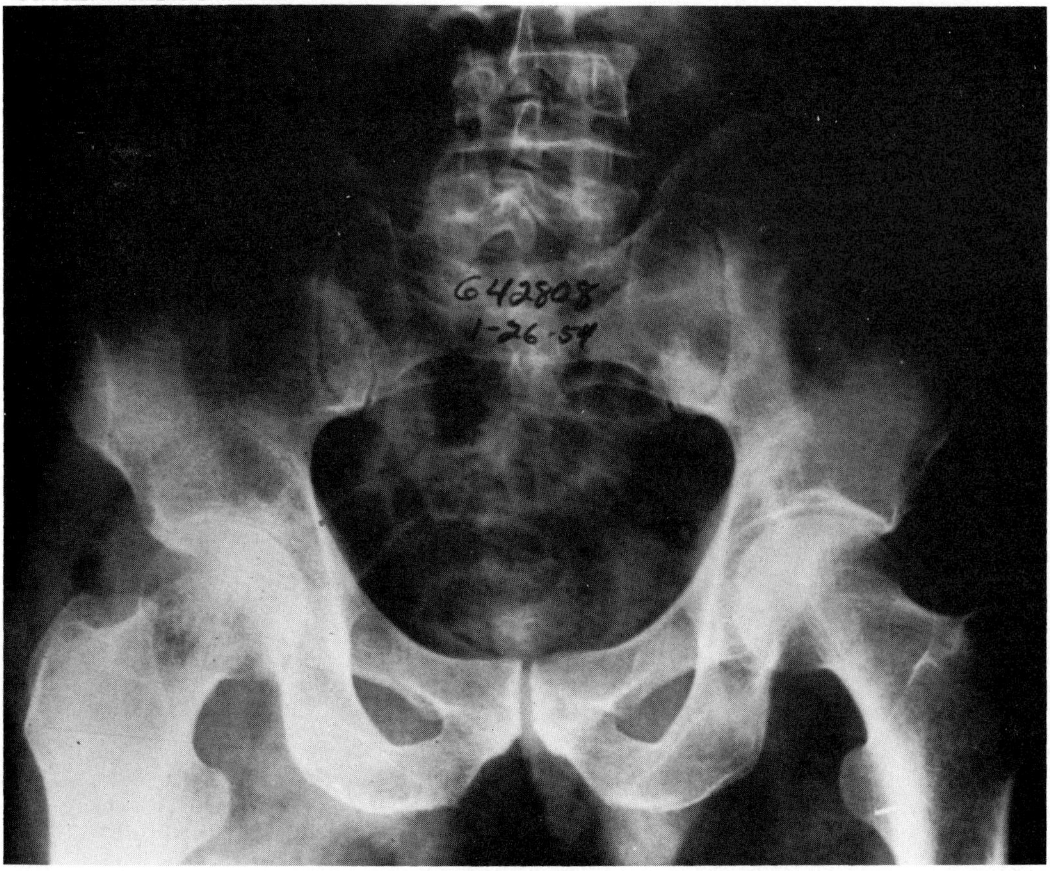

Figure 4–71. *See legend on opposite page.*

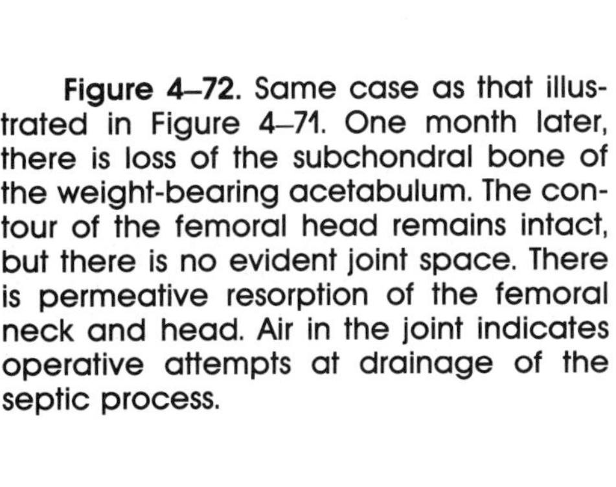

Figure 4–72. Same case as that illustrated in Figure 4–71. One month later, there is loss of the subchondral bone of the weight-bearing acetabulum. The contour of the femoral head remains intact, but there is no evident joint space. There is permeative resorption of the femoral neck and head. Air in the joint indicates operative attempts at drainage of the septic process.

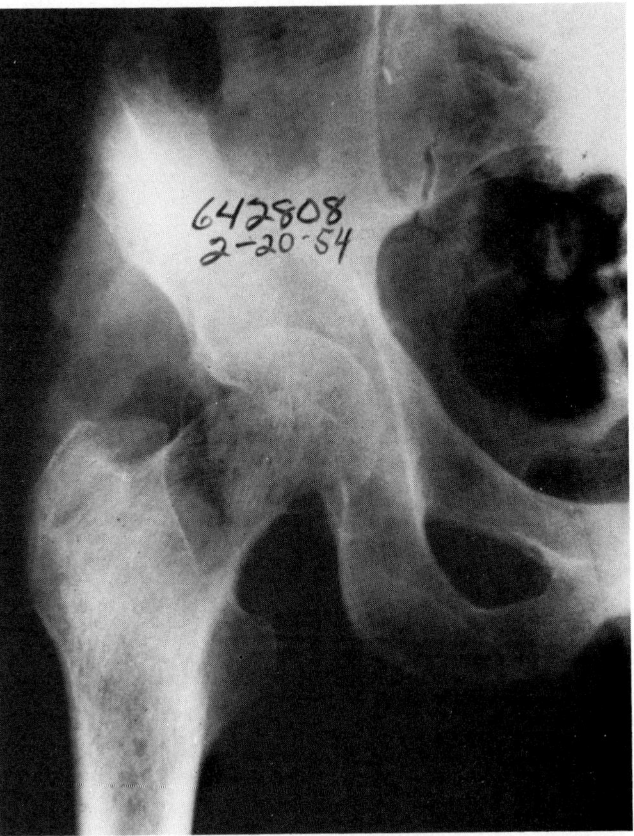

surface ensues (Fig. 4–74). The process of enzymatic cartilage destruction will continue even after the joint is sterilized by antibiotic therapy. Continued use of the joint will then result in rapid disintegration from wear and tear, and radiographically the changes are most pronounced in contact areas (Figs. 4–75 and 4–76). This contrasts with the erosion seen in tuberculosis and rheumatoid arthritis, which is the result of pannus formation and occurs at the non–weight-bearing margins of the joint.

Once the articular surface has worn away, the subchondral bone may also be penetrated, with the infection extending into the metaphysis. Hyperemia causes extensive osteoporosis around the joint. Continued use of this weakened deformed bone will result in gross and microscopic changes of total joint disorganization. Even if the infection is healed at this point, the destroyed joint will not recover. Extensive scar-tissue formation may result in fibrous ankylosis and eventually spontaneous arthrodesis (Figs. 4–77 to 4–82).

Since motion is so detrimental to the damaged cartilage during the acute stage of the infection, it is clinically advisable to rest the infected joint until the process has

Text continued on page 160

Figure 4–70. Same case as that illustrated in the preceding three figures. Six months after the onset, the proximal femur is still repositioned in proximity to the acetabulum. There are multiple changes in the proximal metaphysis suggesting chronic osteomyelitis, and the ossific nucleus for the femoral head remains absent.

Figure 4–71. Anteroposterior radiograph of the pelvis of an adult with osteomyelitis and septic arthritis in the right hip. There is marked thinning of the joint space and radiolucencies in the femoral head and neck.

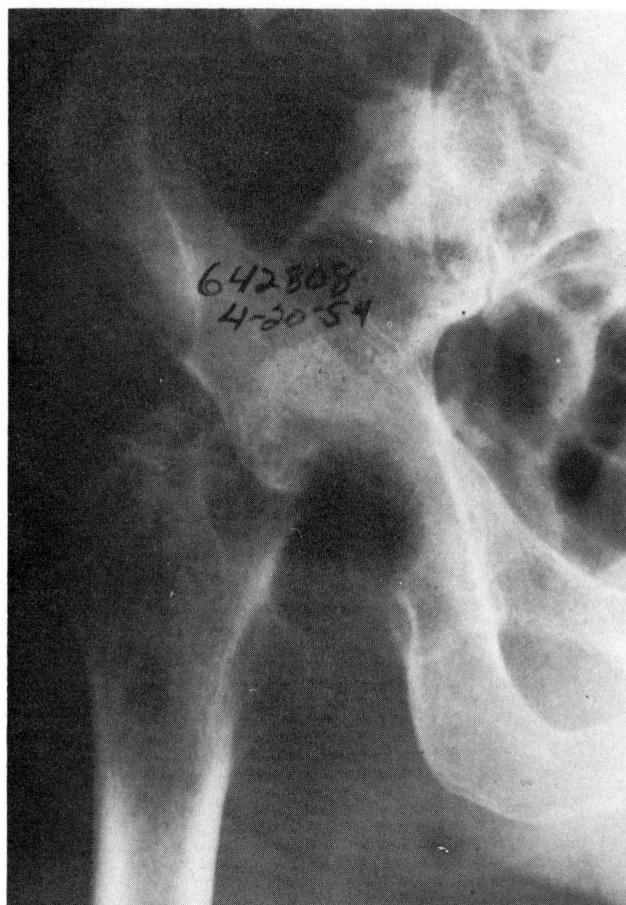

Figure 4–73. Postoperative film following further attempts of débridement of the infected joint. Major portions of the femoral head are gone. The joint is dislocated. There is severe osteoporosis of the entire proximal end of the femur resulting from a combination of inflammation and disuse.

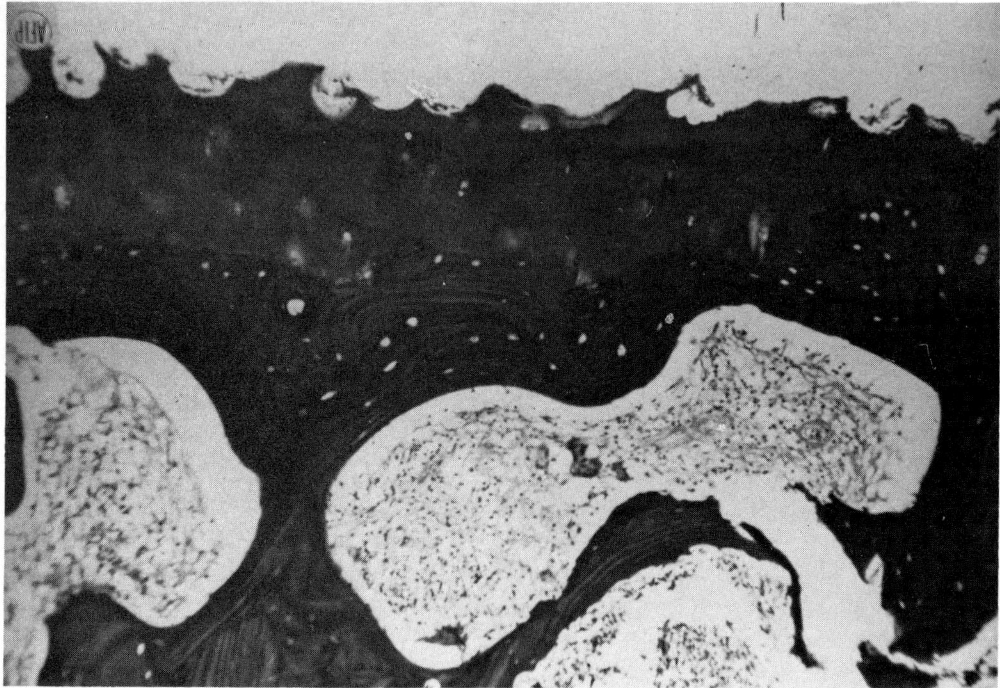

Figure 4–74. Section through the articular surface of a septic hip joint. Note the absence of articular cartilage down to the level of the calcified tide mark. The subchondral bone remains intact. There are inflammatory changes in the subjacent marrow.

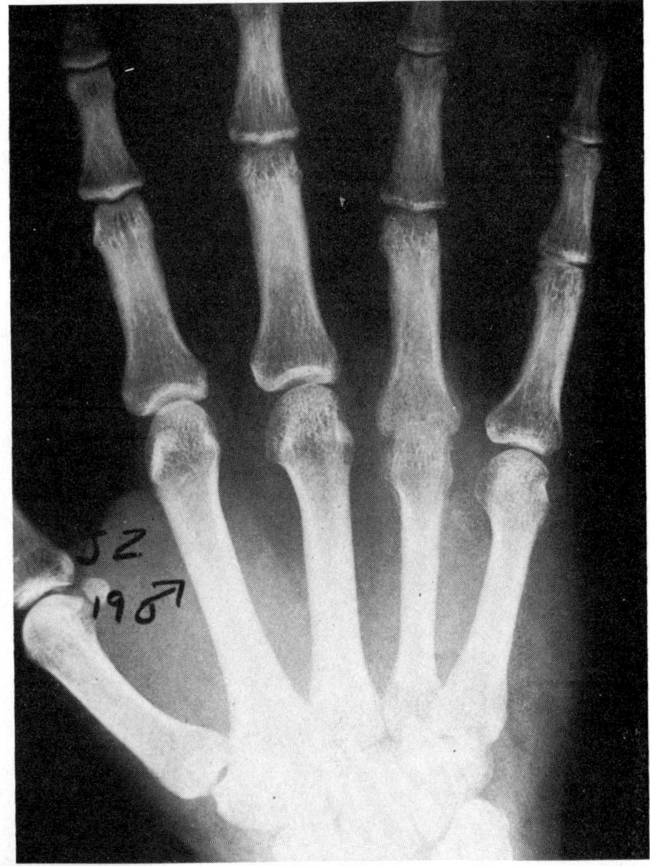

Figure 4–75. Radiograph of the hand of a patient with gonococcal arthritis of the metacarpal-phalangeal joint of the ring finger. Note the para-articular osteoporosis, the virtual disappearance of the joint space and subchondral bony plates, and the soft tissue swelling of the digit.

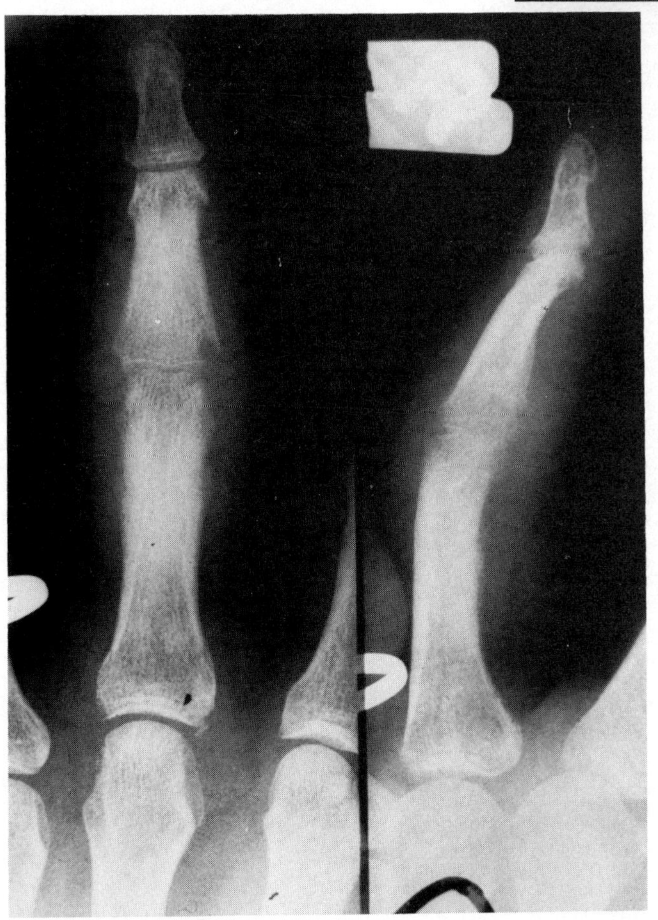

Figure 4–76. Radiograph of a finger with purulent arthritis of the proximal interphalangeal joint. Soft tissue swelling is pronounced, and there is major destruction of the bone on either side of the joint with periosteal new bone formation. There is loss of the joint space and of subchondral bony plates.

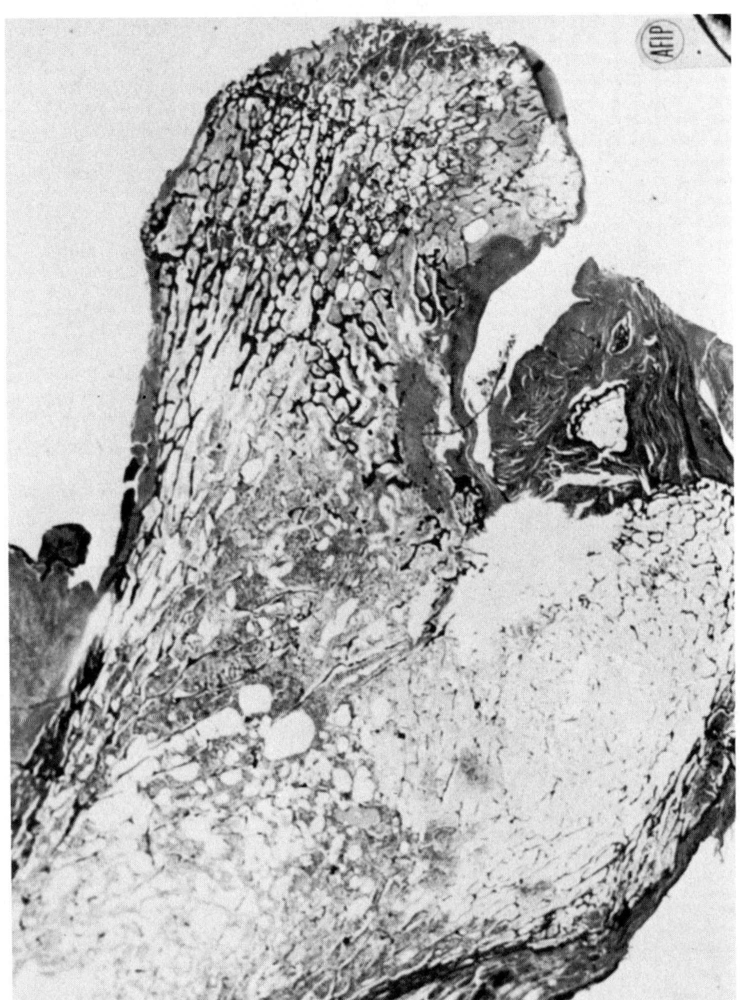

Figure 4–77. Macrosection of the proximal femur following septic arthritis. Note the deformity of the femoral head and the absence of major portions of bone. The articular surface is entirely devoid of cartilage.

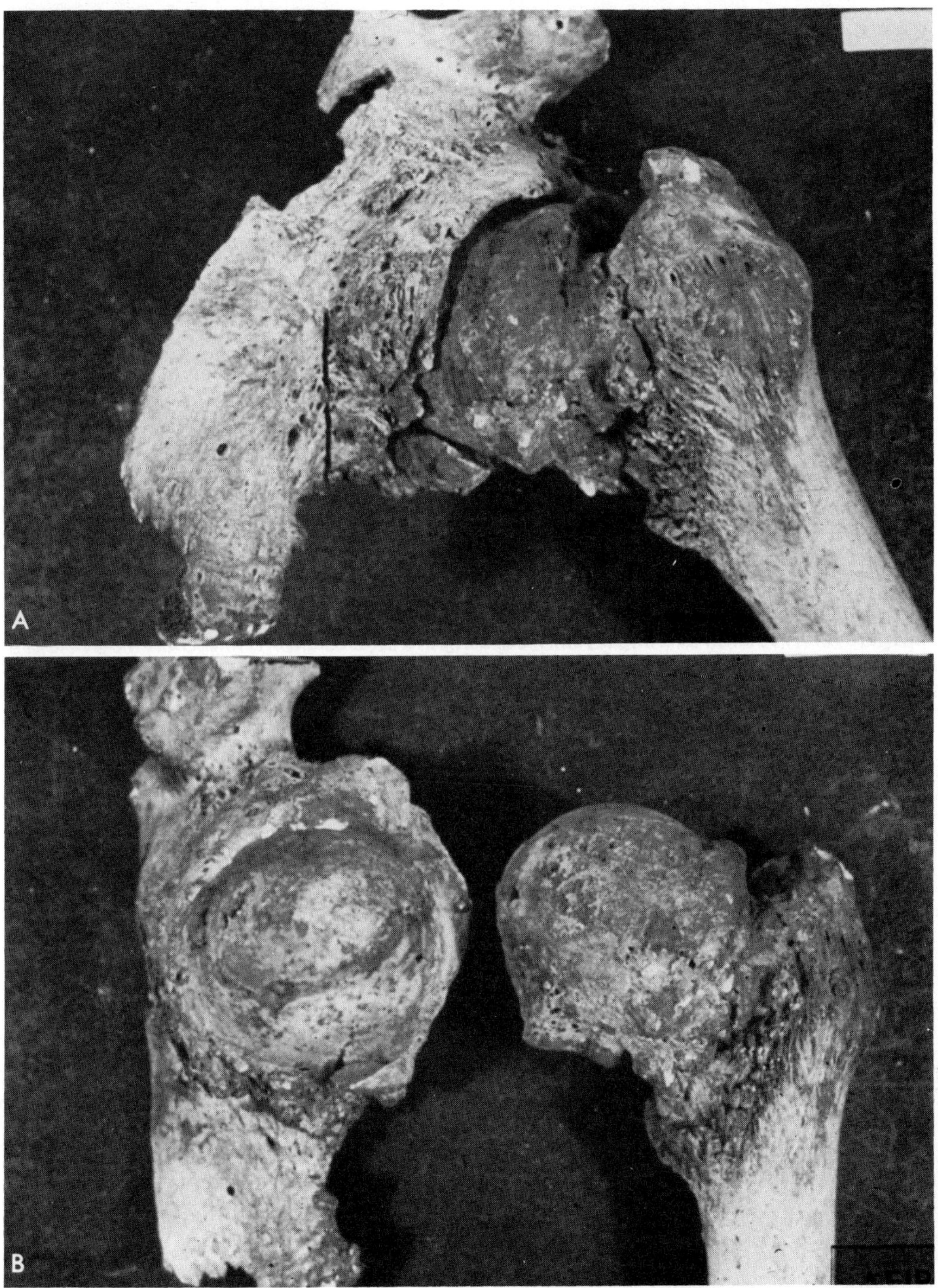

Figure 4–78. Gross specimens of femur and acetabulum dating from the Civil War era. The changes that followed an old infection secondary to a gunshot wound are shown. Trauma is a major cause of joint infections, and antibiotics have not changed this picture. Note the absence of subchondral bone and matching deformities of the head and acetabulum. The process had continued for 1 year before the patient died.

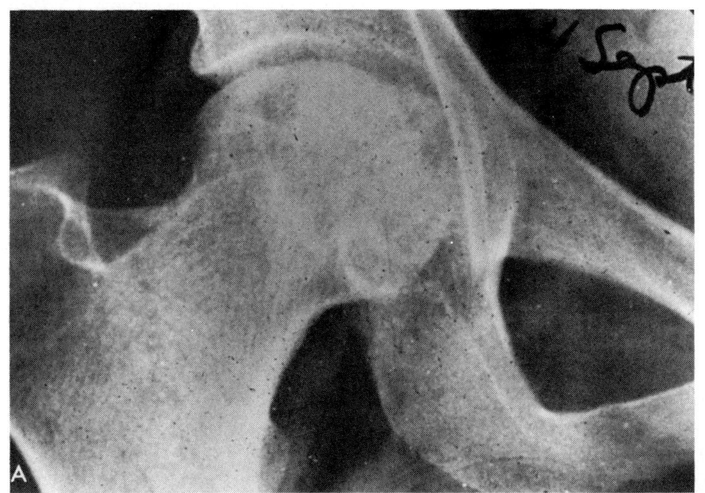

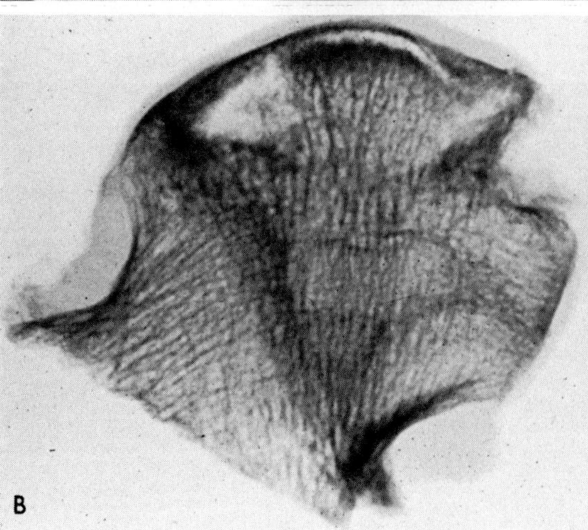

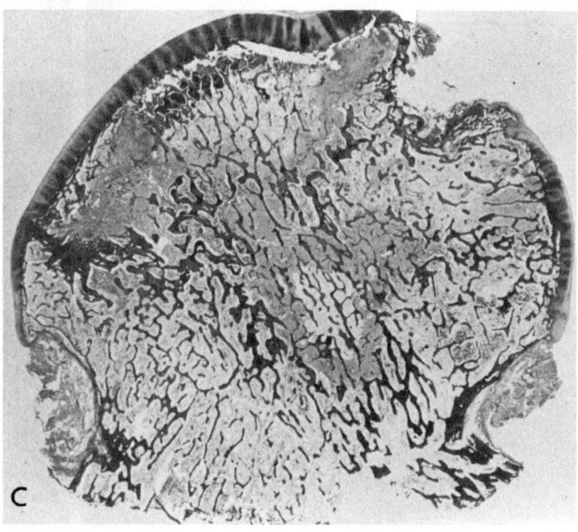

Figure 5–4. Clinical radiograph *(A)*, specimen radiograph *(B)*, and corresponding macrospecimen *(C)* of femoral head from a 26-year-old patient on long-term steroid therapy for idiopathic thrombocytopenic purpura with progressive pain and disability of both hips. Note the crescent sign, a cleft beneath the articular cartilage due to compression fractures of dead trabeculae. Also note the lytic areas in lateral aspect of the femoral head due to revascularization with removal of dead trabeculae and replacement with viable fibrous tissue. Zones of increased density are also evident.

Figure 5–5. Schematic diagram of the femoral head illustrated in Figure 5–4. Articular cartilage is not visible radiographically. The irregular contour of the femoral head is due to impaction of the infarcted trabeculae in the subchondral zone. The sharply circumscribed lytic defect on the lateral margin is due to creeping substitution: ischemic scar tissue removing infarcted trabeculae of bone. This ischemic tissue also extends into the zone in which trabeculae still retain their original density, and further removal of infarcted bone will follow once blood supply is re-established. The pale-staining areas in the center of the ischemic zones, best seen in the macrospecimen, are infarcted areas in which there has been no revascularization. The increased density at the base of the infarct is due to appositional bone growth on existing trabeculae and represents the organism's effort to wall off the infarct. The increased density below the cleft is a result of impaction of infarcted bone fragments. The osteoporotic bone in the neck of the femur is clearly identifiable in the macrospecimen as well as in the specimen radiograph and may be due to either disuse or the osteoclastic effect of steroid therapy.

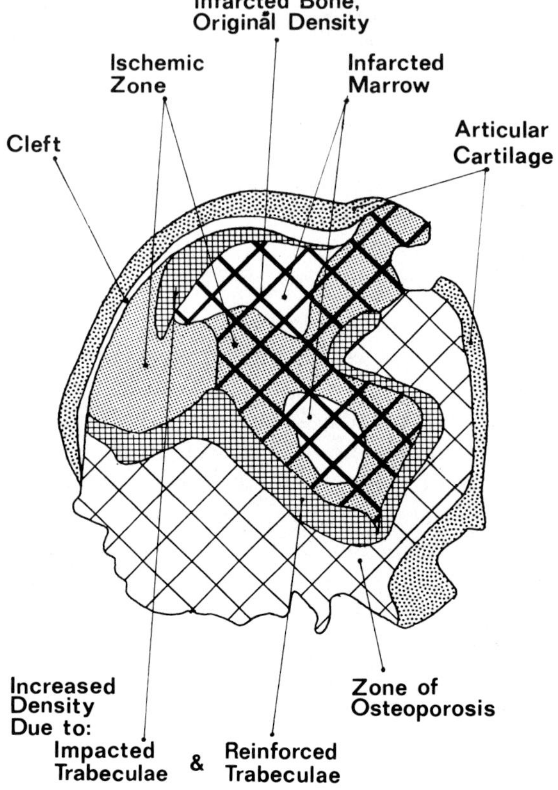

from the periosteum is interrupted, but in most instances periosteal blood supply is maintained, and therefore cortical infarction is rare. Once the marrow is infarcted, the first tissue to disappear is hematopoietic tissue. After a short period, marrow fat cells lose their cellular outline and ultimately succumb to fat necrosis. The osteocytes usually disappear from the lacunae at that point. Prior to the death of the osteocyte, lacunar enlargement may be noted in infarcted bone. This confirms the capability of the osteocyte to resorb bone under appropriate circumstances.

The bone infarct incites the same inflammatory response as that seen with an infarct at any other site within the body (Figs. 5–5 to 5–10). The infarcted tissue is sharply demarcated from surrounding tissue that has maintained its blood supply. In the immediate vicinity of the infarcted zone, there is a zone of variable width in which there is ischemic damage but not complete infarction. This zone contains dense fibrous connective tissue but mature osseous structures are not formed. Outside the ischemic zone, there is a hyperemic reactive zone from which granulation tissue

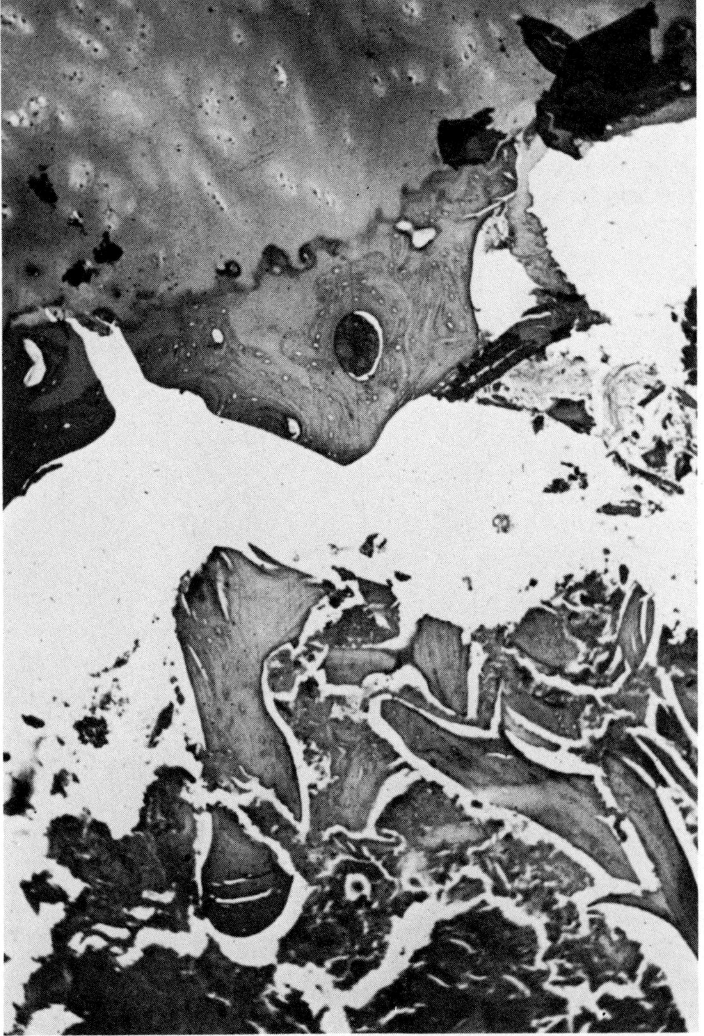

Figure 5–6. Subchondral plate with crescent sign. The cleft is created by dead brittle bone fragments that have become separated from the remainder of the subchondral plate. Notice that the cartilage is viable. (Chondrocytes are not dependent on blood supply.)

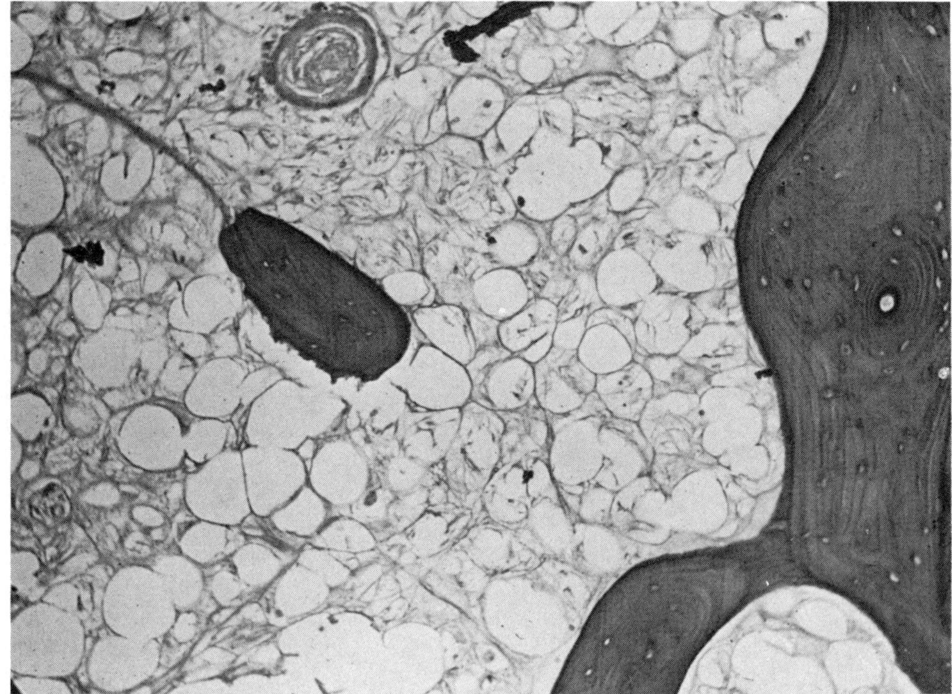

Figure 5–7. Bone from central area of infarction, exhibiting infarcted fatty tissue, obliterated vessels, and infarcted bone. Note absence of either osteoclastic or osteoblastic activity. The trabeculae in this zone have retained their original density.

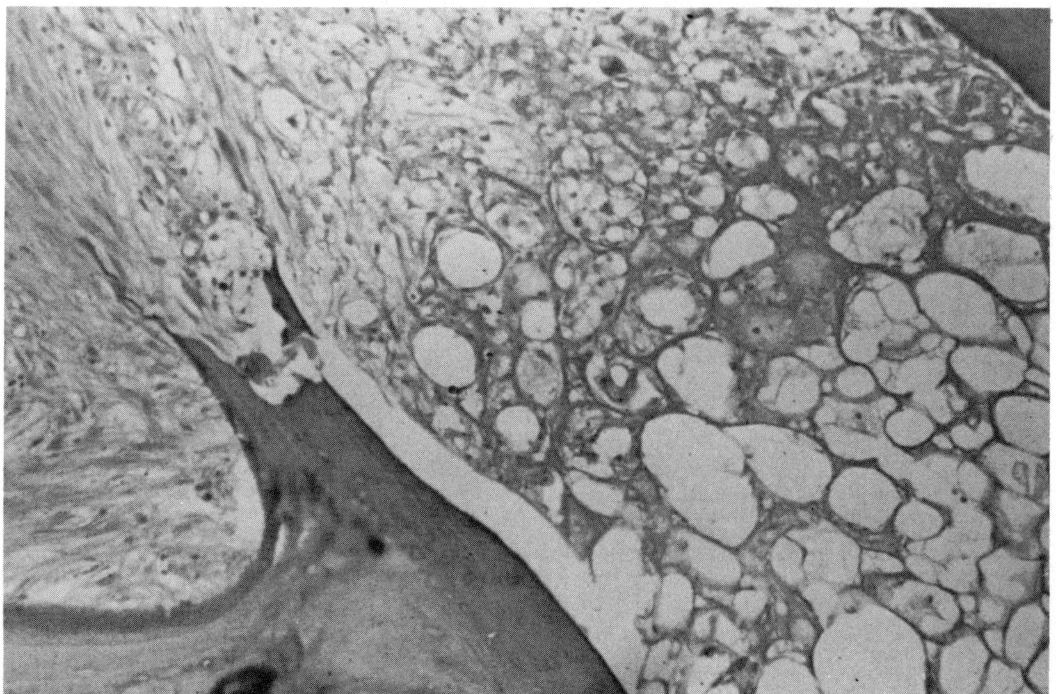

Figure 5–8. Junction of ischemic and infarcted zones. The ischemic zone, on the left side of the photograph, consists of dense fibrous connective tissue. Note that there is some osteoclastic activity at the junction of dead and ischemic tissue, with removal of infarcted fragments of the bone.

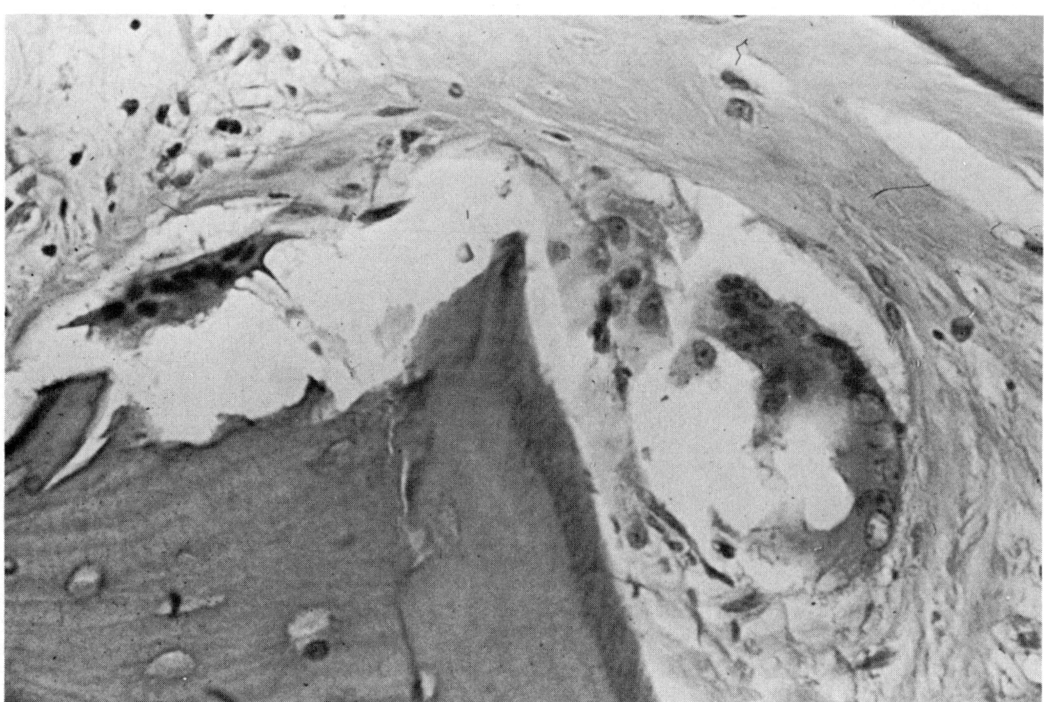

Figure 5–9. Higher magnification of ischemic zone with osteoclasts. The osteoclasts remove the previously infarcted bone fragments, preparing the way for creeping substitution.

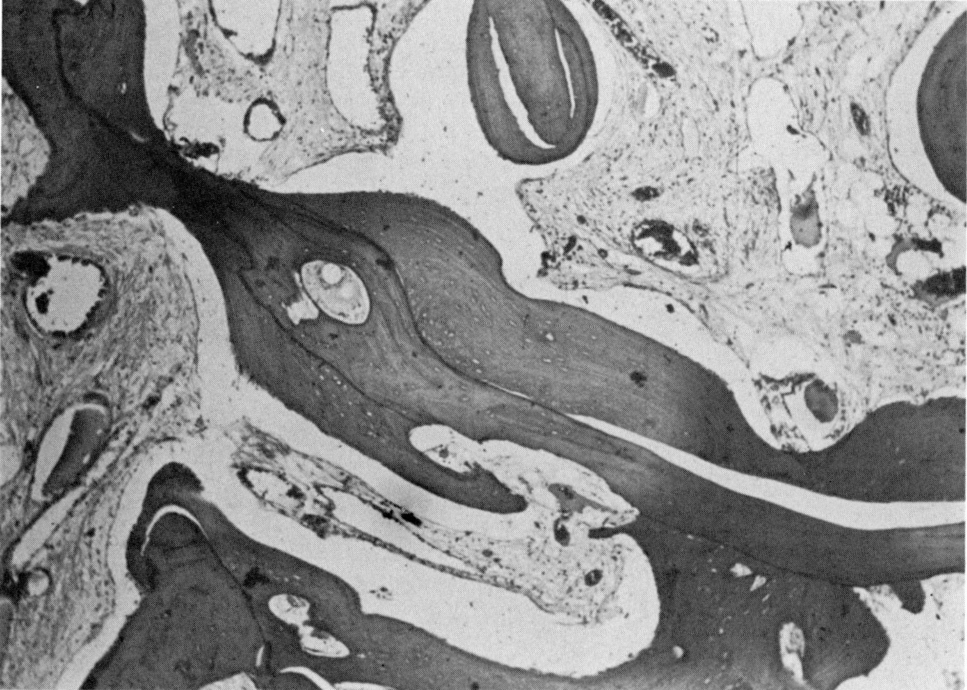

Figure 5–10. Zone of increased density at the base of the infarct as a result of appositional bone growth at the edge of infarcted tissue. The original trabecula can be seen in the center, and well-defined mature appositional lamellae of bone are present on either side of the original trabecula. Ischemic tissue is present on both sides of the reinforced trabeculae, with numerous vascular channels.

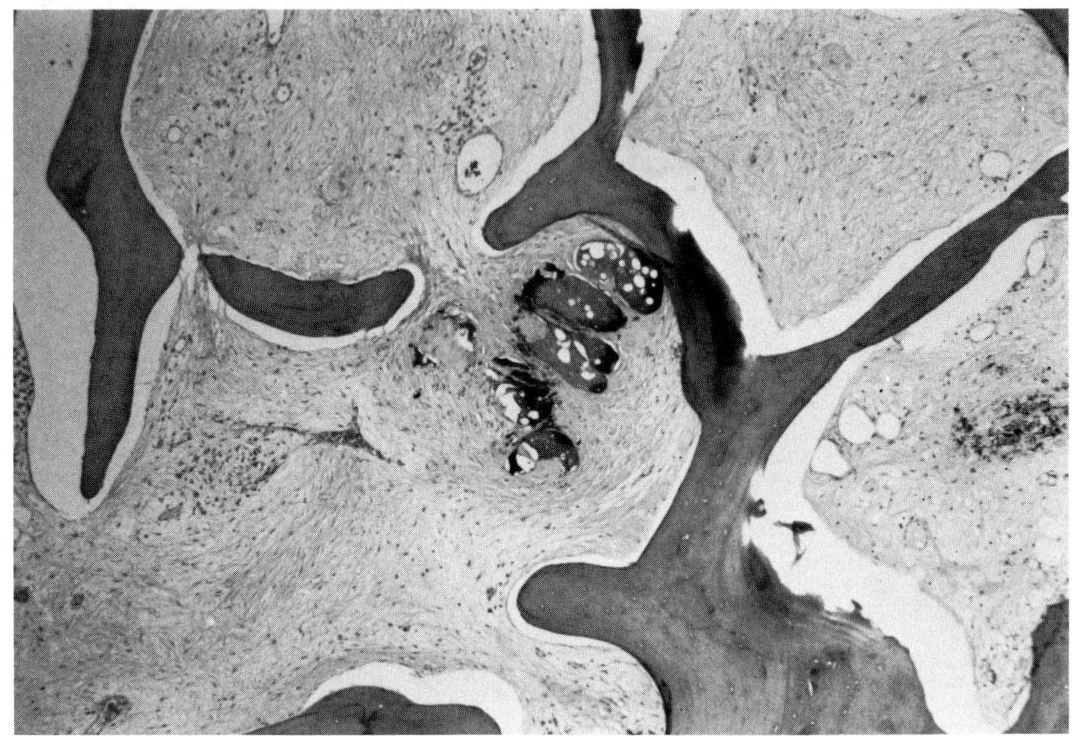

Figure 5–11. Focal area of calcification and saponification of infarcted fat. The saponified fat is surrounded by ischemic marrow replacement tissue.

enters the infarcted zone. Fibrovascular proliferation is noted, and the new blood supply is accompanied by osteoclasts removing dead bone. Osteoblasts also accompany the revascularized tissue; thus, there is not only removal of infarcted bone but also stimulation of new bone formation ("creeping substitution"). Numerous trabeculae of new bone will use the infarcted bone as a scaffold, thus incorporating the infarcted fragments into the reparative process. The ability of granulation tissue to form new bone on the lattice of old infarcted bone is the basis for the success of bone grafts.

If an infarct is of limited size and blood supply can be re-established in a short time, the recovery will occur without any persistent damage to the structural integrity of the bone. If the infarction is of longer duration, not only the bone but also the marrow fat will undergo structural changes. As fat cells are deprived of their blood supply, there is a breakdown into fatty acids and triglycerides, and calcification, or "saponification," will occur. As a rule, the deposition of calcium is not sufficient to increase the radiographic density. (Fig. 5–11).

The consequences of infarction may vary from none to severe degenerative osteoarthritis, depending on the location of the infarct. Dead bone will not resist or transmit stress in the normal manner. Continued use of infarcted bone will result in multiple small fractures of the infarcted trabeculae. This is of particular importance in the subchondral plate of a major weight-bearing bone (Figs. 5–12 and 5–13). With continued use of an infarcted bone, there is impaction of the dead trabeculae that results in more trabeculae per unit area than previously. Radiographically, this is demonstrated by a dense shadow in this particular region. A cleft is created between the impacted trabecular bone and the old subchondral plate because the overlying cartilage rebounds away from the dead bone. This cleft is a prominent radiographic feature, the "crescent sign" (Figs. 5–14 and 5–15).

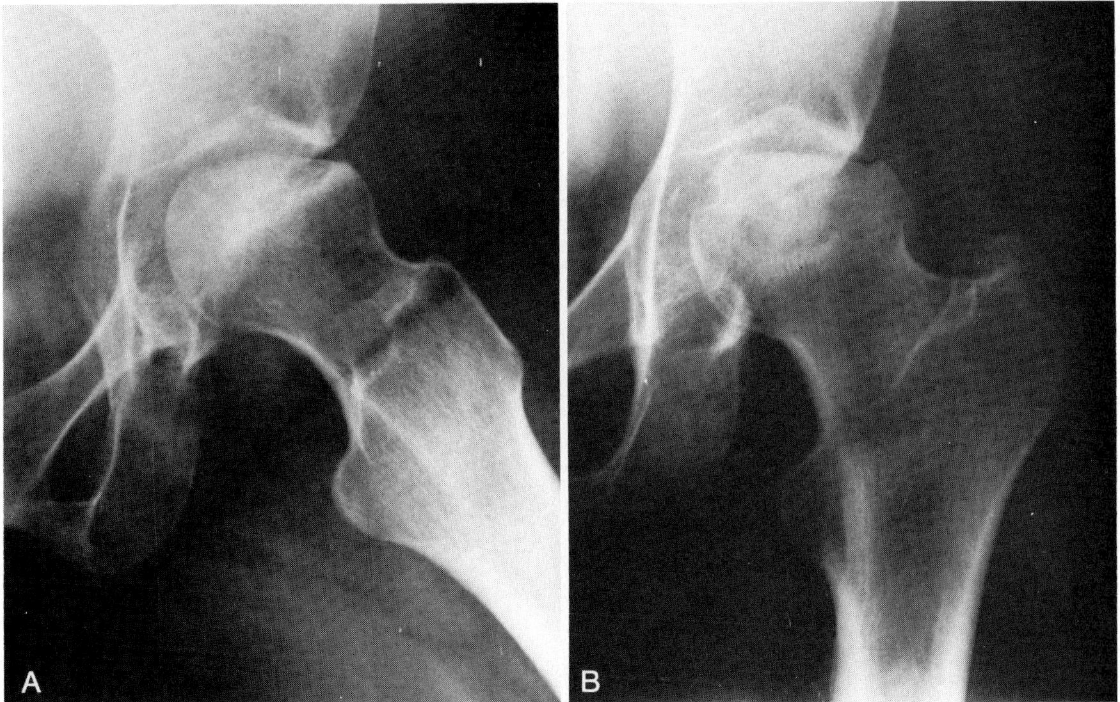

Figure 5–12. Frogleg *(A)* and anteroposterior *(B)* radiographs of patient with collapse of femoral head due to idiopathic avascular necrosis. Areas of trabecular reinforcement demarcate peripheral extent of lesion. Collapse of the head occurs during the healing phase, when removal of dead bone creates loss of support during weight-bearing.

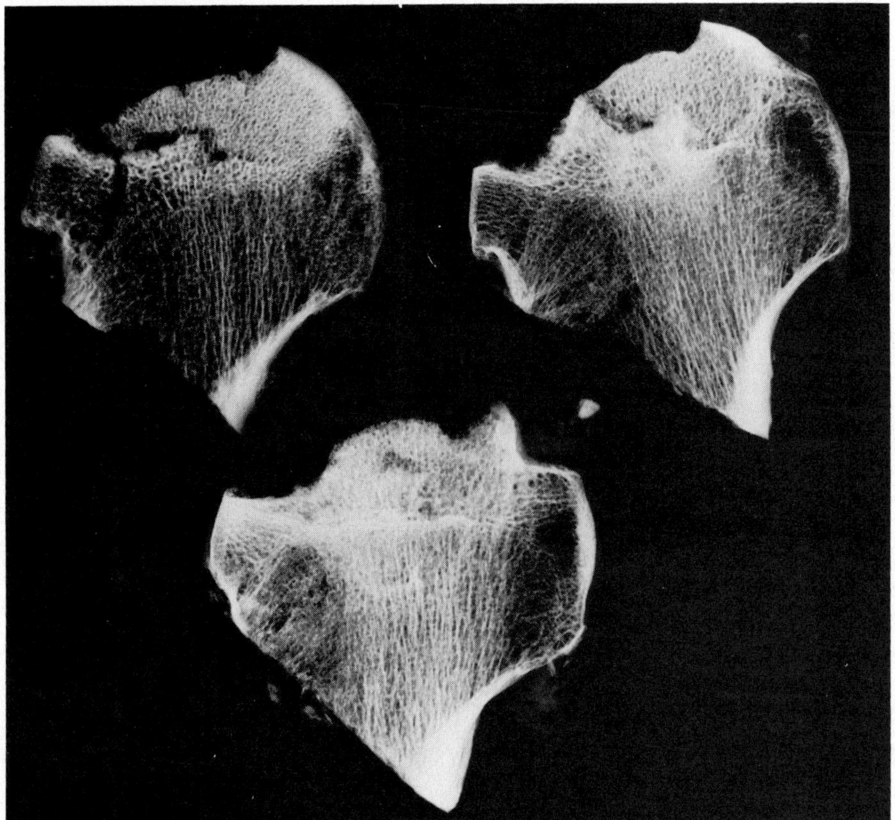

Figure 5–13. Specimen radiograph of slices through femoral head. Zone of trabecular reinforcement in the metaphysis is adjacent to the advancing margin of vascular invasion. Note removal of dead trabeculae and radiographic lucency.

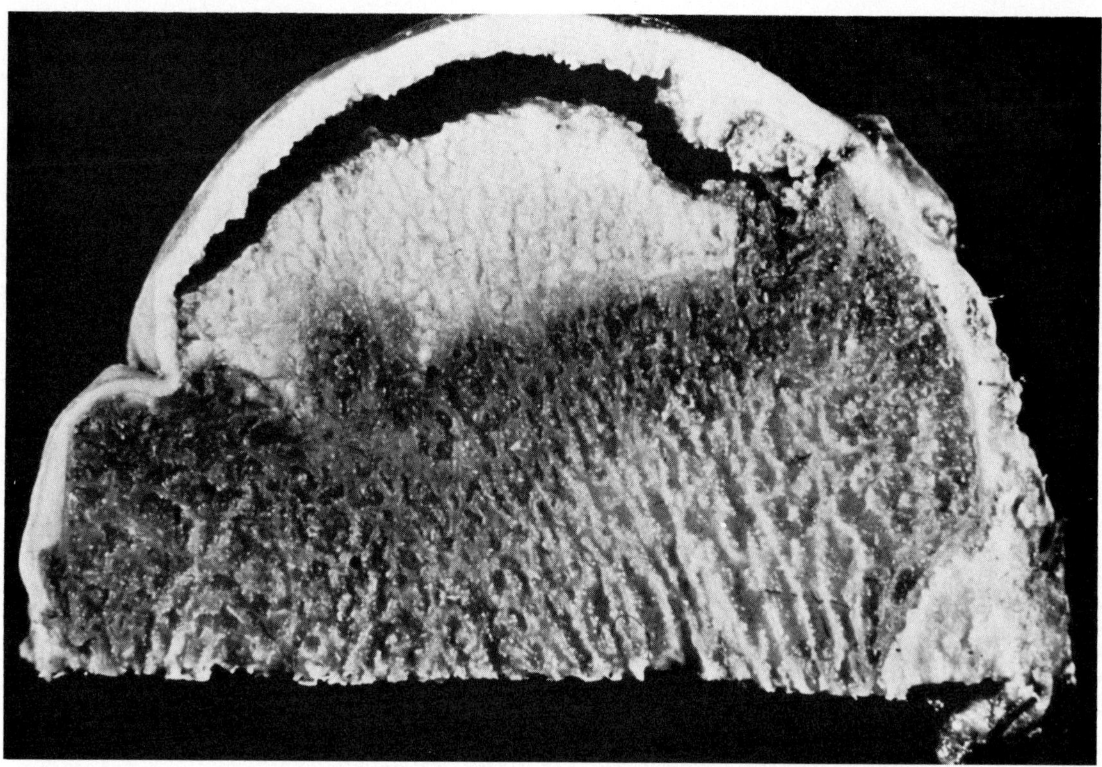

Figure 5–14. Gross specimen of femoral head with infarct. Note subchondral cleft resulting from impaction fractures of dead trabecular bone and rebound of the more elastic cartilage. Dense white bone is dead; adjacent to it is a darker vascular area (hyperemic border). Beyond that is normal bone of metaphysis (femoral neck).

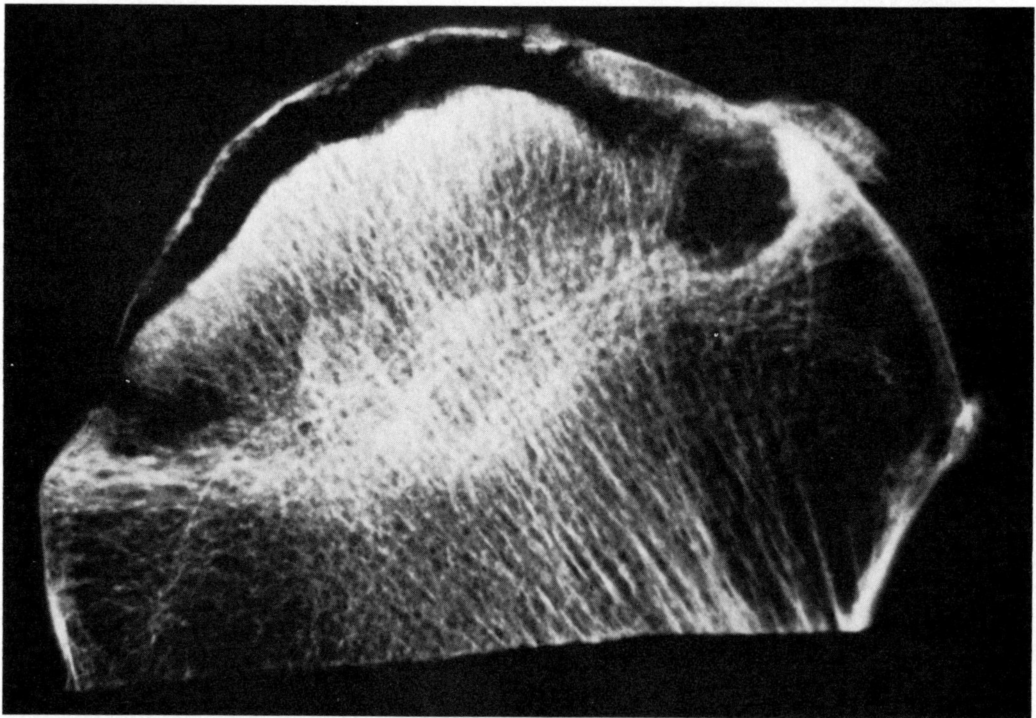

Figure 5–15. Specimen radiograph of the femoral head shown in Figure 5–15. Subchondral cleft is dark owing to absence of bone. At each end is a dark area, also with bone removed but replaced by vascularized fibrous granulation tissue invading and cleaning up the debris of the infarct. Reinforced trabeculae of the infarct margin are well seen.

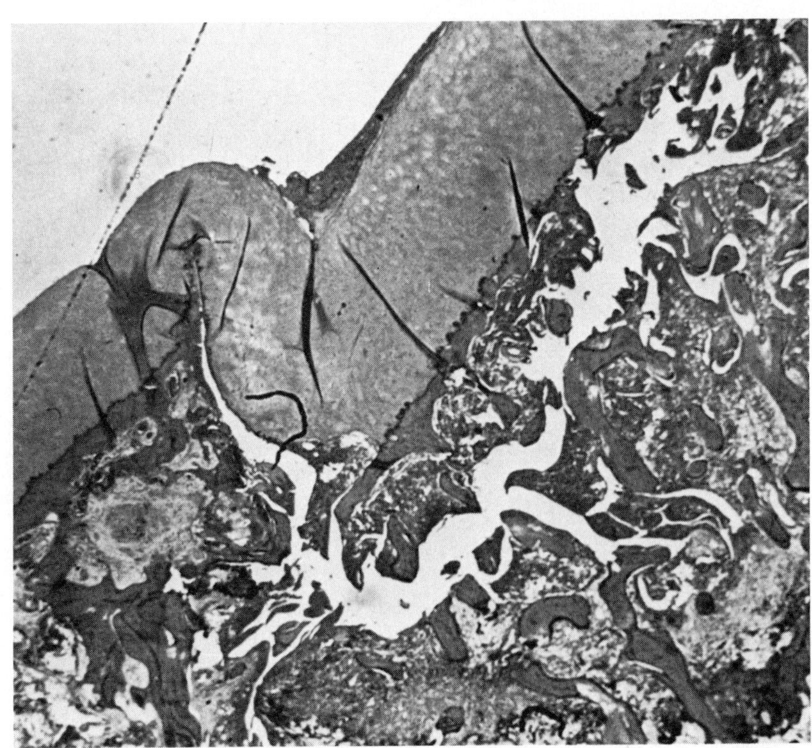

Figure 5–16. Section through articular surface at margin of infarct. Vascular invasion and removal of dead tissue begins at the margins of the infarct. Continued weight-bearing after removal of dead bone and before the replacement with new living bone ("creeping substitution") causes collapse of portions of the articular surface with buckling at the margins. This can be seen grossly as groove in the articular surface.

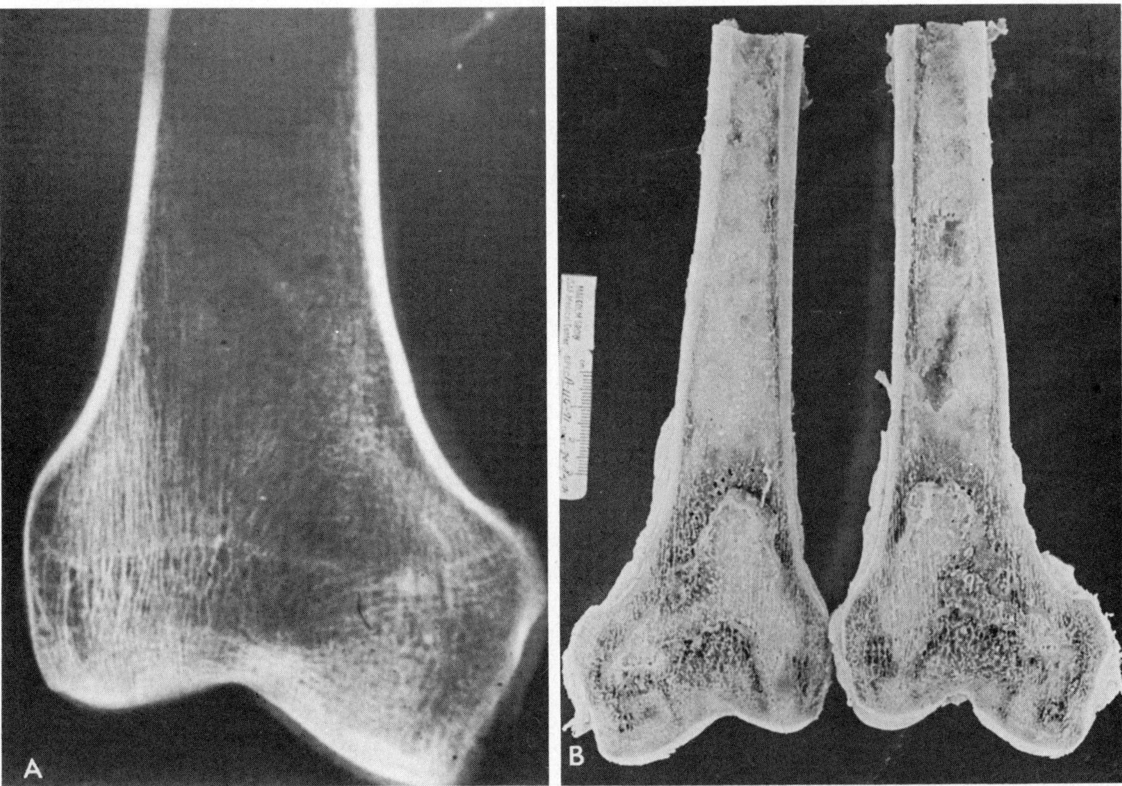

Figure 5–17. Specimen radiograph *(A)* and specimen *(B)* of the distal femur from an asymptomatic patient on long-term steroid therapy for lupus erythematosus. Splitting the femur discloses a large infarct, sharply circumscribed, with a zone of ischemia as well as total infarction. At this stage, no radiographic evidence of the infarct is present. Structural changes will occur only when the repair process replaces infarcted bone, many months after the actual infarct occurs (Lee et al., 1980). If structural changes are severe near a joint, the process may lead to degenerative osteoarthritis.

Cartilage depends on synovial fluid for nutrition, and therefore the superficial layers of articular cartilage are not infarcted when the blood supply to bone is interrupted (Fig. 5–6). The deeper layers will show variable changes.

Reactive margins of infarct are readily demonstrated by the white fibrous zone of connective tissue; however, this zone is not visible radiographically (Fig. 5–17). The impacted zone beneath the subchondral plate is of increased radiographic density; conversely, those areas in which revascularization has already been established and some of the infarcted bone has been removed will demonstrate decreased radiographic density. If the zone of demarcation around the infarct persists for longer periods, it will be characterized by an increased density of bone caused by the appositional bone growth at the edge of the infarct: first granulation tissue, then scar tissue formation, and finally bone formation and delineation of the infarct.

At the moment of infarction, dead bone will not show any radiographic change. Radiographs will indicate the area of infarction only when secondary structural changes occur, long after the infarction has occurred.

The diagnosis is based on changes in density. In general, density of bone may be either unchanged, decreased, or increased. Increased or decreased densities are relative concepts, dependent on what happens to the adjacent viable bone. The diagnosis of a bone infarct is classically made on the basis of the *appearance* of increased density. In reality, the infarcted bone itself is unchanged. Without blood supply, there can be no cellular activity, and there can be no loss or increase in bone substance. The "increased density" of infarction and the "dense" sequestrum of osteomyelitis represent pre-existing bone of *unchanged* density. The active hyperemia of the inflammatory reaction, inducing osteoclastic resorption of the adjacent bone, reduces the density of

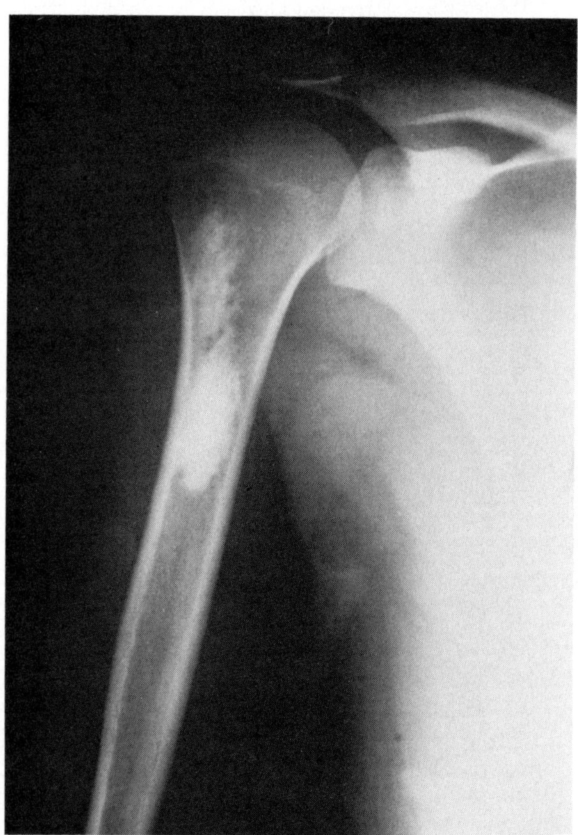

Figure 5–18. Radiograph of humerus of patient with history of deep-sea diving. The sclerotic area represents infarction of the marrow cavity with formation of calcium soaps and new bone from the reparative margins.

the viable bone but leaves the infarcted bone unchanged. Thus, the "increased density" actually represents unchanged density. It is a result of osteoclastic resorption of adjacent structures and delineates the infarcted area.

Actual increased radiographic density is the result of associated conditions: There may be fracture with collapse and impaction of cancellous fragments, saponification of fat (formation of calcium soaps), and appositional bone growth on the trabeculae of bone at the margin of the infarct as part of the inflammatory reaction demarcating the infarct. The first two types of increases in density occur in areas of dead or ischemic bone; the last requires living tissue with intact vascularization.

It is thus clear that failure to change bone density in the presence of developing osteoporosis is evidence of infarction; conversely, decreased density is evidence of vascularization and viable bone, and finally, true increase in density can occur in living or dead bone.

ASEPTIC NECROSIS

The term "aseptic necrosis" refers to infarction of bone; the two terms are interchangeable. "Aseptic" is used to distinguish the septic infarct of osteomyelitis from the aseptic necrosis of infarction. An inflammatory response is characteristic of both conditions.

LEGG-CALVÉ-PERTHES DISEASE

Legg-Calvé-Perthes disease is a peculiar aseptic necrosis of the proximal femur due to infarction. The infarction is localized to the epiphysis prior to the closure of the growth plate (Figs. 5–19 and 5–20). It is presumably due to interruption of the blood supply to the epiphysis, resulting in localized infarction, although other factors may also play a role (Catterall, 1981). The joint space appears widened because of continued growth of articular cartilage that is nourished by joint fluid but not replaced by enchondral ossification in the epiphysis. The secondary ossification center fails to expand and keep pace with cartilage development. The clear areas in the metaphysis usually represent hyperemic tissue removing bone (active hyperemia). In the long run, usually after 4 or 5 years, the head of the femur is reconstituted by slow revascularization. However, the bone is usually deformed, with coxa magna and a short, broad neck. The shortness is due to loss of growth in the epiphysis; the germinal cells have lost their blood supply. The broad neck is secondary to the hyperemia, bone loss, periosteal reaction, and ultimate condensation with inlay bone (Fig. 5–21). The microscopic picture of Legg-Calvé-Perthes disease demonstrates the usual features of infarction of bone, without any characteristics that differentiate it from infarcts due to other etiology. Legg-Calvé-Perthes disease is often bilateral.

OSTEOCHONDROSES

Numerous other entities are often included with the "aseptic necroses" of bone, such as osteochondritis dissecans, Blount's disease, Köhler's disease, Osgood-Schlatter disease, and Scheuermann's disease. Some are avulsion fractures (Katz, 1981; Mital et al., 1980), some are tertiary or irregular epiphyseal growth centers (Langenskiold, 1981), some represent traumatic chondral separation with secondary infarction (Wil-

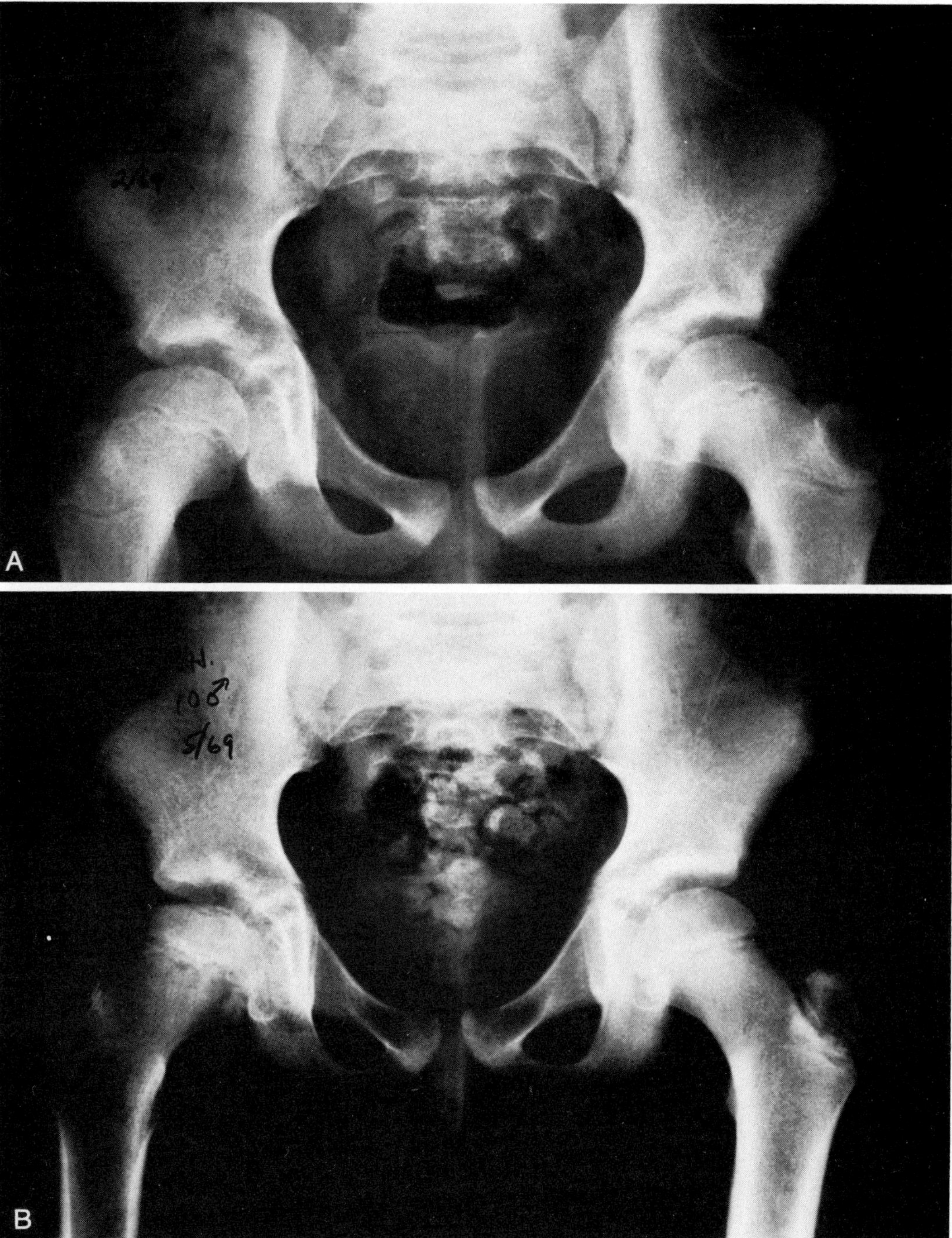

Figure 5–19. Anteroposterior radiographs of pelvis taken 3 months apart in 10-year-old boy hospitalized for "toxic synovitis" of right hip with pain and limited motion that subsided with 8 days of traction. At the time of follow-up film the patient was asymptomatic, but radiographic changes of radiolucent cleft, disparity of density between epiphysis and metaphysis, and widened joint space are all evident here.

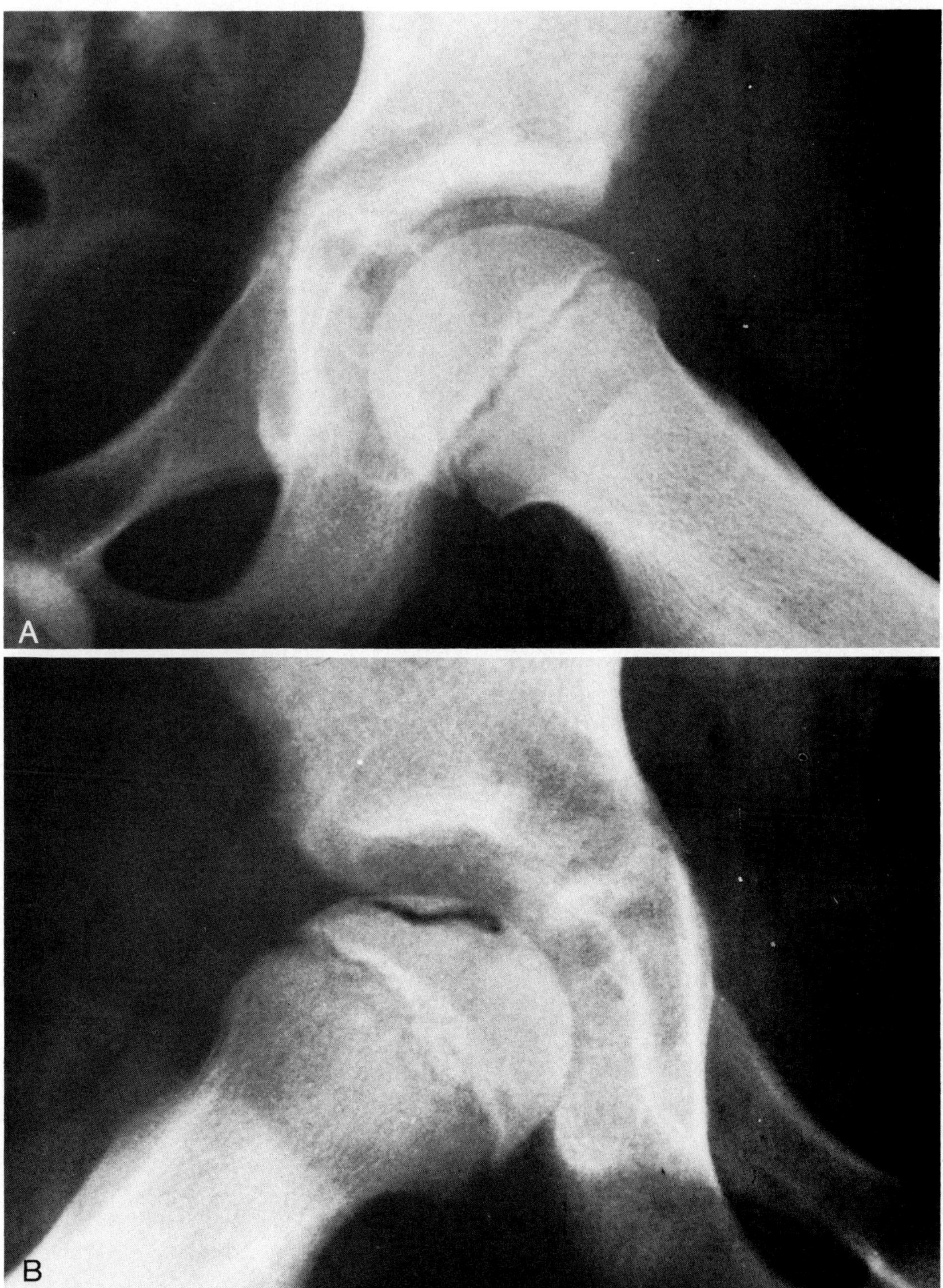

Figure 5–20. Frogleg radiographs of both hips of patient whose pelvis is shown in Figure 5–19. The frogleg view accentuates the subchondral cleft in right hip *(B)* in comparison with often-seen vacuum line in the left joint space *(A)*. Metaphyseal osteoporosis contrasts sharply with retained normal density of epiphysis. Note width of joint space in right hip.

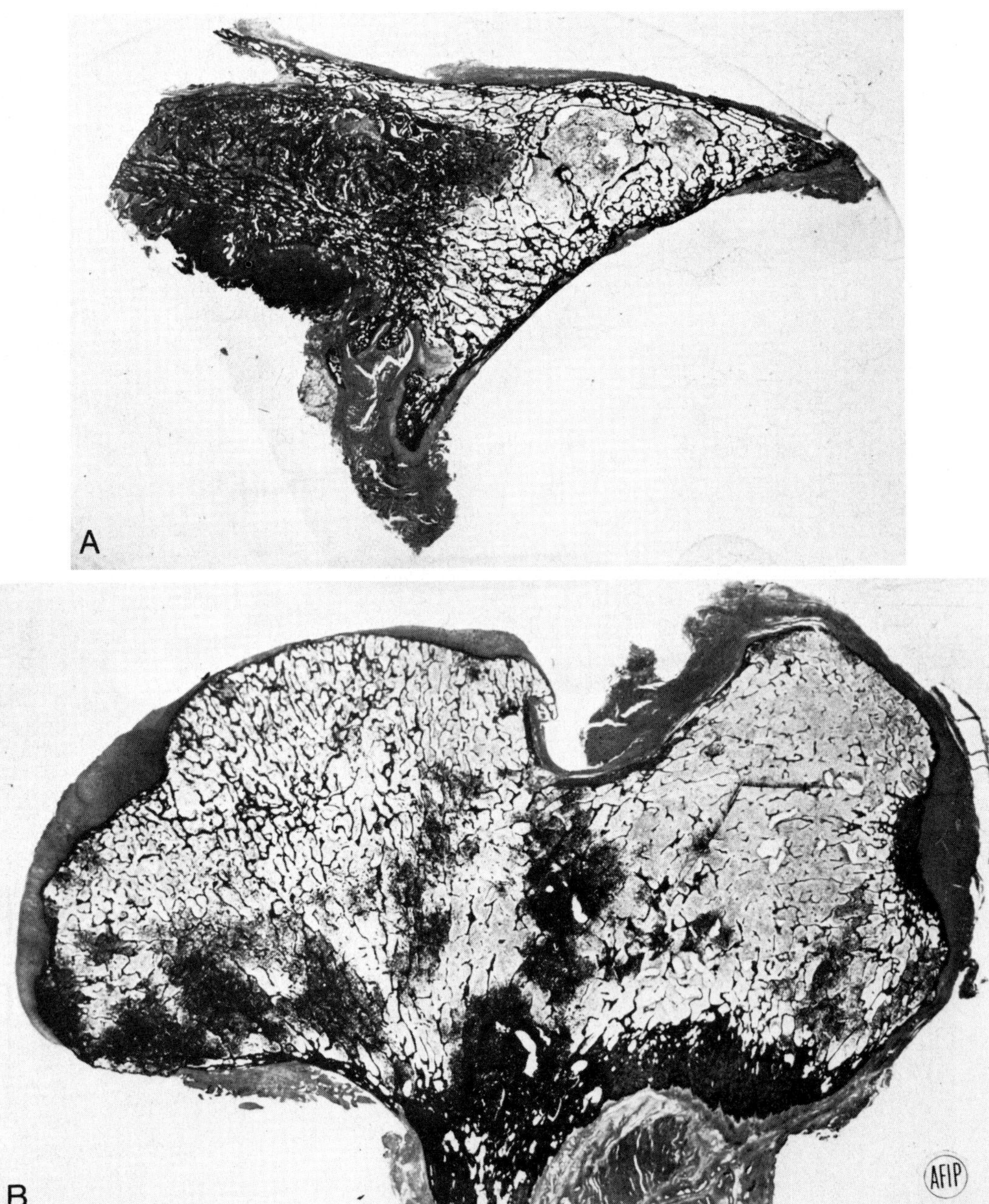

Figure 5–21. Macrosections of acetabulum *(A)* and femoral head *(B)* from old case of Legg-Calvé-Perthes disease. The lesion occurs only in femoral head, but with growth and remodeling the acetabulum will conform to the deformed femoral head.

liams and Cowell, 1981), and some are deformities caused by herniation of disc material (Bradford, 1981). However, except for Freiberg's infarction, none are true infarcts in which the disease process is due to primary loss of arterial blood supply.

Osteochondritis dissecans represents a condition in which a detached fragment of cartilage and bone lies free in the joint space. In the majority of cases, it results as a consequence of trauma to the articular surface. Most of these are osteochondral fractures of a normal epiphysis. Some may represent separation of a tertiary ossification center. Trauma to this relatively avascular area may separate the ossification center

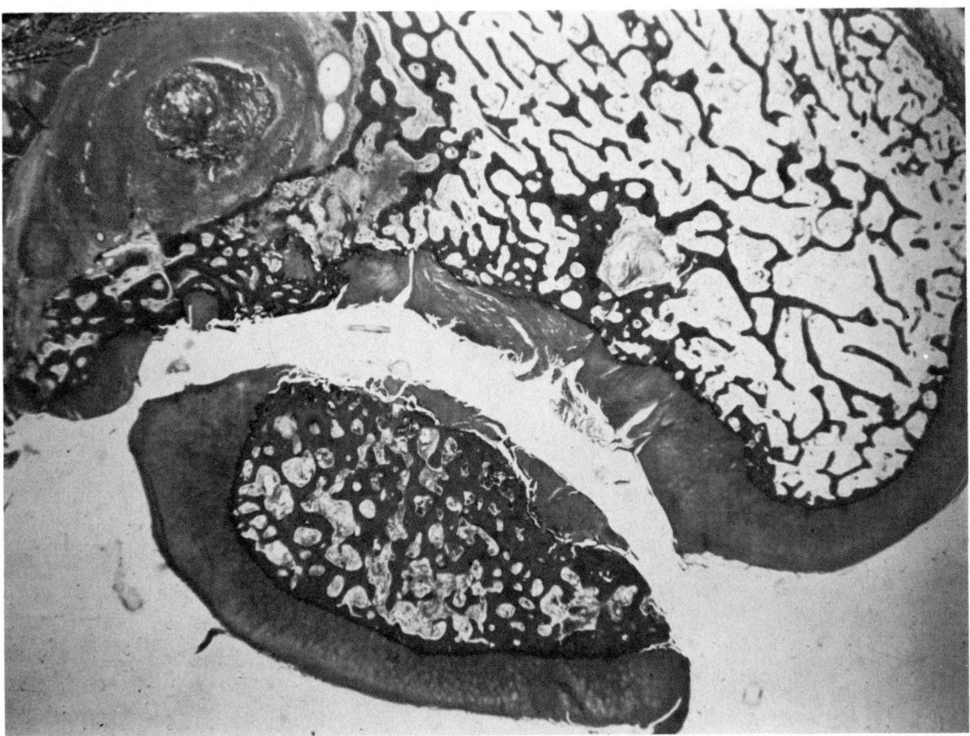

Figure 5–22. Macrospecimen from patient with osteochondritis dissecans exhibiting separation of bone and cartilage fragments from articular surface. Note that the cleavage plane is through the cartilage.

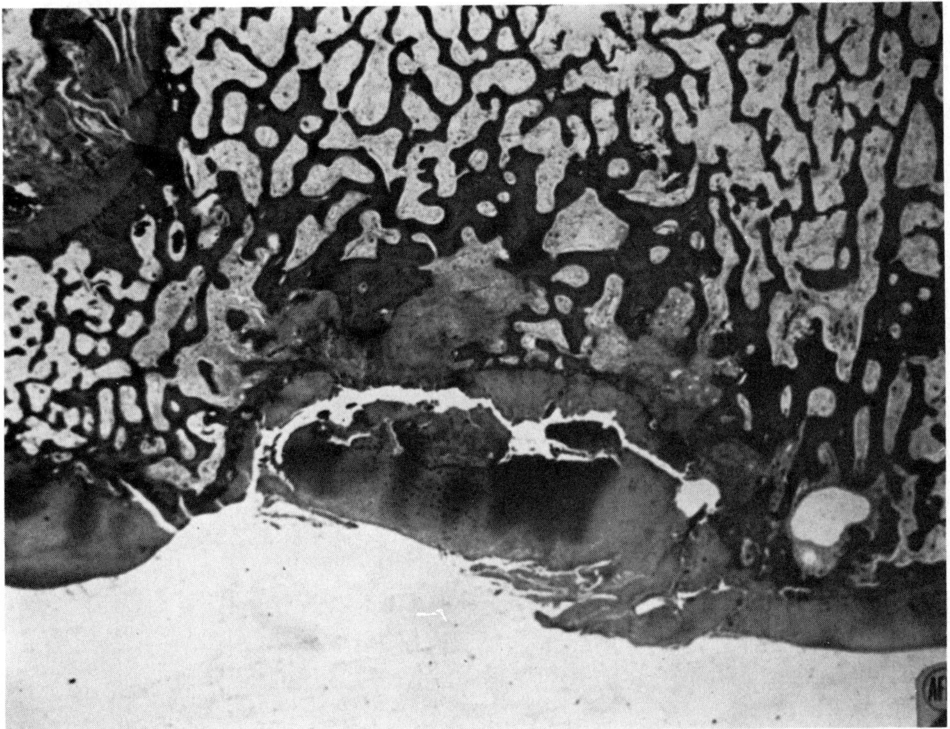

Figure 5–23. Macrospecimen from patient with osteochondritis dissecans exhibiting separation of cartilaginous fragments into the joint space. No bone is present in osteochondritic fragment in this view. The bone contour is irregular, suggesting long-term failure of this portion of the subchondral metaphysis to develop in synchrony with the adjacent areas.

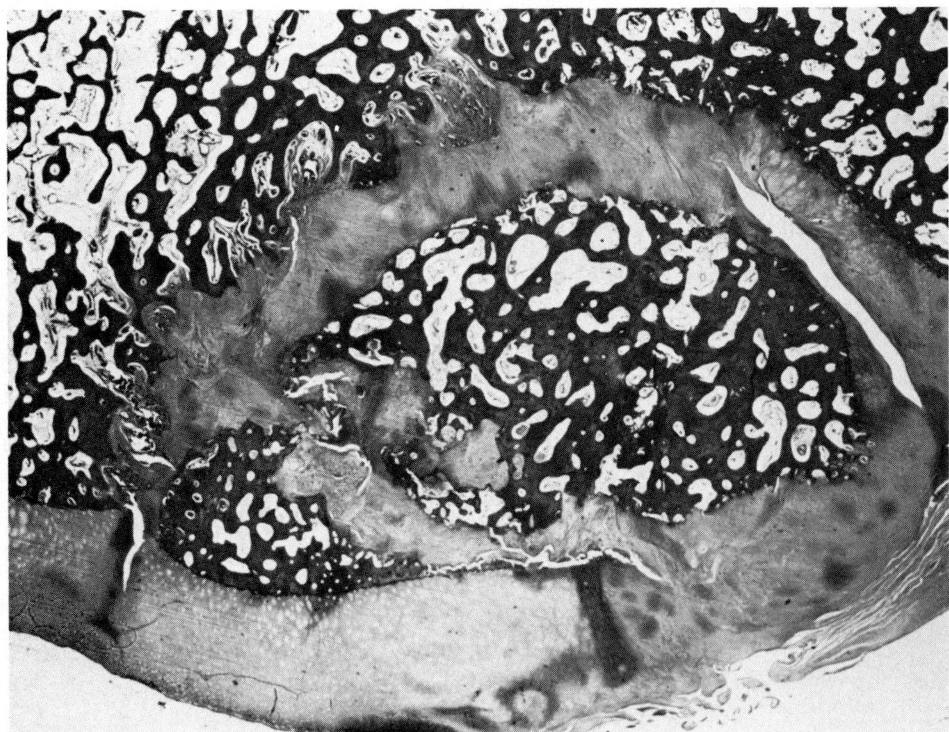

Figure 5–24. Macrosection from patient with osteochondritis dissecans exhibiting cleft formation and partial separation from the underlying bone.

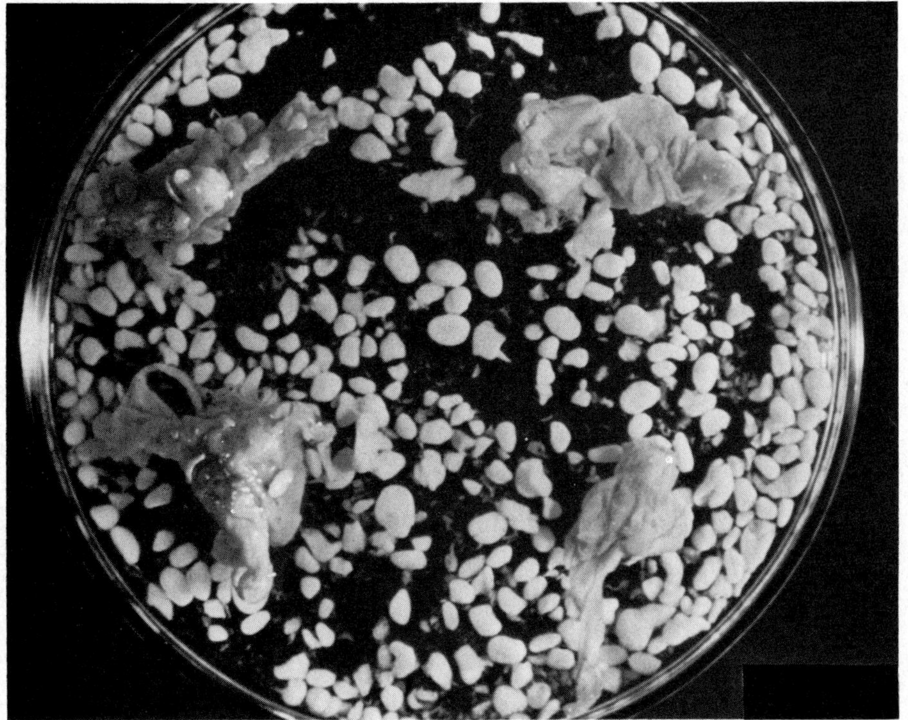

Figure 5–25. Gross specimen of rice bodies representing proliferating cartilage within the joint space. Note fragments of synovium with excrescences that may indicate rheumatoid arthritis.

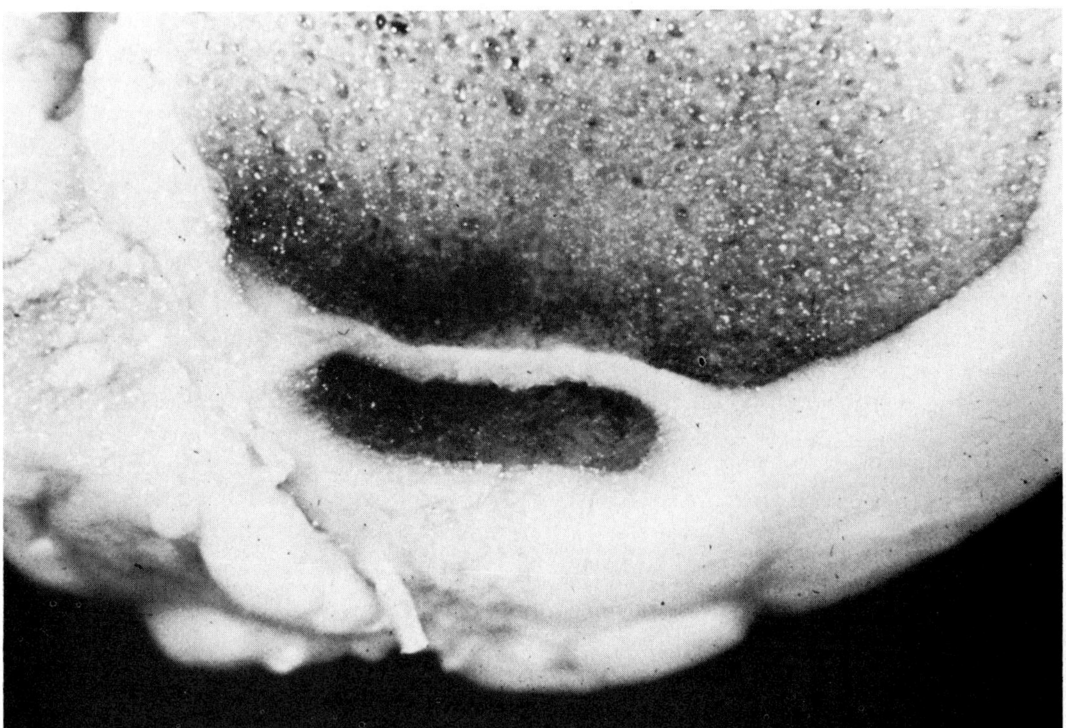

Figure 5–26. Gross photograph of bone of patient with osteochondritis dissecans, taken prior to separation of specimen into joint space. The bone remains viable as long as the blood supply is intact. If the entire fragment is separated into the joint space, the bone becomes infarcted. Cartilage continues to survive when bathed in synovial fluid. Notice irregularity of cartilage contour on articular surface.

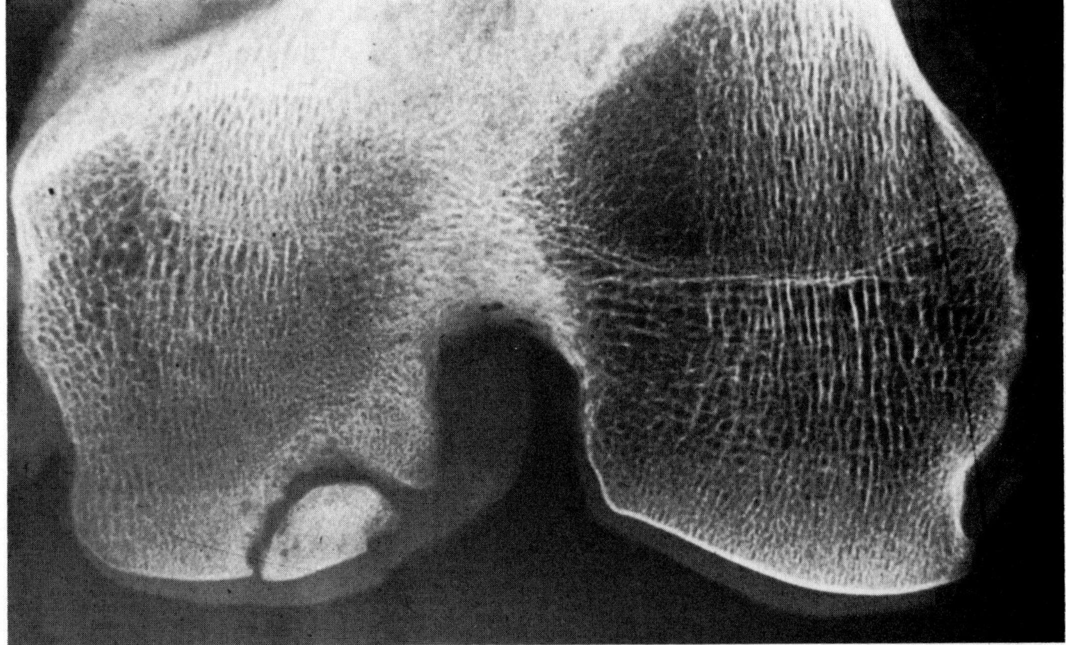

Figure 5–27. Specimen radiograph of osteochondritis dissecans exhibiting the complete separation of bony fragment from the lower end of the femur. It is still entirely encased in cartilage and thus retains its position. This picture is consistent with that of a tertiary epiphysis.

from the parent bone, in which case the center becomes completely isolated from its blood supply (Clanton and DeLee, 1982). In either event the fragment is then separated into the joint space; the cartilage continues to grow because it is nourished by synovial fluid and does not require a blood supply, but the bone becomes infarcted. These free-lying fragments of cartilage surrounding infarcted bone are commonly known as "joint bodies," or "joint mice" (Figs. 5–22 to 5–27).

PAGET'S DISEASE OF BONE

Paget's disease of bone is characterized by repeated irrational episodes of osteoclastic activity followed by excessive repair that produces a weakened deformed skeleton with increased bone mass. The initial lesion is osteoclastic, located in the cortex. A cutting cone of normal osteoclasts is activated, but it removes bone without regard to structural integrity. As the bone is removed, it is replaced by rapidly deposited mesenchymal tissue that is highly vascular with a loose fibrous configuration. Osteoblasts attempt to repair the defect with new bone. The new bone is

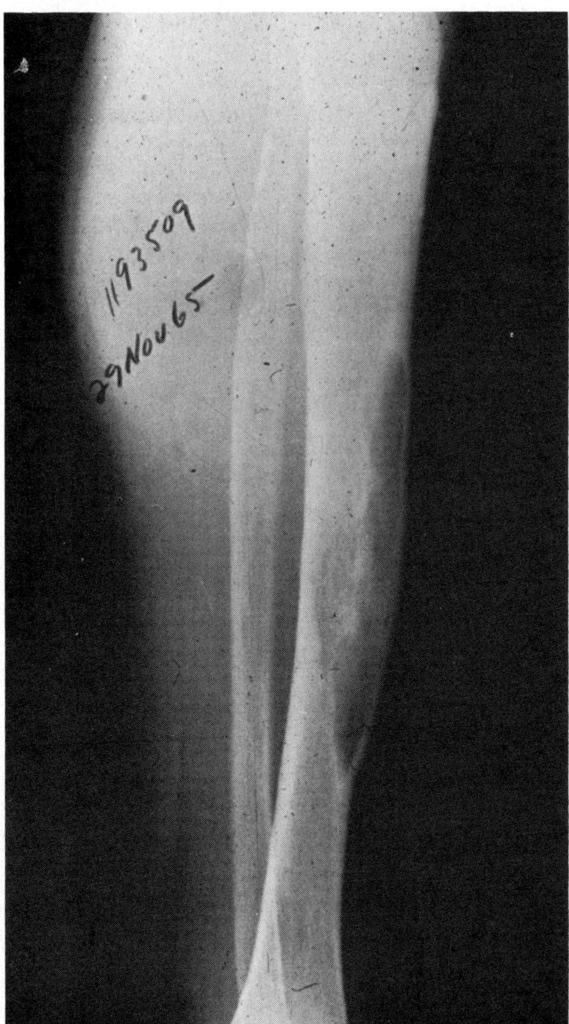

Figure 5–28. Clinical radiograph of the tibia of a patient with Paget's disease exhibiting a "blade of grass," a sharply circumscribed lytic process usually limited to the cortex. This is often the first manifestation of Paget's disease. There is localized expansion of bone diameter in the involved area.

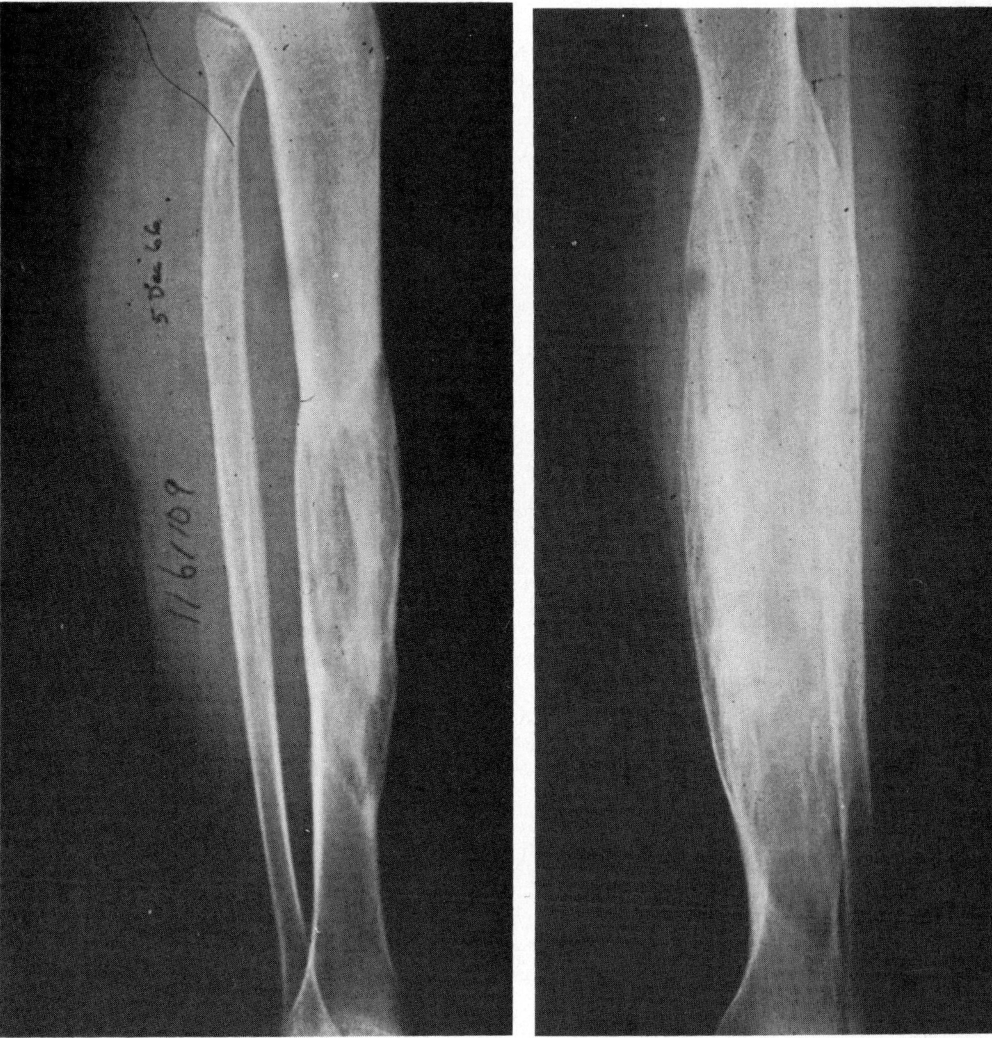

Figure 5–29   Figure 5–30

Figure 5–29. Clinical radiograph of the tibia of a patient with Paget's disease exhibiting lytic destruction of the bone with characteristic "blade of grass" at both margins of the lesion. The sclerotic portions in the center of the radiograph represent replacement of destroyed bone in irregular, nonosteonal patterns.

Figure 5–30. Clinical radiograph from case illustrated in Figure 5–29, approximately 5 years later, exhibiting extensive lytic destruction of the tibia and refill of portions of the destroyed bone with a resulting picture of irregularly intermingled areas of sclerosis and lysis.

deposited in irregular fashion and is abnormal; as soon as it is formed, it is again removed by fresh relays of osteoclasts. This process of resorption and deposition occurs in an irregular manner over many years and causes loss of osteonal structure in the involved cortex. Smaller trabeculae disappear in the osteoclastic process, but the remaining ones become prominent and coarse (Figs. 5–28 to 5–34).

Although the bone has increased skeletal mass, it tends to fracture easily. Fractures are characteristically transverse, and healing is slow with excessive callus formation.

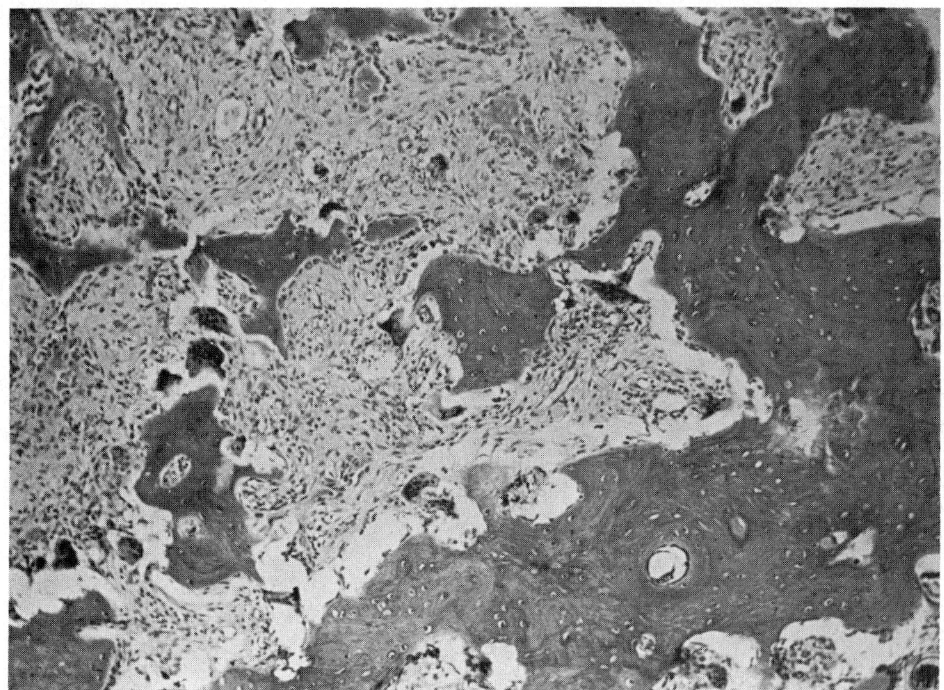

Figure 5–31. Histologic study of Paget's disease. There is extensive osteoclastic resorption in the cortex, without regard to structural integrity. Note the haphazard arrangement of osteoclasts and the extensive replacement of bone. The spaces created are filled by vascular fibrous connective tissue. The haphazard arrangement is characteristic of Paget's disease and differentiates it from hyperparathyroidism, in which there is reinforcement of trabeculae in response to mechanical demands.

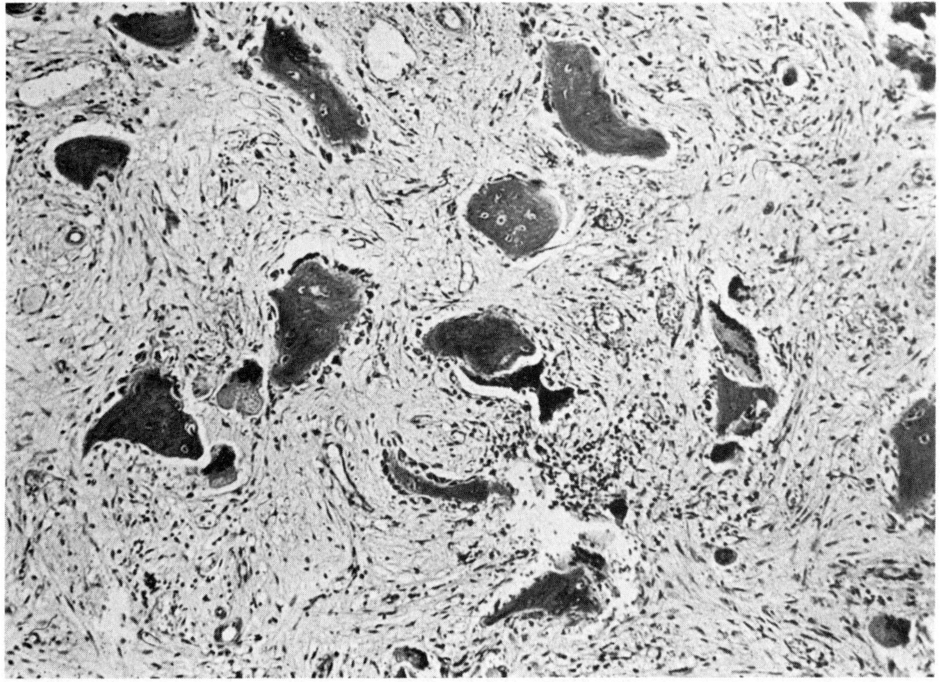

Figure 5–32. Histologic study of Paget's disease illustrating osteoblastic and osteoclastic activity often occurring on the same trabecula. There is removal of bone and replacement by fibrous connective tissue as well as a number of inflammatory cells. The differential diagnosis of the histologic picture must include hyperparathyroidism, fibrous dysplasia, and cortical fibrous dysplasia (ossifying fibroma). The presence of a clearly identifiable osteoblastic seam around each of the newly formed trabeculae is inconsistent with the diagnosis of fibrous dysplasia.

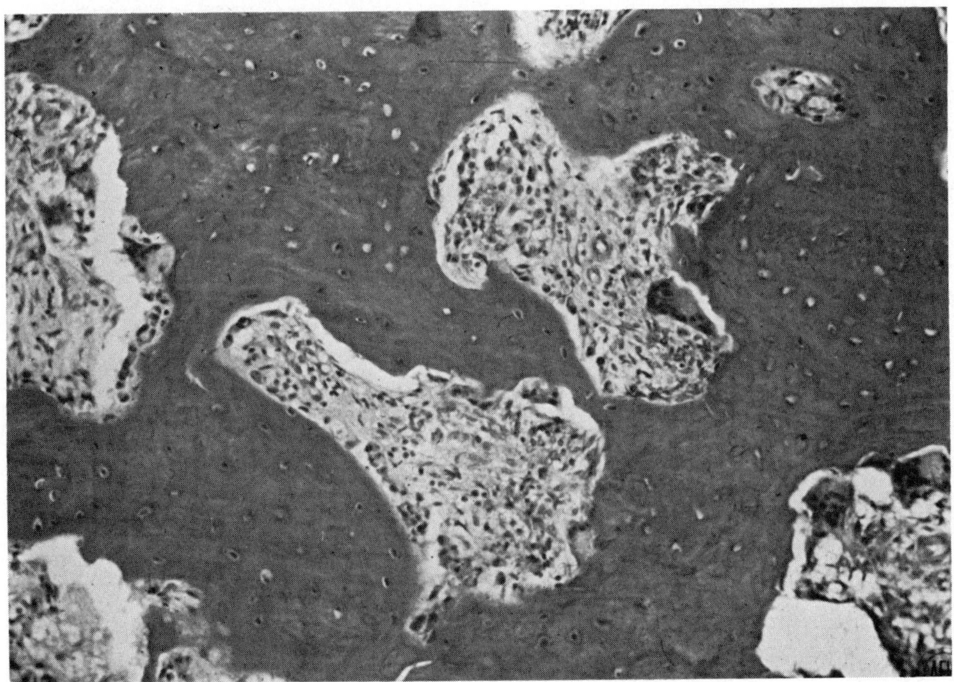

Figure 5–33. Histologic study of bone in Paget's disease with fibrous connective tissue showing extensive osteoclastic and osteoblastic activity.

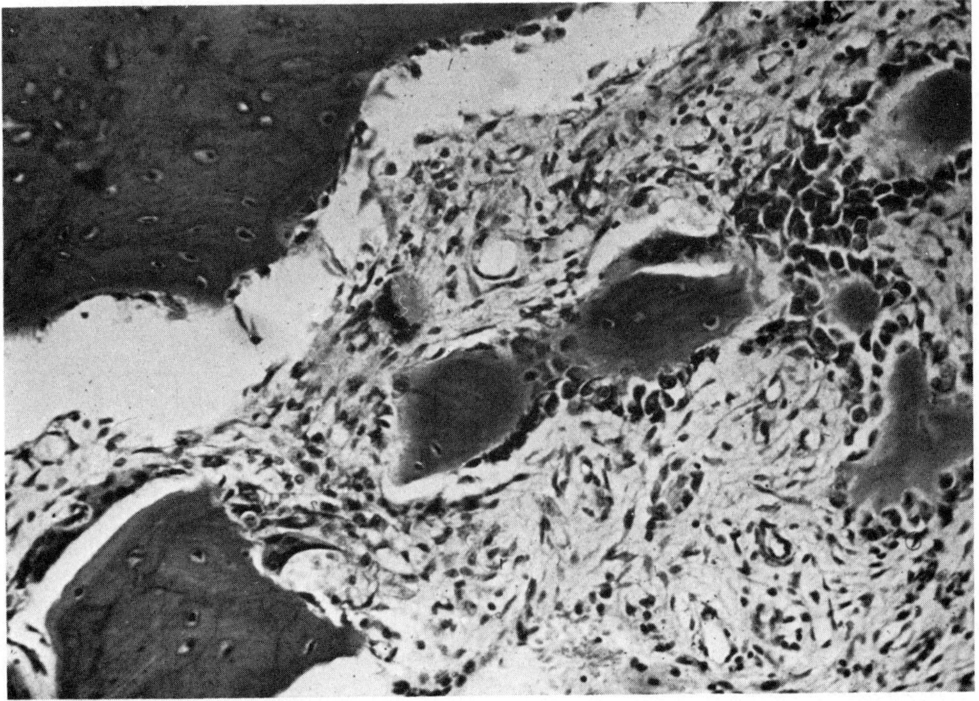

Figure 5–34. Numerous osteoclasts and osteoblasts in a fibrous connective tissue stroma, characteristic of Paget's disease.

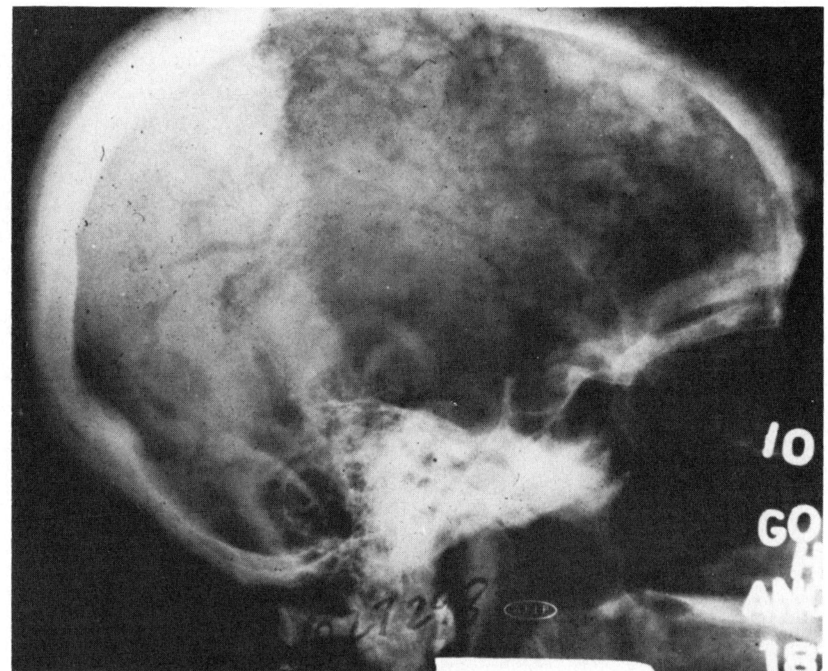

Figure 5–35. Lateral skull radiograph of patient with Paget's disease exhibiting marked osteolytic destruction of skull with patchy refill. Such removal of large areas of skull is termed "osteoporosis circumscripta."

The process appears to be limited and decelerates with time. After cessation of osteoclastic and osteoblastic activity, the bone is left with numerous cement lines, residuals of recurring waves of removal and deposition of new bone. Ultimately, inactive Paget's disease reveals bone with an extensive mosaic pattern, and the fibrous stroma converts back to unremarkable fat tissue (Teitelbaum and Bullough, 1979) (Figs. 5–37 to 5–39).

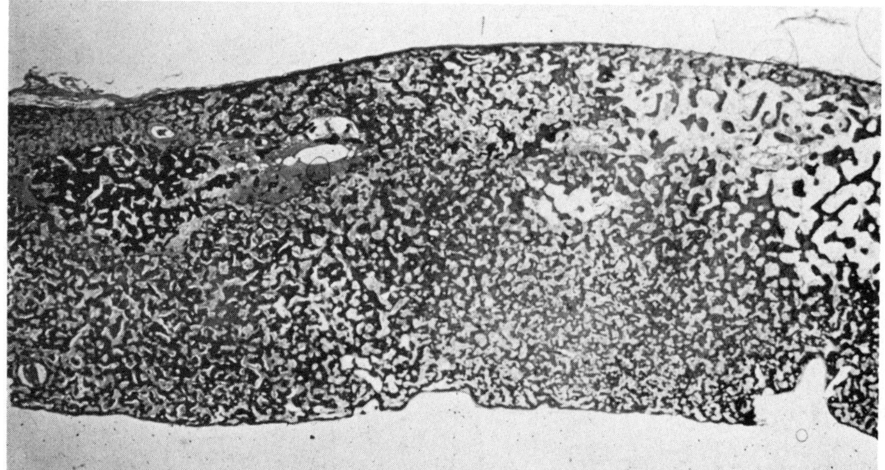

Figure 5–36. Macrospecimen of skull bone exhibiting lytic region in the upper right-hand corner and extensive sclerotic pumice bone in the remaining portion of the specimen. Pumice bone is so termed because the trabeculae formed in Paget's disease are not interconnected with each other as in normal bone, and if soft tissue is removed from the specimen, the bony trabeculae will crumble like volcanic pumice.

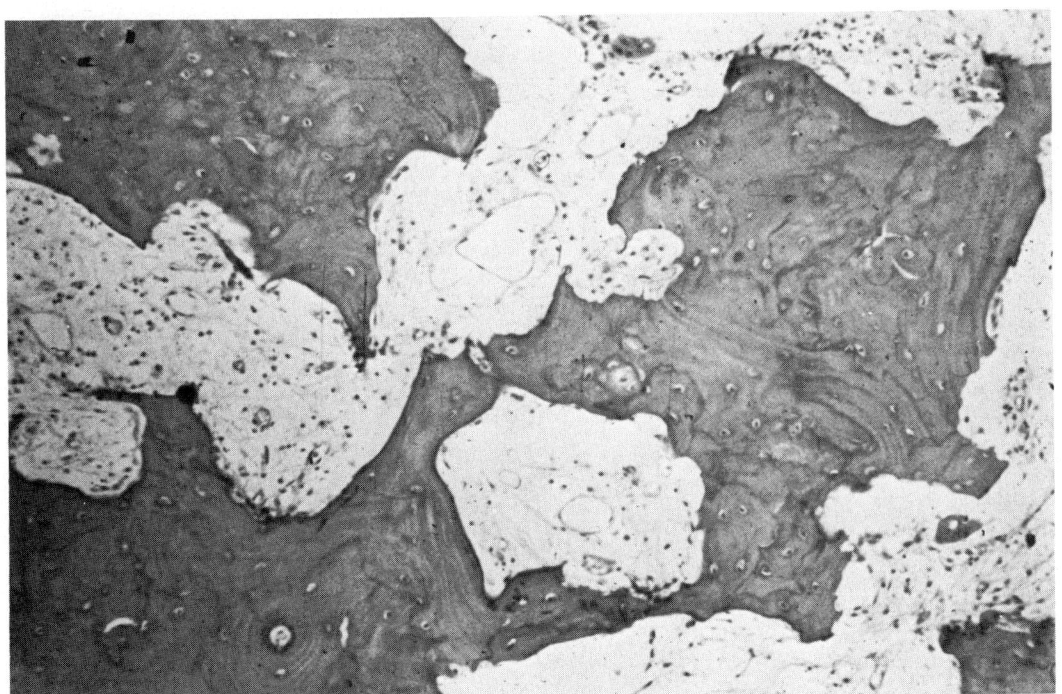

Figure 5–37. Inactive Paget's disease in bone with numerous reversal lines, loose fibrous connective tissue, and occasional inflammatory cells in quiescent marrow. This is a characteristic histologic picture of inactive Paget's disease and should be reflected in normal alkaline phosphatase values.

Neoplastic transformation in Paget's disease is not uncommon and accounts for the heightened incidence of osteosarcoma in older individuals (Unni and Dahlin, 1979; Jacobs et al., 1979) (Fig. 5–40; see also Fig. 9–253). The markedly increased vascularity associated with Paget's disease, readily indicated by extensive sinusoid formation, can cause circulatory difficulties with high-output cardiac failure. The bone lesions behave as if an arteriovenous fistula exists, although morphologic studies have demonstrated no actual fistulas (Putschar, 1972; Rhodes et al., 1972).

CHARCOT'S ARTHROPATHY

Charcot's arthropathy is a condition characterized by traumatization of the articular cartilage and bone with resultant severe structural deformity. It is a response to the loss of normal neurologic response to both pain and proprioceptive sensory perception. Patients afflicted with such neurologic deficits include those suffering from tabes dorsalis, syringomyelia, and advanced diabetes mellitus with peripheral neuropathy, as well as those with congenital insensitivity to pain (Jaffe, 1972). Radiographic features include extensive destruction of bone and disruption of normal joint structure. Histologic features confirm the radiographic findings, and entire fragments of articular cartilage and subchondral bone can be demonstrated within the hypertrophied synovium (Figs. 5–41 to 5–45).

Cellular debris with foreign body material secondary to failed prosthesis may involve synovial tissue in a process similar to that in Charcot's disease. Polyethylene, methyl methacrylate, and other substances generate a typical foreign body reaction (Fig. 5–46).

Text continued on page 190

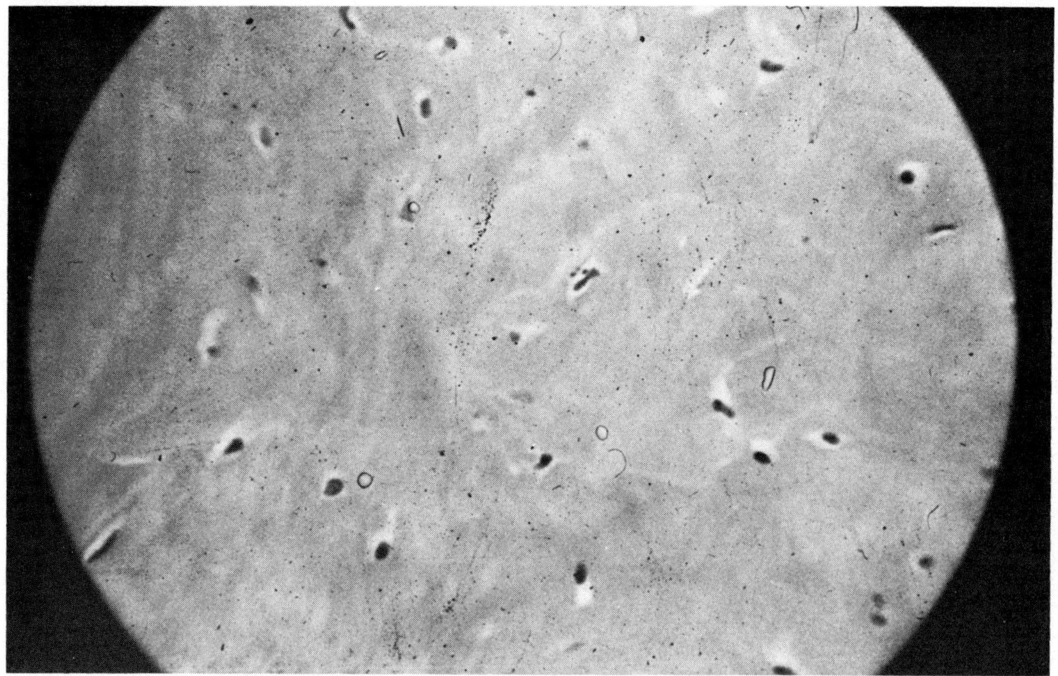

Figure 5–38. Paget's disease, inadequate hematoxylin staining. Demonstration of reversal lines, diagnostic of Paget's disease, requires intense staining with hematoxylin.

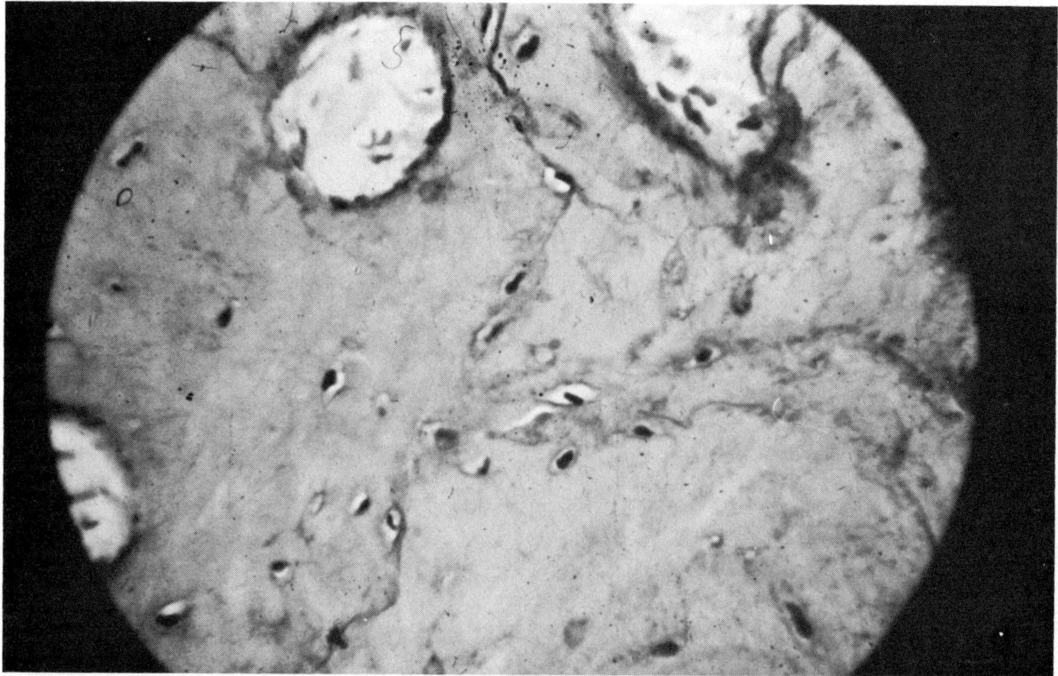

Figure 5–39. Specimen similar to that seen in Figure 5–38. Here, appropriate intense hematoxylin staining demonstrates reversal lines, which represent the place at which osteoclastic activity ceased and osteoblasts deposited a proteoglycan substance as initial substrate on which they then deposit bone. These reversal lines may also be seen in chronic osteomyelitis or other sclerotic processes in which alternate removal and deposition of bone occurs.

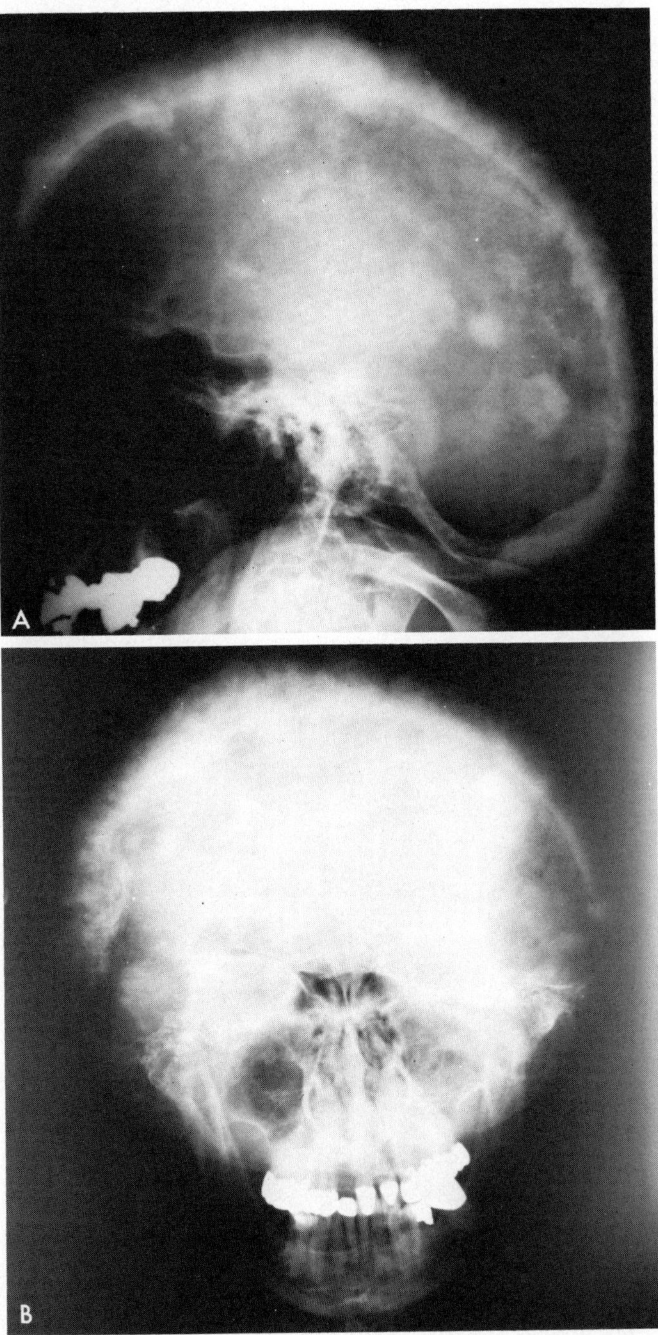

Figure 5–40. Lateral *(A)* and anteroposterior *(B)* views of skull of patient with Paget's disease. Loss of definition of the inner table of the skull indicating active growth of a mass illustrates problem of malignant degeneration in Paget's disease, usually osteosarcoma (as in this case), fibrosarcoma, or giant cell tumor.

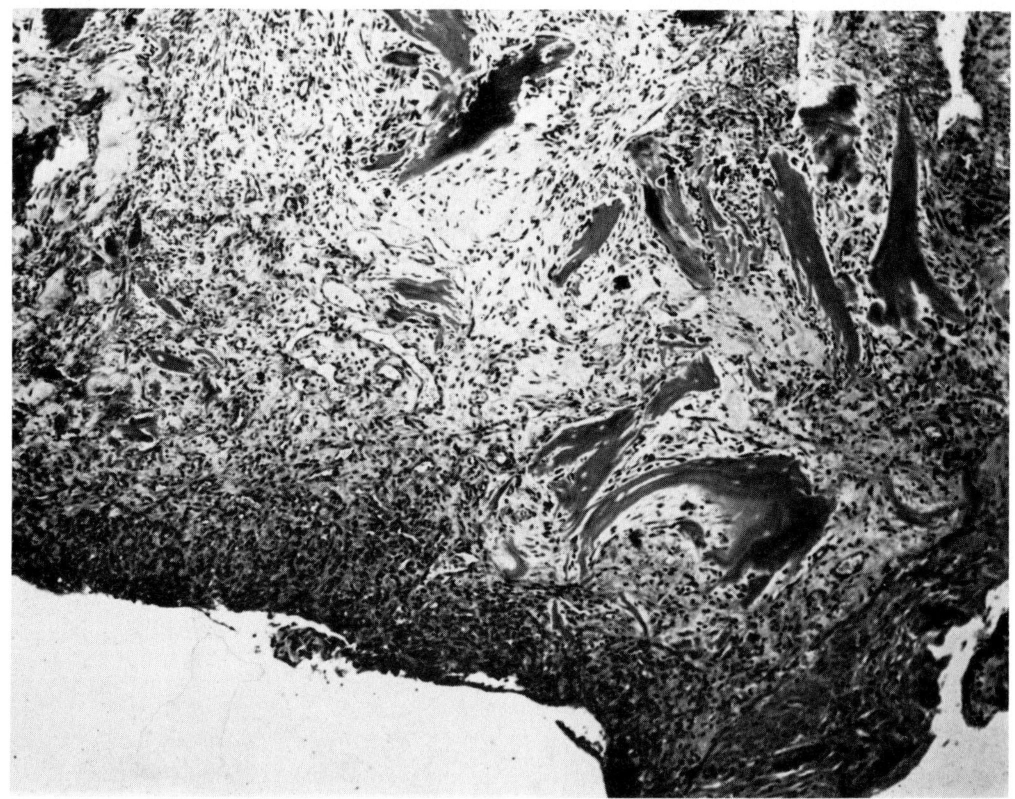

Figure 5–41. Fragments of synovial tissue of patient with Charcot's arthropathy containing shards of infarcted bone and cartilage.

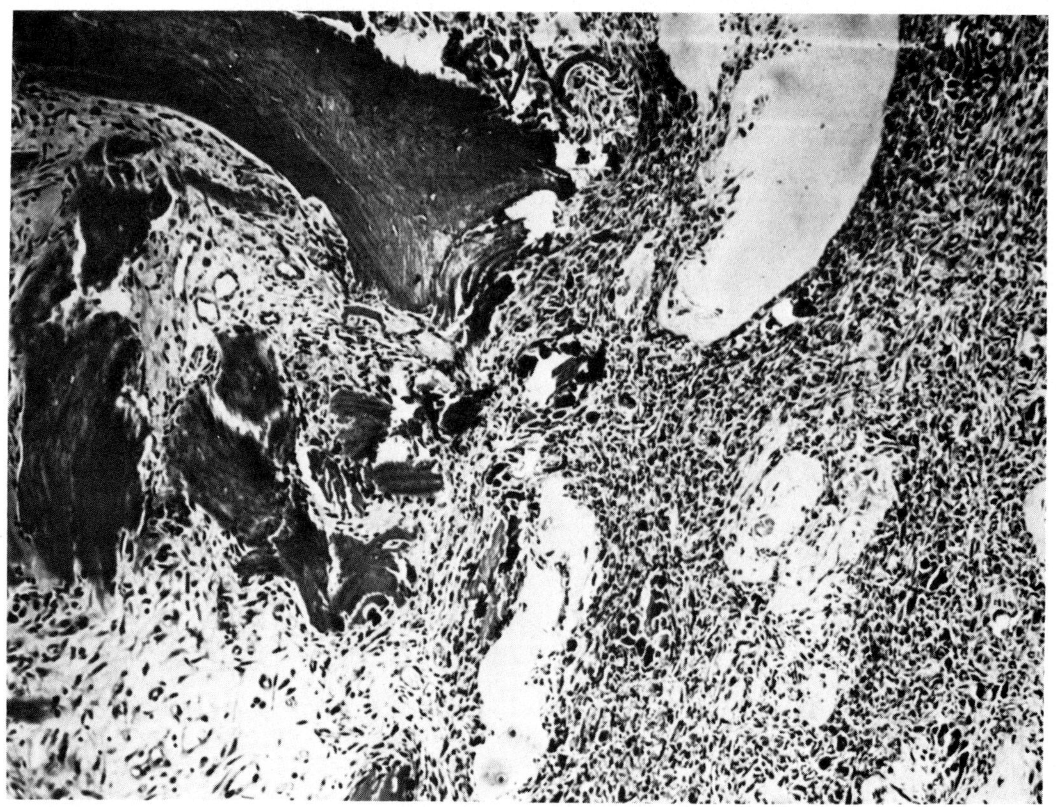

Figure 5–42. Charcot's arthropathy. Higher magnification of tissue shown in Figure 5–41 exhibiting infarcted fragments of bone phagocytosed by hypertrophied synovial tissue containing numerous foreign body giant cells. Fragments of cartilage are also included within the synovium.

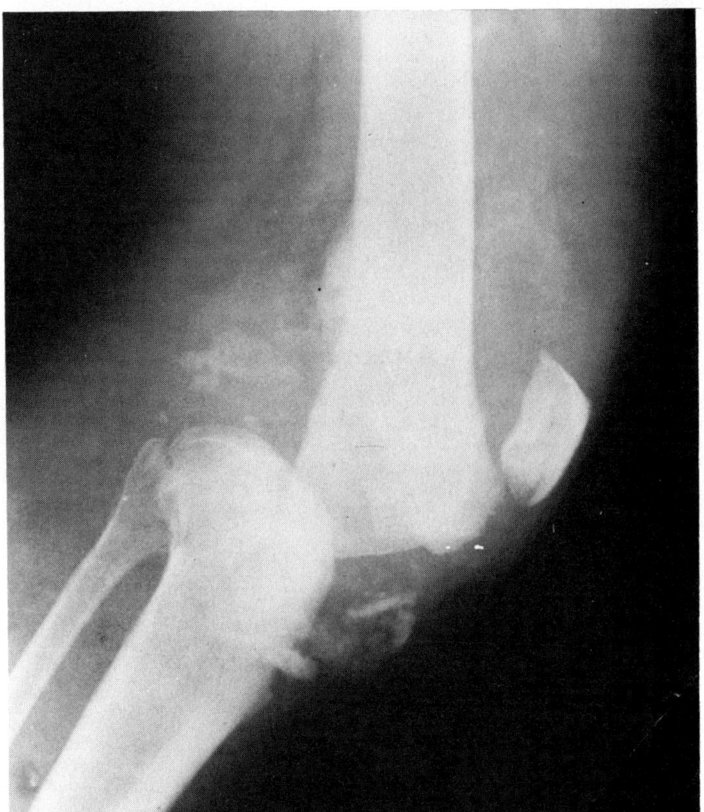

Figure 5–43. Charcot's arthropathy. Radiographic appearance of knee in patient with syphilis exhibiting distortion and avulsion of normal knee joint and presence of numerous fragments within the joint space.

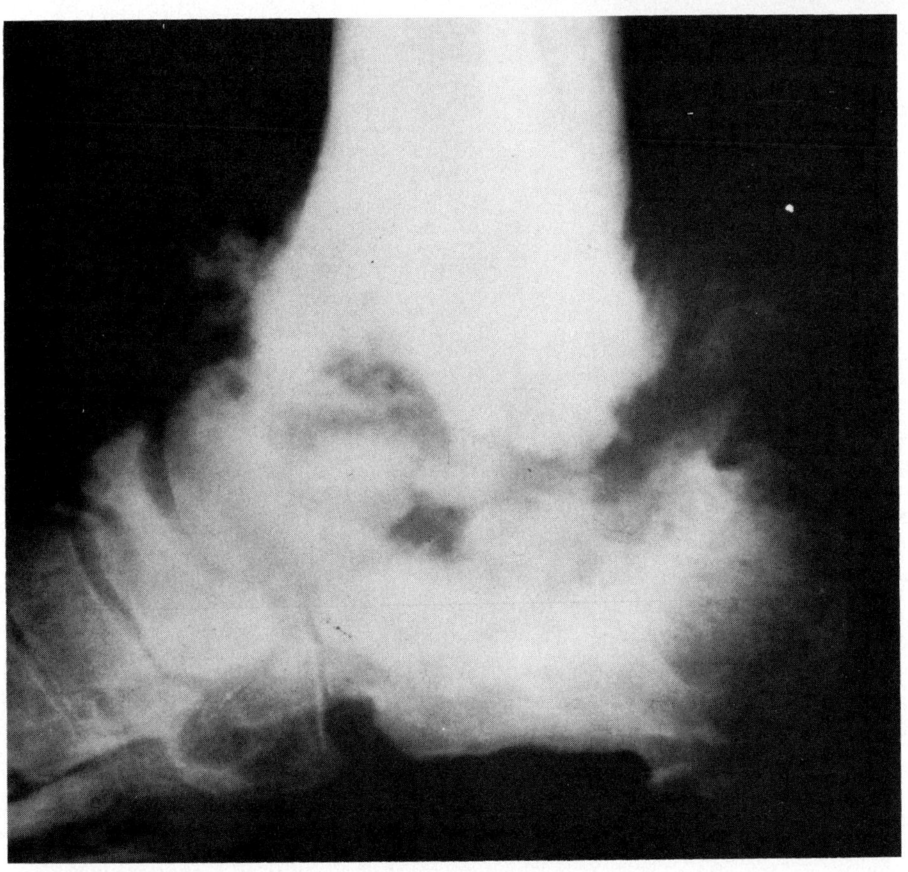

Figure 5–44. Charcot's arthropathy. Radiographic appearance of ankle joint in patient with syphilis exhibiting fragmentation of bone and deposition within the hypertrophied synovium.

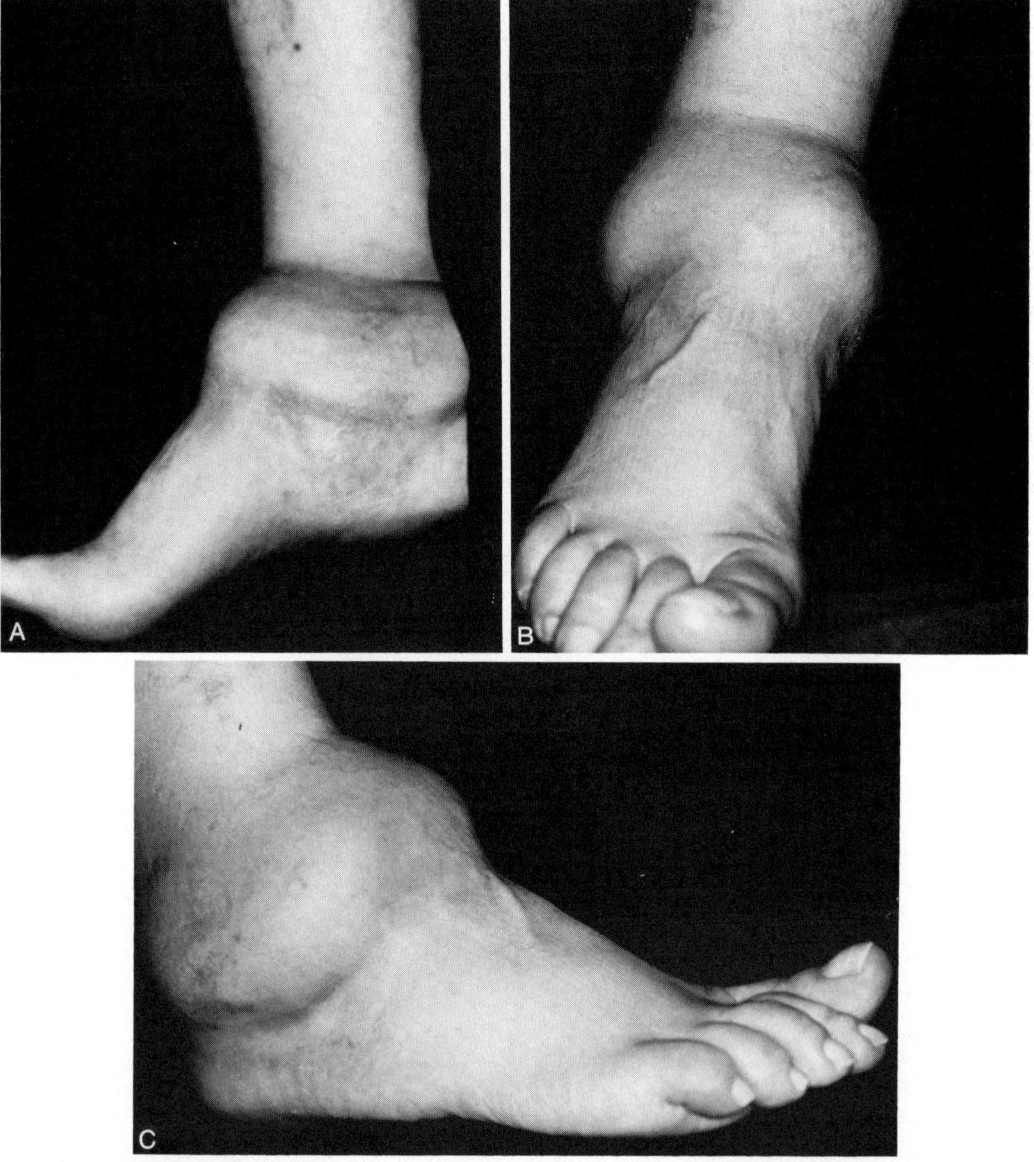

Figure 5–45. Charcot's arthropathy. Clinical photographs of ankle region demonstrating pronounced enlargement and distortion from neuropathic joint changes following minor injury 20 years earlier. There is no evidence of neurologic disease or diabetes mellitus. The ankle is mildly painful.

HEMOGLOBINOPATHIES

Sickle cell disease and the thalassemias place unusual demands on marrow space and therefore interfere with the normal remodeling process. There is lack of metaphyseal funnelization, and normal spongiotic bone is reduced in order to provide room for hematopoietic activity. The radiographic appearance of a patient with thalassemia or fully developed sickle cell disease will thus include widened metaphyses, lack of funnelization, coarse trabeculae, osteoporosis, and a "hair-on-end" appearance of the skull. These morphologic features are simply a reaction to increased demands for marrow space.

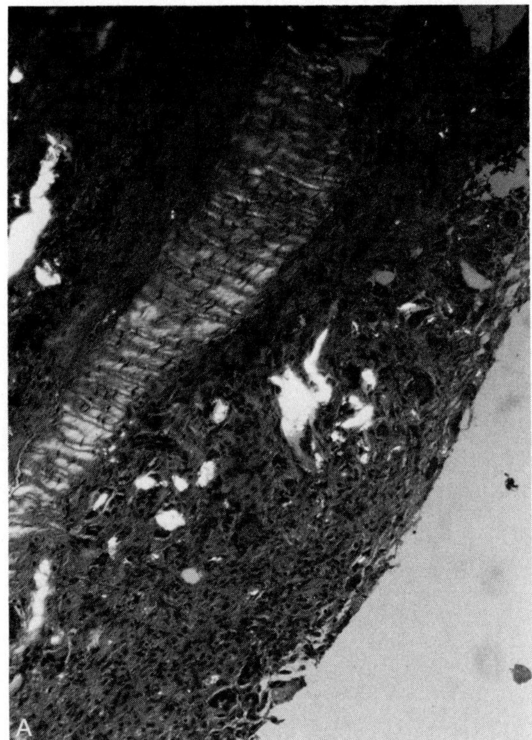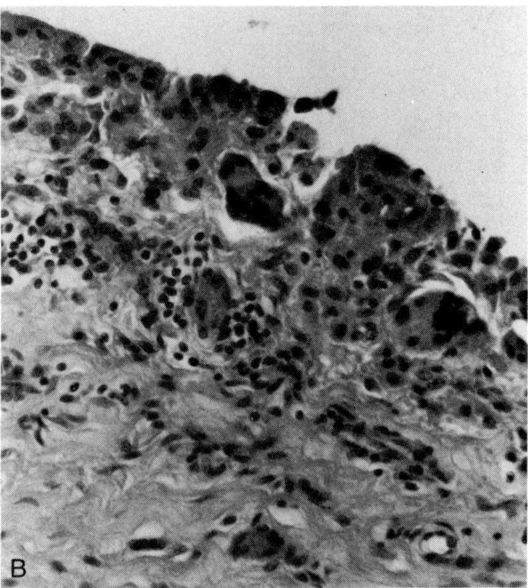

Figure 5–46. Histologic appearance of synovium in patient with failed prosthesis. Note numerous foreign body giant cells and doubly refractile material ingested by synovium.

CITED REFERENCES

Bradford, D. S.: Vertebral osteochondrosis (Scheuermann's kyphosis). Clin. Orthop. *158*:83, 1981.

Catterall, A.: Legg-Calvé-Perthes syndrome. Clin. Orthop. *158*:41, 1981.

Clanton, T. O., and DeLee, J. C.: Osteochondritis dissecans. History, pathophysiology and current treatment concepts. Clin. Orthop. *167*:50, 1982.

Jacobs, T. P., Michelsen, J., Polay, J. S., D'Adamo, A. C., and Canfield, R. E.: Giant cell tumor in Paget's disease of bone: familial and geographic clustering. Cancer *44*:742, 1979.

Katz, J. F.: Nonarticular osteochondroses. Clin. Orthop. *158*:70, 1981.

Langenskiold, A.: Tibia vara: osteochondrosis deformans tibiae (Blount's disease). Clin. Orthop. *158*:77, 1981.

Lee, C. K., Hansen, H. T., and Weiss, A. B.: The "silent hip" of idiopathic ischemic necrosis of the femoral head in adults. J. Bone Joint Surg. *62A*:795, 1980.

Mital, M. A., Matza, R. A., and Cohen, J.: The so-called unresolved Osgood-Schlatter lesion—a concept based on fifteen surgically treated lesions. J. Bone Joint Surg. *62A*:732, 1980.

Putschar, W. G. J.: Circulation in Paget's disease of bone. Editorial. N. Engl. J. Med. *287*:717, 1972.

Rhodes, B. A., Greyson, N. D., Hamilton, C. R., White, R. I., Giargiana, F. A., and Wagner, H. N.: Absence of anatomic arteriovenous shunts in Paget's disease of bone. N. Engl. J. Med. *287*:686, 1972.

Teitelbaum, S. L., and Bullough, P. G.: The pathophysiology of bone and joint disease. Am. J. Pathol. *96*:318, 1979.

Unni, K. K., and Dahlin, D. C.: Premalignant tumors and conditions of bone. Am. J. Surg. Pathol. *3*:47, 1979.

Williams, G. A., and Cowell, H. R.: Köhler's disease of the tarsal navicular. Clin. Orthop. *158*:53, 1981.

GENERAL REFERENCES

Aegerter, E., and Kirkpatrick, J. A., Jr.: Orthopedic Diseases. 4th ed. Philadelphia, W. B. Saunders Co., 1975.

Jaffe, H. L.: Metabolic, Degenerative, and Inflammatory Diseases of Bones and Joints. Philadelphia, Lea and Febiger, 1972.

Springfield, D. S., and Enneking, W. F.: Idiopathic aseptic necrosis. In Ackerman, L. V., Spjut, H. J., and Abell, M. R. (Eds.): Bones and Joints, International Academy of Pathology Monograph. Baltimore, Williams and Wilkins Co., 1976.

Stulberg, S. D., Cooperman, D. R., and Wallensten, R.: The natural history of Legg-Calvé-Perthes disease. J. Bone Joint Surg. *63A*:1095, 1981.

6

DEGENERATIVE JOINT DISEASE: OSTEOARTHRITIS

DEVELOPMENT OF JOINTS

A joint is formed by a rapid, precise sequence of events. Dense condensation of mesenchyme is formed between cartilaginous elements of the skeleton. Cavities appear as a result of genetically determined enzymatic processes. Joints are formed as a consequence of normal embryologic growth and development, but muscular activity and motion are required to maintain the joint space (Figs. 6–1 to 6–3).

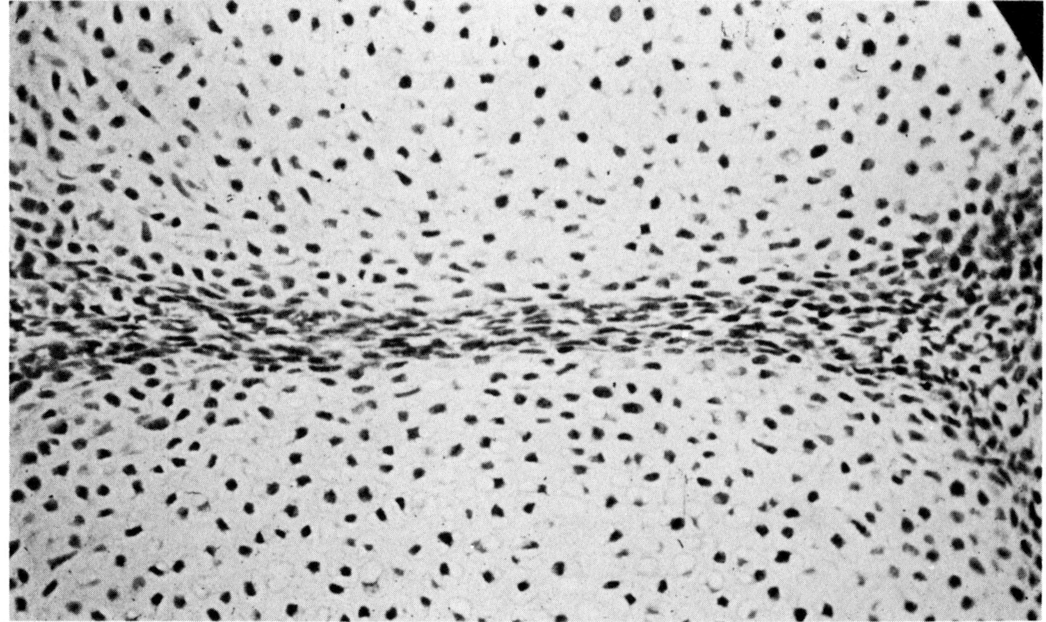

Figure 6–1. Histologic study of fetus, approximately 6 weeks' gestation, depicting early joint formation. Note the identifiable cartilage and the condensed mesenchymal tissue of the interzone destined to become the joint.

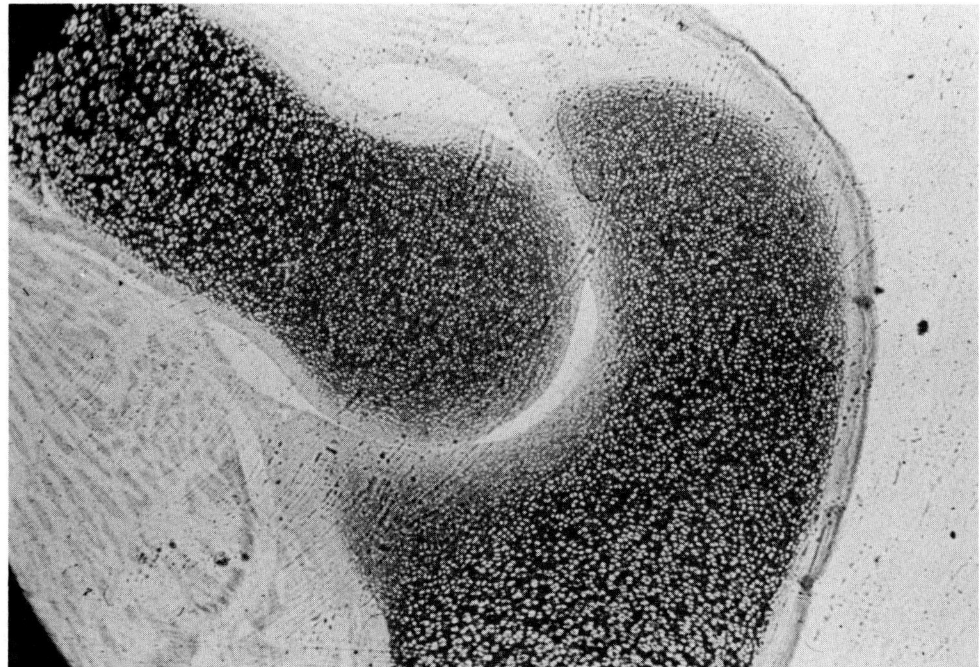

Figure 6–2. Histologic study of fetus, approximately 14 weeks' gestation. Cartilage model of the elbow joint with well-formed joint space. The joint space develops by enzymatic action independent of muscles or passive motion, but it requires motion to be maintained as a space.

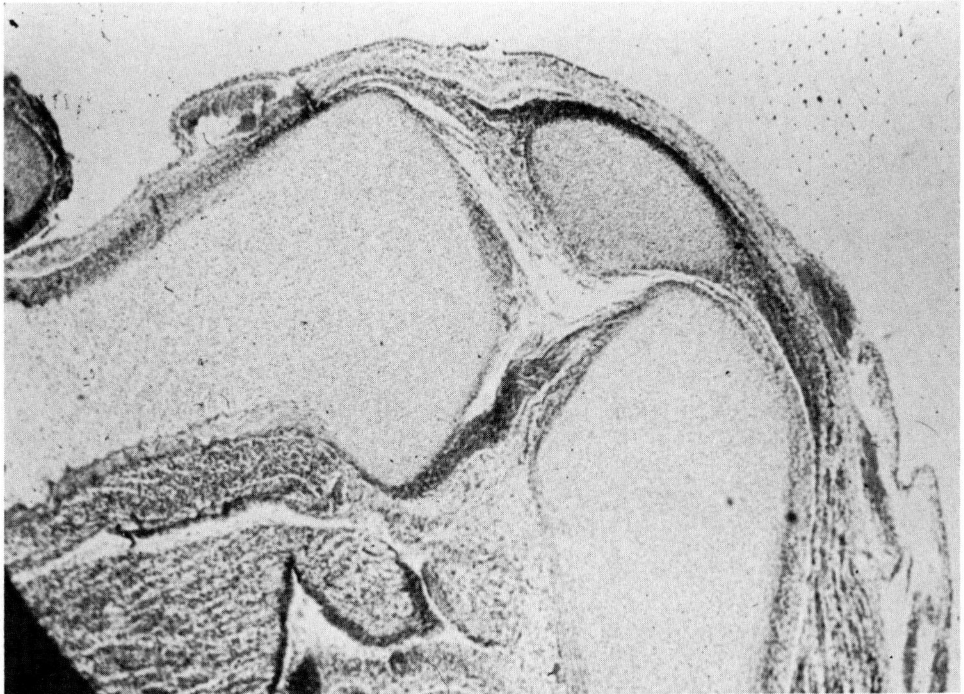

Figure 6–3. Histologic study of the knee joint of a fetus, approximately 14 weeks' gestation, exhibiting the cartilage skeleton, well-formed joint space, cruciate ligaments, tendons, menisci, and joint capsule. These structures develop in situ and are well developed at this gestational age.

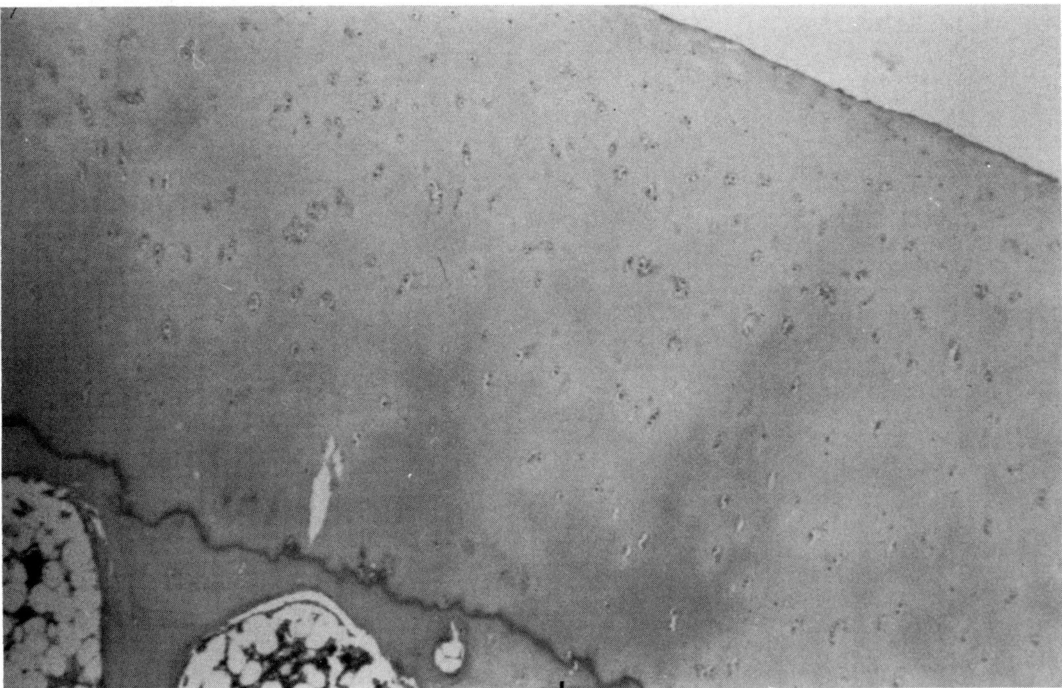

Figure 6–4. Normal articular surface exhibiting superficial gliding zone, transitional zone, a somewhat cellular radial zone, tidemark, and zone of calcification merging into the subchondral plate.

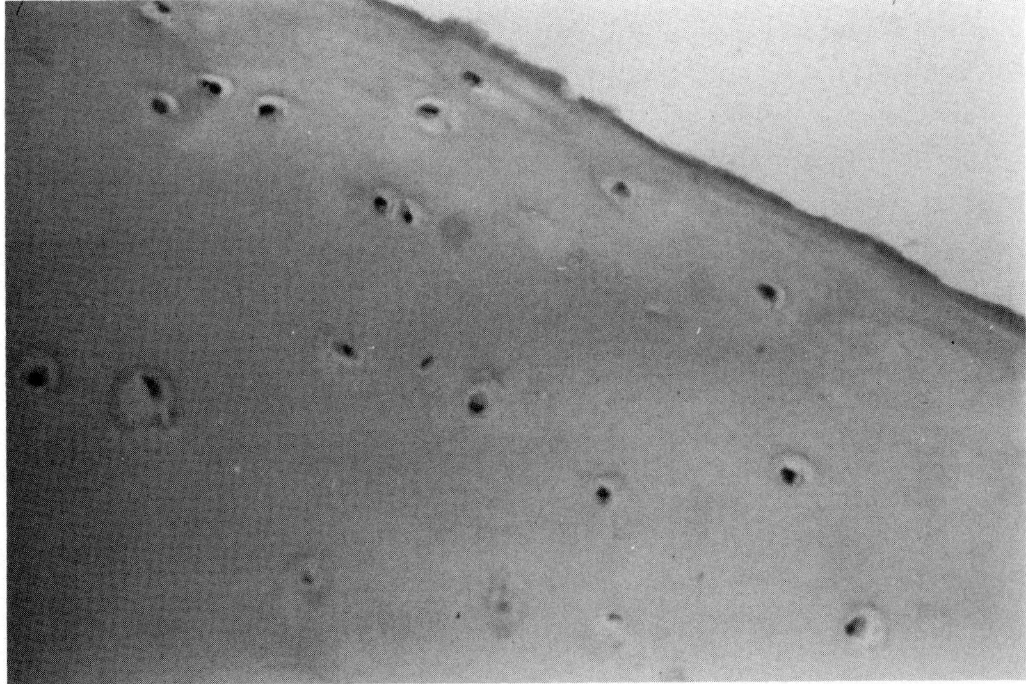

Figure 6–5. Normal articular cartilage, higher magnification of superficial gliding and transitional zones. Chondrocytes are flattened, and a single layer (lamina splendens) is visible at the surface of the articular cartilage. Cartilage cells are shed into the synovial space.

Ligaments, synovium, menisci, and other intra-articular and periarticular structures develop in situ. The menisci at the knee develop as peripherally located semicircular fibrocartilaginous pads. At no stage of development are they ever completely circular.

Normal articular cartilage consists of four layers: the upper tangential (gliding) zone, in which the cartilaginous cells are flattened and shed into the joint fluid; a calcified basal layer adjoining the subchondral bone; and two intermediate layers, the transitional and radial, which serve as shock absorbers (Jaffe, 1972) (Figs. 6–4 to 6–6). At the junction of the upper and middle thirds of the intermediate zone, cloning of cartilage cells can be demonstrated, indicating the equivalent of a "germinal layer" (Mankin, 1974). The question of whether or not cartilage is capable of reproduction at the normal articular surface is a matter of debate. On the one hand, outright mitotic activity cannot be easily demonstrated; on the other hand, clones of cartilage cells are always present in the intermediate zone (Fig. 6–7). Metabolic activity of chondrocytes strongly suggests an internal remodeling process rather than simple matrix maintenance, which in turn would confirm reproductive activity. Regardless of the presence or absence of mitotic activity in normal cartilage, there is no question that cartilage cells can reproduce in pathologic states to the point of recreating functional articular surfaces (Mankin, 1974; Mankin et al., 1971; Sokoloff, 1976; Teitelbaum and Bullough, 1979) (Figs. 6–8 and 6–9). One may therefore assume that some form of mitotic activity is responsible for the clones, even in the normal state.

Clones of cartilage cells migrate slowly toward the joint surface and are shed into the joint space. At the deeper margin, there is always slow and persistent conversion of cartilage to bone. Progressive tidemarks of calcified cartilage document changes of contour at the subchondral plate.

Text continued on page 199

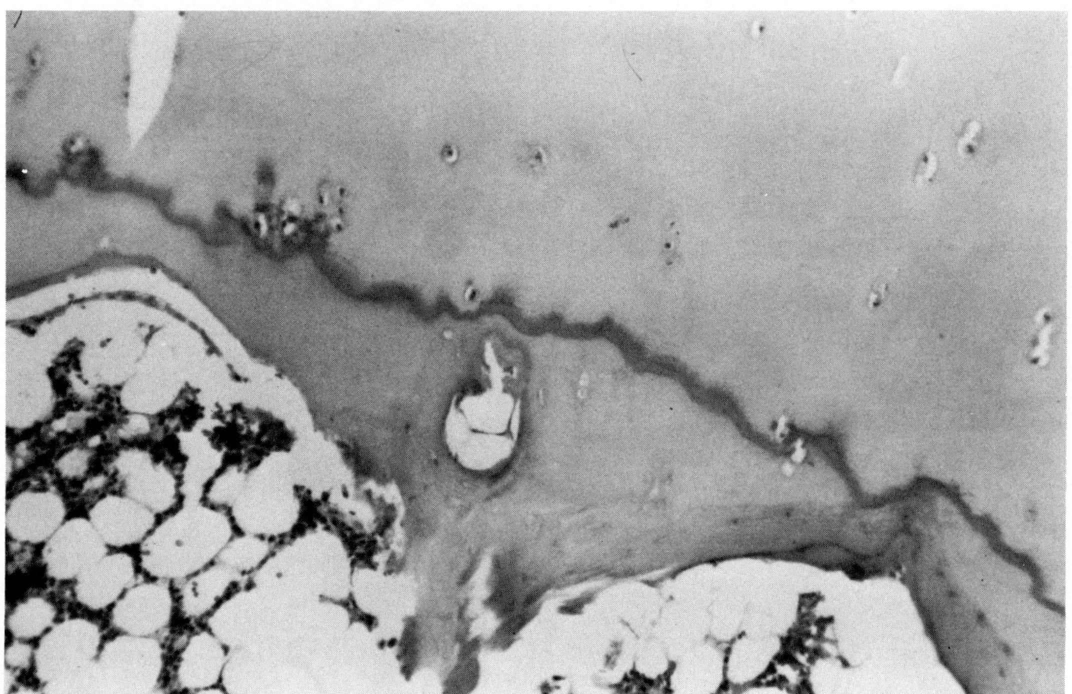

Figure 6–6. Higher magnification of tidemark, calcified cartilage and bone. The tidemark delineates the forward limit of calcification. Calcified cartilage and bone are present beneath the tide mark.

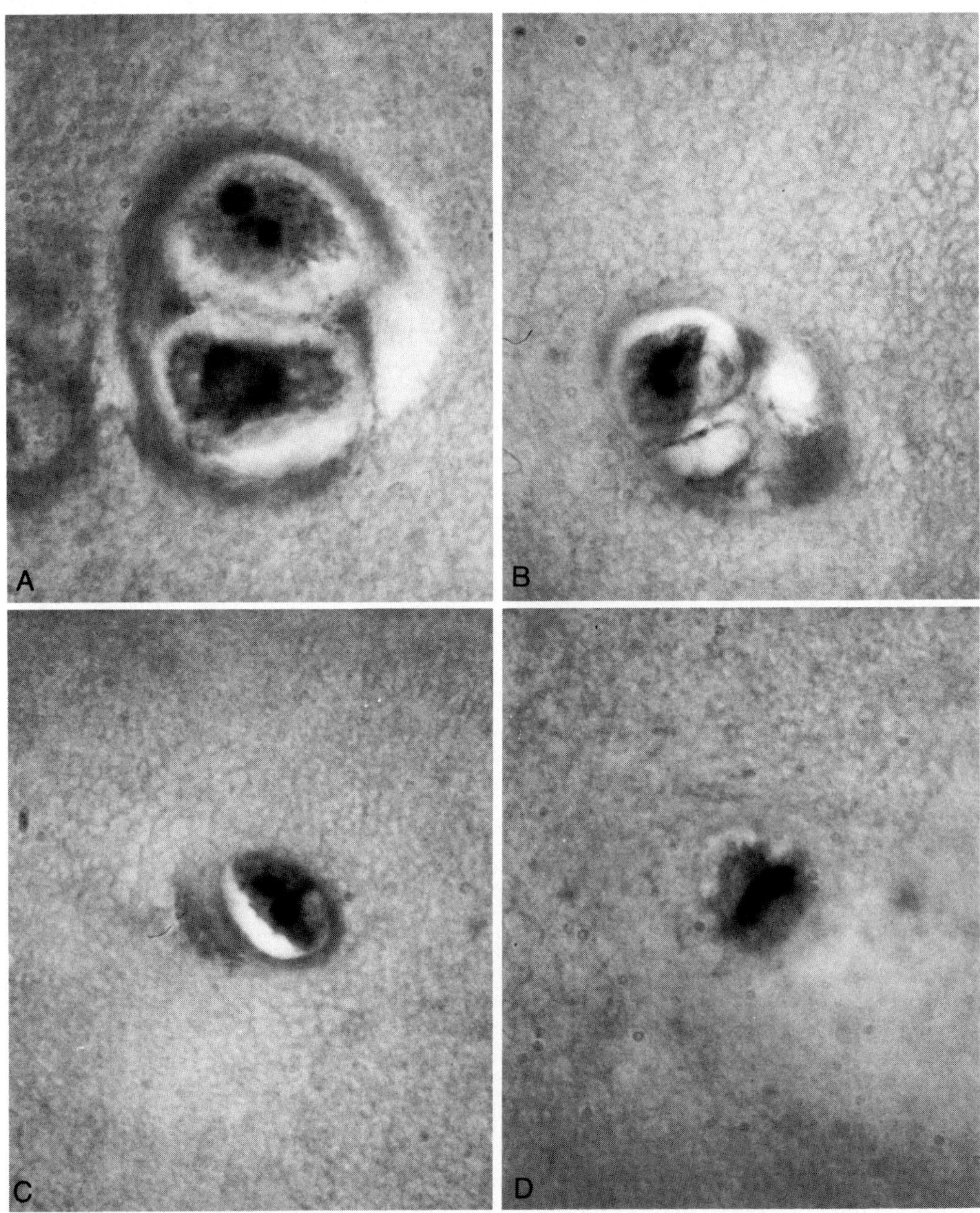

Figure 6–7. Normal articular cartilage exhibiting clones of cartilage cells in the regenerative middle zone. Although mitotic activity cannot be demonstrated, pairs and quadruples of cells are evident.

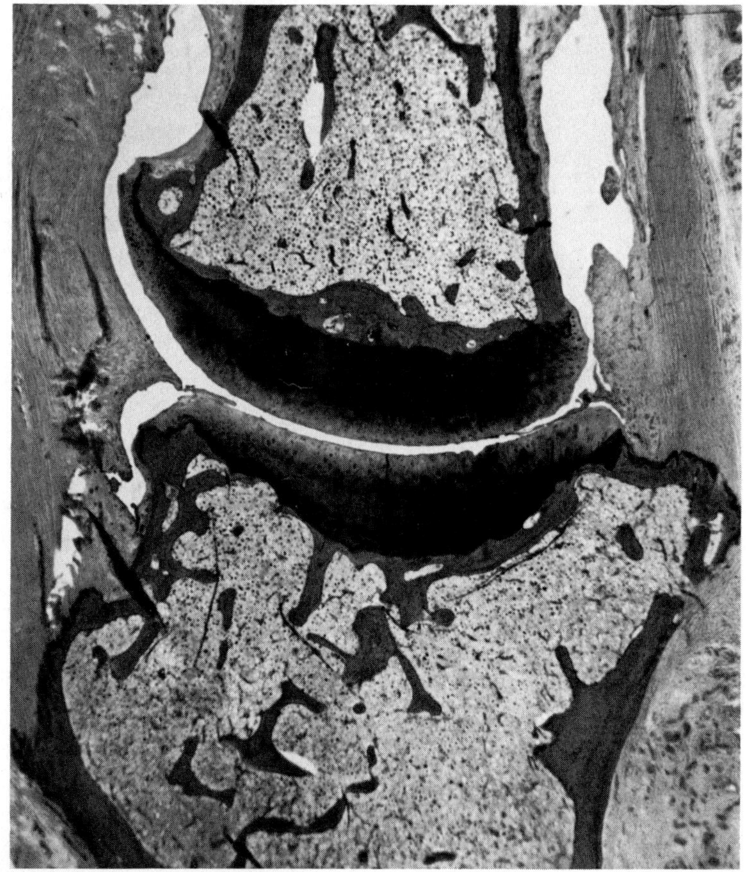

Figure 6–8. Macrospecimen of patient with acromegaly. Note the proliferating articular cartilage, characterized by successive tidemarks. A Heberden node, an example of circumferential remodeling, is present.

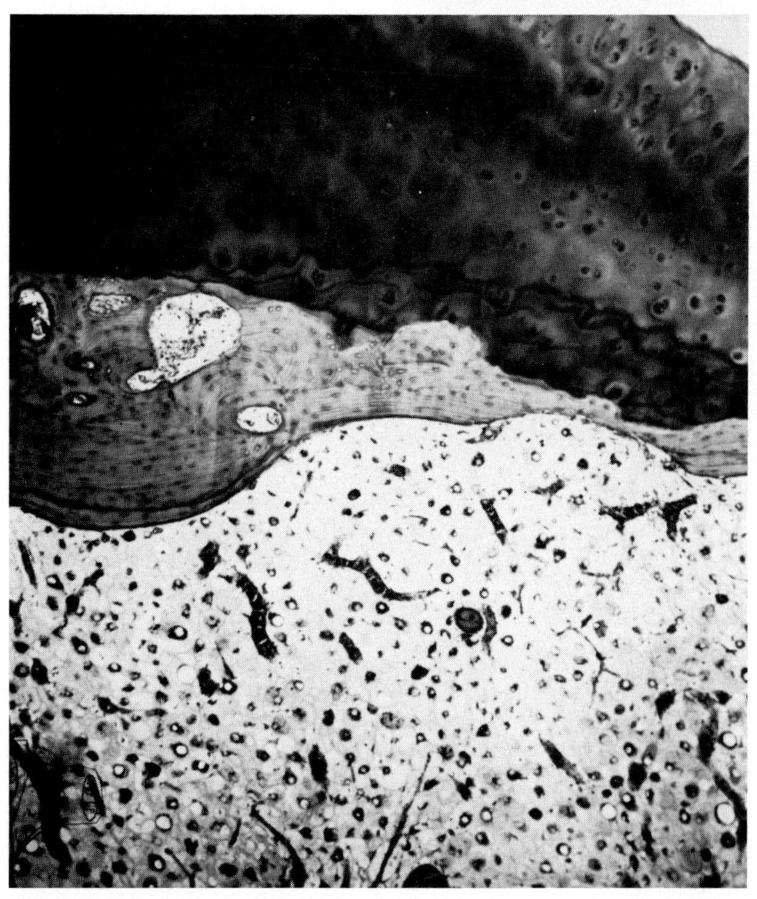

Figure 6–9. Higher magnification of articular cartilage in patient with acromegaly. The successive tidemarks indicate progressive remodeling. The regenerative zone of the cartilage is in the midportion, and clones of cartilage cells migrate upward to be shed into the joint surface. The clones also migrate downward, and there is transformation of cartilage to bone, as evidenced by the successive tidemarks. Acromegaly represents the accentuation of normal processes and is an indication of the growth potential of normal articular cartilage.

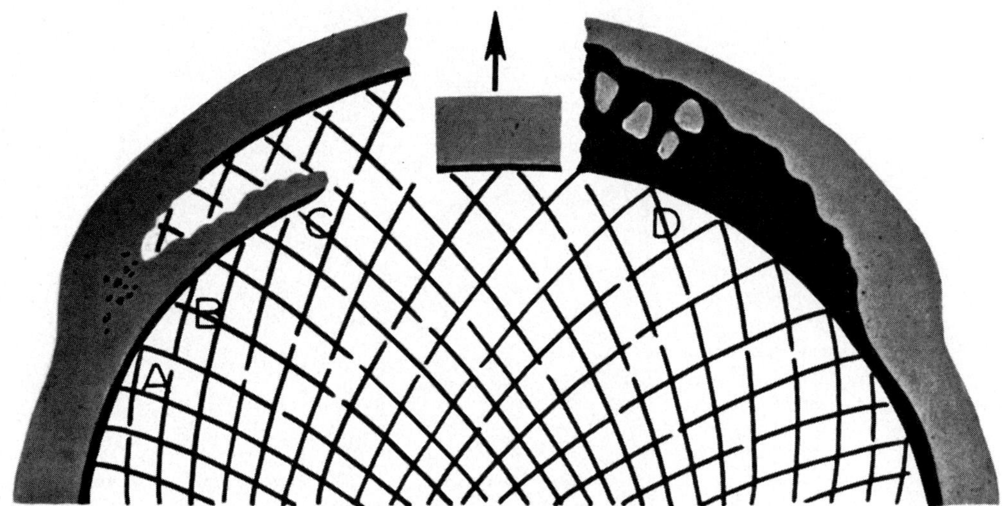

Figure 6–10. Schematic diagram exhibiting the features of progressive remodeling. *A,* Increased height of cartilage is associated with increased diffusion distance, accounting for death of cartilage cells and vascular invasion from subchondral area. Vascular invasion is accompanied by transformation to bone, accounting for a new subchondral plate. *B,* A new subchondral plate is formed, although residuals of the old articular cartilage surface remain. *C,* After remodeling, the old articular cartilage may be removed, and the entire bone has a new contour, with articular cartilage at a more forward position. *D,* The new subchondral plate may be thickened, but remodeling ultimately occurs in response to mechanical demands. (Modified from Johnson, L. C.: J. Am. Vet. Assoc. *141:*1237, 1962.)

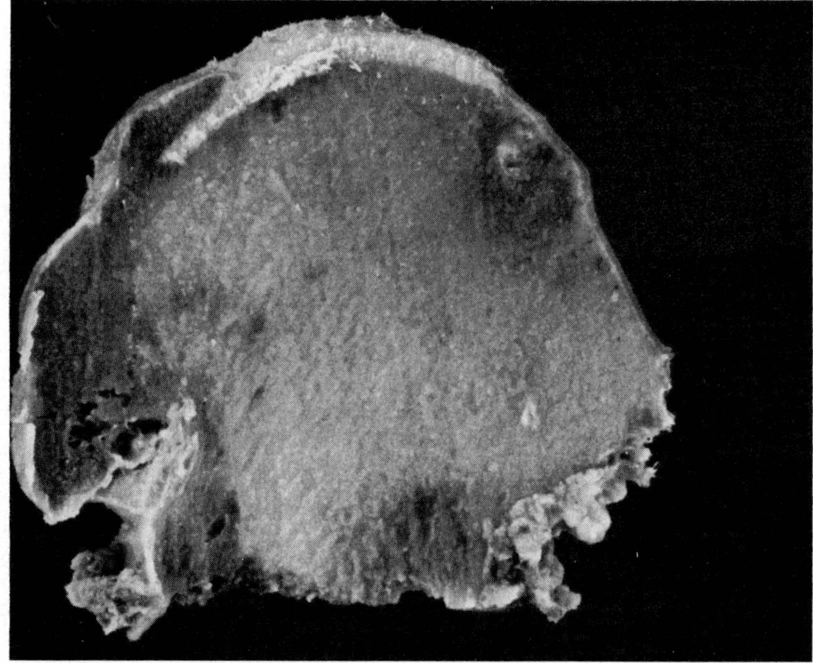

Figure 6–11. Gross photograph of specimen exhibiting progressive remodeling. Note increased height of cartilage, residual articular cartilage beneath the subchondral plate, and irregular contour of femoral head. Compare with Figure 6–10.

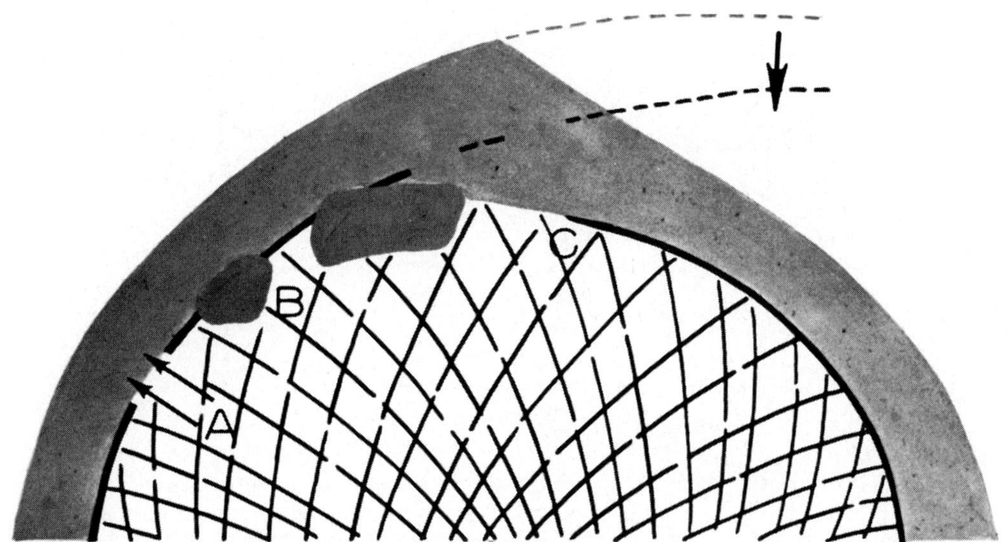

Figure 6–12. Regressive remodeling. *A,* Osteoclasts move in and remove the subchondral plate in response to altered mechanical stresses. *B,* Myxoid material replaces the subchondral plate, and there is formation of cartilage to replace the myxoid material. *C,* A new layer of cartilage is formed, a new subchondral plate is established, and the entire contour of the bone is altered to conform to the new demands. (Modified from Johnson, L. C.: J. Am. Vet. Assoc. *141:*1237, 1962.)

JOINT REMODELING

The contour of joints is subject to continuous change (i.e., "remodeling"). The remodeling is designated "progressive" when it adds to bone length, "regressive" when it subtracts from bone length, and "circumferential" when it adds to the diameter of the bone. Accentuation of this normal remodeling merges into "disease": osteoarthritis. Disease occurs when the remodeling is decompensated or unbalanced or when the patient perceives it as such (Johnson, 1959; Johnson, 1962).

Figure 6–10 illustrates progressive remodeling. Proliferation of interstitial cartilage cells produces increased thickness of the articular cartilage. Conversion of cartilage to calcified cartilage and subsequently to bone can be seen at the base of this thickened cartilage. The subchondral bone becomes thickened. Occasionally, successive layers of subchondral plates are identifiable, with residuals of the original subchondral plate present in the trabecular bone (Fig. 6–11).

Remodeling can also be regressive (Fig. 6–12). It is initiated by osteoclastic resorption of the subchondral plate and adjacent cancellous bone. Myxoid and cartilaginous metaplasia occurs in the adjacent marrow matrix, and there is shedding of the superficial layers of cartilage into the joint. A new subchondral bony plate develops. Examples of regressive remodeling are the Schmorl's node and the "codfish" vertebrae seen in Cushing's disease and osteoporosis.

The third type of remodeling occurs at margins of joints and is called "circumferential remodeling" (Fig. 6–13). It may be due to new periosteal bone formation, ossification of tendons or ligaments, or upward and lateral growth of cartilage with progressive transformation to bone. Osteophyte formation in the spine is a common example of circumferential remodeling and can cause bridging across the joint surface by bone. Formation of Heberden's nodes in the interphalangeal joints is an example of circumferential remodeling carried to excess.

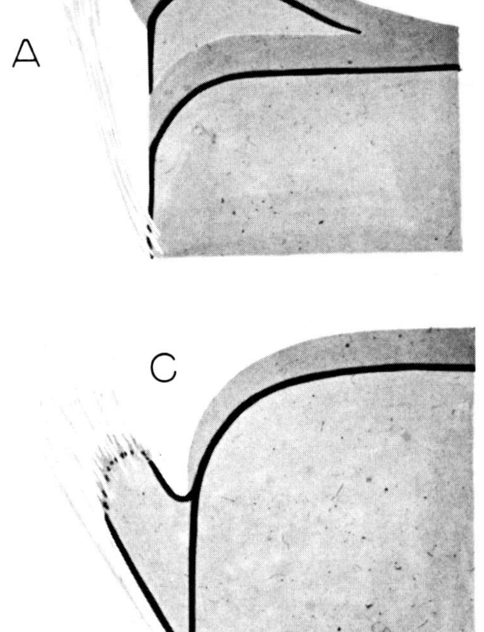
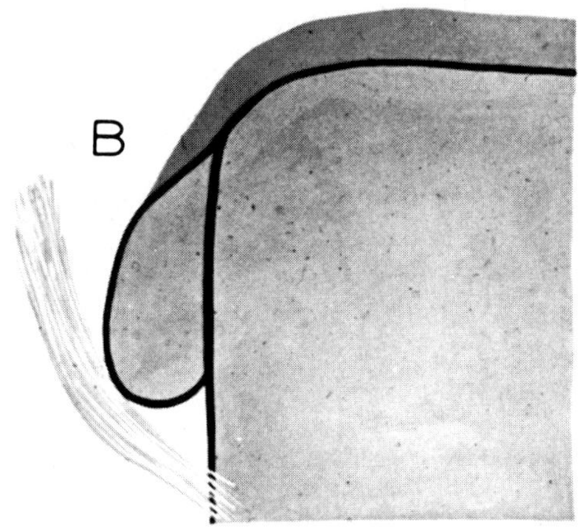

Figure 6–13. Circumferential remodeling. *A,* Successive tidemarks and forward remodeling can elevate the periphery of the joint in response to altered mechanical stimuli. *B,* Lateral growth of the bone and articular cartilage, such as seen in a Heberden's node. *C,* Calcification and ultimately ossification of a tendon insertion can also result in circumferential remodeling. This is characteristic of spinal remodeling processes. (Modified from Johnson, L. C.: Lab. Invest. *8:*1223, 1959.)

OSTEOARTHRITIS

Osteoarthritis, as opposed to physiologic remodeling, is a result of decompensation of the remodeling process.

Unbalanced remodeling can be initiated by numerous factors:

1. Deformities leading to discongruity of the joint surface (slipped capital femoral epiphysis; Legg-Calvé-Perthes disease or other infarctions; fracture through articular cartilage, acute trauma with loss of cartilage layers).

2. Pannus formation, blocking surface diffusion of cartilage (rheumatoid arthritis, tuberculosis).

3. Pyogenic inflammation of joint, with resultant destruction of articular cartilage.

4. Hyperpolymerization of cartilage proteoglycans, leading to brittle cartilage (ochronosis).

5. Depolymerization of proteoglycans resulting in disintegration of cartilage (gout).

6. Extensive changes in the physical and osmotic properties of the synovial fluid, which may inhibit nutritional diffusion with surface cartilage (repeated hemarthrosis in hemophilia).

7. Excessive cartilage proliferation (acromegaly).

Any of these processes will initiate both excessive shearing of the tangential surface layer and unbalanced remodeling. Thus, pure degenerative osteoarthritis is cartilaginous in origin (Sokoloff, 1976). At first, articular cartilage exhibits enlargement and hypertrophy of the cartilage cells. The radiating configuration of the collagen bundles in cartilage is evident when there is metabolic breakdown of the proteoglycan matrix. Fibrillation of the matrix becomes evident (Figs. 6–14 and 6–15). As the collagen fibers become unmasked, they become less resistant to normal wear and tear, and fissures develop. These fissures are irregularly placed and eventually extend into the basal layers of the articular cartilage and subchondral bone (Fig. 6–16). Separation of fragments of cartilage may occur, and chunks of cartilage break off into the joint. When the entire articular cartilaginous surface becomes separated, myxoid changes occur in the overlying bone, and eburnation results. The eburnated bone requires reinforcement of the trabeculae beneath the surface to allow bone to perform its weight-bearing function. Myxomatous changes occur that lead to cyst formation in the subchondral marrow. Such cyst formation may also be at some distance from the joint and is probably related to the altered metabolic factors in the nutrition of the cartilage. These cysts may become quite extensive and may precede the actual destruction of the cartilaginous surface (Figs. 6–19 to 6–28).

Radiographically, the earliest evidence of osteoarthritis is pointing or sharpening of the articular margins, a sign associated with gradual narrowing of the joint space due to thinning (shedding) of the articular cartilage (Fig. 6–29). Subsequent changes include sclerosis of the subchondral bone, development of osteophytes, erosion of the opposing articular bony surface, and cyst formation.

Osteoarthritis is the end result of any condition that causes unbalanced remodeling or interference with normal cartilage physiology. Trauma, cartilage derangements from infections, rheumatoid arthritis, gout, ochronosis, and hypertrophic synovitis all eventually terminate in manifestations of degenerative osteoarthritis. The etiologic factors are not always identifiable.

It should be emphasized that severe degenerative changes are not always perceived as "disease" by the afflicted, and little if any functional impairment or pain may be associated with what are obviously severe morphologic alterations (Figs. 6–30 to 6–41).

Text continued on page 216

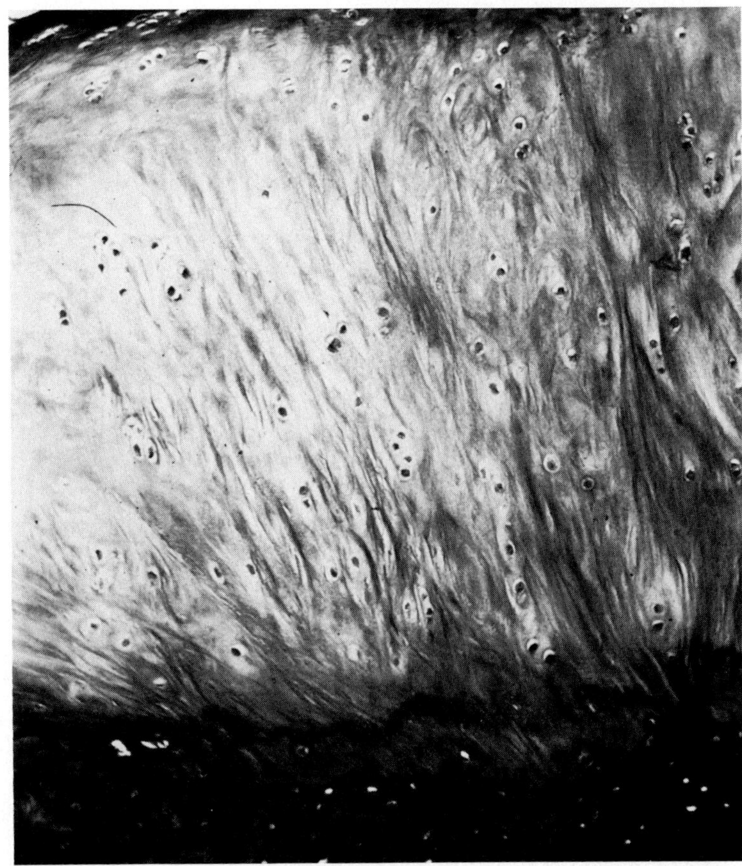

Figure 6–14. Osteoarthritis. Note fibrillation of the surface cartilage layers with unmasking of the fiber structure. Even though the fibers are identifiable and the arcade structure is unmasked, no fissures are present. The fibrillary pattern indicates dehydration, possible calcification, and brittle structure. There is extension of cloning through the full depth of cartilage instead of the normal limitation to a single stratum.

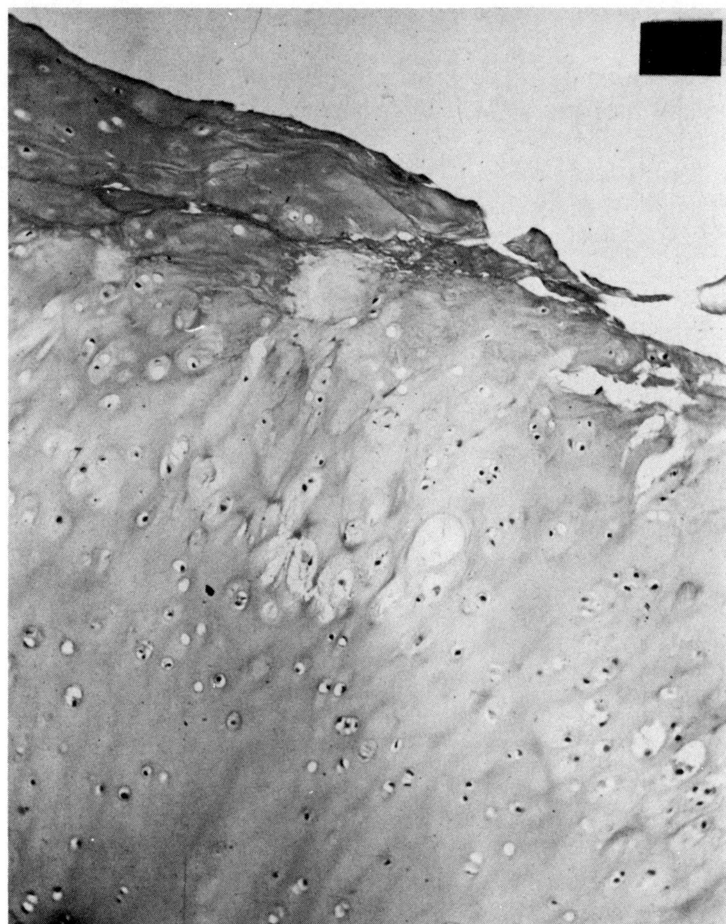

Figure 6–15. Osteoarthritis. More advanced fibrillary degeneration of cartilage with formation of Weichselbaum lacunae. These represent secretory activity and lacunae formation by the increased proliferative activity of the articular cartilage. Fragmentation of the surface layer is evident.

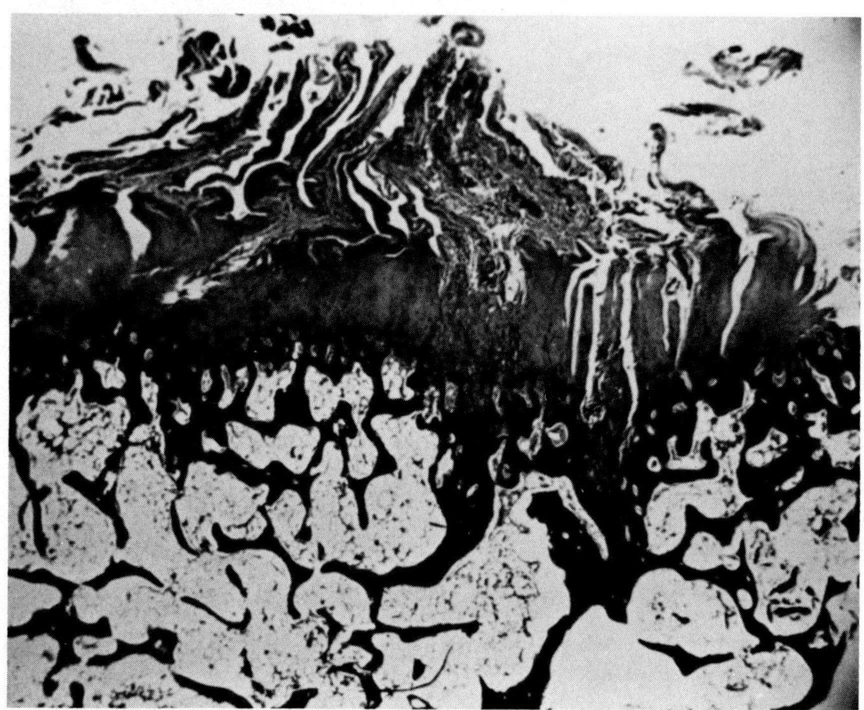

Figure 6–16. More advanced stage of articular cartilaginous degeneration exhibiting extensive fissure development, with some fissures extending into the subchondral plate. Mild sclerosis of subchondral bone is present.

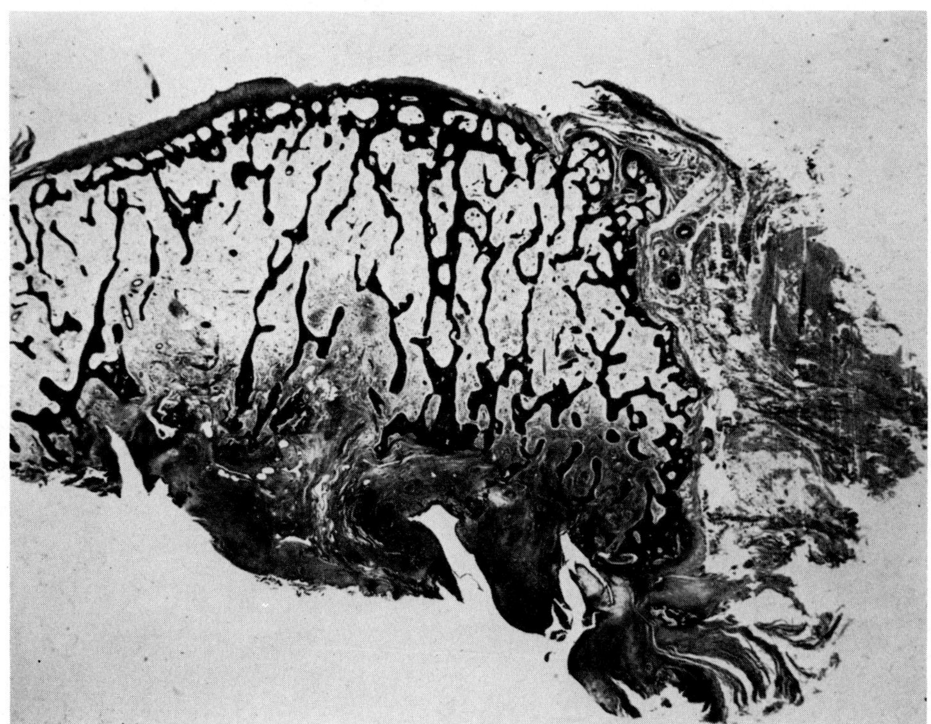

Figure 6–17. Macrosection exhibiting progressive remodeling as a result of active hyperemia. The patient, suffering from tuberculosis, exhibits the effects of active hyperemia: osteoporosis and accentuation of the progressive remodeling process. Two successive subchondral plates are identifiable. Tuberculous synovitis is present at the lateral margin with extension into the metaphyseal portion of the bone.

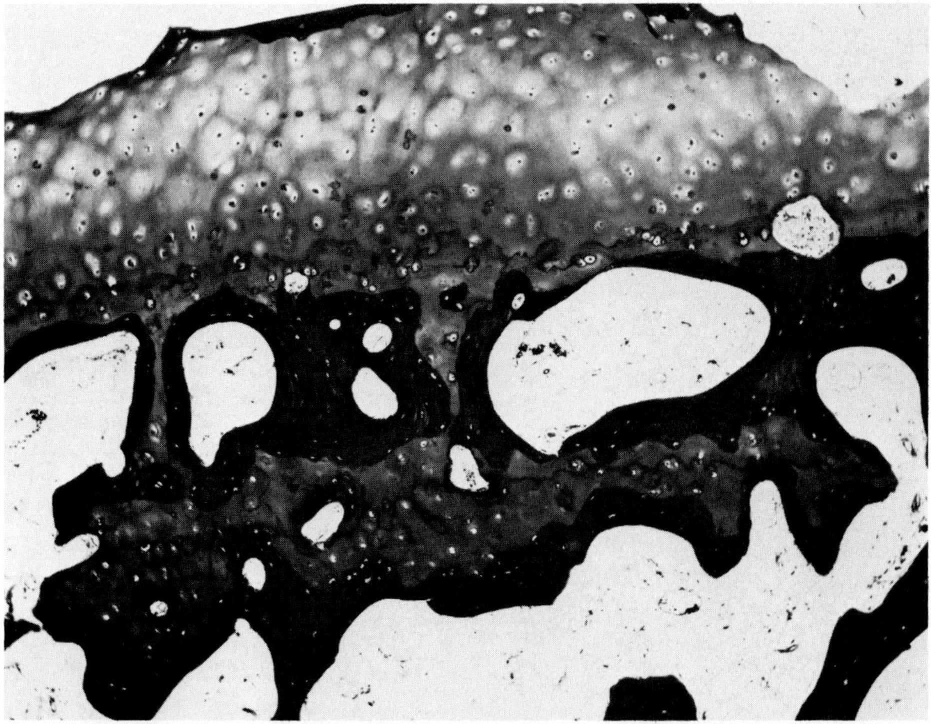

Figure 6–18. Higher magnification of macrospecimen shown in Figure 6–17. Note the articular cartilage at the surface, subchondral plate formation, and the residual articular cartilage beneath the subchondral plate. The progressive remodeling process proceeds at a rapid rate so that the cartilage is not completely absorbed. Compare with Figures 6–10 and 6–11.

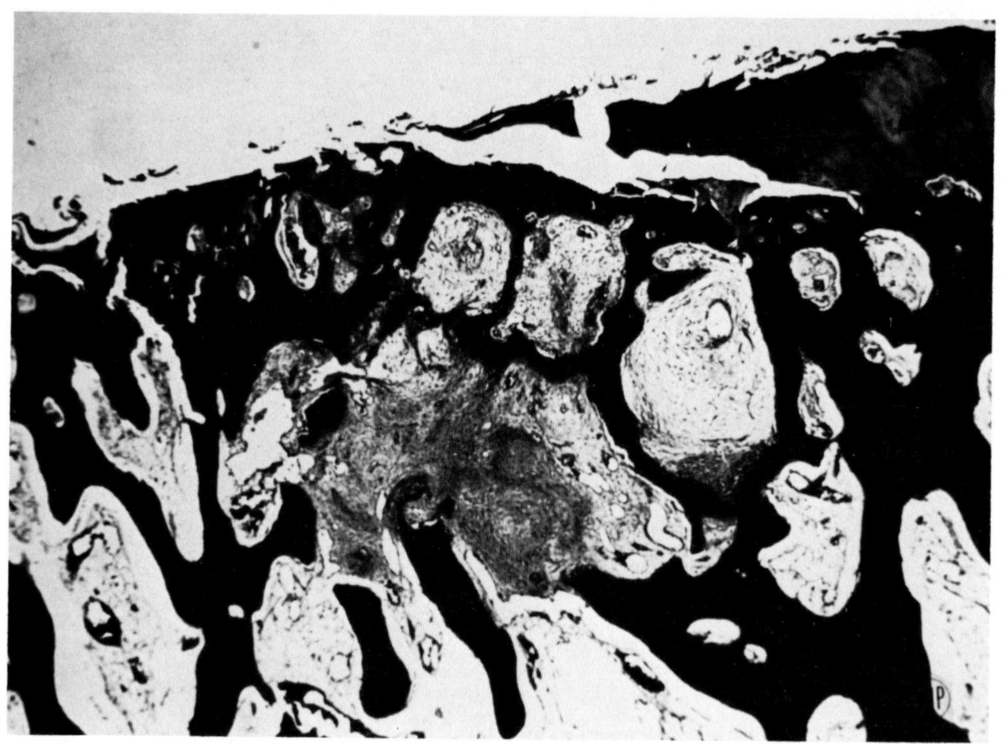

Figure 6–19. Eburnated bone showing formation of chondrogranuloma. Numerous inflammatory cells and myxoid chondroid material are present beneath the sclerotic reinforced subchondral bone.

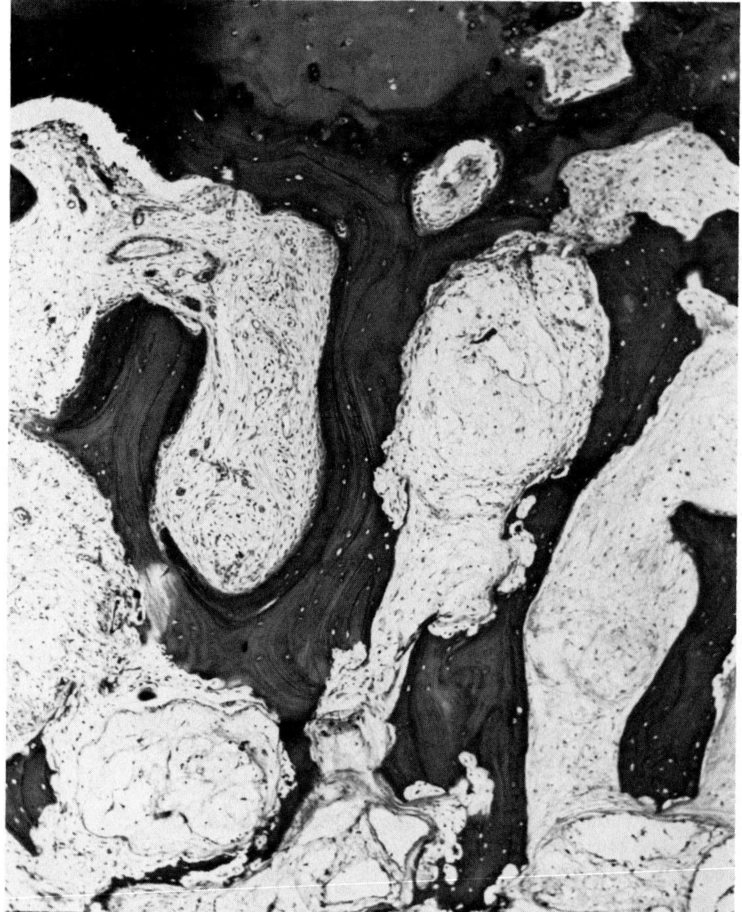

Figure 6–20. Subchondral area of patient with osteoarthritis. Early formation of chondrogranuloma in subchondral area. Note accumulation of fibrous connective tissue, myxoid stroma, early cyst formation, and extensive remodeling activity as well as appositional bone formation and numerous Howship's lacunae.

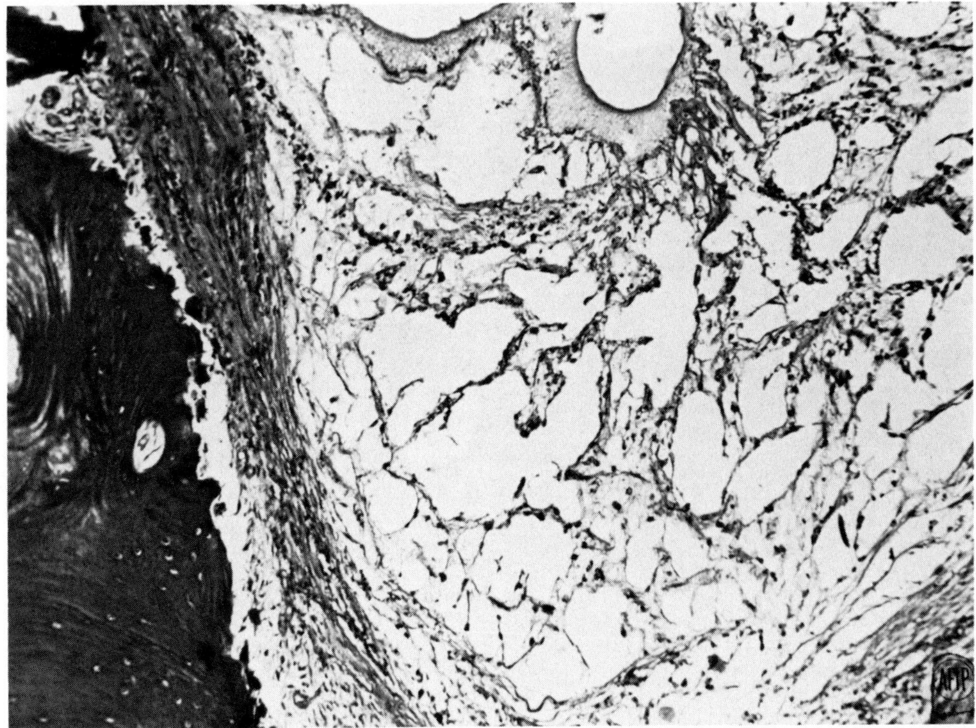

Figure 6–21. Cyst. Early cyst formation in subchondral area. Note the reinforced bone and loose myxoid stroma with formation of cystic cavities.

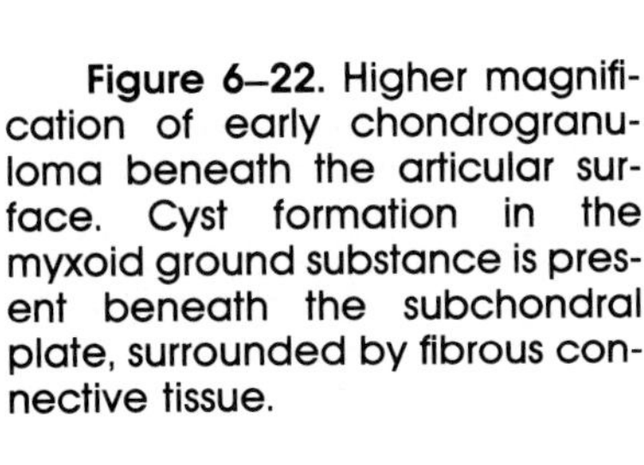

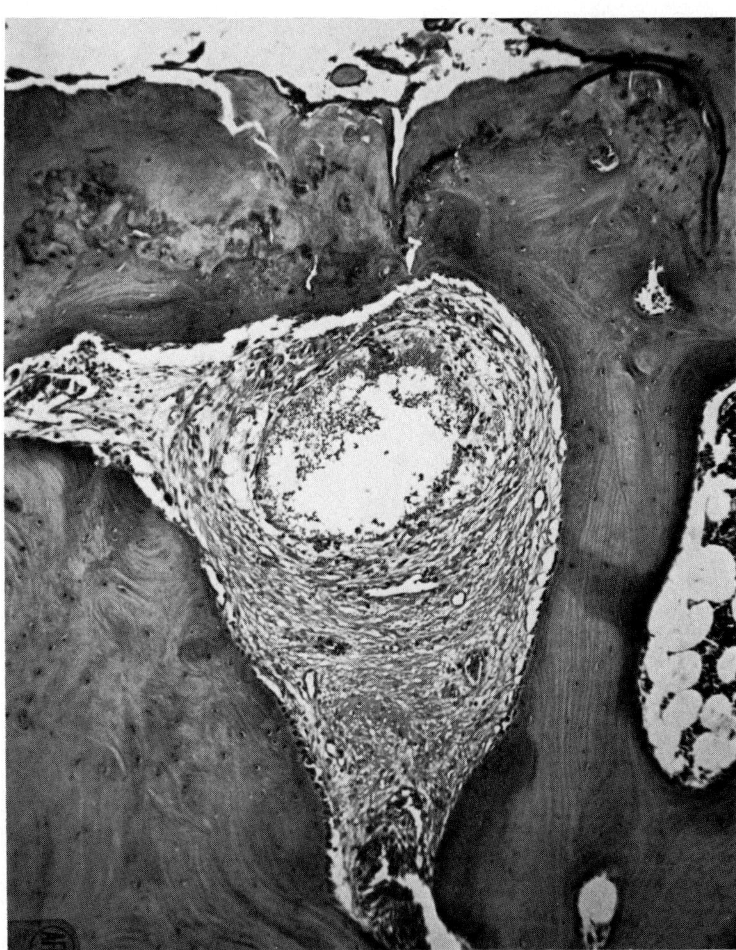

Figure 6–22. Higher magnification of early chondrogranuloma beneath the articular surface. Cyst formation in the myxoid ground substance is present beneath the subchondral plate, surrounded by fibrous connective tissue.

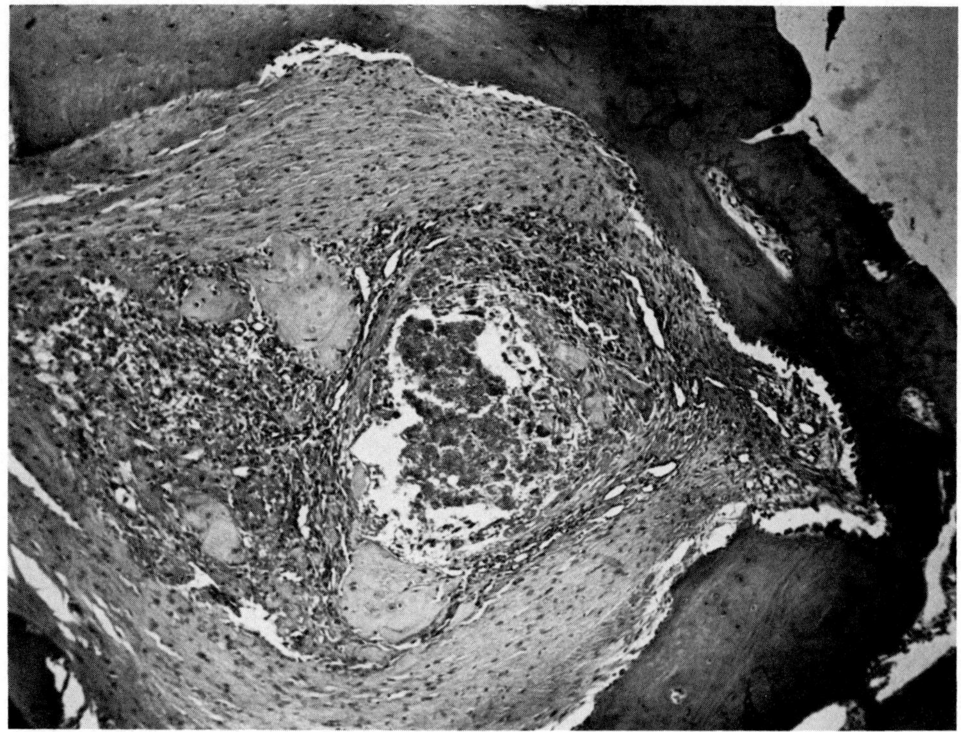

Figure 6–23. Subchondral plate exhibiting fragments of intact cartilage, myxoid material, cystic degeneration of myxoid material, and fibrous connective tissue surrounding the cartilaginous degenerative products.

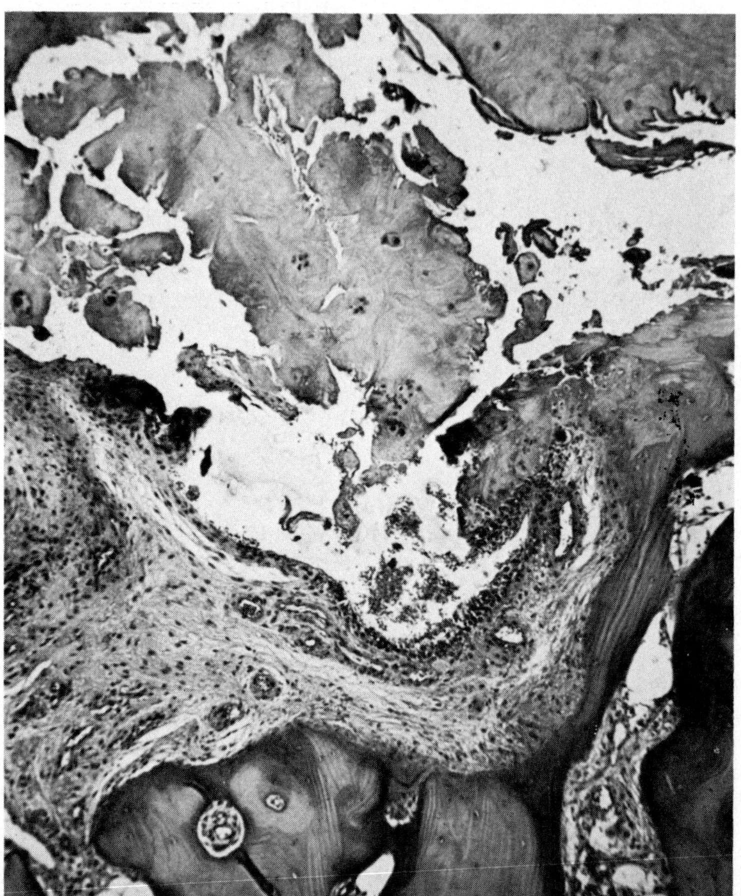

Figure 6–24. Fragments of cartilage within the subchondral cyst, surrounded by fibrous connective tissue. Note the early formation of a synovium-like epithelium surrounding these intact cartilage fragments.

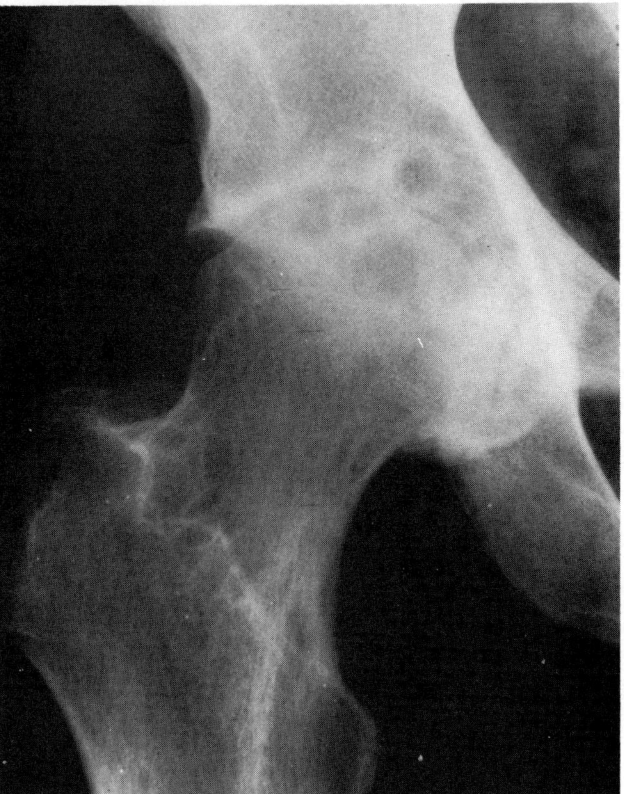

Figure 6–25. Radiographic manifestation of subchondral cyst formation in patient with advanced osteoarthritis. Radiolucencies surrounded by bony reinforced trabeculae are visible in the neck of the femur and acetabulum.

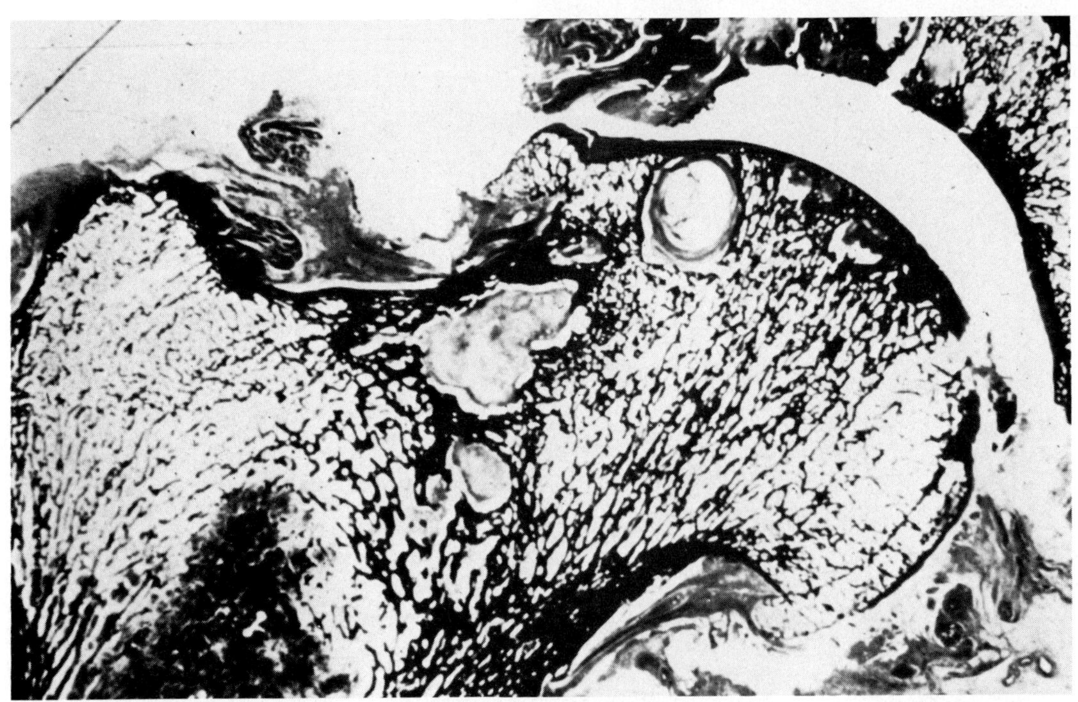

Figure 6–26. Macrosection of the femoral head and acetabulum exhibiting progressive, regressive, and circumferential remodeling. Numerous cysts are present in the subchondral bone. Notice the cyst formation deep within the metaphysis of the femur as well as the acetabulum. The degenerative products of the cartilage may extend deep into the bony structure, even when the surface articular cartilage is still intact. Cyst formation is evidence of regressive remodeling. The medial portion of the femoral head shows progressive remodeling with an advancing articular surface. Circumferential remodeling is indicated at the lateral margin of the femoral head by osteophyte formation. The combination of these remodeling processes changes the shape of the femoral head and acetabulum.

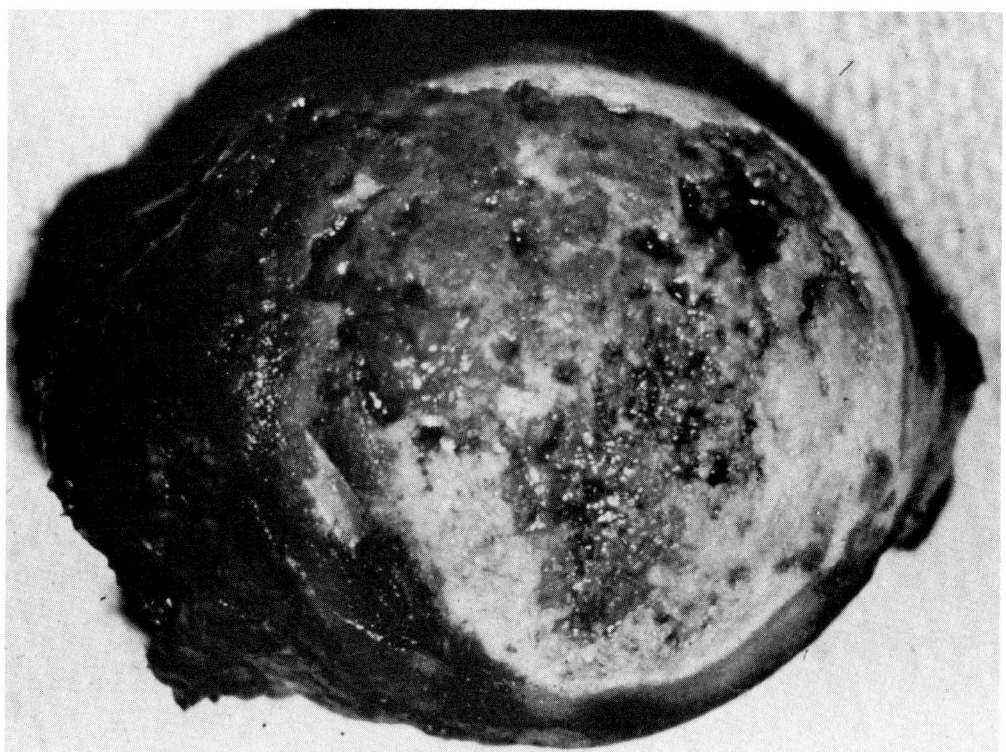

Figure 6–27. Gross appearance of femoral head in severe osteoarthritis. Note eburnated bone with complete loss of normal articular cartilage. The ground substance forms myxoid material in order to maintain a gliding surface.

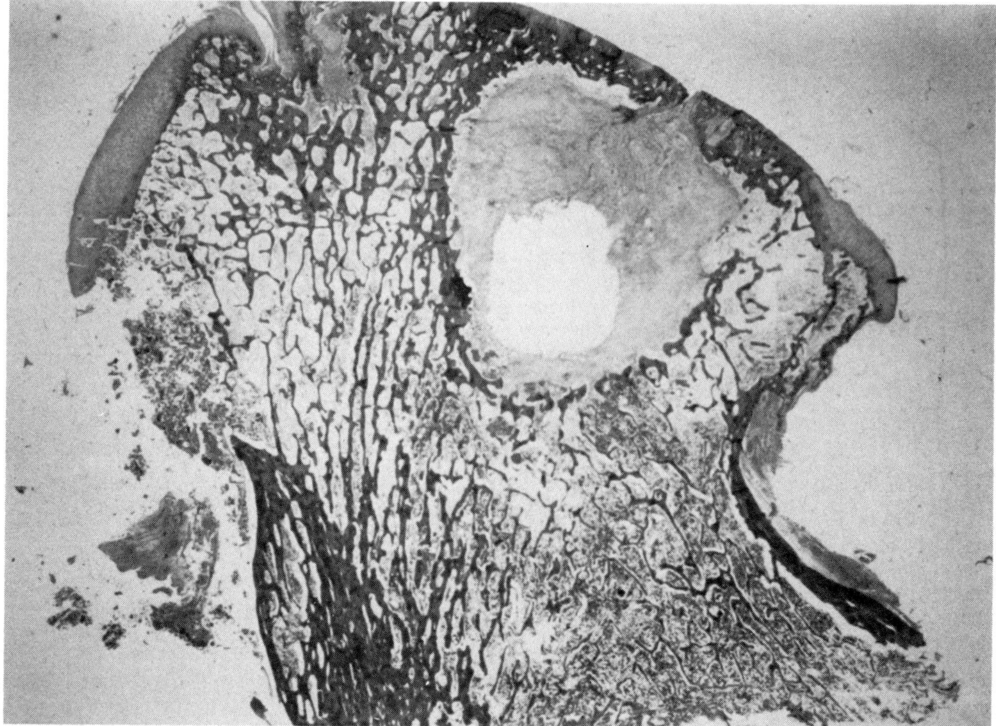

Figure 6–28. Large cyst in the subchondral area, secondary to osteoarthritis. These cysts usually, but not invariably, connect to the surface. Although they are radiographically lucent, it is clear that many of these "cysts" are not actually filled with fluid but rather contain varying amounts of tissue.

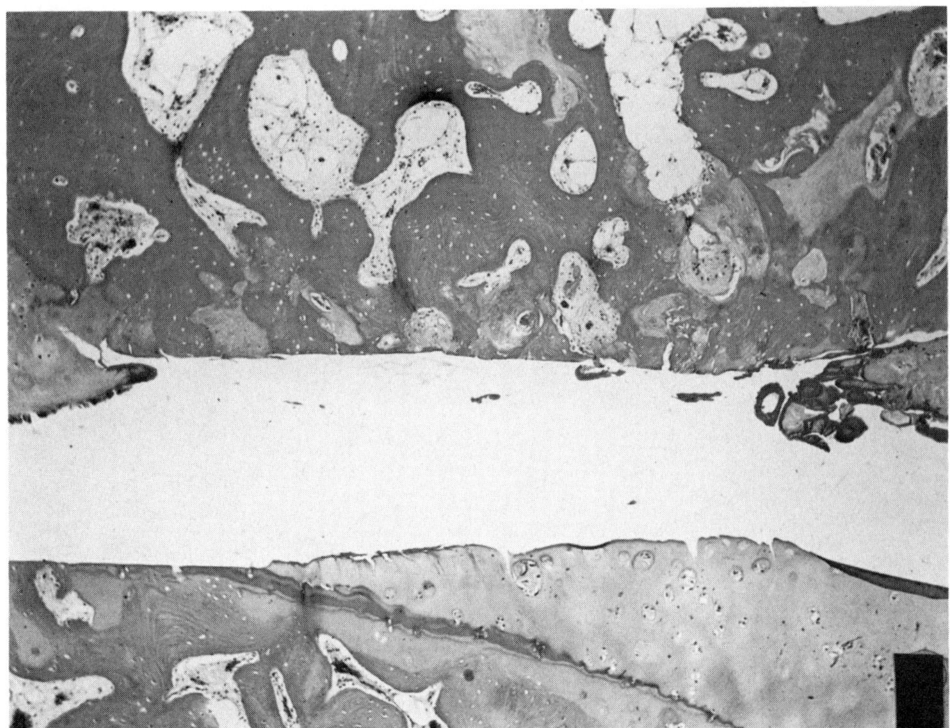

Figure 6–29. Microscopic appearance of opposing articular surfaces in severe osteoarthritis. Note the eburnated bone with formation of mucoid ground substance at the surface, sclerotic reinforcement of the subchondral plate, and erosion of the remaining articular cartilage. Note the progressive tidemarks in the articular cartilage.

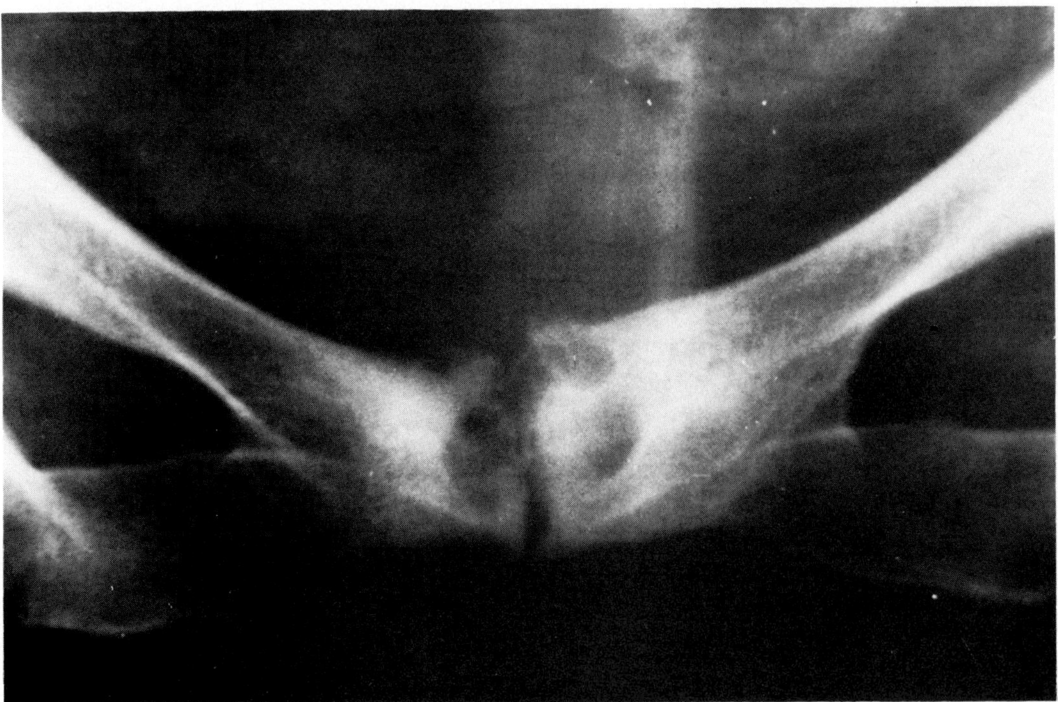

Figure 6–30. Radiograph of symphysis pubis showing numerous subchondral cysts. Degenerative osteoarthritis of the symphysis is associated with multiple pregnancies. It is also seen in professional soccer players.

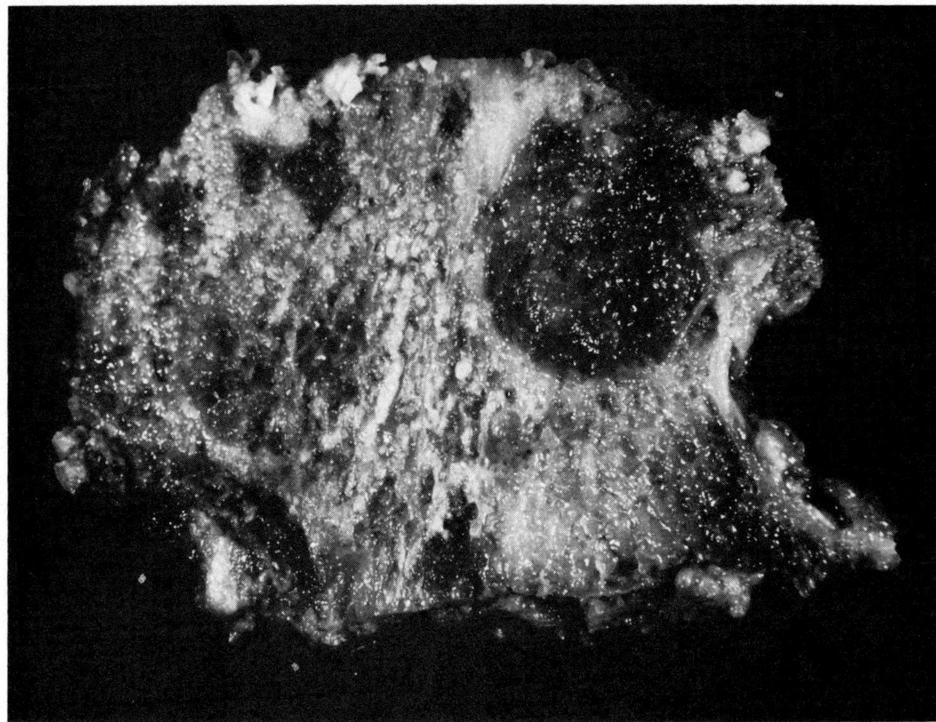

Figure 6–31. Gross specimen of femoral head exhibiting formation of large subchondral cyst. The cyst content is mucoid and gelatinous but contains identifiable cartilage fragments.

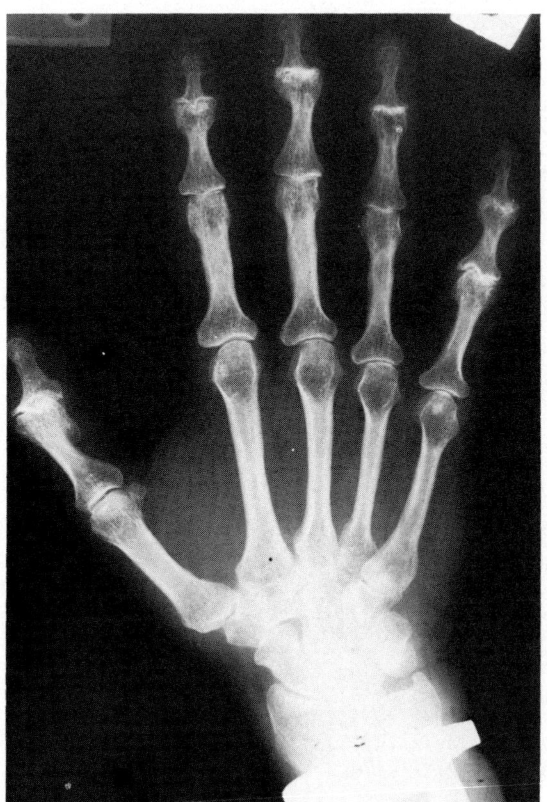

Figure 6–32. Radiograph of the hand of a patient showing moderate degenerative changes. Notice the loss of joint spaces, particularly in the interphalangeal joints. Circumferential remodeling has caused the formation of osteophytes at joint margins. Osteoarthritis typically attacks the interphalangeal joints, as opposed to rheumatoid arthritis, which attacks the metacarpophalangeal joints more severely.

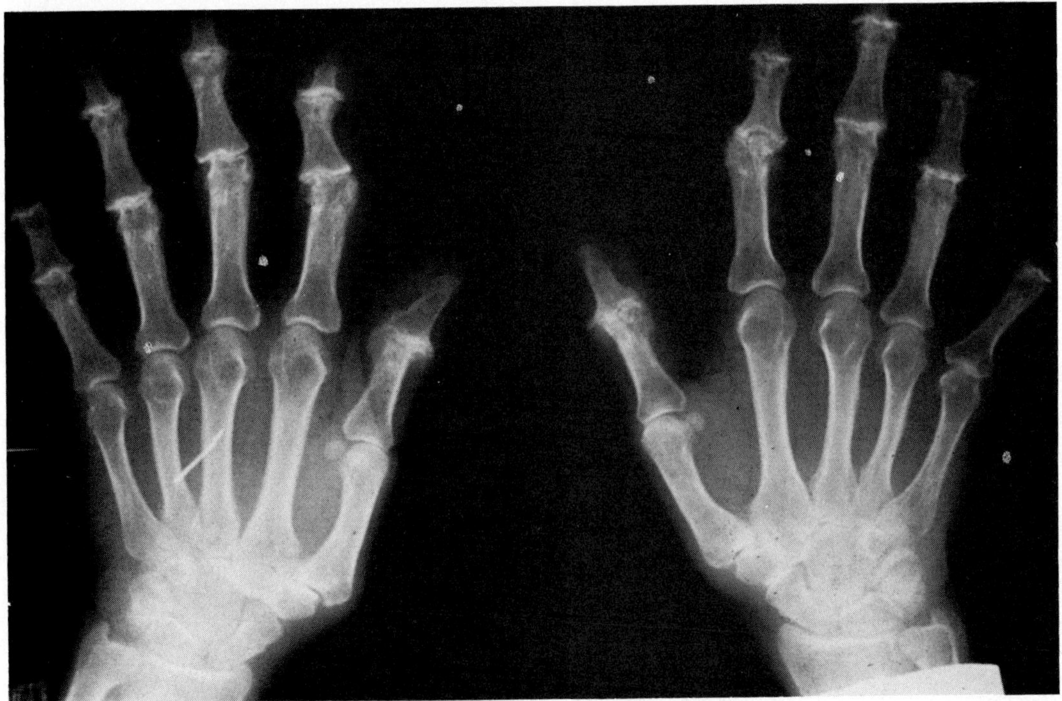

Figure 6–33. Radiographic manifestation of morphologically severe alterations corresponding to changes unusually encountered in osteoarthritis. The patient is a secretary who is able to type more than 100 words per minute without significant complaints. Morphologic alterations are not necessarily associated with disease.

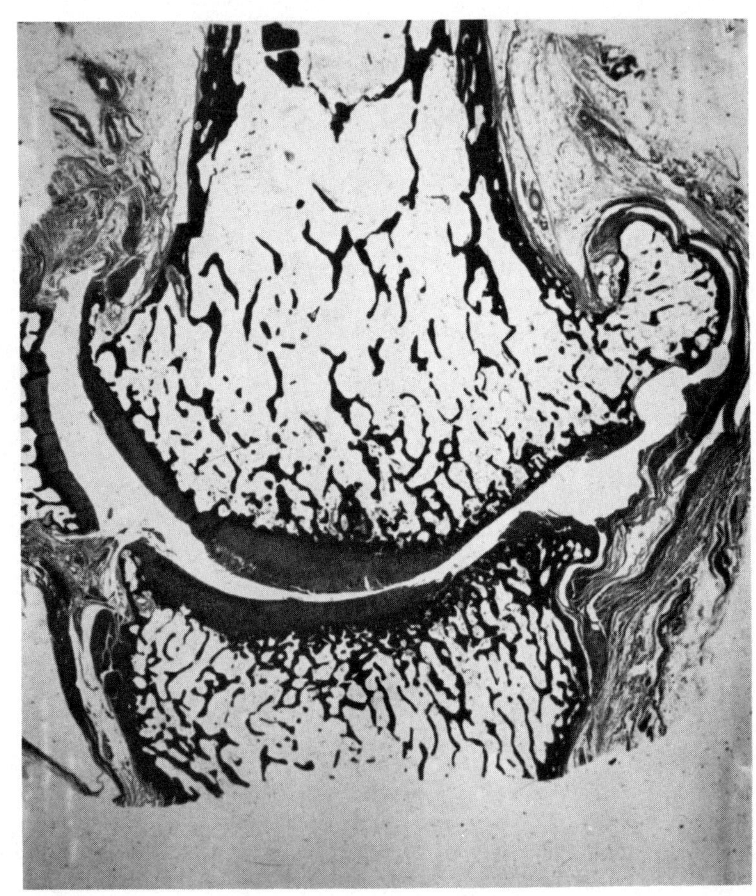

Figure 6–34. Macrospecimen from a patient with degenerative osteoarthritis in the metatarsophalangeal joint of the great toe. Note the exophytic circumferential remodeling process, the great variation in the articular cartilaginous surface, and the eburnation of the joint surfaces at the periphery. (From Syllabus: Revised Clinical Slide Collection on Rheumatic Diseases. Atlanta, Arthritis Foundation, National Office, 1981.)

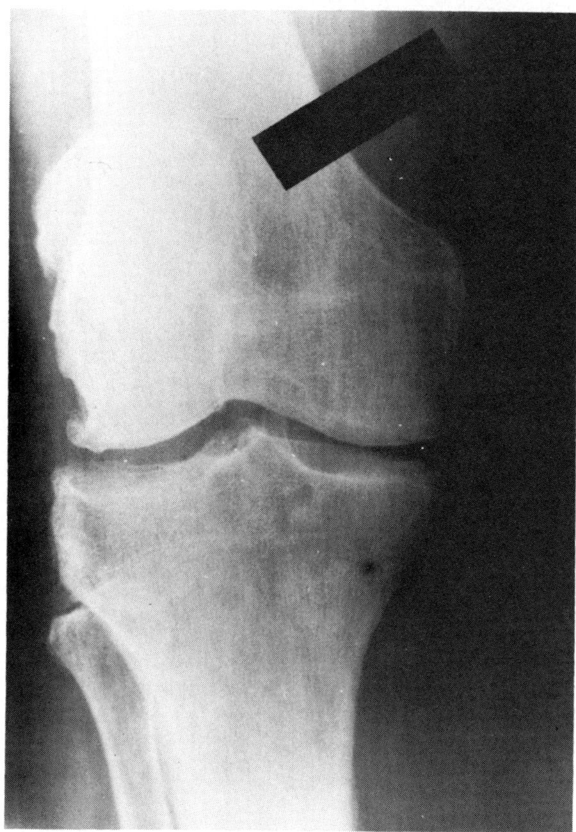

Figure 6–35. Anteroposterior radiograph of knee in patient with osteoarthritis. Note the irregular contour of the subchondral bone and the osteophyte formation at the lateral margins. These are the earlier signs of osteoarthritis and precede actual narrowing of the joint space.

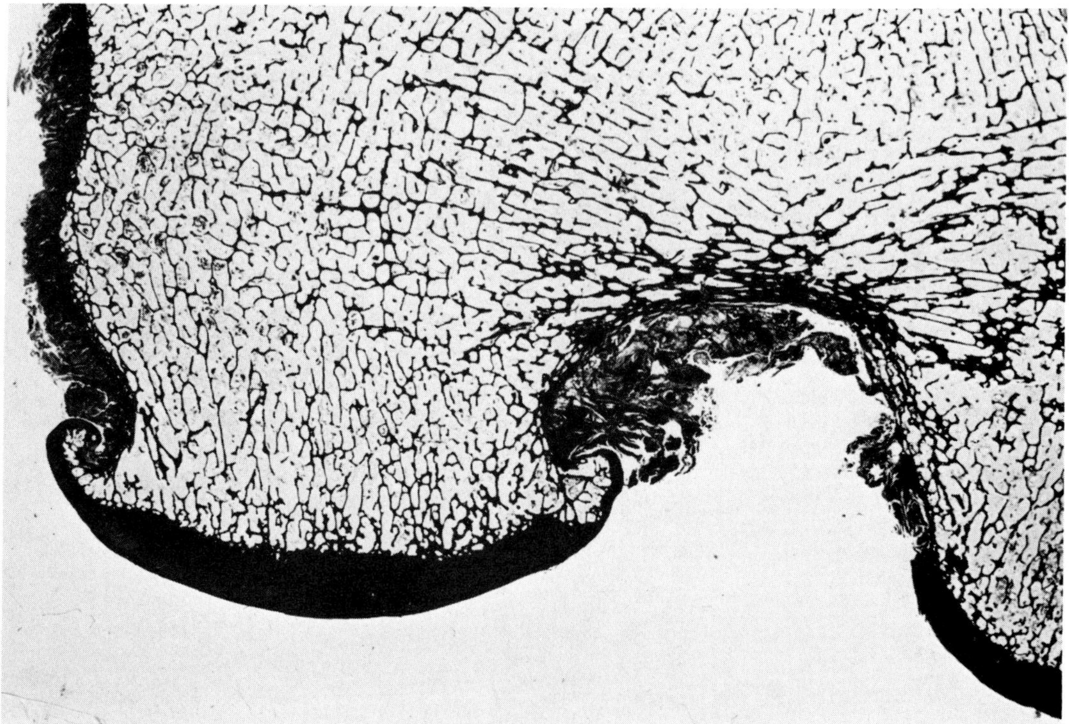

Figure 6–36. Macrospecimen of lower femur exhibiting osteophyte formation on the lateral surfaces of the condyle. This circumferential remodeling is an early sign of osteoarthritis and precedes changes in the articular cartilage.

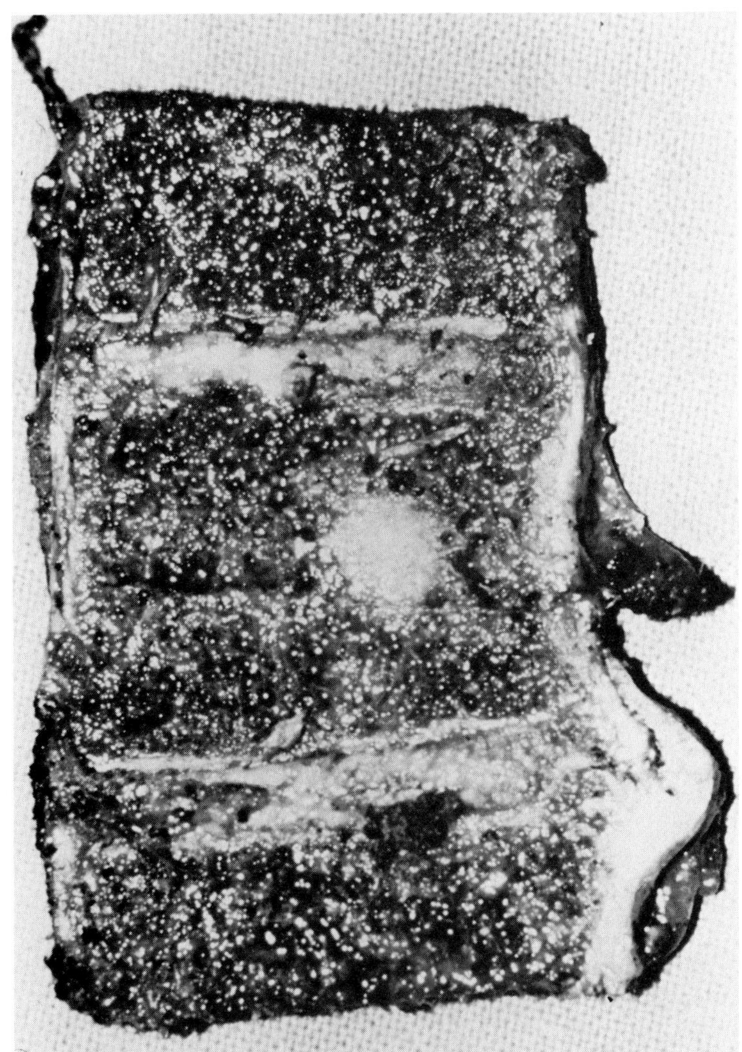

Figure 6–37. Gross specimen of vertebral bodies with circumferential remodeling and osteophyte formation. Rigidity of the spine may result as a consequence of extensive osteophyte formation.

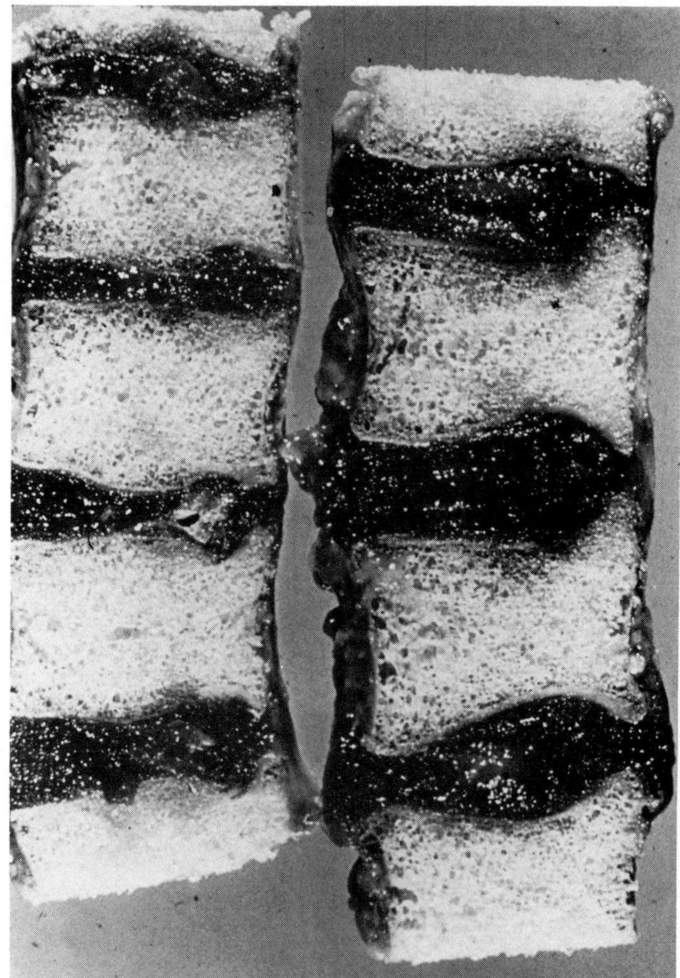

Figure 6–38. Gross specimen of spine exhibiting extensive regressive remodeling. The formation of biconcave vertebrae results in expansion of the discs. Note early Schmorl-node formation, a consequence of regressive remodeling.

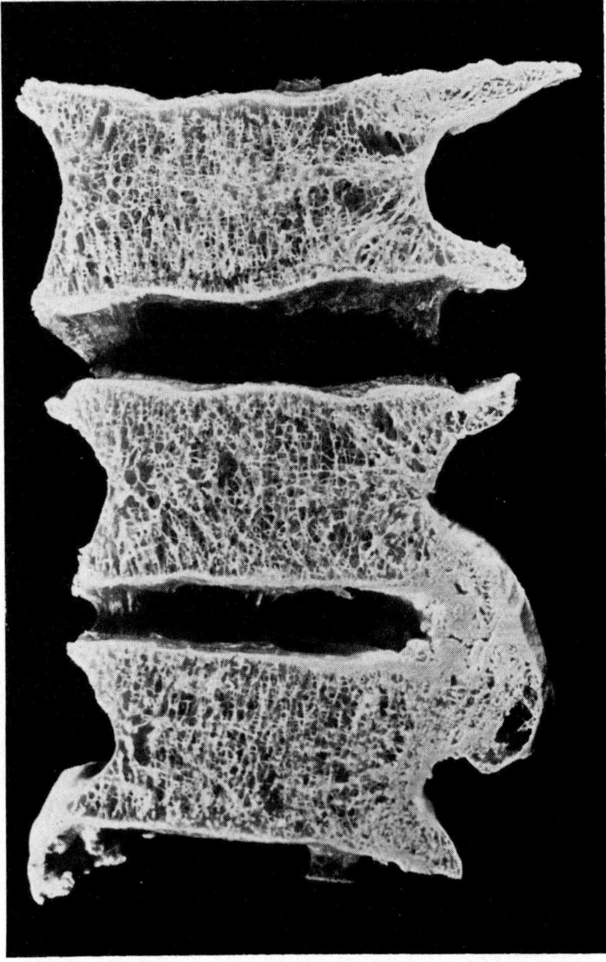

Figure 6–39. Macerated specimen of vertebral bodies exhibiting fusion of osteophytes to form an osseous bridge between adjacent vertebral bodies. This picture contrasts with that of Marie-Strümpell disease, in which calcification of ligaments leads to secondary ossification and osseous fusion. Osteoarthritis is therefore characterized by prominent osteophyte formation; rheumatoid spondylitis does not exhibit osteophytes.

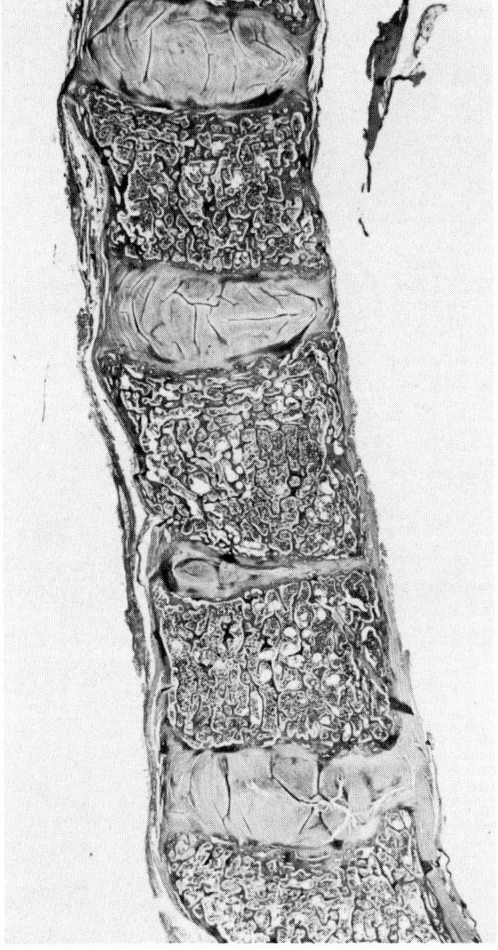

Figure 6–40. Macrospecimen of vertebral bodies with moderate osteoporosis and regressive remodeling. There is expansion of the intervertebral discs secondary to the remodeling process.

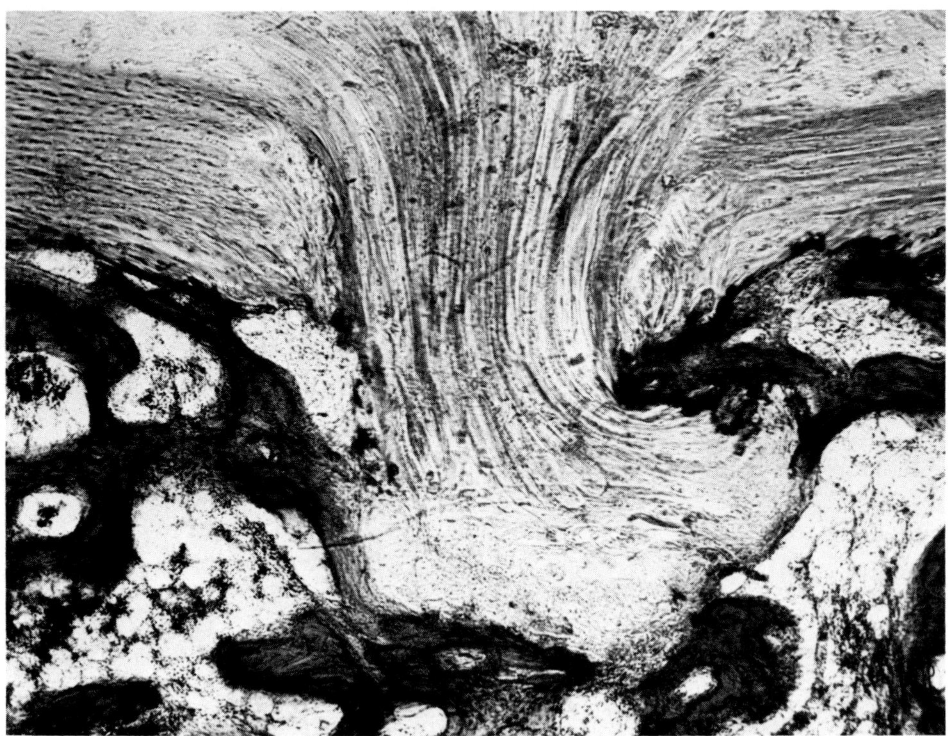

Figure 6–41. Higher magnification of expanded intervertebral discs with extension of disc material into the subchondral plate. This herniation is known as a "Schmorl's node."

CITED REFERENCES

Jaffe, H. L.: Metabolic, Degenerative, and Inflammatory Diseases of Bones and Joints. Philadelphia, Lea and Febiger, 1972, pp. 87–88.

Johnson, L. C.: Kinetics of osteoarthritis. Lab. Invest. 8:1223, 1959.

Johnson, L. C.: Joint remodeling as the basis for osteoarthritis. J. Am. Vet. Med. Assoc. 141:1237, 1962.

Mankin, H. J.: The reaction of articular cartilage to injury and osteoarthritis. N. Engl. J. Med. 291:1285; 1335, 1974.

Mankin, H. J., Dorfman, H., Lipiello, L., and Zarins, A.: Biochemical and metabolic abnormalities in articular cartilage from osteoarthritic human hips. J. Bone Joint Surg. 53A:523, 1971.

Teitelbaum, S. L., and Bullough, P. G.: The pathophysiology of bone and joint disease. Am. J. Pathol. 96:331, 1979.

GENERAL REFERENCES

Bullough, P. G.: Pathology changes associated with the common arthritides and their treatment. Pathol. Annu. 14:69, 1979.

Jaffe, H. L.: Metabolic, Degenerative, and Inflammatory Diseases of Bones and Joints. Philadelphia, Lea and Febiger, 1972.

Sokoloff, L.: Osteoarthritis. *In* Ackerman, L. V., Spjut, H. J., and Abell, M. R. (Eds.): Bones and Joints, International Academy of Pathology Monograph. Baltimore, Williams and Wilkins Co., 1976.

7

RHEUMATOID ARTHRITIS

Rheumatoid arthritis is of particular interest to the orthopaedic surgeon because its effects can be clearly demonstrated in the various components of the locomotor system of the body. Locomotion depends on a functional balance between the muscle-tendon motor units and the bone-joint lever arm. Rheumatoid arthritis distorts this functional balance by attacking both the muscle-tendon and bone-joint portions, resulting in deformity and disability.

Synovitis is the first step in the progressive structural changes encountered in rheumatoid arthritis. An undefined antigen localizes in the synovial tissue and is phagocytosed by type A synovial cells. Portions of this antigen diffuse into the synovial fluid, where the antigen is bound to B lymphocytes. This induces their transformation to plasma cells. Antibodies are produced, including the rheumatoid factor. Antibody production by lymphocytes produces an antigen-antibody complex that initiates the full-scale inflammatory reaction, including activation of complement and the kinin-forming system as well as attraction and activation of granulocytes and macrophages to produce collagenases, elastases, and hydrolases, which degrade the molecular structure of the articular cartilage. The initial confinement of the process to the synovium and synovial fluid results in a proliferative synovitis. The morphologic changes within the synovium are relatively nondiagnostic and are often reported as chronic nonspecific synovitis by the pathologist. They consist of increase in the number of villi, thickening of the villi and infiltration with inflammatory cells, vasculitis, edema, and synovial epithelial proliferation at the surface, including the formation of giant cells (Figs. 7–1 to 7–4). The edema and swelling of the synovium create redundant synovial tissue with a fibrinous surface exudate (Fig. 7–12). Increas-

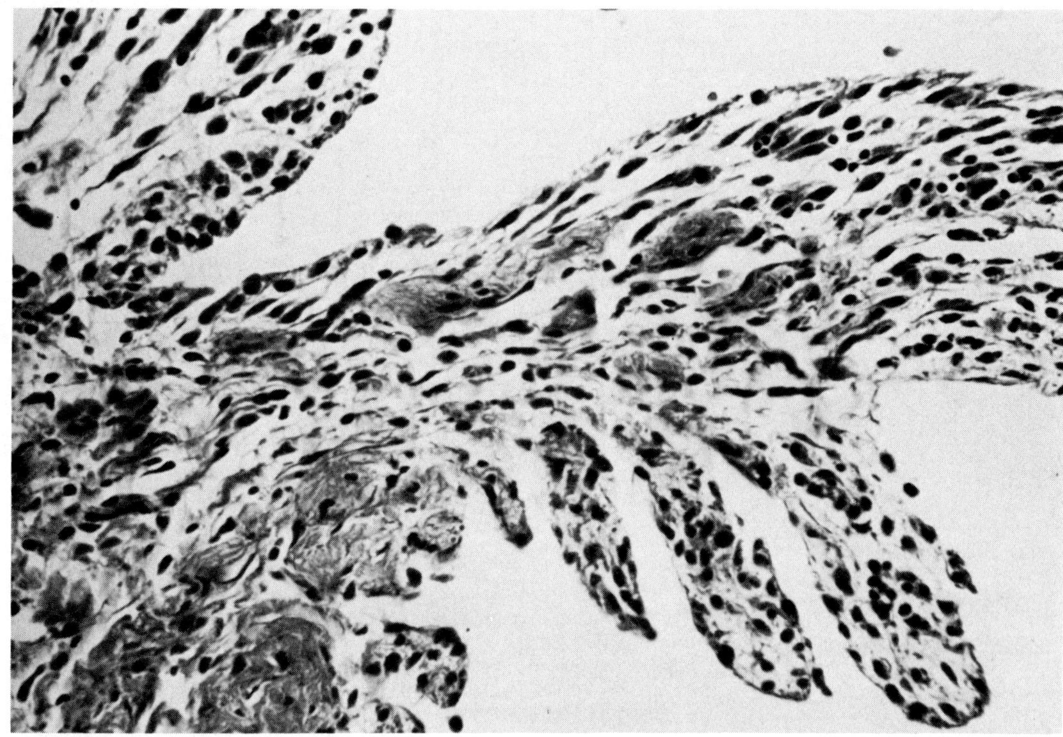

Figure 7–1. Histologic study of normal synovium. Villi have filamentous fronds that are covered by a cellular layer, varying in thickness. Numerous type A and occasional type B synovial lining cells are present. The synovial lining is characterized by the absence of a basement membrane. The central core of synovial villi contains loose fibrous stroma and small vessels.

ing the quantity and thickness of the synovial tissue interferes with the normal nutrition of the articular cartilage; direct contact with the cartilage surface ultimately results in loss of cartilage followed by loss of bone. These features are manifested radiographically by erosion. In the hand, the early visible changes of rheumatoid arthritis are erosion of the phalanges adjacent to the collateral ligament attachments and erosion of the lateral portions of the metacarpal and phalangeal heads (Resnick, 1976) (Figs. 7–5 to 7–8). As the process continues, major destructive changes occur in the cartilage and underlying bone. Loss of cartilage and stretching of ligaments result in dislocation of the metacarpophalangeal joint; the inflammatory hyperemia and loss of function result in severe osteoporosis.

Muscle and tendons are also involved in the rheumatoid vasculitis with eventual fibrosis. The extensive vascular inflammation is a significant feature of rheumatoid disease (Fig. 7–31).

Although the destructive process is progressive, intelligent therapy can prevent crippling (Ehrlich, 1974). If untreated, the process results in subluxation, osteoporosis, cystic degeneration of proximal ends of the phalanges, and, finally, ankylosis of the opposing bone fragments due to complete loss of cartilage.

The rheumatoid process involves the substance of the bone by means of vascular reaction. The hyperemia of the inflammatory process is associated with severe osteoporosis. Under unusual circumstances, dissolution of major portions of the phalanges due to abnormal vascular shunting occurs and results in the so-called "opera glass fingers" (Figs. 7–9 to 7–11).

Text continued on page 230

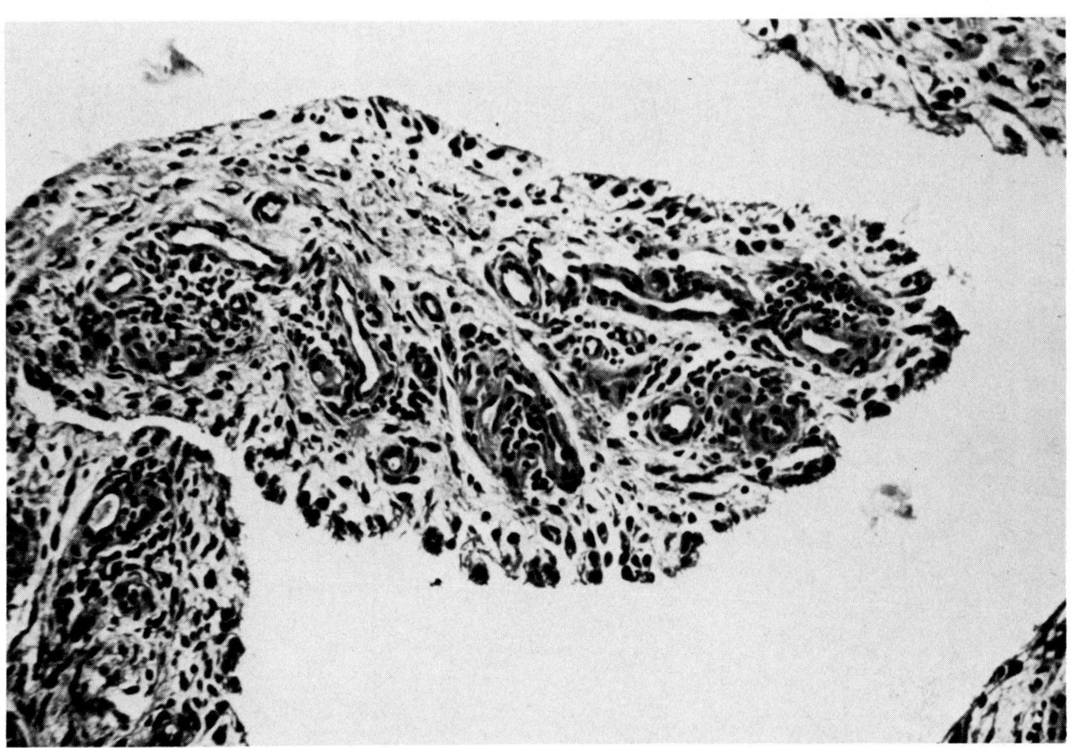

Figure 7–2. Early synovitis. Perivascular infiltration of inflammatory cells and mild edema in the center of the villous frond are evident.

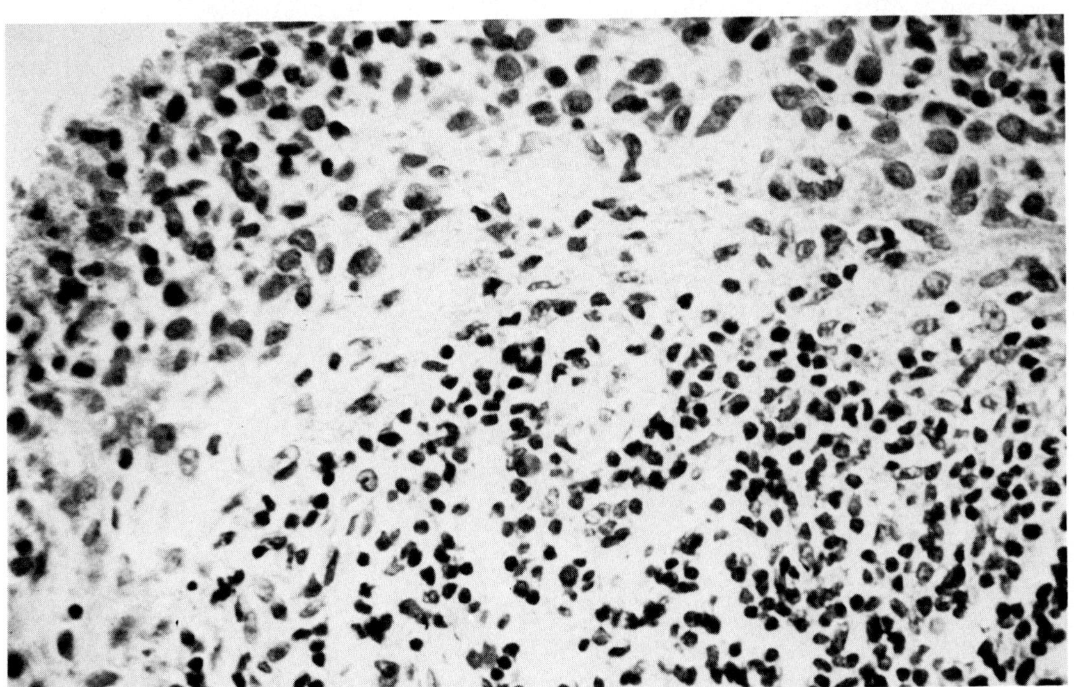

Figure 7–3. With more frequent attacks of longer duration, the number of inflammatory cells increases markedly. Edema and perivascular inflammation persist. There is multiplication of the lining cells that results in a thickened covering membrane, which makes it difficult for nutrients to pass back and forth from the joint space to the vessels. The inflammatory cells are responsible for formation of antibody and proteolytic enzymes.

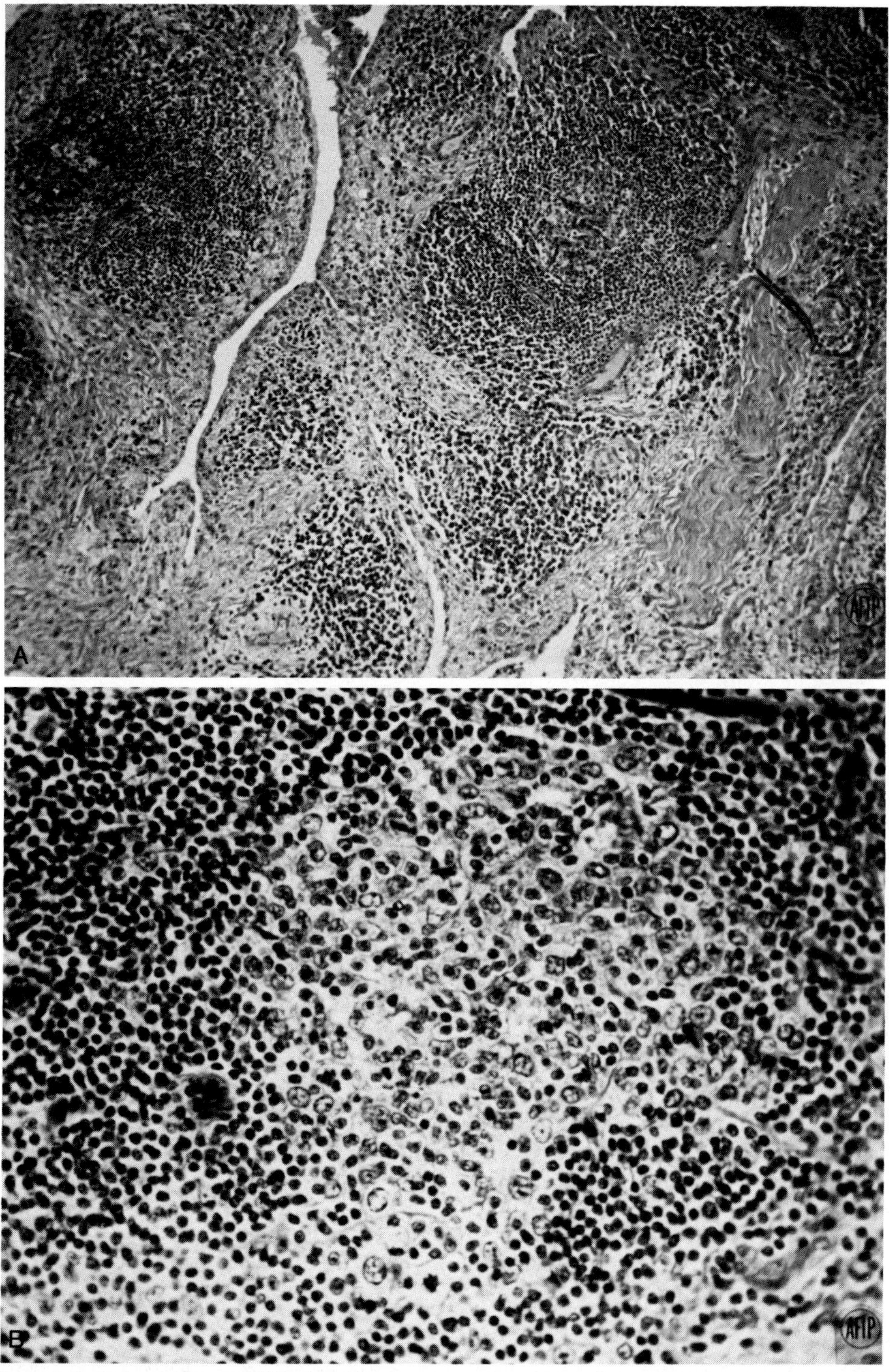

Figure 7–4. Low-power *(A)* and high-power *(B)* views of synovium in chronic case of rheumatoid arthritis. In long-standing disease, the synovium becomes hypertrophied and there are extensive accumulations of lymphocytes and plasma cells. Lymphocytes form germinal centers within the synovium. Note collagen fiber formation, evidence of chronic disease.

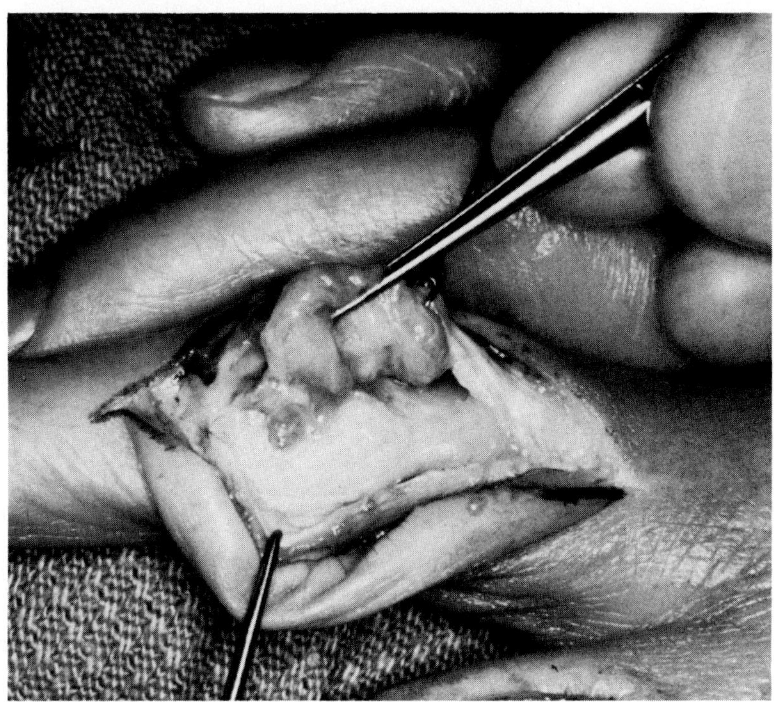

Figure 7–5. Intraoperative photograph of the hand of a patient with rheumatoid arthritis. The upper forceps holds the hypertrophied synovium while the lower hook exposes the swollen ligament. Cell multiplication, dilated capillaries, and perivascular edema results in stretching of ligaments by intra-articular pressure as well as ligamentous remodeling due to the inflammatory hyperemic synovium.

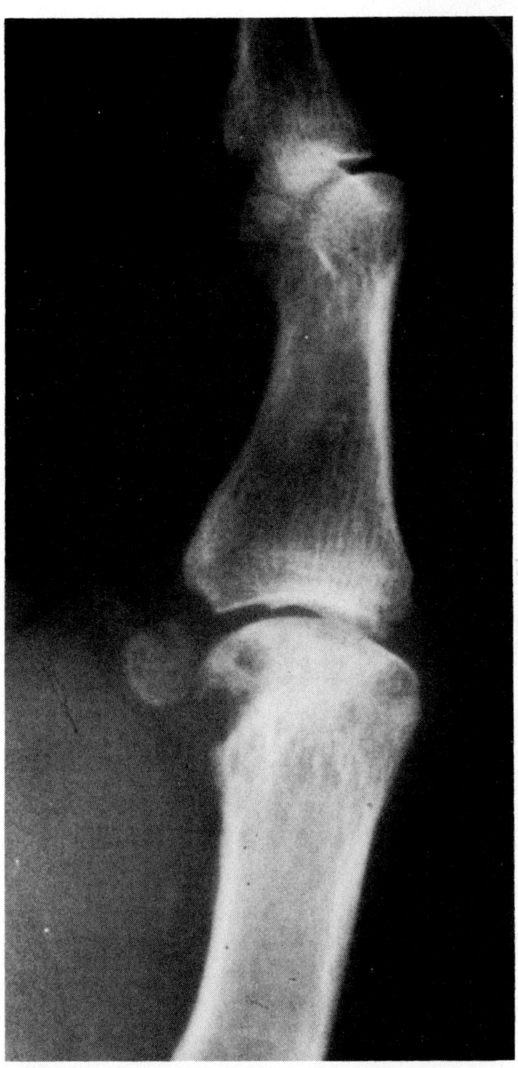

Figure 7–6. In the synovial recesses, where the synovium is in direct contact with areas of bone not covered by cartilage, the active hyperemia will induce resorption of bone and para-articular erosions.

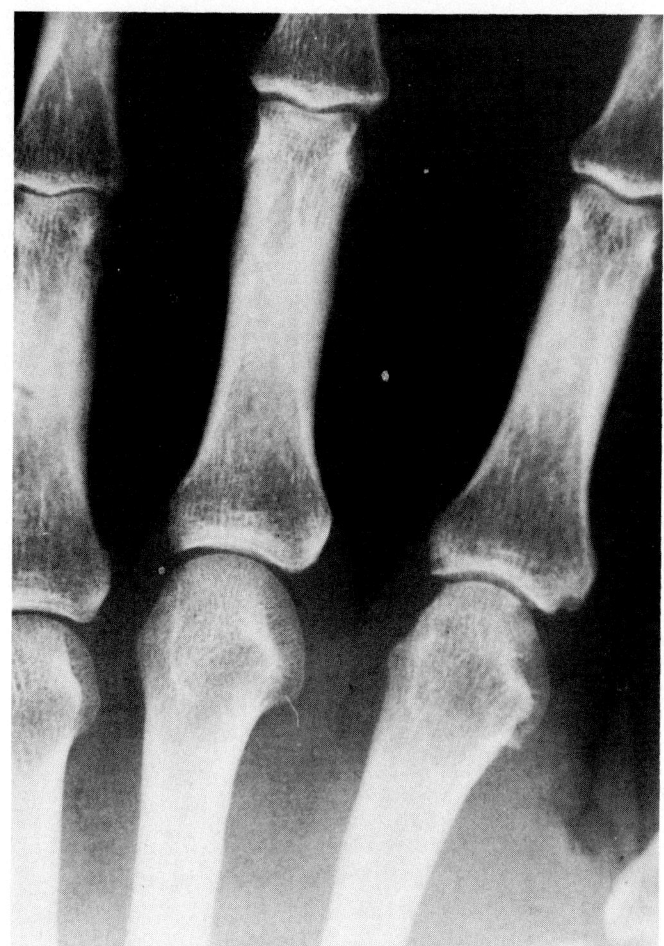

Figure 7–7. Radiograph of fingers in a hand with early rheumatoid arthritis exhibiting erosions of the proximal phalangeal bases. The erosions are also present on the metacarpal head but do not show well unless special views are obtained. Collateral ligaments attach close to the edge of the joint, so there is only a small synovial recess distally. Erosions occur only where synovium is in direct contact with bone. Because of the small recess, the erosions on the proximal phalanx tend to be small.

Figure 7–8. Resorption of bone is a function of surface area exposed to blood vessels. Spongiotic bone and the relatively thin epiphyseal cortex undergo more rapid bone resorption than the thick diaphyseal cortex. Although the process involves the entire bone, the osteoporosis is more severe and readily apparent in the epiphyseal portions.

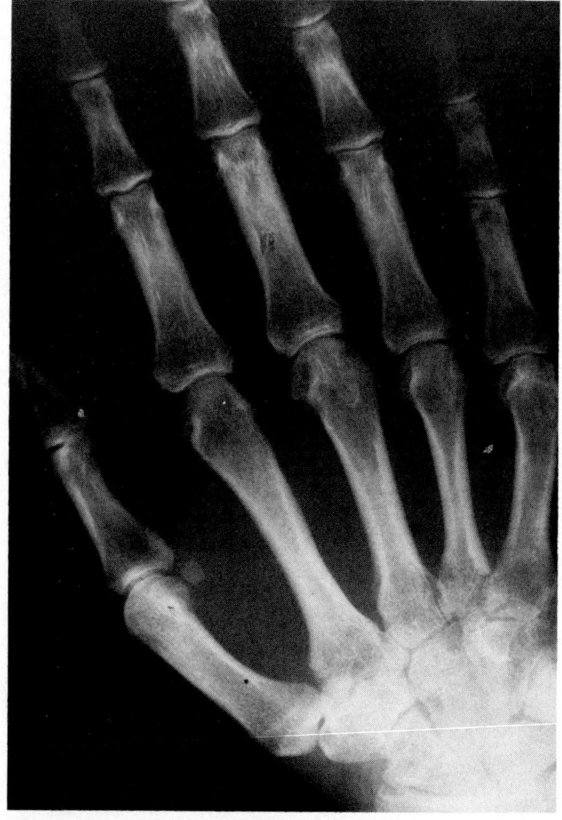

Figure 7–9. Radiograph of a hand in a more advanced case of rheumatoid arthritis. The osteoporosis is severe and involves the diaphyses of all of the metacarpals and phalanges. The metacarpophalangeal (MP) joint spaces are reduced in thickness owing to cartilage loss. There is subluxation of the ring and index finger MP joints. There are pronounced changes in the thumb, with characteristic flexion of the MP joint and hyperextension of the interphalangeal (IP) joint. Dorsal erosions of the proximal phalanx indicate long-standing deformity. The wrist joint shows pronounced changes with marked destruction of the distal radioulnar and radiocarpal joints. The scaphoid and lunate are no longer evident, indicating severe resorption of bone with displacement of the wrist in a volar and ulnar direction. The distal radial articular surface is extensively eroded, and the carpus is settling into the radius. All these changes are consequences of marked resorption of bone.

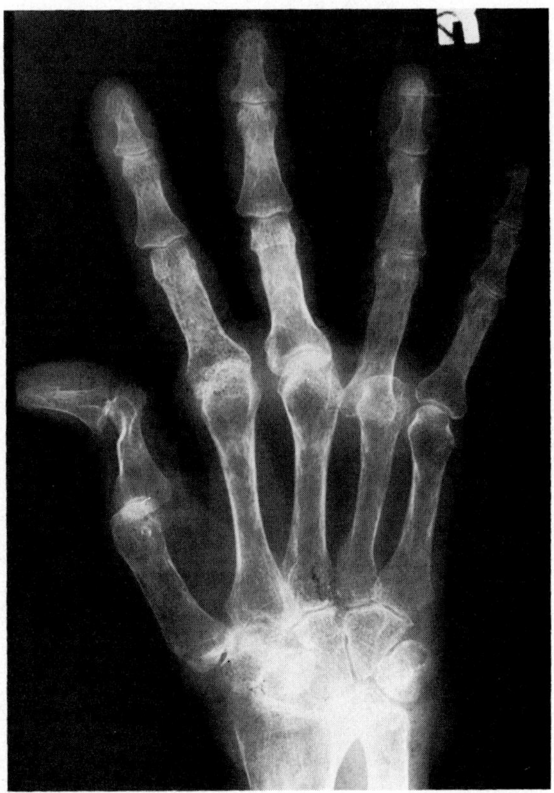

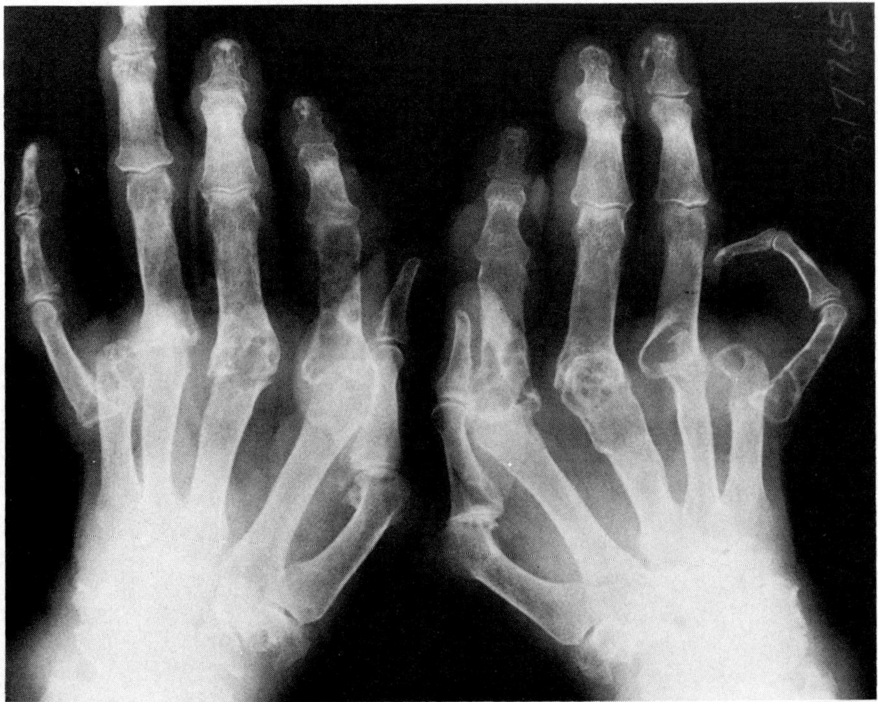

Figure 7–10. Radiograph of both hands of a patient with long-standing rheumatic arthritis. Osteoporosis in all bones is marked. The wrist joints show advanced destruction. There is dislocation of the metacarpophalangeal joints of all fingers. Steroid therapy causes expansion of metacarpals and phalanges secondary to changes in the marrow fat (steroid lipomatosis).

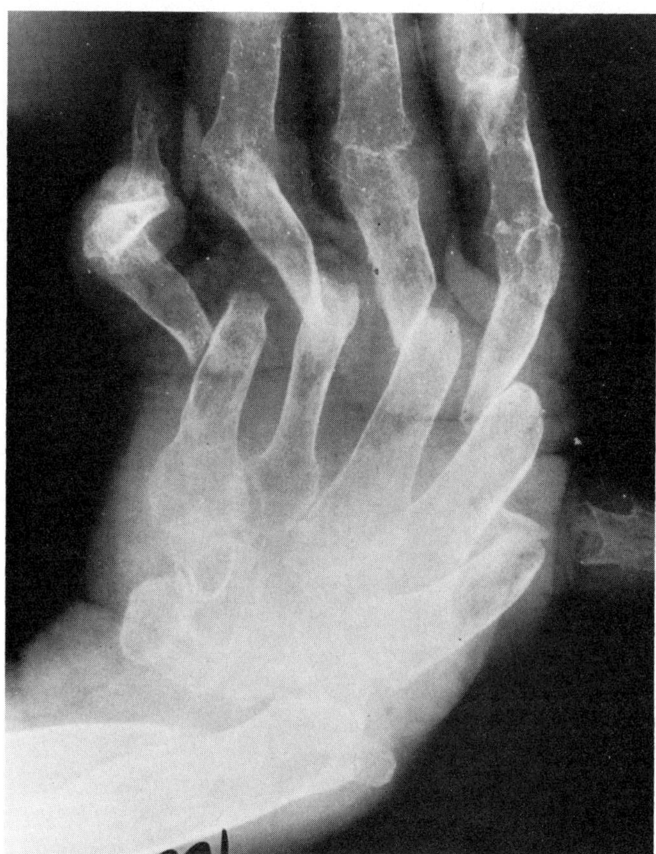

Figure 7–11. Radiograph of the left hand of a patient with severe rheumatoid arthritis. The wrist joint is totally dislocated with marked resorption of the distal radius and ulna. There is severe resorption of the metacarpals and phalanges, producing a loose hand with almost no possible stability for any normal functional activity.

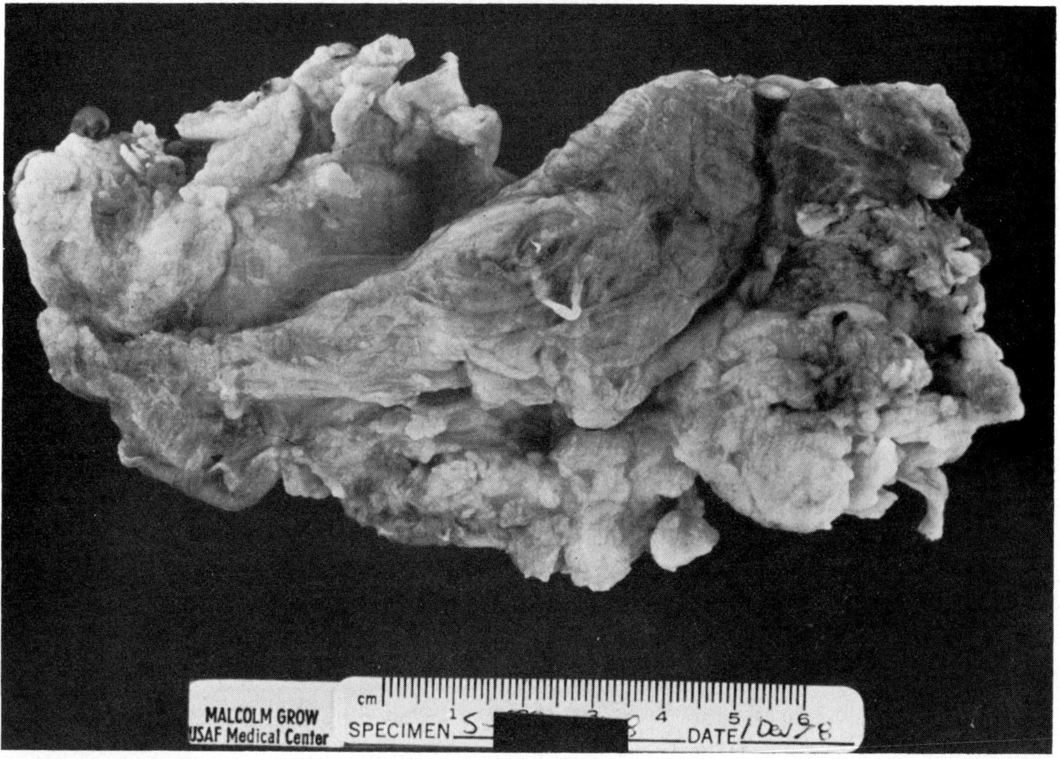

Figure 7–12. Large mass of boggy, swollen synovium removed from a knee joint. The surface is irregular with numerous edematous villi.

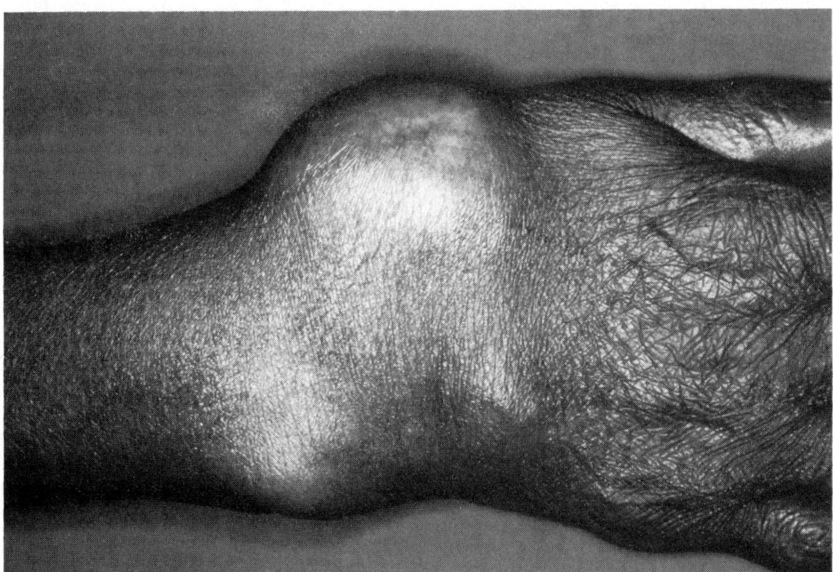

Figure 7–13. Photograph of the right wrist in a patient with severe rheumatoid arthritis. The marked hypertrophy of the synovium with accompanying extensive fluid production causes increased pressure that will force fluid through areas of weakened capsule and create large tenosynovial cysts. Note that the wrist has shifted towards the radial side, and the distal ulna is subluxed dorsally.

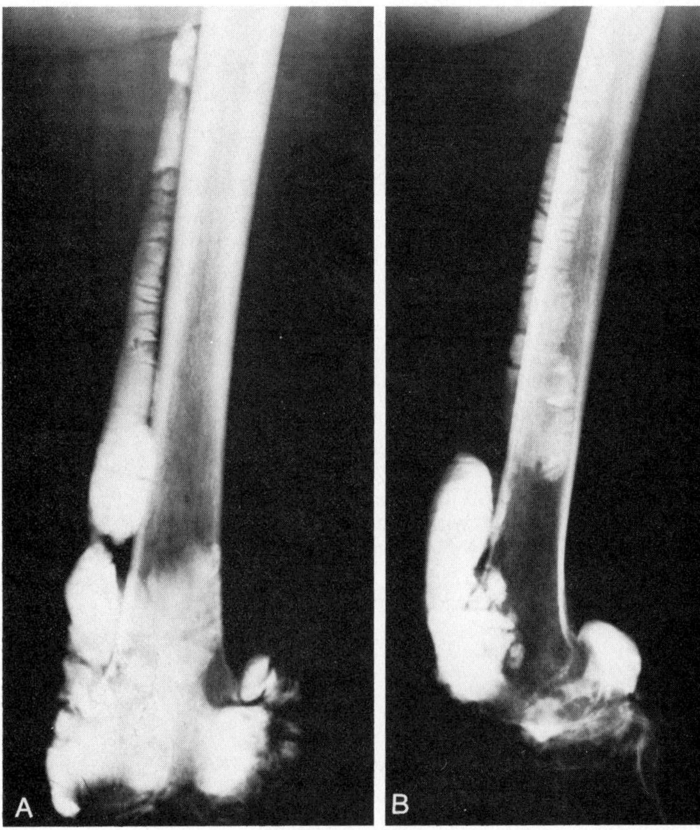

Figure 7–14. Anteroposterior *(A)* and lateral *(B)* radiographs of the distal thigh following an arthrogram of the knee. The patient has developed a large rheumatoid cyst that has dissected up the medial aspect of the thigh almost to the groin. Such cysts are relatively common about the knee, but more often they dissect distally into the calf and present as a tender mass mimicking a tumor.

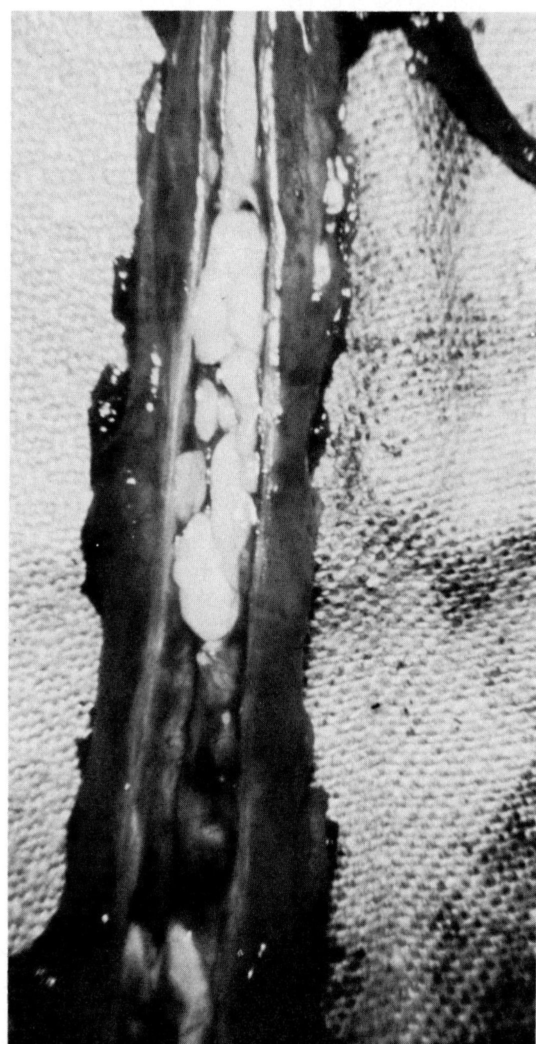

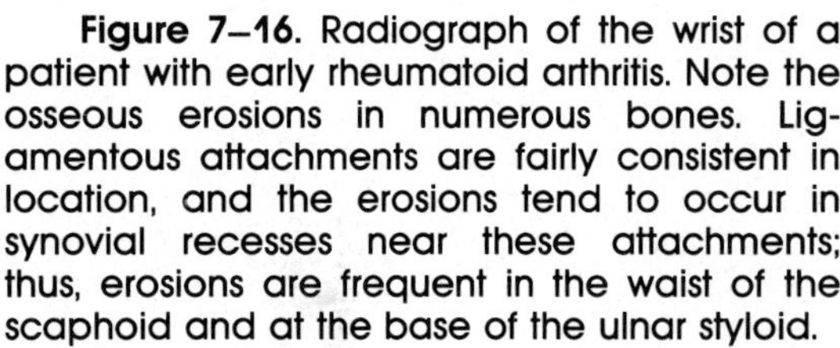

Figure 7–16. Radiograph of the wrist of a patient with early rheumatoid arthritis. Note the osseous erosions in numerous bones. Ligamentous attachments are fairly consistent in location, and the erosions tend to occur in synovial recesses near these attachments; thus, erosions are frequent in the waist of the scaphoid and at the base of the ulnar styloid.

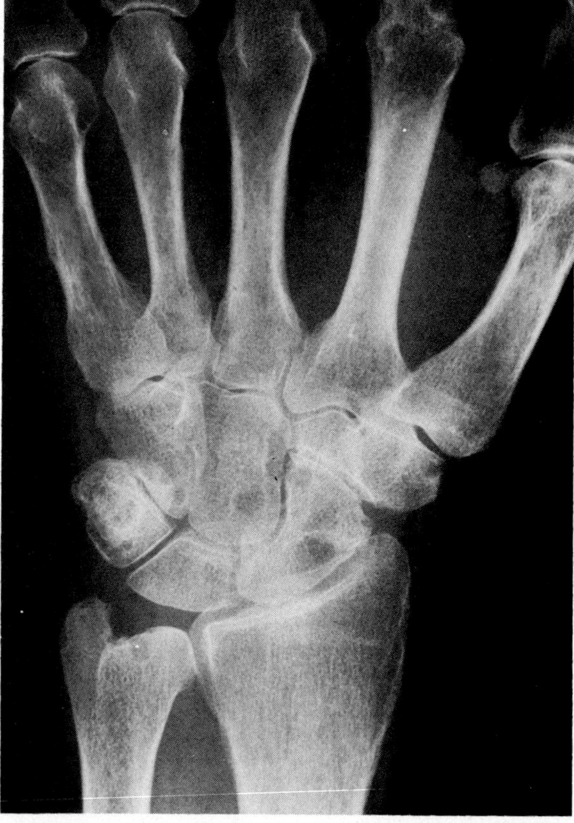

Figure 7–15. Elongated rheumatoid cyst removed from the thigh shown in the preceding figure. Numerous rice bodies are contained within the cyst.

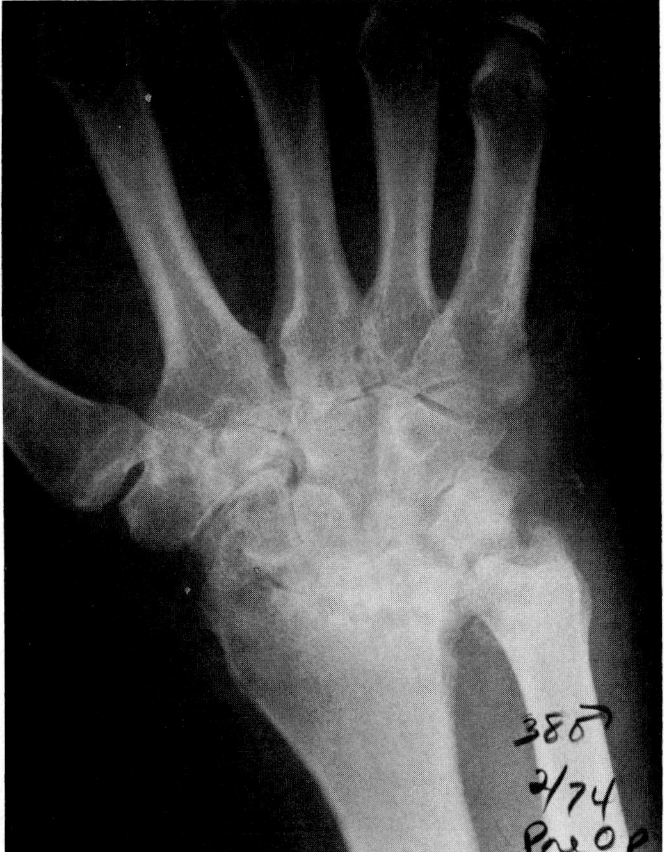

Figure 7–17. More advanced erosive disease of the wrist joint. A combination of bone and cartilage loss with ligamentous stretching results in subluxation of the joints in this fairly characteristic manner.

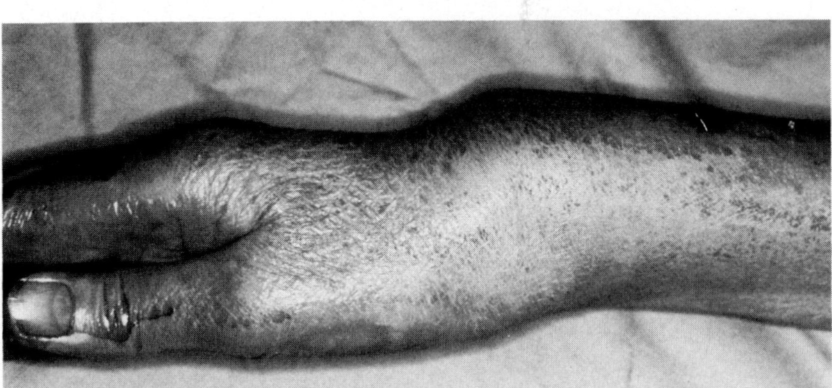

Figure 7–18. Lateral photograph of a hand and wrist of a patient with subluxation of the wrist joint in volar and proximal direction. The subluxation is due to forces of gravity and muscular pull acting on the hand over a period of time. The swollen, eroded joint is no longer able to resist normal forces generated during use.

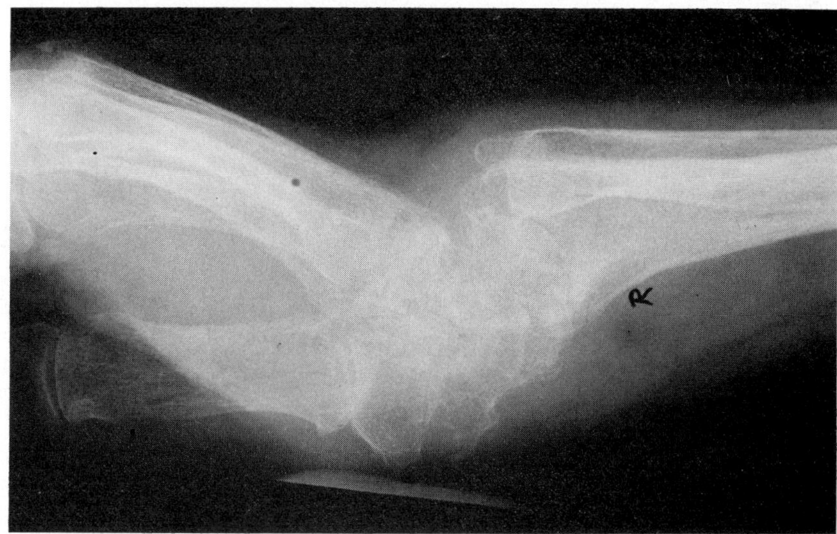

Figure 7–19. Lateral radiograph of the hand of a patient with advanced rheumatoid arthritis demonstrating total collapse of the intercarpal and radiocarpal joints with volar dislocation of the wrist.

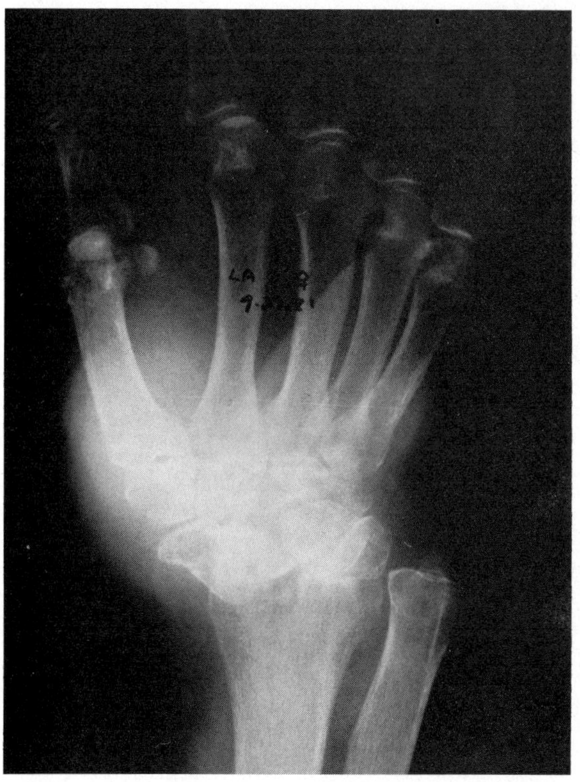

Figure 7–20. Oblique radiograph of the same hand as that seen in Figure 7–13 with a large tenosynovial cyst demonstrated by the soft tissue swelling. There is major destruction of the carpal bones with dislocation of the wrist and overlapping of the proximal carpus and the distal radius. Note that the distal radioulnar joint is dislocated.

Figure 7–21. Lateral *(A)* and anteroposterior *(B)* radiographs of the elbow joint in a patient with advanced rheumatoid arthritis. Destructive erosion of articular surfaces has resulted in severe bone loss with marked instability of the joint.

Figure 7–22. Plantar *(A)* and dorsal *(B)* views of the foot of a patient with rheumatoid arthritis with characteristic dislocation of all toes, which tend to drift off into marked hallux valgus with dorsal displacement of the phalanges onto the metacarpals. The metacarpal heads become very prominent in the sole of the foot, and large painful callosities are common.

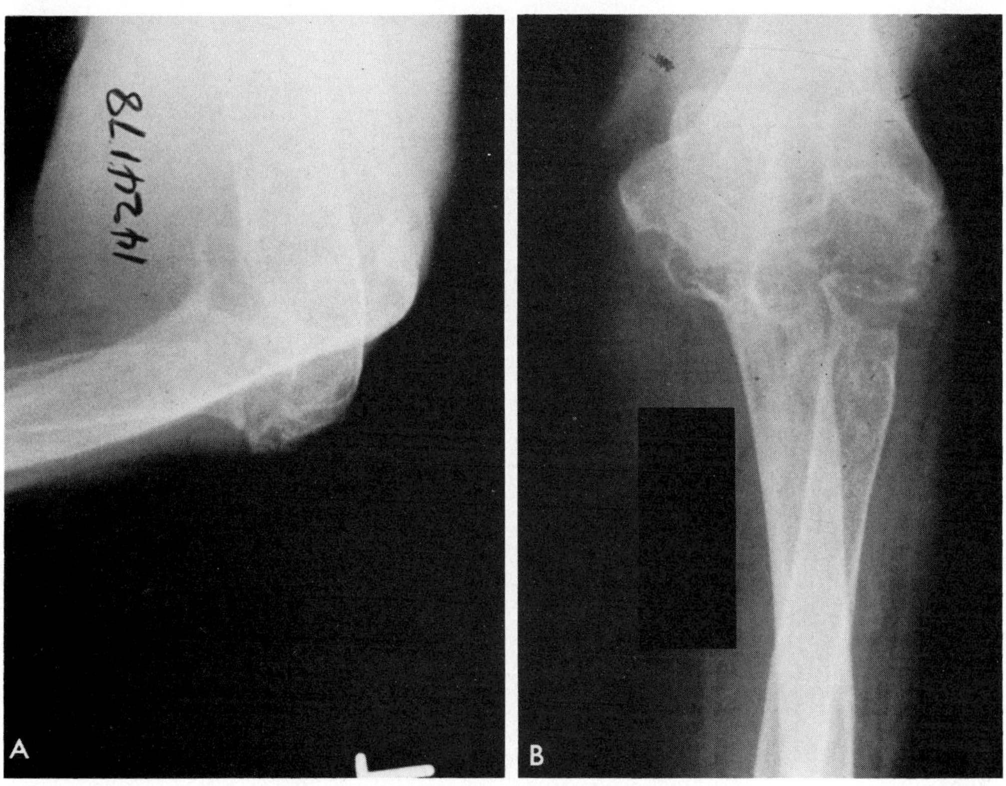

Figure 7–21. *See legend on opposite page*

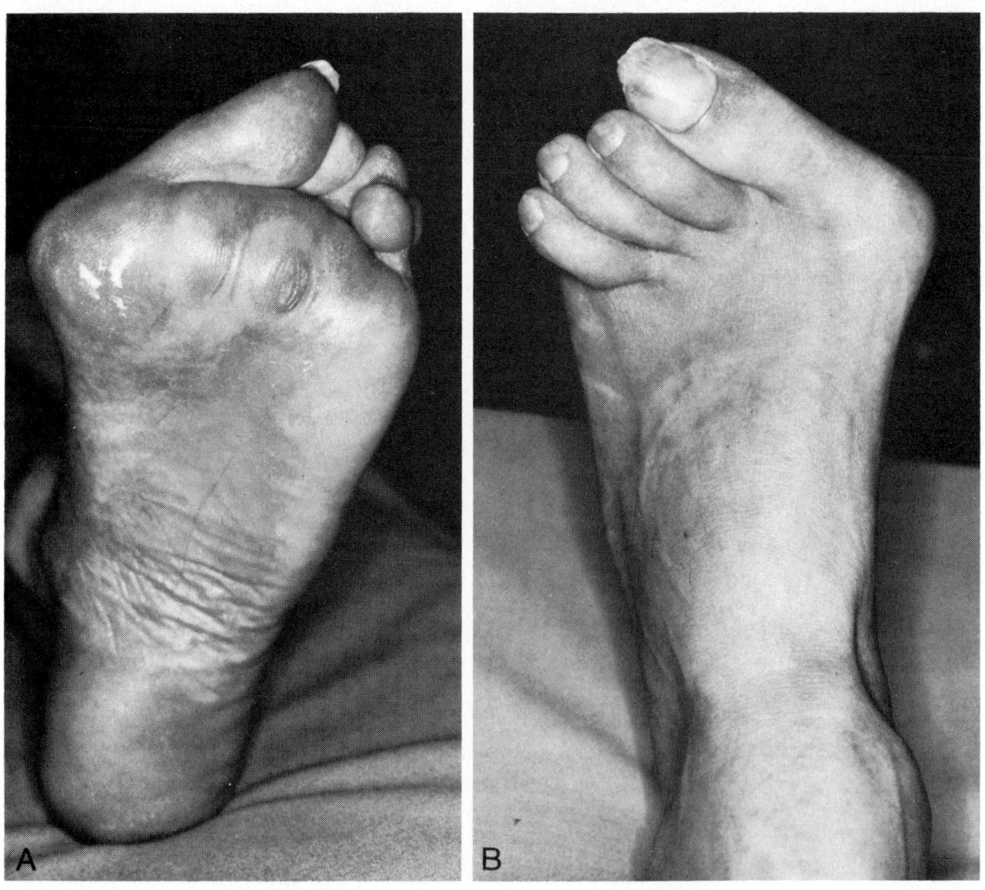

Figure 7–22. *See legend on opposite page*

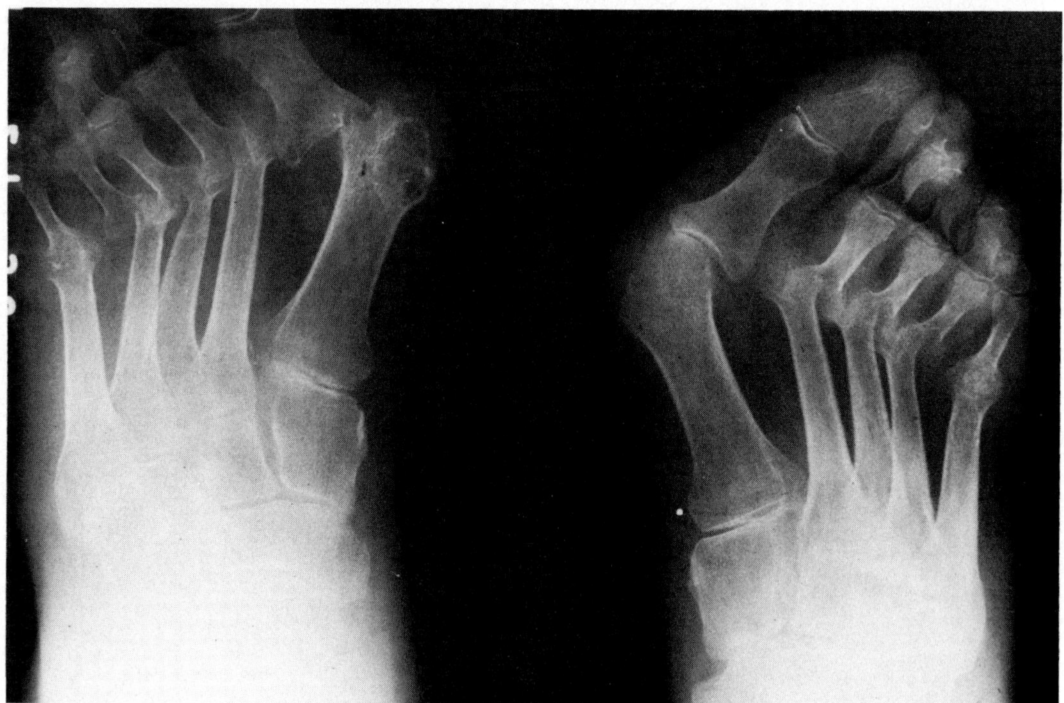

Figure 7–23. Anteroposterior radiographs of both feet in rheumatoid arthritis. Note the marked erosive changes of the ends of the metacarpals on the left foot with dislocations of all the metacarpophalangeal joints. The bony destruction is not as prominent in the right foot, but the joints are dislocated.

In association with the joint changes, subcutaneous nodules appear throughout the body. These are prominent around joints because there is less subcutaneous tissue and the nodules are more readily detected (Fig. 7–32). Their gross appearance is gray; histologically, they have necrotic areas surrounded by histiocytes that form a characteristic palisading structure at the periphery of the necrosis (Figs. 7–33 and 7–34). This granulomatous process must be differentiated from tuberculosis and the gumma of syphilis. It is virtually impossible to differentiate the process from granuloma annulare, except by observation of the latter's more superficial location in the skin.

Rheumatoid nodules occur in 20 to 25 per cent of patients with rheumatoid arthritis but are seldom seen in ankylosing spondylitis, Still's disease, or psoriatic arthritis. Although there are obviously major differences in the clinical manifestations of these last three disease processes, there are no major identifiable morphologic differences between them and classic rheumatoid arthritis (Peter, 1978) (Figs. 7–36 to 7–39).

Text continued on page 240

Figure 7–24. Diagram *(A)* and section *(B)* of a finger joint of a patient with rheumatoid arthritis. The marked synovitis is evident in the synovial recesses with erosions into the bone on both sides of the articular surface (long curved arrows). The pannus is beginning to encroach on margins of the joint (short arrows). Although the cartilage retains its normal appearance in the center of the joint, the proteoglycan structure is affected by the altered synovial fluid. It is susceptible to rapid removal by wear and tear as well as by the encroaching pannus. Since the pannus grows in from the margins, the earliest radiographic erosions are seen at the margins, and the contact surfaces are spared until relatively late.

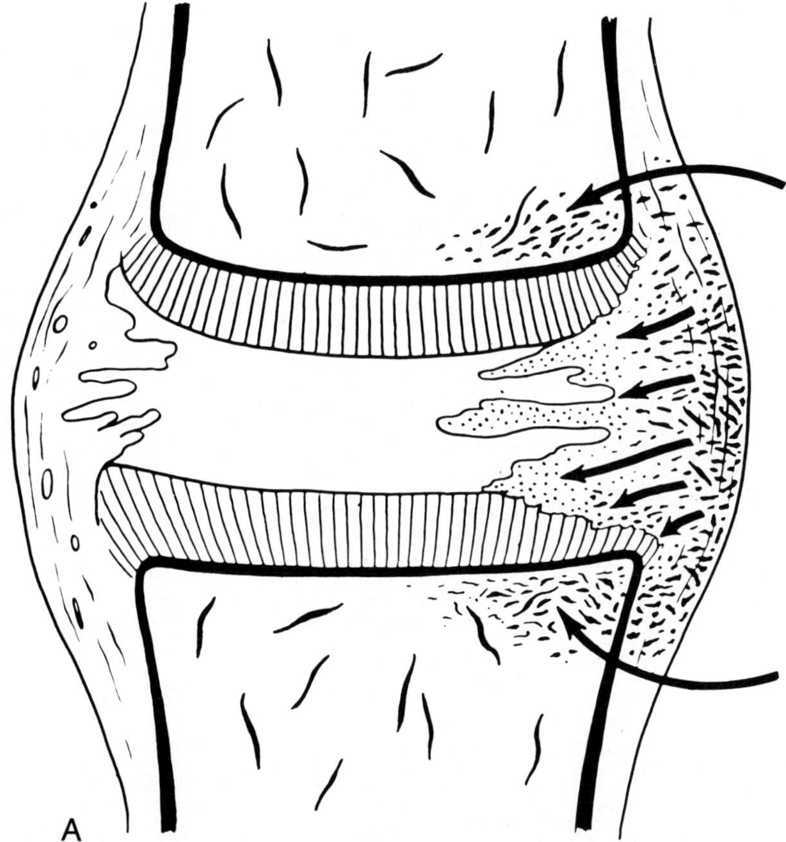

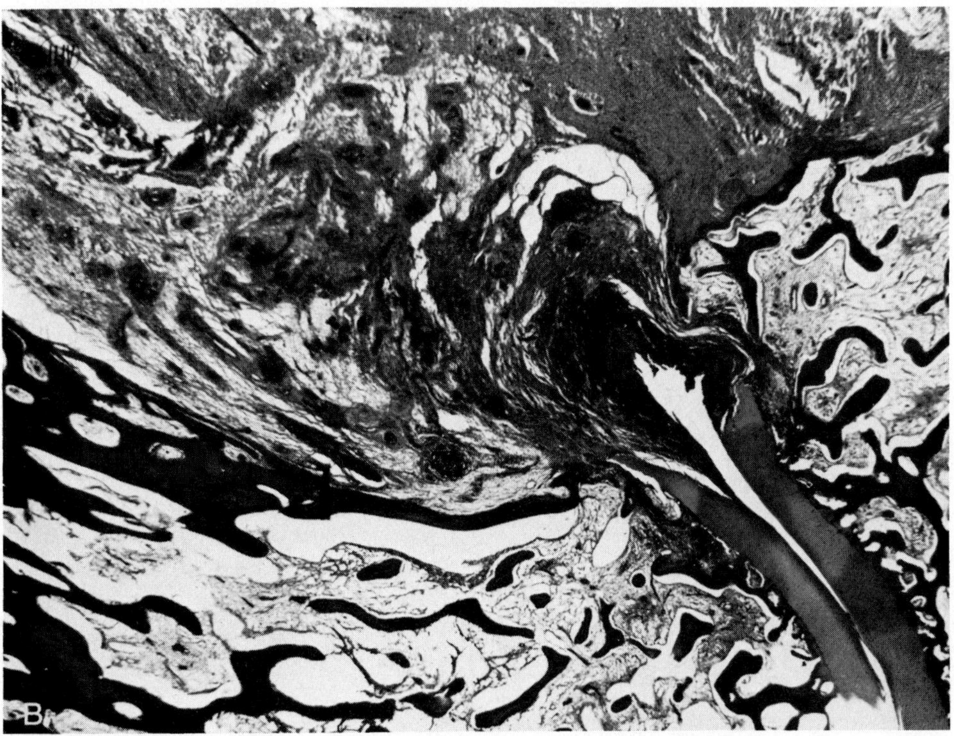

Figure 7–24. *See legend on opposite page*

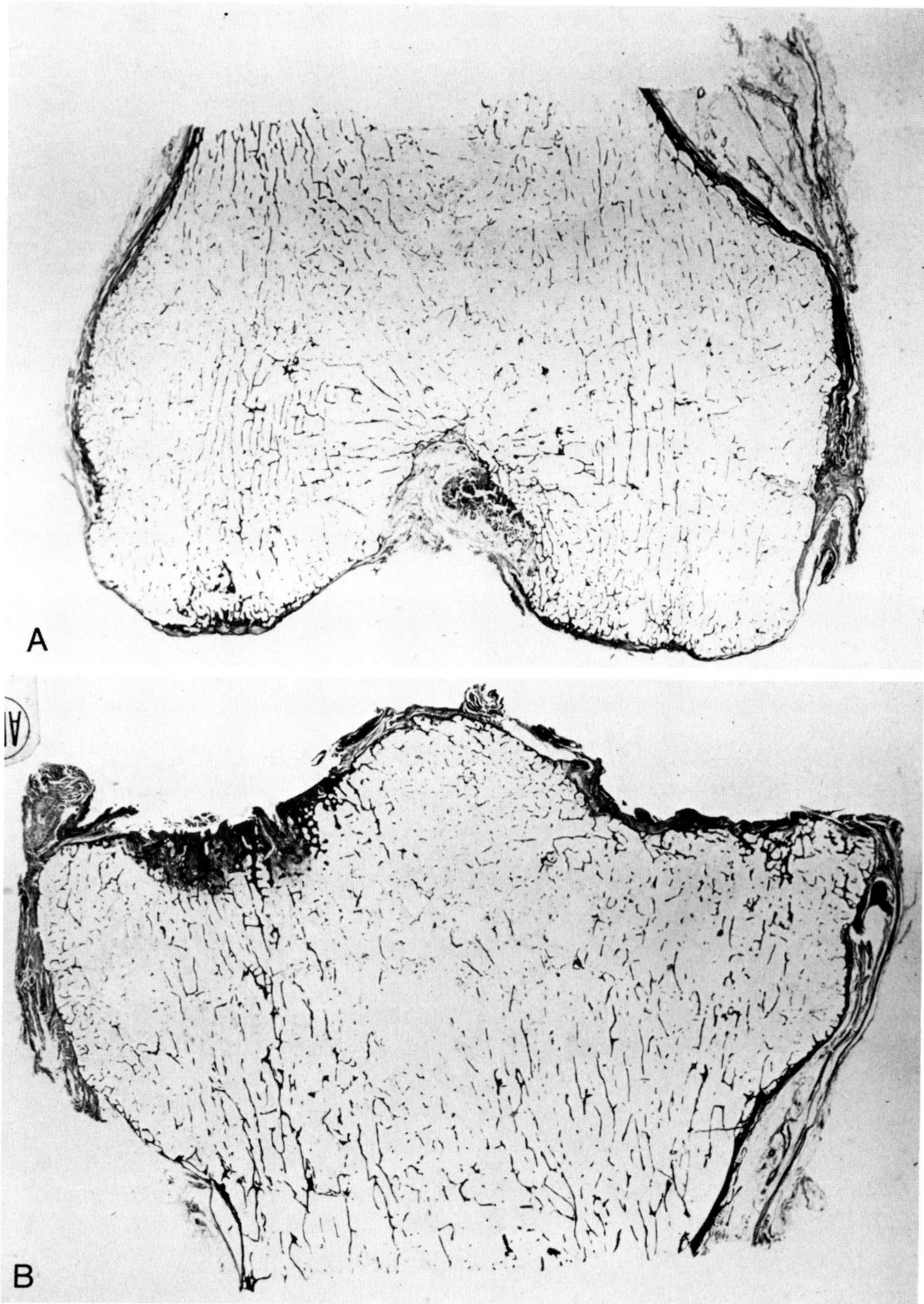

Figure 7–25. Macrosections of distal femur *(A)* and proximal tibia *(B)* in a patient with long-standing rheumatoid arthritis. There is marked osteoporosis. Articular cartilage is lost, and the process extends through portions of the subchondral plate.

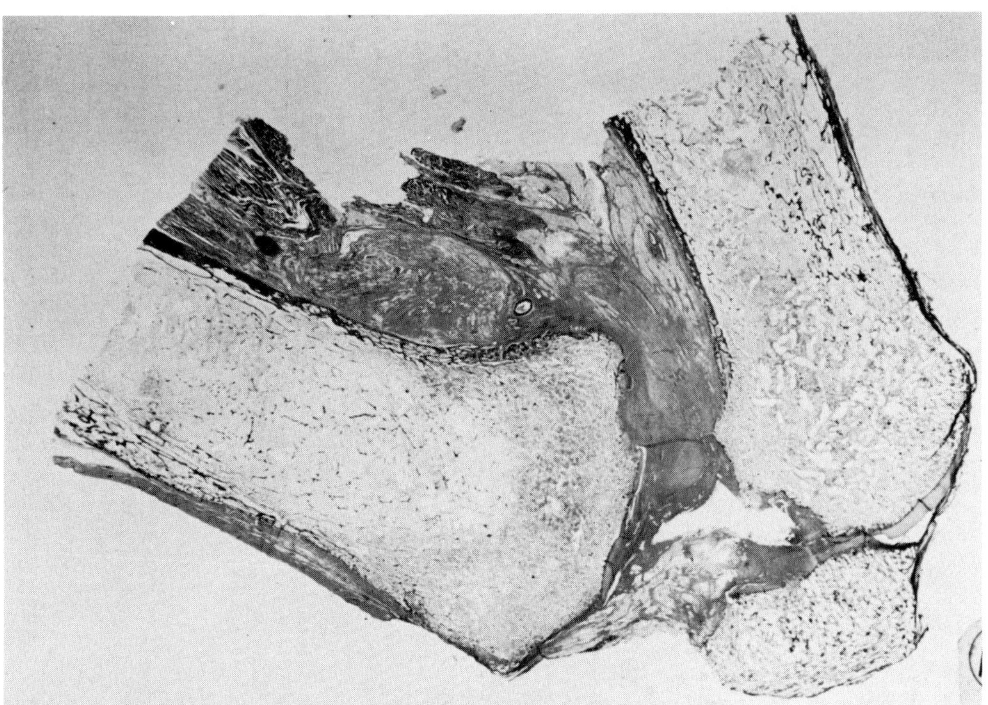

Figure 7–26. Macrosection of knee joint in a patient with long-standing rheumatoid arthritis. There is extensive pannus formation covering the entire joint surface with destruction of the articular cartilage. Note the severe osteoporosis.

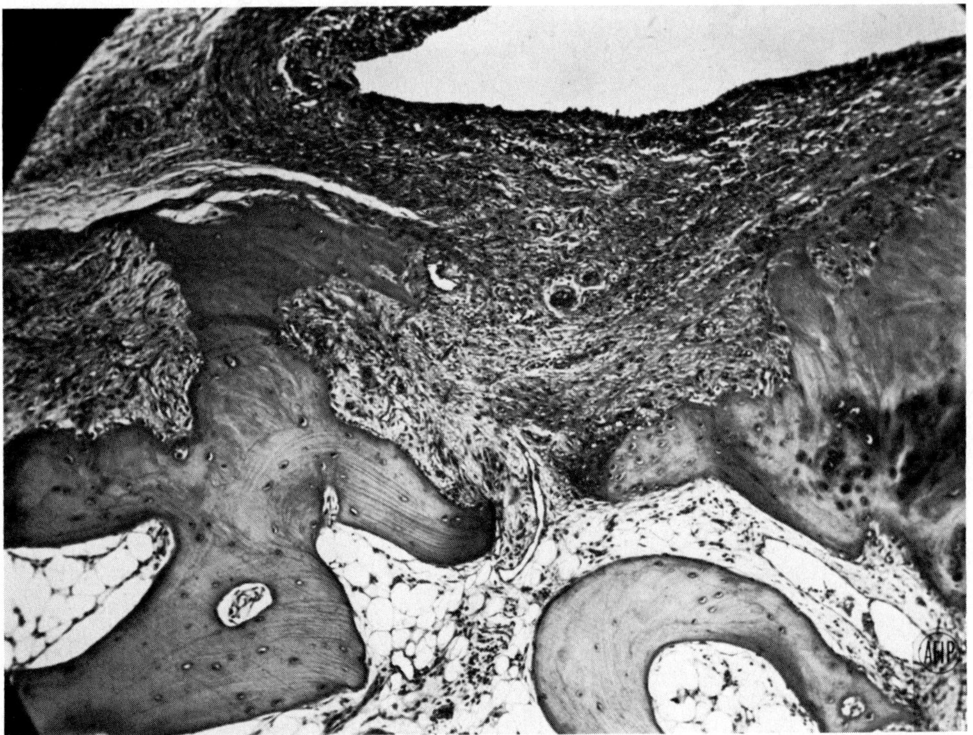

Figure 7–27. Histologic view of finger joint in a patient with long-standing rheumatoid arthritis. The articular surfaces are completely gone. The inflammatory process and fibrous tissue cover the ends of the bone, and there is marked fibrosis in the corners of the joint. With increased production of fibrous tissue the surfaces join together, totally obliterating the joint space and resulting in a fibrous ankylosis.

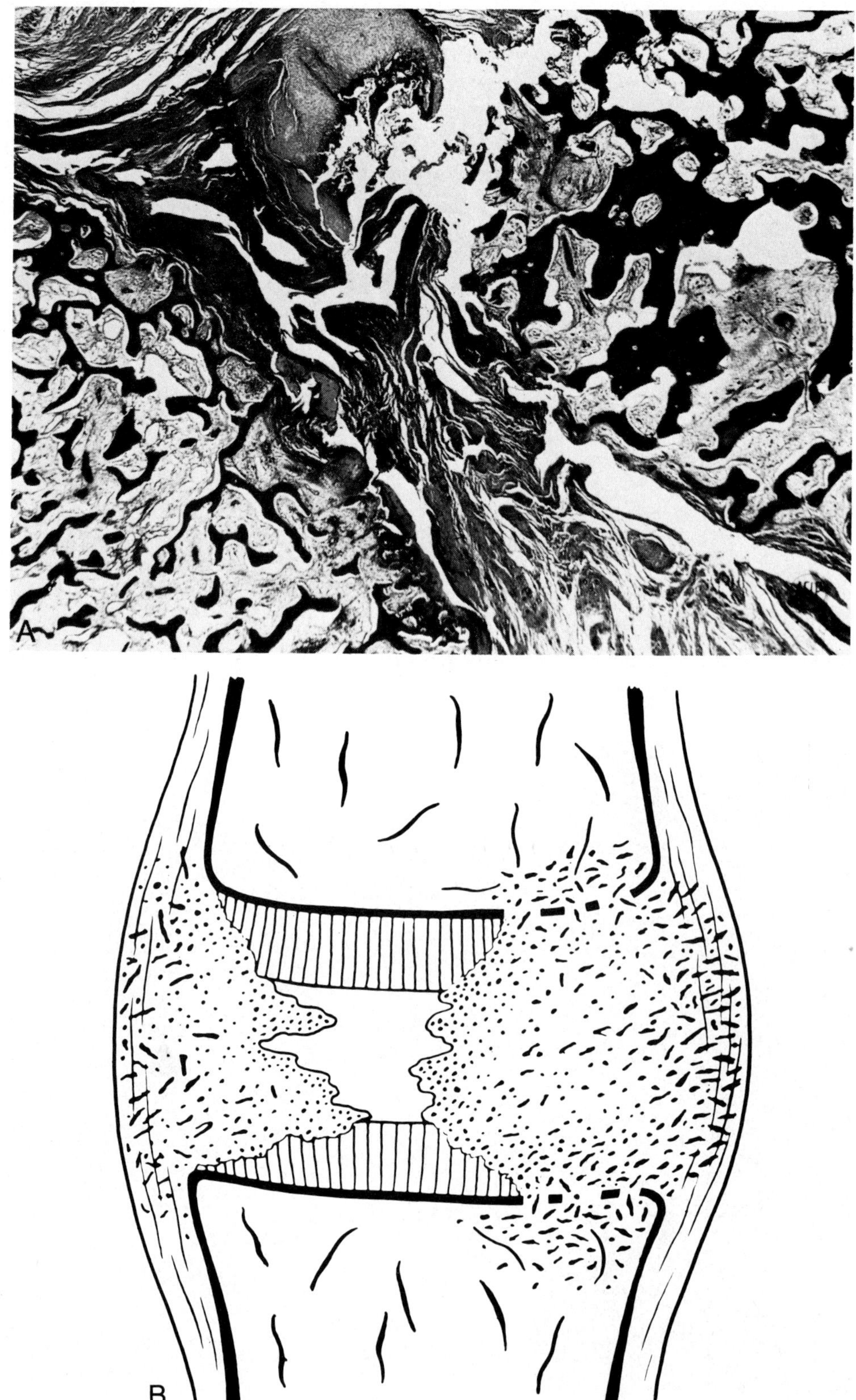

Figure 7–28. Histologic view *(A)* and diagram *(B)* of the corner of a joint at which the synovial tissue erodes the bony surface. There is no articular cartilage left, and the bony plate is breached by the inflammatory process, with extension into the metaphyseal marrow spaces.

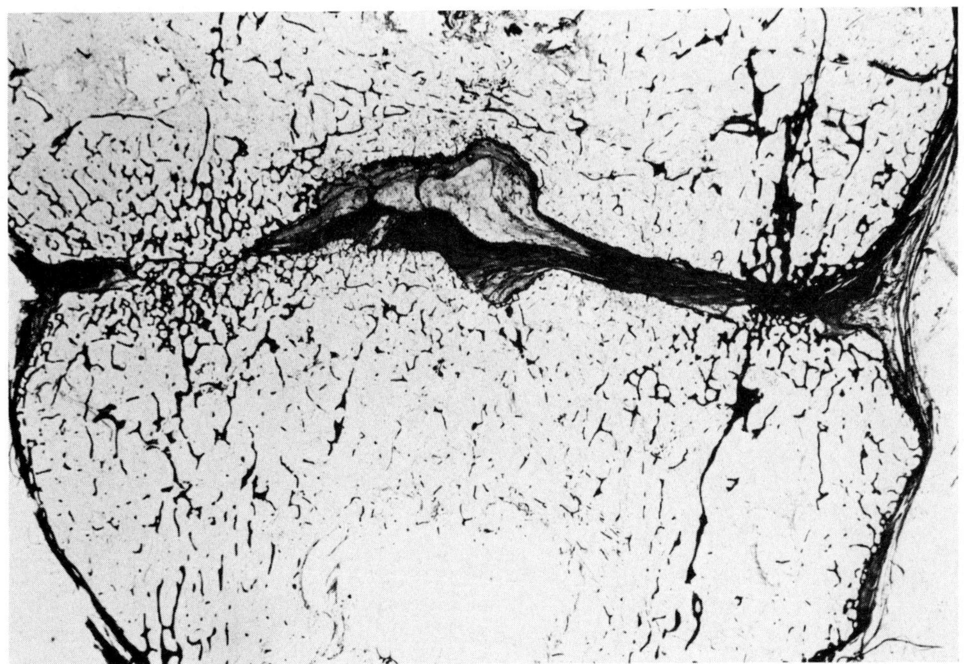

Figure 7–29. Macrosection of a knee joint exhibiting arthrodesis across the obliterated joint space on one side. There is fibrous ankylosis on the opposite side. Note the marked osteoporosis.

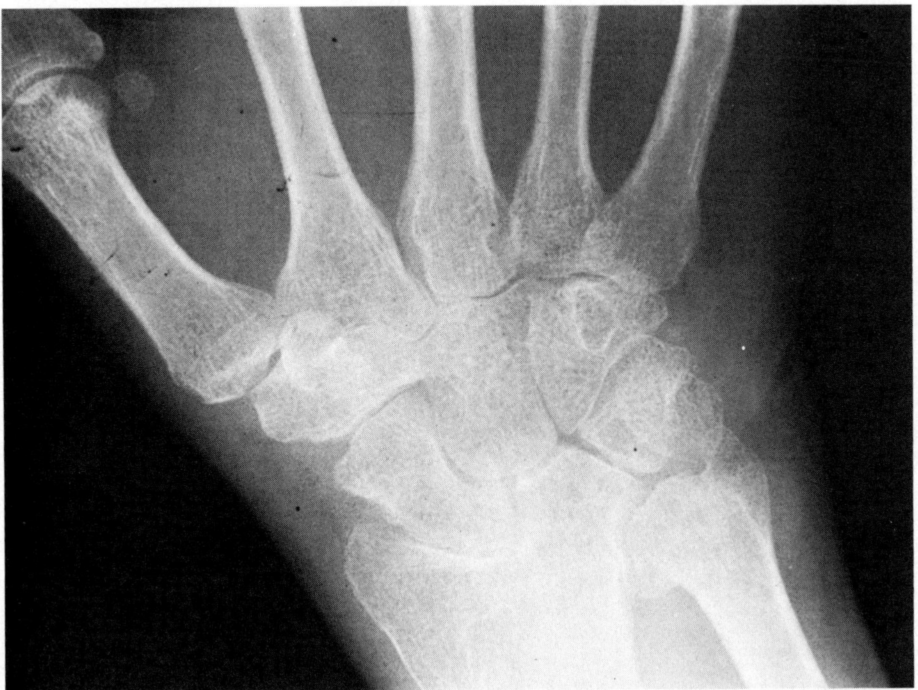

Figure 7–30. Anteroposterior radiograph of the wrist showing erosion of the scaphoid into the distal radius. There is spontaneous arthrodesis of the lunate to the distal radius, which provides a measure of stability to the joint and keeps it from dislocating.

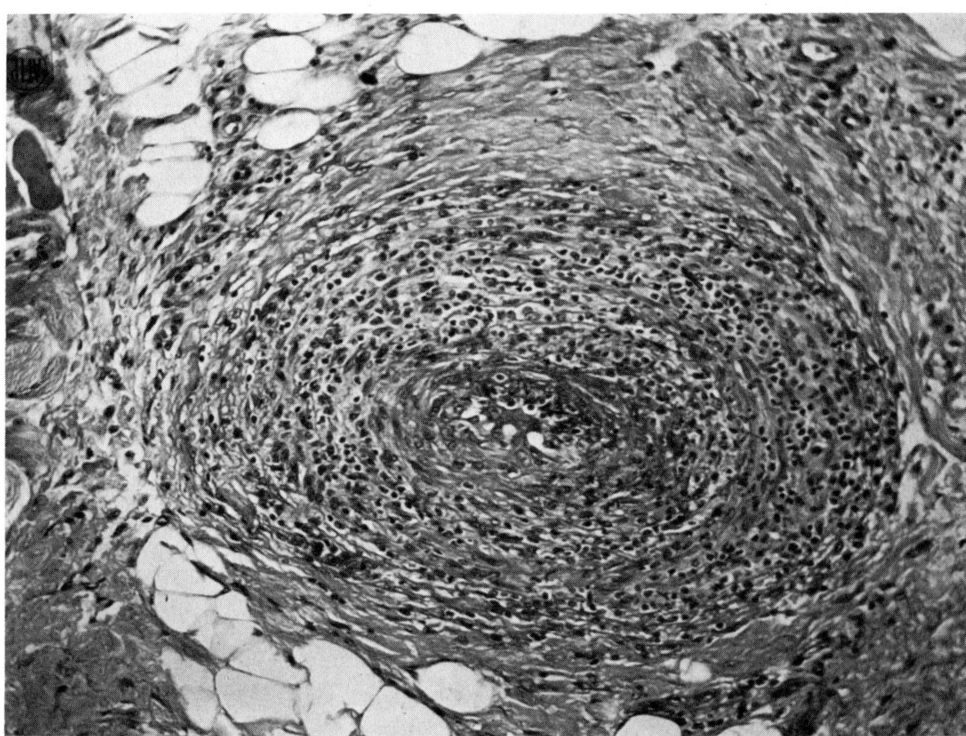

Figure 7–31. Rheumatoid arthritis is a diffuse disease involving connective tissue, muscle, and tendon as well as synovium and bone. Vasculitis is a regular feature of the disease, as illustrated in this section of a small artery surrounded by a chronic inflammatory infiltrate with necrosis of the vessel wall.

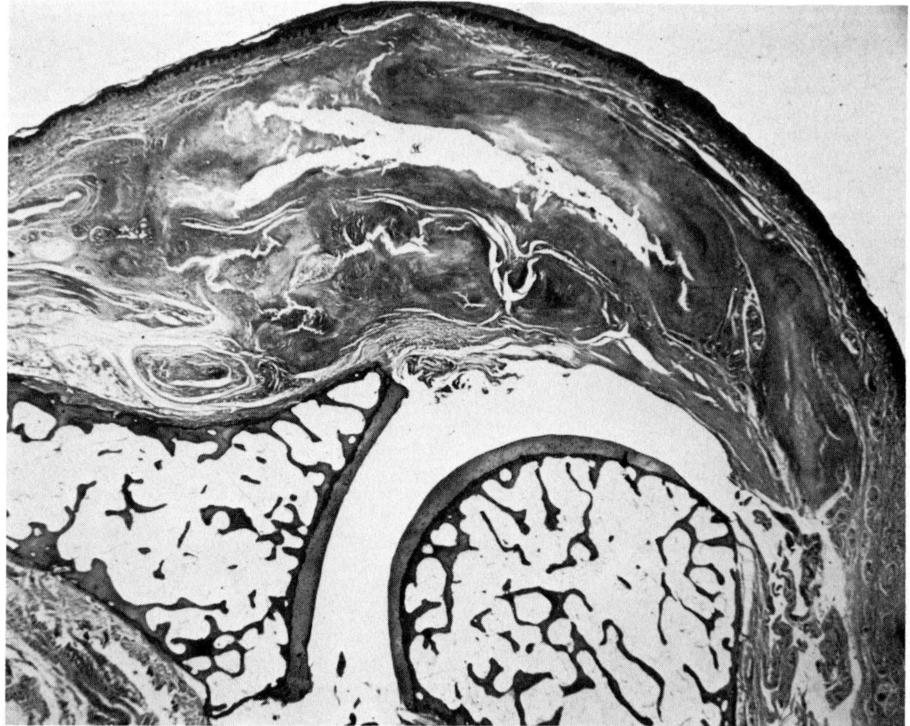

Figure 7–32. Macrosection of a finger joint exhibiting a rheumatoid nodule on the dorsal surface of the joint that fills the entire space between bone and skin and blends with the extensor tendon.

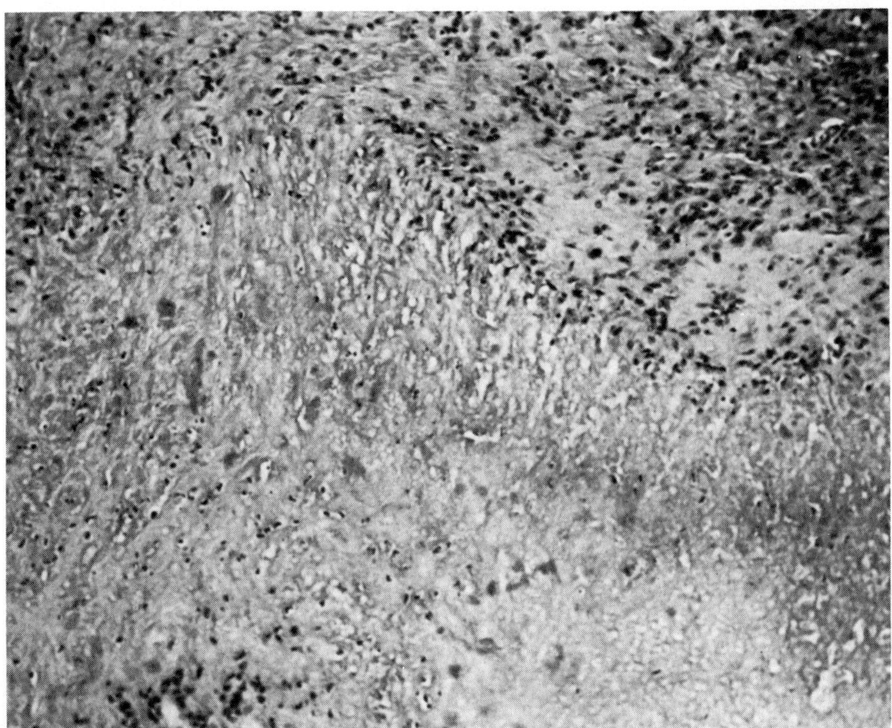

Figure 7–33. Section of a rheumatoid nodule showing a central area of necrosis surrounded by a zone of histiocytes and chronic inflammatory cells. This section exhibits the characteristic palisading of histiocytes at the edge of the necrosis.

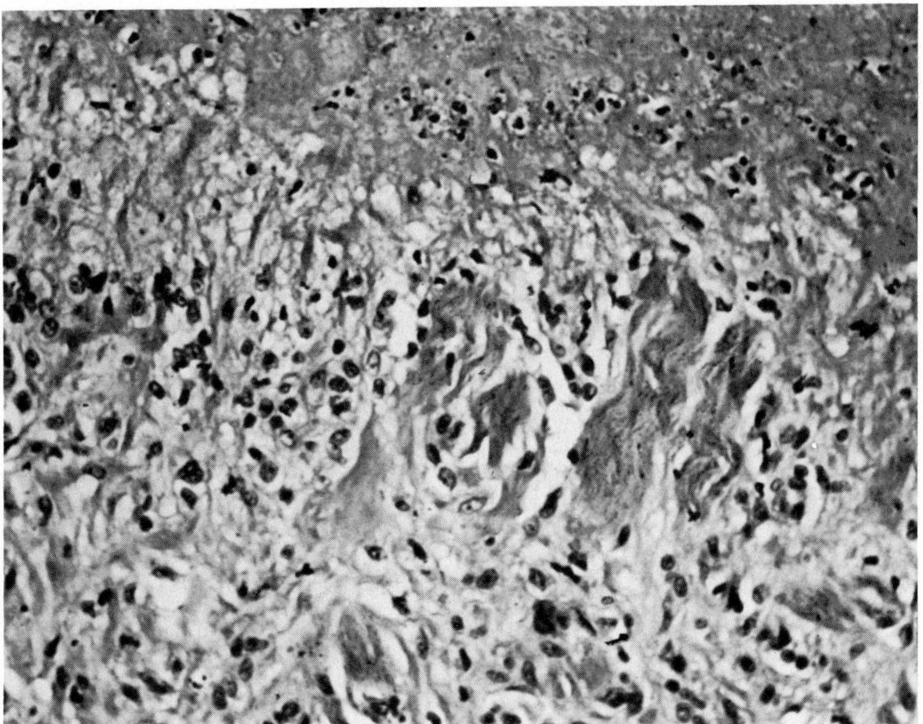

Figure 7–34. Higher magnification of a rheumatoid nodule exhibiting a large number of histiocytes oriented at right angles to the central area of necrosis. In rheumatoid nodules, Langhans' giant cells are infrequent, but the necrosis is similar to the caseation necrosis of tuberculosis.

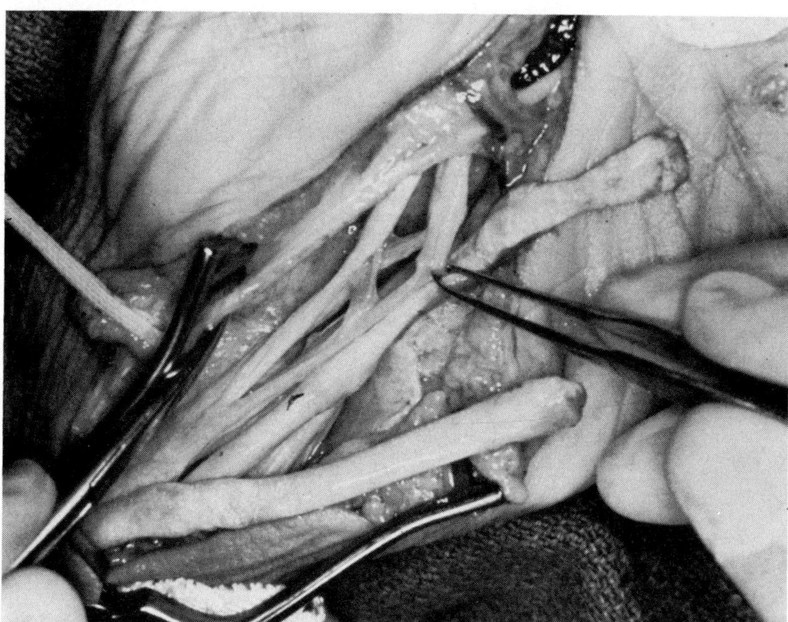

Figure 7–35. Photograph of the carpal canal of a patient with rheumatoid arthritis. Since the disease attacks synovial tissue of tendons as well as joints, rupture of tendons is very common in areas in which they pass through a restricted space. The increased volume of the synovium causes interference with the nutrition of the tendon and can actually cause infarction. Tendons can also rupture when infiltrated by rheumatoid nodules or by rubbing on the raw surface of bone that has eroded through the joint capsule.

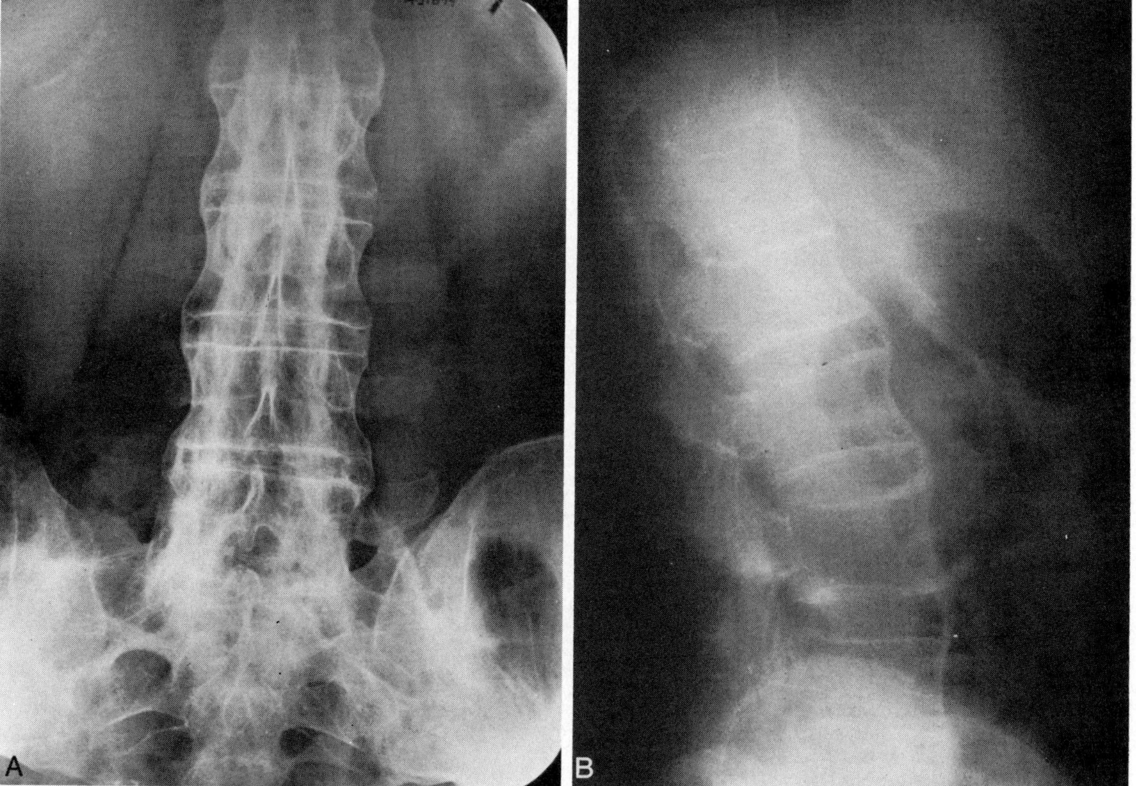

Figure 7–36. Anteroposterior *(A)* and lateral *(B)* radiographs of the lumbosacral spine of a patient with rheumatoid spondylitis. The vertebrae are joined by bridges of bone extending around the outer circumference of the margins of the discs. Note the arthrodesis of the sacroiliac joints with obliteration of the joint space and trabecular bridging. Although osteoarthritis may also lead to fusion of vertebral bodies (see Fig. 6–39), it is always secondary to circumferential remodeling processes and therefore associated with osteophyte formation. Rheumatoid spondylitis is a result of calcification in ligaments and does not exhibit osteophyte formation.

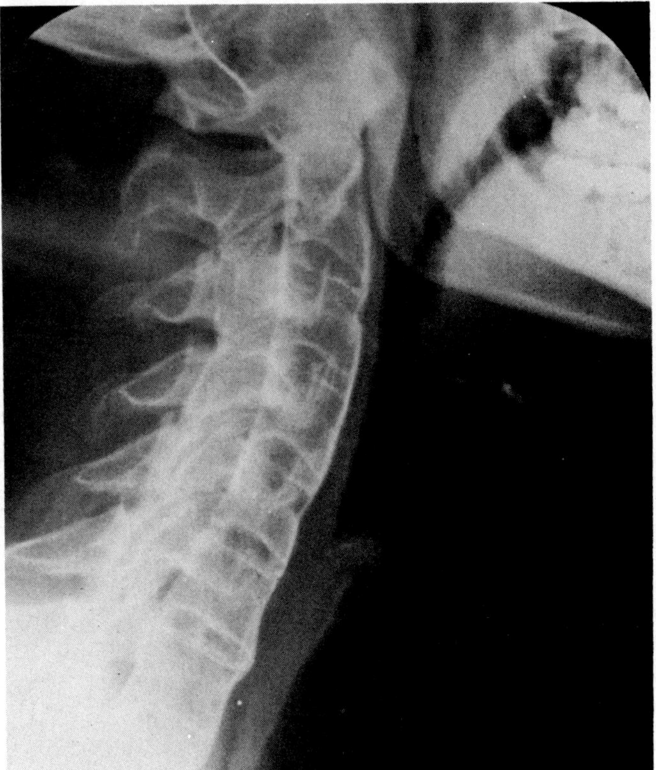

Figure 7–37. Lateral radiograph of the cervical spine of a patient with rheumatoid spondylitis. Usually, the process begins in the lower vertebral column and slowly extends upward. In long-standing or more severe cases, it may involve the cervical spine, and the patient becomes locked into a rigid posture.

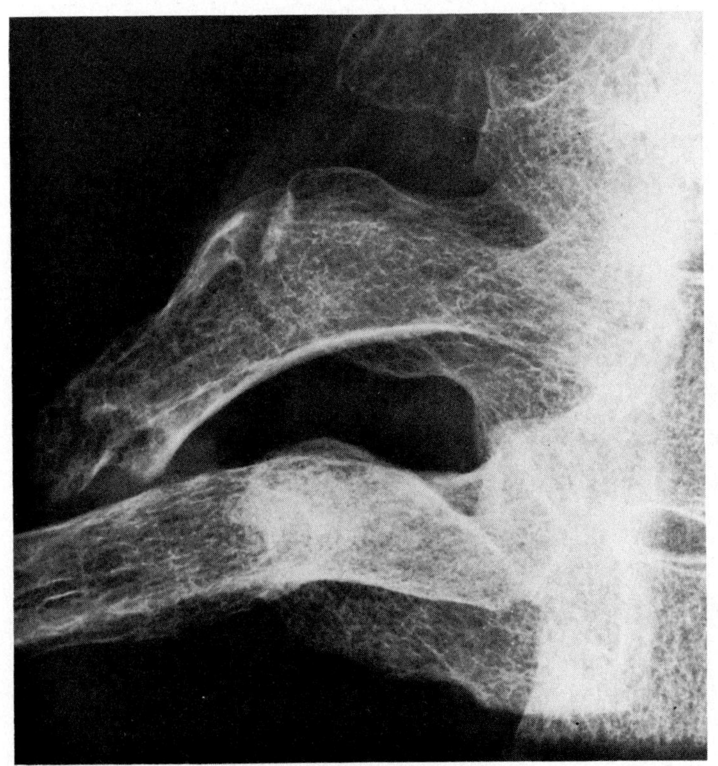

Figure 7–38. Specimen radiograph of the ribs of a patient with rheumatoid spondylitis. The costovertebral joints frequently fuse, resulting in marked restriction of respiratory excursion of the ribs.

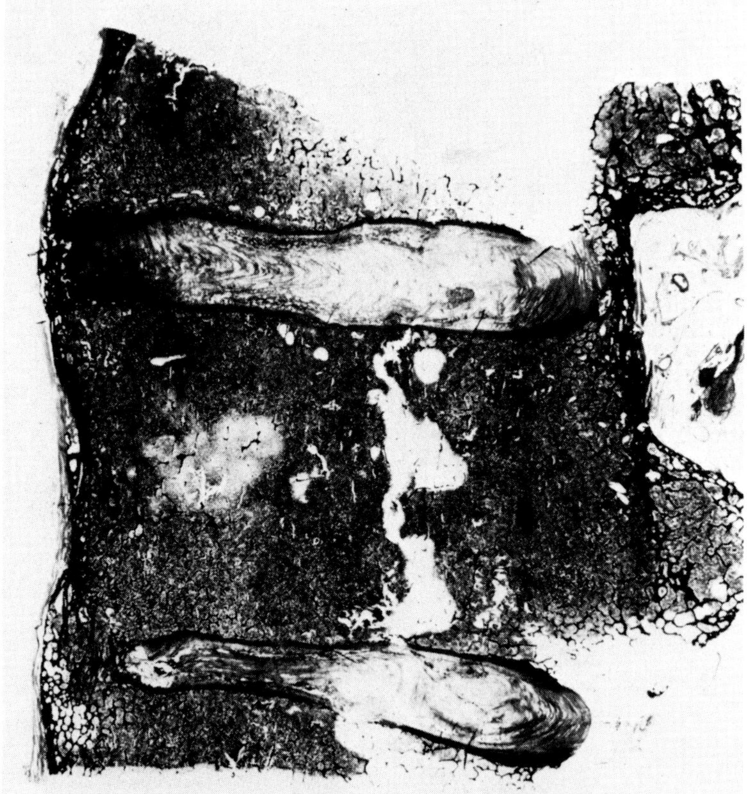

Figure 7–39. Macrosection of vertebrae and two discs in a patient with rheumatoid spondylitis. Notice that the bony bridges are extending from one vertebra to the other around the edge of the disc.

For a more extensive discussion of rheumatoid disease, the reader is referred to the text published by Jaffe, which is based on many years of experience accumulated in a major center for the treatment of rheumatoid disease at a time when these diseases were more prevalent than they are today (Jaffe, 1972).

CITED REFERENCES

Ehrlich, G. E.: Treatment of rheumatoid arthritis. J.A.M.A. *228*:94, 1974.
Peter, J. B.: The major varieties of arthritis. Diagnostic Medicine, August 1978, pp. 67–80.
Resnick, D.: Rheumatoid arthritis of the wrist—the compartmental approach. Med. Radiogr. Photogr. 52:50, 1976.

GENERAL REFERENCES

Jaffe, H. L.: Metabolic, Degenerative, and Inflammatory Diseases of Bones and Joints. Philadelphia, Lea and Febiger, 1972, pp. 781–806.
Resnick, D., and Niwayama, G.: Diagnosis of Bone and Joint Disorders, with Emphasis on Articular Abnormalities. Philadelphia, W. B. Saunders Co., 1981.

8

METABOLIC DISEASES OF BONE

Metabolic diseases of bone are characterized by failure of matrix production, mineralization, or maintenance. The metabolic defect may be acquired or inherited. It is a generalized defect and therefore involves all bones in the body. The etiology includes endocrine disturbances, nutritional disturbances, genetic mutations, and toxins. The specific effect produced in the skeleton may be failure or excessive production of one or more components, inadequate or excessive removal of one or more components, or a combination of production and removal errors. Bone has limited capability to react to any insult, so there is considerable similarity in the pattern of response to diseases of different etiology.

Metabolic disease of bone may become manifest in the growing skeleton and result in structural abnormality. Once the skeleton is fully formed, structural manifestations of metabolic disease occur during normal remodeling. Thus, some degree of osteoporosis must always precede morphologic manifestations of any metabolic bone disease.

OSTEOPOROSIS

Osteoporosis is simply a quantitative loss of bone. Numerous conditions cause osteoporosis. There may be nothing more than the "normal" loss of bone with aging, especially in slender women; nutritional factors, lack of exercise, decreasing muscle mass, loss of gravity (Pace, 1977), estrogen secretion, alcohol, and steroids have all been implicated (Jowsey, 1977). Regardless of etiology, the bone that remains is morphologically intact and exhibits no abnormality. It is simply reduced in volume and caliber.

Osteoporosis affecting cortical bone will reduce the thickness of the cortex by progressive resorption of the inner surface, with replacement of bone by marrow tissue. This progressive transformation of cortical bone to slender bone and marrow constituents is called "trabeculization of the cortex." The resorption of the inner surface is accompanied by some deposition of bone on the outer surface of the cortex, but the net effect is loss of bone. Trabeculae in lines of stress are maintained although reduced in number. The number of trabeculae that remain compared with the normal number can be used as a useful index of the degree of osteoporosis. At least 30 per cent of the bone must disappear before any radiographic evidence of osteoporosis is present (Figs. 8–1 to 8–4).

In fully developed disease, the trabeculae of bone within the medullary cavity are markedly thin and reduced in number, and they are surrounded by fat and hematopoietic tissue.

The vertebral bodies are often the site of severe osteoporosis. Regressive remodeling with the creation of "codfish vertebrae" is common. Although many conditions may lead to a single vertebral body collapse, simple, pure osteoporosis must not be forgotten when one is attempting to determine etiology.

Radiographic appearance of osteoporosis is simply one of thin bone. The density differential between the endosteal cortical margin and the medullary cavity becomes indistinct. The trabeculae become more prominent. The prominence is due to the sharp contrast between the few remaining trabeculae and soft tissue density but does not imply thickened structure (Figs. 8–5 to 8–8).

Text continued on page 247

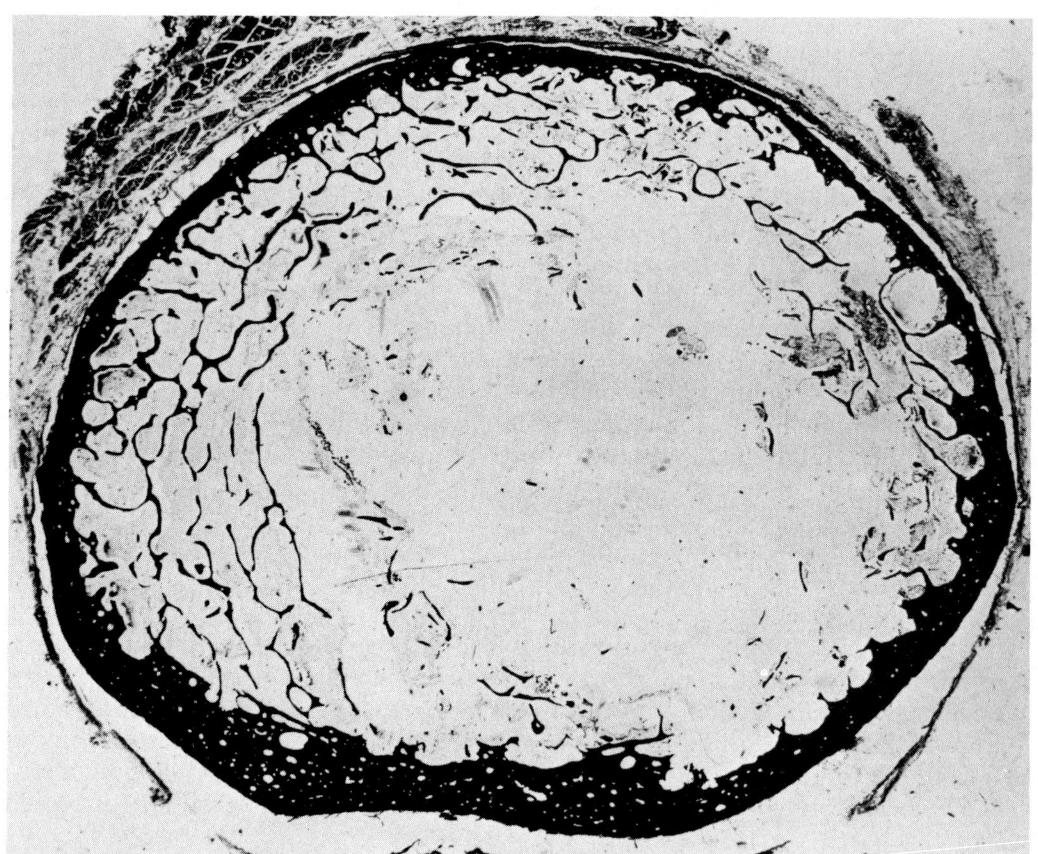

Figure 8–1. Osteoporosis. Cross section of distal femur with reduction of cancellous bone and loss of cortical thickness. Note replacement of cortical bone and trabeculization of cortex.

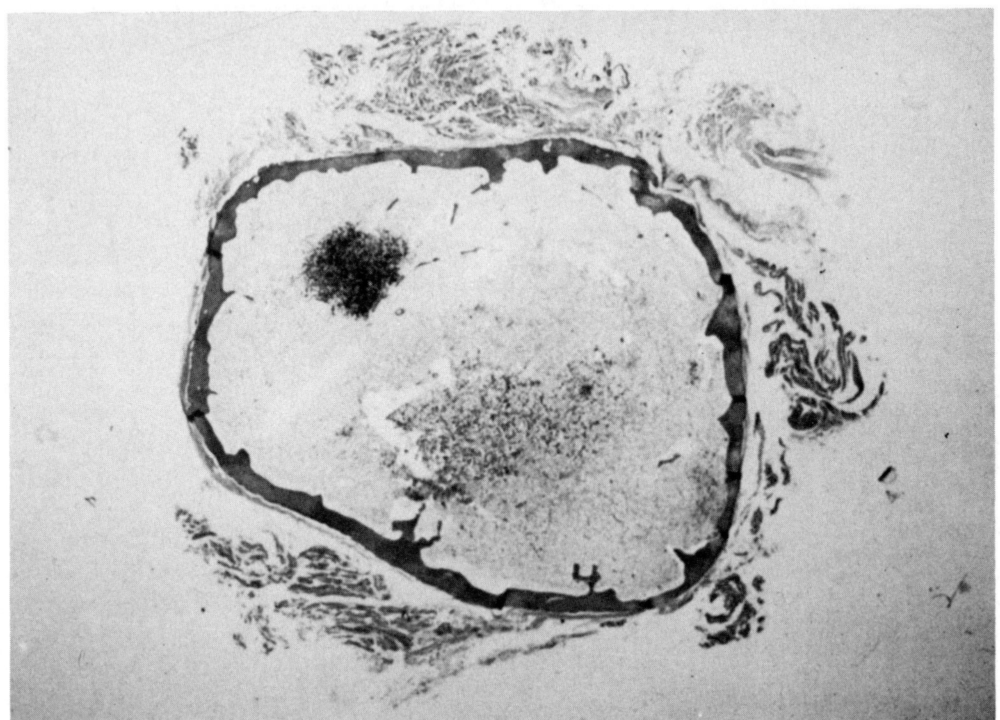

Figure 8–2. Cross section of distal femur exhibiting severe osteoporosis. Virtually no cancellous bone remains, and there is extensive replacement of the marrow cavity by xanthomatous fat. The cortex is markedly thinned.

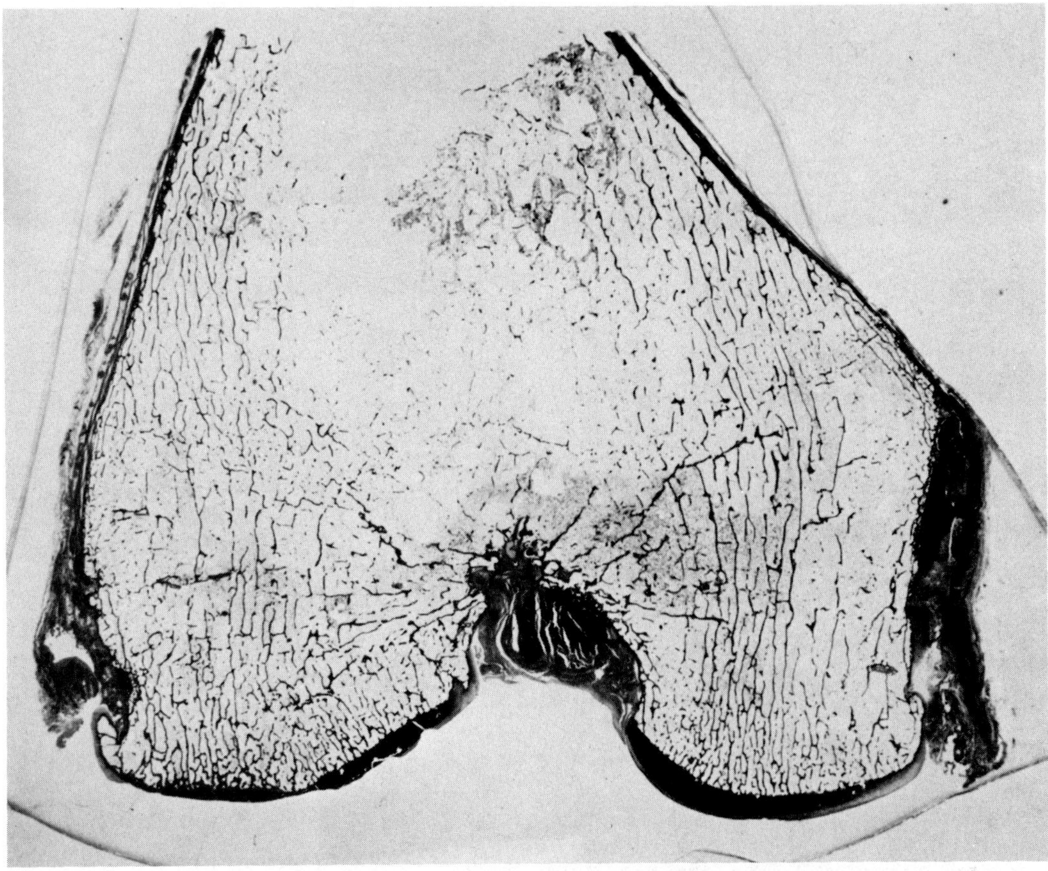

Figure 8–3. Macrosection of distal femur exhibiting severe osteoporosis. Notice trabeculization of cortex (replacement of inner cortex with trabecular bone), thin trabeculae, and major loss of trabeculae in the medullary cavity.

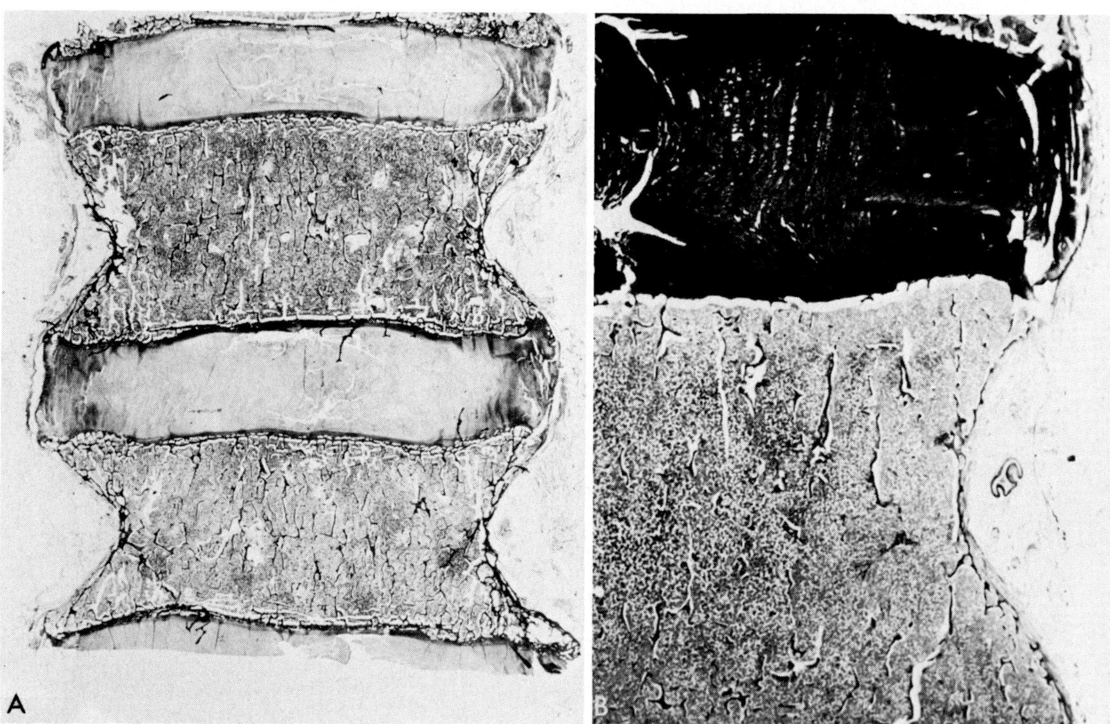

Figure 8–4. Macrosections of spine showing severe osteoporosis of the vertebral bodies. The number of trabeculae is reduced, and the cortex is thin. There is no change in the shape of the bone.

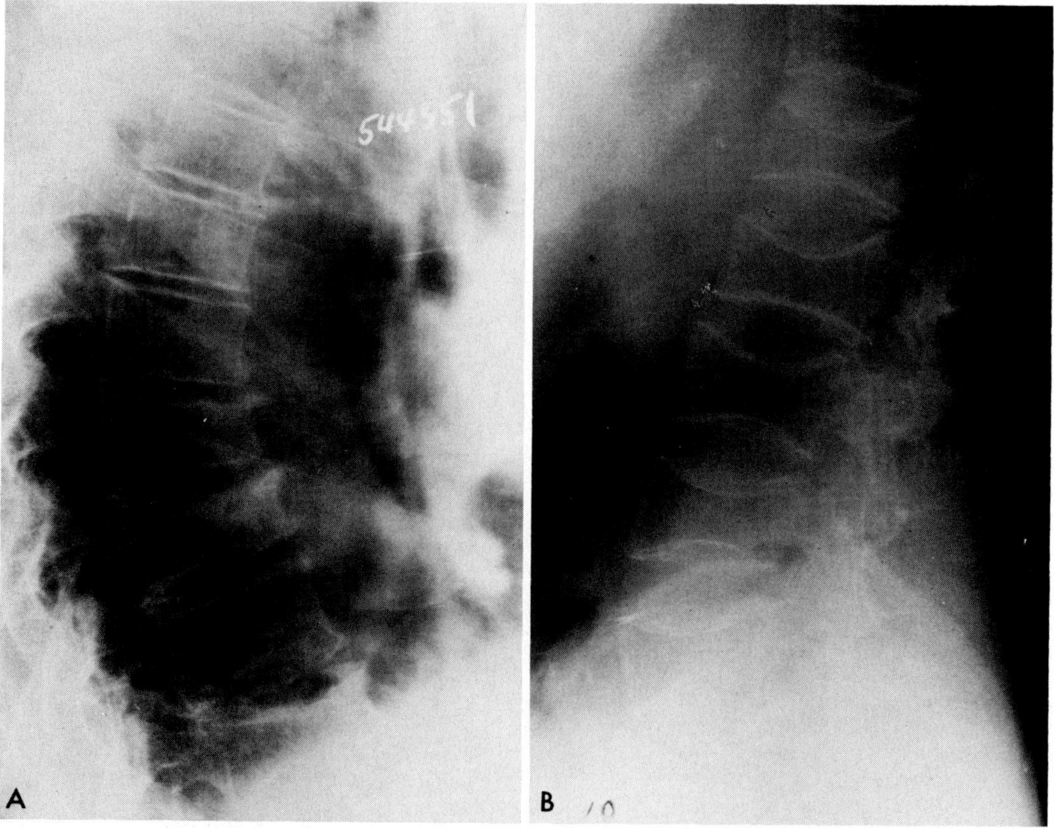

Figure 8–5. Radiographs of spine showing osteoporosis. Cortical bone appears accentuated by contrast with osteopenic marrow. Longitudinal trabeculae also appear accentuated because smaller transverse trabeculae are absent. Anterior wedging and end-plate compression are present. In the more severe case (*B*), regressive remodeling results in the formation of classic "codfish" vertebrae.

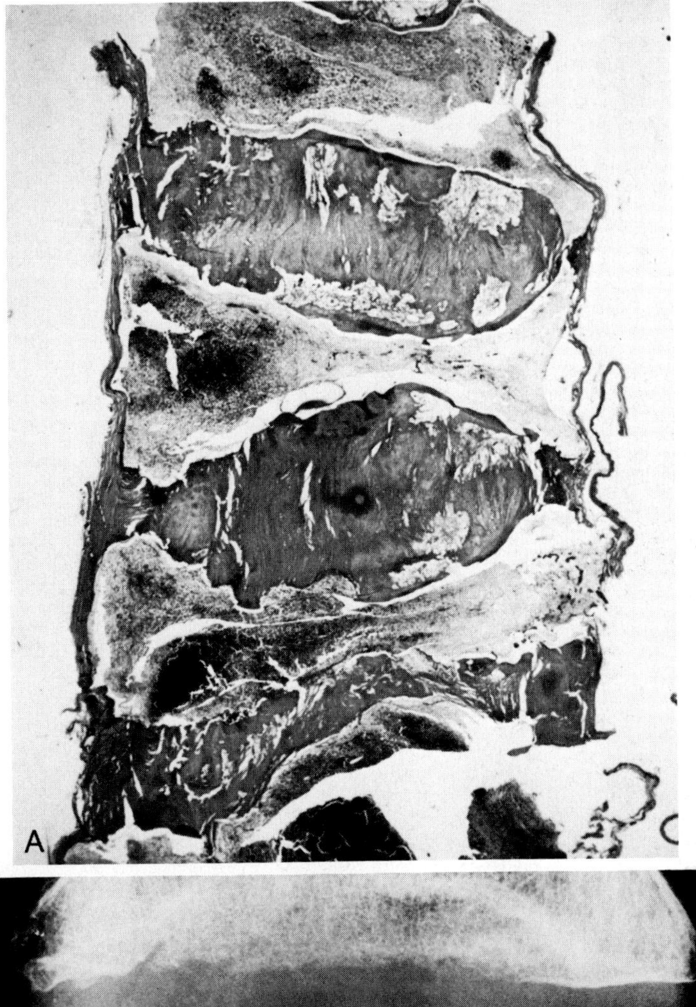

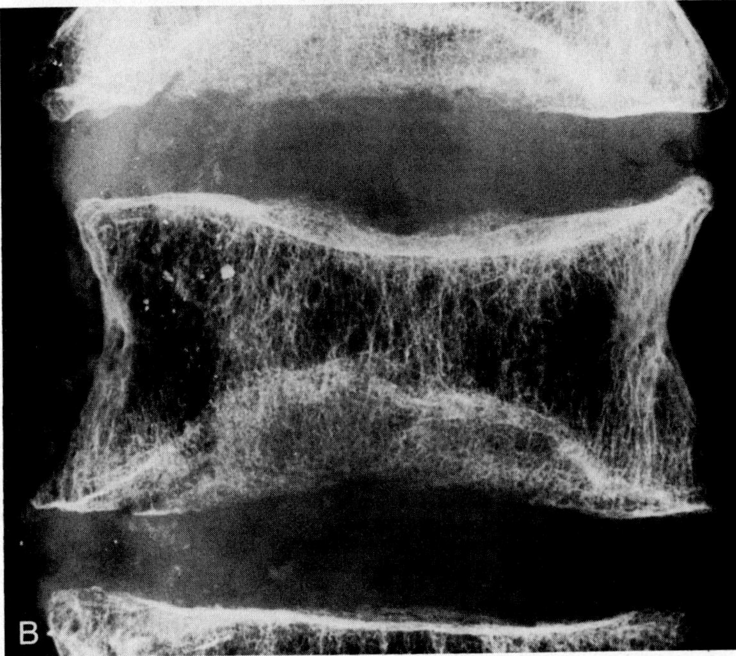

Figure 8–6. Macrosection (*A*) and specimen radiograph (*B*) of vertebral bodies exhibiting severe regressive remodeling of vertebral end-plates associated with osteoporosis. Regressive remodeling results in diminished height of vertebral bodies, with expansion of the intervertebral discs due to their intrinsic expansile pressure. Such severe changes are more commonly seen in hyperadrenalism than in ordinary osteoporosis. Microfractures may be a factor in collapse of the end plates.

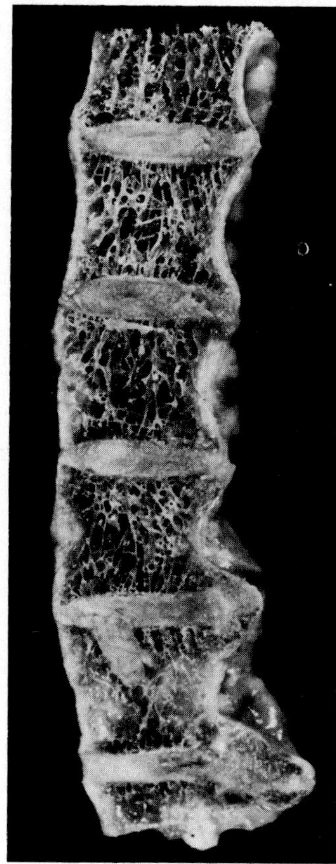

Figure 8–7. Partially macerated specimen of spine of patient with moderate osteoporosis exhibiting reduction in the number of trabeculae. There is no regressive remodeling, and the cortex appears relatively normal.

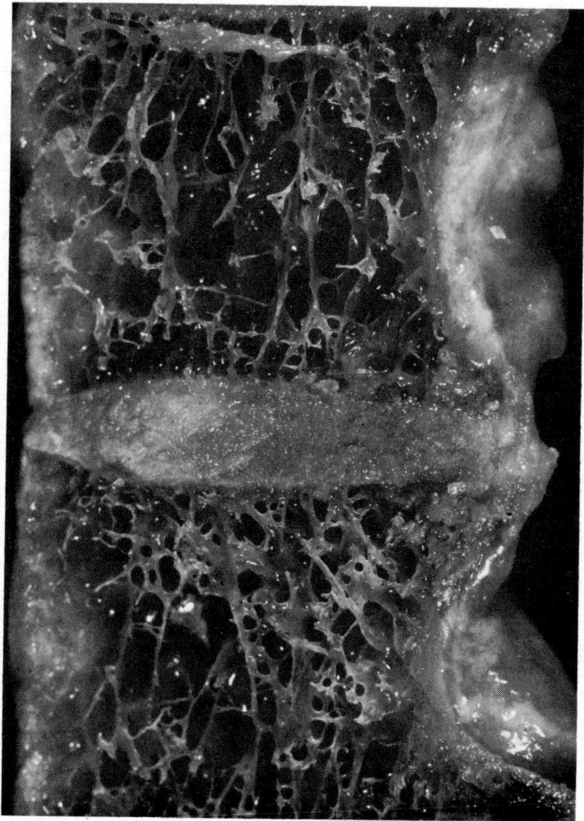

Figure 8–8. Higher magnification of specimen exhibiting osteoporosis, with the number of smaller transverse marrow trabeculae diminished. The longitudinal trabeculae appear more prominent, even though they are not increased in number or size.

When the conditions leading to osteoporosis are corrected, additional bone can be formed on existing trabeculae. The formation of new trabeculae requires "blastema" formation, and blastema will not be formed unless the appropriate stimulus is present, such as fracture callus. Thus, the patient whose osteoporosis is corrected forms appositional bone on *existing* trabeculae but cannot form *new* trabeculae. The radiographic picture will be one of coarse, thick, prominent trabeculae, reduced in number.

Histologic examination of pure osteoporosis reveals thin but normal trabeculae of bone and normal marrow. As a rule, there is no significant osteoblastic or osteoclastic activity, but detailed morphometric studies may identify increased or decreased activity (Lane, 1983).

HYPERPARATHYROIDISM

Excessive circulating parathyroid hormone stimulates mobilization of calcium into the blood stream. Bone is removed by osteoclasts and replaced by primitive mesenchymal connective tissue (Figs. 8–9 to 8–14).

Although osteoblasts are inhibited by the parathyroid hormone, continued osteoblastic activity is necessary to maintain structural integrity. Osteoclasts remove bone, and osteoblasts form bone in response to stress. Cancellous trabeculae are hollowed out and replaced with mesenchymal connective tissue; the remaining lateral margins of the trabeculae are actually widened by osteoblasts. Despite concurrent activity by osteoclasts and osteoblasts, the net result is a loss of bone and liberation of calcium salts into the blood stream.

Cortical bone is also lost, both by extensive tunneling and by reduction in the

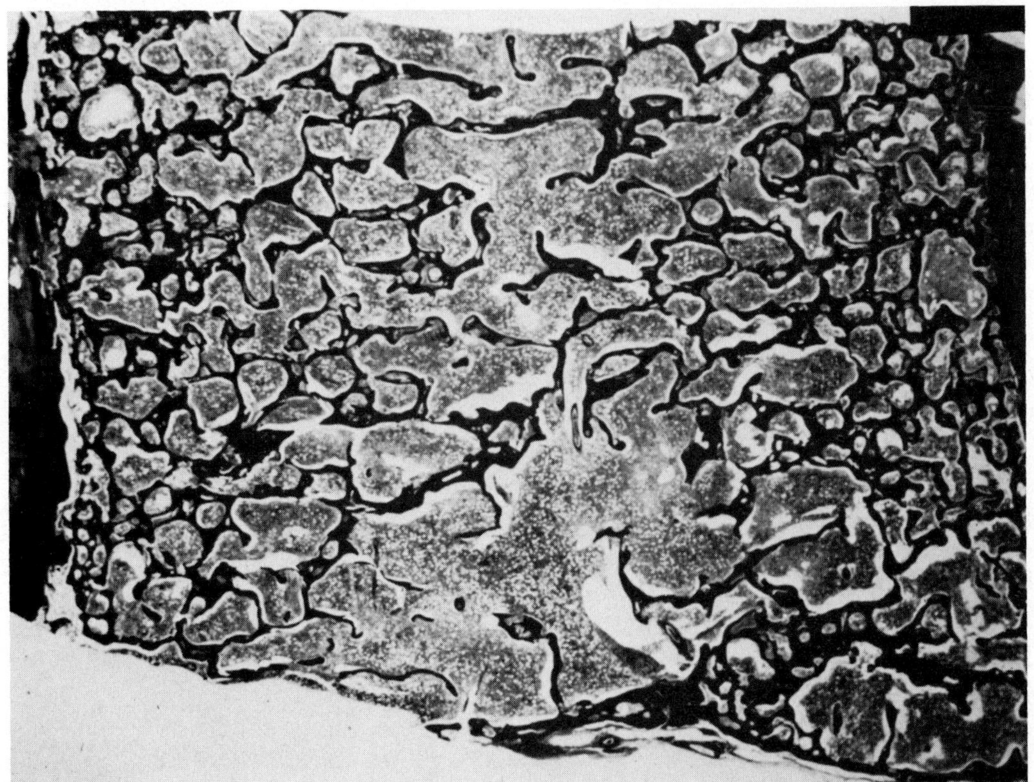

Figure 8–9. Hyperparathyroidism. Macrosection of vertebral body exhibiting erosion of trabecular bone from within individual trabeculae. The space created is filled with mesenchymal tissue distinct from normal marrow.

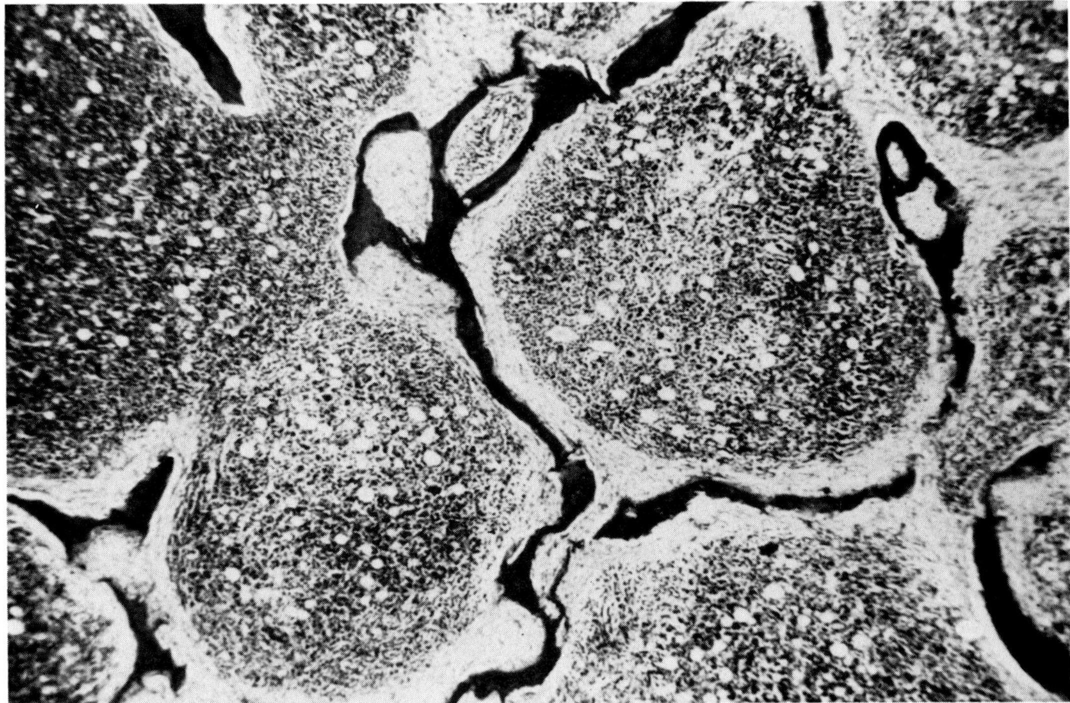

Figure 8–10. Hyperparathyroidism. Histologic section exhibiting mesenchymal connective tissue replacing the normal marrow next to the trabeculae of bone. Notice the generalized osteoporosis due to diminished trabecular size. Numerous osteoclasts are present but are difficult to recognize at this magnification.

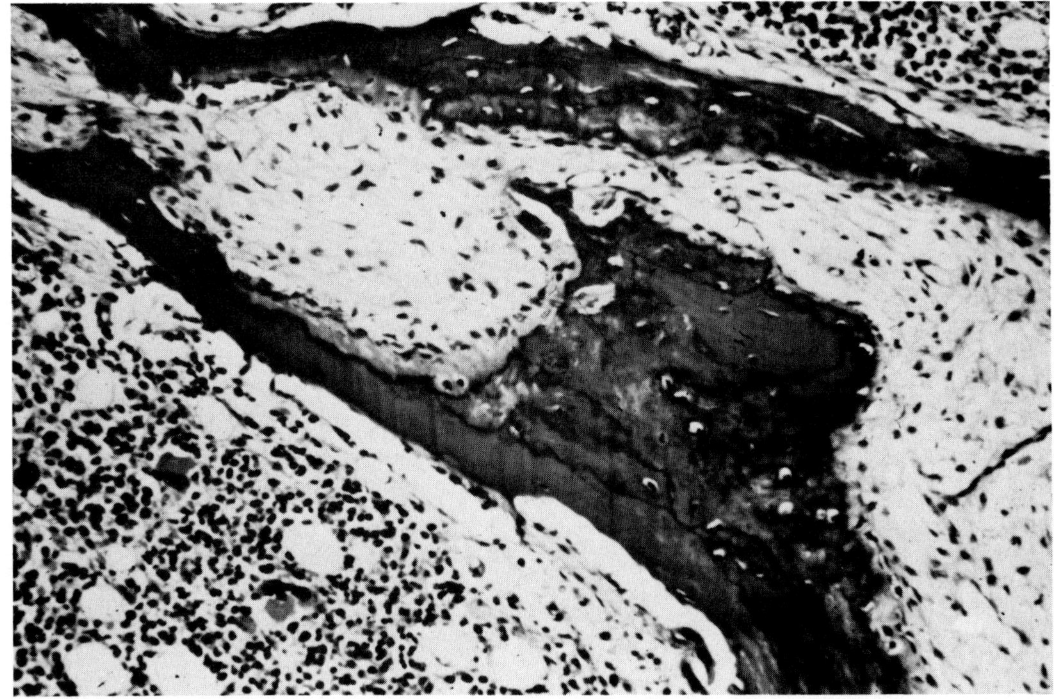

Figure 8–11. Hyperparathyroidism. "Railroad track" formation due to removal of the central portion of a trabecula ("dissecting osteitis"). Mesenchymal connective tissue replaces bone in a longitudinal manner, leaving two parallel spicules of bone instead of a single trabeculum. Note persistence of osteoblastic and osteoclastic activity.

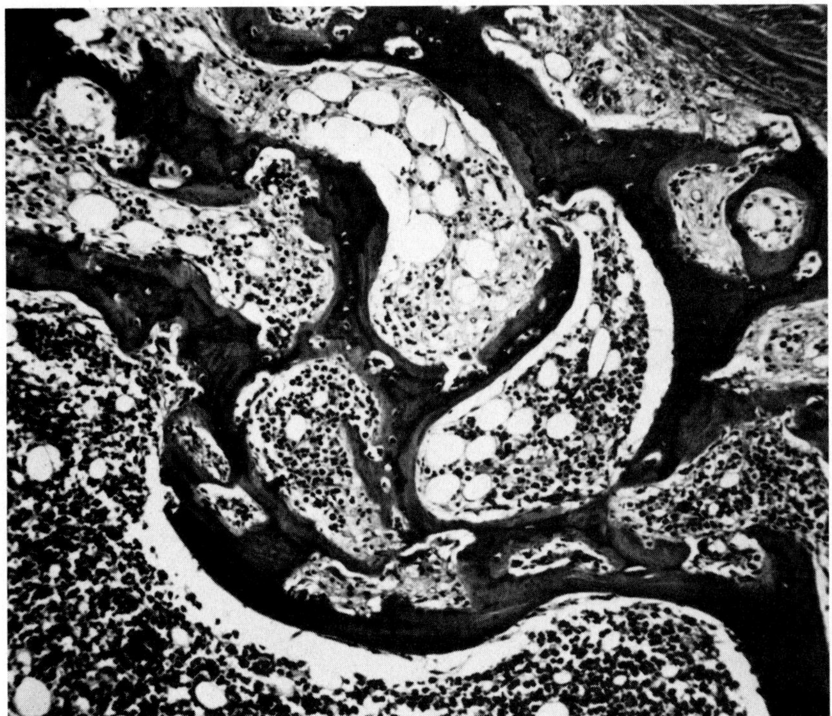

Figure 8–12. Histologic appearance of hyperparathyroidism, with mesenchymal tissue replacing bone.

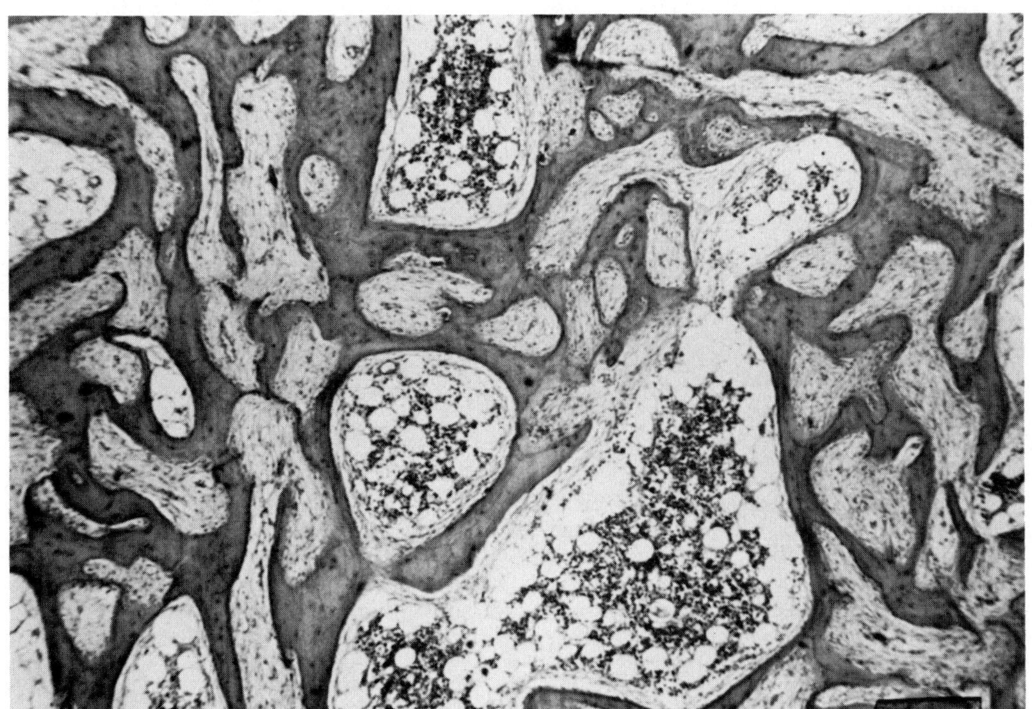

Figure 8–13. Histologic section of more extensive dissecting osteitis in trabecular bone. Note the adjacent normal marrow, separated from the fibrovascular replacement tissue.

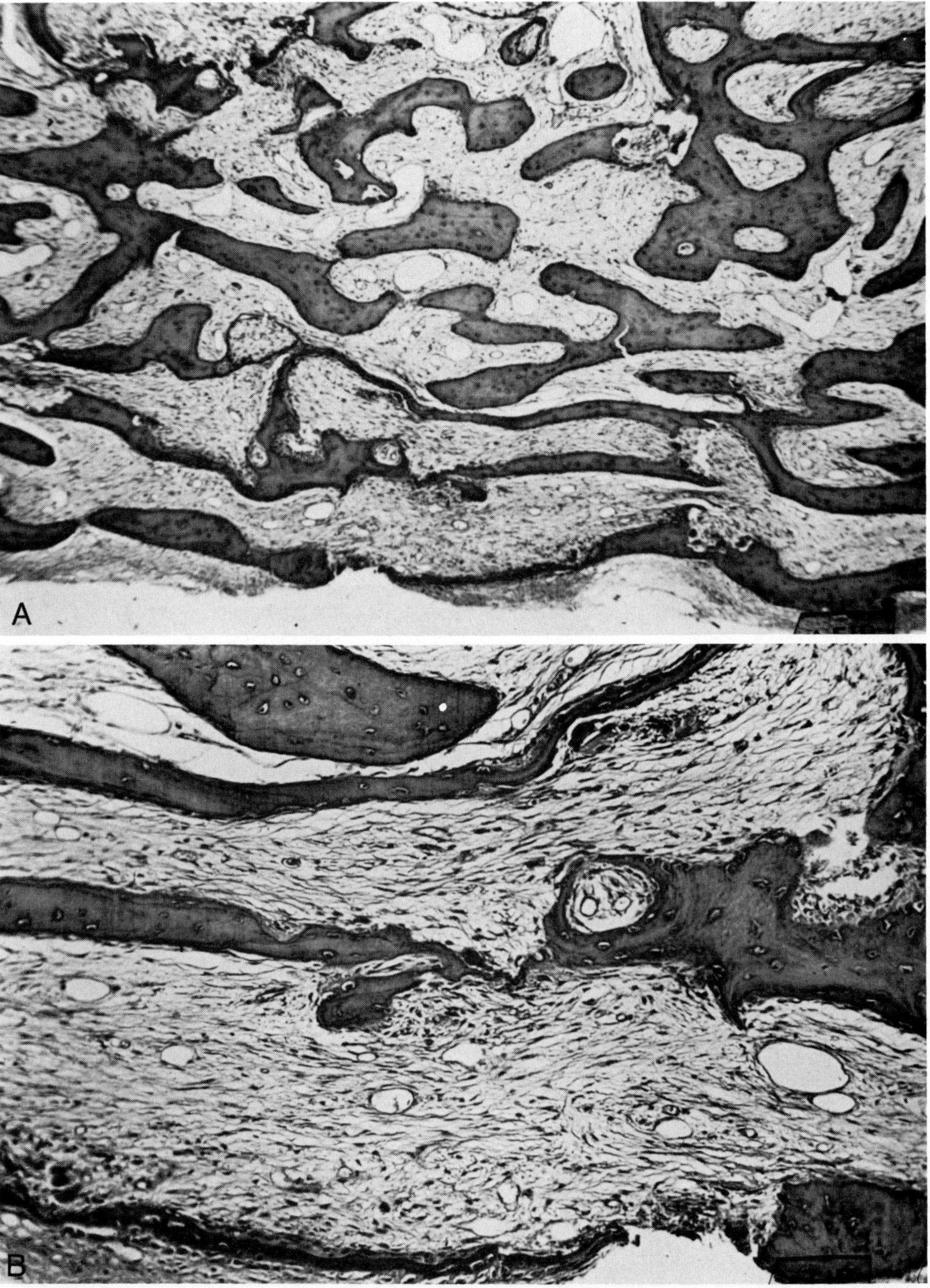

Figure 8–14. Low-power (*A*) and high-power (*B*) views of hyperparathyroidism, with extensive replacement of trabecular bone by mesenchymal tissue. In these sections, all normal marrow is replaced. If the mesenchymal fibrovascular replacement becomes more extensive, a brown tumor will result.

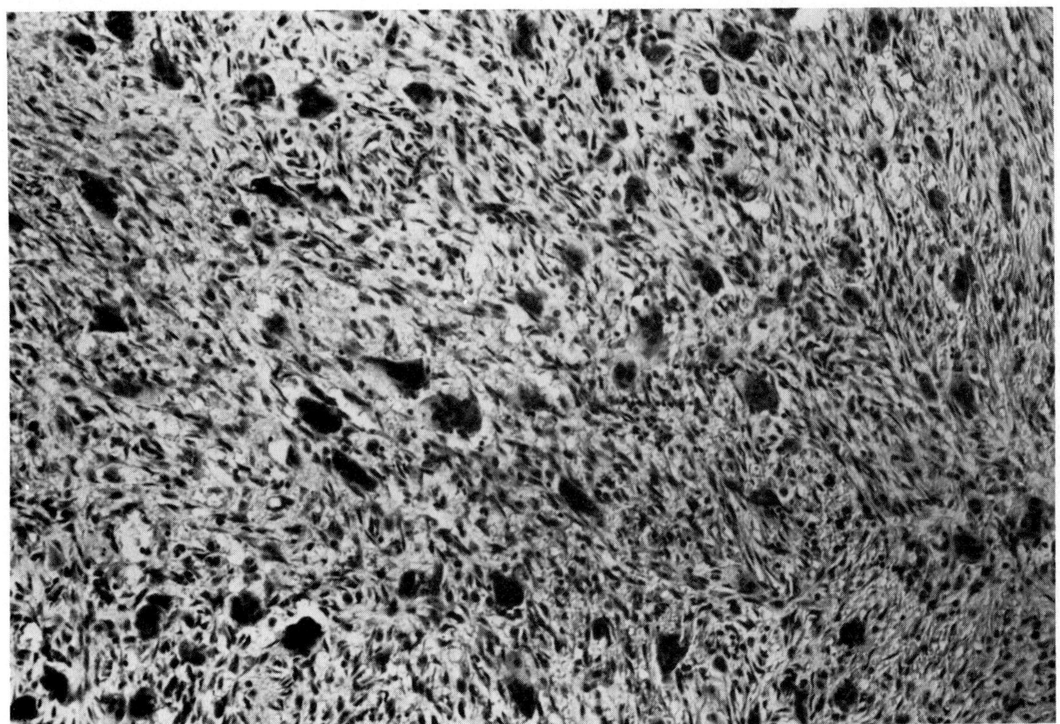

Figure 8–15. Hyperparathyroidism. Low-power view of brown tumor exhibiting numerous giant cells set in a spindled stroma. Although this section is from the medullary cavity, all bone has been removed.

thickness of the cortex, a process essentially similar to that seen in pure osteoporosis, but one that occurs at a faster rate. Trabeculization of the cortex is a common phenomenon in hyperparathyroidism, and the endosteal margin is indistinct. The periosteal margin exhibits active resorption of bone with characteristic fuzzy borders, particularly in the phalanges.

The excessive removal of bone may lead to large spaces filled with both osteoclasts and primitive mesenchymal connective tissue, the so-called "brown tumor" of hyperparathyroidism. These brown tumors are often confused with giant cell tumors of bone; the spindled appearance of the stromal component should serve to differentiate a brown tumor from a bona fide giant cell tumor of bone (Figs. 8–15 to 8–19).

The histologic appearance of hyperparathyroidism consists of marked osteoclastic activity with replacement of bone by loose mesenchymal connective tissue. If the stimulus of excessive parathyroid hormone secretion disappears, the mesenchymal cells will again resume osteoblastic activity and replace the bone that has been previously removed.

The differential diagnosis of hyperparathyroidism must include myelofibrosis, Paget's disease of bone, fibrous dysplasia, and ossifying fibroma (cortical fibrous dysplasia). Hyperparathyroidism is a diffuse disease process involving all portions of skeleton, whereas fibrous dysplasia, cortical fibrous dysplasia, and Paget's disease are localized. Myelofibrosis is associated with myelosclerosis and adds to the thickness of bone; the fibrotic process will always occur at the periphery of the bone spicule rather than hollow out its interior. Paget's disease is characterized by removal and simultaneous replacement of bone, without regard to lines of stress or functional requirements in bone (see Chap. 11).

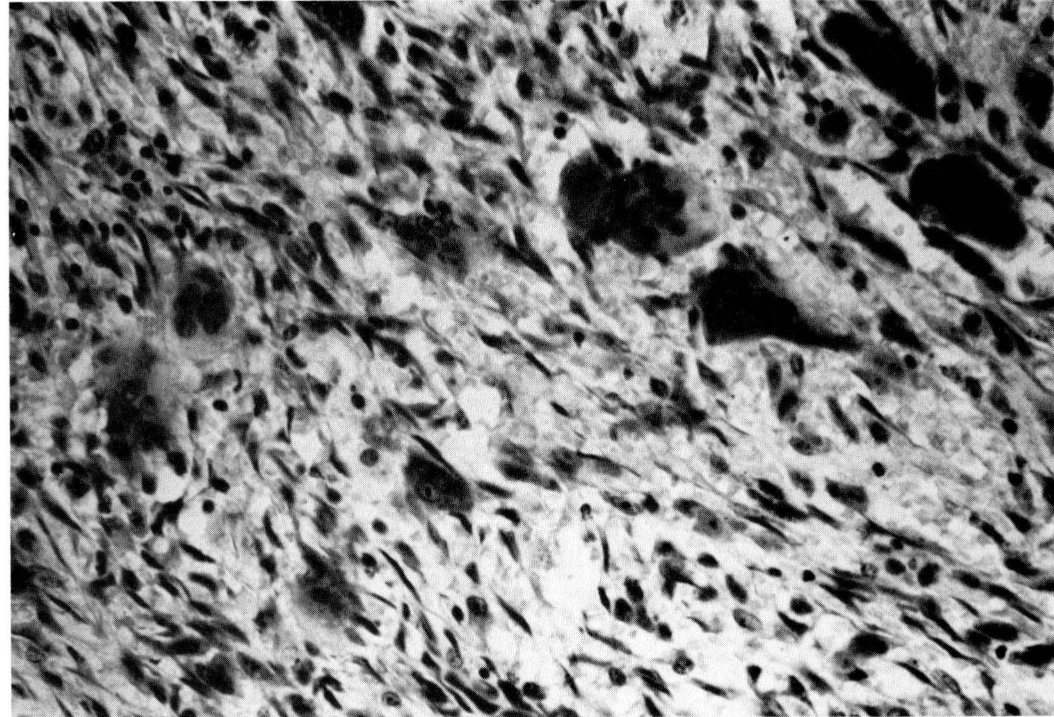

Figure 8–16. Hyperparathyroidism. High-power view of brown tumor with numerous giant cells and spindled stromal cells. The appearance of the spindled cell should cause the pathologist to suspect hyperparathyroidism rather than a bona fide giant cell tumor.

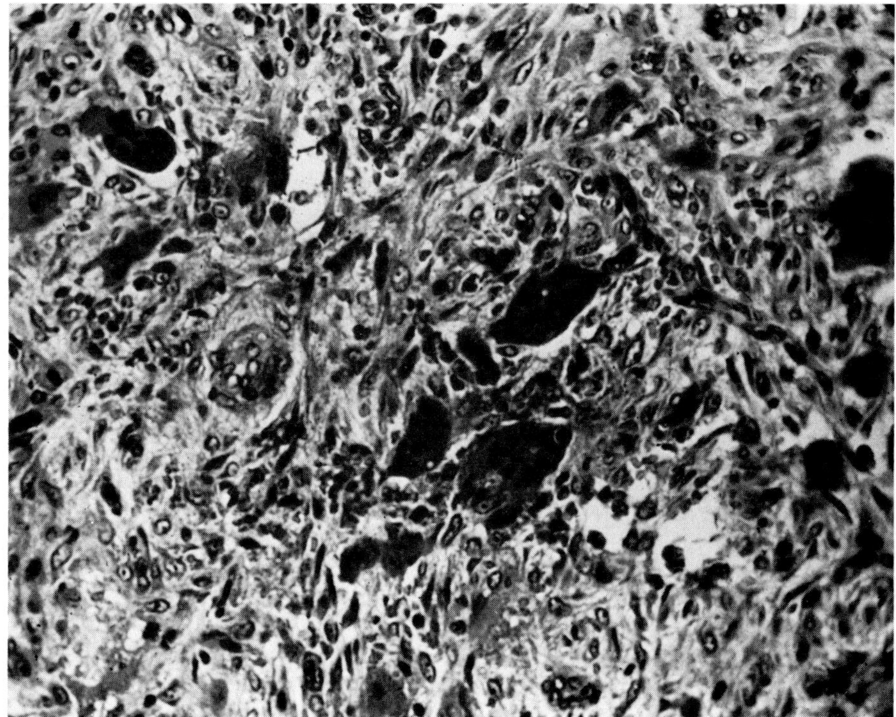

Figure 8–17. Hyperparathyroidism. Fairly pleomorphic appearance of giant cells and stromal cells in a patient with a brown tumor. True giant cell tumor may appear in a patient with hyperparathyroidism and can persist unresolved after the normal parathormone level is restored.

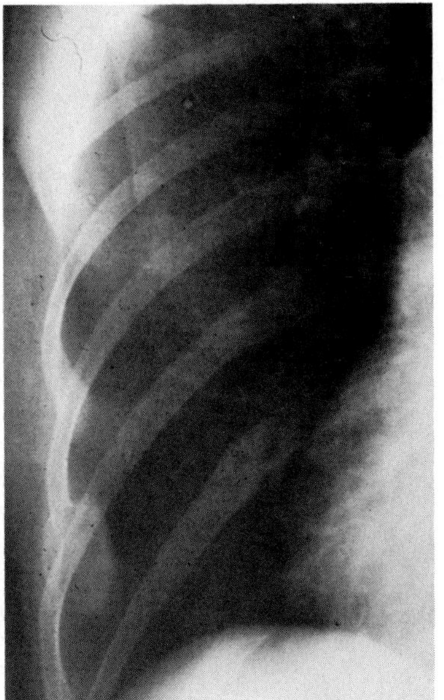

Figure 8–18. Hyperparathyroidism. Brown tumor of a rib in an 80-year-old patient. The lesion was discovered on routine chest film. Evaluation led to discovery of extensive hyperparathyroidism, and a parathyroid adenoma was removed.

The radiographic appearance of hyperparathyroidism has been extensively described in various texts. It consists of severe osteoporosis, trabeculization of cortex (Figs. 8–20 to 8–26), and creation of cystic cavities corresponding to the brown tumor. Hyperparathyroidism is best indicated by lines of subperiosteal resorption in those bones that can be easily visualized, particularly the lateral surface of the middle phalanx of the second and third fingers (Fig. 8–23).

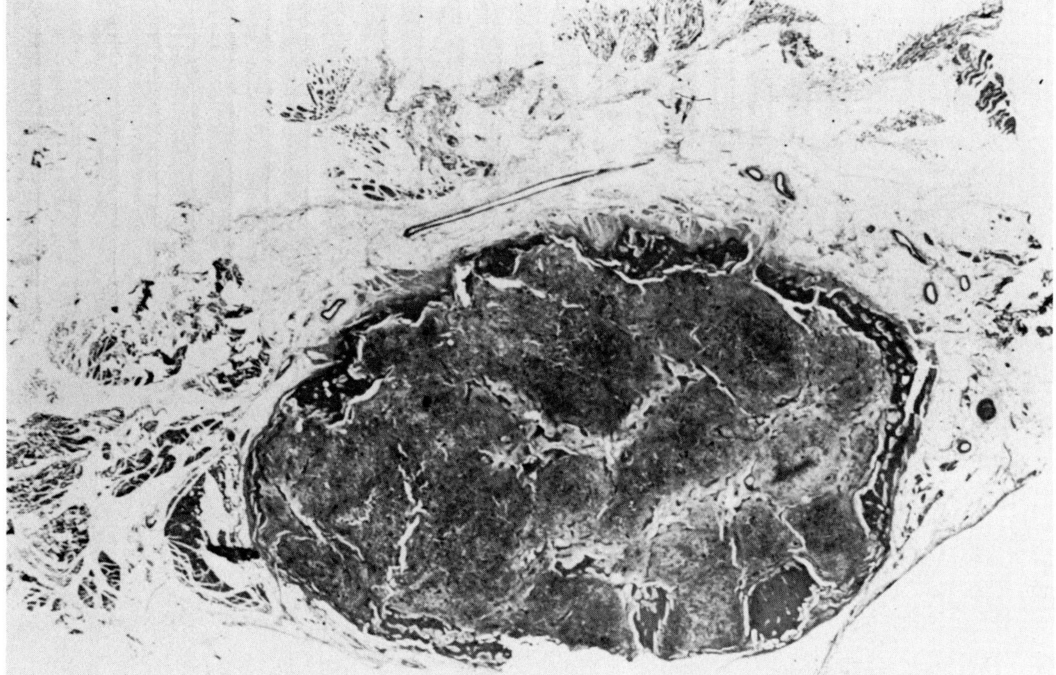

Figure 8–19. Macrosection of the brown tumor shown in Figure 8–18. Note the erosion and removal of residual bone at the periphery of the lesion. There is no periosteal new bone formation.

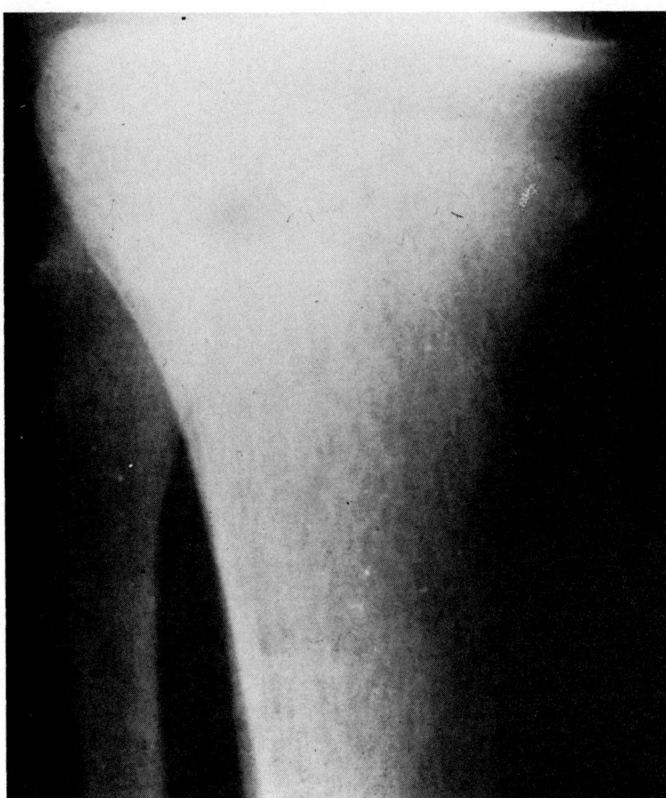

Figure 8–20. Radiograph of tibia with osteoporosis due to hyperparathyroidism. Resorptive tunneling of the cortex is evident, with no major discernible difference in the thickness of cortical or medullary bone. Severe osteoporosis is present in the metaphyseal-diaphyseal area, with subperiosteal resorption in the cutback zone of the medial metaphysis.

Figure 8–21. Hyperparathyroidism. Macrosection of femur exhibiting cancellization of the cortex. Severe osteoporosis is present, with markedly diminished number of trabeculae following lines of stress. Large resorption tunnels are present in diaphyseal cortex.

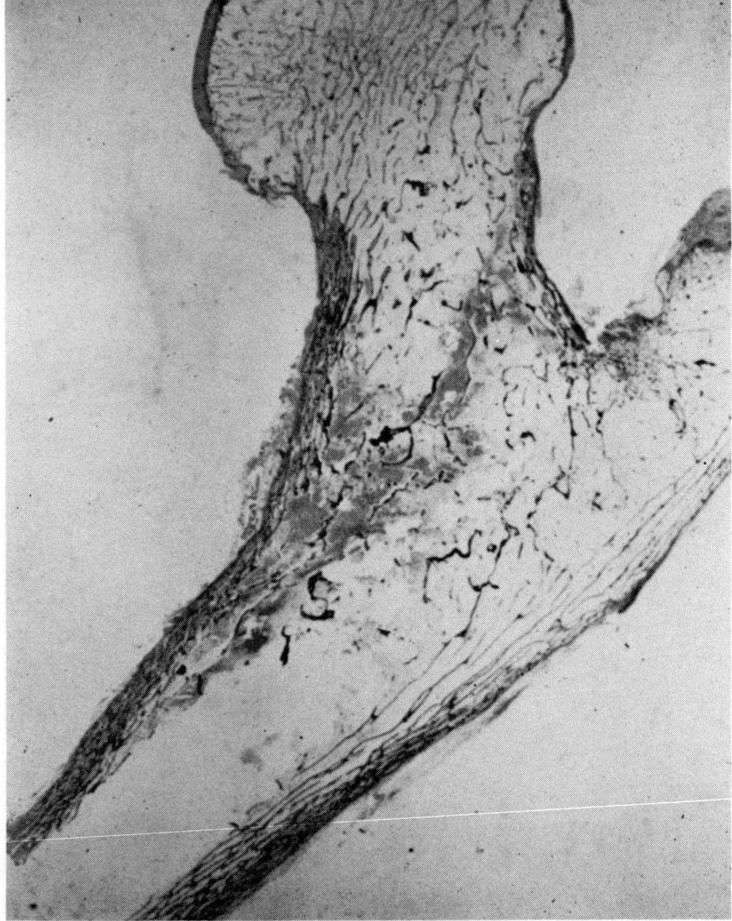

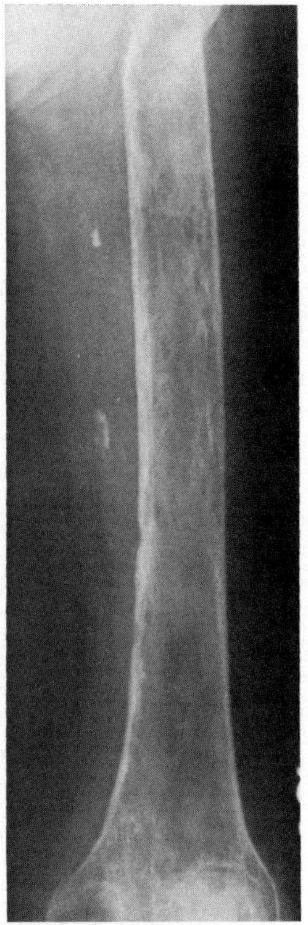

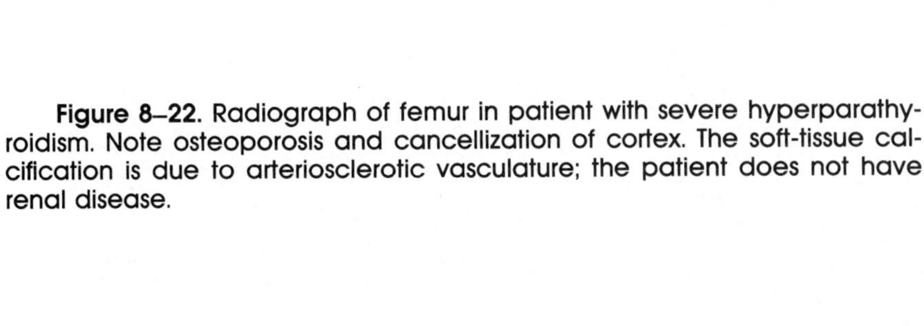

Figure 8–22. Radiograph of femur in patient with severe hyperparathyroidism. Note osteoporosis and cancellization of cortex. The soft-tissue calcification is due to arteriosclerotic vasculature; the patient does not have renal disease.

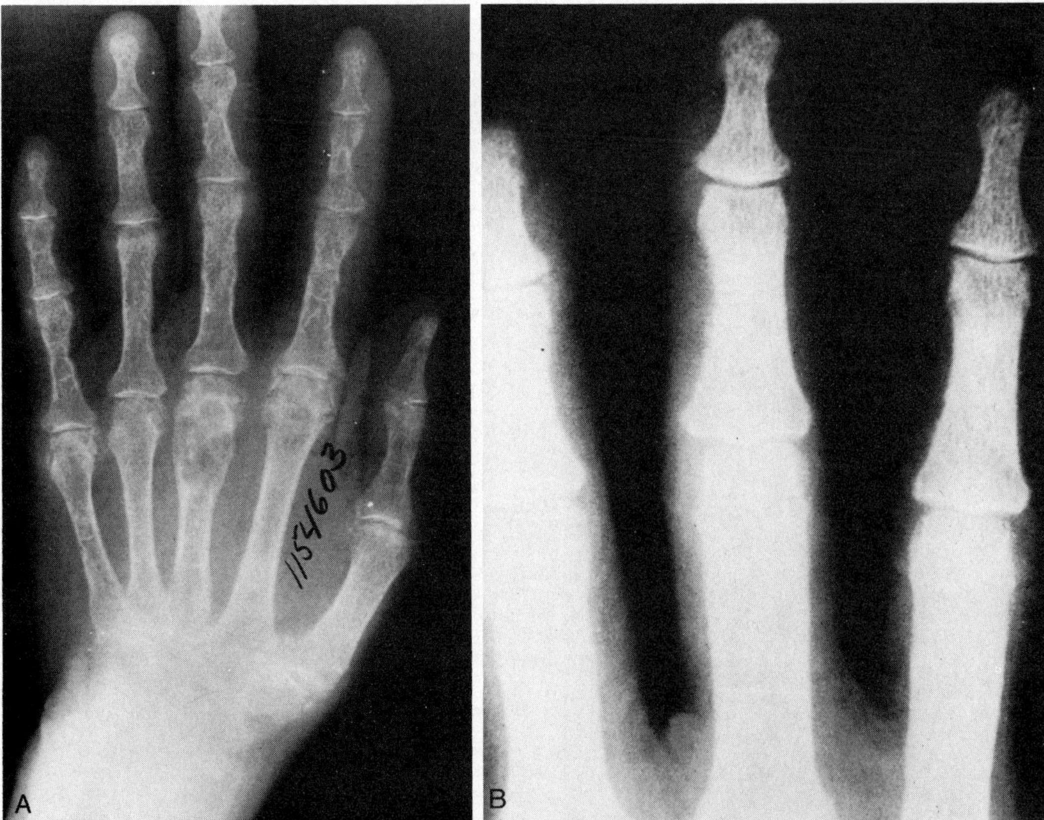

Figure 8–23. Hyperparathyroidism. Radiographs of the hand (*A*) and fingers (*B*) with extensive subperiosteal resorption of numerous phalanges. Note the fuzzy margin, which reflects subperiosteal bone formation and removal. The cyst-like expansion in the third metacarpal is a brown tumor. Subperiosteal resorption of the phalanges is a classic, easily demonstrable bony manifestation of parathyroid disease.

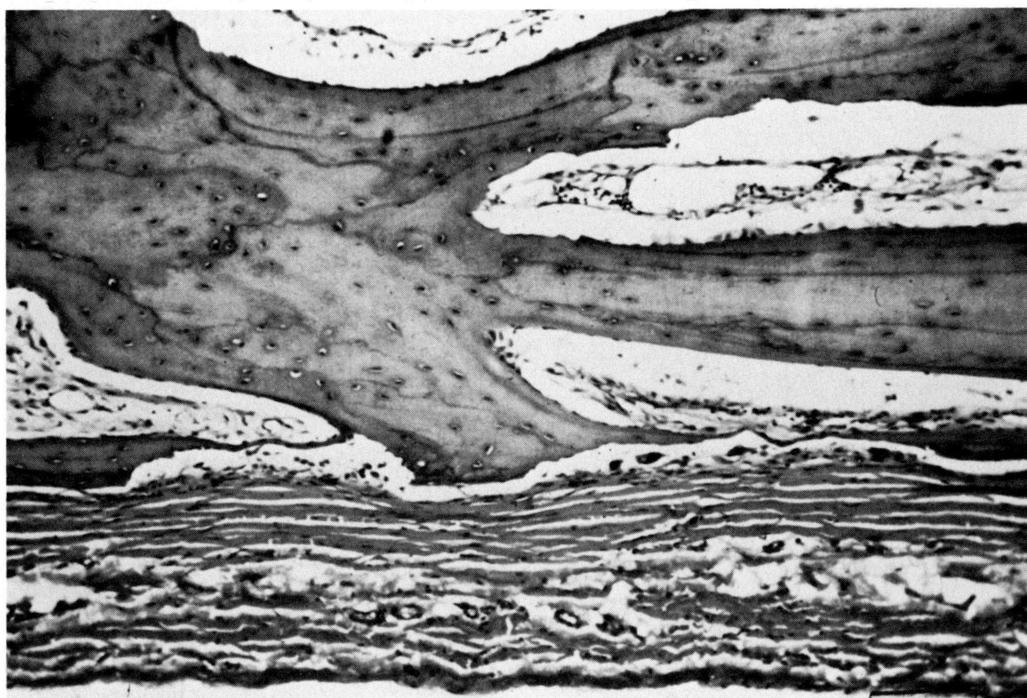

Figure 8–24. Hyperparathyroidism. Histologic appearance of subperiosteal bone. There is mesenchymal connective tissue replacement of cortical bone with numerous reversal lines, indicating continuous formation and removal. This activity is characteristic of hyperparathyroidism and accounts for the fuzzy outline of the bone in the areas of subperiosteal resorption.

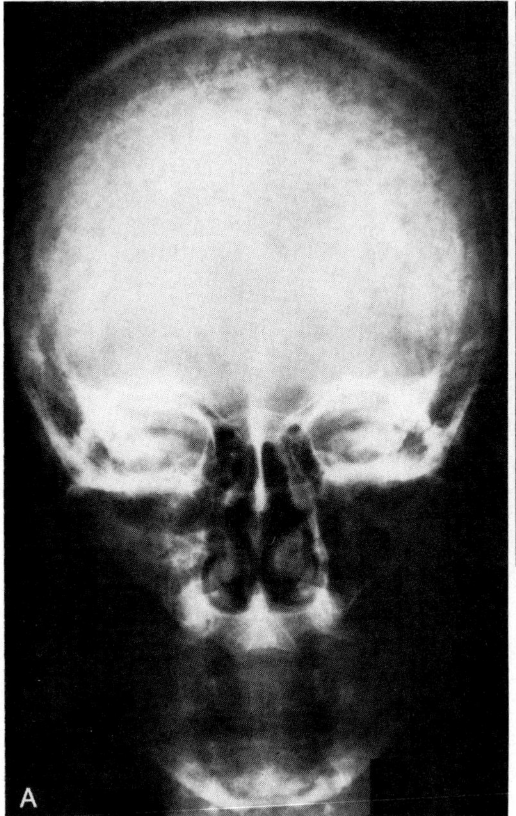

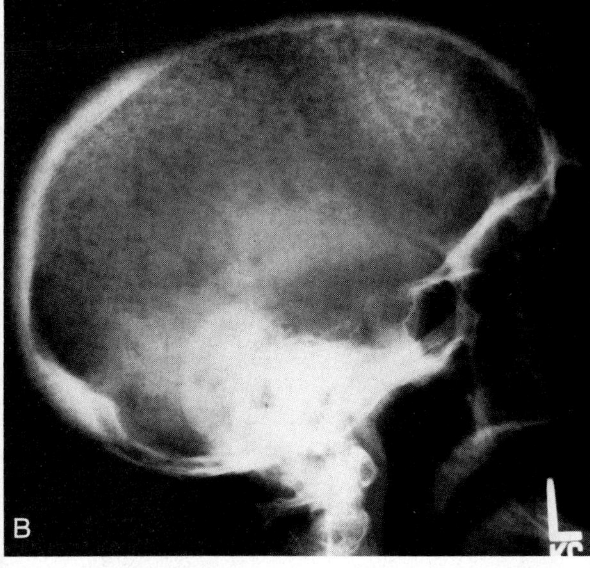

Figure 8–25. Anteroposterior (*A*) and lateral (*B*) radiographs of "salt and pepper" in the skull of a patient with hyperparathyroidism. Alternating waves of increased and decreased activity of parathormone are reflected in alternating waves of osteoclastic and osteoblastic activity.

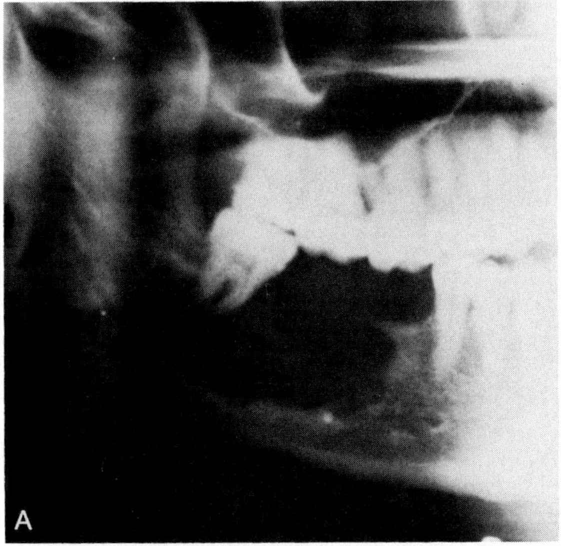
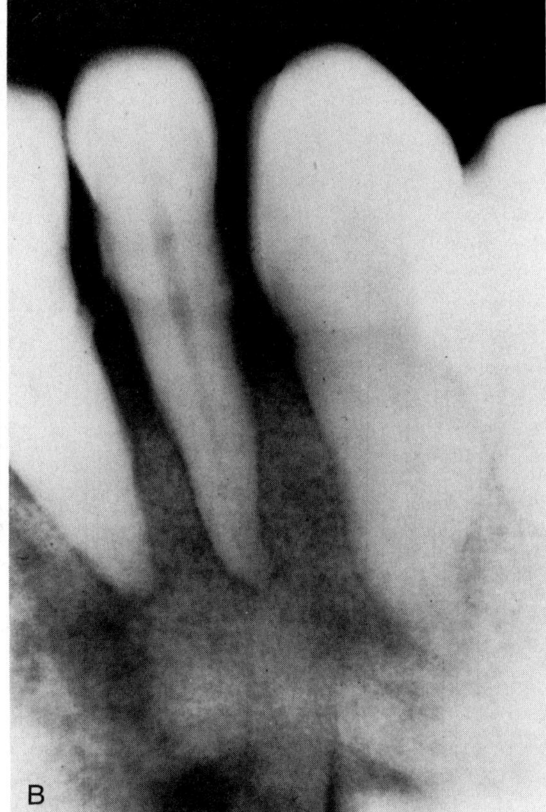

Figure 8–26. Radiographs of mandible with large lytic defect and loss of lamina dura due to primary hyperparathyroidism. The biopsy of the mandibular lesion exhibited a brown tumor. The patient's serum calcium was 13 mg per dl.

On the basis of histologic appearance, there is no difference between primary and secondary hyperparathyroidism. Osteomalacia may accompany hyperparathyroidism secondary to renal failure and thus indicate the underlying disease process. However, the histologic features of osteoclastic resorption, replacement by spindled mesenchymal connective tissue, brown-tumor formation, and severe osteoporosis are identical in primary and secondary hyperparathyroidism.

RICKETS

Rickets is osteomalacia in the growing skeleton. It is characterized by an inability to calcify matrix and thus involves not only bone but also cartilage. In normal maturation of the growth plate, the cartilage matrix secreted by the proliferating cartilage cells dehydrates and then calcifies. In vitamin-D deficiency or rickets due to any other cause, the maturation of cartilage and calcification is abnormal. Once the first step in the maturation process is deranged, all subsequent steps are also abnormal. Columnization by cartilage is irregular—the zone of hypertrophy does not form in a consistent pattern, and there is poor and spotty mineralization in the zone of provisional calcification. In the absence of calcified cartilage bars, osteoid is not produced and primary trabeculae are not formed. Because the patients with rickets can mineralize neither osteoid nor cartilage matrix, the bone and cartilage are pliable and bow easily. These children have grossly deformed long bones, characterized by severe bowing (Figs. 8–27 to 8–32).

Radiographically, the growth plate appears widened with indistinct margins. Reproduction of cartilage is responsible for the normal enlargement of epiphysis in

Text continued on page 262

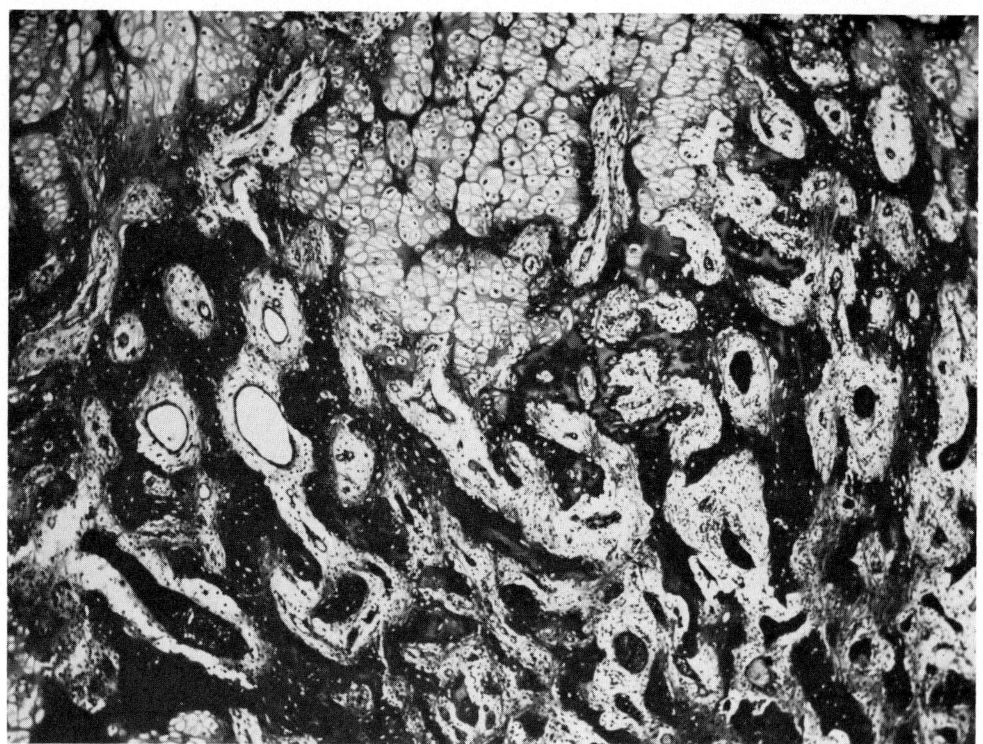

Figure 8–27. Epiphyseal growth plate of patient with rickets exhibiting disorganization and lack of maturation of epiphyseal cartilage, with irregular cartilage column formation. The osteoid that is formed is of poor quality and irregular in shape, and it does not calcify properly.

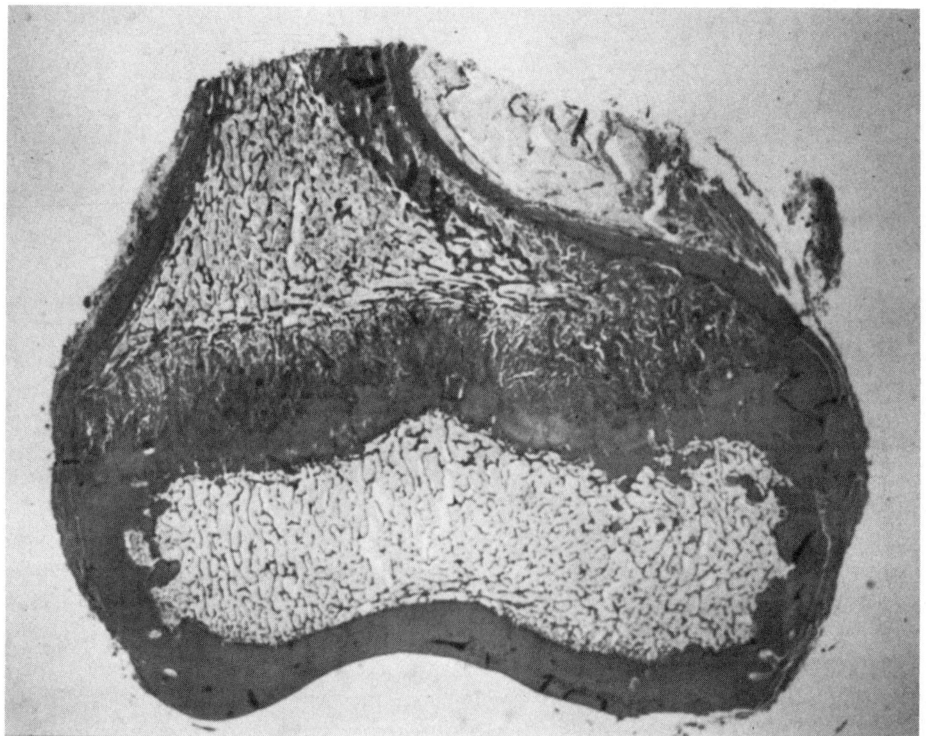

Figure 8–28. Rickets. Macrosection of distal femur. The overall shape of the bone is nearly normal. The cartilage portion of growth plate blends with grossly smudged, irregular deposits of osteoid in metaphysis. The unmineralized osteoid does not appear on the radiograph and is not removed by osteoclasts. Continued production of this material results in an irregular zone of radiolucency.

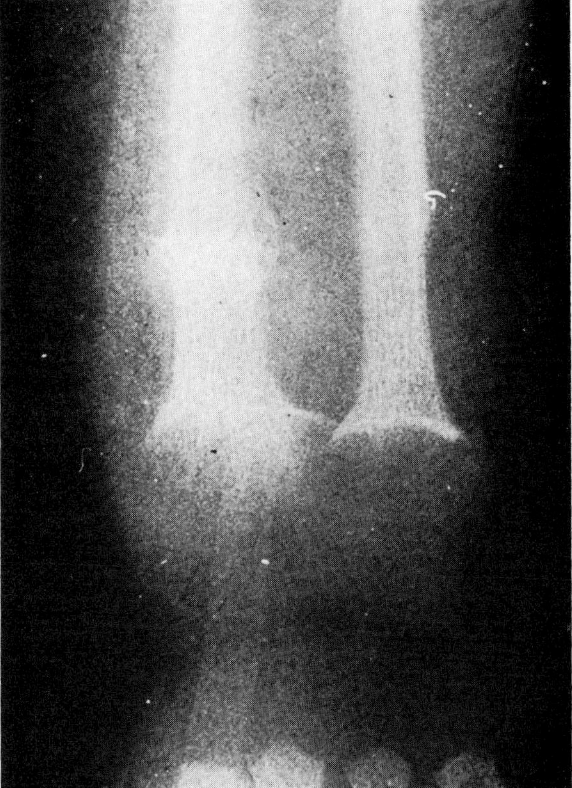

Figure 8–29. Radiograph of wrist of child with active rickets exhibiting the irregular widened zone of provisional calcification that is replaced by abnormal osteoid. The cartilage masses are not visible, but the widened epiphyseal growth plate and irregular calcification are readily seen. Note pathologic fracture of radial shaft.

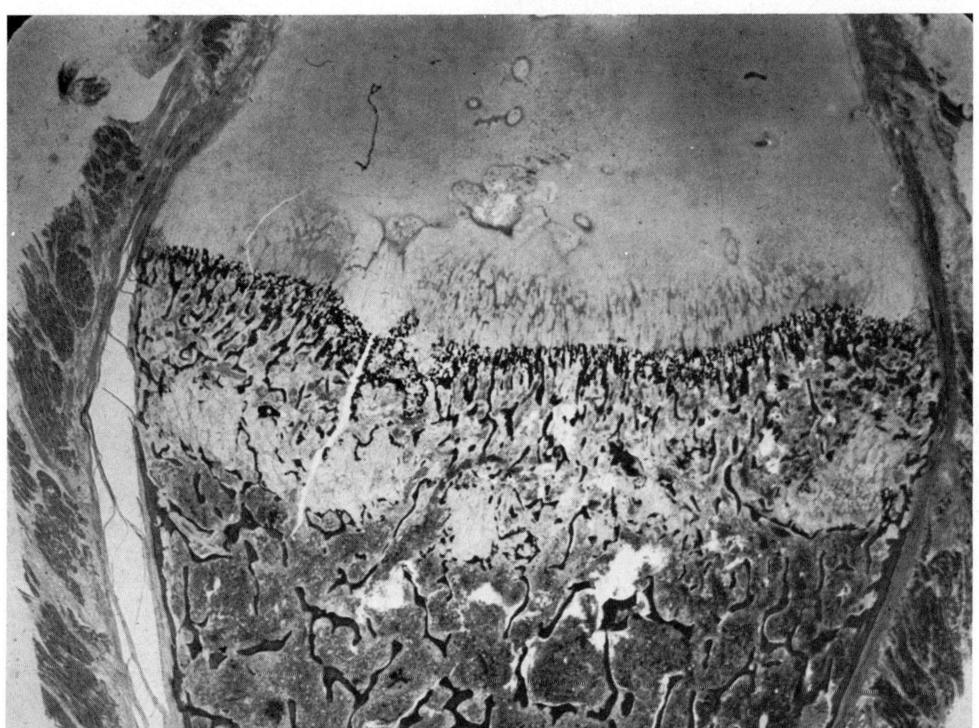

Figure 8–30. Macrosection of rachitic rib responding to therapy. The line of cartilage bars in the zone of provisional calcification exhibits extensive calcification. Note the large masses of cartilage that were formed earlier. They have not matured and persist between the growth plate and bone formed prior to the onset of rickets.

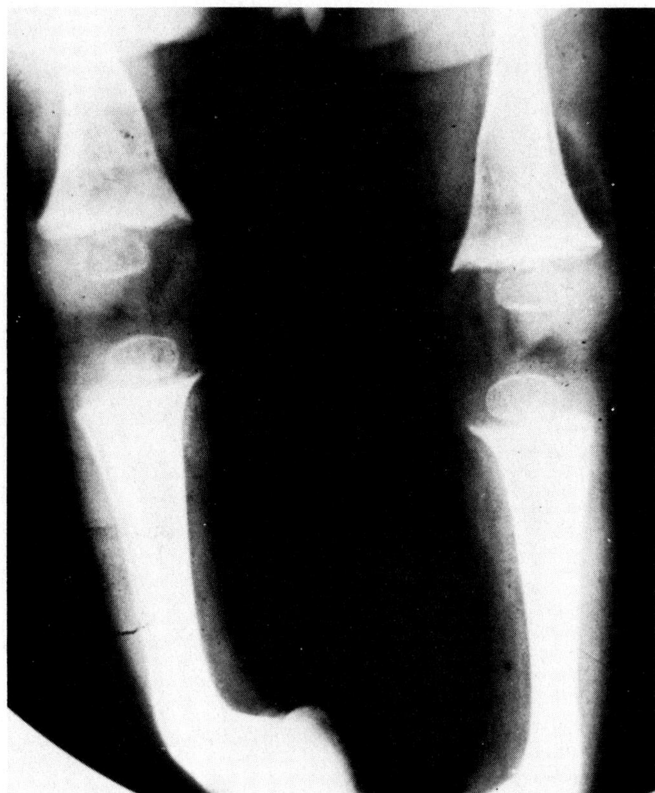

Figure 8–31. Radiograph of patient with healing rickets. Note the metaphyseal flare, irregular contour, and cupping of growth plate with the epiphysis settled into the metaphysis. Calcification of newly formed bone is evident, with a lucent area from a period of inactivity persisting in the metaphysis.

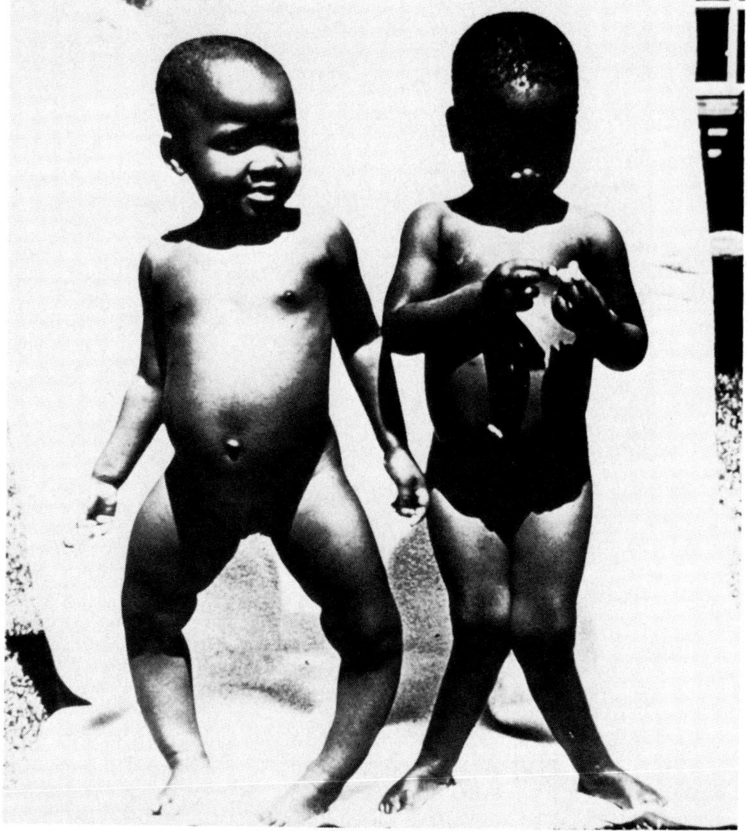

Figure 8–32. Two patients with residual rachitic deformities of lower extremity.

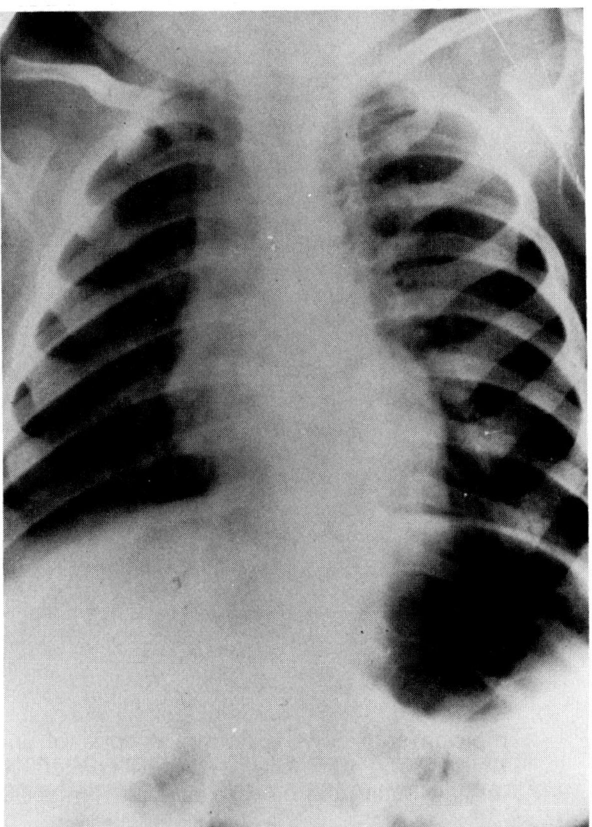

Figure 8–33. Chest radiograph showing classic rachitic rosary at the costochondral junction.

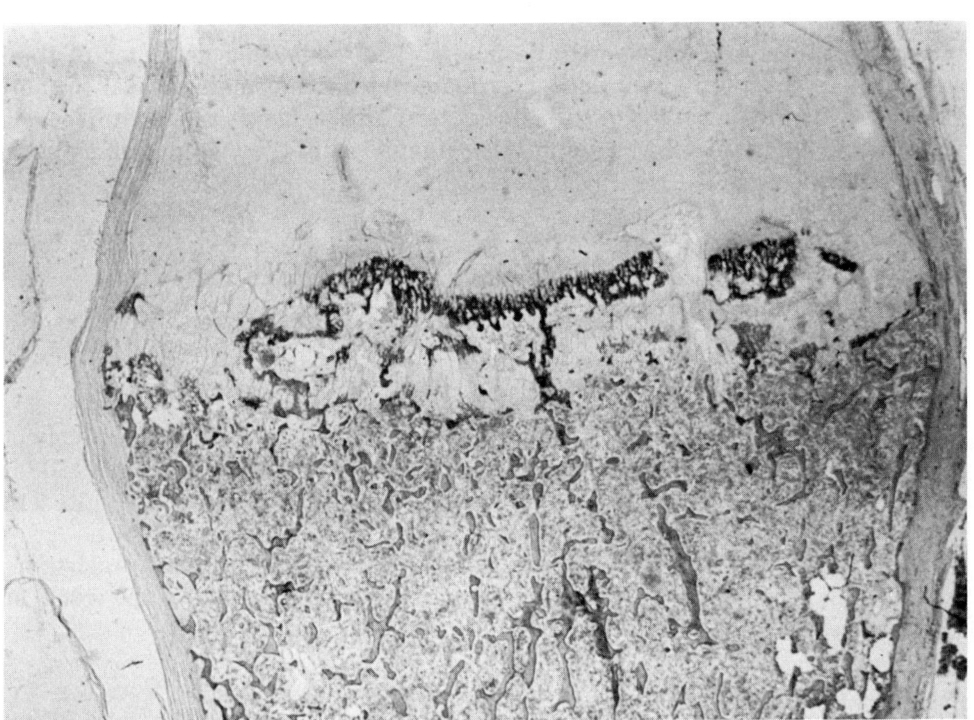

Figure 8–34. Histologic section of rickets responding to therapy. Bone is deposited at the site in which the most recently formed cartilage matures and mineralizes (i.e., nearest to the epiphysis). Cartilage formed during the active disease remains unmineralized. It demonstrates that the disease process is due to a defect in matrix formation rather than to a lack of calcium. Neither the cartilage nor the osteoid matrix is calcifiable.

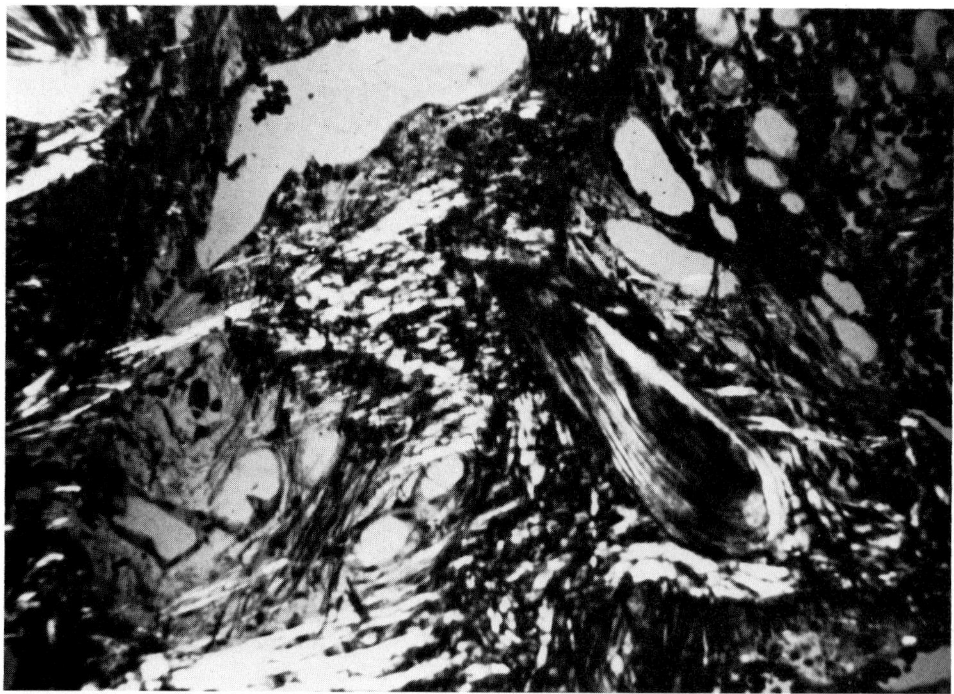

Figure 8–38. Osteomalacia. Section of bone under polarized light exhibiting disorganization of pattern. The central portion of the photograph exhibits residual osteonal bone. Other areas of osteoid are not well mineralized and exhibit an immature woven bone pattern. The collagen fibers are essentially unremarkable and exhibit normal characteristics under polarized light.

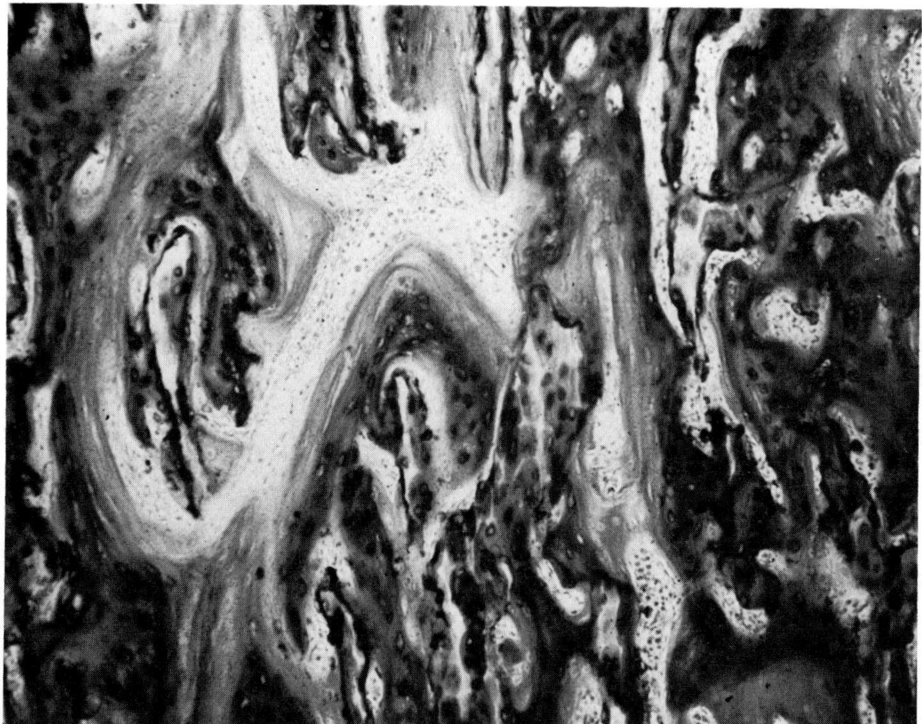

Figure 8–39. Histologic section demonstrating severe osteomalacia. Note the broad unmineralized osteoid seams on the surface of bone spicules that form earlier and exhibit mineralization.

phatemia, primary hypocalcemia (Marie et al., 1982), and secondary deficiencies associated with renal disease and intestinal malabsorption. An adult patient who is forming osteoid is doing so in response to normal remodeling with previous removal of bone; it therefore follows that osteomalacia occurs as a consequence of absolute or relative osteoporosis.

The collagen matrix is not mineralized and is therefore malleable. The natural consequence of osteomalacia is a tendency for bowing. Distorted vertebral columns, kyphosis, scoliosis, and other deformities of this nature occur. In its minor form, osteomalacia is associated with small stress fractures at typical locations. These are identified as Milkman's fractures, or Looser's transformation zones (Figs. 8–36 and 8–40).

The characteristic histologic feature of osteomalacia is the formation of osteoid without mineralization. This is classically identified in undecalcified tissue sections, although the decalcified material also exhibits wide osteoid seams, often twice as wide as the calcified central core, and absence of osteoclastic resorption. Osteoclasts remove calcified material, and therefore osteomalacic bone cannot be removed until it becomes mineralized (Figs. 8–36 to 8–39).

Radiographically, the bone will exhibit osteoporosis, but instead of the sharp contour and clear outline of bone, the deposition of unmineralized osteoid on existing trabeculae causes a hazy, indistinct outline (Figs. 8–40 to 8–42).

Correction of the underlying condition is a prerequisite to the resolution of osteomalacia.

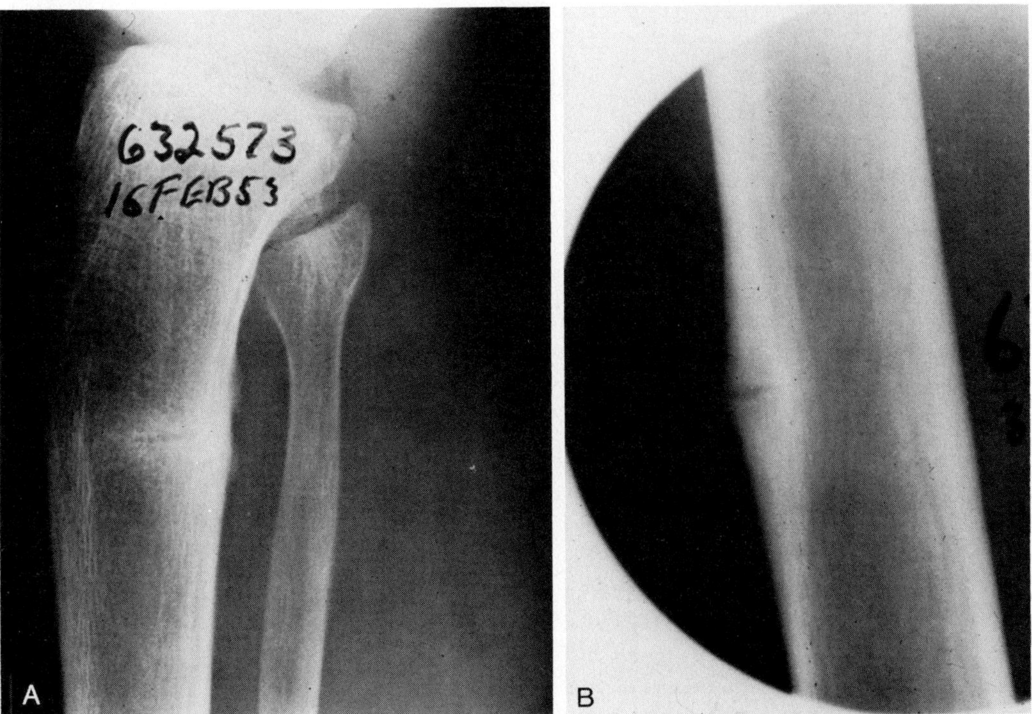

Figure 8–40. Osteomalacia. Radiographs showing Looser's transformation zone. These lines appear at sites in which stress fractures would occur. Stress of normal use incites remodeling with removal of bone. In normal individuals, the removed bone is replaced by normal osteons. In persons with osteomalacia, the removed bone is replaced with abnormal osteoid, which fails to mineralize and leaves a linear radiolucency that may persist for years.

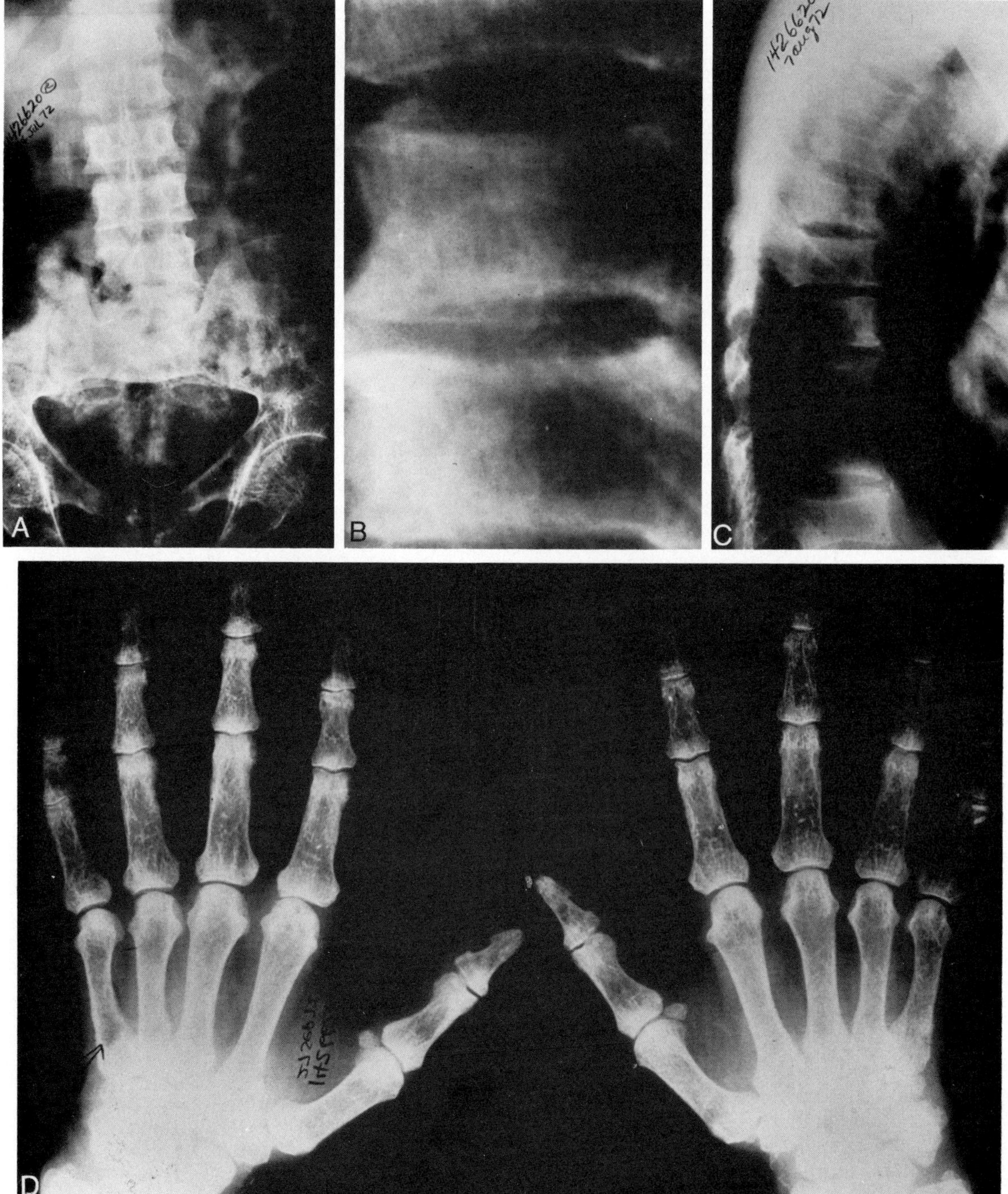

Figure 8–41. Multiple radiographs of a patient with severe osteomalacia exhibiting the classic blurring of trabecular outline and bowing deformities of the vertebral column and pelvis.

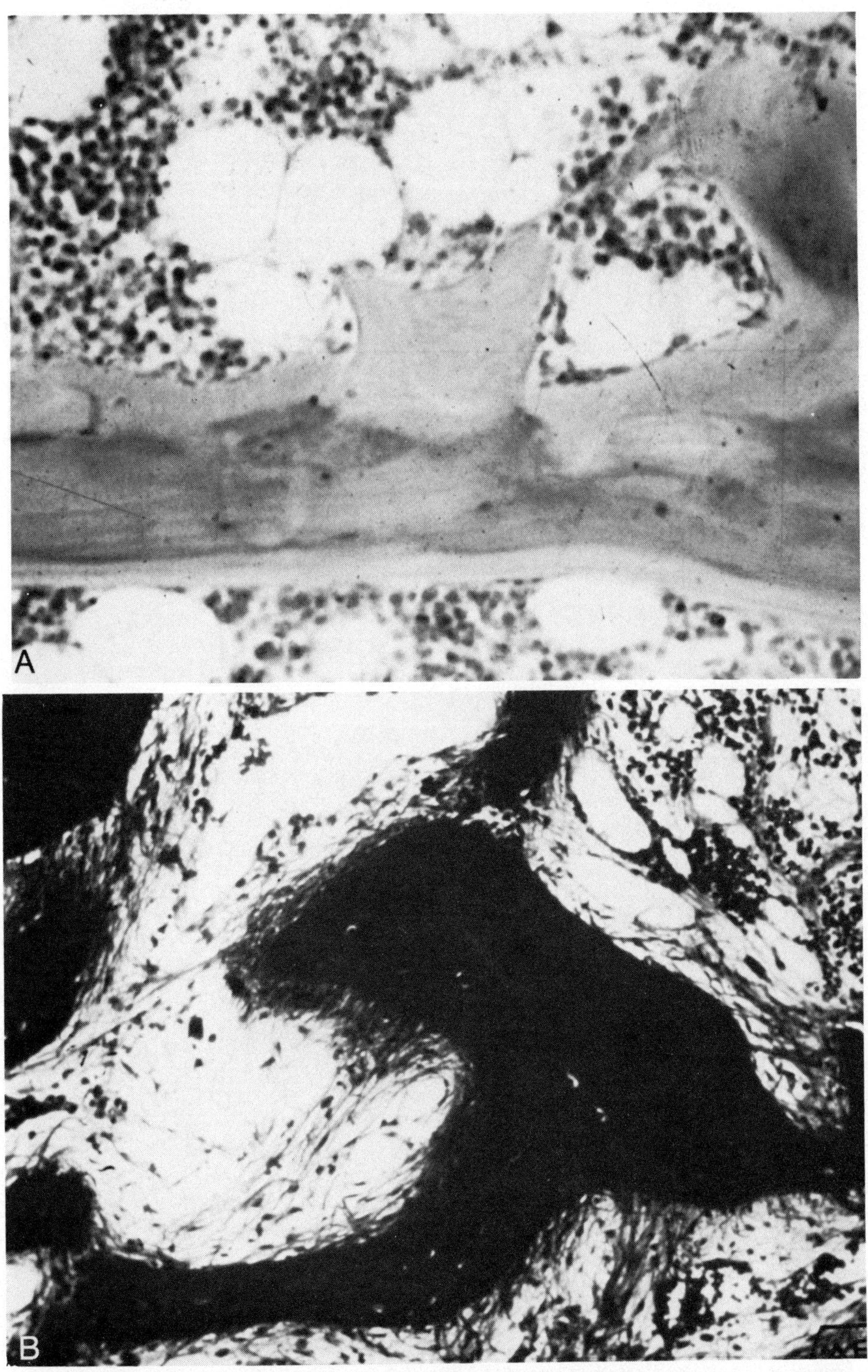

Figure 8–42. Osteomalacia. Histologic sections showing disorganized bone production and partial mineralization with wide osteoid seams. Note the vascular fibrous marrow, where the process is most active. The fuzzy outline of the newly formed unmineralized osteoid is characteristic of the process.

RENAL OSTEODYSTROPHY

Renal tubular disease is associated with loss of phosphate and results in radiographic and histologic pictures indistinguishable from those of classic rickets and pure osteomalacia. When glomerular failure is superimposed, phosphate excretion is impaired, and hyperphosphatemia results. Hypocalcemia accompanies the excess

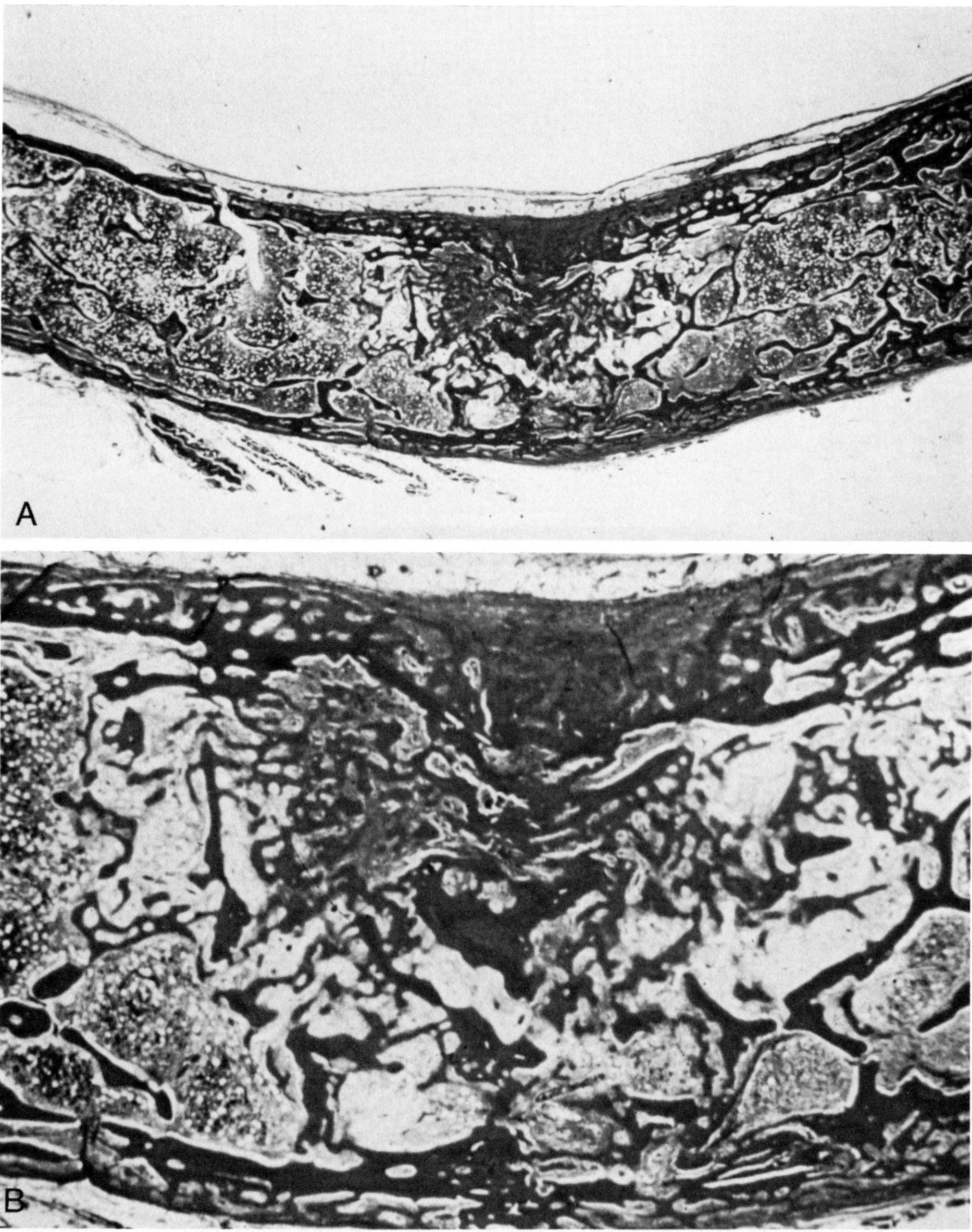

Figure 8–43. Renal osteodystrophy. Low-power (*A*) and high-power (*B*) views of a macrosection of a fractured rib healing with the formation of osteomalacic bone. Despite the formation of osteoid, the lesion appears radiolucent because mineralization is absent (Looser's transformation zone). Note extensive resorption of cortical bone and replacement with fibrous tissue, a feature of hyperparathyroidism that is not present in pure osteomalacia (see Fig. 8–36). The combined histologic alterations of hyperparathyroidism and osteomalacia are diagnostic of renal osteodystrophy.

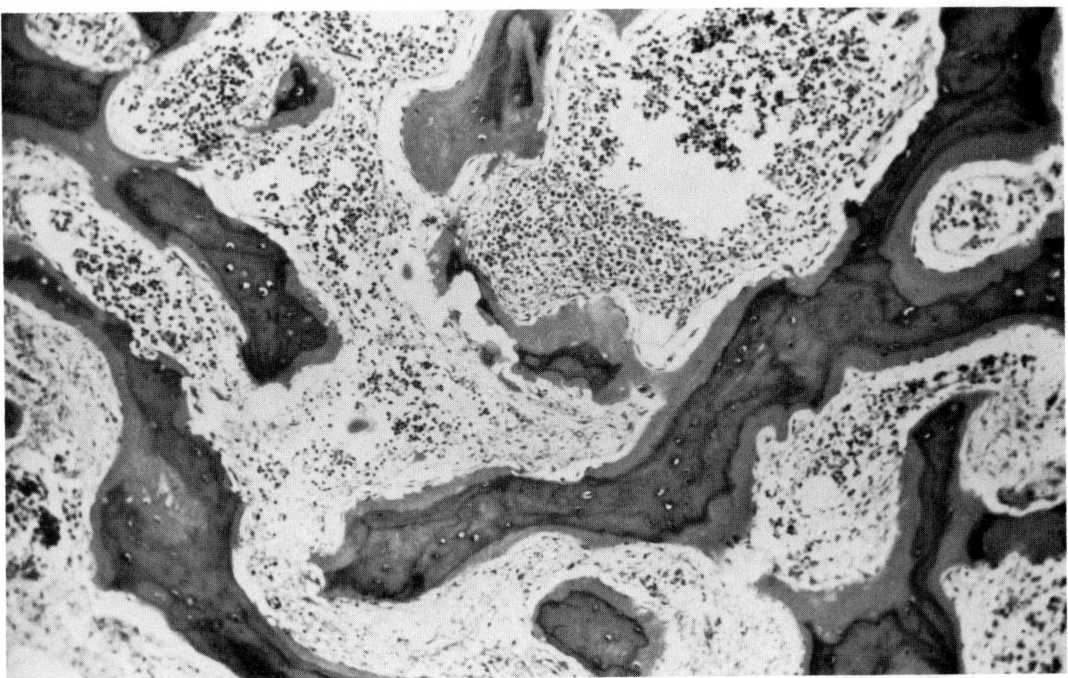

Figure 8–44. Renal osteodystrophy. Histologic section of bone exhibiting wide osteoid seams. These are seen in patients with primary renal disease, but they are not present in patients with primary hyperparathyroidism because the osteoid produced in primary hyperparathyroidism is normal.

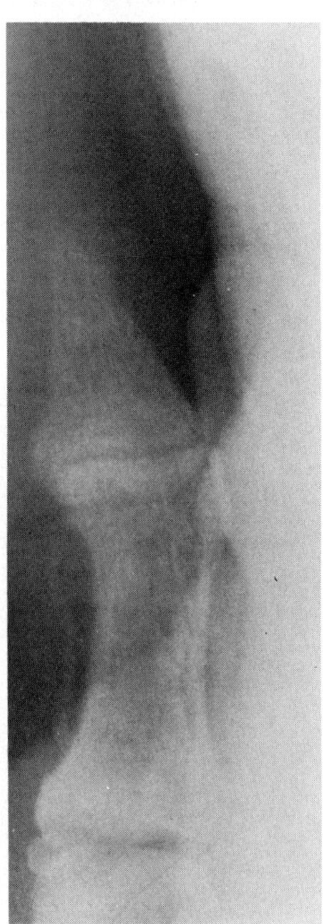

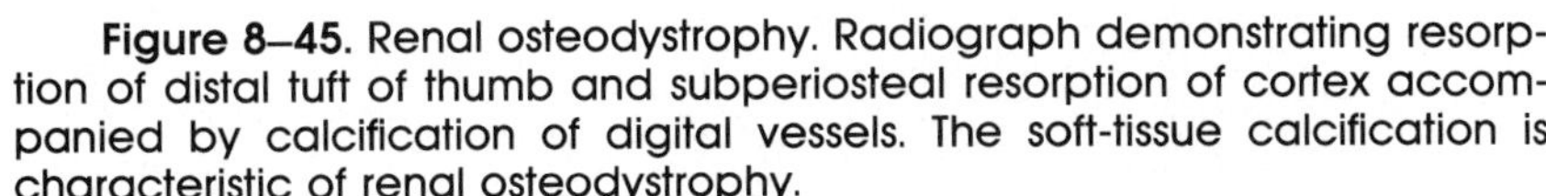

Figure 8–45. Renal osteodystrophy. Radiograph demonstrating resorption of distal tuft of thumb and subperiosteal resorption of cortex accompanied by calcification of digital vessels. The soft-tissue calcification is characteristic of renal osteodystrophy.

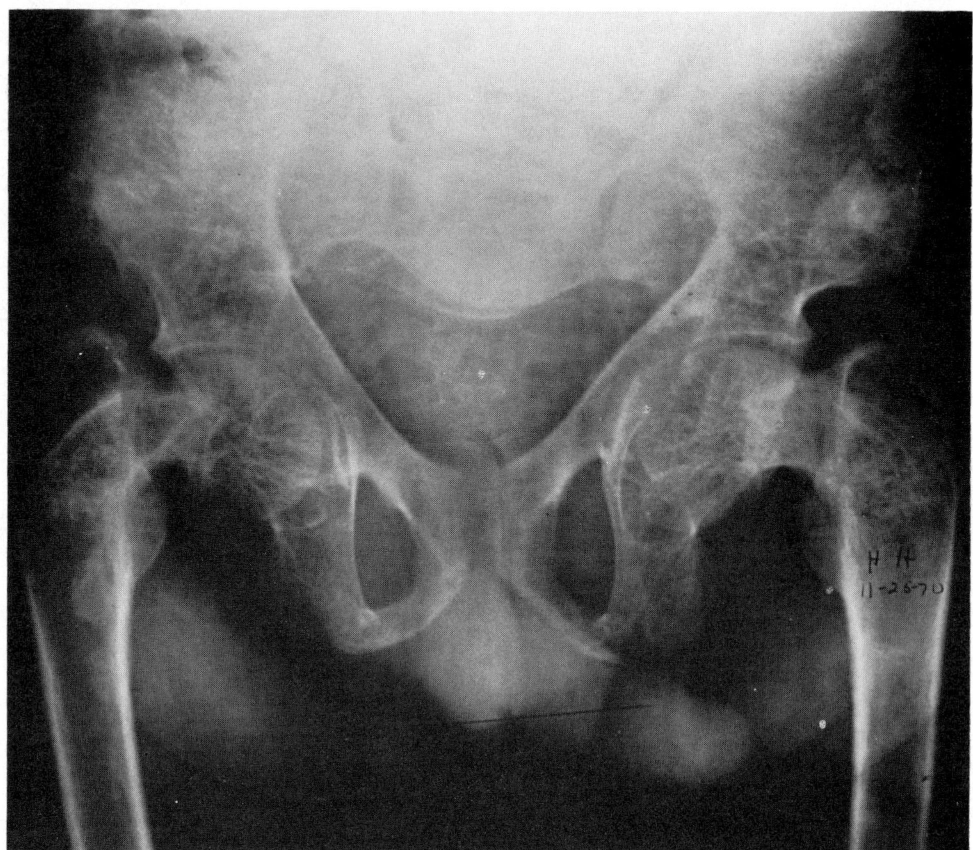

Figure 8–46. Radiograph of patient with long-standing renal osteodystrophy. Marked osteoporosis due to secondary hyperparathyroidism is evident. There is bowing of the proximal femurs, marked lordosis, and pelvic tilt. The deformity of the pelvis is commonly seen in osteomalacia, but it does not usually occur in primary hyperparathyroidism.

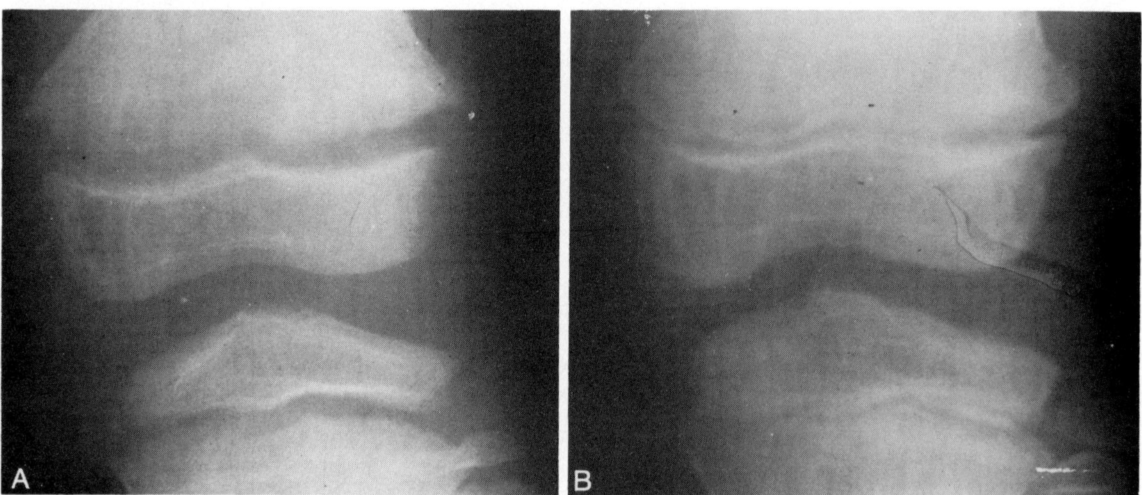

Figure 8–47. Renal osteodystrophy. Radiographs of knee joint before *(A)* and after *(B)* therapy.

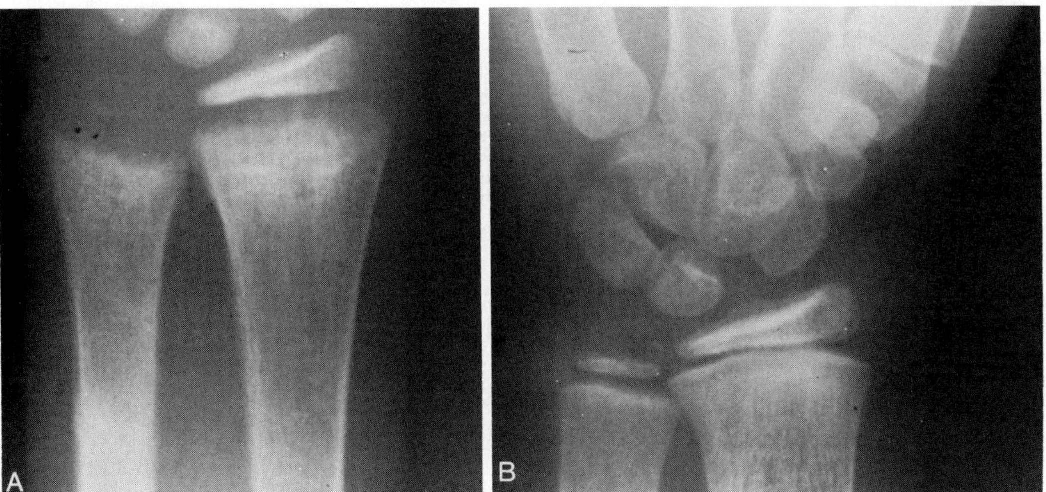

Figure 8–48. Renal osteodystrophy. Radiographs of wrists before *(A)* and after *(B)* therapy. Note the widened growth plate with minor irregularities, corrected after therapy. The radius is osteoporotic owing to secondary hyperparathyroidism.

phosphate retention and stimulates parathyroid hormone secretion. This secondary hyperparathyroidism mobilizes calcium from bone. The histologic features of hyperparathyroidism are thus added to the underlying osteomalacia (Figs. 8–43 to 8–46). The morphologic features of rickets, osteomalacia, and hyperparathyroidism remain unchanged, regardless of whether disease is primary or secondary (Figs. 8–47 to 8–48).

SCURVY

The primary defect in scurvy is an inability to convert proline to hydroxyproline. All collagen formation is thus affected, and in bone there is an inability to form the osteoid matrix. Calcification is not affected. The deficiency in collagen formation extends to other connective tissue as well, resulting in increased blood-vessel permeability, tendency for mucosal bleeding, easy bruising, and gingival hemorrhage. Subperiosteal hemorrhage results in elevation and separation of periosteum from the underlying cortex (Figs. 8–54 to 8–58).

In the growing skeleton, failure to form normal mineralized osteoid results in persistence of the provisional calcified cartilage formed by the growth plate. Primary trabeculae are not formed. The calcified cartilage is brittle, and continued weight-bearing, stress, or motion will cause microfractures and debris formation in the metaphysis. The resulting instability at the growth plate can cause lateral slippage of the epiphysis following metaphyseal fracture, a common complication of infantile scurvy (Figs. 8–49 to 8–53).

The ring of Ranvier, normally formed adjacent to the side of the maturing cartilage, also depends on the formation of normal osteoid. Without normal osteoid formation, the ring is absent, and the cartilage of the growth plate tends to grow laterally. Settling of the epiphysis onto the metaphysis gives the appearance of spur formation at the margin of the growth plate.

Certain characteristic radiographic features are associated with scurvy. The Trümmerfeld zone, or zone of debris, is an area of microfracture of the cartilage bars in the metaphysis. Ringing of the epiphysis is due to the relatively increased

Text continued on page 276

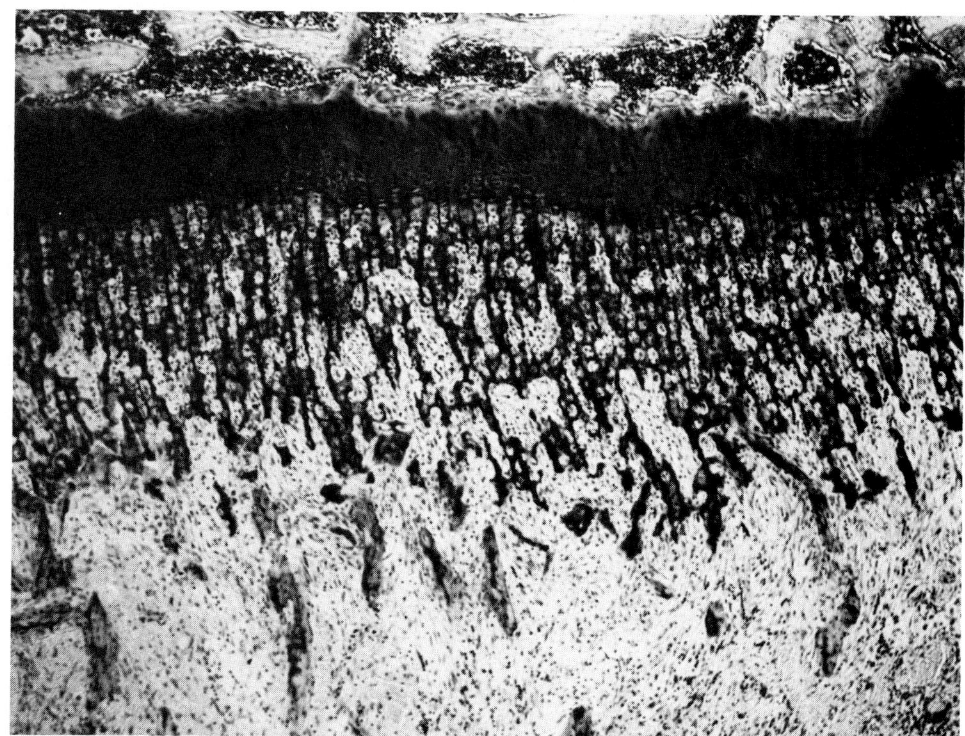

Figure 8–49. Histologic appearance of growth plate in experimental scurvy. Cartilage maturation is normal, the zone of provisional calcification is extended, and there is no osteoid formation. The longer zone of calcified cartilage matrix is radiographically visible as a prominent calcified line at the site of the growth plate.

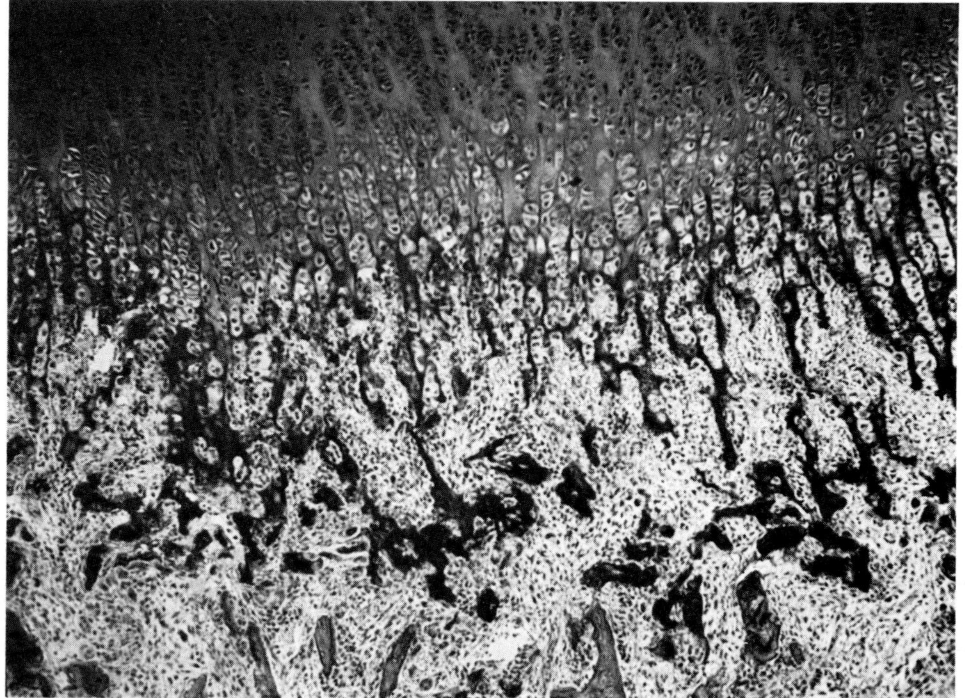

Figure 8–50. Growth plate in experimental scurvy exhibiting normal cartilage and numerous calcified cartilage bars extending into the metaphysis. The abnormal cellular component in the marrow space beneath the growth plate is a feature of the disease process. These cells are capable of forming bone when vitamin C is restored to the diet. Note the normal bone beneath the Trümmerfeld zone.

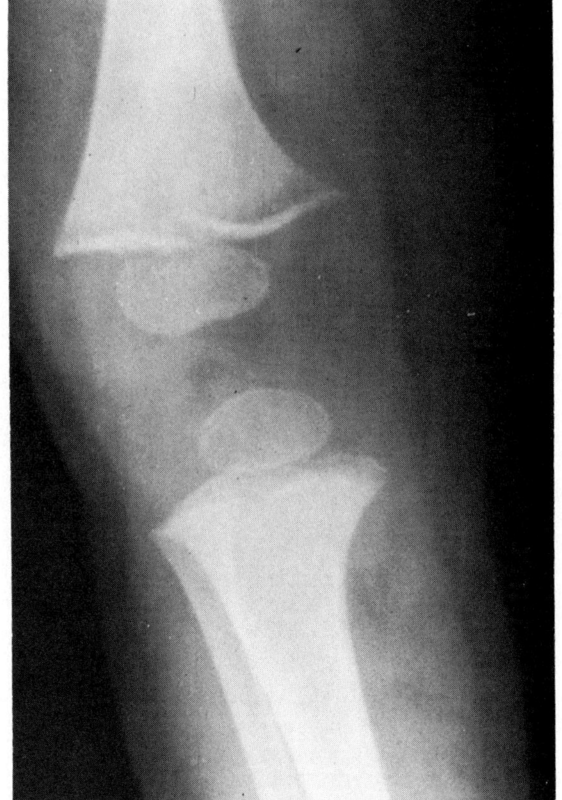

Figure 8–51. Radiographic appearance of knee joint of patient with scurvy exhibiting the very prominent zone of provisional calcification in the growth plate. The zone of radiolucency is the region in which bone forms in the metaphysis of a normal growth plate. Lack of bone in this region makes it vulnerable to collapse or fracture through the metaphysis.

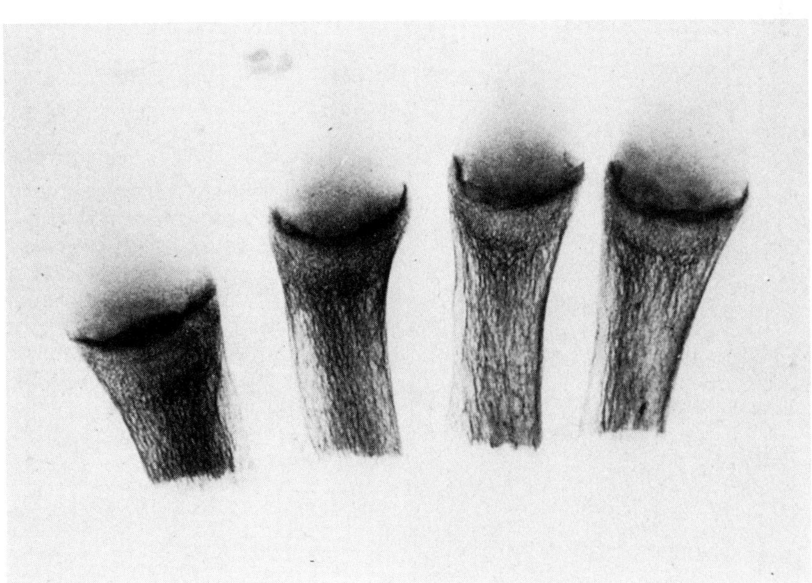

Figure 8–52. Scurvy. Specimen radiograph of ribs exhibiting the dense zone of persistent calcified cartilage and the lytic zone of diminished bone formation, respectively.

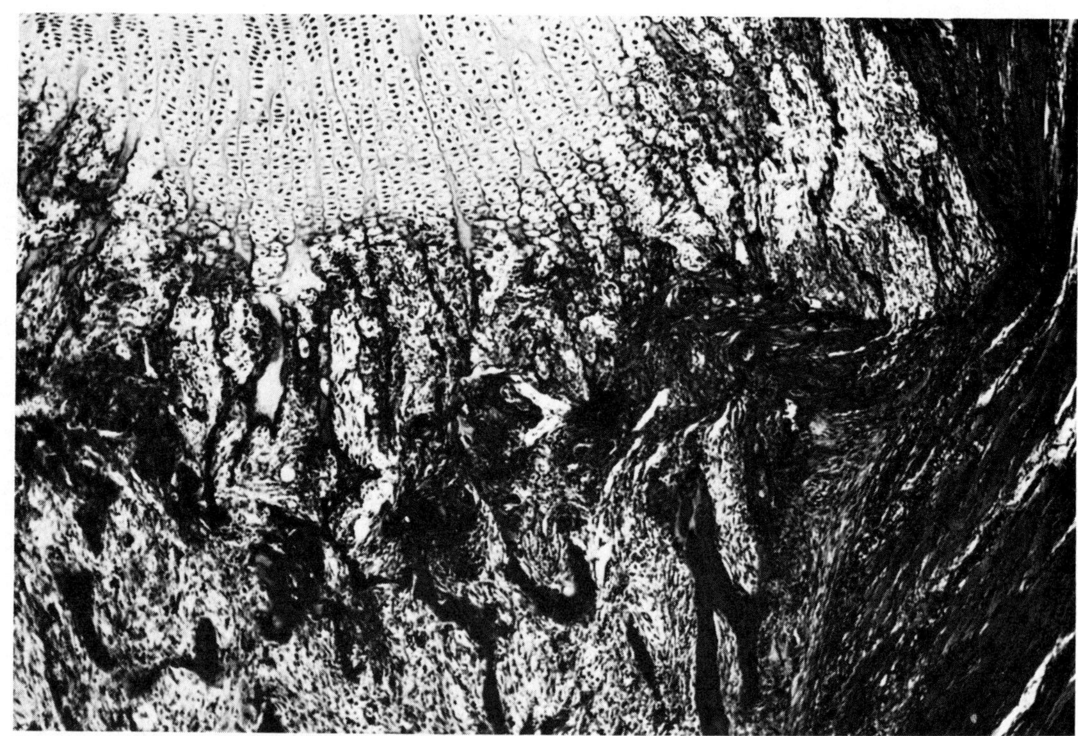

Figure 8–53. Scurvy. Histologic appearance of Pelkan's spur. Calcified cartilage is seen on the lateral margin and will be apparent radiographically as a spur. Traumatic collapse of zone in which bone fails to form (Trümmerfeld zone) brings the epiphyseal cartilage, including the zone of provisional calcification, onto the end of the narrowed metaphysis. It produces the appearance of lateral projection of calcified material, due not to growth but rather to failure of bone production with metaphyseal fracture.

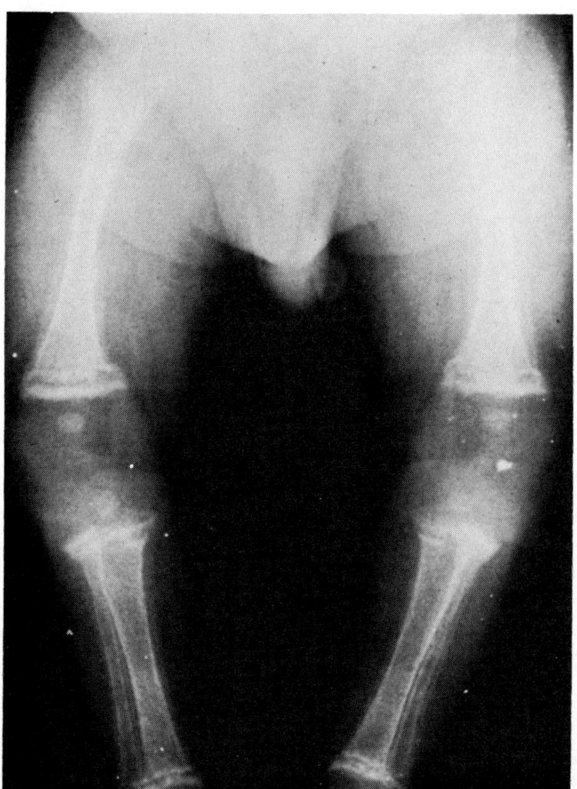

Figure 8–54. Treated scurvy. Radiograph of a 2-month-old infant showing classic manifestations of scurvy. Note the calcified zone with the clear zone beneath and the early calcification of the secondary epiphyseal centers. The patient is beginning to heal, as demonstrated by the early calcification of the uniformly elevated periosteum as well as double zone of provisional calcification.

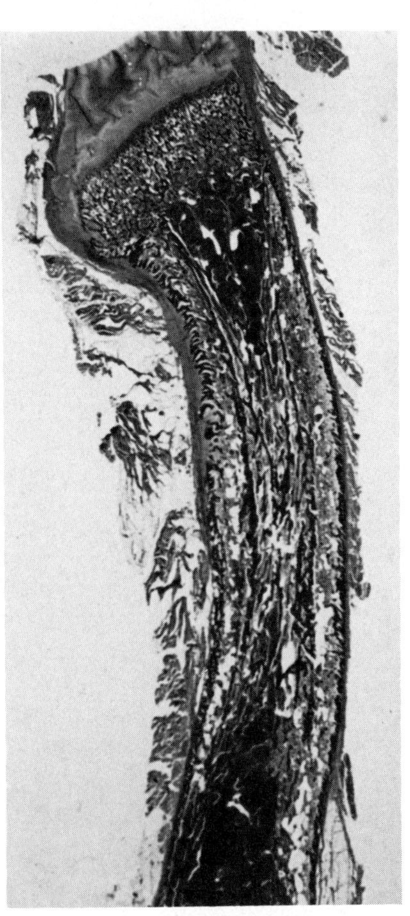

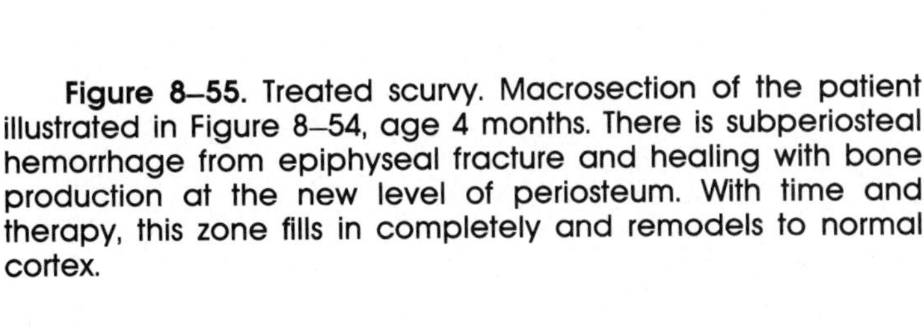

Figure 8–55. Treated scurvy. Macrosection of the patient illustrated in Figure 8–54, age 4 months. There is subperiosteal hemorrhage from epiphyseal fracture and healing with bone production at the new level of periosteum. With time and therapy, this zone fills in completely and remodels to normal cortex.

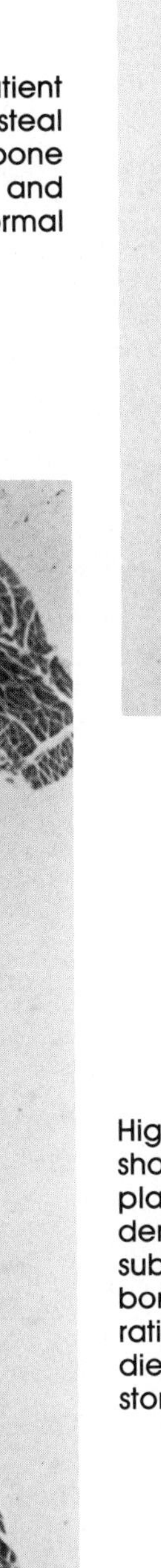

Figure 8–56. Treated scurvy. Higher magnification of specimen shown in Figure 8–55 exhibiting displaced epiphysis. There is no evidence of recent slippage or recent subperiosteal hemorrhage. Normal bone formation occurs after restoration of essential vitamin C to the diet. The growth plate has been restored to normal.

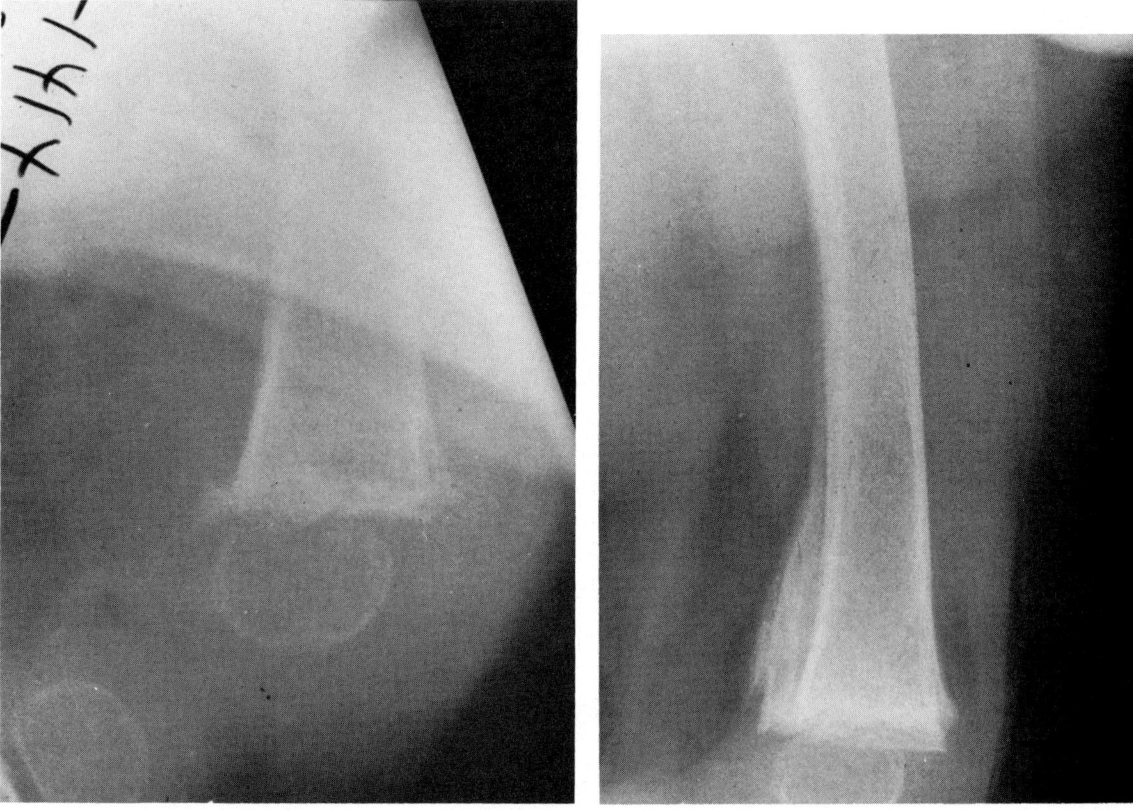

Figure 8–57   **Figure 8–58**

Figure 8–57. Radiograph of patient with scurvy and fracture of the metaphysis with formation of Pelkan's spur. Pelkan's spur is due to compression and apposition of calcified cartilage zone onto the narrower metaphysis.

Figure 8–58. Scurvy. Radiograph of patient in preceding figure, obtained after therapy. The periosteal elevation becomes apparent as new bone is formed.

radiographic density that occurs when a large number of calcified cartilage bars persist without the appropriate remodeling and bone formation. It is accentuated by the contrast between previously normal bone and osteopenia in the zone of debris.

Rickets and scurvy have a tendency to be associated with each other. They are both due to multiple nutritional deficiences and can be instigated in experimental animals through selective dietary restriction. The disease is extremely rare in the Western Hemisphere, but understanding its mechanism aids in comprehending the morphologic consequences of metabolic derangements.

STORAGE DISEASES

Gaucher's disease is a congenital metabolic disturbance caused by deficiency of glucocerebrosidase with resultant excessive deposition of glucocerebroside within the marrow. Radiographically, there is evidence of replacement of marrow space and subsequent enlargement of the bone. Filling of the marrow space causes interference

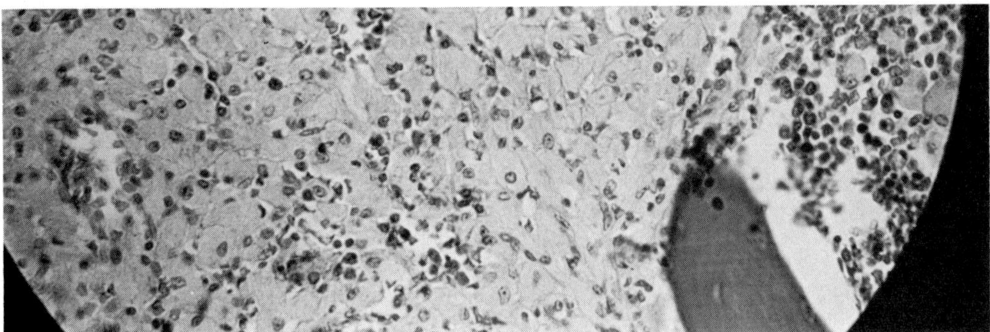

Figure 8–59. Gaucher's disease. Bone and bone marrow, with extensive replacement of all normal marrow components by numerous Gaucher's cells.

with the normal cutback mechanism of metaphyseal remodeling, resulting in an Erlenmeyer-flask appearance.

Major skeletal problems are due to morphologic complications of aseptic necrosis of bone, secondary to interference with normal vascularity. The histologic picture of the lesion is well known to pathologists: numerous cerebroside-laden histiocytes that fill the marrow space.

Niemann-Pick disease is a similar disturbance. It is caused by deficiency of sphingomyelinase, resulting in deposition of abnormal quantities of sphingomyelin and cholesterol in the mesenchymal tissues of the body. The changes within the osseous structures are secondary to marrow infiltration.

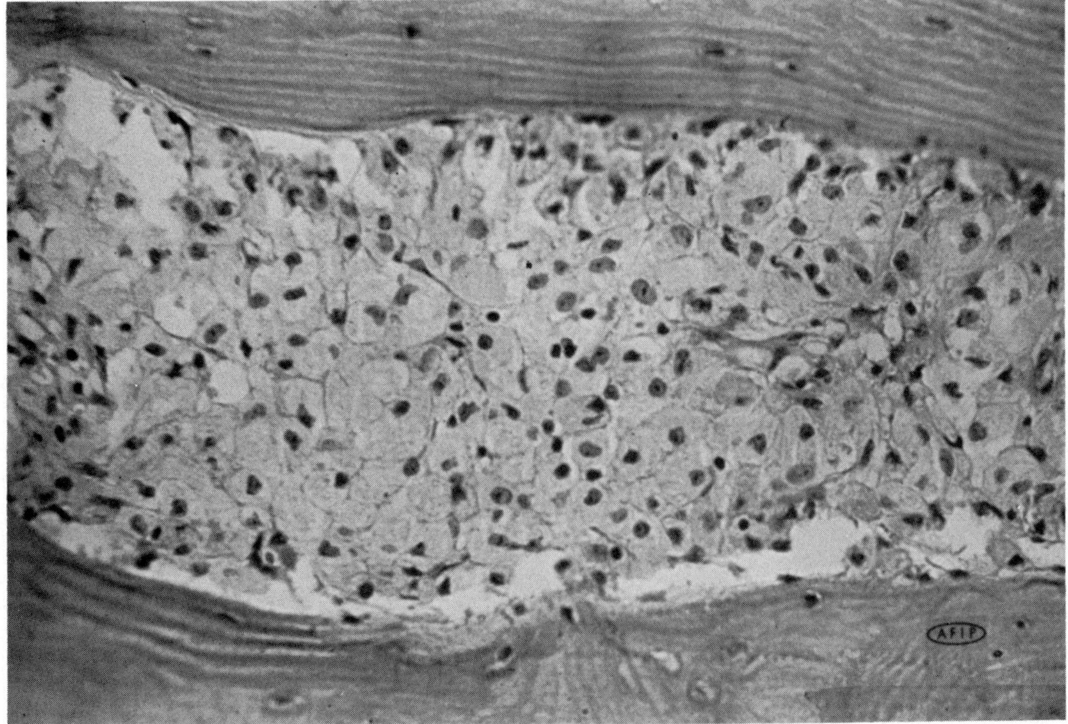

Figure 8–60. Gaucher's disease. Higher magnification of marrow exhibiting almost total replacement of marrow components by characteristic Gaucher's cells, which are distinguished by their histiocytic appearance with cytoplasm-containing glucocerebroside.

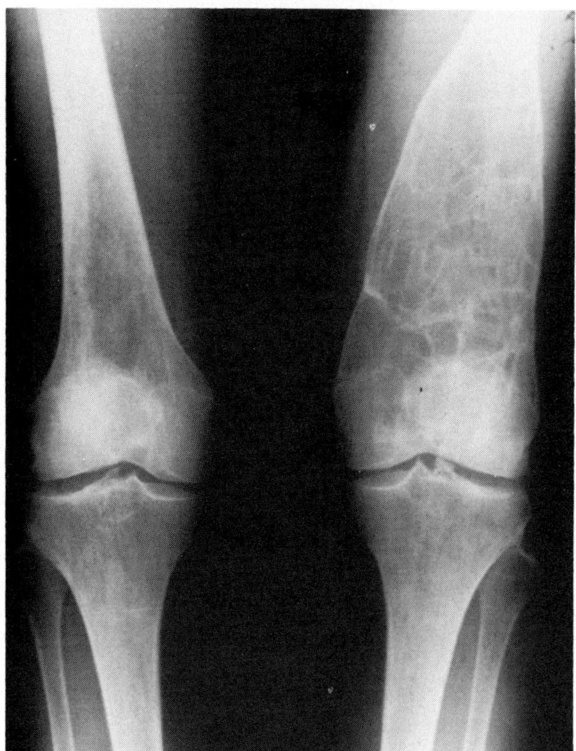

Figure 8–61. Gaucher's disease. Radiograph of Erlenmeyer-flask deformity of the femur. This malformation is due to interference of the cutback mechanism (funnelization) during growth. The replacement of the normal marrow by Gaucher's cells prevents normal remodeling.

Figure 8–62. Long-standing Gaucher's disease in a 57-year-old male. Radiograph exhibits severe degenerative changes with aseptic necrosis of the humeral head. Large numbers of abnormal cells in the marrow interfere with normal circulation. Infarcts are common in Gaucher's disease. The infarct and subsequent degenerative osteoarthritis may require operative therapy.

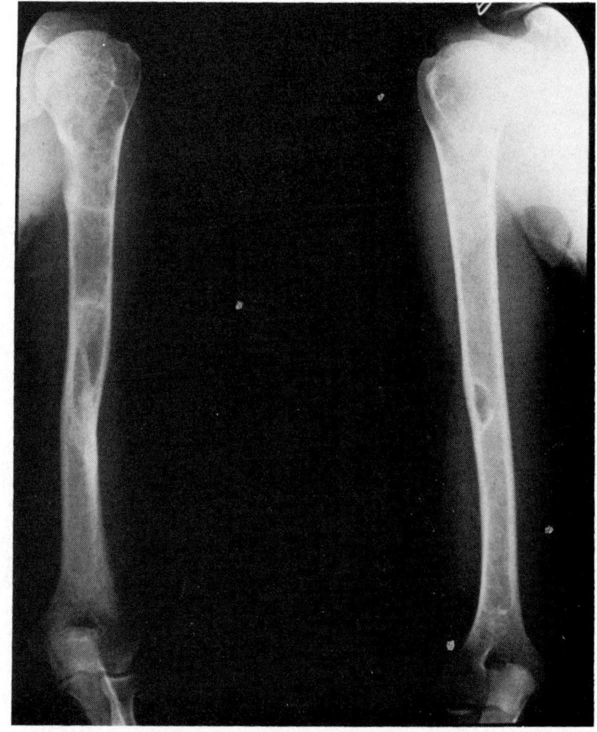

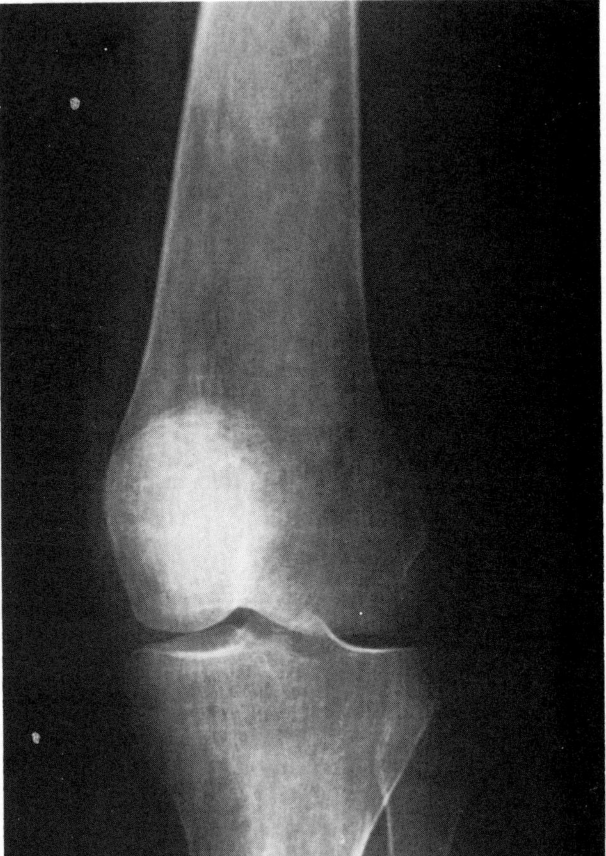

Figure 8–63. Radiograph of distal femur in a 53-year-old female patient. The presence of severe osteoporosis is due to replacement of trabecular bone and marrow by the abnormal infiltrate.

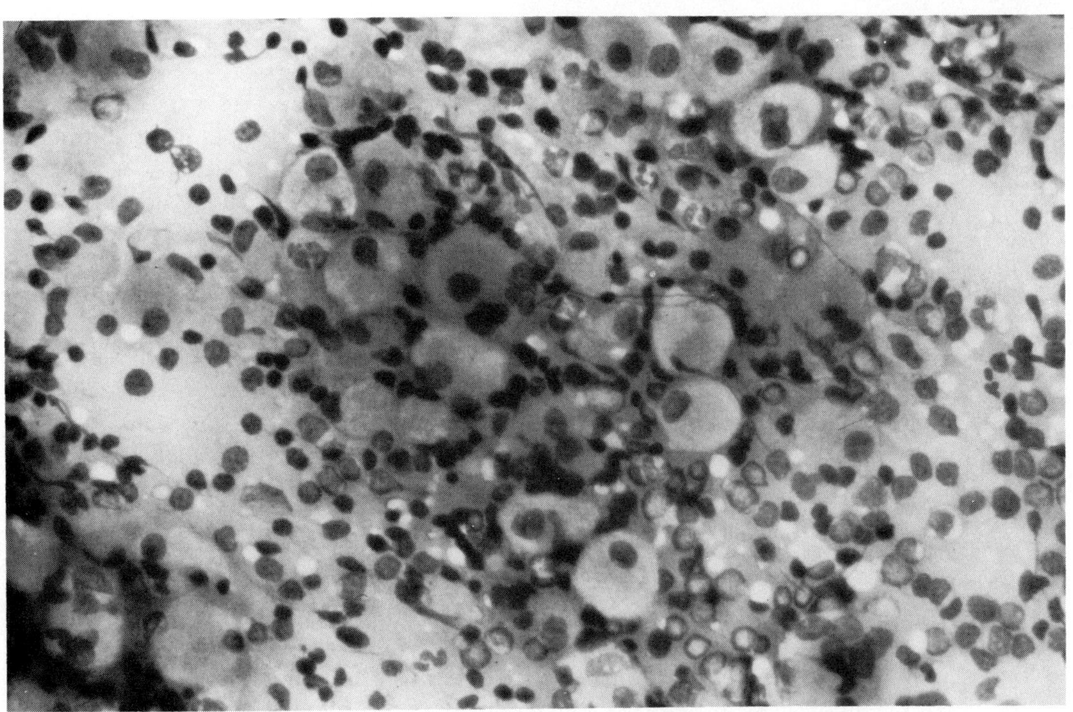

Figure 8–64. Bone-marrow aspirate demonstrating Gaucher's disease. The Gaucher's cell is characterized by the prominent, somewhat feathery cytoplasm in the histiocyte.

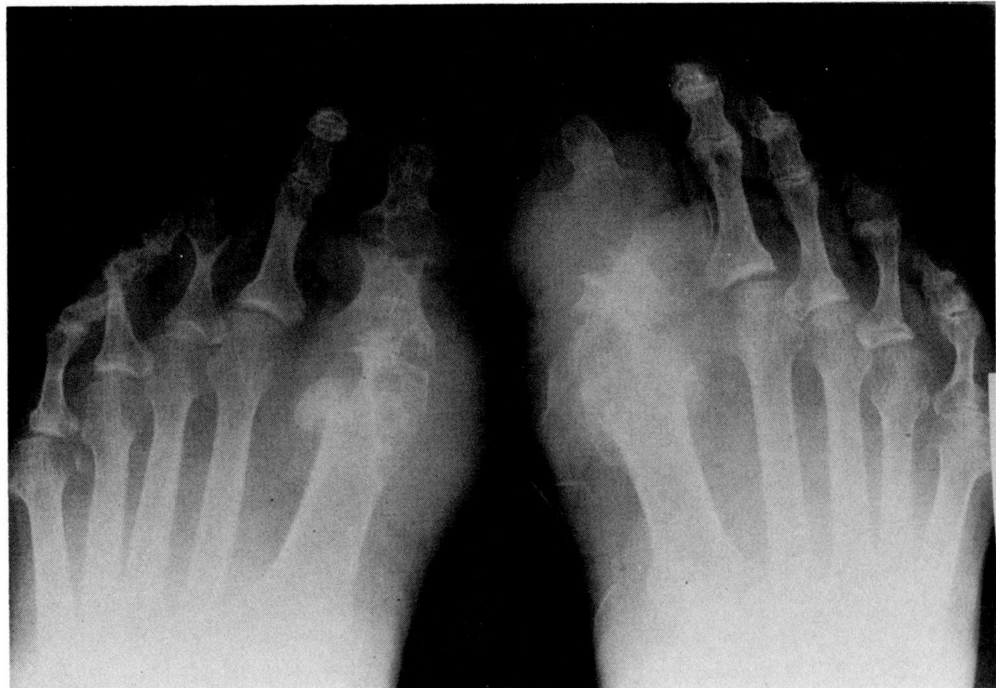

Figure 8–65. Radiographic appearance of patient with gout exhibiting multiple sharply circumscribed defects. Severe degenerative changes are present in the interphalangeal joints of the feet.

GOUT

Gout is a constitutional and frequently hereditary disease of purine metabolism that is characterized by hyperuricemia. The urates and metabolites are produced in amounts exceeding the body's ability to eliminate them. There are retention and deposition of urate material in various portions of the body. Urates have a high affinity for areas that contain proteoglycan. Urate crystals are therefore deposited on and in the articular cartilage (Fig. 8–73) and cause depolymerization of the proteoglycan ground substance. The articular cartilage is fragmented, and pieces break off into the joint space and deposit within the adjacent synovial recesses (Fig. 8–66). The acute gouty attack is a response to this destruction, consisting of an intense, extremely painful vascular reaction and a microurate synovitis.

The material shed into the synovium and into the subchondral bone space is recognized by the body as foreign material, and a foreign-body reaction is created around it (Figs. 8–67 and 8–68). Destruction of the articular cartilage and subchondral bone results (Fig. 8–66). Ultimately, degenerative osteoarthritis occurs.

The characteristic radiographic appearance consists of punched-out areas, involving many joints, with little bony reaction (Fig. 8–69A). The classic location is the metatarsophalangeal joint of the first toe, but any joint may be involved, including the spine.

The tophaceous deposits of urate crystals in the soft tissue are a late manifestation of gout and are not painful, although they may be quite destructive.

Urates are water-soluble. The deposits can be visualized only if the tissue is fixed in absolute alcohol. The needle-like structure of the crystal is readily apparent (Fig. 8–69B), either in properly alcohol-fixed tissue or in synovial fluid.

Text continued on page 293

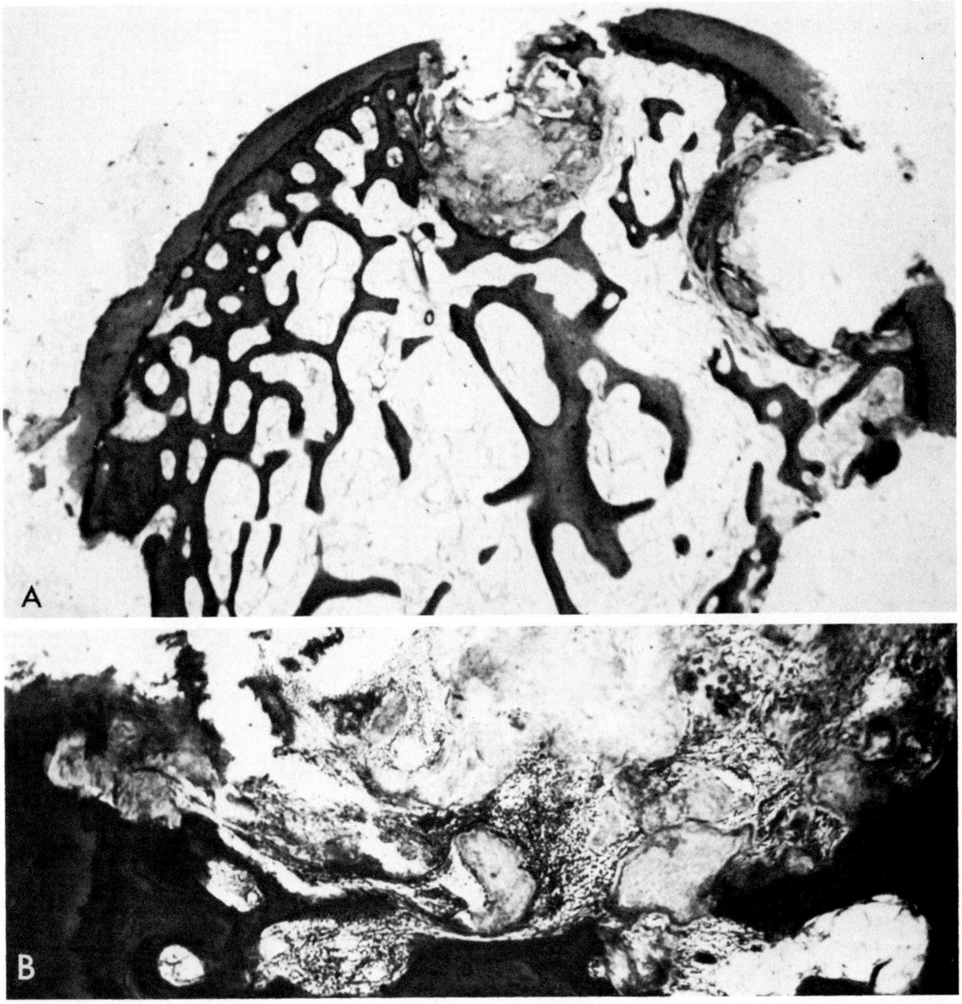

Figure 8–66. Gout. Articular cartilage on the surface has been eroded by subarticular deposits of urate crystals, and there is a sharply circumscribed defect in the joint space. These features produce the radiographic signs that are characteristic of gout.

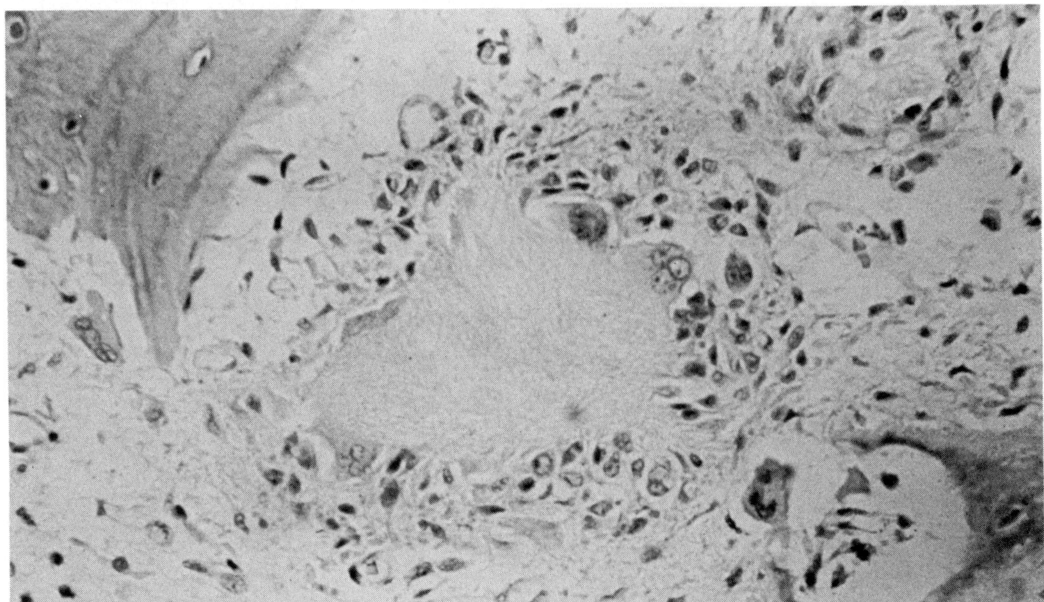

Figure 8–67. Gout. Histologic appearance of the margin of a tophus exhibiting acellular material surrounded by foreign-body giant cells. The deposition of urate salts in the tissue and the proteinaceous material produced in response to them elicit a foreign-body reaction. Crystals have been removed in the preparation of the sections.

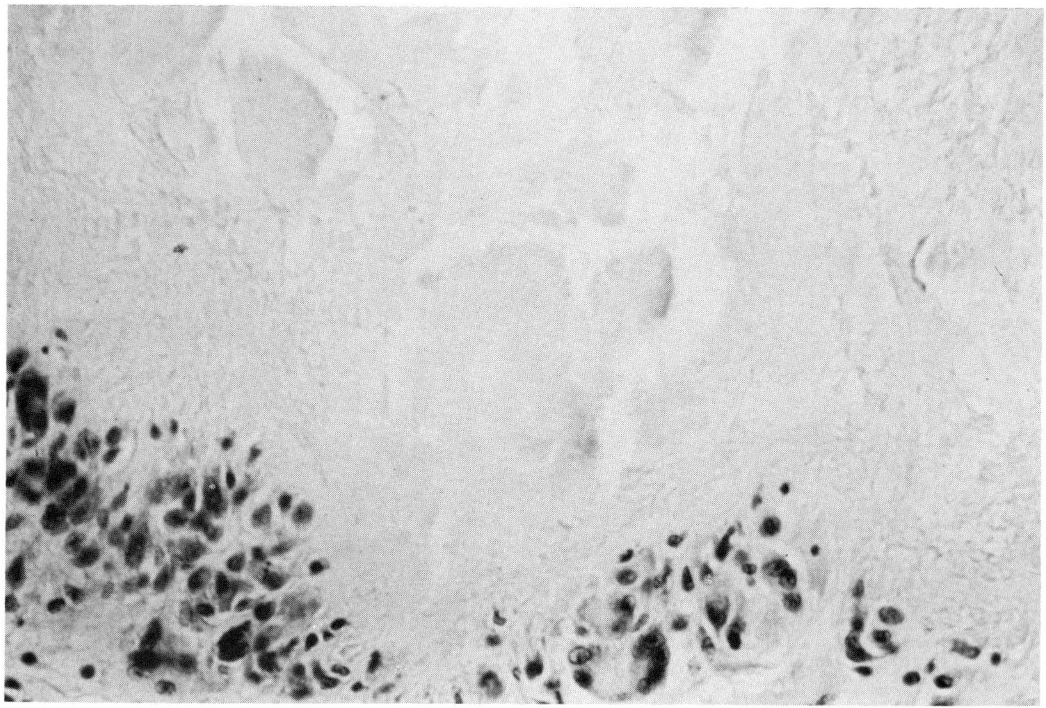

Figure 8–68. Gout. High-power view of a tophus within the bone showing foreign-body giant cells. The outline of the needle-like crystal is identifiable within the center of the tophus.

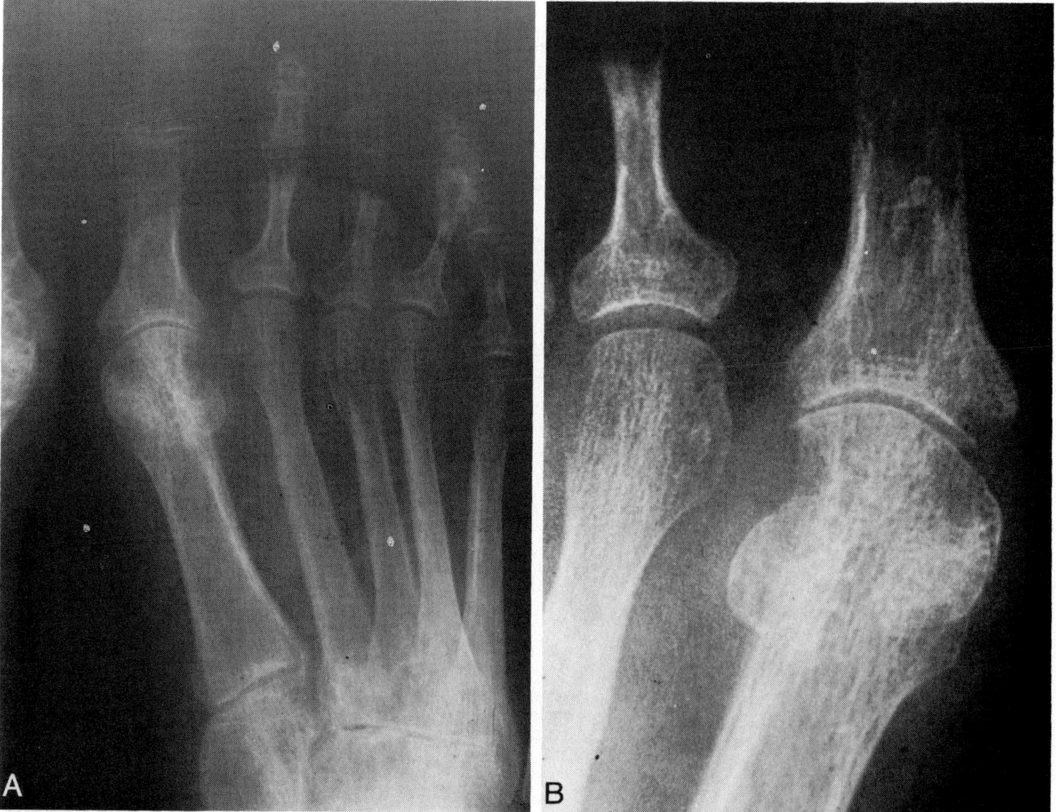

Figure 8–69. Radiographic appearance of a patient with gout. There are erosions at the lateral margins of the interphalangeal joints, with moderate to severe osteoporosis. Some involvement of the articular surface is apparent.

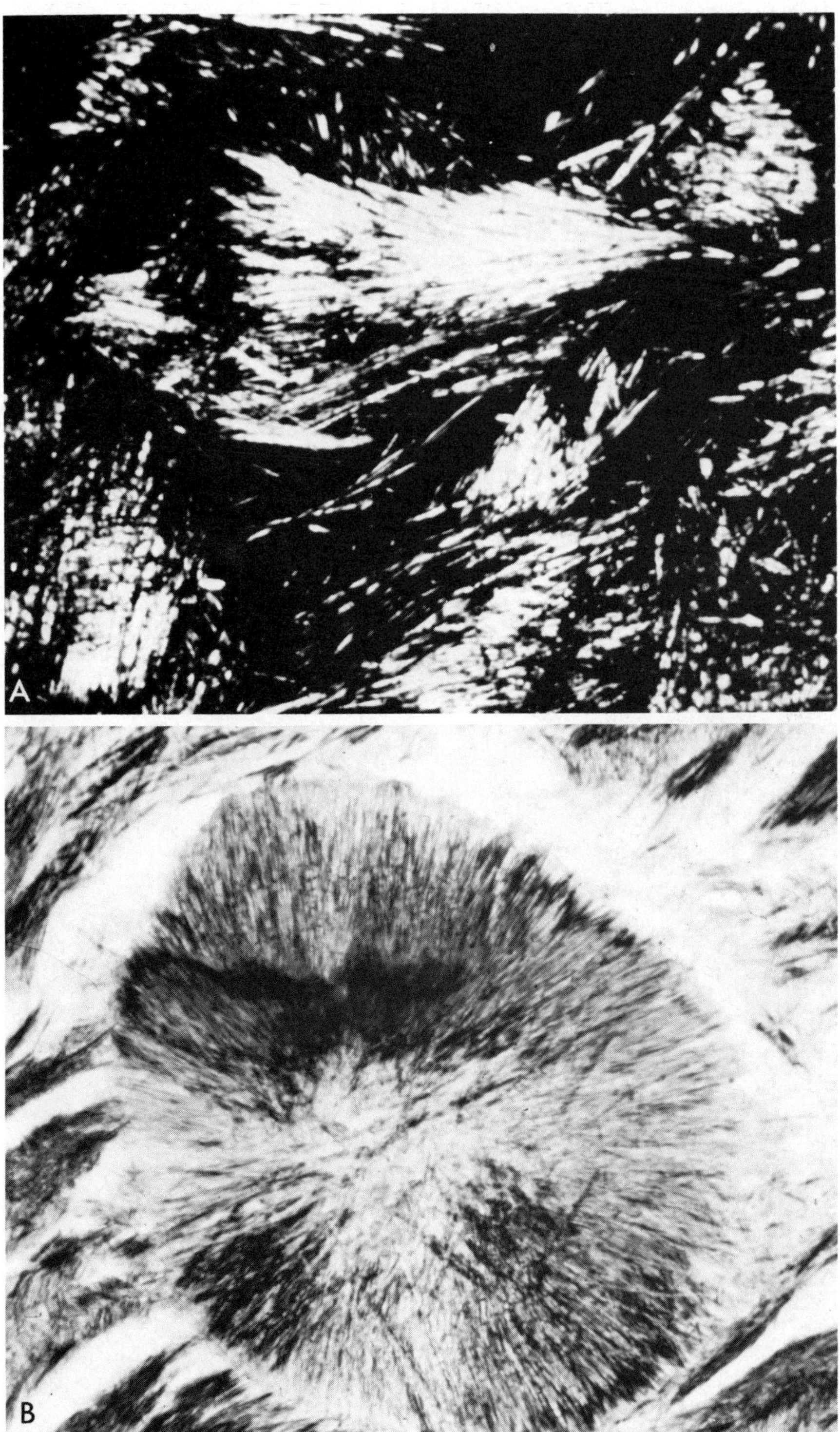

Figure 8–70. Gout. Histologic appearance of the uric-acid crystal viewed under polarized light. The needle-shaped crystalline pattern is characteristic.

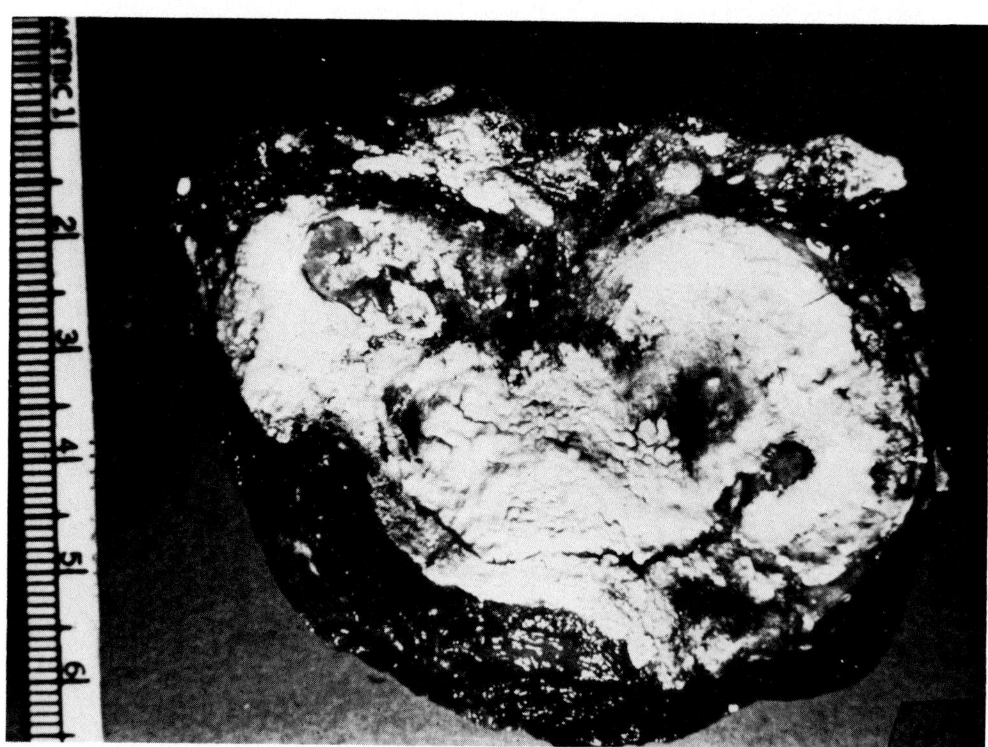

Figure 8–71. Proximal tibial articular surface of patient with chronic gout demonstrating coating of the articular cartilage surface by sodium urate salts.

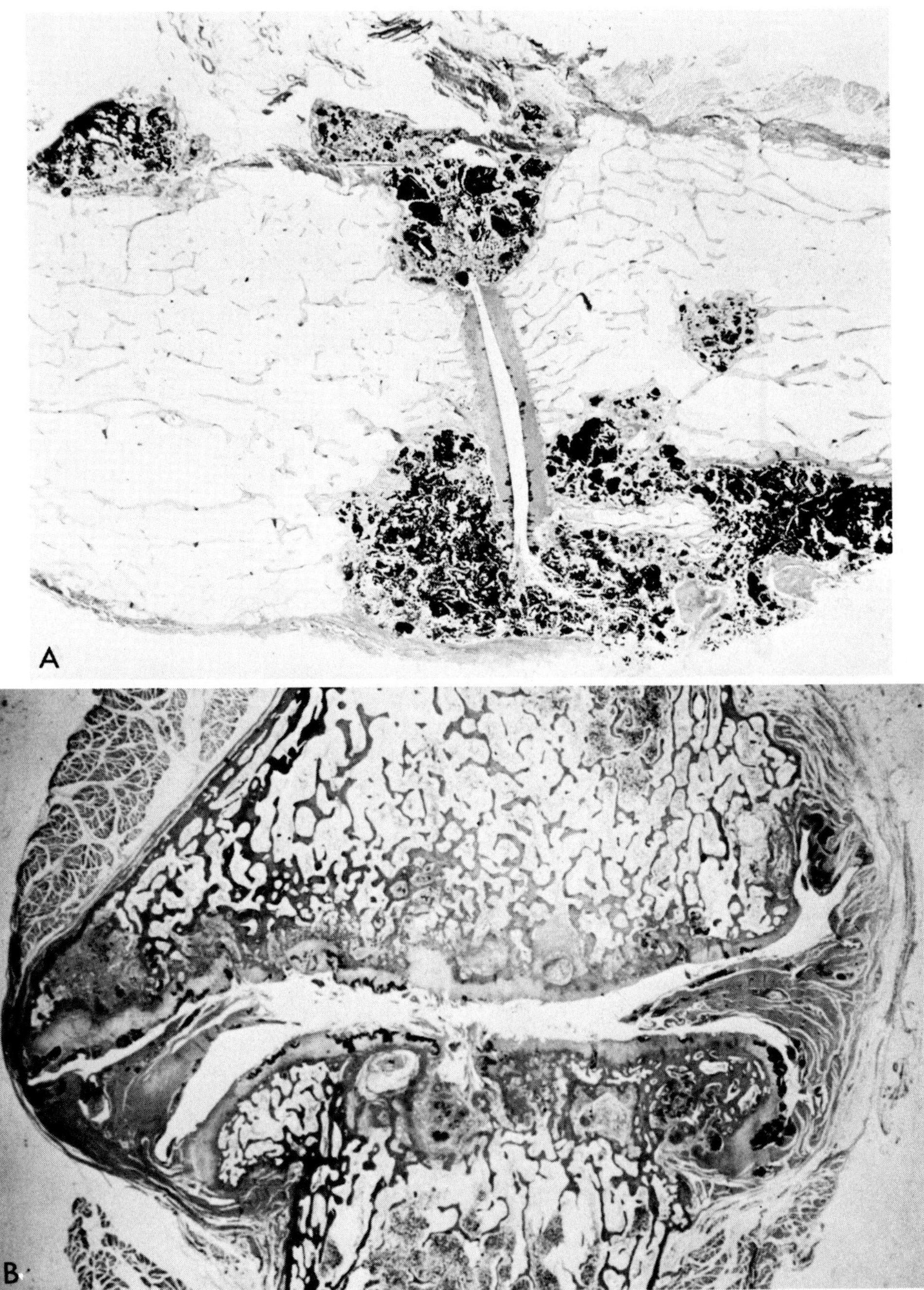

Figure 8–72. Macrosections of a patient with gout exhibiting deposition of sodium urate salts in the synovium, articular cartilage surface, and subchondral areas within the substance of the bone. The urate salt establishes itself as a foreign body and is surrounded by foreign-body granulation tissue. Crystals plus cartilage fragments deposit in a synovial recess and elicit inflammation with erosion into the subchondral area at the joint margins. Direct erosion through the articular surface occurs. The process terminates in severe destructive osteoarthritis.

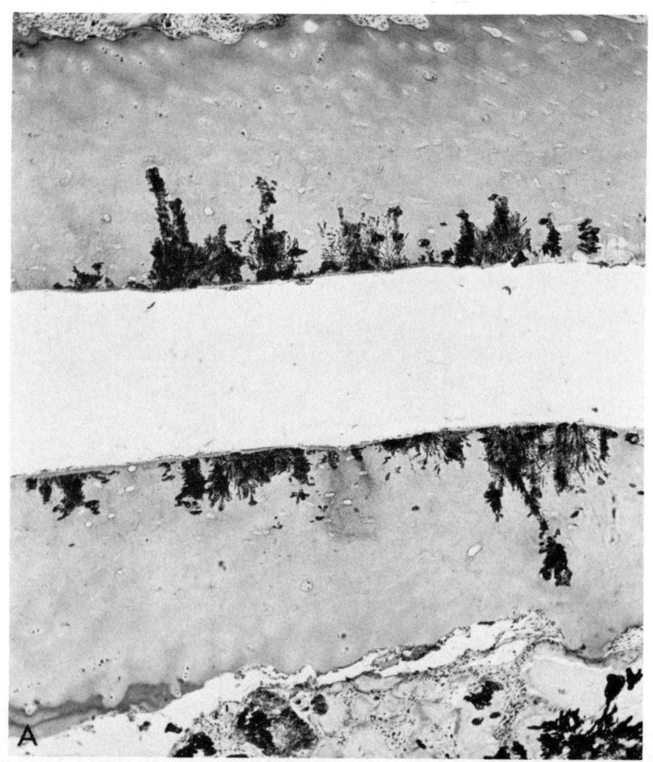

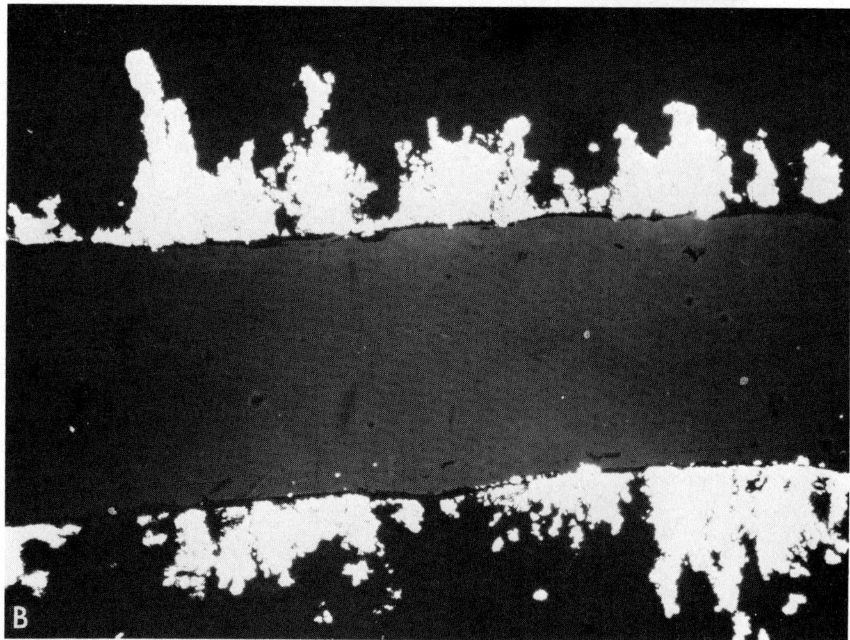

Figure 8–73. Gout. Macrosections of urate deposits on and in the articular cartilage. Identical sections visualized with (*B* and *D*) and without (*A* and *C*) polarized light.

Illustration continued on opposite page

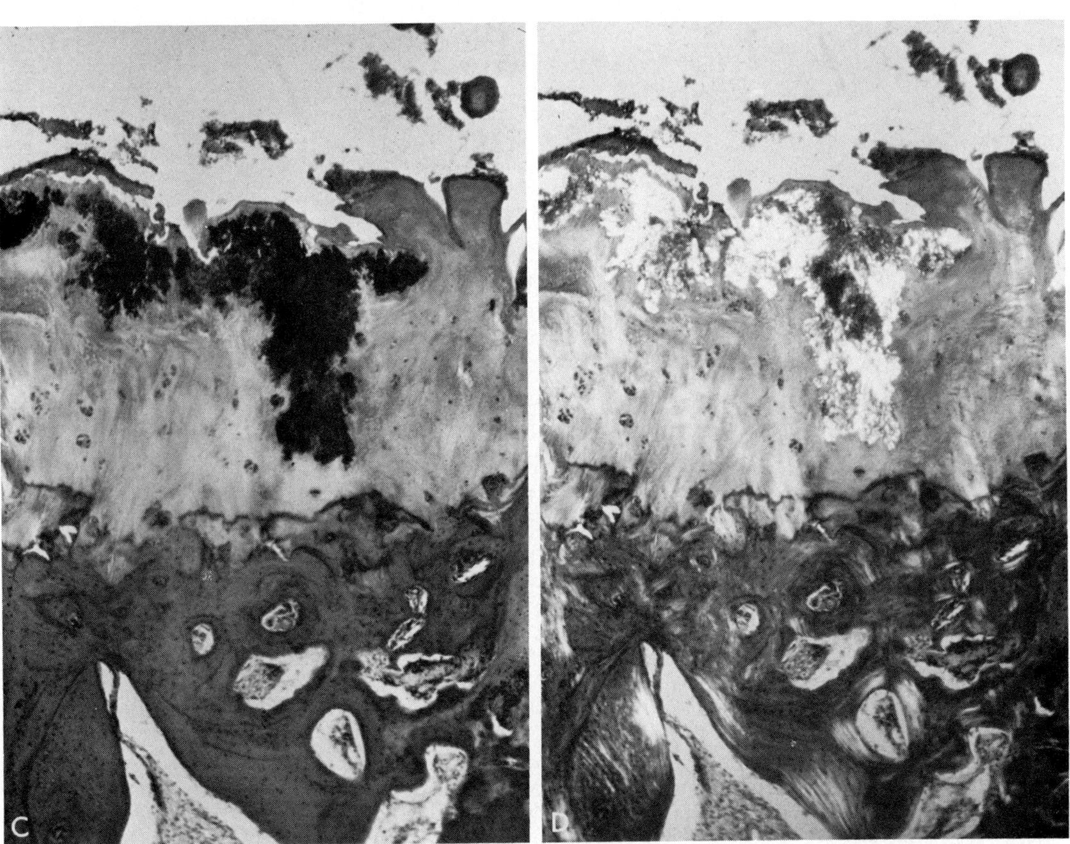

Figure 8–73 *Continued*

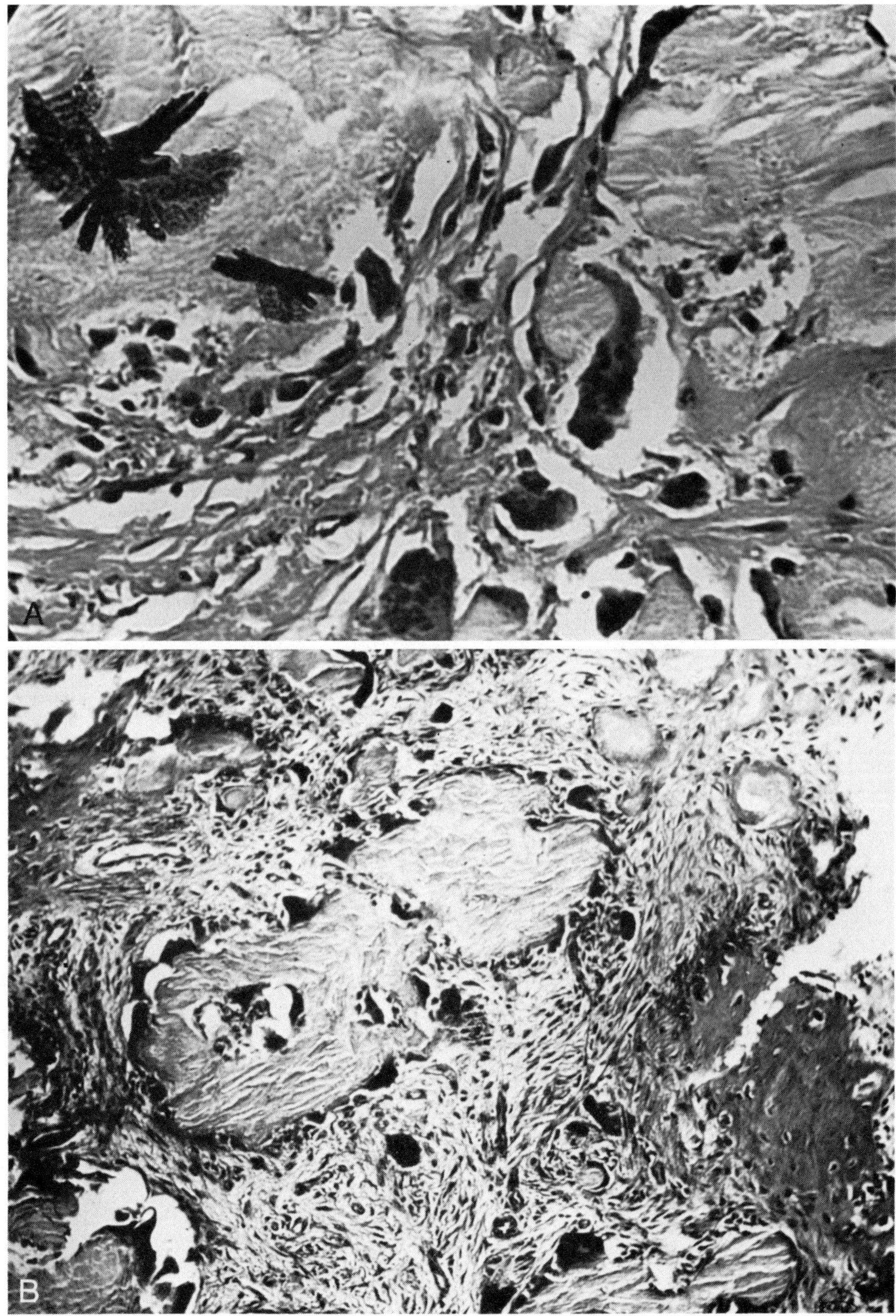

Figure 8–74. Gout. Histologic sections of a tophus with foreign-body giant cells and amorphous crystalline material. The crystalline substance accounts for a small portion of the total volume of the tophus; the remainder is composed of the cellular and proteinaceous material.

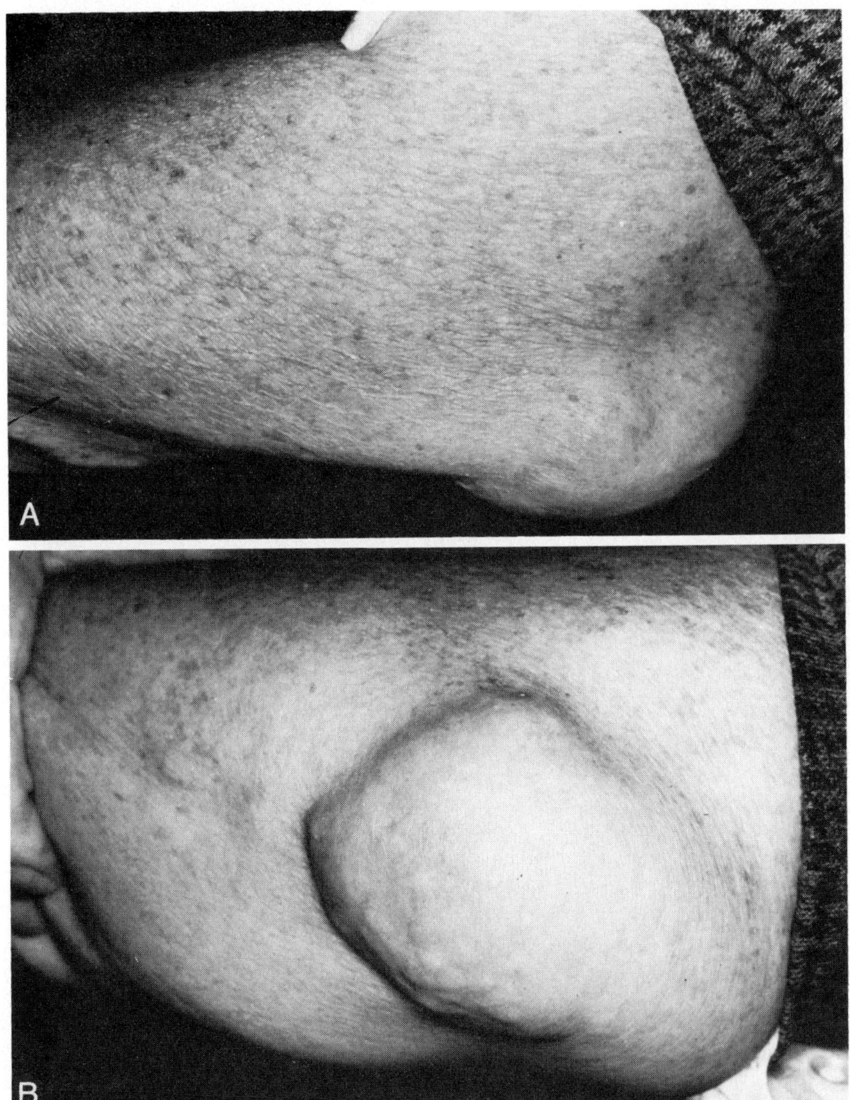

Figure 8–75. Gout. Photographs of a tophus in a common location: the olecranon bursa. Poor vascularity within the lesion and surrounding tissue can cause severe problems if the skin ulcerates over the tophus.

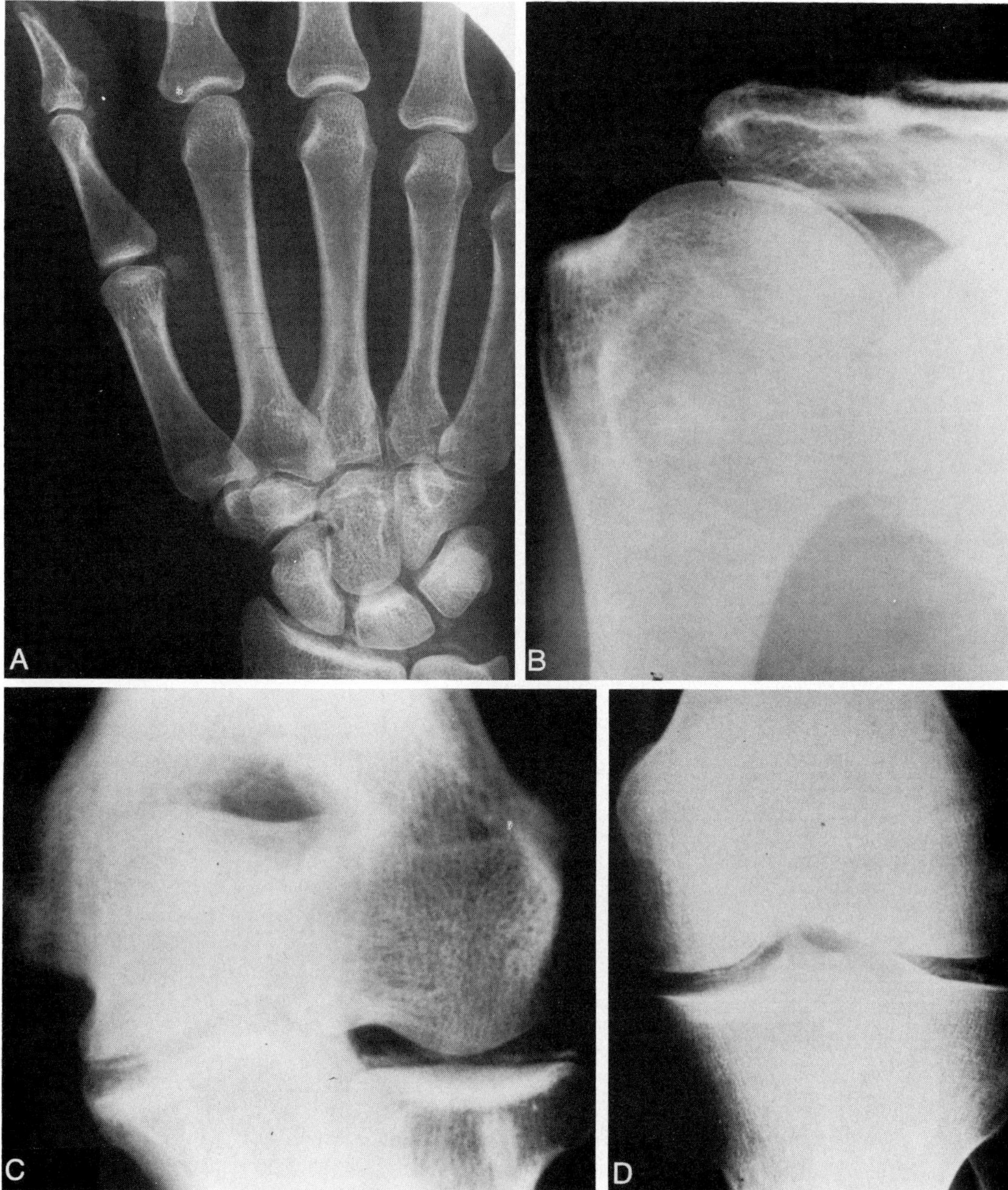

Figure 8–76. Radiographs of the hand *(A)*, shoulder *(B)*, elbow *(C)*, and knee *(D)* of patients with chondrocalcinosis. Notice the deposition of calcium salts onto the articular cartilage surface. The process is similar to that of gout, but the calcium salts remain confined to the cartilage surface. Acute symptoms may mimic gouty attacks, but the calcium deposition does not elicit a foreign-body reaction; no tophus is formed.

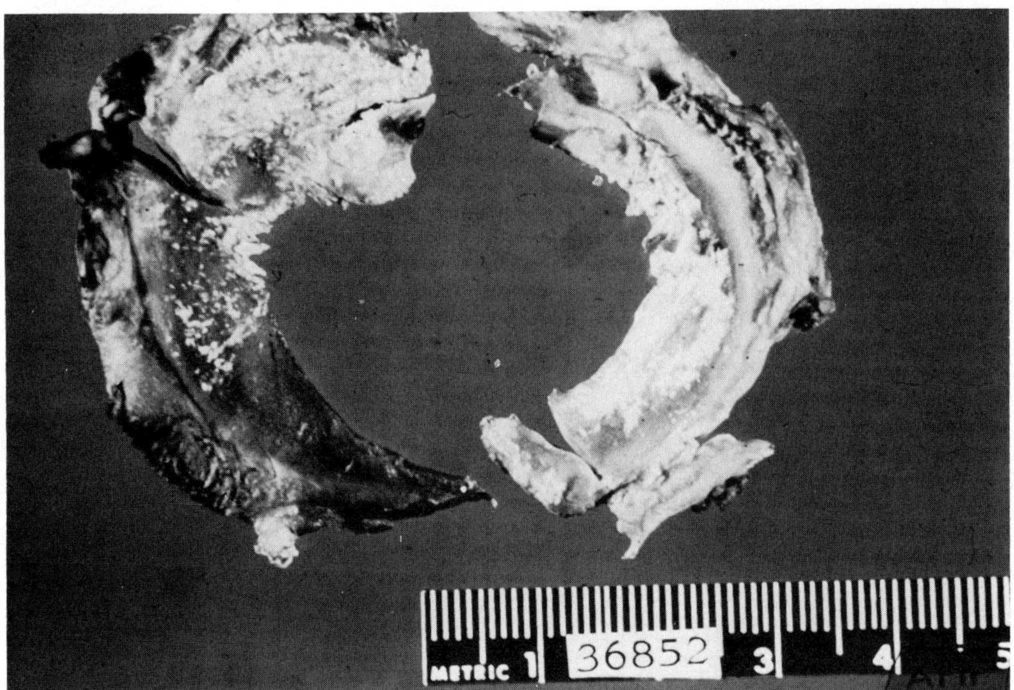

Figure 8–77. Gross appearance of a meniscus in a patient with chondrocalcinosis. Note the deposition of crystalline material onto the surface of the meniscus.

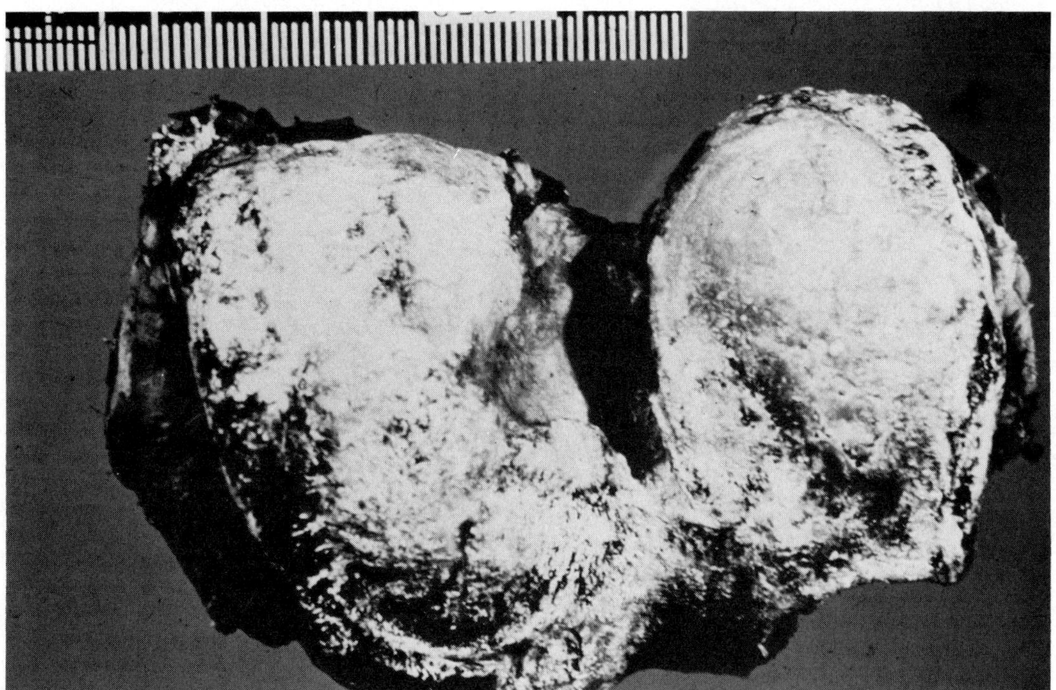

Figure 8–78. Gross appearance of knee joint in patient with chondrocalcinosis. Note the extensive deposition of calcium pyrophosphate crystal on the surface of the articular cartilage. This deposition of crystalline material is similar to what occurs in gout, but there is no tophus (see Fig. 8–71).

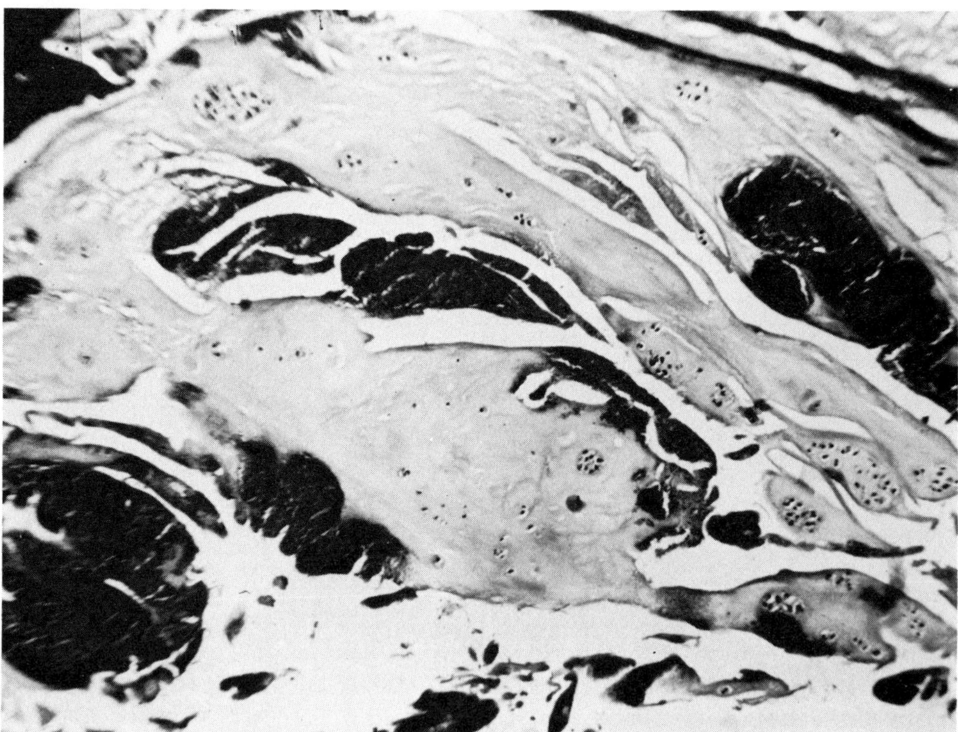

Figure 8–79. Histologic section of dystrophic calcification within the meniscus in a patient with chondrocalcinosis. Note the deposition of shards of abnormal material on the surface and within the substance of the meniscus.

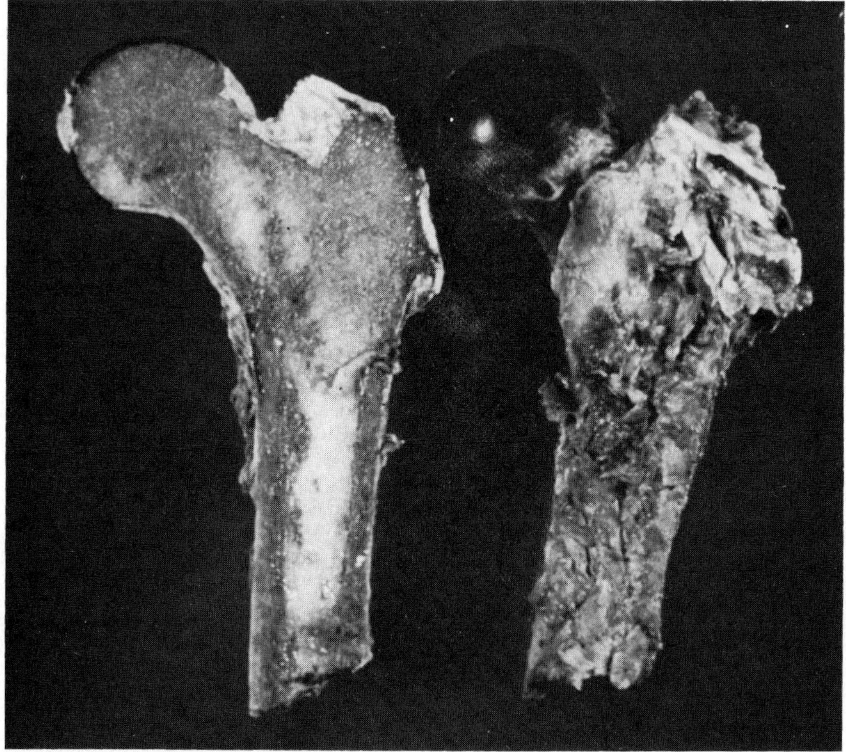

Figure 8–80. Ochronosis. Gross specimen of femoral head exhibiting the black discoloration of the articular cartilage surface.

OCHRONOSIS

Ochronosis is a hereditary error of protein metabolism. The patient is unable to oxidize homogentisic acid, a metabolite of phenylalanine and tyrosine. The homogentisic acid is excreted into the tissues, and it has a high affinity for proteoglycan, similar to uric acid. The chemical reaction results in hyperpolymerization of the cartilage. This material is brittle and readily fractured, and fragments are shed into the joint cavity. The articular cartilage surface is destroyed, and the fragmented cartilage is phagocytosed by the synovium. Homogentisic acid is black when oxidized, and this discoloration of ear lobes, conjunctivae, and all cartilaginous surfaces is readily recognized (Figs. 8–80 to 8–84).

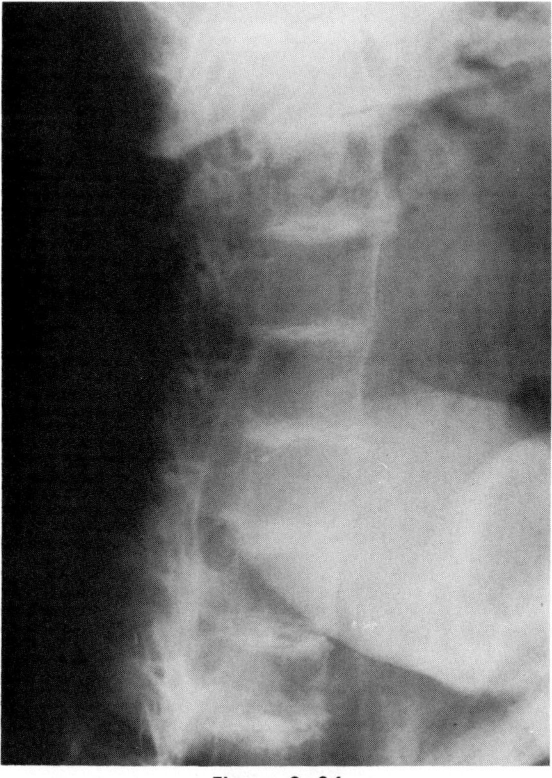

Figure 8–81

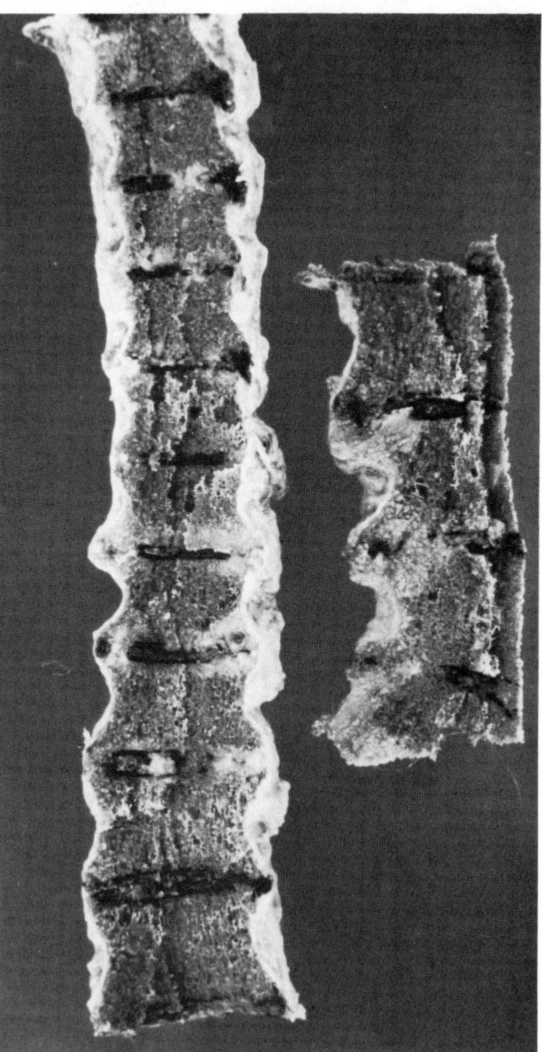

Figure 8–82

Figure 8–81. Radiograph of the spine of a patient with ochronosis exhibiting marked calcification and degeneration of the intervertebral discs. The degeneration of the intervertebral discs with dysplastic calcification results in severe thinning and ultimate disappearance of the disc space.

Figure 8–82. Gross appearance of vertebral bodies in a patient with ochronosis. Notice the diminution of the intervertebral discs, black discoloration of the cartilage components, virtual disappearance of all joint spaces, and bony bridging.

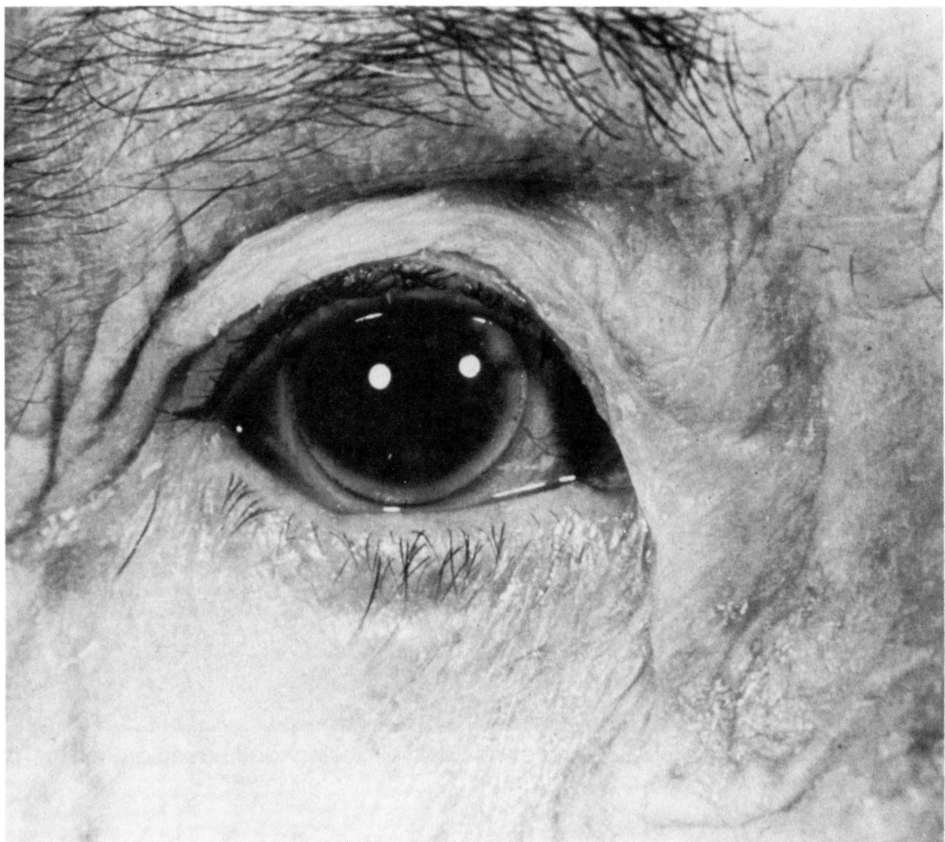

Figure 8–87. Characteristic pigmented conjunctiva in patient with ochronosis. The pigmentation may also be noted on ear lobes.

The radiographic appearance is one of diffuse osteoarthritis involving *every* articular surface. The histologic appearance is one of destruction of the cartilage with deposition of black homogentisic acid on the remaining cartilaginous structures.

CITED REFERENCES

Lane, J. M., and Vigorita, V. J.: Osteoporosis. J. Bone Joint Surg. 65A:274, 1983.
Marie, P. J., Pettifor, J. M., Ross, F. P., and Glorieux, F. H.: Histological osteomalacia due to dietary calcium deficiency in children. N. Engl. J. Med., 307:584, 1982.
Pace, N.: Weightlessness: a matter of gravity. N. Engl. J. Med., 297:32, 1977.

GENERAL REFERENCES

Jowsey, J.: Metabolic Diseases of Bone. Philadelphia, W. B. Saunders Co., 1977.
Sissons, H. A.: Osteoporosis and osteomalacia. In Ackerman, L. V., Spjut, H. J., and Abell, M. R., (Eds.): Bones and Joints, International Academy of Pathology Monograph. Baltimore, Williams and Wilkins Co., 1976.
Teitelbaum, S. L., and Bullough, P. G.: The pathophysiology of bone and joint disease. Am. J. Pathol., 96:341, 1979.

9

ANOMALIES AND NEOPLASMS

GENERAL PRINCIPLES

In this text the differential diagnosis of neoplasms and anomalies of bone is based on the field theory, proposed by Dr. Lent C. Johnson and published in 1953. Paraphrased liberally, the theory states that the mesenchymal cell will modulate and differentiate into a component of the mature osseous structure, depending on the field in which it is placed. Mesenchymal cells are totipotential, but it is the field rather than the cell itself that determines its ultimate function. A mesenchymal cell located in the epiphysis will become a chondroblast, whereas the same cell located in the metaphysis will become a chondrocyte. Tumors or anomalies will mimic the field in which they arise; epiphyseal cartilage tumors are chondroblastomas, whereas metaphyseal tumors are chondrosarcomas. As cancellous bone gives way to the relatively bone-free marrow cavity of the diaphysis, skeletogenic cells become fibroblasts and undifferentiated round cells when they overgrow as neoplasms. Thus, Ewing's sarcoma is usually a diaphyseal tumor. The predominant cell of the tumor matches the normal cell activity of the field in which the tumor arises (Diagram 9–1).

Tumors also occur in proportion to the rate of activity. The fastest growing bone ends and those of largest mass (lower end of femur and upper tibia) are more likely to develop a tumor than those of lesser mass and slower growth.

These general principles hold true in a majority of cases, and although exceptions may be found, they do not invalidate the basic underlying concept. The theory therefore provides the logical conceptual support for presumptive diagnosis based on location within bone.

The radiographic differential diagnosis is based on rapidity of growth. Malignant neoplasms grow rapidly, whereas benign neoplasms progress slowly. Evidence for rapid or slow growth is based on the character of the advancing margin and the nature of the periosteal reaction. A slower-growing tumor erodes the adjacent surface gradually and allows the osteoblasts sufficient time to reinforce the margin. Benign lesions are therefore sharply circumscribed and may have a sclerotic margin. A rapidly growing tumor penetrates the adjacent bone, bypassing existing trabecular structures. It will therefore have a poorly defined moth-eaten or permeative-destructive pattern (Madewell et al., 1981; Diagrams 9–2 and 9–3).

297

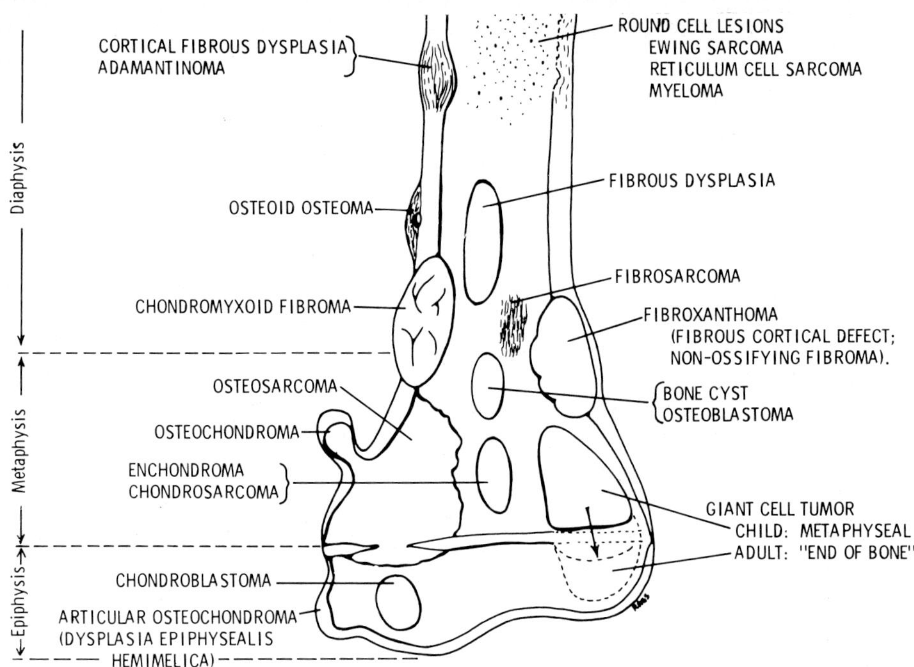

Diagram 9–1. Composite diagram illustrating frequent sites of bone tumors. The diagram depicts the end of a long bone that has been divided into the epiphysis, metaphysis, and diaphysis. The typical sites of common primary bone tumors are labeled. Bone tumors tend to predominate in those ends of long bones that undergo the greatest growth and remodeling and hence have the greatest number of cells and amount of cell activity (shoulder and knee regions). When small tumors, presumably detected early, are analyzed, preferential sites of tumor origin become apparent within each bone, as shown in this illustration. This suggests a relationship between the type of tumor and the anatomic site affected. In general, a tumor of a given cell type arises in the field in which the homologous normal cells are most active. These regional variations suggest that the composition of the tumor is affected or may be determined by the metabolic field in which it arises (Johnson, L. C.: Bull. N.Y. Acad. Med. *29*:164, 1953). (Illustration from Madewell, J. E., et al.: Radiol. Clin. North Am. *19*:715, 1981.)

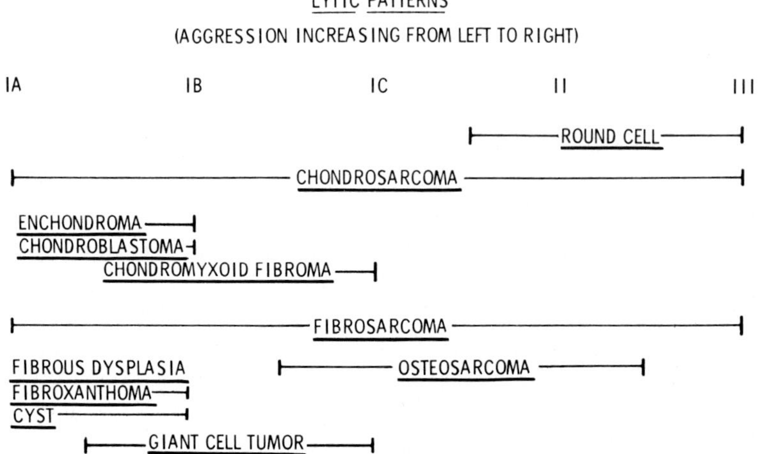

Diagram 9–2. This diagram delineates common bone tumors and their typical patterns of bone destruction. *IA*, Well-defined geographic destruction with sclerosis in the margin. *IB*, Well-defined geographic destruction without sclerosis in the margin. *IC*, Geographic destruction with ill-defined margin. *II*, Moth-eaten (regionally invasive) destruction. *III*, Permeative (diffusely invasive) destruction. Note that most benign tumors occur on the left-hand side, from IA to IC, whereas most malignant tumors occur on the right-hand side, from IC to III. This illustrates the general principle that the biologic activity and probability of malignancy increase from left to right. Chondrosarcoma and fibrosarcoma can present with any of the five patterns. They frequently arise in pre-existing benign lesions. In such cases, the radiographic pattern may lag behind the histologic activity, producing a radiographic discrepancy (slow-appearing lesion with malignant histology). (From Madewell, J. E., et al.: Radiol. Clin. North Am. *19*:715, 1981.)

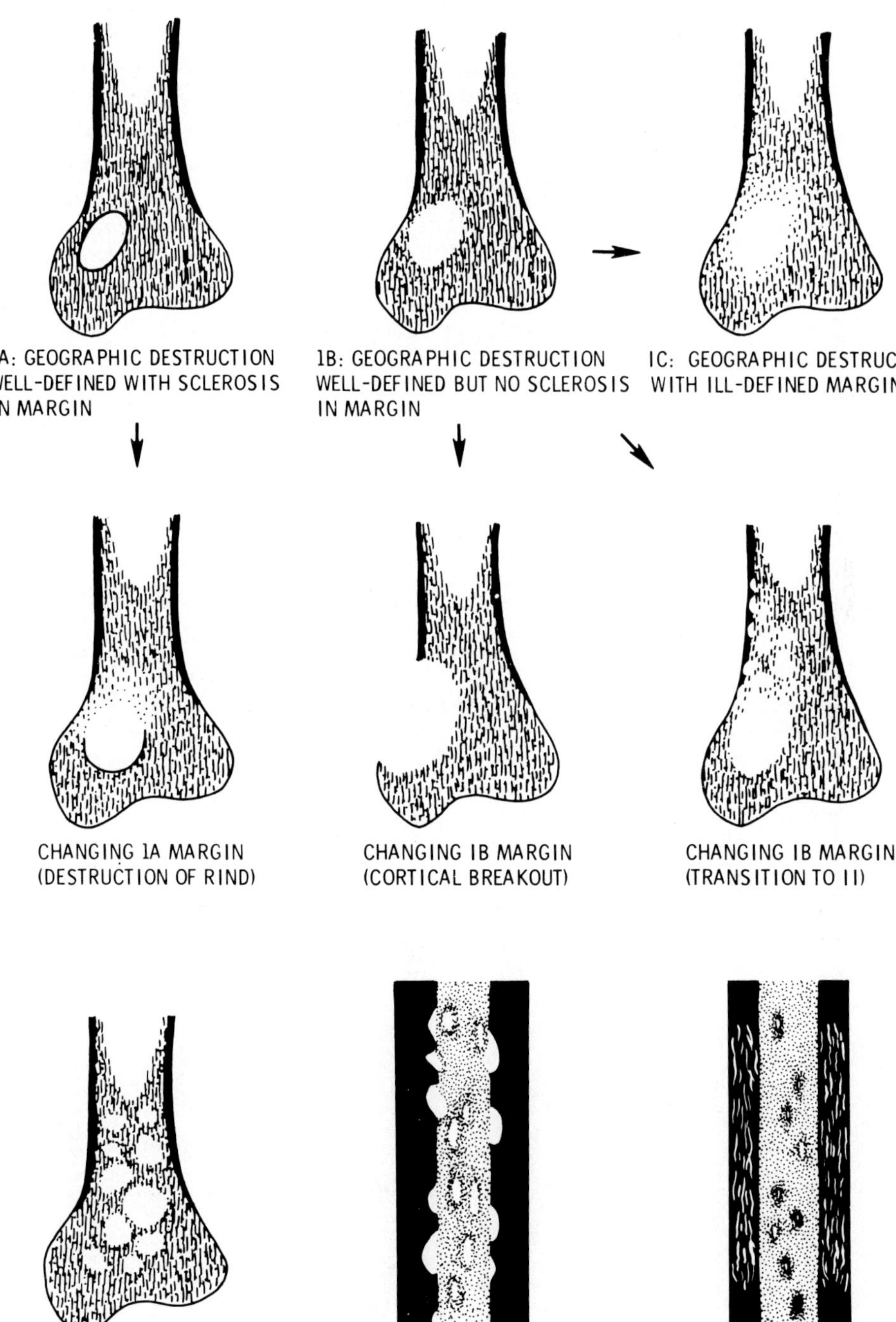

Diagram 9–3. Schematic diagram of patterns of bone destruction (types IA, IB, IC, II, and III) and their margins. Arrows indicate the most frequent transitions or combinations of these margins. Transitions imply increased activity and a greater probability of malignancy. (From Madewell, J. E., et al.: Radiol. Clin. North Am. *19:*715, 1981.)

The periosteal reaction is a similar barometer of slow-versus-fast growth. "Expansion" of bone is actually reinforcement of the outer surface that occurs while the neoplasm erodes the inner surface. It is slow because bone formation keeps pace with destruction on the inner surface. Rapid destruction weakens the cortex and results in a periosteal reaction, either a spiculated "hair on end" or a laminated "onion peel." Rapid destruction will also result in a thin hairline periosteal reaction at the edge of the neoplasm, the Codman's triangle. Slow growth will give osteoblasts enough time for bone formation and results in buttress formation (Ragsdale et al., 1981; Diagram 9–4).

The flocculent calcification of cartilage can be differentiated from the fine, linear calcification of osteoid. A purely destructive lytic pattern indicates soft-tissue density, without calcifiable matrix formation (Sweet et al., 1981; Diagram 9–5).

PERIOSTEAL REACTIONS

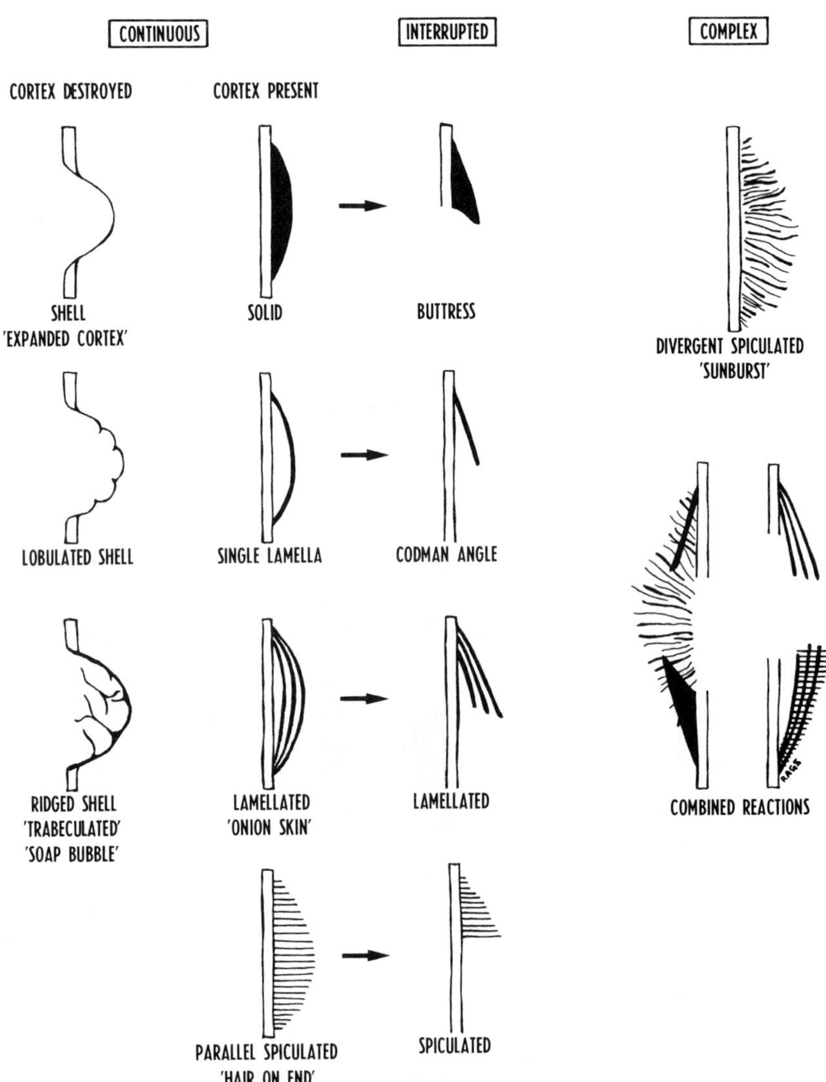

Diagram 9–4. Schematic diagram of periosteal reactions. The arrows indicate that the continuous reactions may be interrupted. (From Ragsdale, B. D., et al.: Radiol. Clin. North Am. *19*:749, 1981.)

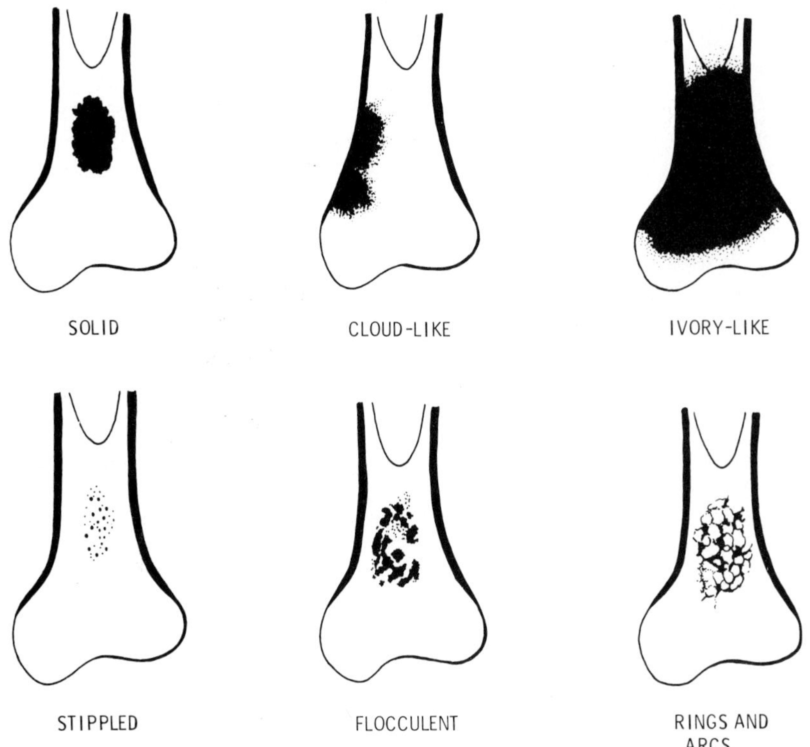

Diagram 9–5. Schematic diagram of mineralized matrix patterns. Tumor osteoid appears as increased density with a solid (sharp-edged) or cloud-like to ivory-like (ill-defined edge) pattern. Tumor cartilage creates stippled, flocculent, and solid density patterns. Rings and arcs represent bony rims about tumor cartilage lobules. Dystrophic mineralization and ischemic osteoid tend to mimic the stippled, flocculent, or patchy solid density pattern. (From Sweet, D. E., et al.: Radiol. Clin. North Am. *19*:785, 1981.)

Ultimately, the diagnosis is made on the basis of accurate interpretation of histologic material. In most instances, preoperative evaluation permits reasonable assessment of the lesion's biologic potential and will determine the sequence of events leading to the appropriate diagnostic preoperative studies (Mankin et al., 1982; Simon, 1982). These include computerized axial tomography, arteriography, and bone scans. Evaluation of the results determines both the biopsy site and the technique. The biopsy must be planned with extreme care. The skin incision should not compromise the subsequent definitive surgical procedure. As a rule, a transverse incision on an extremity prevents subsequent en-bloc excision.

A decision as to whether to use an open or closed biopsy depends on consultation among the radiologist, the pathologist, and the surgeon. Closed needle biopsies are advantageous because they do not create a large defect in bone, spillage of tumor into adjacent tissue is avoided, possible radiation therapy is not delayed, there is little hematoma, and the possibility of infection is minimized. However, the accuracy of the closed biopsy depends on appropriate sampling of the neoplasm and is, at best, a matter of chance. Reactive tissue at the margin of the neoplasm may prompt an erroneous diagnosis. A negative biopsy, in view of positive radiographic findings, should therefore be followed with either open biopsy or repeat closed biopsies until the surgeon, the radiologist, and the pathologist are satisfied that the lesion has been truly sampled.

If possible, a lesion should be biopsied outside the cortex. Even though the accuracy of diagnosis may be diminished, pathologists can usually identify the underlying nature of the neoplasm. Biopsy outside the cortex minimizes the risk of subsequent pathologic fracture, reduces the extent of the hematoma, and minimizes tumor spillage into adjacent tissue.

Frozen sections should be attempted in open biopsies. As a rule, sufficient soft tissue is present to confirm the suspected diagnosis and guide the surgeon in the appropriate therapy. At worst, the pathologist is unable to process or diagnose the tissue, but the surgeon is at no greater disadvantage than without the attempt, and he is assured that adequate viable tissue is available for an ultimate diagnosis.

The surgeon bears the ultimate responsibility for the care of the patient and therefore must be satisfied with the validity of the preoperative studies, the accuracy of the interpretation of these studies, and the choice of the biopsy process. If there is disagreement among the pathologist, radiologist, and surgeon in the interpretation of the findings, additional consultation should be sought. If the degree of expertise at any institution is insufficient or if the definitive therapy cannot be performed at the institution, then the preoperative studies, staging, and biopsy should also be referred to the tertiary care center.

The discussion of the anomalies and tumors that follows is brief and designed to outline for the reader the salient histologic and radiographic features of these lesions without attempting to be encyclopedic. Authoritative and complete discussion of modern diagnosis and therapy can be found in the texts by Huvos (1979), Mirra (1980), and Schajowicz (1981); the reader is also referred to the classic volumes by Jaffe (1958) and Dahlin (1978).

FIBROUS AND FIBROCYSTIC LESIONS

Included in the group of fibrous lesions of bone are (1) fibrous dysplasia of bone, (2) cortical fibrous dysplasia of bone (ossifying fibroma), (3) nonossifying fibroma of bone (fibroxanthoma of bone, fibrous cortical defect), (4) the unicameral bone cyst (and the uncommitted metaphyseal lesion), (5) aneurysmal bone cyst, (6) angioma, (7) lipoma, (8) desmoplastic fibroma, (9) fibrosarcoma of bone, and (10) fibrous histiocytoma. Although the first four can be classified as "congenital anomalies," they behave as benign neoplasms of bone, and they do have rare malignant counterparts.

FIBROUS DYSPLASIA

Fibrous dysplasia is characterized by the replacement of normal trabecular bone and marrow elements by fibrous tissue. It is a congenital anomaly and may involve either one bone (monostotic fibrous dysplasia) or many bones (polyostotic fibrous dysplasia). The early lesion of fibrous dysplasia is strictly fibrous, composed of spindle-cell nuclei and a connective tissue stroma. As the lesion becomes more mature, metaplasia of the fibrous connective tissue occurs with the formation of bone. It is not uncommon to have fragments of cartilage within the connective tissue, and occasionally a cartilaginous neoplasm may arise in a focus of fibrous dysplasia.

Histologically, the mature lesion exhibits trabeculae of bone arising directly out of the fibrous connective tissue stroma. Characteristically, no osteoblasts are noted, although a few fibroblasts may line up along the osteoid margin. The trabeculae thus formed have a peculiar slender, curlicue shape, reminding one of "alphabet soup." Under polarized light, the collagen pattern is one of immature woven bone. The pattern does not change, and the bone remains immature. The characteristic slender curved forms are usually seen in long bones; the ribs or flat bones may exhibit flat fragments of bone formed directly from the fibrous connective tissue. The osteoid matrices thus formed are calcified and, if sufficient numbers are present, contribute to the radiographic "ground-glass" density of the bone. In the initial stage, however, during the pure fibrous phase, the lesion is radiographically lytic.

Fibrous dysplasia arises beneath the growth plate, usually involving the entire metaphysis and extending into the diaphyseal portion of the bone as well. The lesion may infiltrate the epiphysis after the growth plate fuses. The replacement of cancellous bone by the dysplastic process weakens the structure and causes bowing and deformity. At the edge of the fibrous dysplastic lesion, the remaining bony trabeculae are reinforced, resulting in sclerotic margination.

These lesions are often found in the skull and ribs. Atypical patterns may represent fracture and healing admixed with fibrous dysplasia of the rib (Schlumberger, 1946).

Patients with fibrous dysplasia may suffer from complications, particularly hemorrhage. Evidence of low-grade hemorrhage is always provided by the identifiable hemosiderin pigment within the lesion. Massive hemorrhage may cause excessive pressure and pain and may present as a markedly lytic lesion with periosteal reaction, simulating a malignant neoplasm.

Albright's syndrome should not be confused with polyostotic fibrous dysplasia, even though both have similiar histologic features within the osseous structures. Albright's syndrome is associated with precocious puberty, abnormality of ovarian development, and osseous lesions. In polyostotic fibrous dysplasia, however, there is no evidence of precocious puberty, and there are no histologic features to differentiate

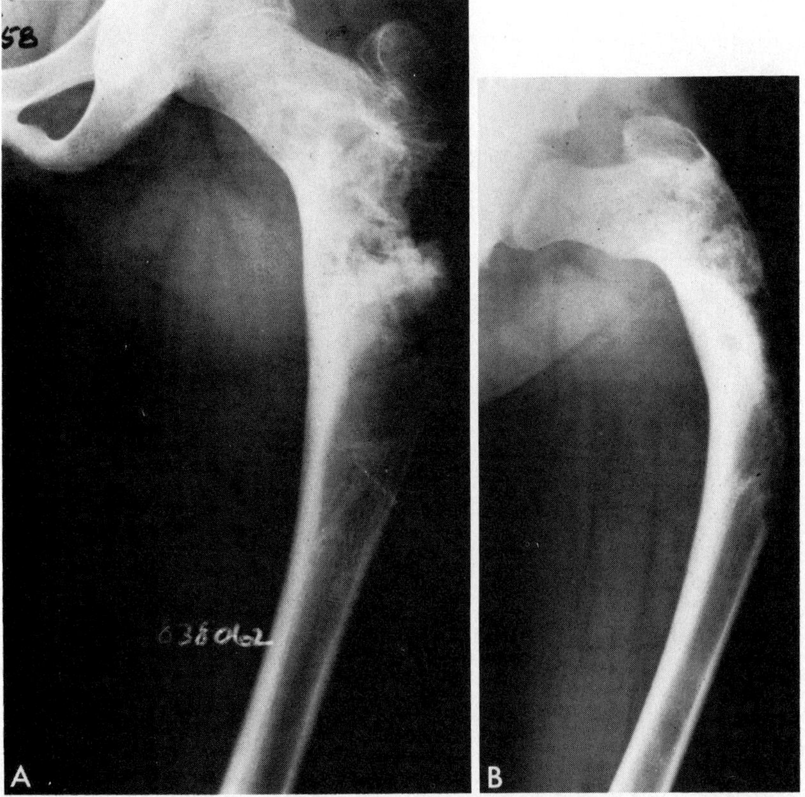

Figure 9–1. Fibrous dysplasia. Radiographic appearance of fibrous dysplasia. In *A*, note expansion of the cortex, with lytic defect and calcification within the lesion. The lesion is located in the metaphysis and is slow-growing. Radiographic evidence of this slow growth consists of a sharply defined margin, expansion of the cortex, absence of permeative destruction, and absence of periosteal reaction. The second film *(B)* shows progression of the lesion, with increased expansion and distortion of bone. Weakness due to replacement of normal bone by fibrous tissue leads to the shepherd's-crook deformity.

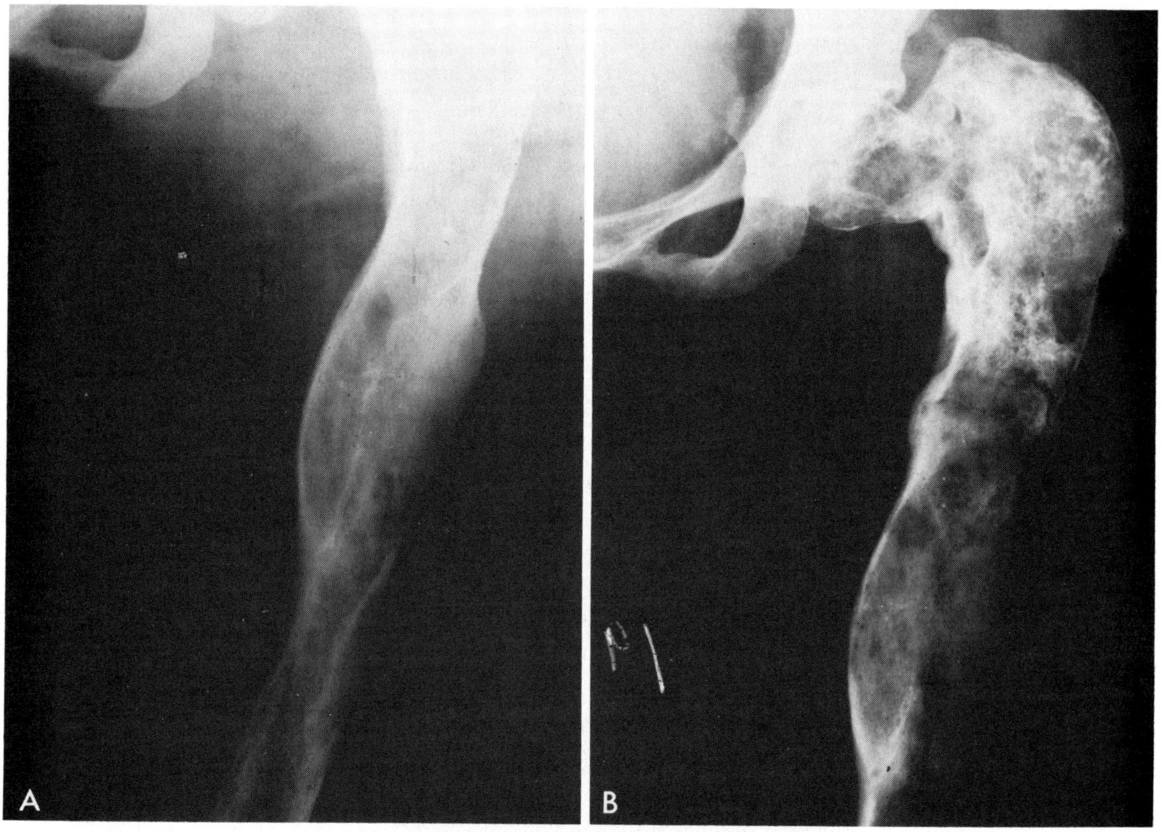

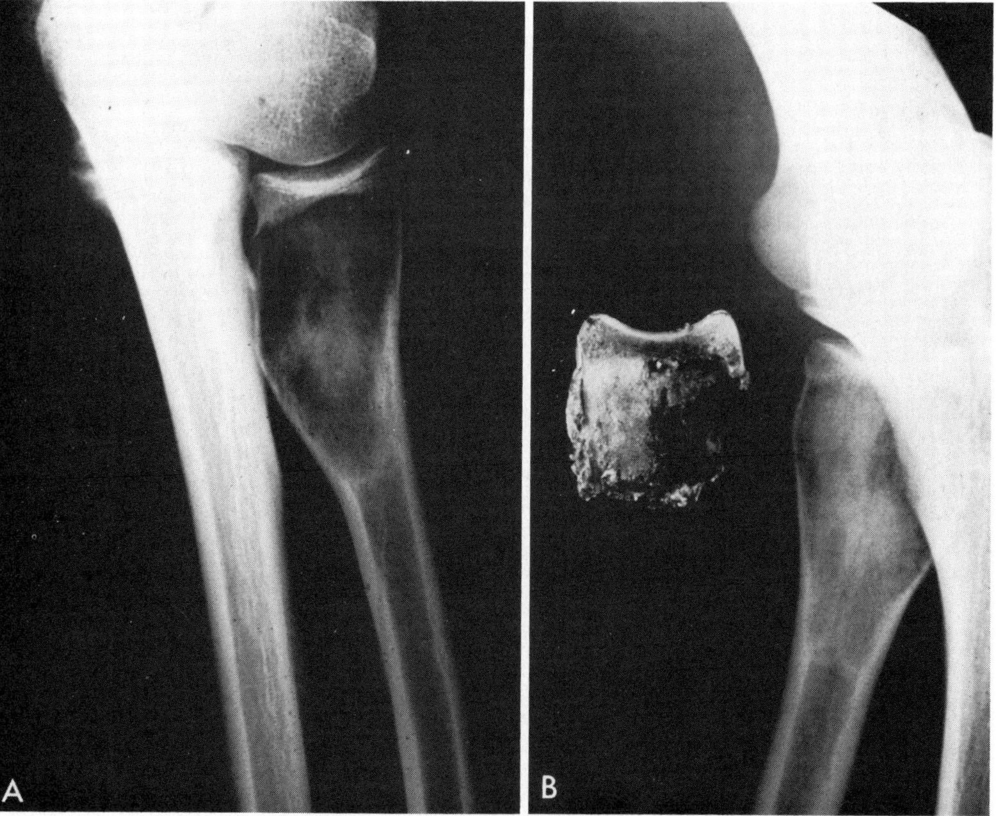

Figure 9–2. *See legend on opposite page*

Figure 9–3. *See legend on opposite page*

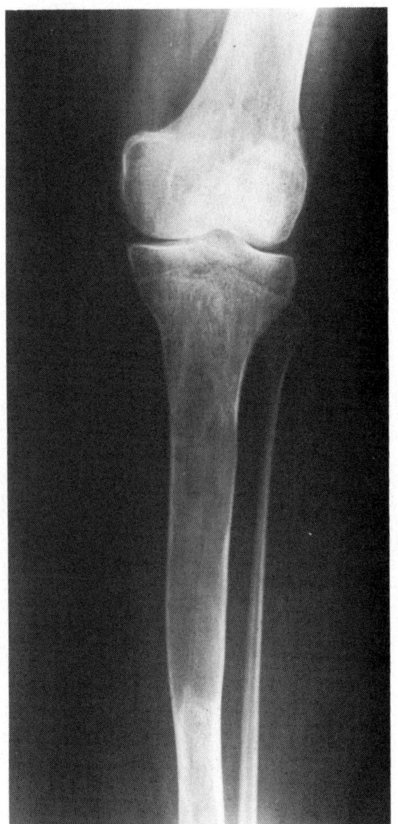

Figure 9–4. Fibrous dysplasia. The lesion involves the full width of the metaphysis and diaphysis. There is expansion and classic ground-glass density within the lesion. Sharp demarcation and absence of periosteal reaction indicate a benign process.

it from the usual monostotic fibrous dysplasia. Abnormal skin pigmentation may be present in both fibrous dysplasia and Albright's syndrome.

On the basis of histology alone, the differential diagnosis of fibrous dysplasia of bone should include nonossifying fibroma of bone, hyperparathyroidsm, and Paget's disease of bone. A well-differentiated osteosarcoma, particularly parosteal osteosarcoma, exhibits a similar histologic picture (Unni et al., 1976). Correlation with radiographs should easily resolve the problems of differential diagnosis. The characteristic radiographic appearance of fibrous dysplasia is an oval lesion, involving the full width of the bone as well as the diaphysis, rather than a sharply circumscribed eccentric circular lesion such as one finds in a nonossifying fibroma of bone. Differentiating the lesion from the well-differentiated osteosarcoma requires attention to histologic detail, particularly the variability and pleomorphism of the cellular elements (variability in size, staining characteristics, and shape of cells, as well as mitotic activity).

Text continued on page 313

Figure 9–2. Fibrous dysplasia. Radiographic appearance of a patient with more extensive fibrous dysplasia and marked deformity involving metaphysis and diaphysis of femur. In *A*, note expansion of bone and ground-glass appearance. The second film *(B)*, obtained 3 years later, shows extensive progression of the lesion with marked deformity of the femoral neck, shepherd's-crook deformity with extensive sclerosis secondary to bowing.

Figure 9–3. Fibrous dysplasia. Radiograph and gross specimen exhibiting expansile lesion involving epiphysis and metaphysis of proximal radius. Note sharply circumscribed lytic area adjacent to proximal ulna; the patient complained of sudden onset of pain. The specimen reveals focal area of hemorrhage within the fibrous dysplasia. Pressure from hemorrhage can cause sudden pain, with erosion and subsequent periosteal reaction.

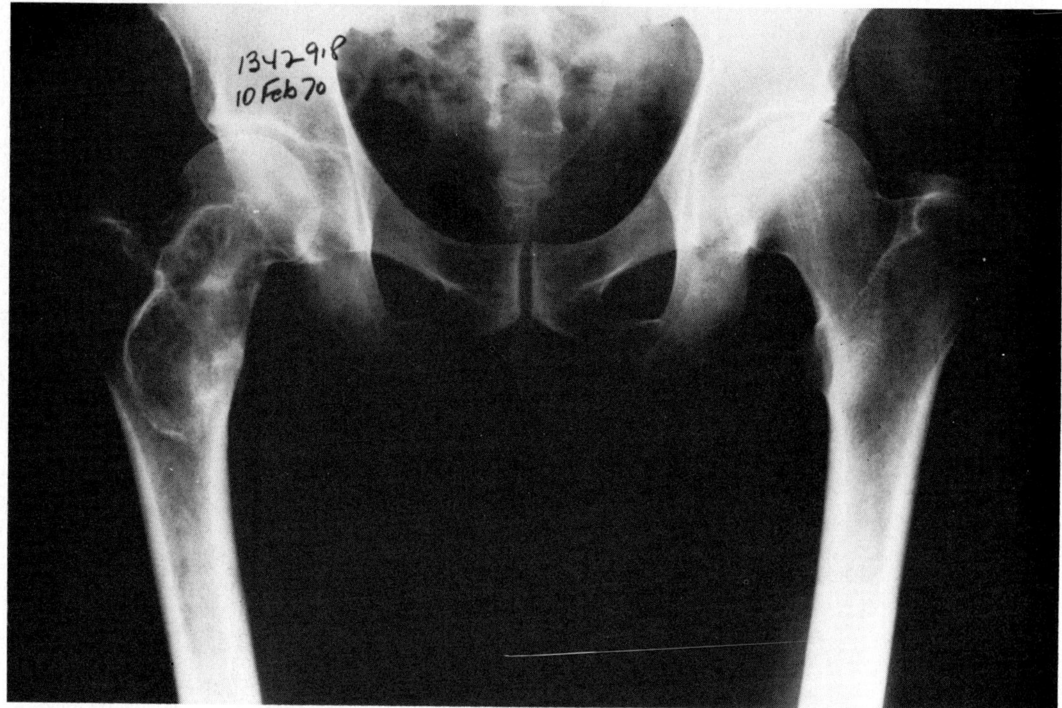

Figure 9–5. Fibrous dysplasia. Radiograph of hip with circumscribed metaphyseal defect, lytic, with focal ground-glass density in the defect. There is no distortion of the femur, but the lesion may progress into the characteristic shepherd's-crook deformity. The margins of the lesion are sharply circumscribed. Reinforcement of the trabeculae results in a sclerotic bony rim, which may contain the abnormal cells of the fibrous dysplasia. Complete excision must include the rim of the lesion to prevent recurrence.

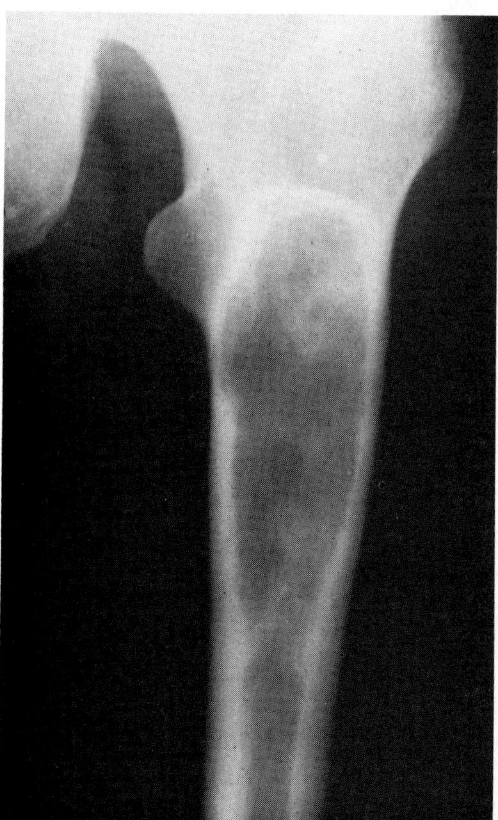

Figure 9–6. Fibrous dysplasia. Sharply circumscribed metaphyseal defect. The sclerotic margin and the increased matrix mineralization with classic ground-glass appearance indicate a long-standing process.

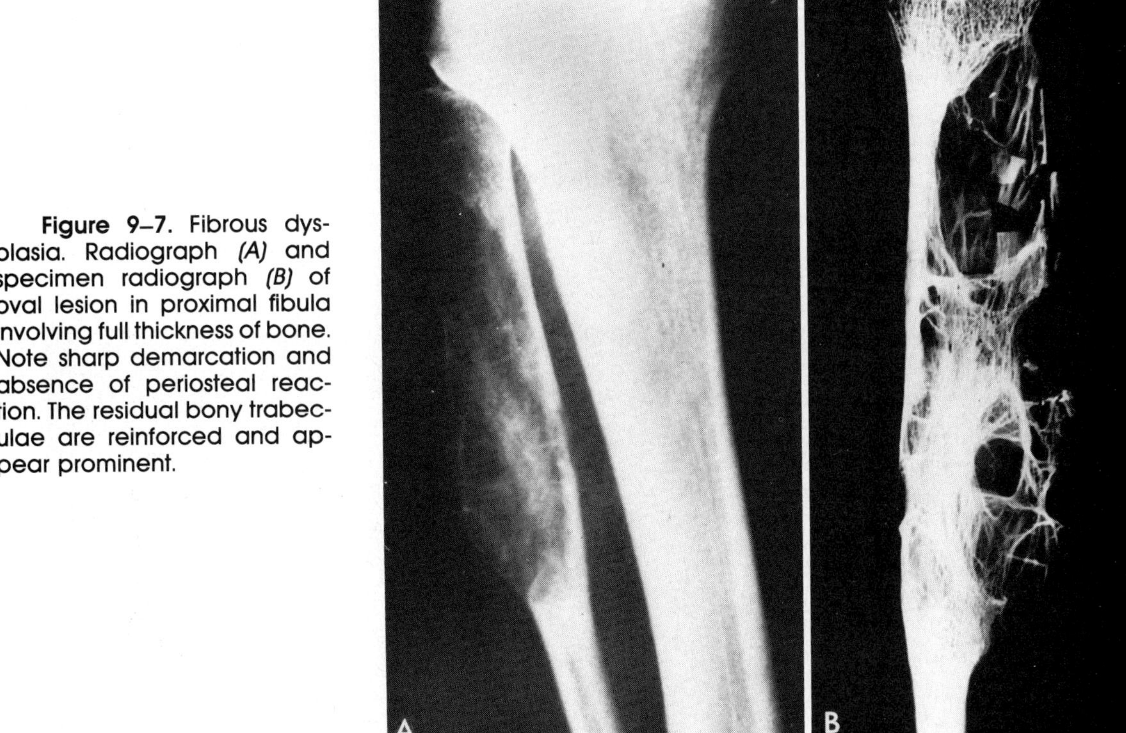

Figure 9–7. Fibrous dysplasia. Radiograph *(A)* and specimen radiograph *(B)* of oval lesion in proximal fibula involving full thickness of bone. Note sharp demarcation and absence of periosteal reaction. The residual bony trabeculae are reinforced and appear prominent.

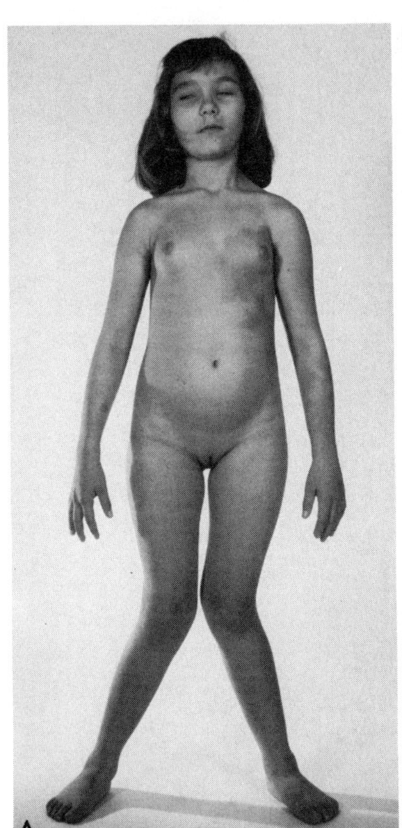

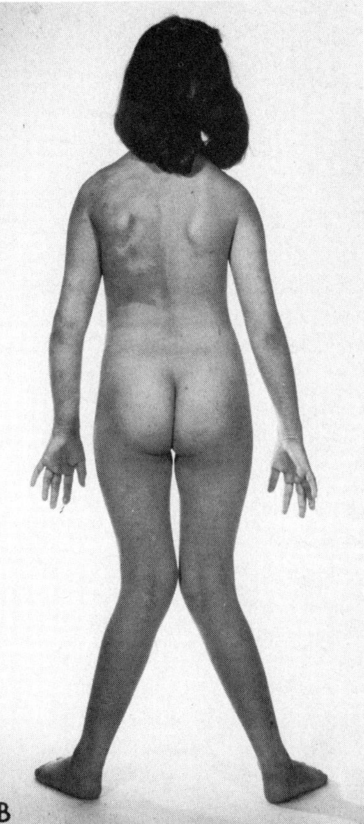

Figure 9–8. Fibrous dysplasia. Multiple deformities in a 13-year-old girl without endocrine disturbances. Note the pigmentation changes in the left hemithorax, occasionally associated with polyostotic fibrous dysplasia. Note asymmetry of face, indicating facial bone involvement.

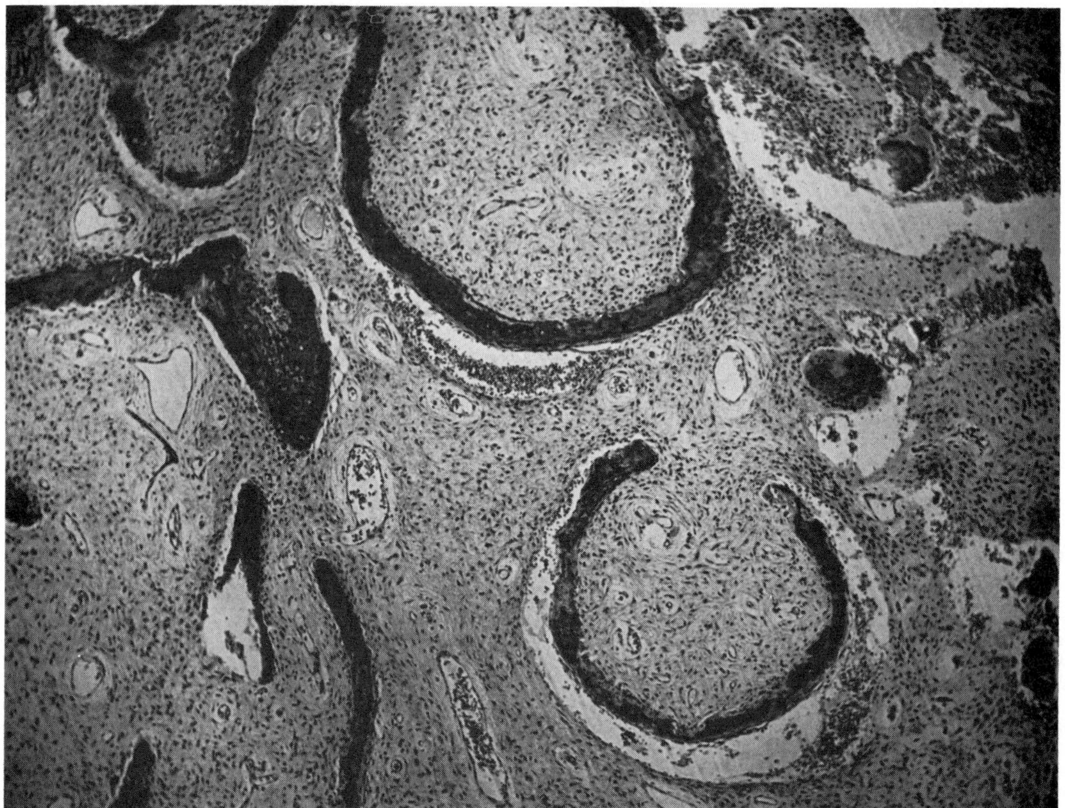

Figure 9–9. Fibrous dysplasia. Fibrous connective tissue and dysplastic bone formation are present. Slender, elongated curlicues form so-called "alphabet soup."

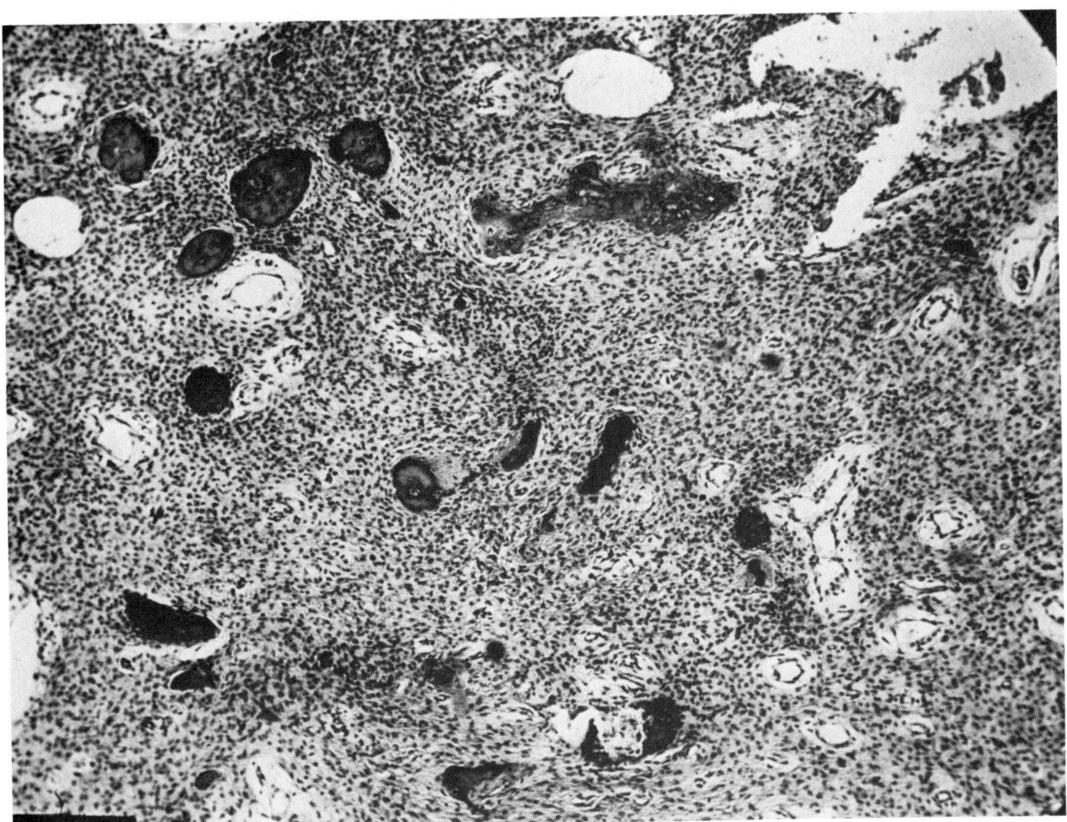

Figure 9–10. Fibrous dysplasia. Fibrous connective tissue with formation of small circular fragments of bone rather than the elongated curlicues. These smaller bone fragments are more commonly seen in the flat bones.

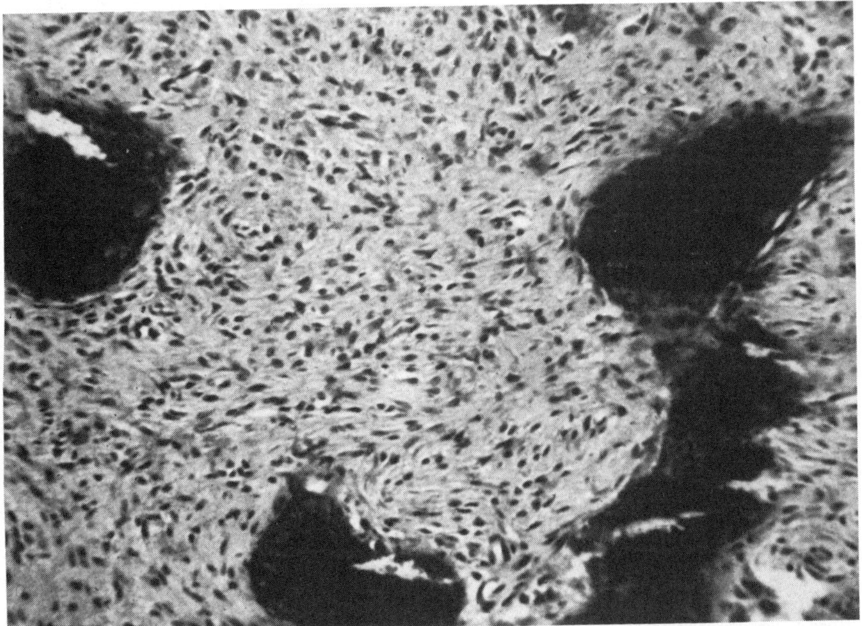

Figure 9–11. Fibrous dysplasia. Higher magnification in relatively early cellular lesion. Despite the cellularity, the fibrous connective tissue consists of spindled cells with little pleomorphism or mitotic activity. The differential diagnosis must include well-differentiated intraosseous osteosarcoma.

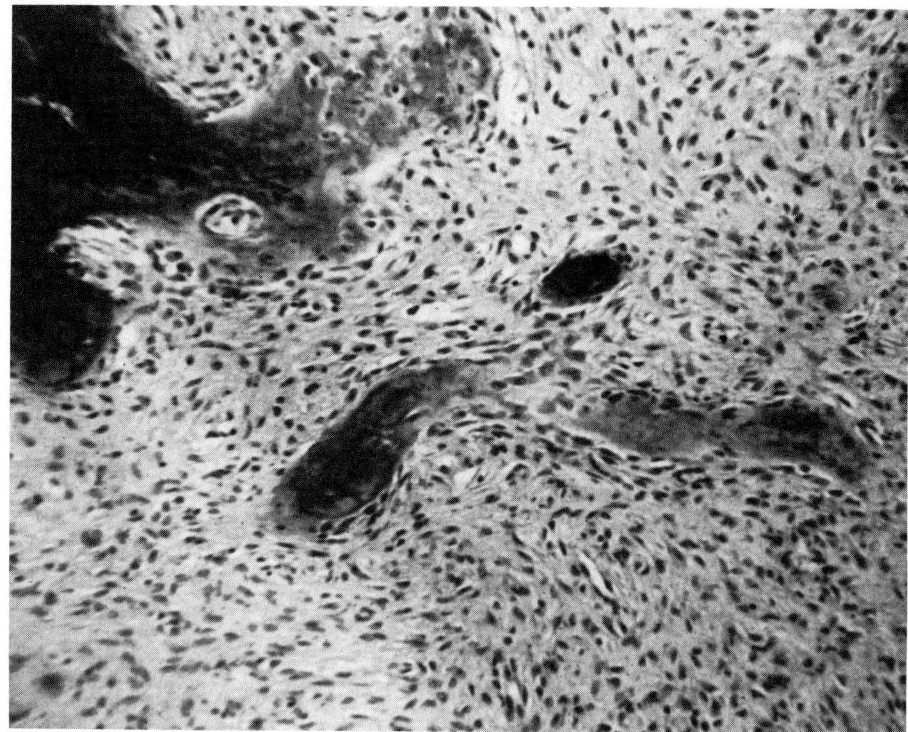

Figure 9–12. Fibrous dysplasia. Dysplastic bone formation from connective tissue. Osteoblasts are not identifiable. The bone that is formed consists of relatively immature woven bone and does not mature to form osteonal structures.

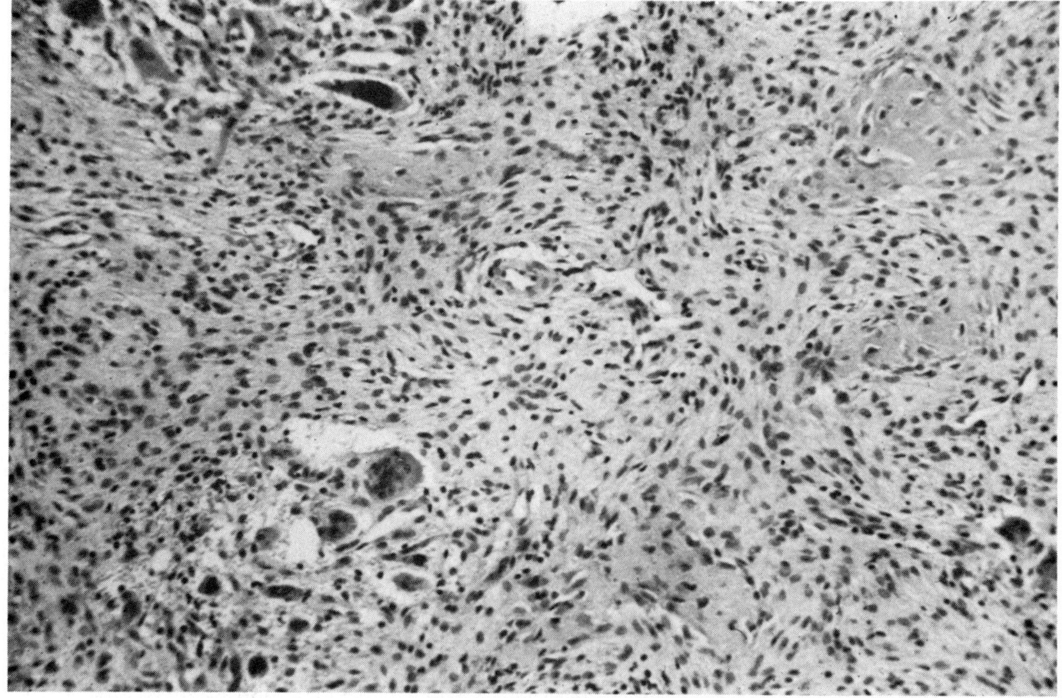

Figure 9–13. Fibrous dysplasia. Giant cells may be present in portions of the lesion.

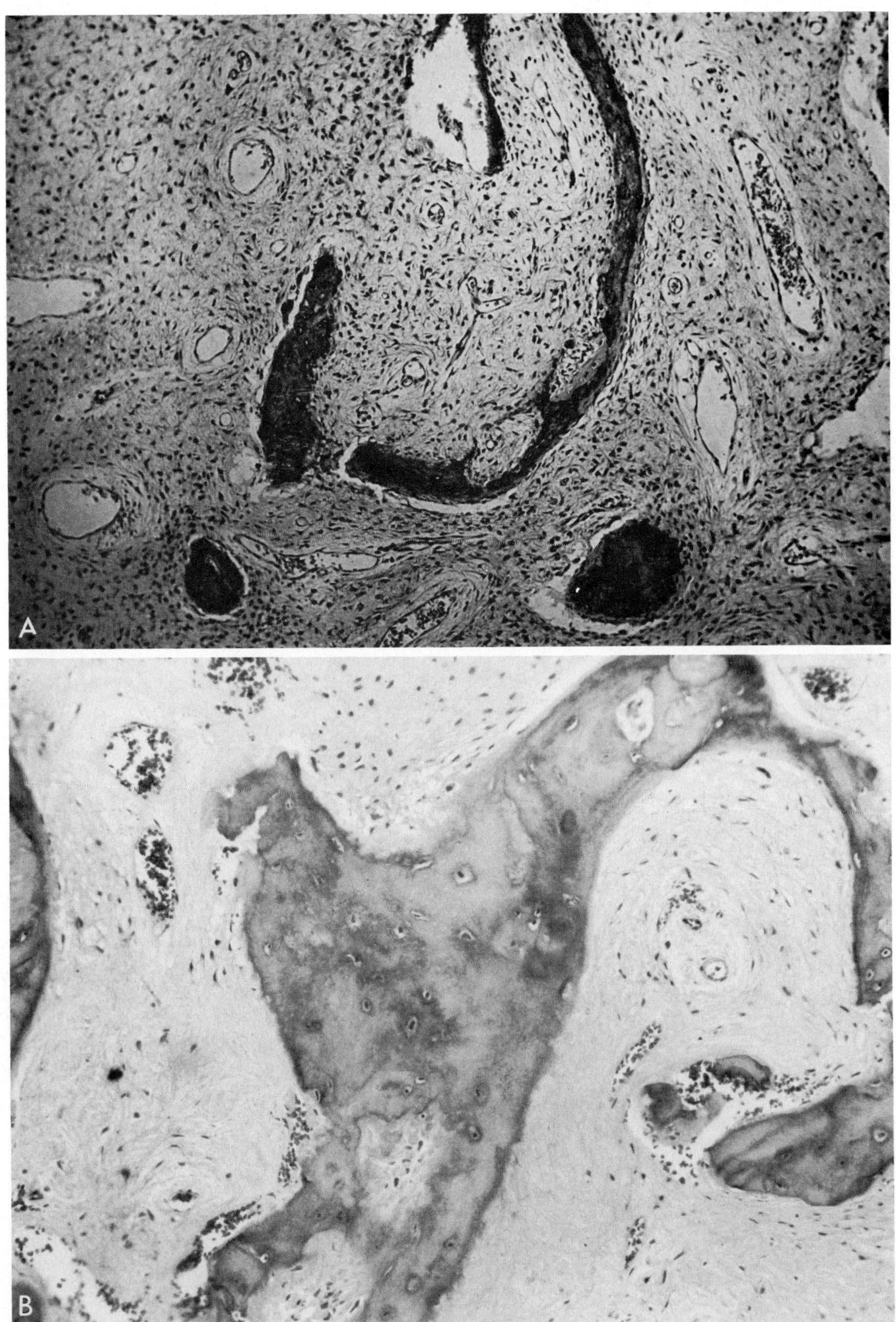

Figure 9–14. Fibrous dysplasia. Histologic sections of older lesions, which exhibit progressively less cellularity with age. A biopsy of a lesion from a 70-year-old patient is shown in *B* (Ruth et al., 1982).

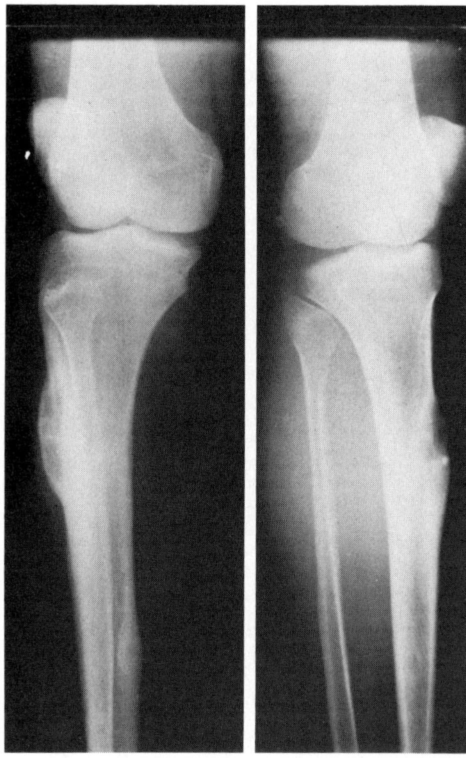

Figure 9–15. Cortical fibrous dysplasia. Radiographs of tibia exhibiting a lytic defect localized to the diaphyseal portion of the cortex. The lesion is sharply circumscribed, with some reactive bone formation at each margin.

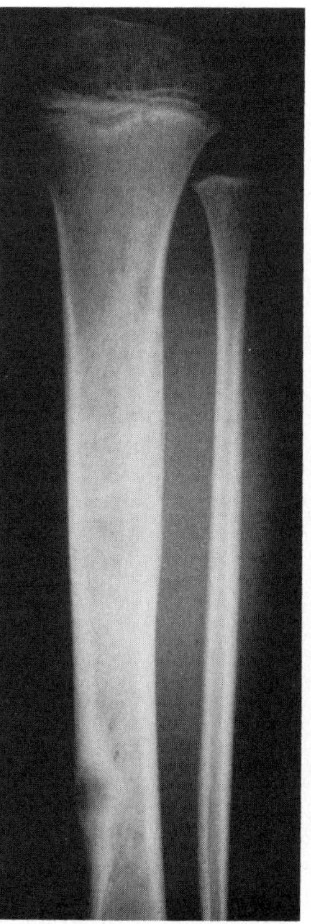

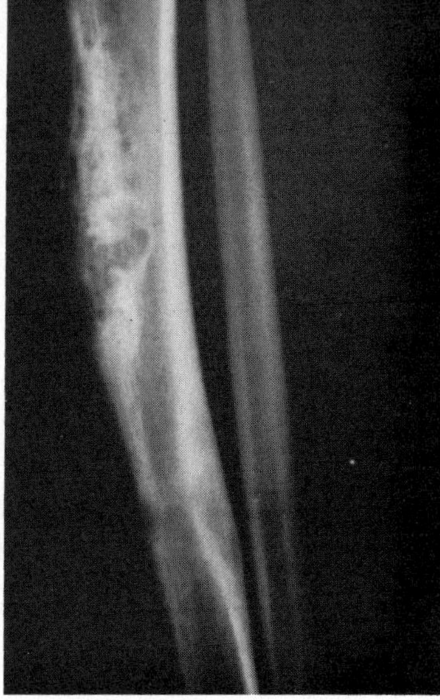

Figure 9–16. Cortical fibrous dysplasia. Radiograph of patient with cortical fibrous dysplasia in the metaphyseal-diaphyseal cortex. Note the expansion of the external and endosteal cortical surface. The defect is sharply circumscribed, lytic and intracortical.

Figure 9–17. Cortical fibrous dysplasia. Radiograph of a patient with more advanced intracortical fibrous dysplasia. Multiple lesions are present on both cortical surfaces. The pattern of destruction indicates a more aggressive tumor. The radiographic appearance of the lesion is difficult to differentiate from that of adamantinoma of long bone. The lesions are intracortical, and expansion of the endosteal surface is visible in both lesions.

Figure 9–16   Figure 9–17

CORTICAL FIBROUS DYSPLASIA (OSSIFYING FIBROMA OF LONG BONE, INTRACORTICAL FIBROUS DYSPLASIA)

Cortical fibrous dysplasia is characterized by the intracortical location of the dysplastic process. A characteristic osteoblastic seam is seen lining the trabeculae of bone (Fig. 9–21). Bony trabeculae and fibrous tissue are otherwise similar to those found in fibrous dysplasia. The association of this lesion with adamantinoma of long bone has been described (Markel, 1978; Johnson L. C., personal communication).

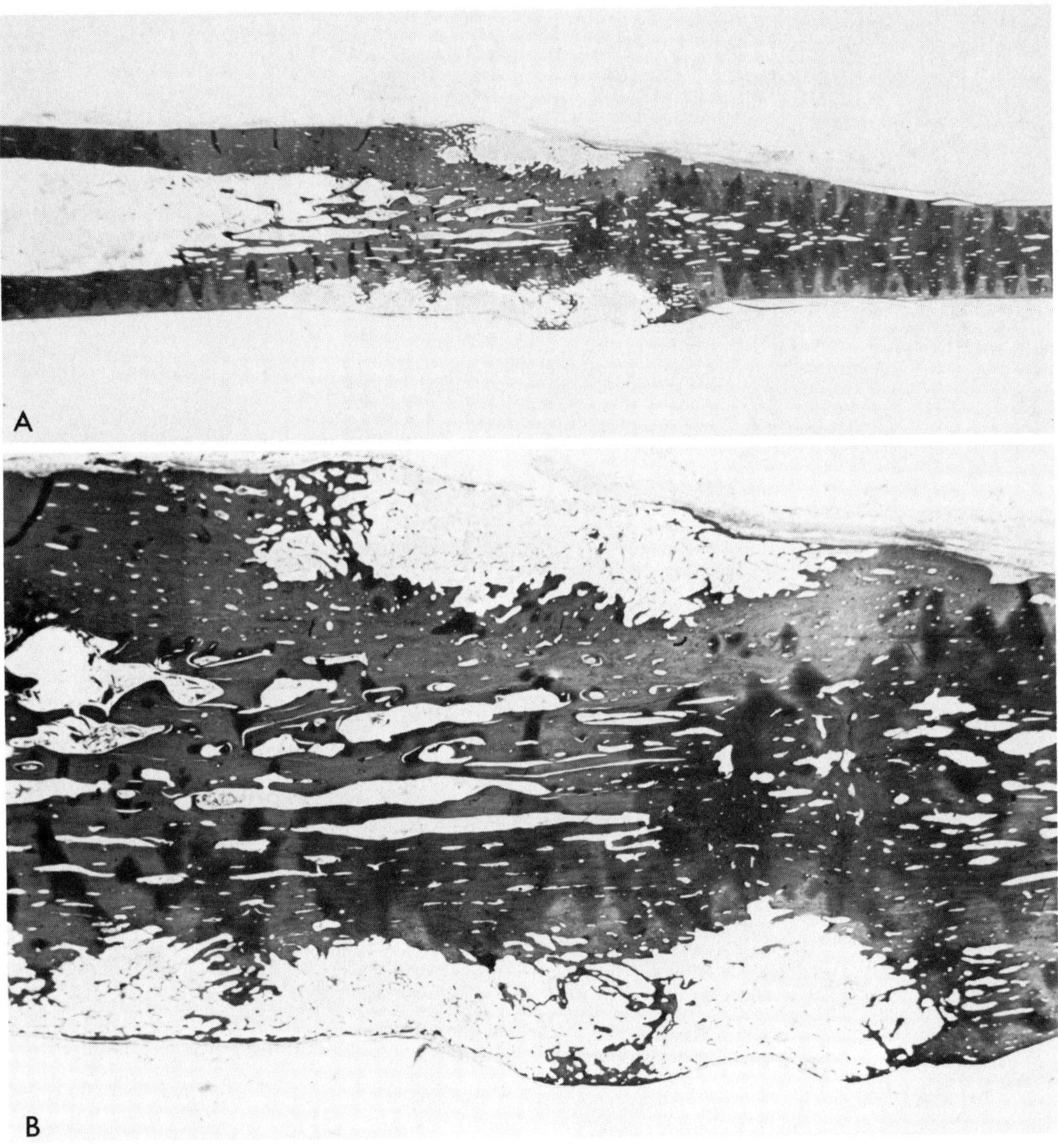

Figure 9–18. Cortical fibrous dysplasia. Low *(A)* and higher *(B)* magnification of macrosection of the lesion shown in Figure 9–17. Note fibrous replacement of the cortex on both surfaces and the reactive sclerosis of the medullary cavity in response to the removal of cortical bone.

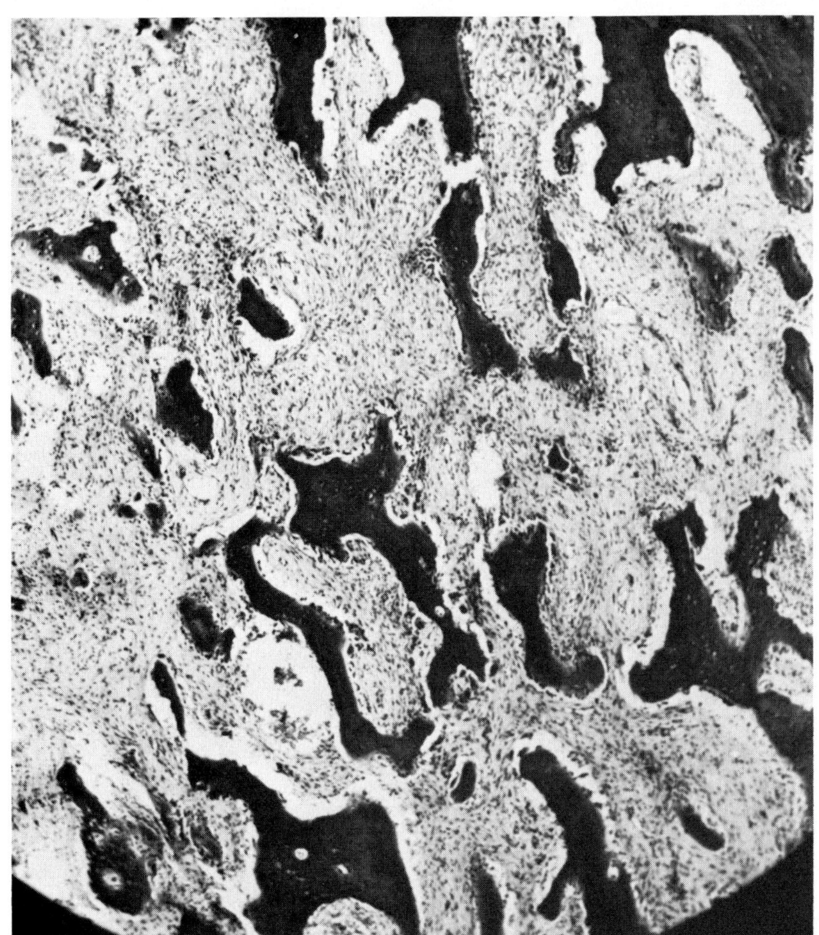

Figure 9–19. Cortical fibrous dysplasia. Fibrous replacement of bone with formation of trabeculae.

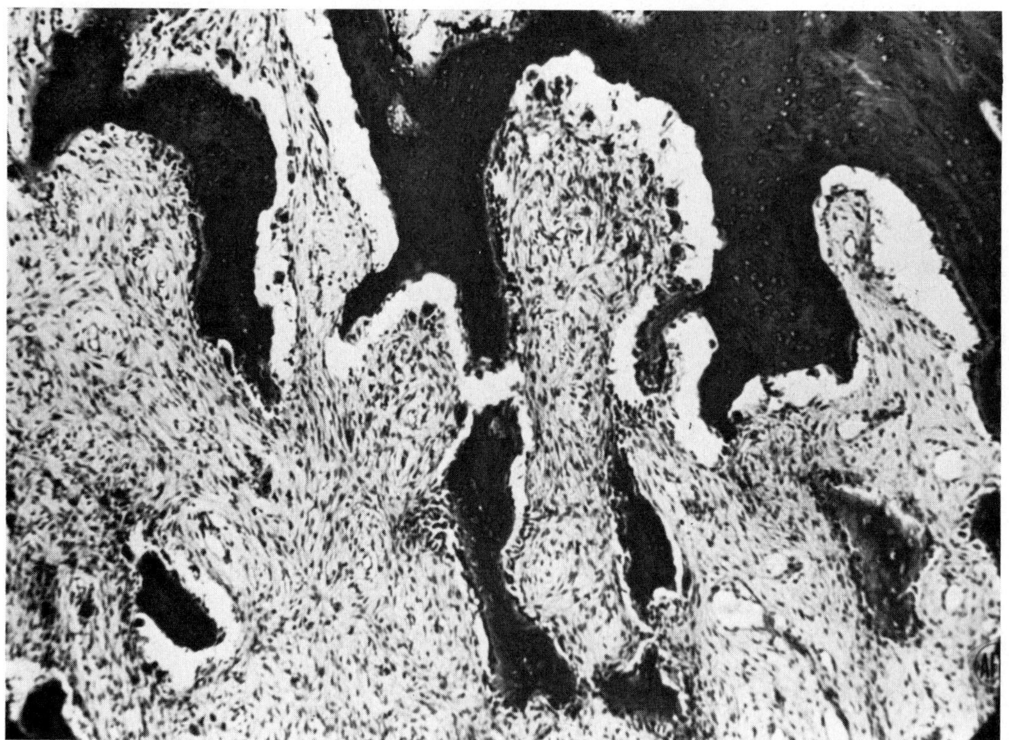

Figure 9–20. Cortical fibrous dysplasia. Slightly higher magnification exhibiting fibrous replacement of bone, osteoblasts, and osteoclasts. There is superficial similarity to intramedullary fibrous dysplasia as well as Paget's disease of bone.

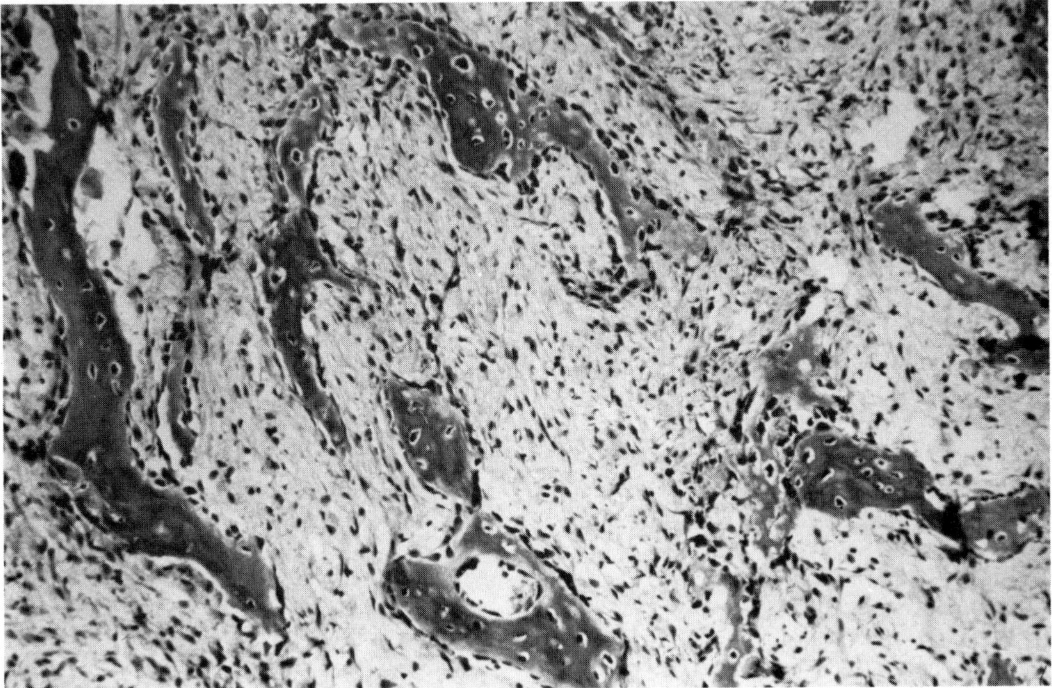

Figure 9–21. Cortical fibrous dysplasia. Fibrous replacement of bone and bone formation. Note the prominent rim of osteoblasts forming trabeculae. This prominence is not present in the usual intramedullary fibrous dysplasia.

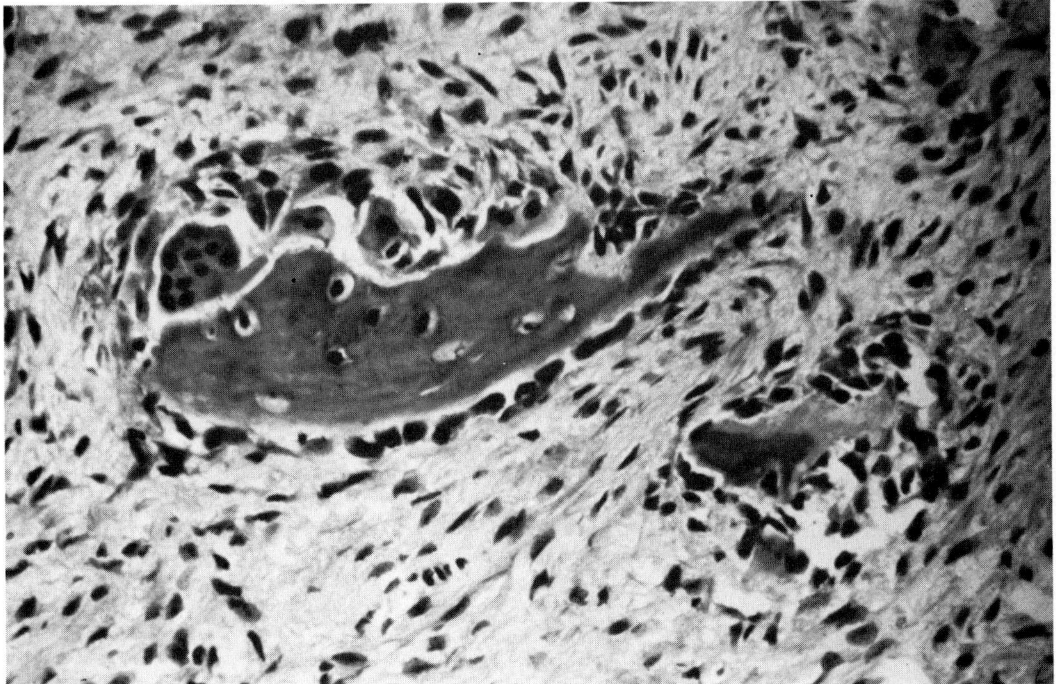

Figure 9–22. Cortical fibrous dysplasia. Prominent seam of osteoblasts and osteoclasts forming and removing trabeculae of bone. The differential diagnosis must include the lytic phase of Paget's disease.

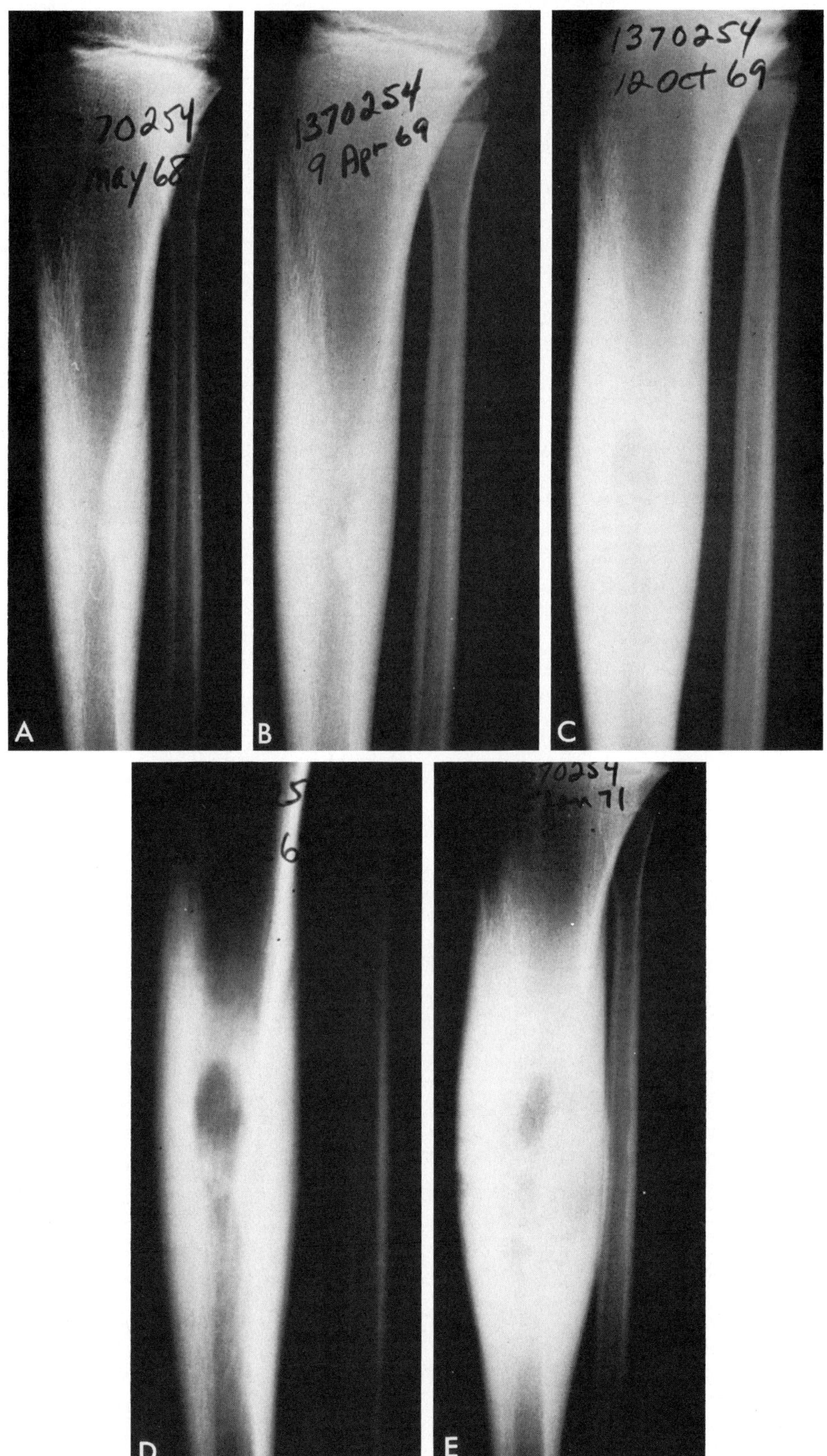

Figure 9–23. Adamantinoma. Progressive radiographic appearance of adamantinoma followed for a period of 2 years. The lesion is characteristically located in the diaphyseal portion of the tibia. It involves the cortex as well as the medullary portion of bone. There is no associated periosteal reaction, indicating a moderate rate of growth.

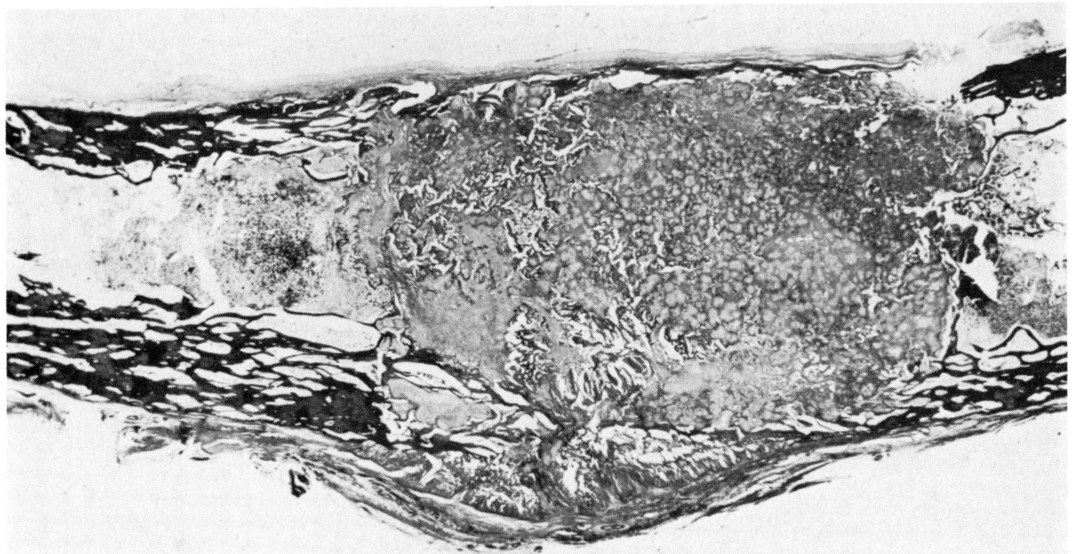

Figure 9–24. Adamantinoma. Macrospecimen of lesion shown in Figure 9–23. The tumor involves both cortical margins and the medullary cavity, and there is erosion of one cortical surface.

ADAMANTINOMA OF LONG BONE

Adamantinoma of long bone is an extremely rare tumor, most often localized in the tibia and composed of a biphasic histologic pattern, consisting of epithelioid clusters and spindled stroma. The lesion is of intermediate malignancy, and exhibits a moderately aggressive radiologic appearance. The adamantinoma is almost always diaphyseal in location, with indistinct margins, some expansion of the cortex, and no identifiable calcification of matrix. Periosteal reactions are rare, indicating slow progression of the lesion (Unni et al., 1974).

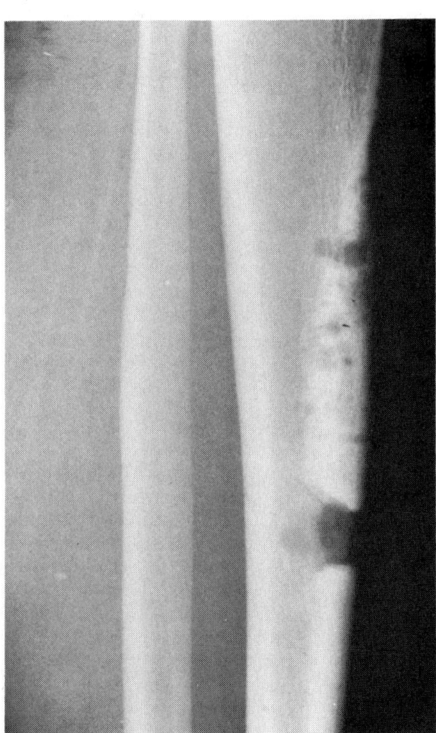

Figure 9–25. Adamantinoma. Radiograph of adamantinoma of long bone. The larger distal defect represents biopsy site, and the remainder of the lytic and sclerotic lesions represent the adamantinoma. Note the similarity to cortical fibrous dysplasia (Fig. 9–17).

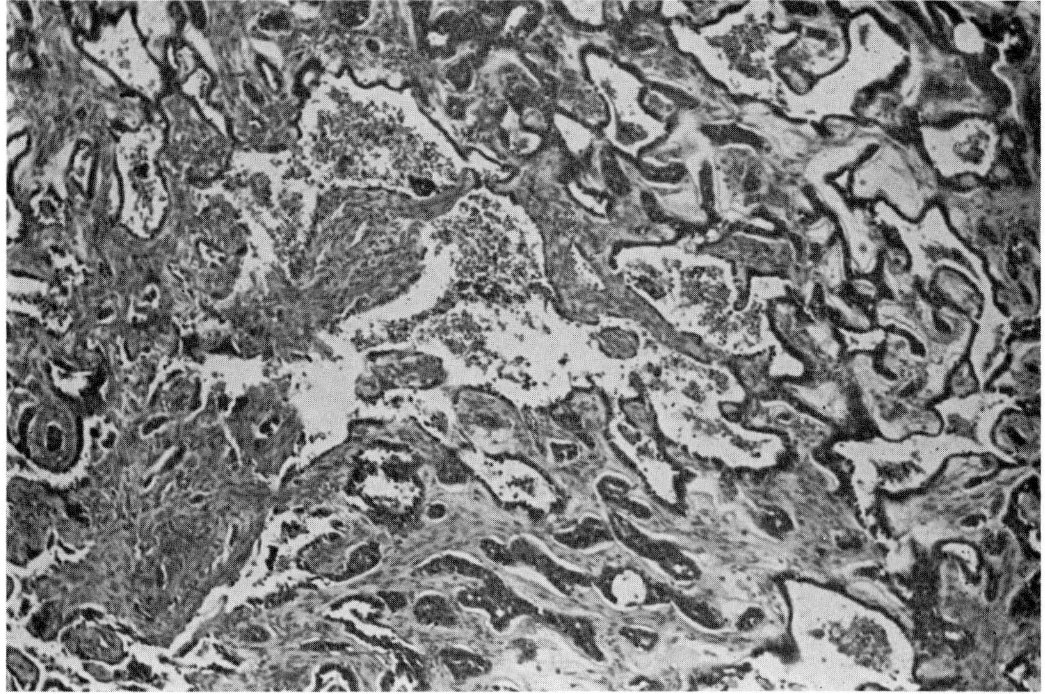

Figure 9–26. Adamantinoma. Section of the adamantinoma of a long bone illustrating the characteristic biphasic pattern. The tumor is composed of both fibrous and epithelioid components. Bone formation is absent.

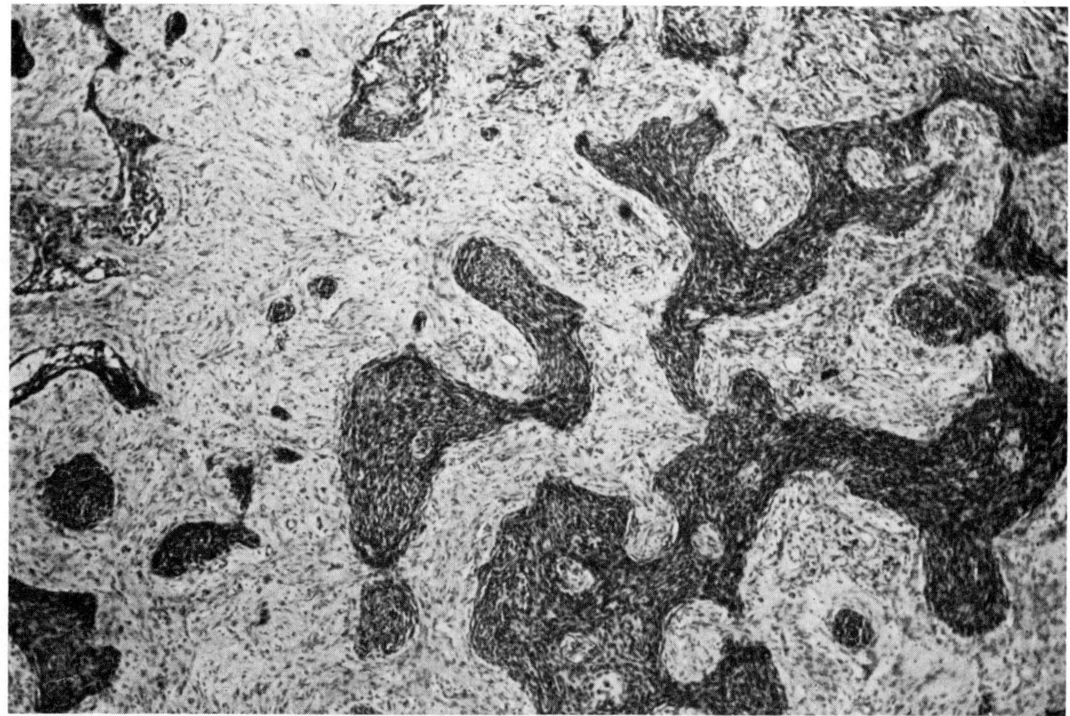

Figure 9–27. Adamantinoma. Characteristic biphasic pattern of adamantinoma with more prominent epithelioid component.

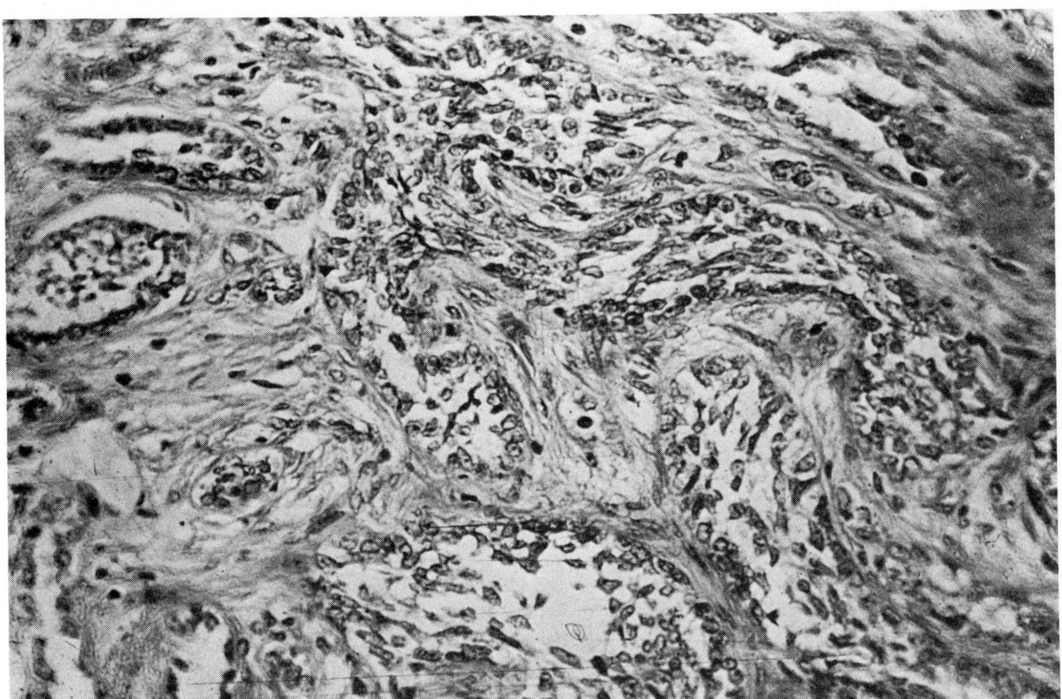

Figure 9–28. Adamantinoma. Higher magnification exhibiting the biphasic pattern. The fibrous component surrounds spaces lined by scattered cells of the epithelioid component. It has been suggested that the slits in the epithelioid component represent primitive vascular spaces.

NONOSSIFYING FIBROMA OF BONE (FIBROXANTHOMA OF BONE, FIBROUS CORTICAL DEFECT)

The nonossifying fibroma of bone is a very common, sharply circumscribed lesion that always arises in the metaphysis. It is eccentrically located in the bone and is histologically identical with the "fibrous cortical defect," but it has no relationship to the cortical desmoid (see Chap. 3, p. 93). The lesion may start as a cortical lesion, but as the cortex extends laterally during growth the lesion remains, located in the metaphyseal portion of the cancellous bone. The eccentric location on one side of bone is characteristic but is not always identifiable in some of the thinner bones, particularly fibula or rib. There is almost invariably a clear zone between the nonossifying fibroma and the epiphyseal growth plate. The gross appearance of the lesion is yellow because numerous xanthoma cells are present. This appearance contrasts with that of fibrous dysplasia, which is white. There may also be areas of red or brown discoloration, indicating recent or more remote hemorrhage.

The histologic pattern shows a whorled spindle-cell pattern with fibrous tissue and numerous xanthoma cells. Occasional giant cells are seen within the nonossifying fibroma; giant cells may be present in any lesion of bone. The lesion is relatively stable, with sharp demarcation apparent at the growing edge. The rind is caused by sclerotic bone at the margin of the growing edge. The lesion may expand the cortex, with buttress formation. Periosteal reactions are rare. However, pathologic fractures through a nonossifying fibroma are common, and the resultant mixture of the fibrous stroma and callus may cause difficulties in diagnosis (Arata et al., 1981).

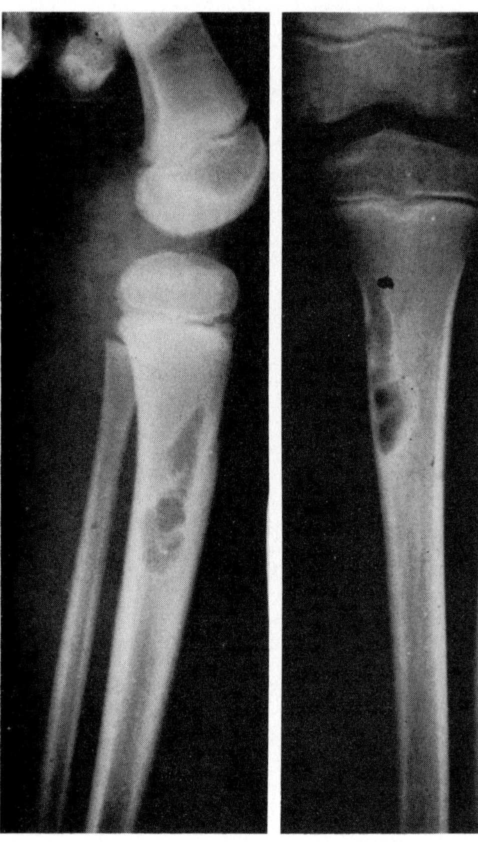

Figure 9–29. Nonossifying fibroma. Radiographs of tibia containing a nonossifying fibroma. Eccentric location in the metaphysis, lytic defect with sharply circumscribed sclerotic rim, and separation from the epiphyseal growth plate are characteristics that make the radiographic diagnosis almost absolute.

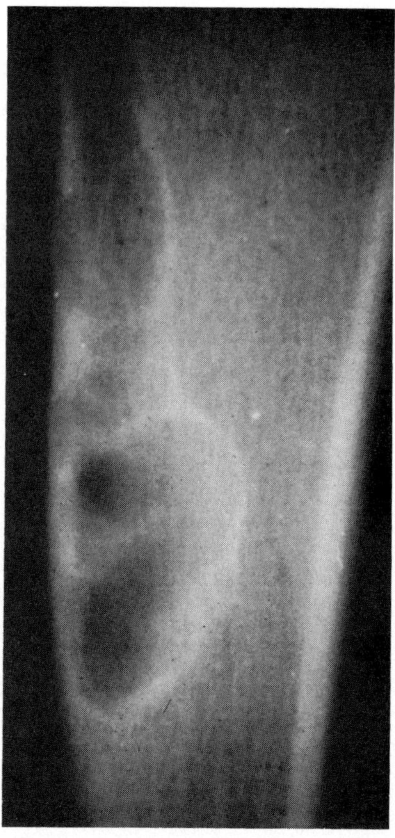

Figure 9–30. Nonossifying fibroma. Closer view of above illustrating the sharply circumscribed lytic defect with sclerotic rim about the lesion. These features indicate a benign process. The metaphyseal location, at some distance from the growth plate, is characteristic of nonossifying fibroma.

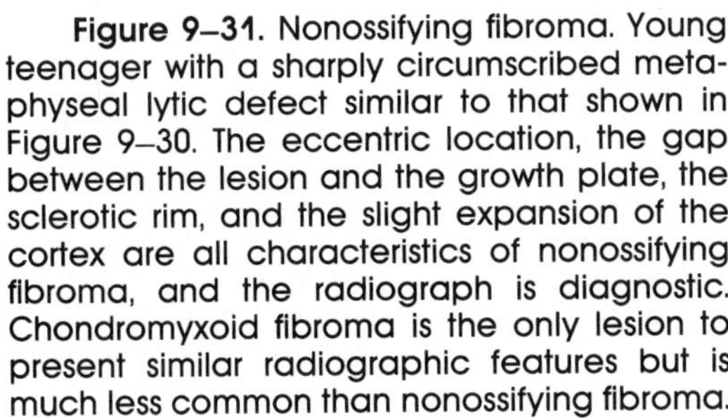

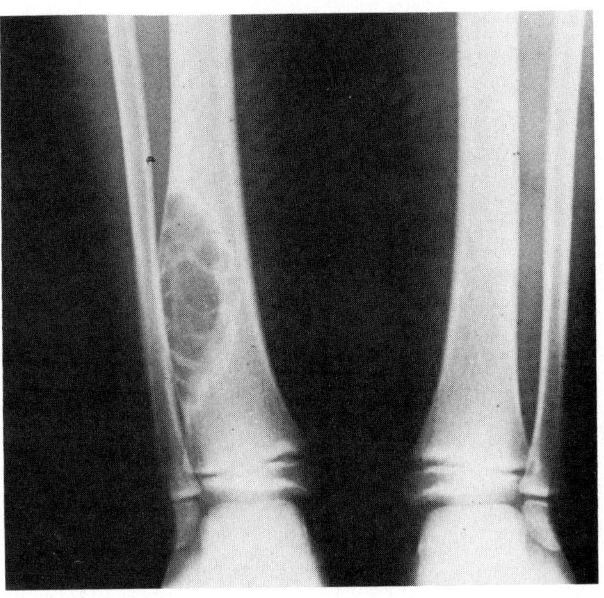

Figure 9–31. Nonossifying fibroma. Young teenager with a sharply circumscribed metaphyseal lytic defect similar to that shown in Figure 9–30. The eccentric location, the gap between the lesion and the growth plate, the sclerotic rim, and the slight expansion of the cortex are all characteristics of nonossifying fibroma, and the radiograph is diagnostic. Chondromyxoid fibroma is the only lesion to present similar radiographic features but is much less common than nonossifying fibroma.

One can easily ascertain the diagnosis radiographically by noting the typical metaphyseal lesion, sharply circumscribed, eccentric, often with a radiographic "rind," as opposed to the more oval-shaped lesion of fibrous dysplasia, which usually involves the entire diameter of the bone. The nonossifying fibroma may heal by ossifying from its diaphyseal end until the entire lesion is eventually ossified. Remodeling causes the lesion to merge into the normal bone structure.

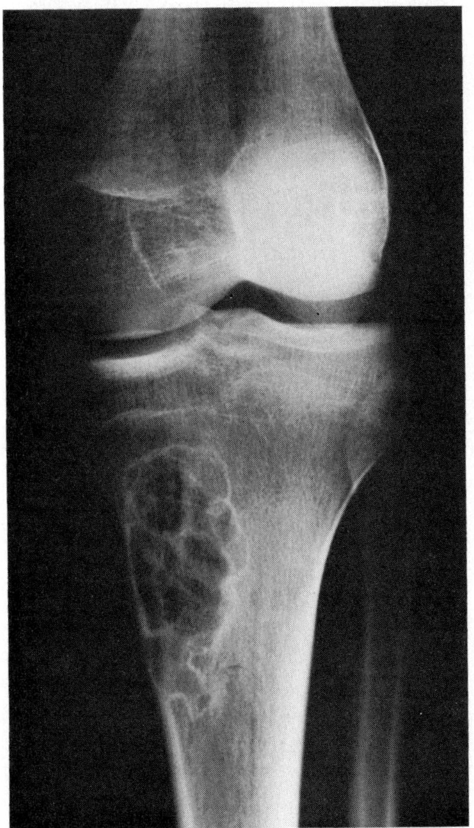

Figure 9–32. Nonossifying fibroma. The lesion is in the tibia of a 16-year-old girl who experienced pain after physical exertion. Note the circumscribed eccentric lytic defect with the sclerotic rim. The soap-bubble appearance is due to ridges on the inner surface of the cortex and the bony "rind." The size of this and the preceding lesion makes surgical removal advisable. If the lesion extends across more than 50 per cent of the diameter of the metaphysis, the danger of pathologic fracture should be considered, and prophylactic curettage is recommended.

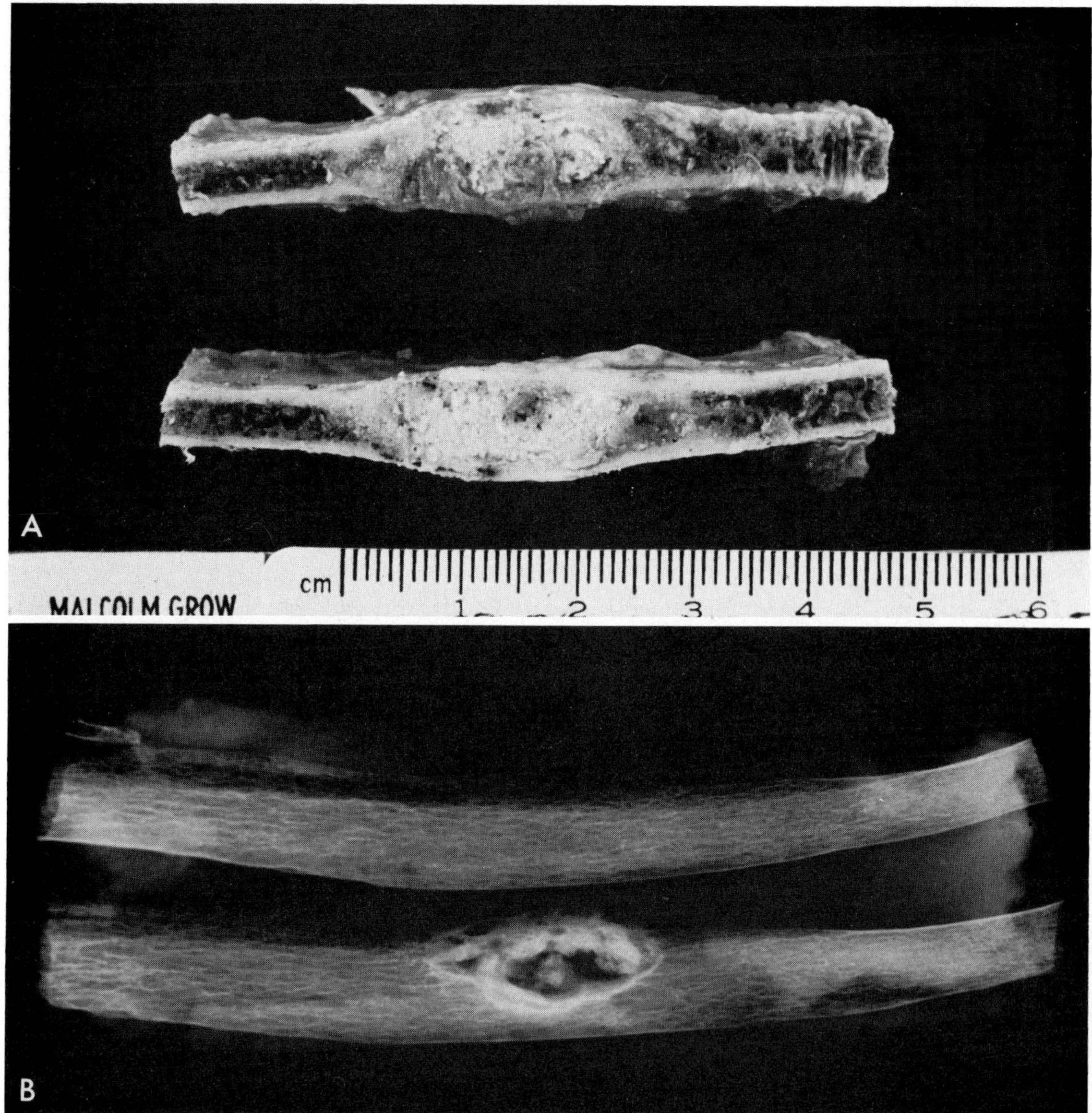

Figure 9–33. Nonossifying fibroma. Sharply circumscribed eccentric lesion in the rib of a patient in his mid thirties; incidental finding on a routine chest film. Note sclerosis with calcification. The older lesions of nonossifying fibroma exhibit secondary ossification. On gross examination, the yellow appearance of the lesion is characteristic and reflects the extensive xanthomatous content.

The lesions are so common and so readily diagnosed on radiographic grounds alone that they can be safely watched without therapy. Intervention is necessary when there is danger of pathologic fracture. As a rule, pathologic fracture is a realistic risk when more than 50 per cent of the cross-sectional diameter of the bone is involved. Simple curettage to include the sclerotic "rind" is adequate therapy.

Malignant transformation of nonossifying fibroma of bone is rarely described (Unni and Dahlin, 1979) but may be more common than is generally appreciated (Fig. 9–94). The malignant counterpart is either fibrosarcoma or malignant fibrous histiocytoma of bone. It is difficult to document pre-existing benign components.

Figure 9–34. Nonossifying fibroma. Note the focal matrix calcification in the diaphyseal portion of the otherwise typical nonossifying fibroma. Radiographic sclerosis and secondary ossification constitute the natural sequence of events in this lesion. Remodeling of the ossified material results in ultimate disappearance of the lesion.

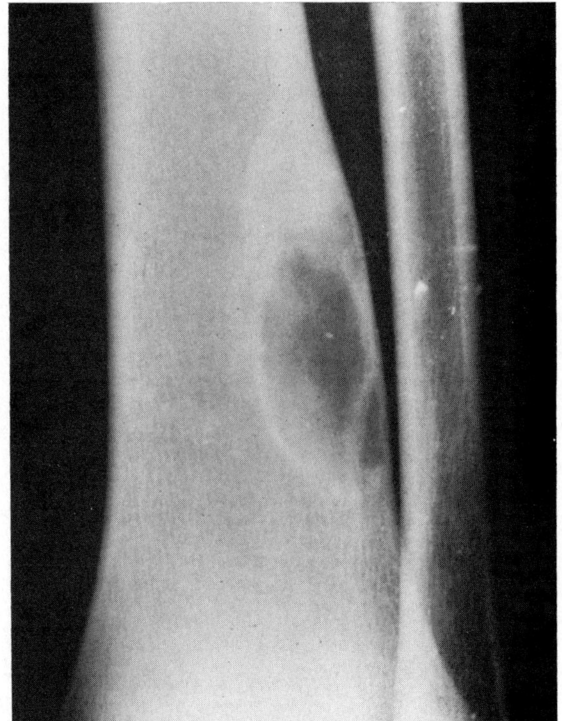

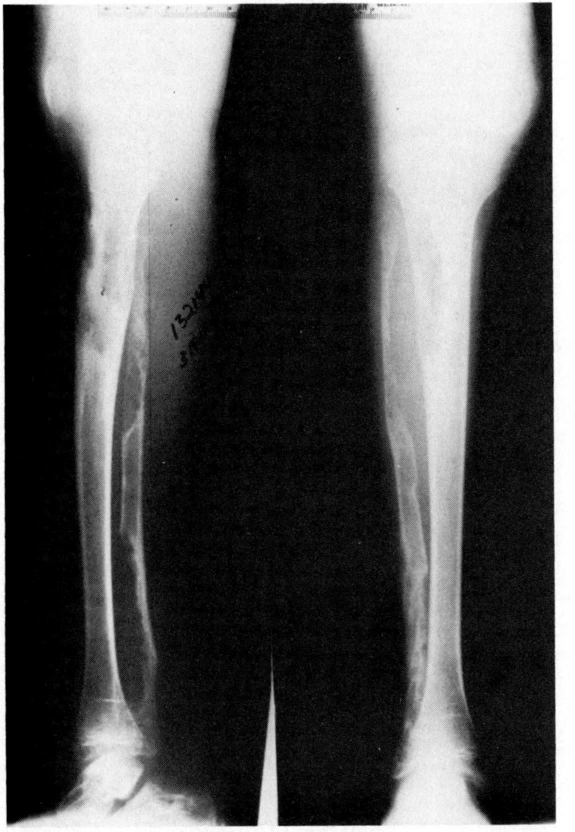

Figure 9–35. Nonossifying fibroma. On rare occasions, multiple nonossifying fibromas occur as part of a disseminated anomaly.

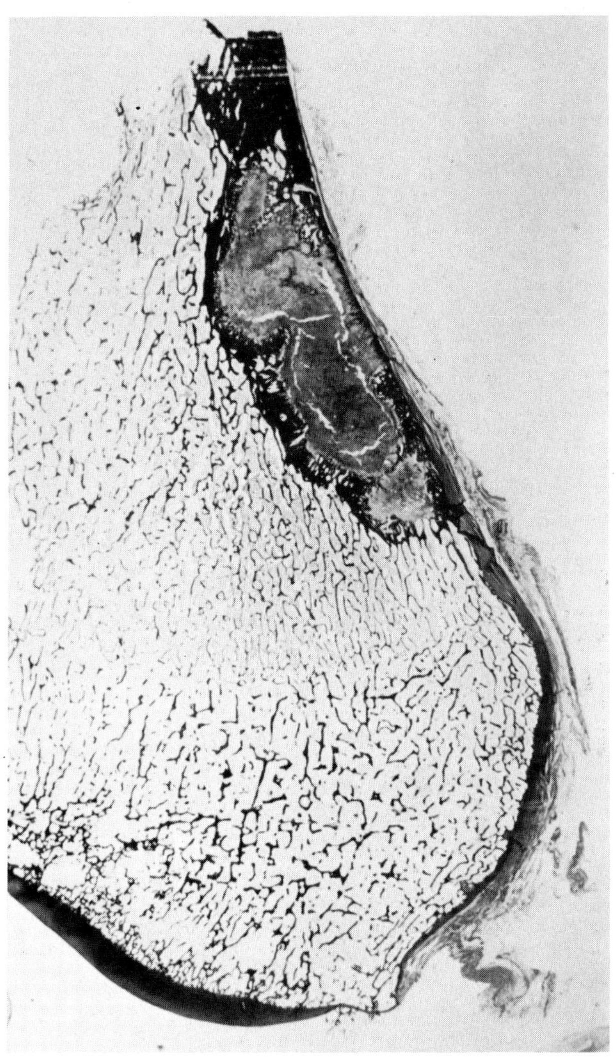

Figure 9–36. Nonossifying fibroma. Macrosection of a lesion with characteristic location in the metaphyseal portion of bone. Note the sclerotic rim around the lesion.

Lesions in cranial bones have the tendency for greater calcification and ossification at an earlier age. It is difficult to differentiate fibrous osteoma and ossifying fibroma of skull bones from fibrous dysplasia or the nonossifying fibroma of long bone. It is possible that these lesions are simply expressions of the same disease process in the bones of the skull, with the tendency for ossification greater at an earlier stage of the lesion. Fibrous dysplasia of the jaw is not uncommon; leontiasis ossea of the facial bones is an expression of multiple nonossifying fibromas in the skull bones, and the osteomas that may arise in the skull may or may not be associated with variable degrees of fibrous proliferation, depending on the nature of the disease process. There is no point in differentiating these lesions of the skull from nonossifying fibroma and fibrous dysplasia of the axial skeleton. The astute orthopaedic surgeon, however, should be aware of the differences of opinion regarding the etiology of these lesions, particularly in the dental profession. Use of the term "osteoma" is justified only when the entire lesion consists of nothing but bone. All other lesions are probably examples of either nonossifying fibroma with secondary calcification and ossification or fibrous dysplasia with extensive osseous metaplasia.

Text continued on page 329

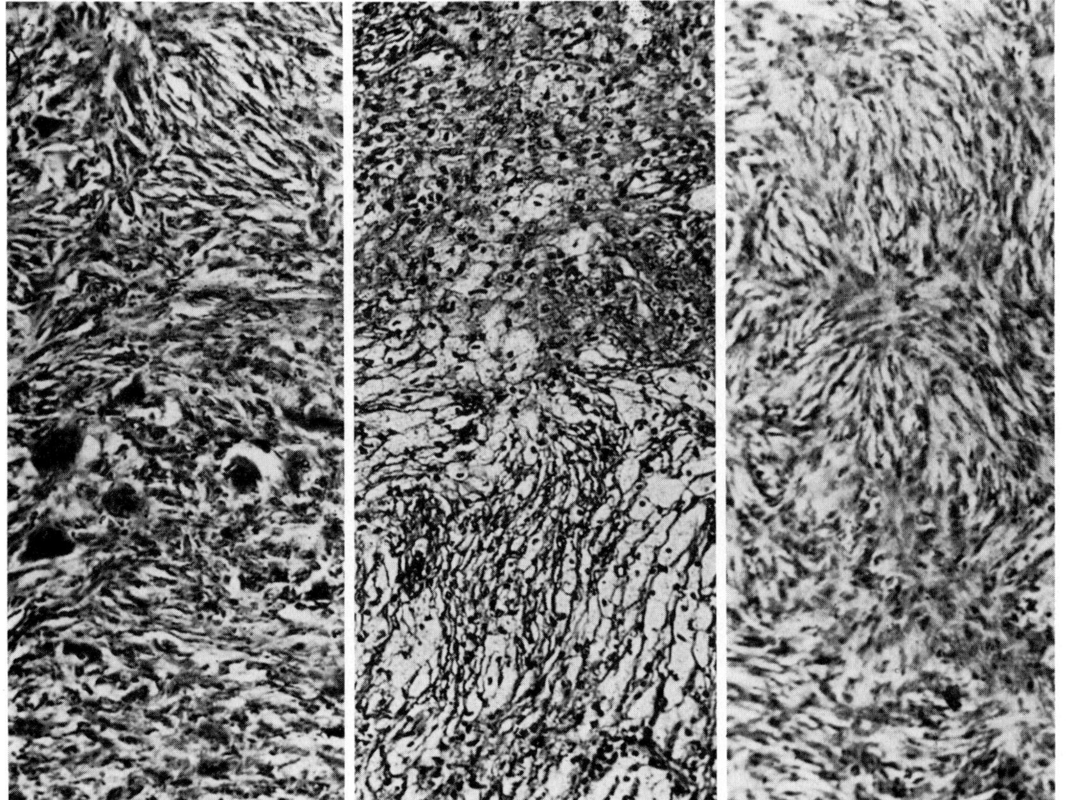

Figure 9–37. Nonossifying fibroma. The characteristic histologic picture includes a storiform fibrous pattern with a tendency toward cartwheel formation; xanthoma cells and occasional giant cells may be present.

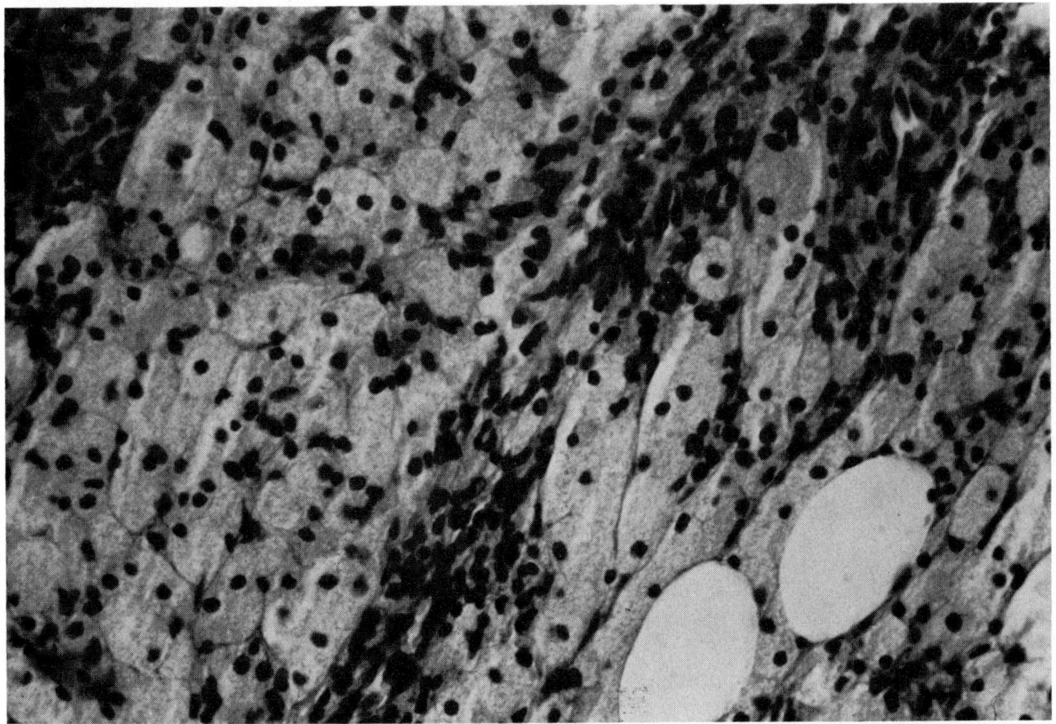

Figure 9–38. Nonossifying fibroma. The xanthomatous component is always present. Xanthoma cells are characterized by a fine-bubble pattern. The fat is usually dissolved in the organic solvents used in tissue processing, leaving a fine, granular to clear cytoplasm. The presence of fat in the xanthoma cell gives the lesion its characteristic yellow appearance. The nuclei are small and dark, and they are located centrally within the cell.

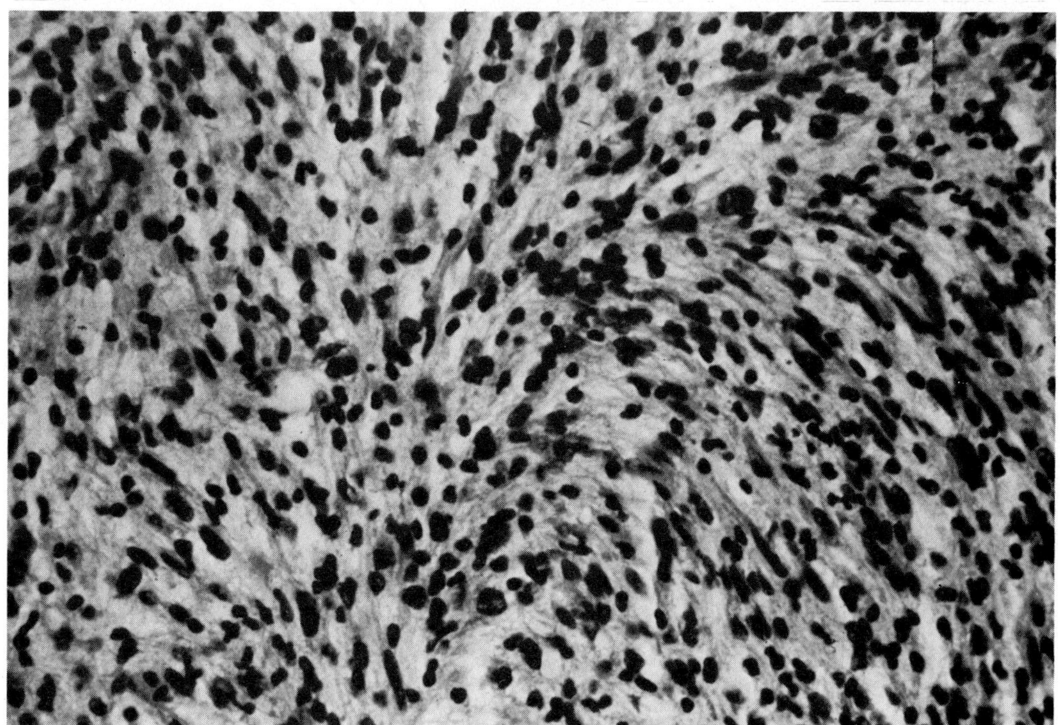

Figure 9–39. Nonossifying fibroma. Histologic appearance of lesion illustrated in Figure 9–32. The spindle-cell component may be cellular and somewhat plump, but despite the moderate pleomorphism the lesion is benign. Note the typical whorled pattern.

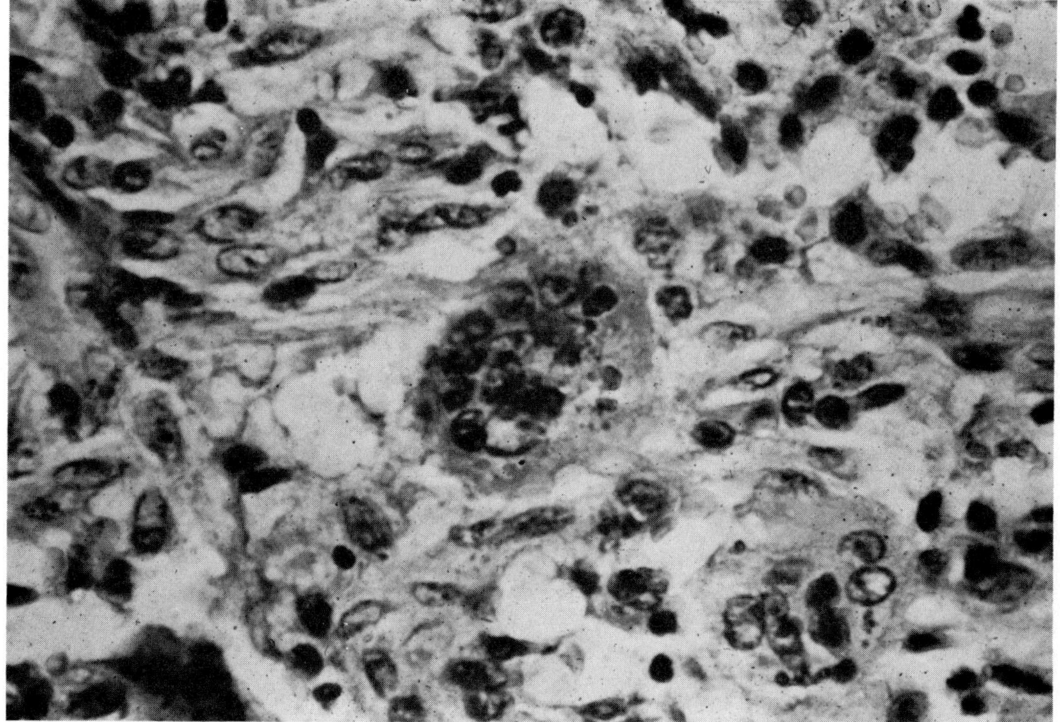

Figure 9–40. Nonossifying fibroma. Giant cells are occasionally encountered in nonossifying fibroma. Note the difference between the giant cell and the stromal cell in this lesion, as opposed to their similarity in the bona fide giant cell tumor (see Fig. 9–277).

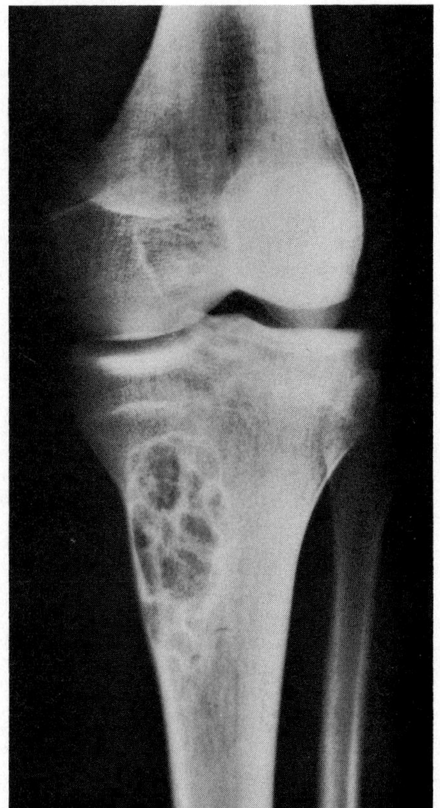

Figure 9–41. Nonossifying fibroma. Older patient with characteristic radiographic appearance of nonossifying fibroma in the tibia. Note sclerosis in the distal portion of the lesion. The oldest portion (distal) ossifies first.

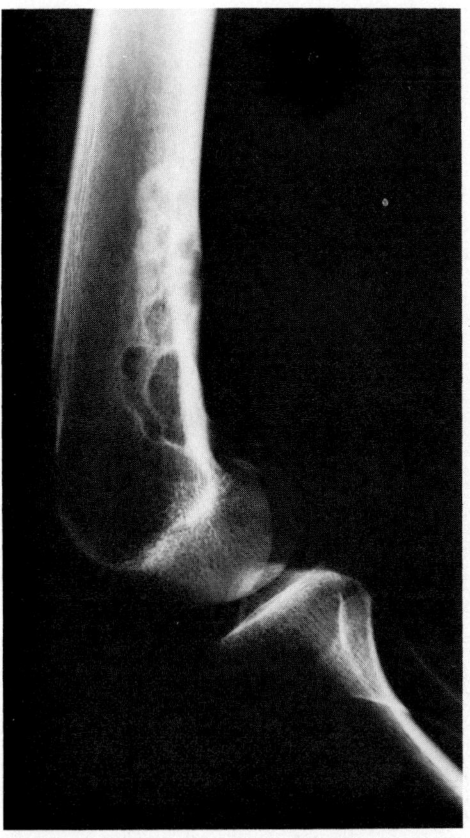

Figure 9–42. Nonossifying fibroma. Similar characteristic nonossifying fibroma in older patient, distal femur. Note the extensive ossification in the proximal (older) portion of the lesion.

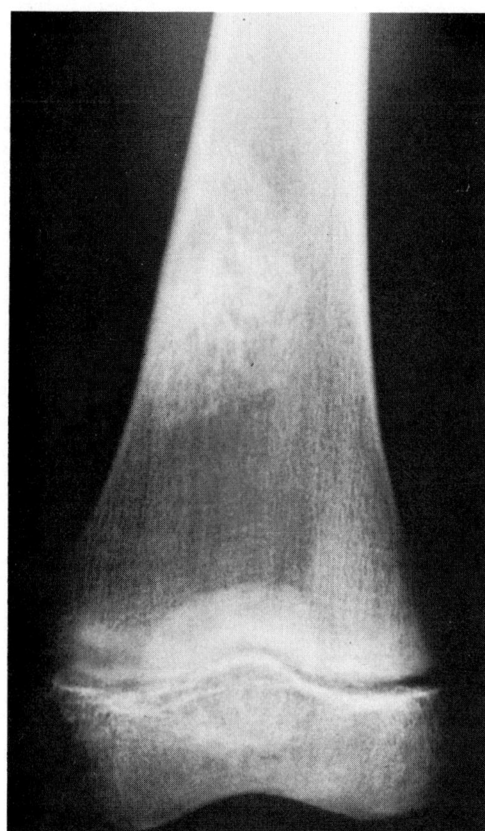

Figure 9–43. Nonossifying fibroma. Radiographic appearance of a fully ossified lesion in the characteristic location, lower femur.

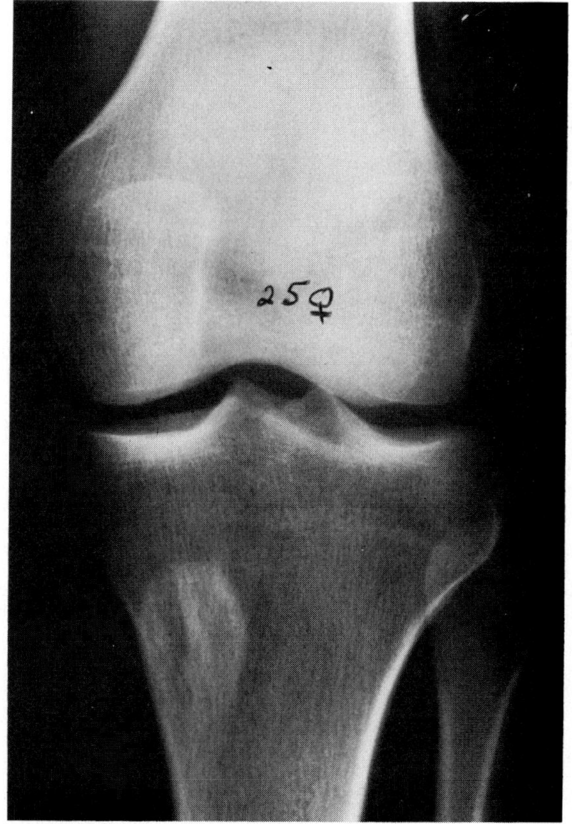

Figure 9–44. Nonossifying fibroma. Radiograph of similar complete ossification. Smaller lesions are remodeled and ultimately blend with the cortical and medullary bone, leading to their "disappearance."

UNICAMERAL BONE CYST

The simple unicameral bone cyst is a fluid-filled cavity located in the metaphyseal portion of the growing long bone. The lining of the cyst consists of fibrous connective tissue with a mesothelial surface and a layer of reactive bone reinforcing the cavity margin. Multiple smaller spaces are often noted at the periphery of the larger central cyst. These are embedded in the adjacent connective tissue, are similarly lined by single-layered flattened mesothelium, and are the source of the "recurrent" cysts if not removed at the time of excision. The fibrous lining of the cyst is capable of metaplasia into osseous structures (cementum-like product), a change that suggests fibrous dysplasia. Myxoid tissue, giant cells, and cholesterol clefts may be present, and tissue from the cyst lining may occasionally become malignant (Johnson et al., 1962).

The cysts are usually metaphyseal in location. The lesion is radiolucent, with minimal evidence of matrix formation. At the time of its origin, the cyst involves the full width of the long bone, abutting against the epiphysis, occasionally with expansion of the cortex. As the lesion matures, the epiphyseal growth plate may grow away from the cysts, leaving it in a metaphyseal or even diaphyseal location. Although thickened

Text continued on page 337

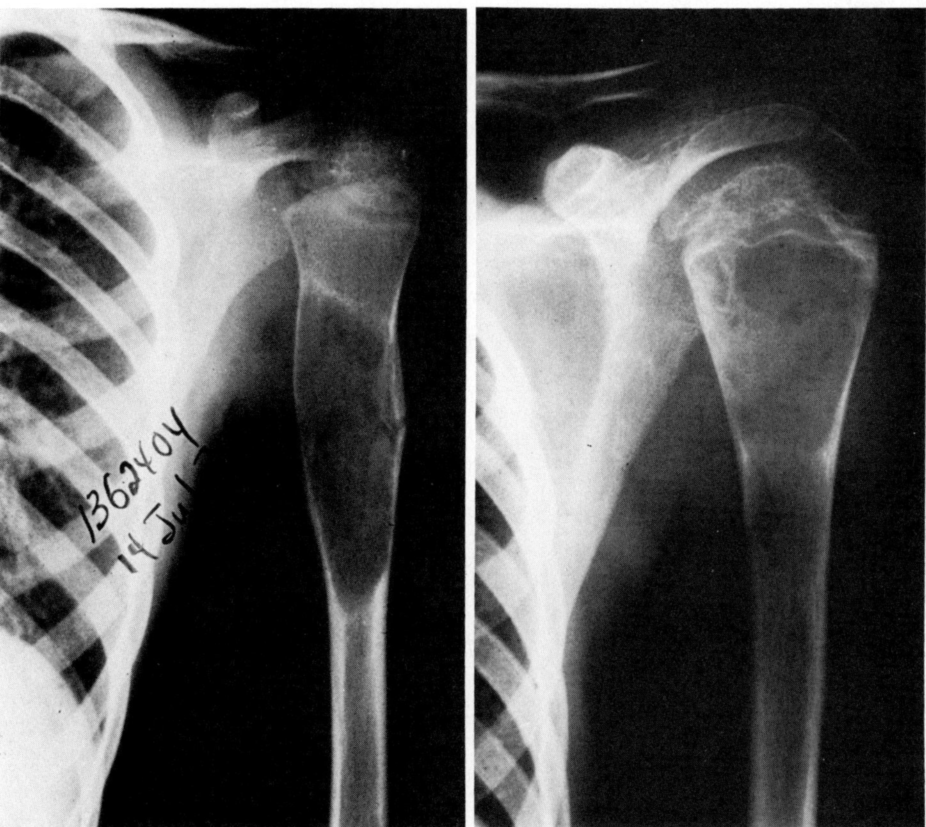

Figure 9–45

Figure 9–46

Figure 9–45. Unicameral bone cyst. The lesion involves the full width of the metaphyseal portion of the humerus, with pathologic fracture. Note slight expansion of bone, sharp demarcation at superior and inferior margins, and lytic destruction without periosteal reaction, all characteristic of the unicameral bone cyst.

Figure 9–46. Unicameral bone cyst. The cyst abuts against the epiphyseal growth plate.

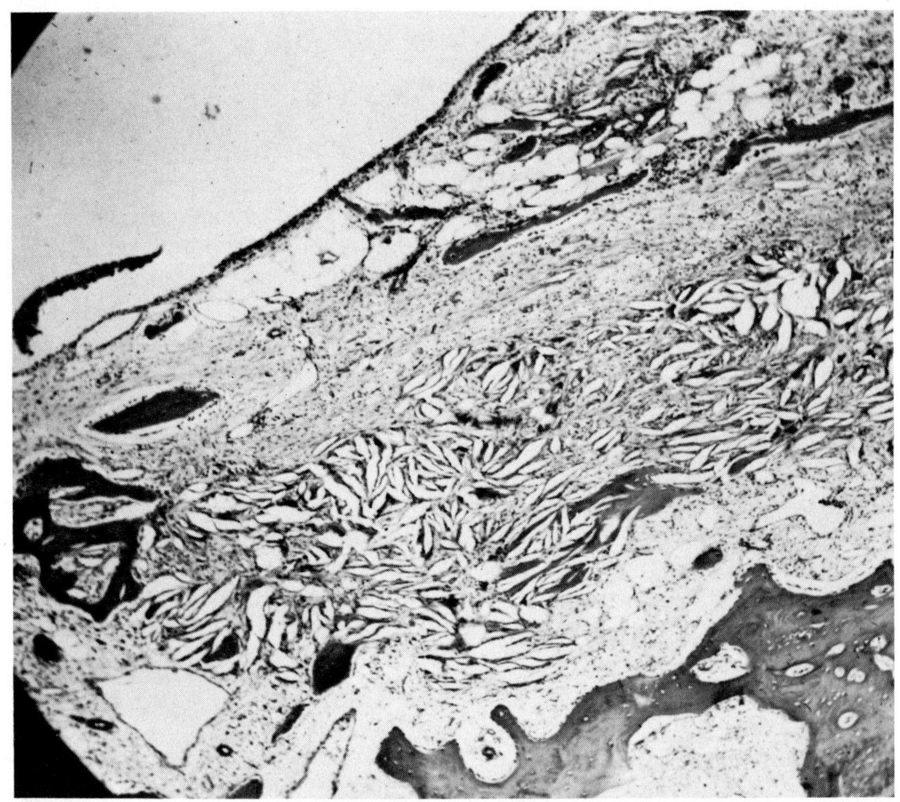

Figure 9–47. Unicameral bone cyst. Section through a cyst wall exhibiting cholesterol clefts, fibrous stroma with curlicues of bone similar to those seen in fibrous dysplasia, mesothelial cyst lining, and reinforced bone at the edge of the cyst.

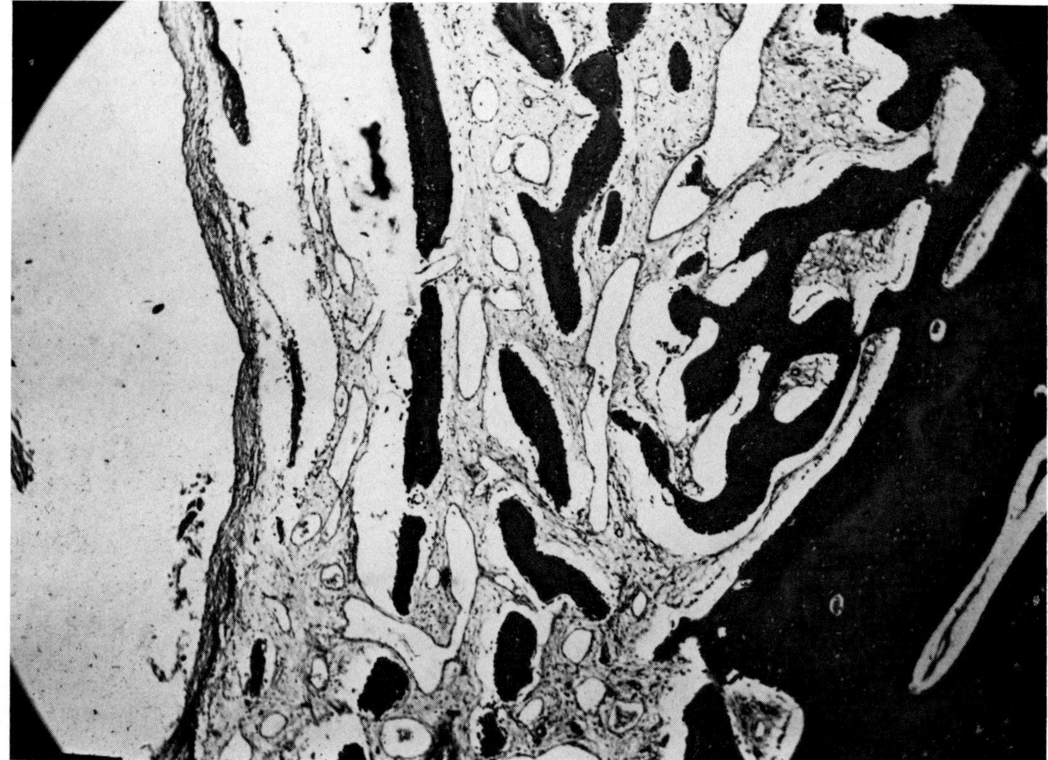

Figure 9–48. Unicameral bone cyst. Section through a cyst wall with thin fibrous lining of cyst cavity. Note reactive bone formation and numerous vascular spaces in the connective tissue lining the main cavity.

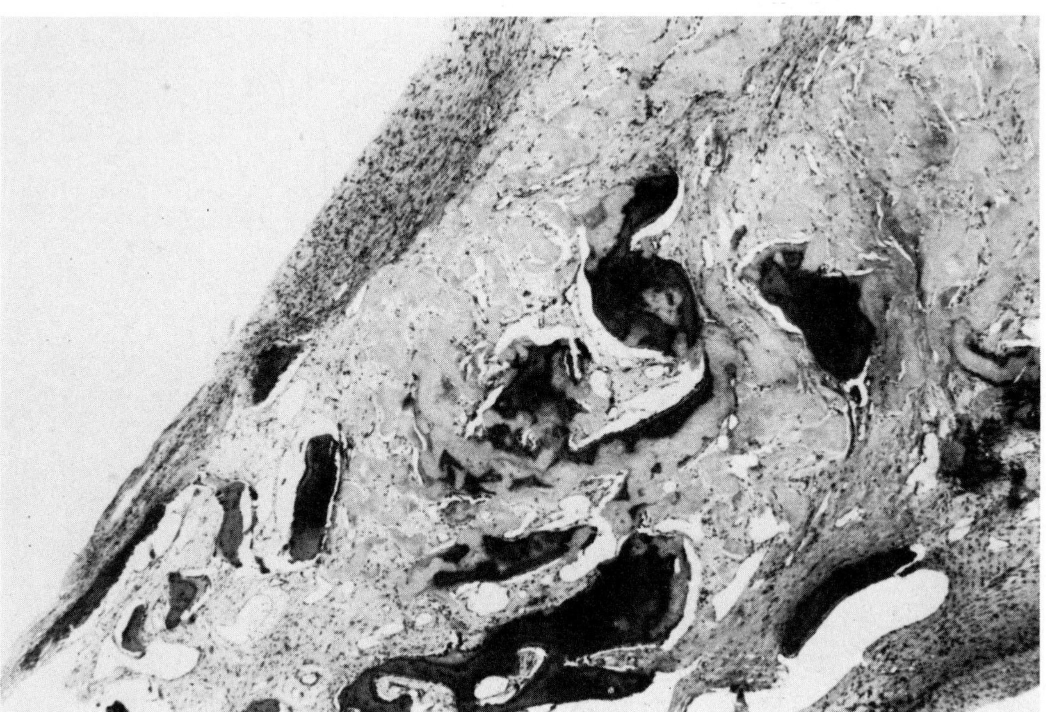

Figure 9–49. Unicameral bone cyst. Histologic section of a cyst wall exhibiting thicker fibrous lining tissue on the surface. Bony trabeculae and primitive cementum-like osteoid are in the wall of the cyst.

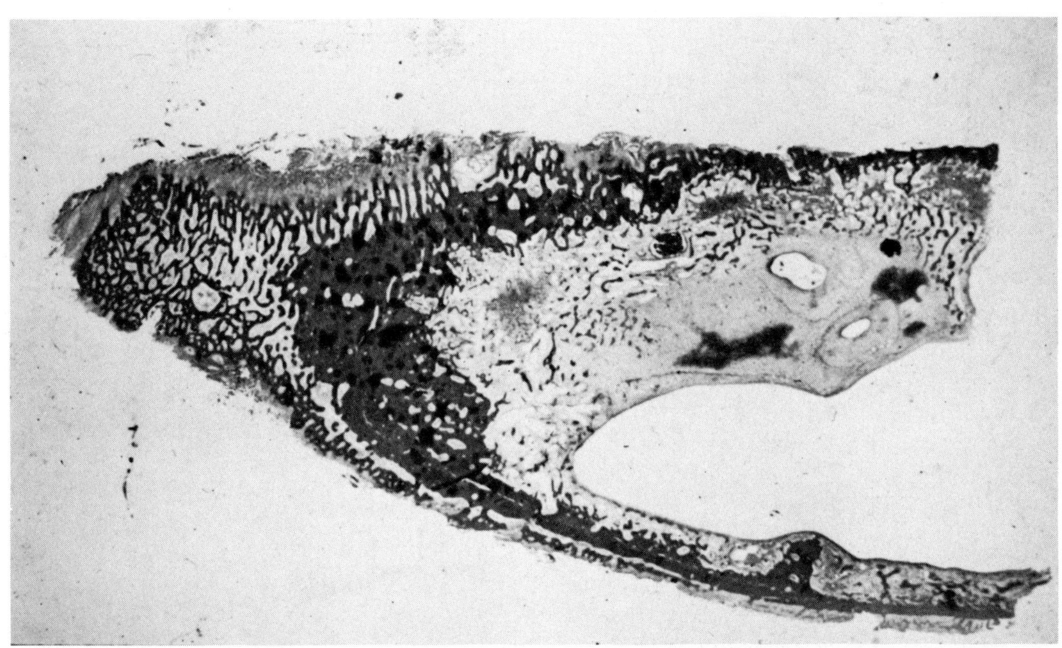

Figure 9–50. Unicameral bone cyst. Macrosection of a cyst exhibiting a large central space and numerous smaller cystic spaces in the lining of the main cavity. Fibrous connective tissue containing spicules of bone is surrounded by a rim of bony reinforcement, which can be demonstrated as a sclerotic rim on radiographs.

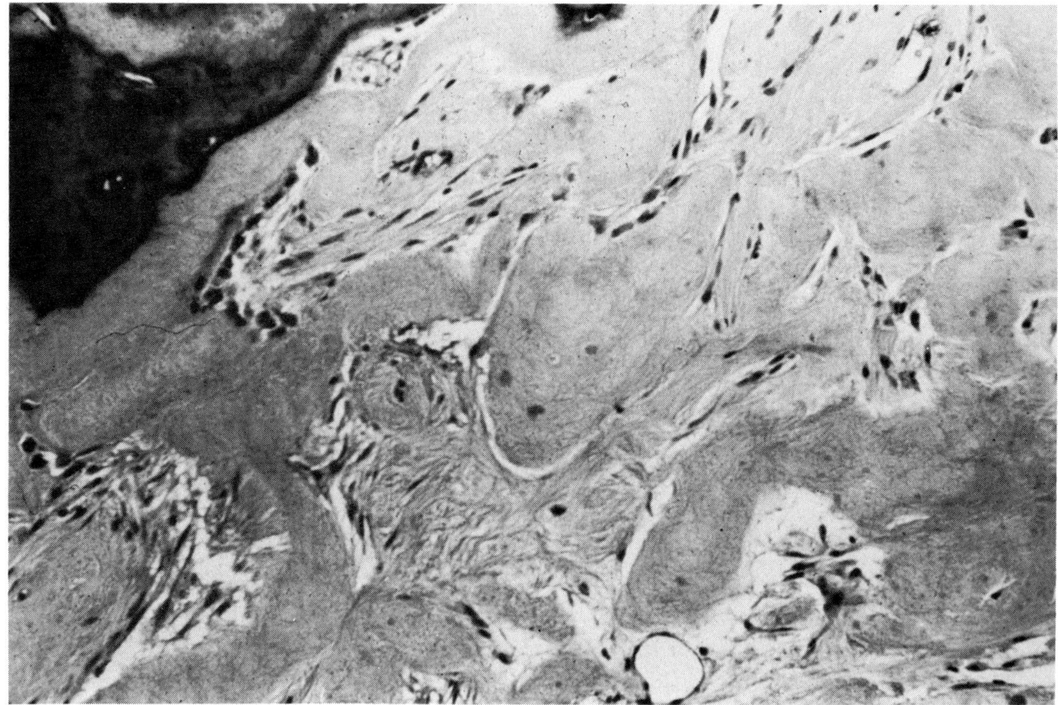

Figure 9–51. Unicameral bone cyst. Note the cementum-like osteoid, often found within the cyst wall.

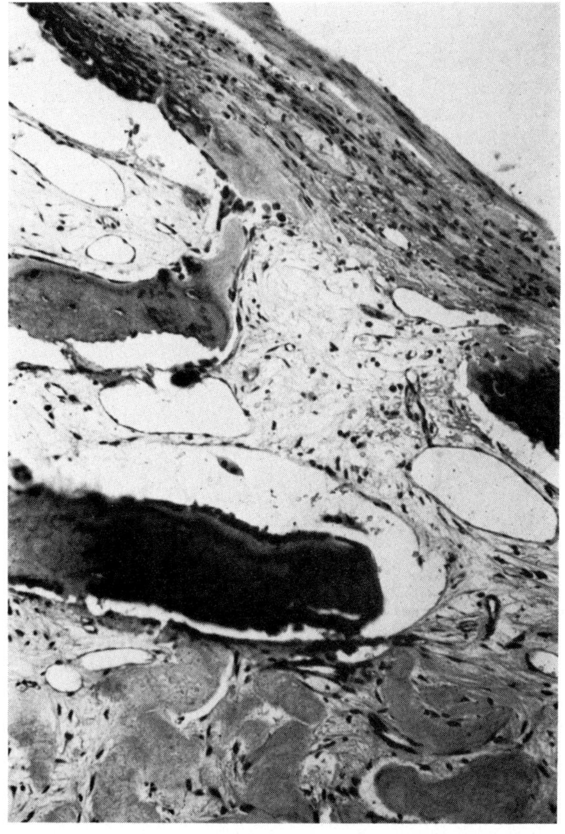

Figure 9–52. Unicameral bone cyst. Cementum-like osteoid is in the cyst wall. The material may actually calcify and thus produce radiographically opaque densities (see Fig. 9–53). Note the numerous sinusoidal vessel spaces of irregular size and contour.

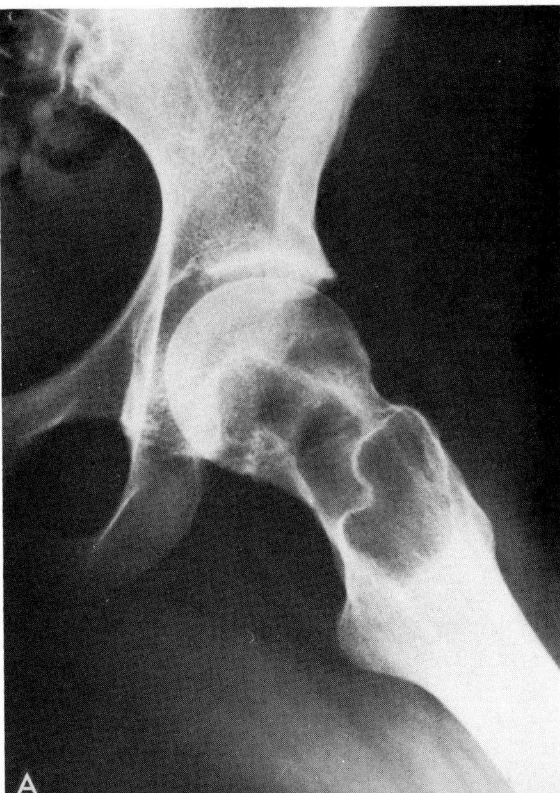

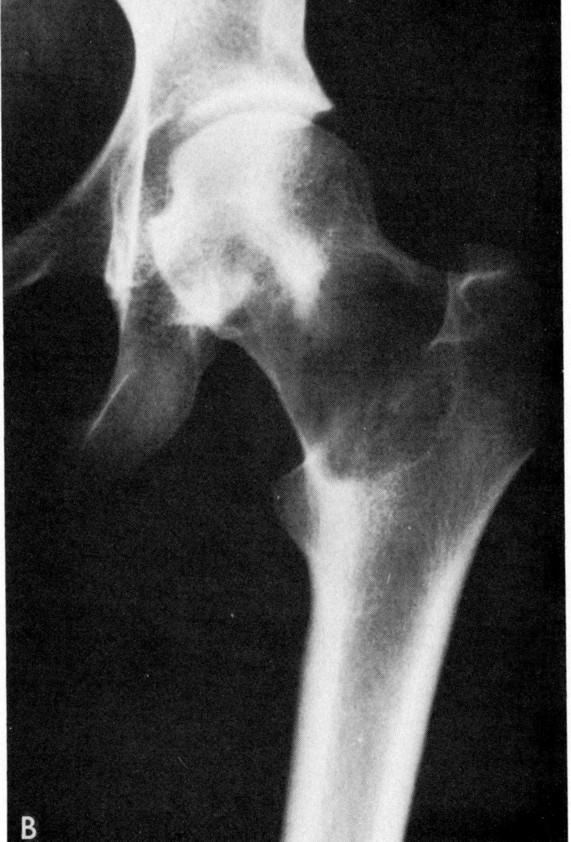

Figure 9–53. Unicameral bone cyst. Metaphyseal defect, full thickness, sharply circumscribed, with focal bone density within the cyst secondary to calcification of primitive osteoid in the wall.

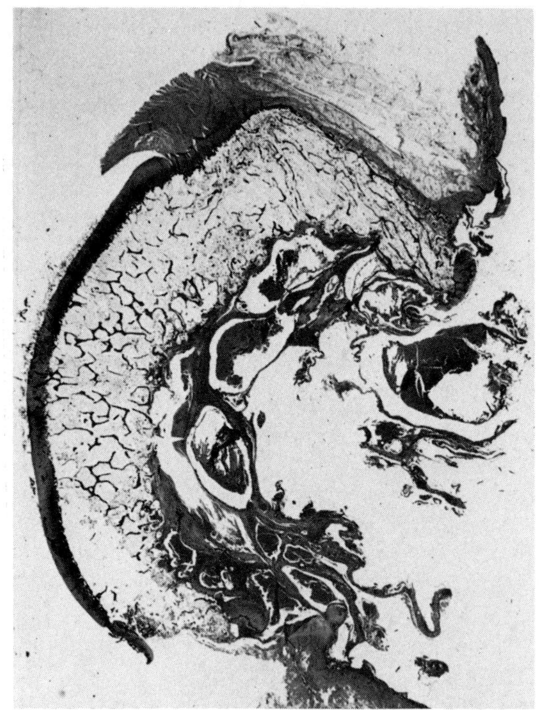

Figure 9–54. Aneurysmal bone cyst. Macrosection of the aneurysmal bone cyst illustrated in Figure 9–55. The lesion exhibits rapid "blowout"; note the sharp demarcation of lesion from the normal bone. The large, irregular blood-filled spaces are not lined by endothelial cells and serve to differentiate the aneurysmal bone cyst from a true vessel.

Figure 9–55. Aneurysmal bone cyst. Radiograph of the aneurysmal bone cyst secondary to a unicameral bone cyst in a 16-year-old girl. Marked expansion of the lesion is evident. Periosteal new bone formation cannot keep pace with the rapid destruction of bone secondary to the increased intraosseous pressure. Note the sharp demarcation between hemorrhagic core and residual bone at the distal margin, indicating a slow rate of growth at the distal end of the defect.

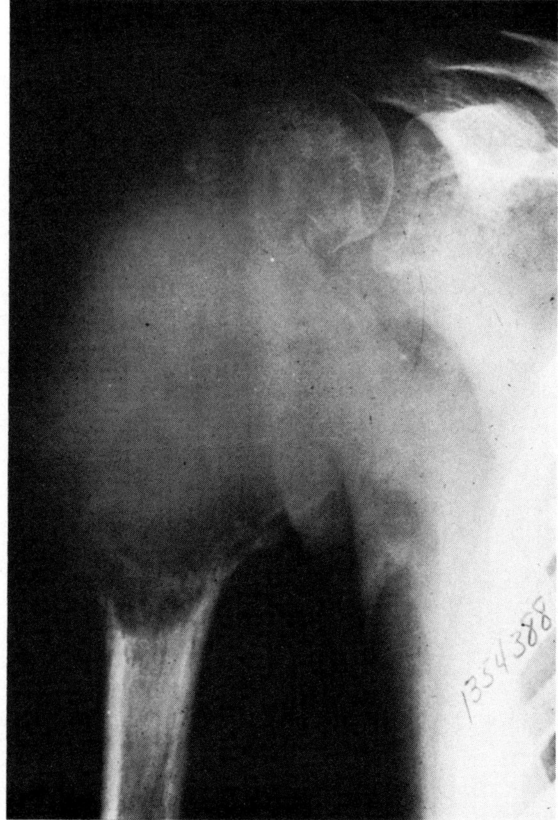

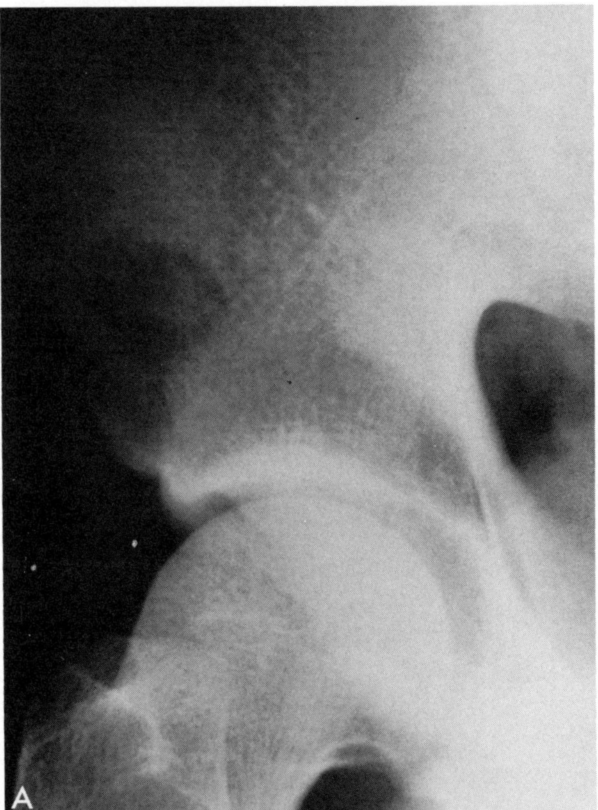
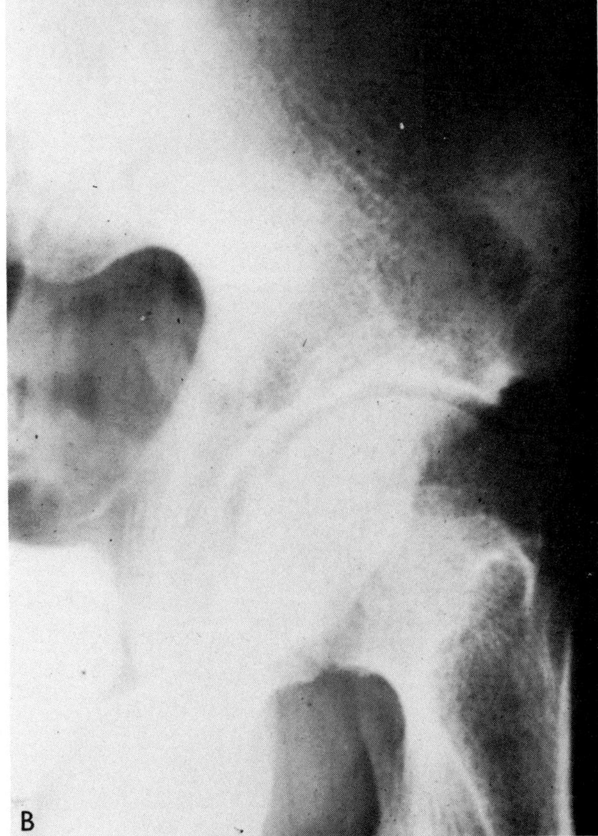

Figure 9–56. Radiographs of hips in two patients. Note the sharply circumscribed lytic defects above the acetabulum, discovered as incidental findings in these otherwise asymptomatic patients. Excision of the lesion reveals cystic spaces lined by thin-layered, flattened mesothelial cells, an appearance similar in all respects to that of a unicameral bone cyst. These lesions may represent degenerative cysts in the subarticular portion of a joint, secondary to increased turnover rate of subarticular bone (regressive remodeling). The histology may be identical with that of the unicameral bone cyst, or there may be myxoid material in varying amounts. Such lesions are often called "intraosseous ganglia." The development of these structures in this location is unexplained.

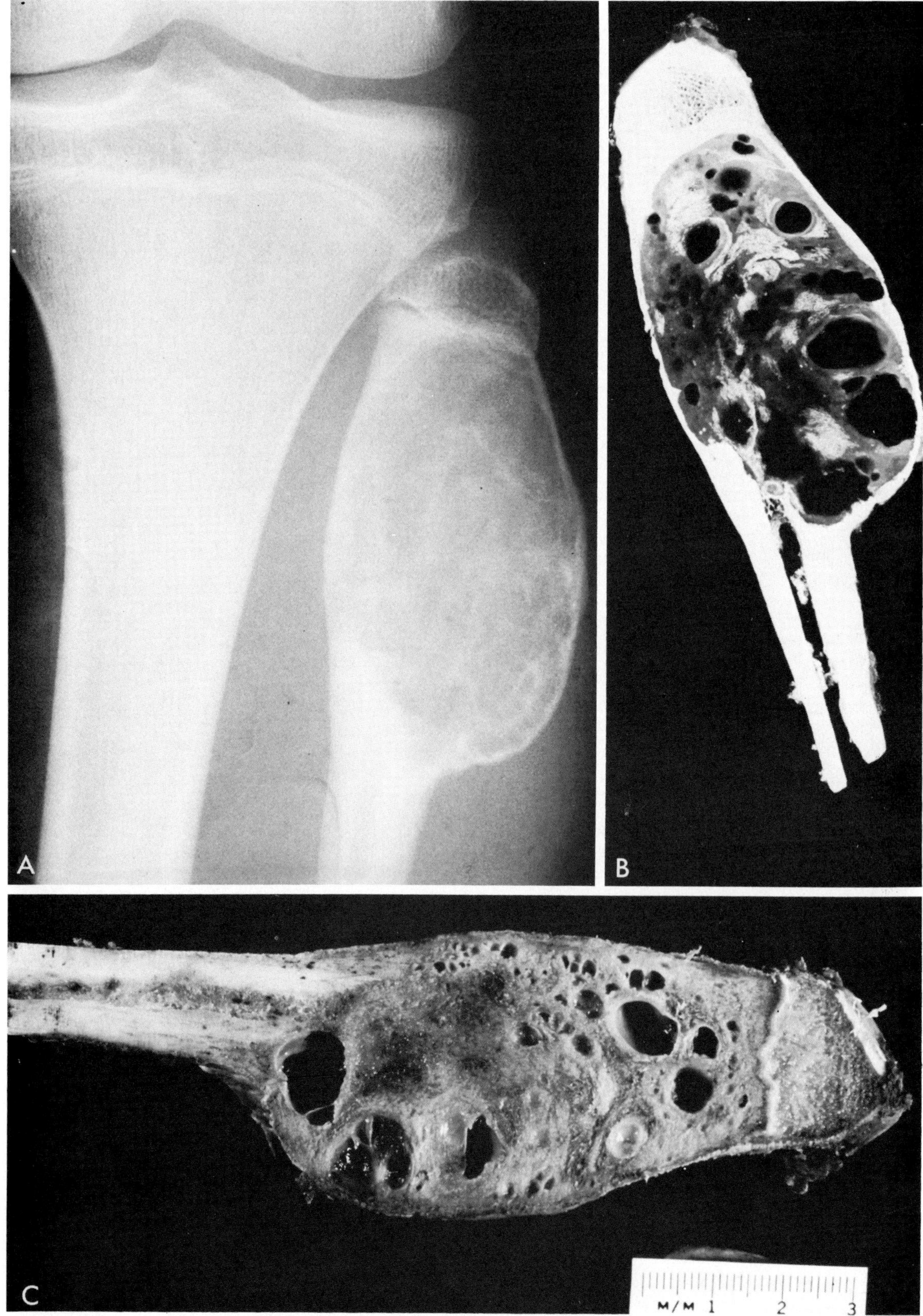

Figure 9–57. *See legend on opposite page*

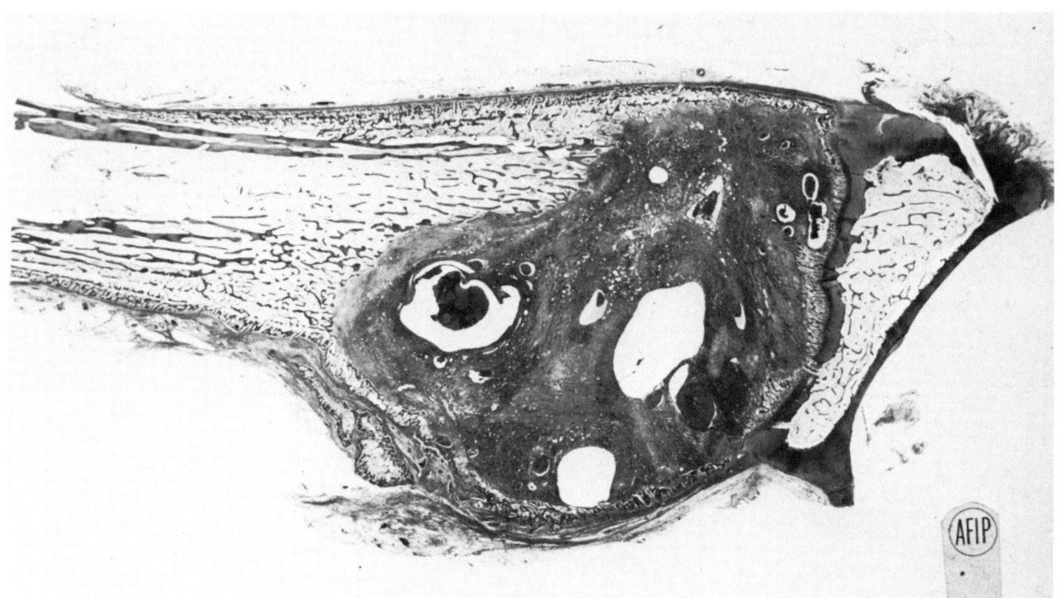

Figure 9–58. Uncommitted metaphyseal lesion. Macrospecimen of a lesion that is similar to that seen in Figure 9–57 located in the immediate subepiphyseal metaphysis. The lesion is expansile and consists of cystic spaces as well as solid-tissue components. These lesions are characteristically seen in young children whose growth plate is open.

trabeculae within the cyst may be visible radiographically, they represent reinforcement of the rim of cortical bone rather than true trabeculae within the cyst.

Pathologic fracture is extremely common in a unicameral bone cyst. The resultant callus must not be confused with neoplastic bone.

When excising a cyst, one must remove the fibrous component of the cyst lining completely, or recurrence is likely. This fibrous tissue may extend behind the rim of the reinforced trabeculae; curettage must therefore remove the shell of bone as well as the underlying tissue. Therapy with intracavitary injection of steroids has been successful in obliterating the cavity (Capanna et al., 1982).

Text continued on page 344

Figure 9–57. Uncommitted metaphyseal lesion. Radiograph (*A*), specimen radiograph (*B*), and specimen (*C*) of an uncommitted metaphyseal lesion. This defect is in proximity to the growth plate and consists of cystic as well as solid components.

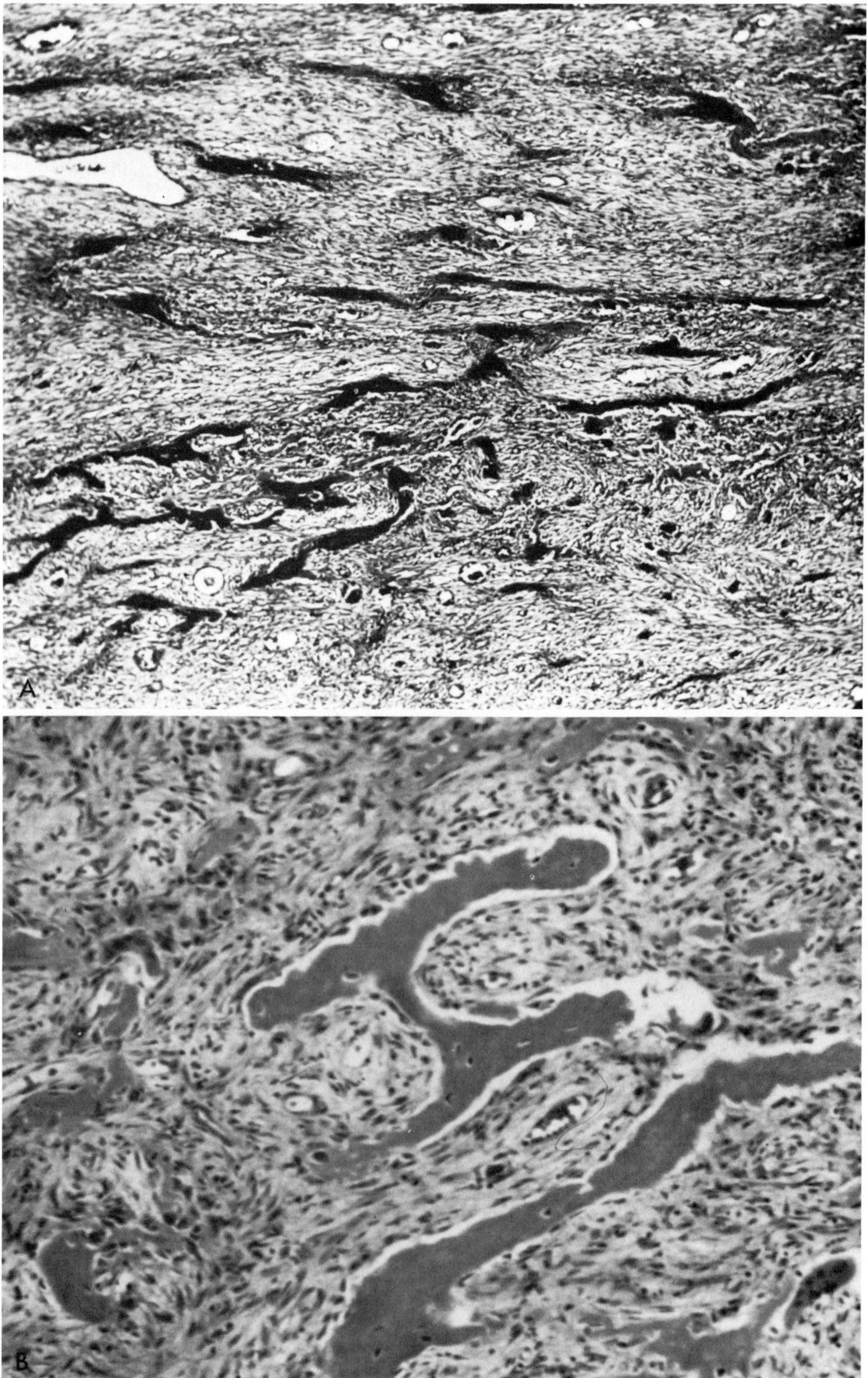

Figure 9–59. Uncommitted metaphyseal lesion. Histologic appearance of tissue removed from an uncommitted metaphyseal lesion. A wide variety of histologic patterns are noted. There is a whorled-fiber pattern similar to that seen in nonossifying fibroma (*F*); bone formation is present (*A* and *B*); cystic spaces are identifiable (*G* and *H*) and presumably are the forerunners of an ultimate unicameral bone cyst; giant cells (*C* and *D*) and vascular components are evident (*E*).

Illustration continued on opposite page

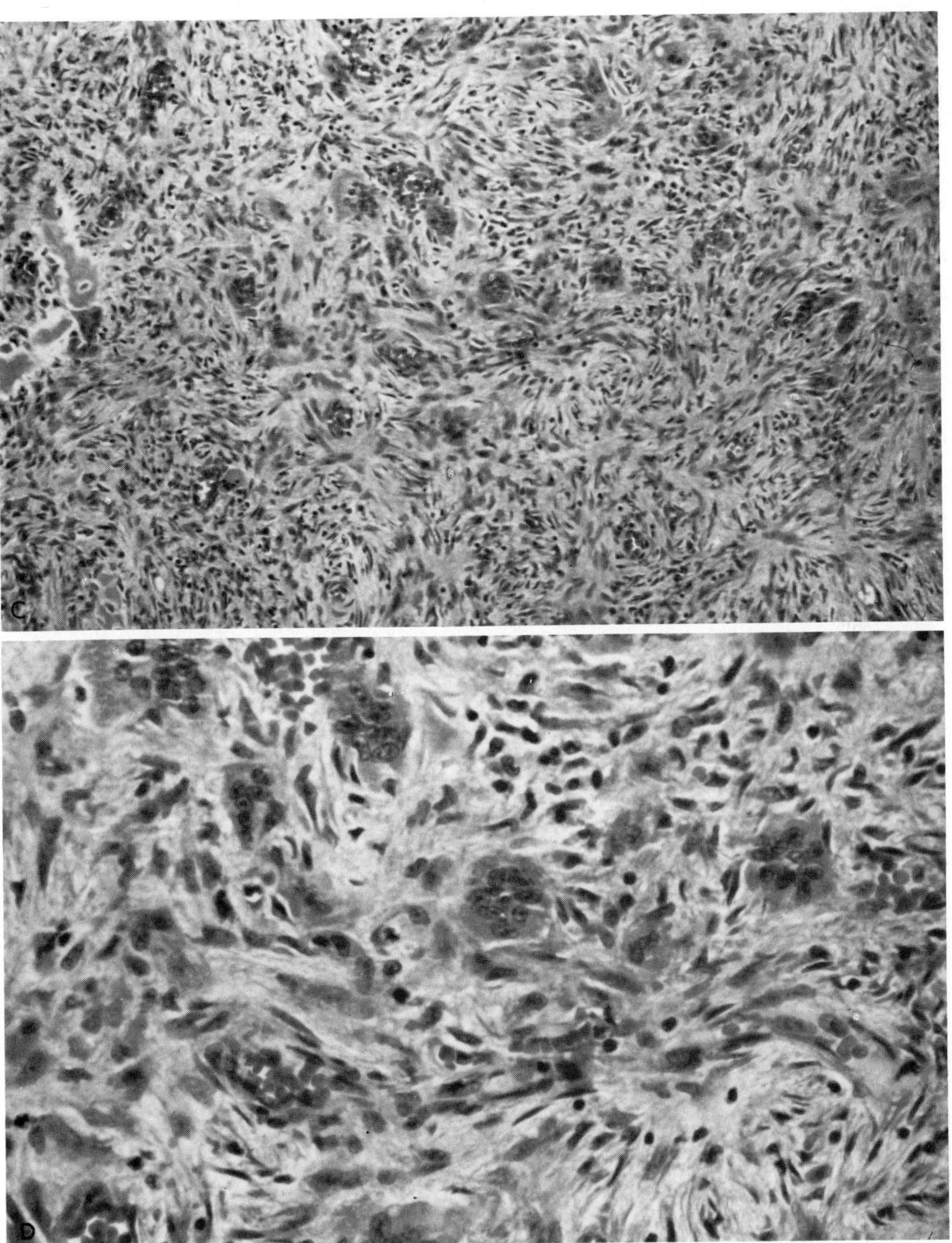

Figure 9–59 *Continued*

Illustration continued on following page

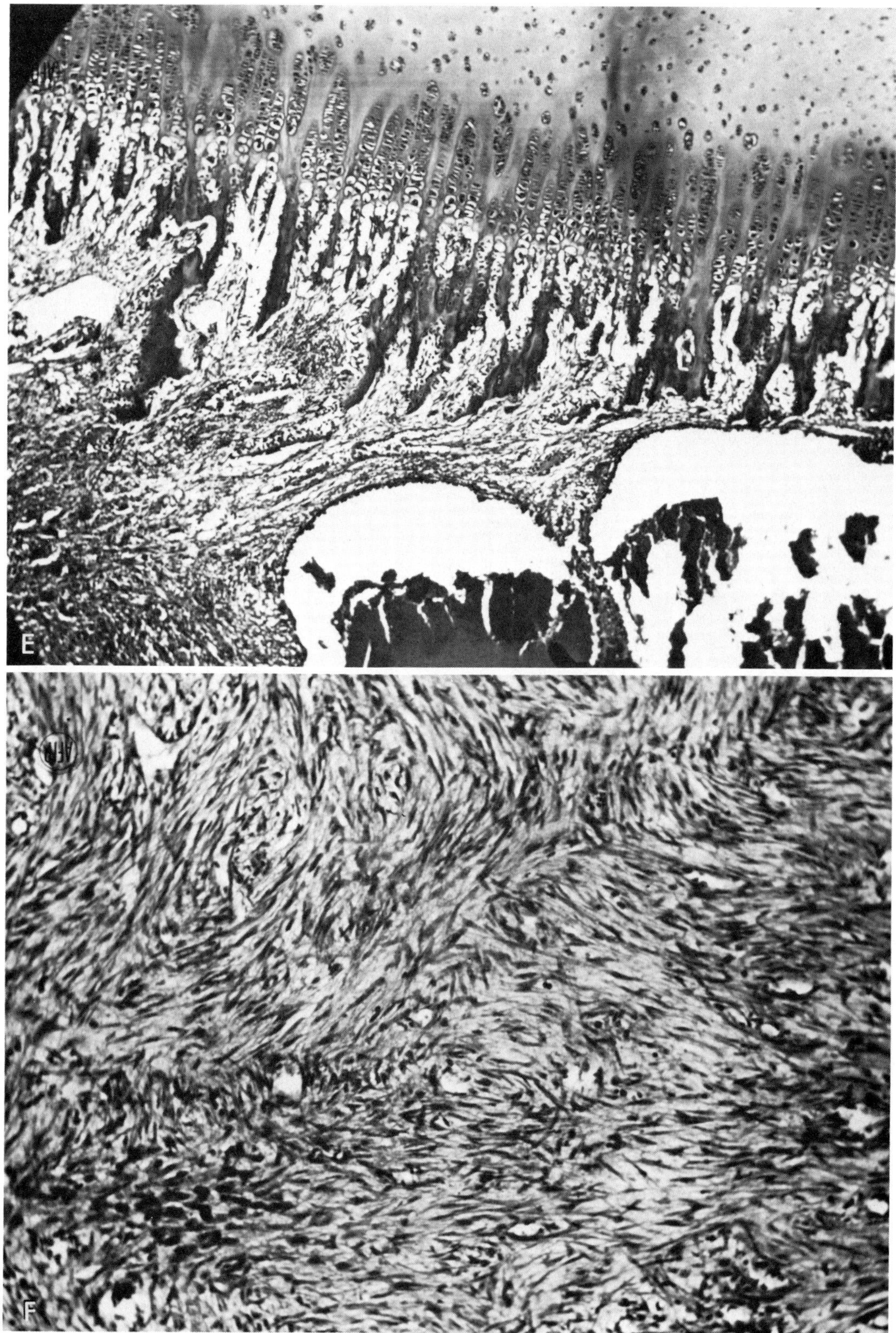

Figure 9–59 *Continued*

Illustration continued on opposite page.

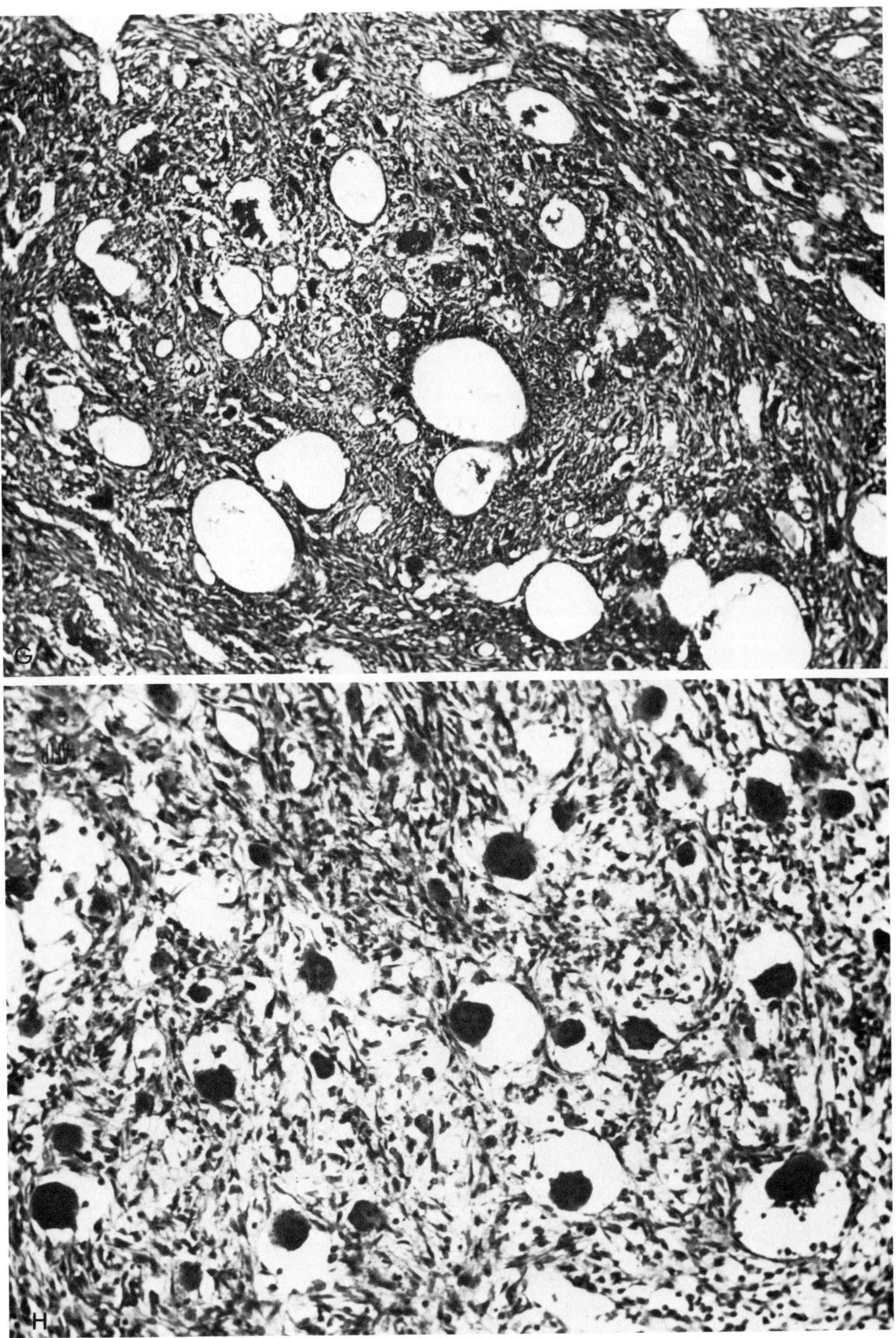

Figure 9–59 *Continued*

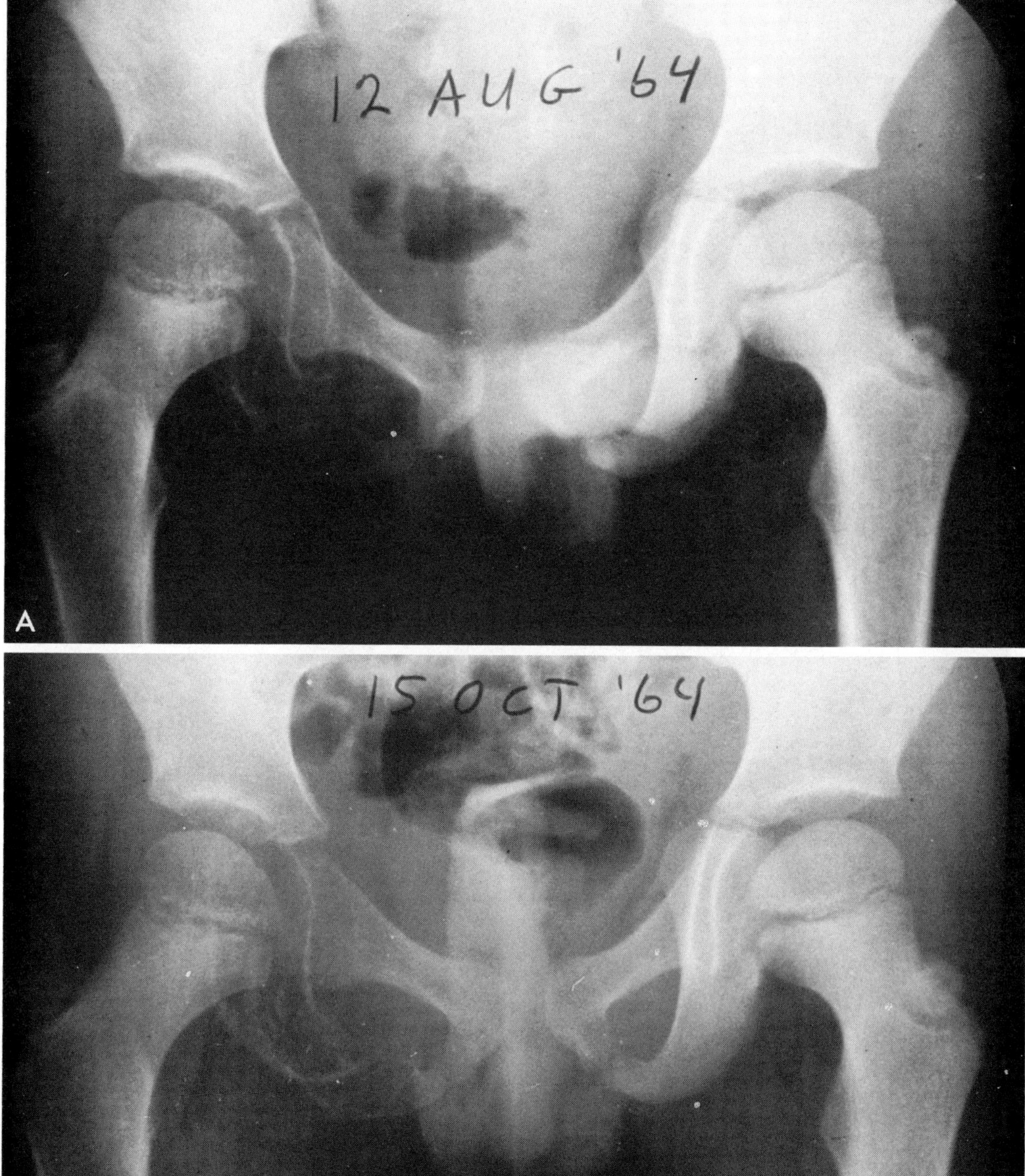

Figure 9–60. Aneurysmal bone cyst. Anteroposterior radiographs of the pelvis of an adolescent male with progressive changes in the right ischium. The initial film (*A*) shows radiolucency and expansion of the inferior ramus of the pubis, the ischial tuberosity, and the inferior ramus of the ischium. The films taken 2 months later (*B*) show expansion of the lesion. There is some periosteal new bone production that outlines the lesion somewhat better. In *C*, the film obtained 6 months after the first one shows a better outline of the lesion. It indicates that growth of the lesion has slowed and there is healing with periosteal new bone production. There has been no treatment in this interval.

Illustration continued on opposite page

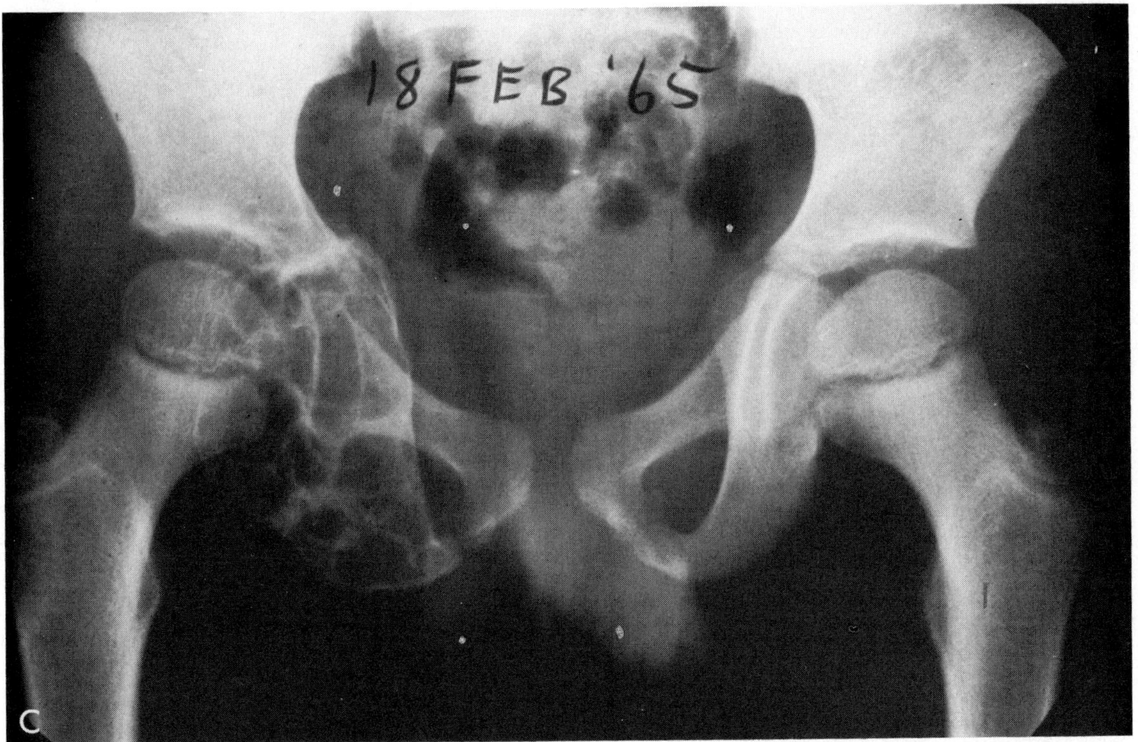

Figure 9–60 *Continued*

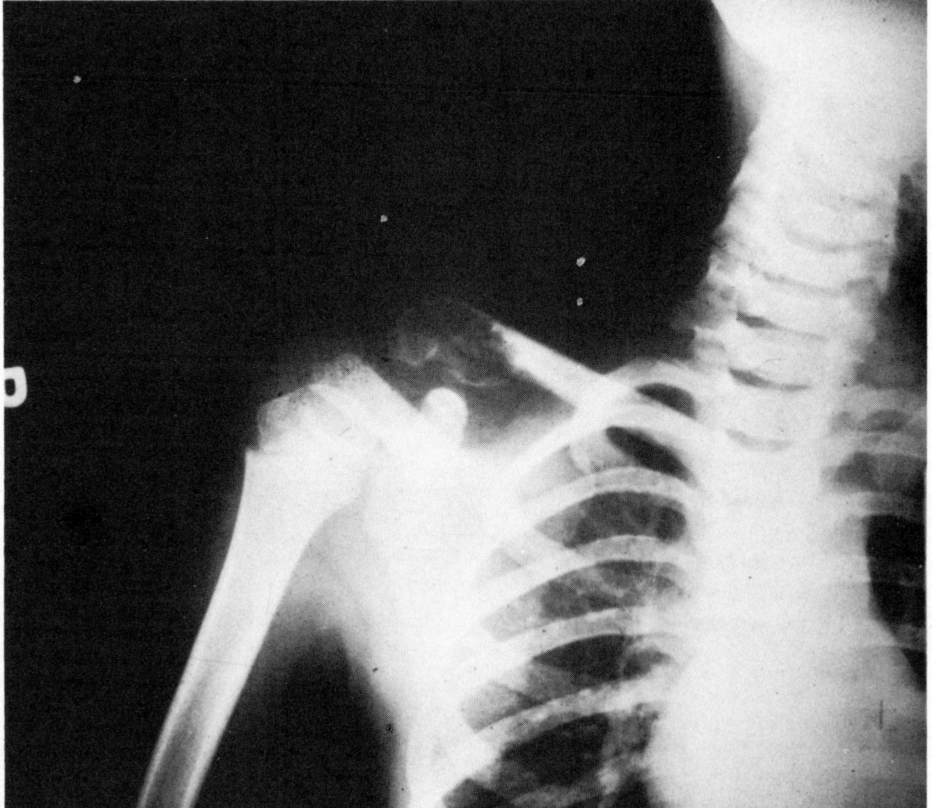

Figure 9–61. Aneurysmal bone cyst. Rapidly expansile lesion of the distal clavicle in a 7-year-old child. Periosteal new bone production keeps pace with the destructive lesions.

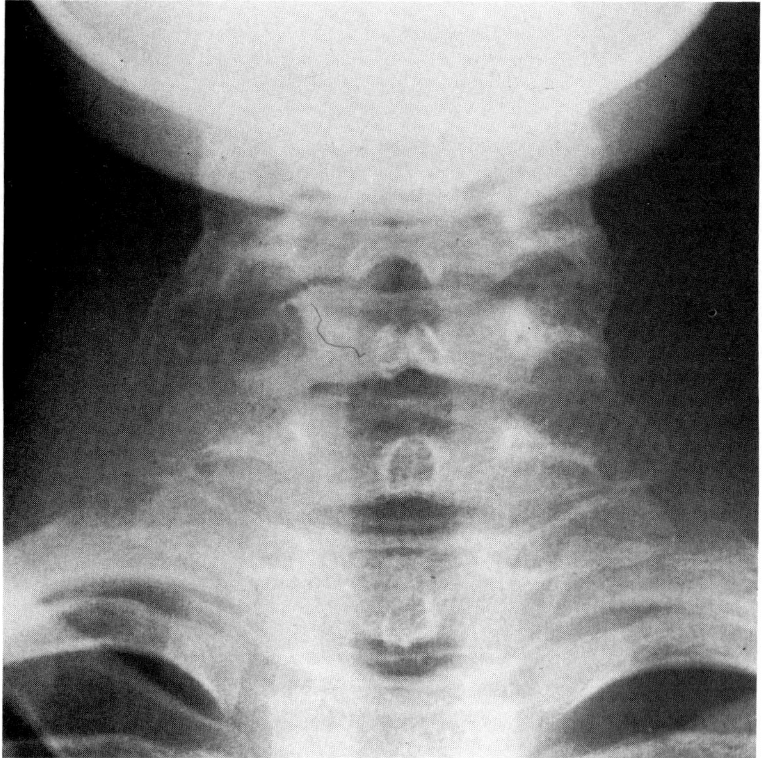

Figure 9–62. Aneurysmal bone cyst. Expansile lesion involving transverse process and lateral portion of the body of C-6. The combination of multiple muscles, tendons, and bony surfaces may contribute to the production of this type of lesion around the spine following injury. In the posterior elements of the vertebrae, this type of vascular change is more common than the solid giant cell tumor of bone or osteoblastoma.

ANEURYSMAL BONE CYST

Aneurysmal bone cyst is a radiographic entity due to vascular malformation. It represents a proliferation of the vascular component of the marrow, with removal of bone and cyst formation secondary to pressure on the adjacent osseous structures. Although this remains a matter of controversy, in our opinion the aneurysmal bone cyst is not a primary lesion of bone but rather always a secondary lesion (Biesecker et al., 1970; Levy et al., 1975). The histologic finding are extremely variable but always include blood-filled lacunae, areas of loose myxoid connective tissue, numerous giant cells, and reactive bone formation. Careful search of the entire lesion will usually demonstrate some evidence of the primary process.

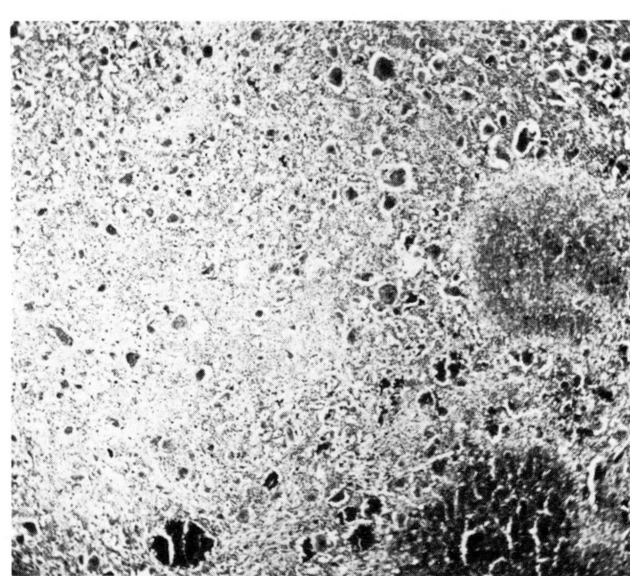

Figure 9–63. Aneurysmal bone cyst. Section of a giant cell tumor with areas of hemorrhage and cyst formation.

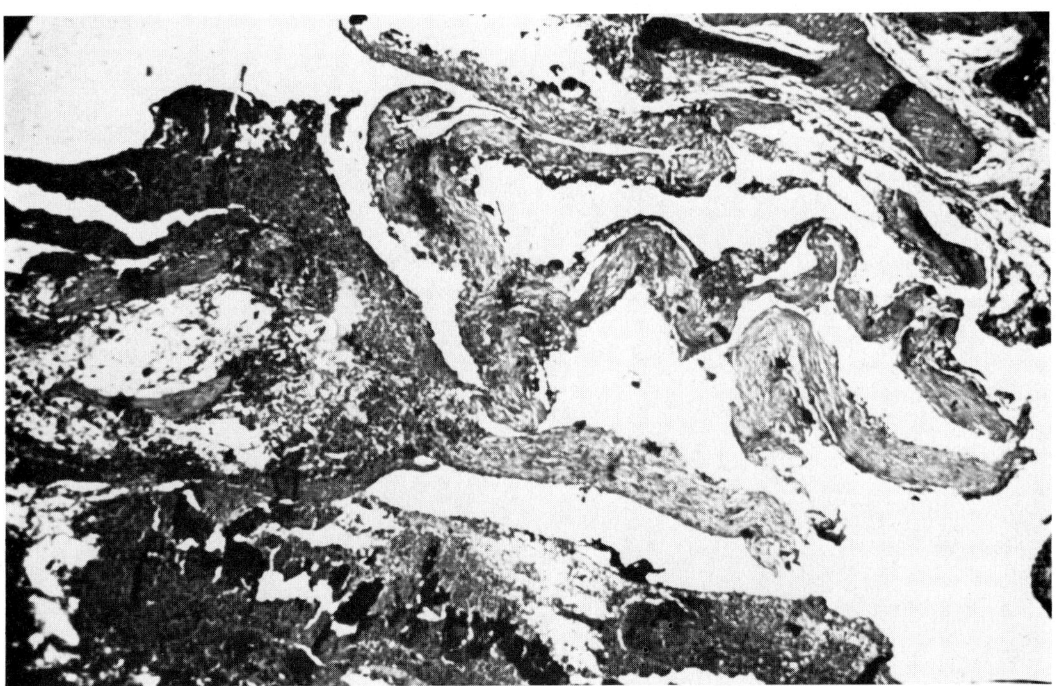

Figure 9–64. Aneurysmal bone cyst. Further progression of the vascular changes in an underlying giant cell tumor. The vascular spaces are lined by the tumor and fibrous stroma. As opposed to normal vessels, these spaces are not lined by endothelial cells.

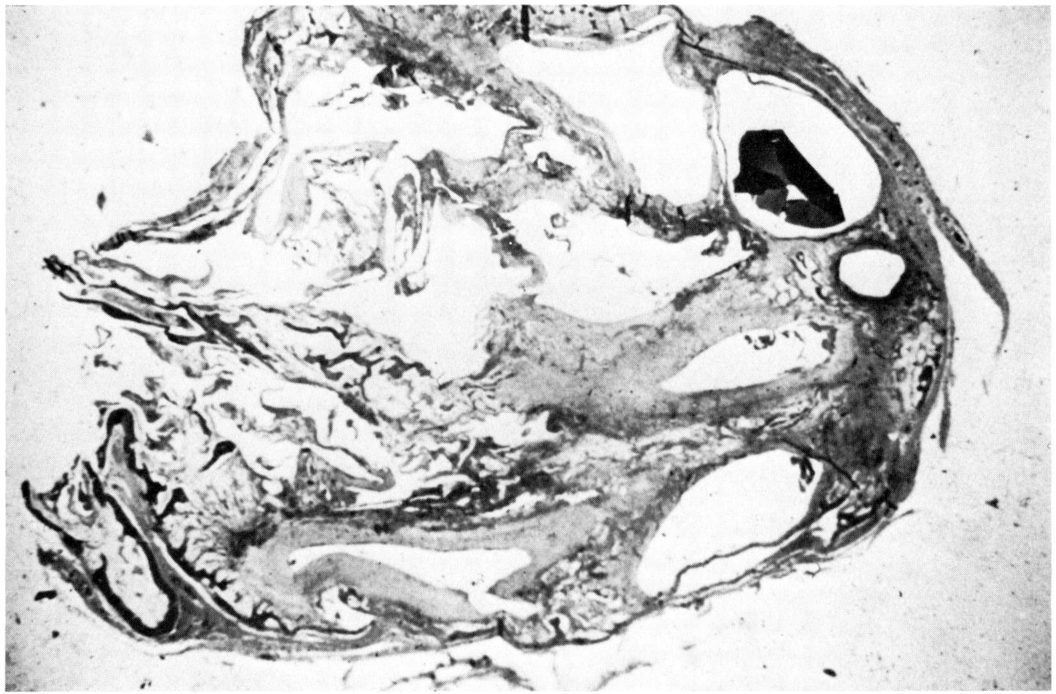

Figure 9–65. Aneurysmal bone cyst. A well-developed aneurysmal bone cyst. The diagnosis of the basic lesion has to be made on the material intervening between the empty spaces.

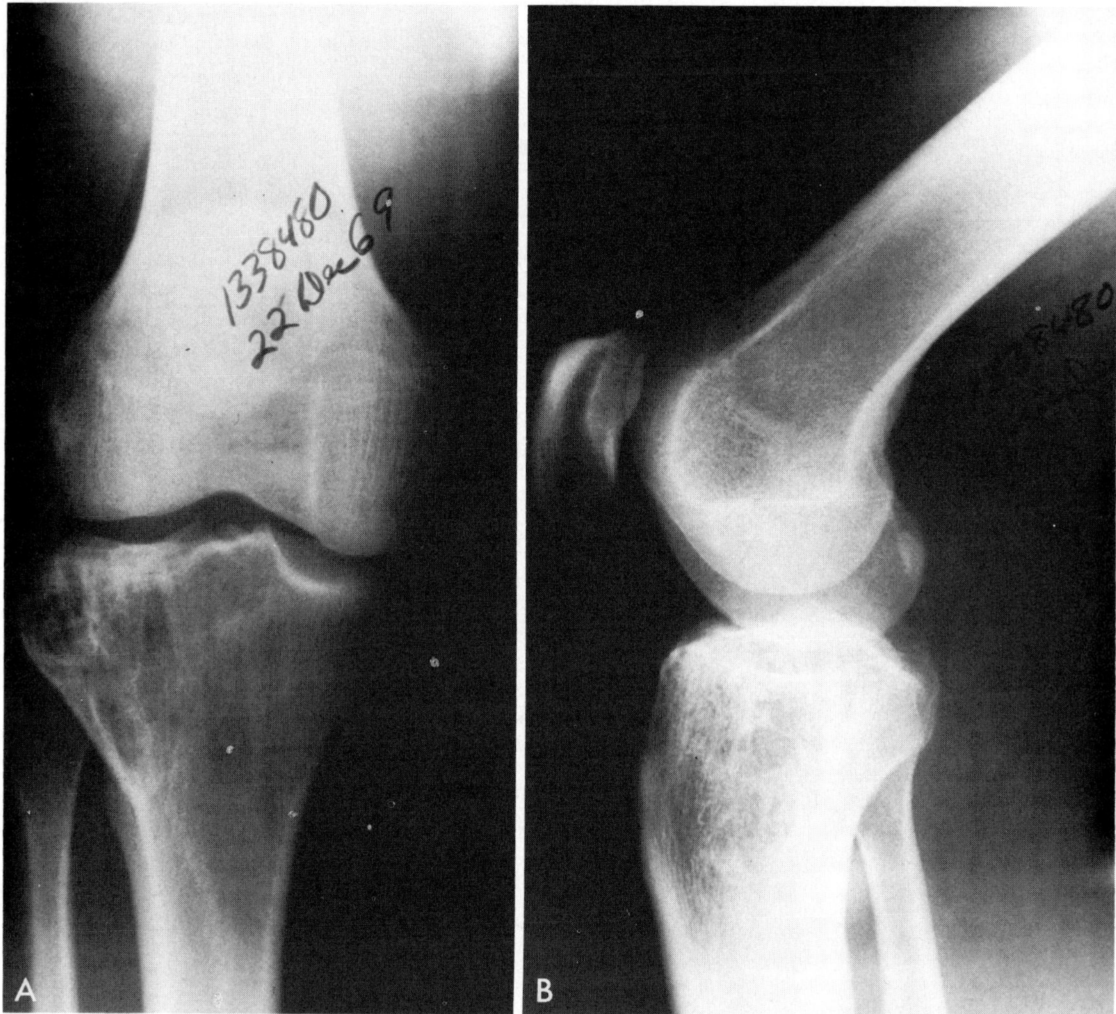

Figure 9–66. Angioma. Anteroposterior (*A*) and lateral (*B*) radiographs of the knee joint of a patient containing a large hemangioma in the proximal tibia. The lesion is eccentric, involving epiphysis and metaphysis and abutting on the subchondral bone of the lateral tibial condyle. There is no periosteal reaction or expansion of bone. Some augmented trabeculae extend through the lesion, but the process is basically a lytic defect.

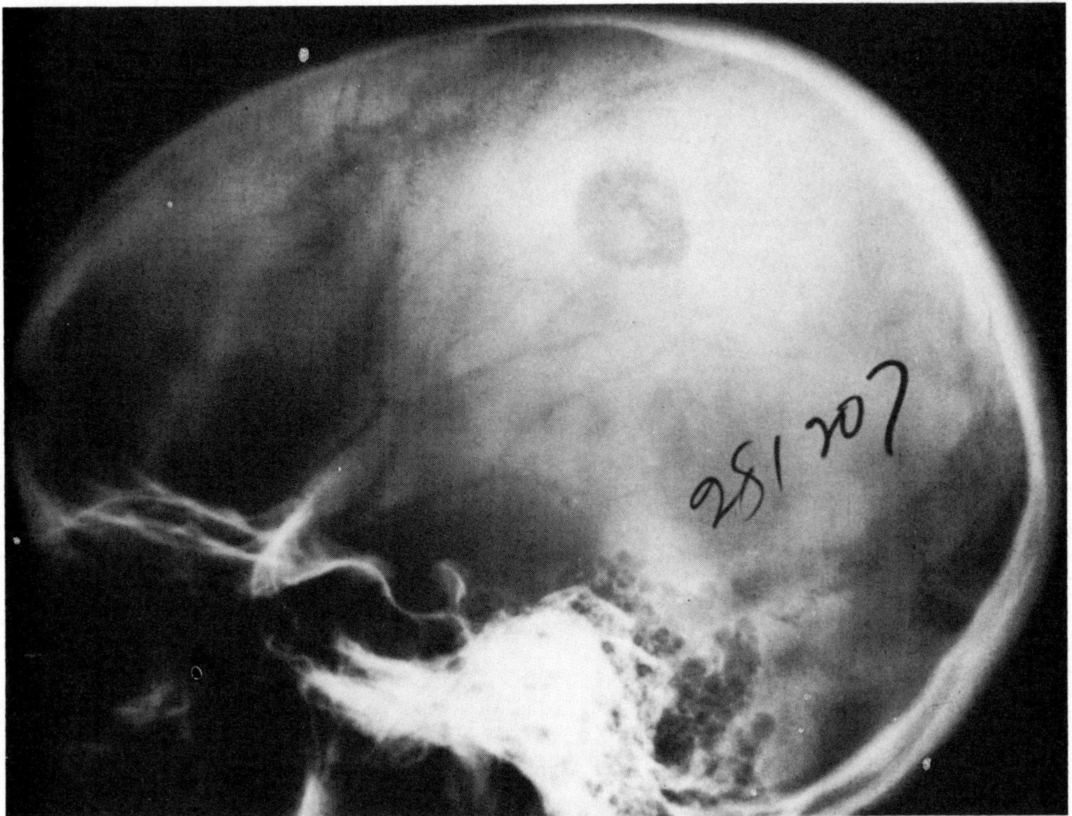

Figure 9–67. Angioma. Lateral radiograph of the skull of a patient with a hemangioma. Note the wide area of bony reaction around the periphery of the lesion. There is an apparent sclerotic nidus in the center of the lesion. Radiating spiculation of bone is common in hemangiomas of the skull.

ANGIOMA OF BONE

Angiomas of bone are benign anomalies that consist of large, thin-walled vessels or small vessels of varying thickness and size. The lesions are stable and usually asymptomatic. Although they may be found in any bone, they are common in the vertebral column. Occasionally, they are multiple and tend to cluster around a joint. Pathologic fracture is an infrequent complication.

Text continued on page 357

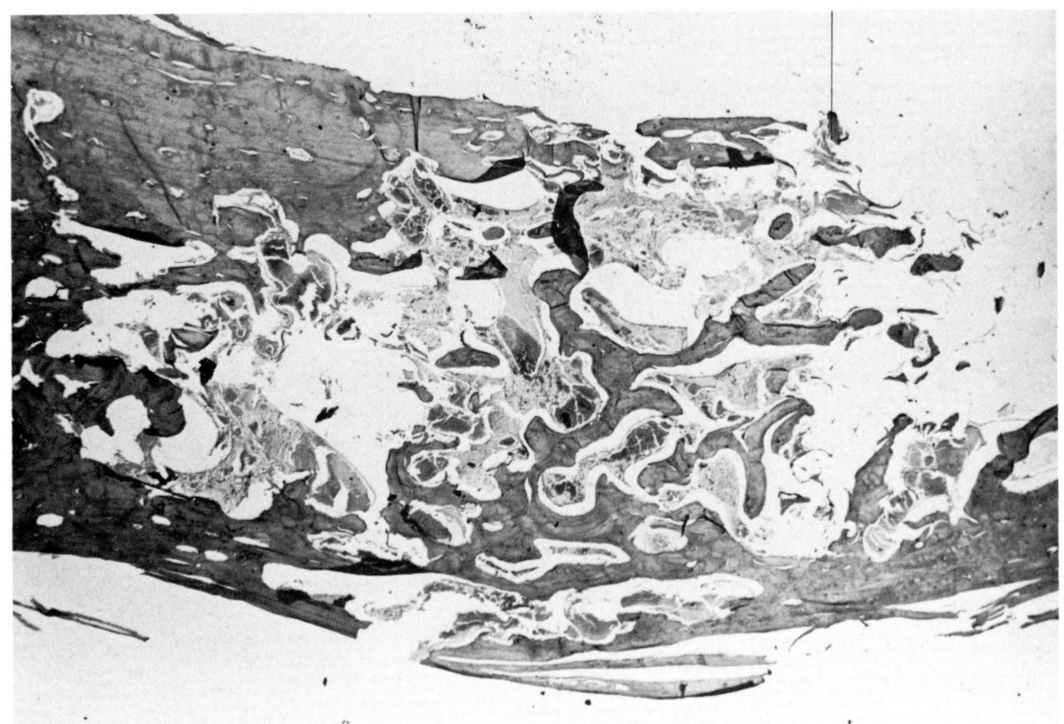

Figure 9–68. Angioma. Section of the hemangioma of the skull illustrated in Figure 9–67. On the left-hand side of the figure, the blood-filled calvarial tables are intact; in the center, they have been extensively removed and replaced with dilated, filled vessels of various sizes and shapes. There is an intervening fibrous stroma.

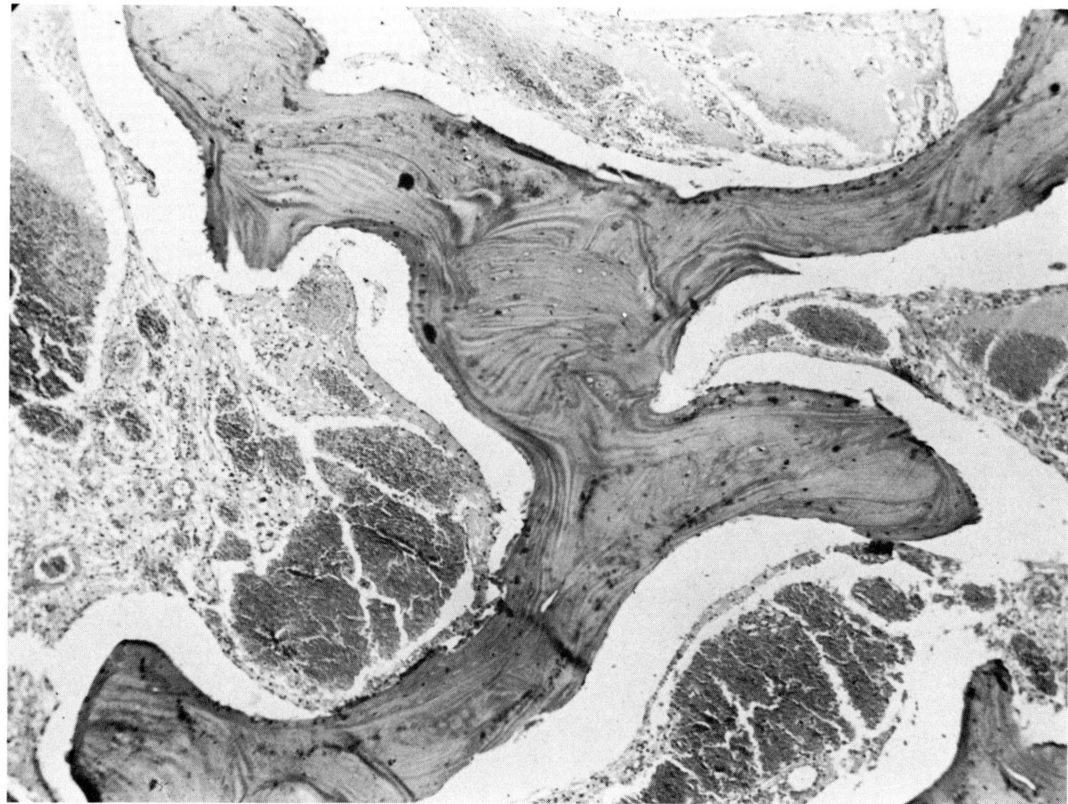

Figure 9–69. Angioma. Higher-power view of the same section shown in Figure 9–68. Note the dilated sinusoidal vessels. There has been augmentation of the bony trabeculae in response to the passive hyperemia.

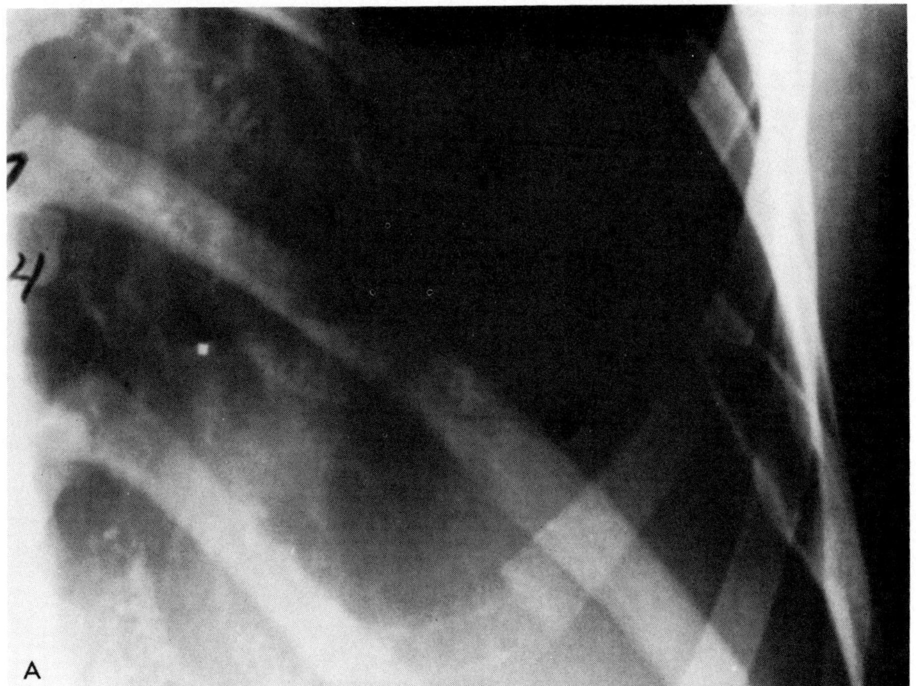

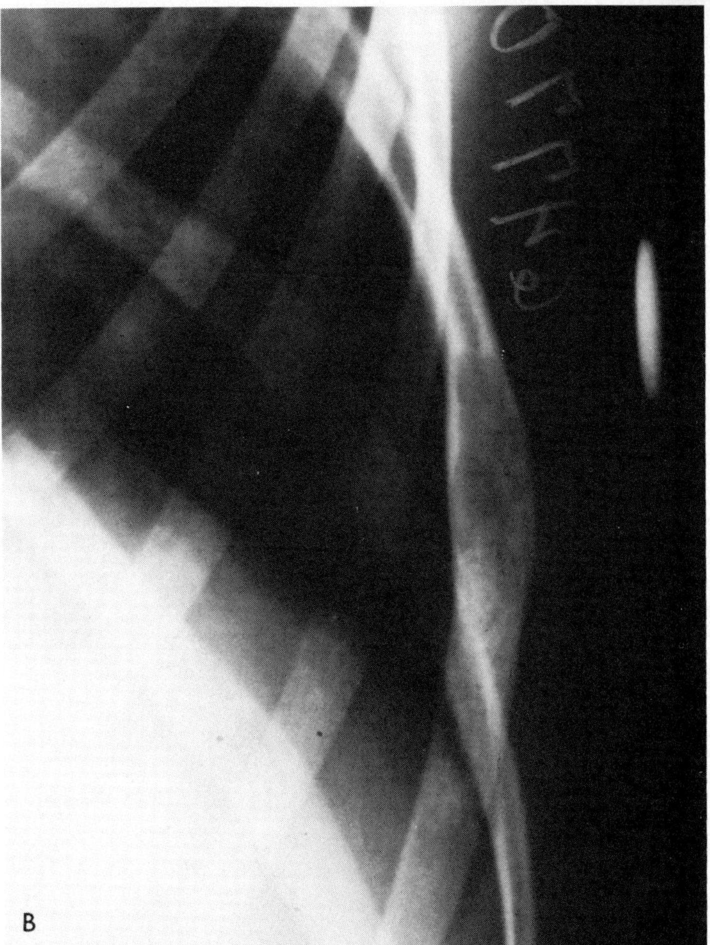

Figure 9–70. Angioma. Views of hemangioma in rib of two patients found on routine chest radiographs. In *A,* the lesion is almost purely lytic with slight expansion of the bone, but there is no evidence of any matrix calcification or ossification. In *B,* the lesion is also expansile and somewhat longer, and it has a ground-glass consistency indicating numerous spicules of bone present throughout the lesion.

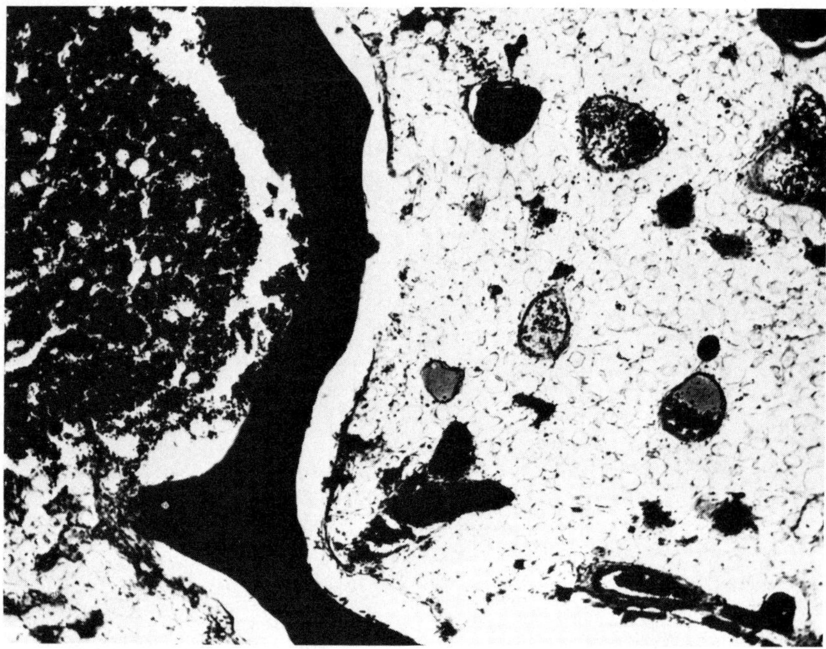

Figure 9–71. Angioma. Histologic appearance of an angioma in bone. Note the numerous vessels of different sizes and shapes in the medullary cavity. Most are quite thin-walled, sinusoidal vessels.

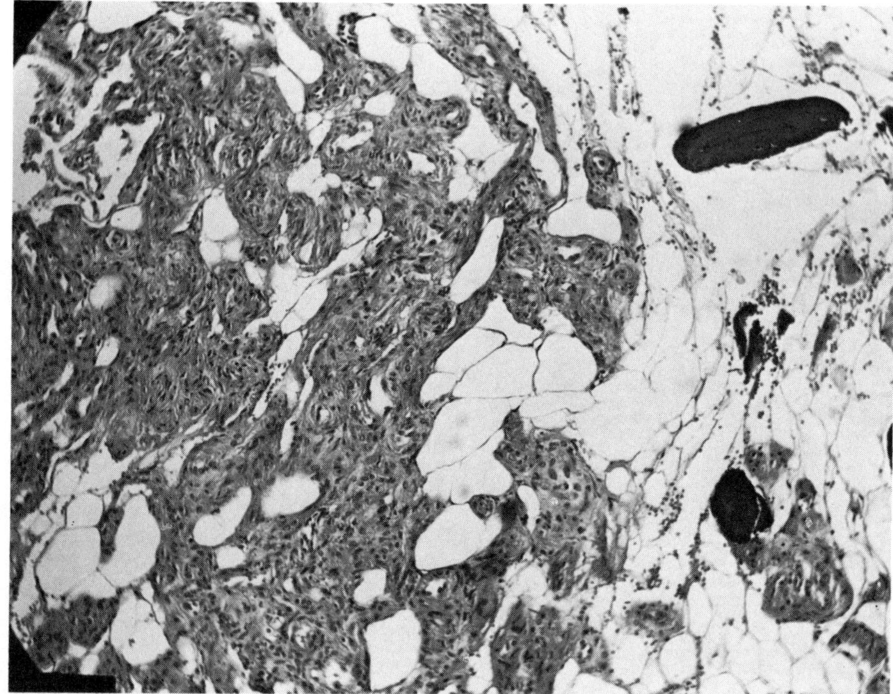

Figure 9–72. Angioma. The fatty marrow has been invaded by cellular tissue rich in vessels of various sizes and shapes.

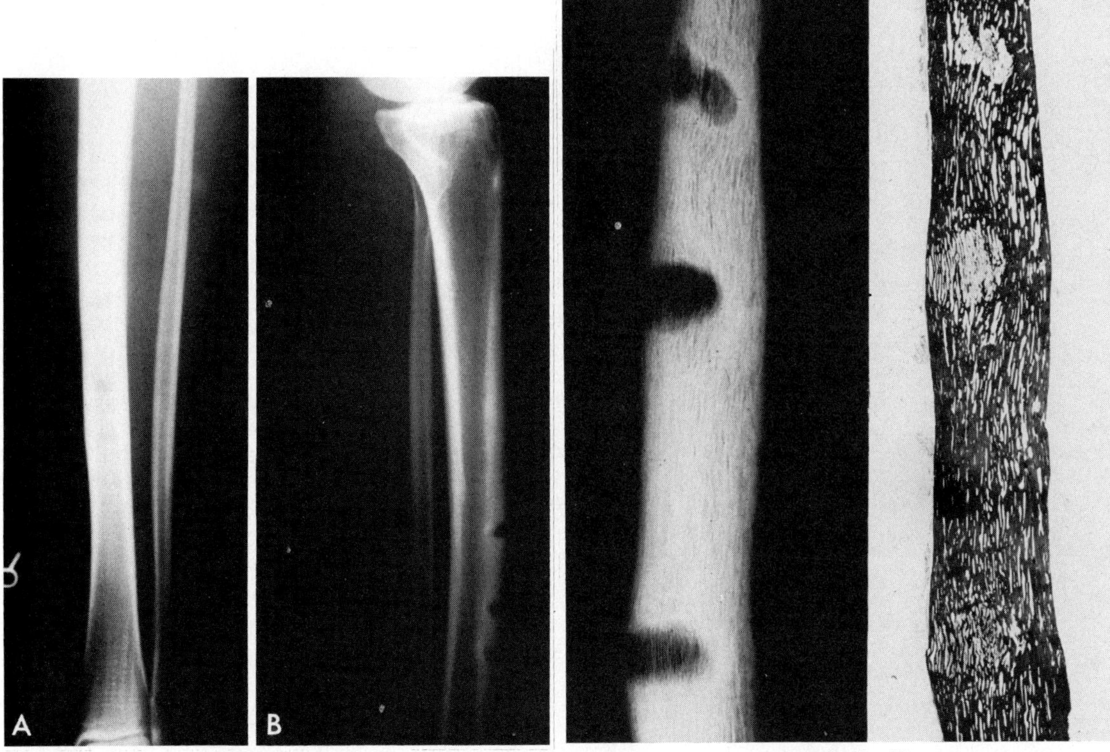

Figure 9–73   **Figure 9–74**

Figure 9–73. Angioma. Anteroposterior (*A*) and lateral (*B*) radiographs of the tibial shaft of a 38-year-old woman who has a 15-year history of lumps on her leg that are often painful, tender to the touch, and quite warm. She has nodules on each leg that are readily palpable. Bone scan in this region shows three discrete "hot spots."

Figure 9–74. Angioma. Specimen radiograph (*A*) and macrosection (*B*) of the tibial cortex shown in Figure 9–73. In *A*, the cortex is reinforced by increased bone, and there are three discretely punched-out lesions in the anterior tibial cortex that created a defect in the bone that was palpable through the skin. In *B*, three defects in this sclerotic bone with thin trabeculae of bone passing through each defect are visible.

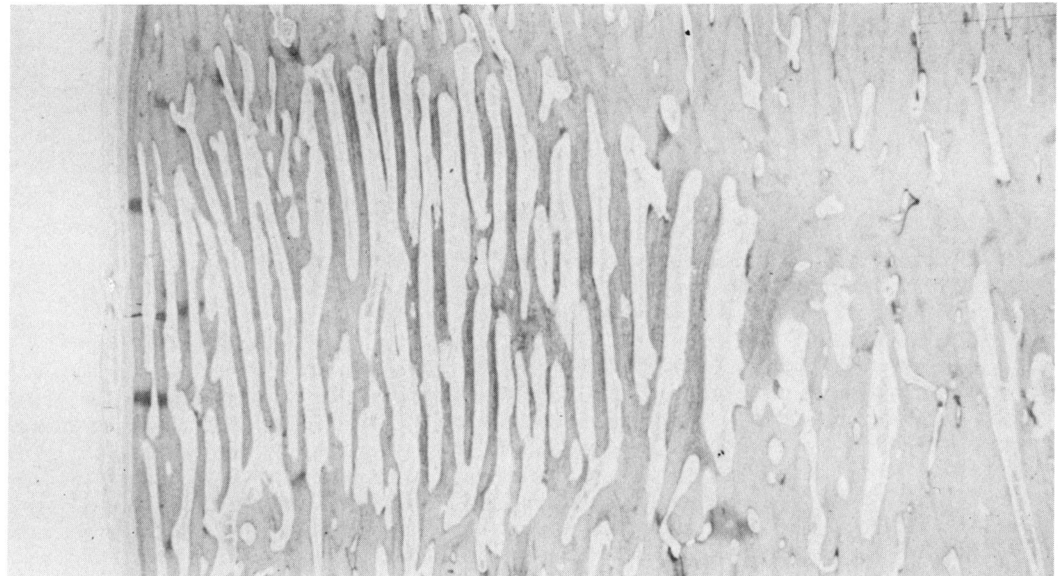

Figure 9–75. Angioma. Section through the bony defect seen in Figure 9–74. Note the long, slender laminae of bone extending across the defect. The spaces are filled with vessels of varying sizes and shapes.

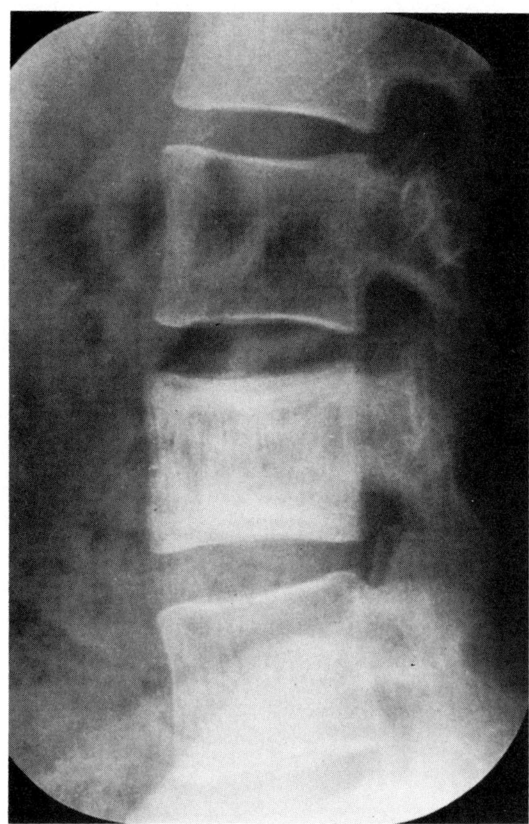

Figure 9–76. Angioma. Lateral radiograph of lumbar spine with a hemangioma in the body of the fourth lumbar vertebra. Note the accentuation of the vertical trabeculae. These are more evident because of both increased bone deposition in response to stress and removal of the smaller horizontal trabeculae. There is augmentation of the vertebral end-plates. Note that the lesion extends into the pedicles posteriorly.

Figure 9–77. Angioma. Radiographs of the lumbar spine of a 36-year-old woman with hemangioma in the second lumbar vertebra. *A* was taken shortly following a normal pregnancy and delivery, after which the patient suffered a fall that caused a compression fracture of the vertebra. The symptoms cleared after several weeks. *B* was taken over 2 years later, after another normal pregnancy and delivery. The patient fell and had severe pain, but neurologic examination was negative. More severe osteoporosis of the vertebra is recognized. There is extension into the pedicle posteriorly, and there is a fracture of a weakened area of the body anteriorly. CT scan shows no invasion of soft tissue around the vertebra. *C* was taken 4 months later. There was no intervening treatment. There is healing of the fracture with reinforcement of the bone anteriorly. *D* shows an anteroposterior view of an arteriogram in which the second lumbar artery was cannulated. Injection of dye into this area filled the defect in the body of L-2, and there are numerous irregular vessels of varying sizes and shapes with some "puddling" of the dye, suggesting proliferation of blood vessels.

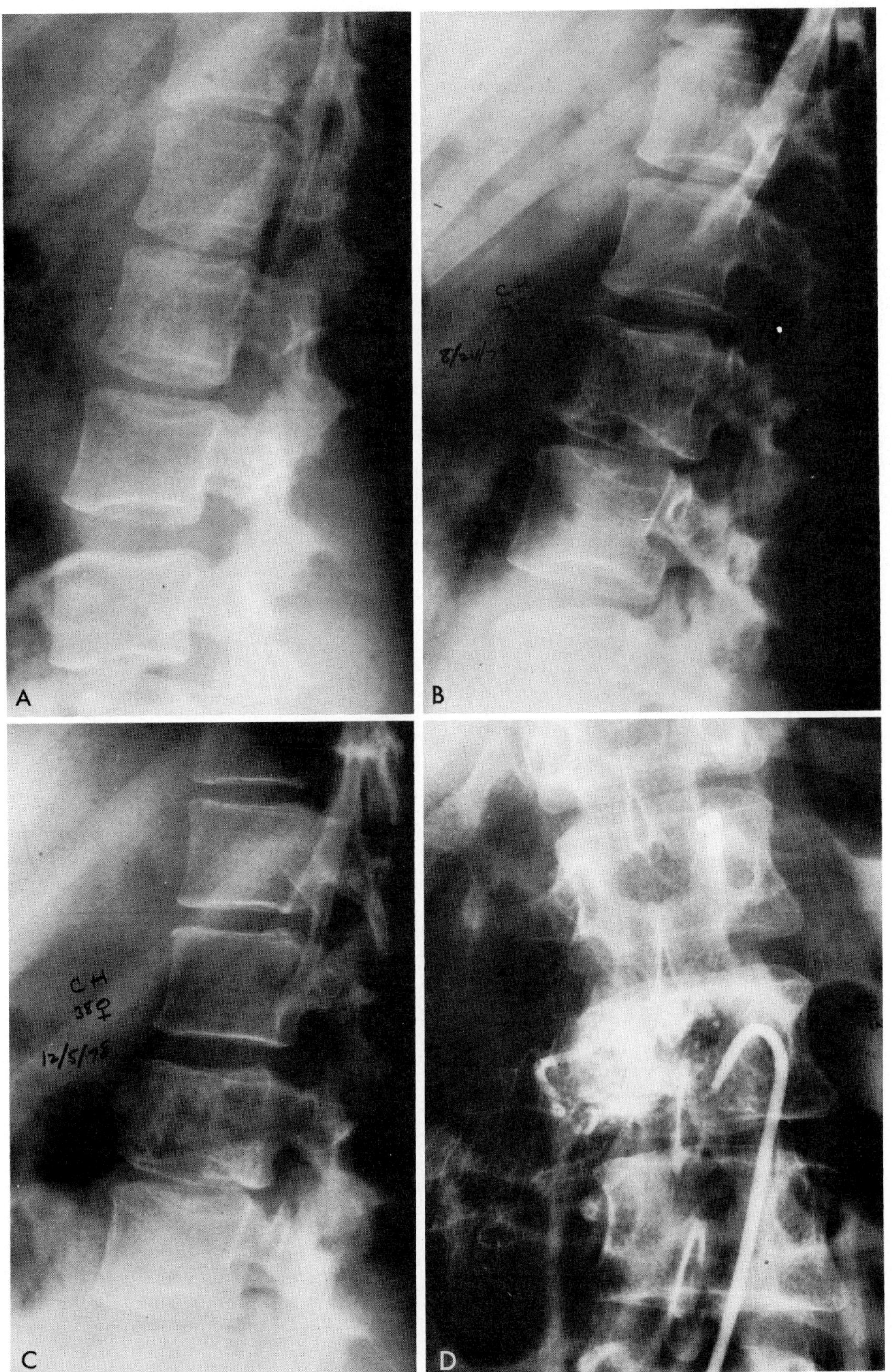

Figure 9–77. *See legend on opposite page*

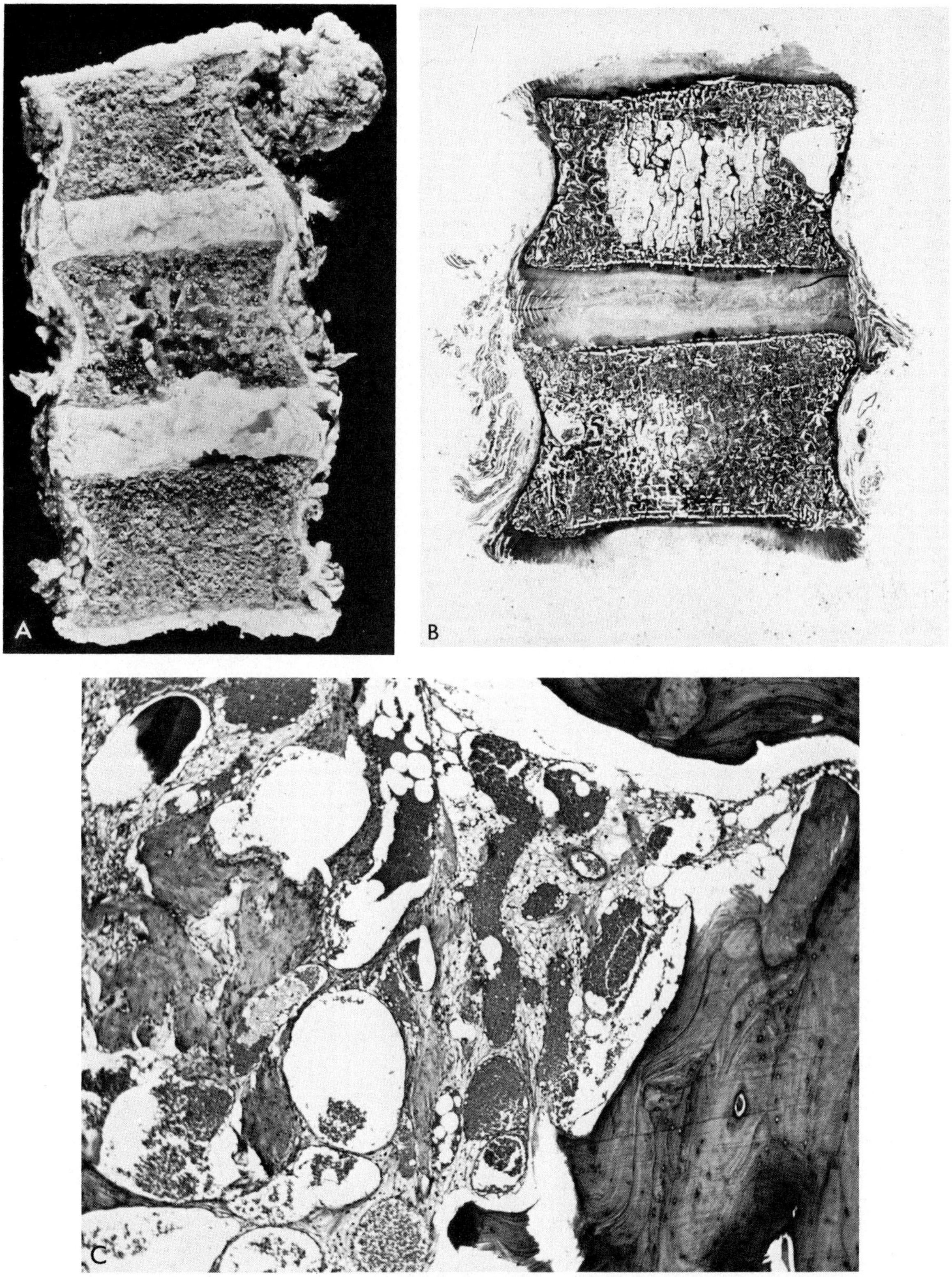

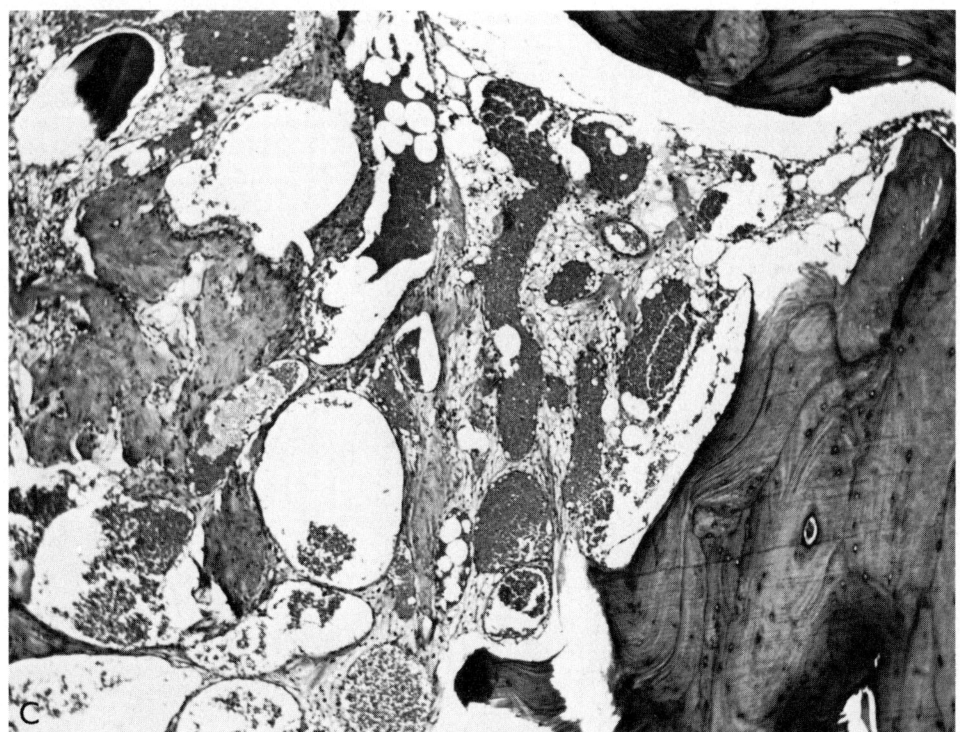

Figure 9–78. Angioma in vertebral body. *A,* Gross specimen of a vertebra containing an angioma in the center of the body. Note the large dilated spaces with prominent vertical orientation of the trabeculae. *B,* Macrosection of this same vertebra, with removal of the smaller horizontal trabeculae and augmentation of the vertical ones. There is normal marrow around the central focus of the angioma. *C,* Section through the angioma represented in *A* and *B.* The marrow has been replaced by thin-walled, dilated vascular channels.

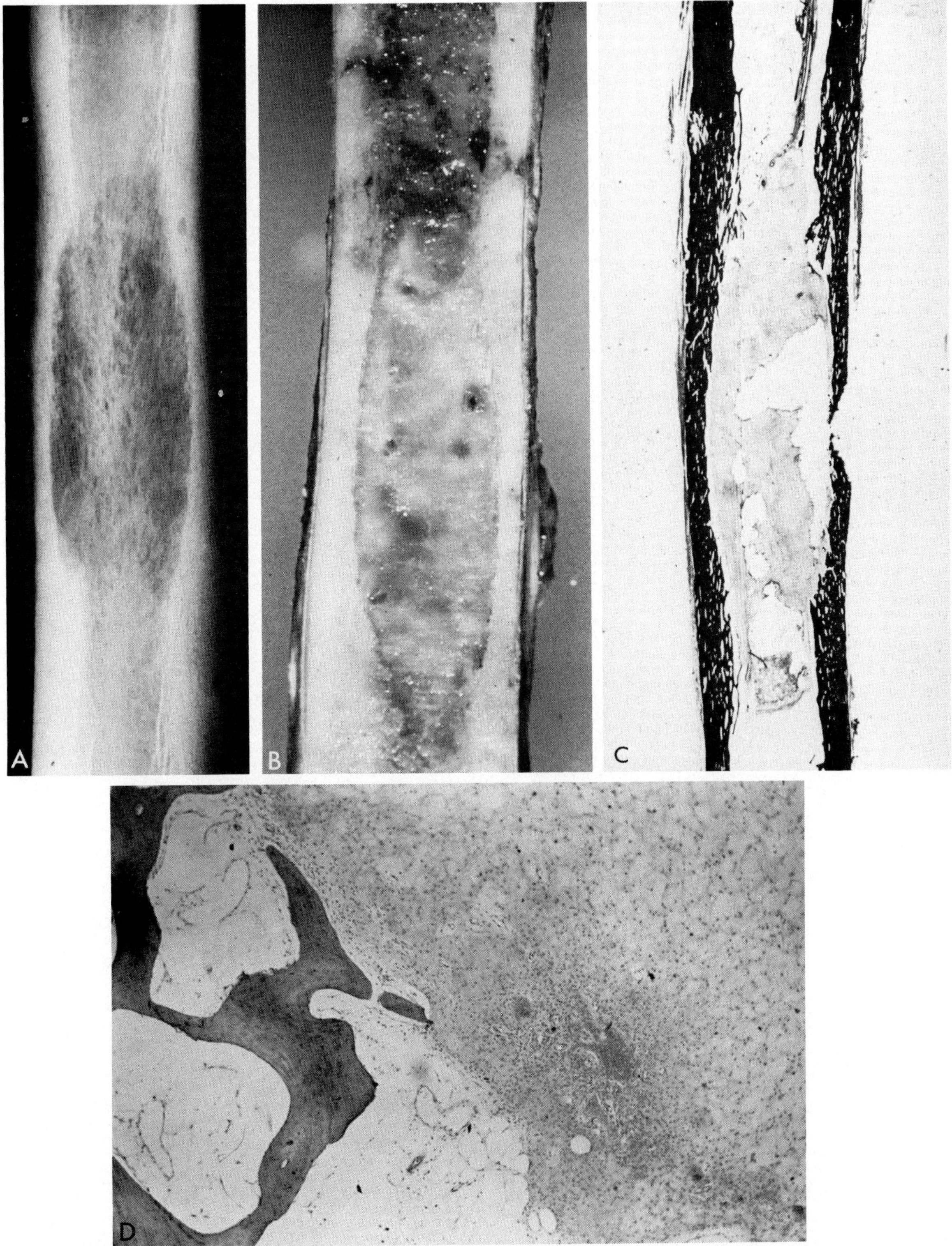

Figure 9–79. Lipoma. Incidental finding in the tibia of a 20-year-old male who required a hip disarticulation for osteosarcoma of the femur. *A,* Sharply outlined lytic defect in the tibial diaphysis. There is removal of cortex from the inner aspect but no significant expansion or periosteal reaction. The bone has not produced a sclerotic intramedullary rim around the lesion. *B,* Gross photograph of the sharply outlined bright yellow lipoma in the middiaphysis of the tibia. *C,* Macrosection of the lesion. There is some resorption occurring in the cortex adjacent to the lesion, but there is no reaction by the bone to this benign process. *D,* Histologic appearance of the lesion, composed of fat cells of varying sizes, shapes, and maturity. The lesion is well demarcated from the normal marrow fat, which lies between the bony trabeculae. Notice the absence of bone in the lesion itself.

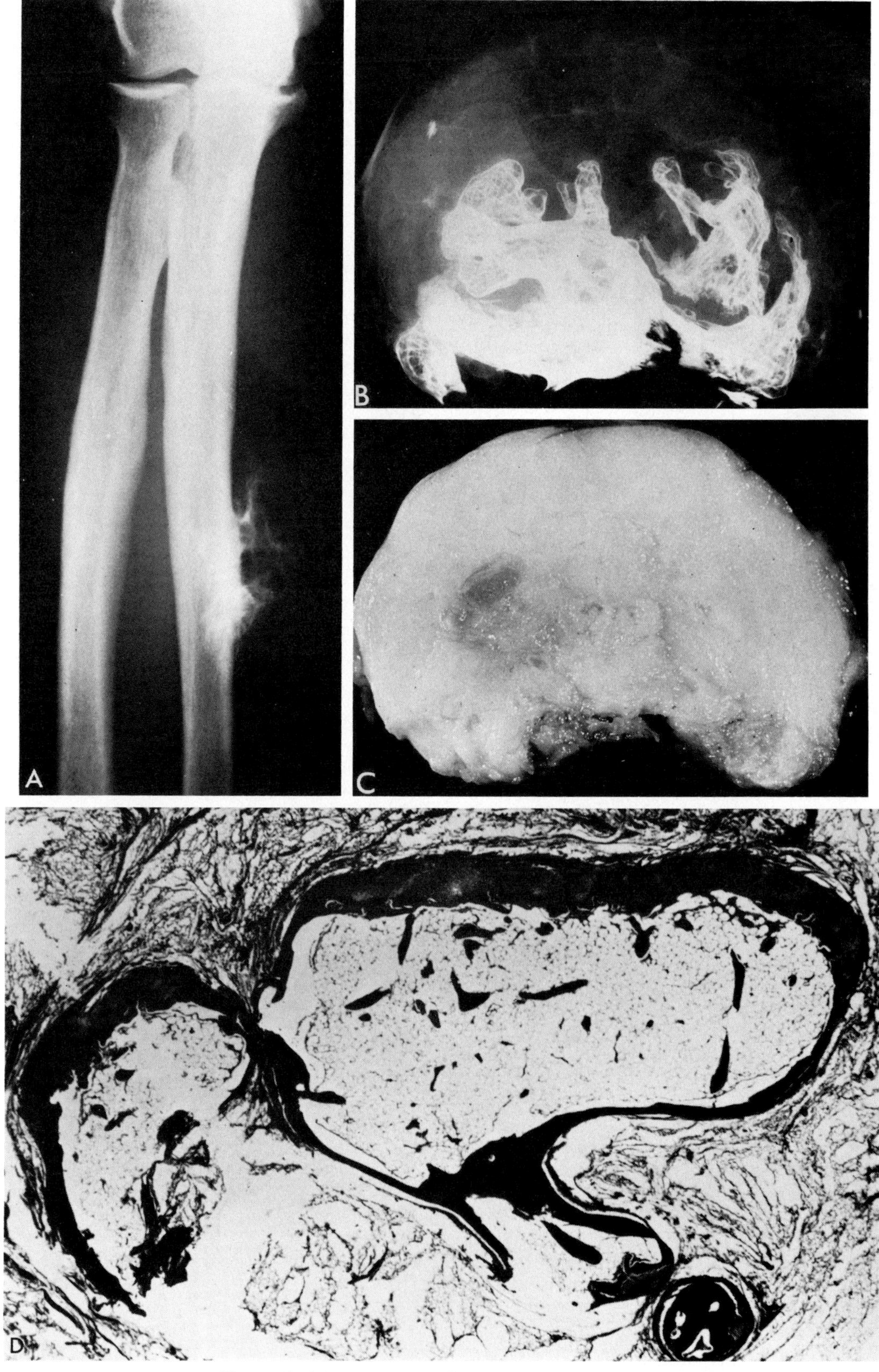

Figure 9–80. *See legend on opposite page*

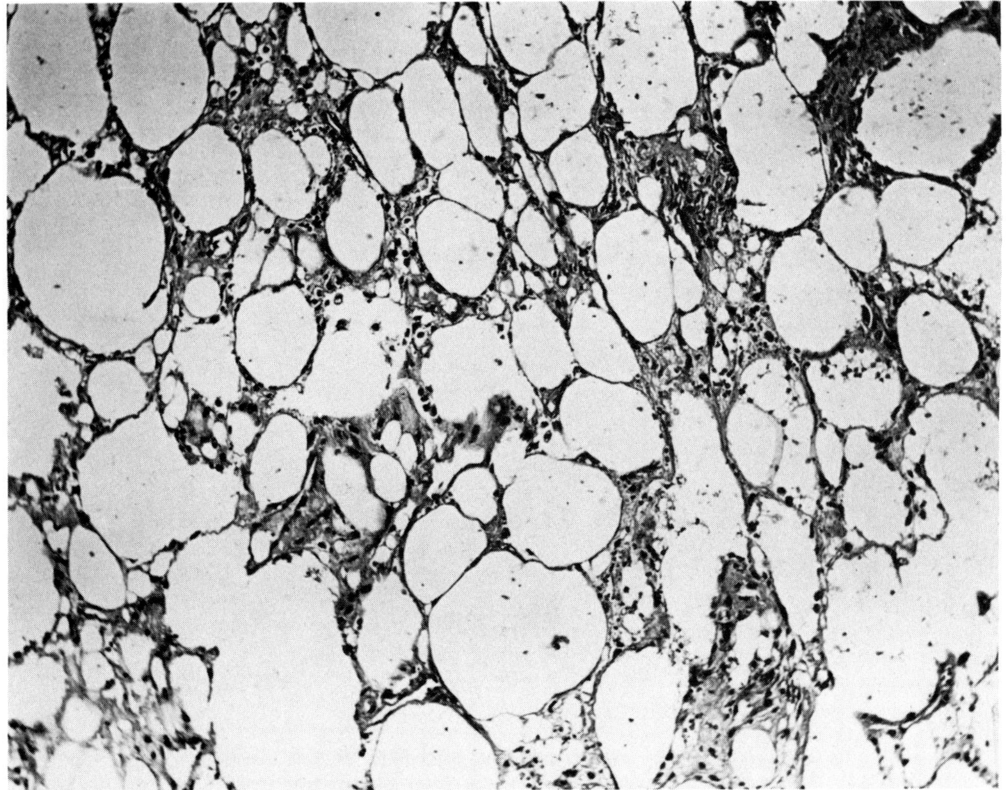

Figure 9–81. Lipoma. Typical histologic appearance of a lipoma showing great variability in size and shape of the fat cells. There is no pleomorphism of the nuclei to suggest malignancy.

LIPOMA OF BONE

The few well-documented lipomas in bone exhibit a well-differentiated fatty tumor, usually discovered as an incidental finding. In many instances the tumor expands, and infarction of portions of the tumor results. Calcification is then observed within the well-defined lesion, and secondary bone formation may result. Although pure lipomas are rare, well-defined lesions with foci of calcification or ischemic bone formation are more frequent, and malignant tumors are described arising from such foci. The precise nomenclature for these lesions is under debate; some observers classify them as fibrous histiocytomas or osteosarcomas when they become malignant.

Text continued on page 365

Figure 9–80. Lipoma. Periosteal lipoma in a 37-year-old male. The lesion was asymptomatic except for the presence of a mass. *A,* Anteroposterior radiograph of the forearm illustrating irregular ossific projection from the surface of the middiaphysis of the ulna with a clearly defined soft-tissue mass of fatty density intimately involved with the bony projection. *B,* Specimen radiograph illustrating the irregular ossification extending outward into the soft-tissue mass, which is clearly outlined. *C,* Photograph of a cross section through the mass. It is bright yellow with irregular bone areas in the base and center of the lesion. *D,* Macrosection through the involved area demonstrates a bony stalk and shell with a narrow cartilage cap on the surface of the bone. This cartilage cap blends in directly with the overlying fatty tissue, which composes 90 per cent or more of the bulk of the lesion.

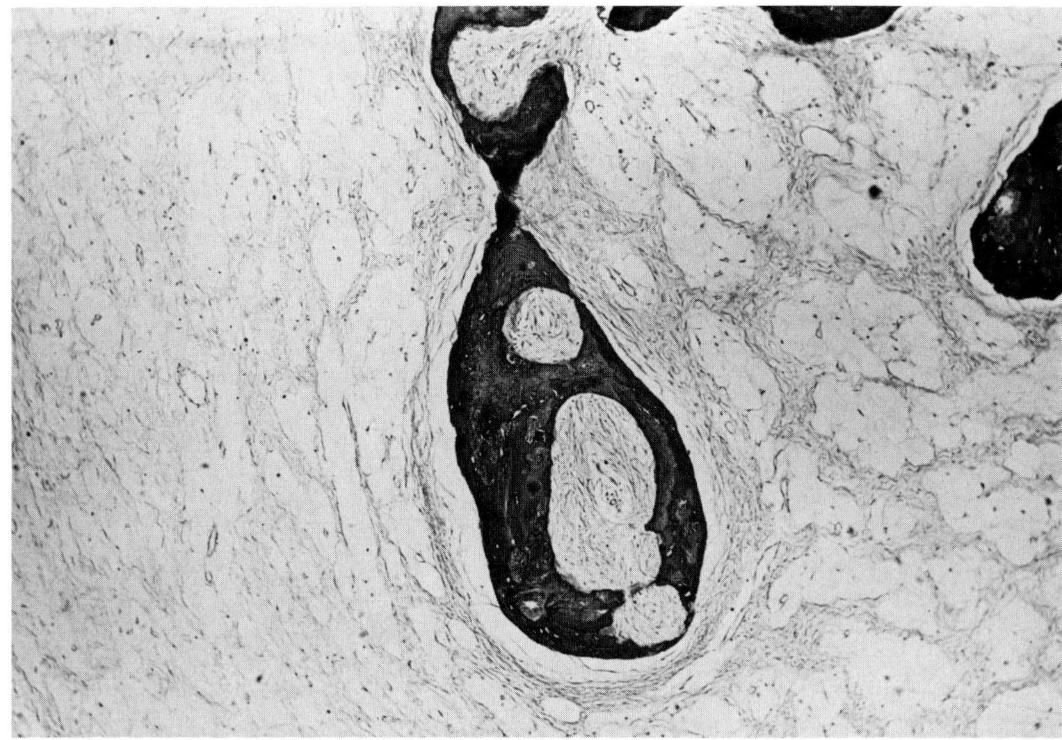

Figure 9–82. Lipoma. Numerous irregularly shaped fatty lobules surround the remaining spicules of bone in the medullary cavity. The bone is viable and is undergoing resorption in portions of the trabecula.

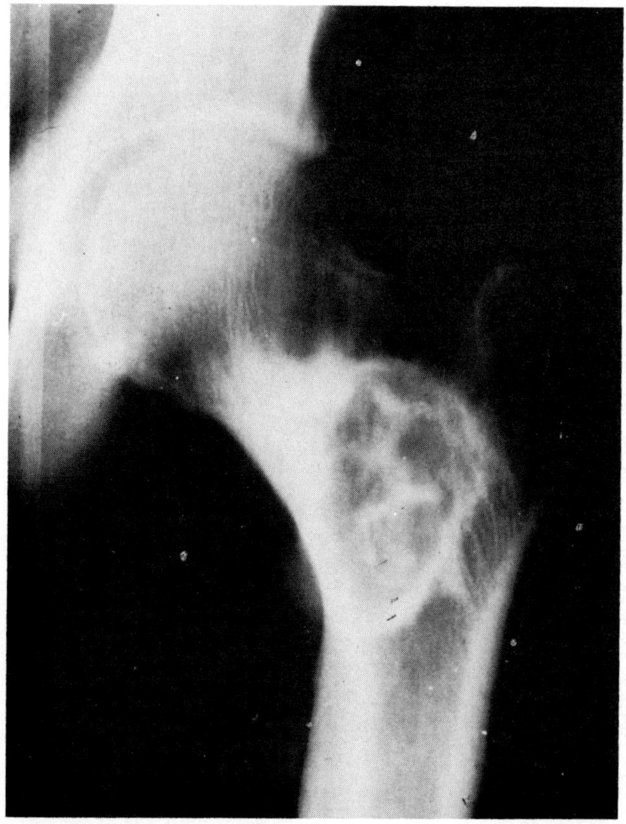

Figure 9–83. Lipoma. Anteroposterior tomogram through the proximal femur. There is a well-defined lesion with a markedly sclerotic rim and evidence of ossification within the matrix. Weight-bearing may be a factor in producing sclerotic reinforcement of bone, located around the lesion where lines of stress pass from the head to the shaft.

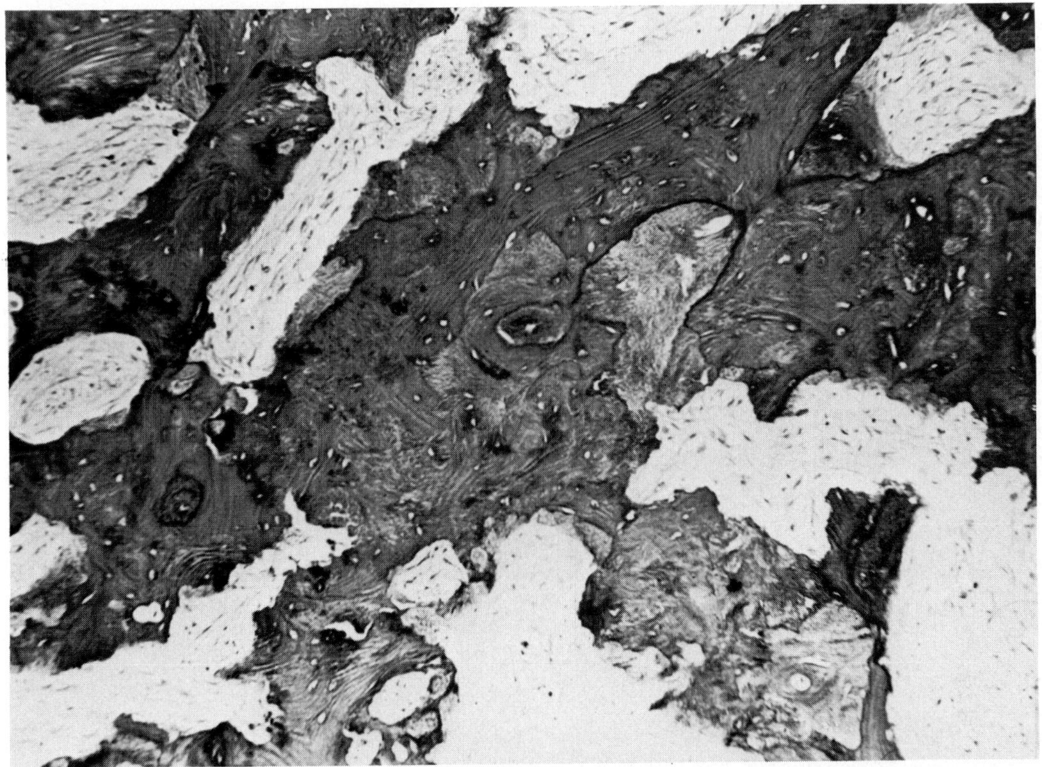

Figure 9–84. Lipoma. Histologic appearance of a sclerotic focus of bone production in a lipoma. Numerous reversal lines suggest haphazard removal and replacement of bone similar to that seen in Paget's disease or chronic osteomyelitis.

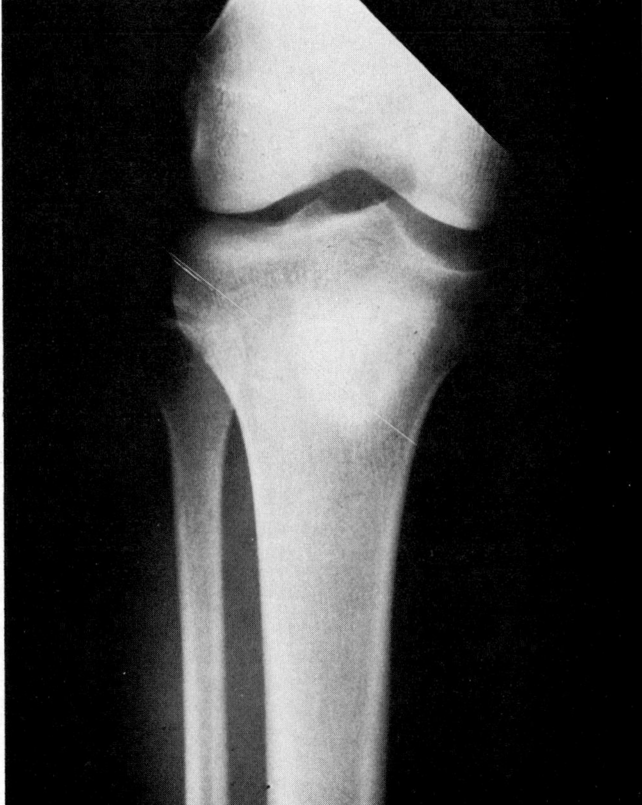

Figure 9–85. Lipoma. Anteroposterior radiograph of the proximal tibia showing sclerotic focus of increased bone production in the tibial metaphysis. The patient had experienced pain for 2 months. Biopsy exhibits lipoma with a large amount of irregular bone production.

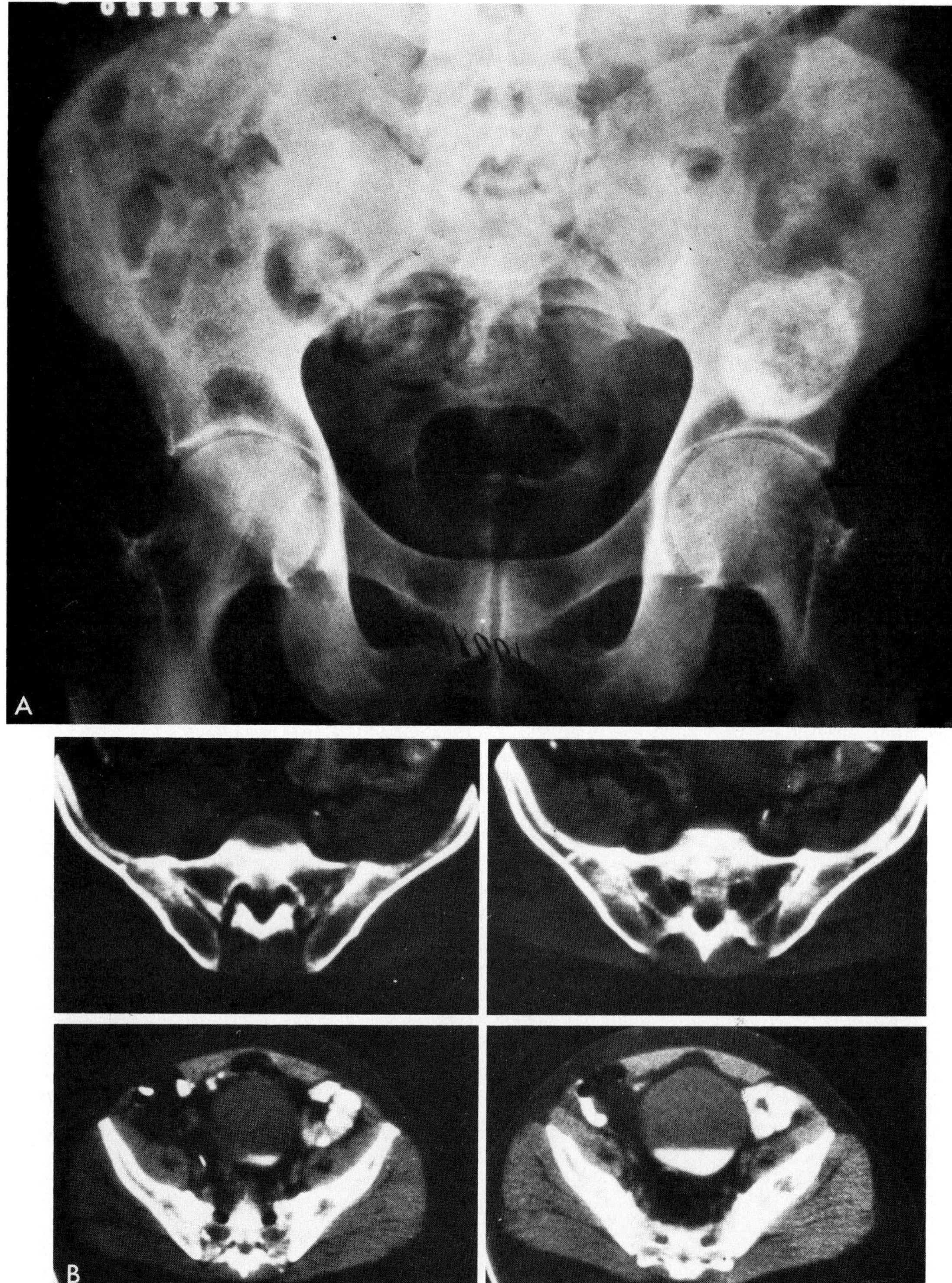

Figure 9–86. Lipoma. Ossifying lipoma in the ilium. *A,* Anteroposterior radiograph of the pelvis with a large, rounded, ossific density above the acetabulum. The center of the lesion is predominantly lucent, but there is extensive bone production at the periphery. *B,* CT scans through the ilium confirm the presence of a lytic defect with extensive bone production around it.

Illustration continued on opposite page

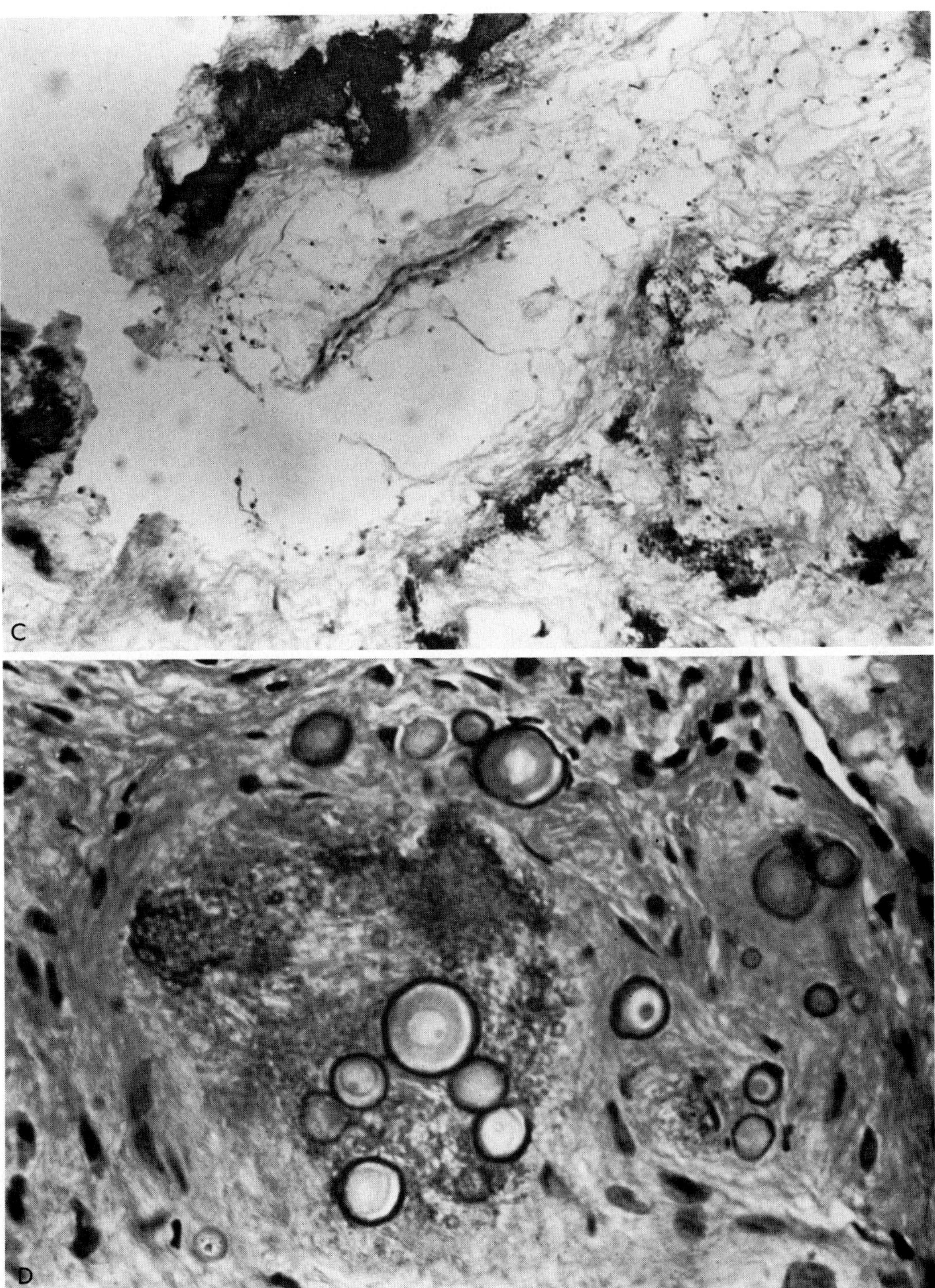

Figure 9–86 (*Continued*) *C*, Section through the tumor showing fatty tissue with cells of irregular shape and size. There is bone production of a peculiar type commonly seen in ischemic areas and around infarcts and bone tumors. *D*, Section of a collagenous area in the lipoma with numerous psammoma bodies.

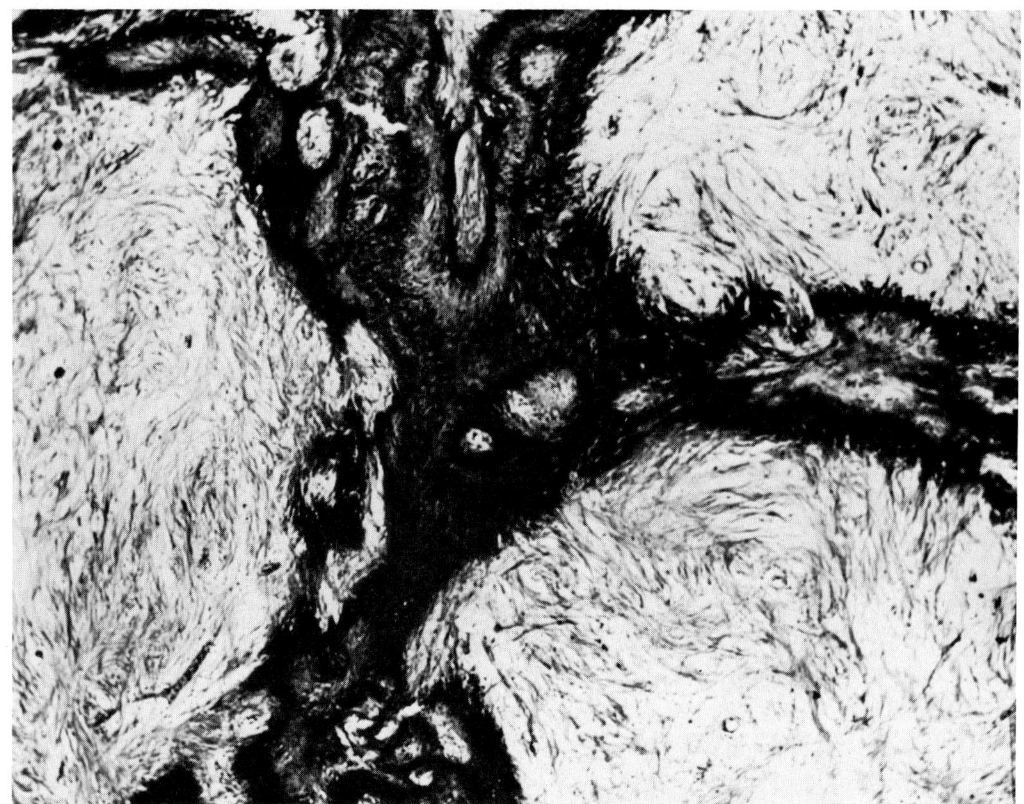

Figure 9–87. Lipoma. Focus of calcification in a somewhat fibrotic portion of a lipoma. This peculiar calcified material (ischemic bone) is commonly seen in these tumors.

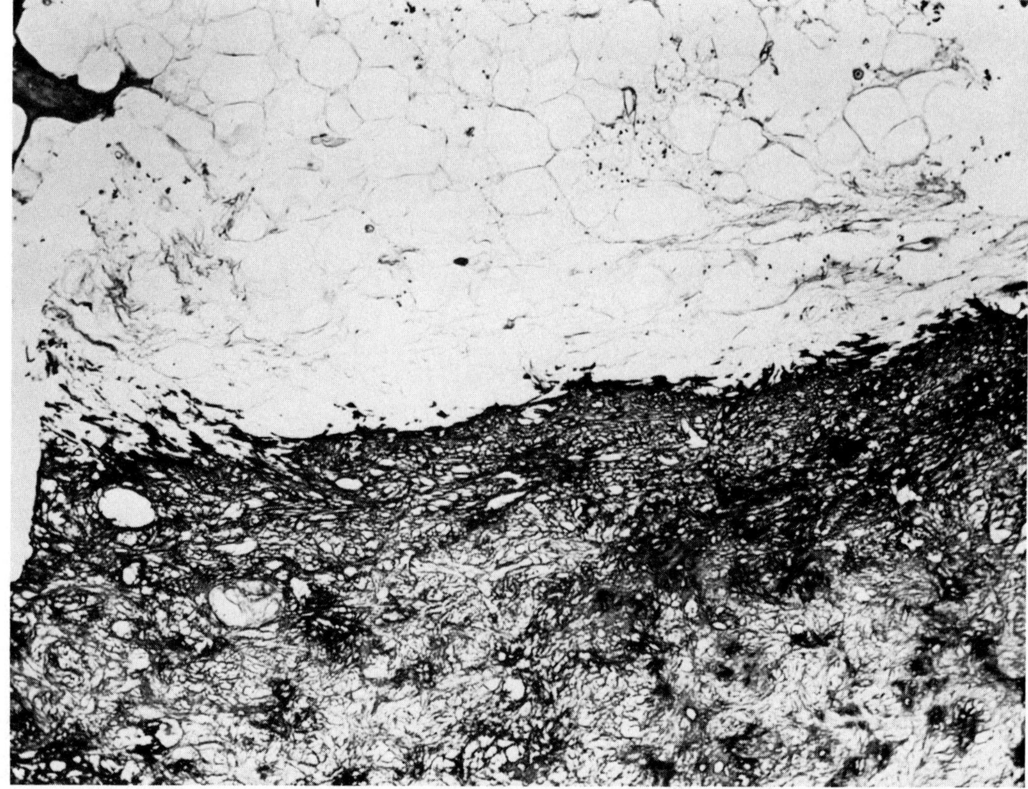

Figure 9–88. Lipoma. Focus of ischemic bone and calcified matrix in a lipoma.

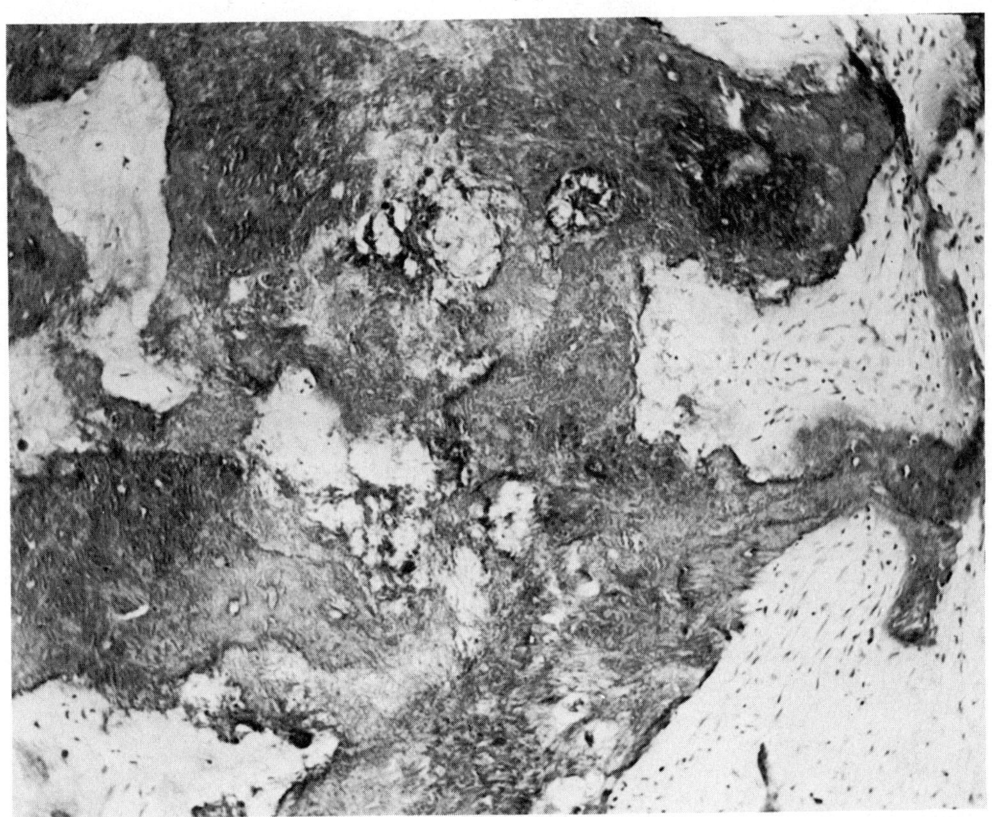

Figure 9–89. Lipoma. More mature but still abnormal ischemic bone produced in a lipoma. It is mineralized and exhibits radiopaque matrix density, but the normal structure of bone is absent.

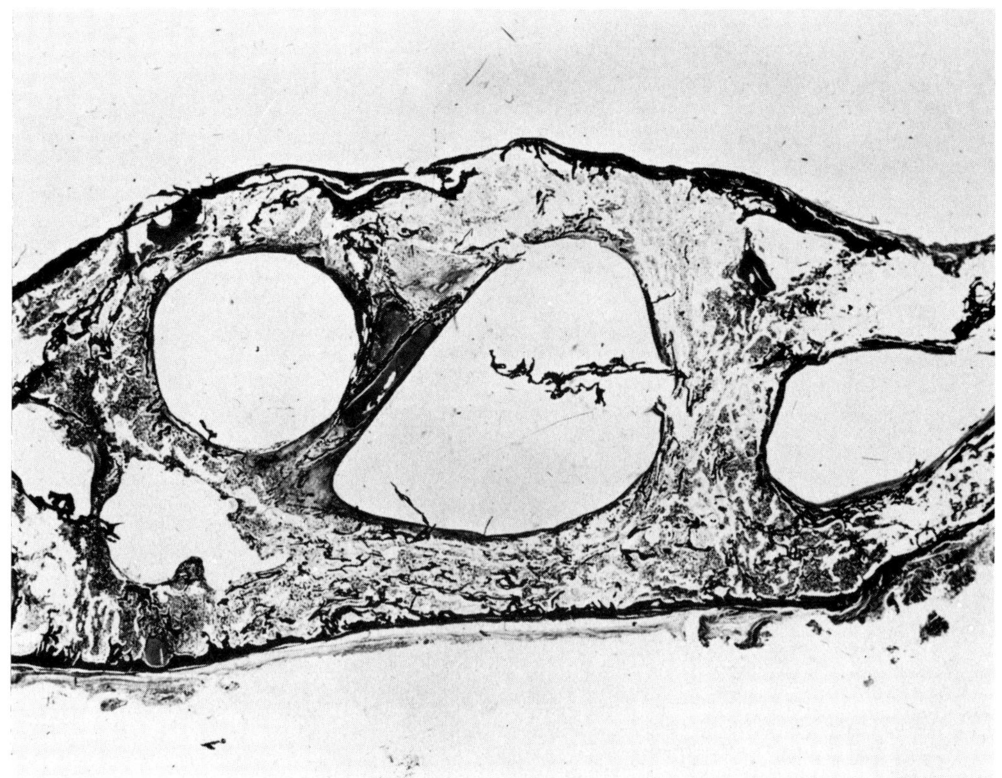

Figure 9–90. Lipoma. Macrosection of a lipoma in a rib. Areas of necrosis result in cyst formation. This is common in such tumors and may be the source of some bone cysts.

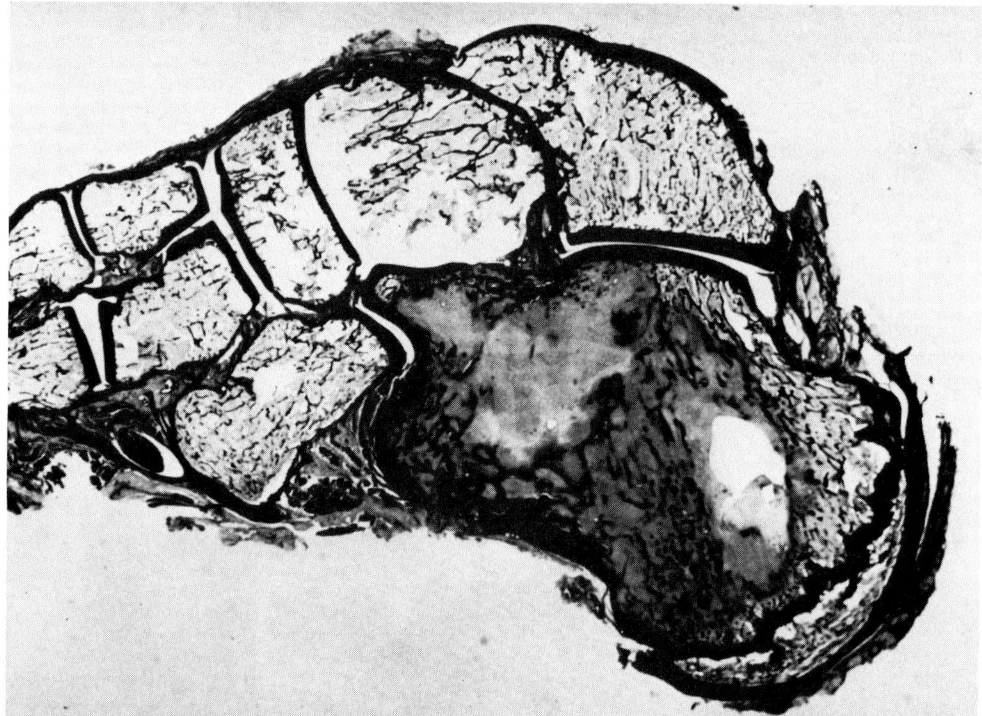

Figure 9–91. Lipoma. Macrosection of a lipoma in an os calcis. Note areas of bony reinforcement outlining the tumor. There is an area of cystic degeneration in the posterior aspect of the os calcis.

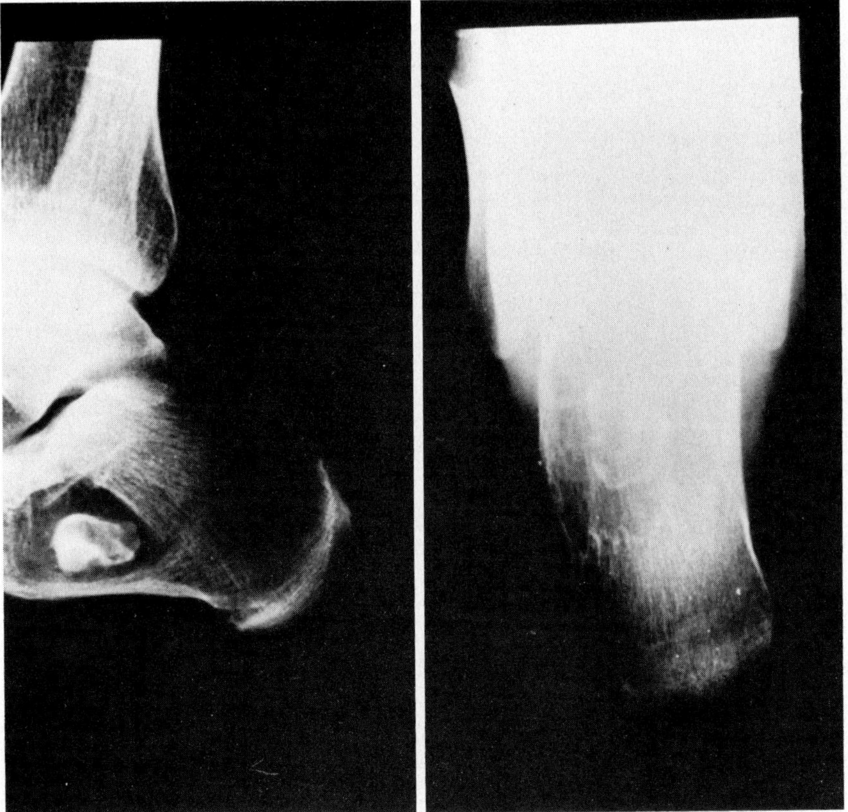

Figure 9–92. Radiographs of a lipoma containing a large calcified nidus in an os calcis. Most of the lesion is solid lipoma. There are areas of cystic degeneration in the lesion, and the calcified body "floats" in the cystic cavity.

DESMOPLASTIC FIBROMA

The intraosseous desmoplastic fibroma is a tumor of bone characterized by extensive collagen formation. It consists of dense fibrous connective tissue that replaces the normal osseous structures of bone, and no bone formation is demonstrated. The margin of this lesion may be somewhat indistinct, the cortex can be ruptured, and the lesion can extend outside the bone. The histologic features of the pure desmoplastic fibroma exhibit little pleomorphism, mitotic activity, or variability in the nuclear structure, so these lesions are not considered malignant at the time of excision. There is neither osseous nor chondroid matrix formation by the tumor, but the desmoplastic fibrous connective tissue may calcify, thus leading to increased radiographic density. The lesion is difficult to differentiate from low-grade fibrosarcoma of bone.

Text continued on page 370

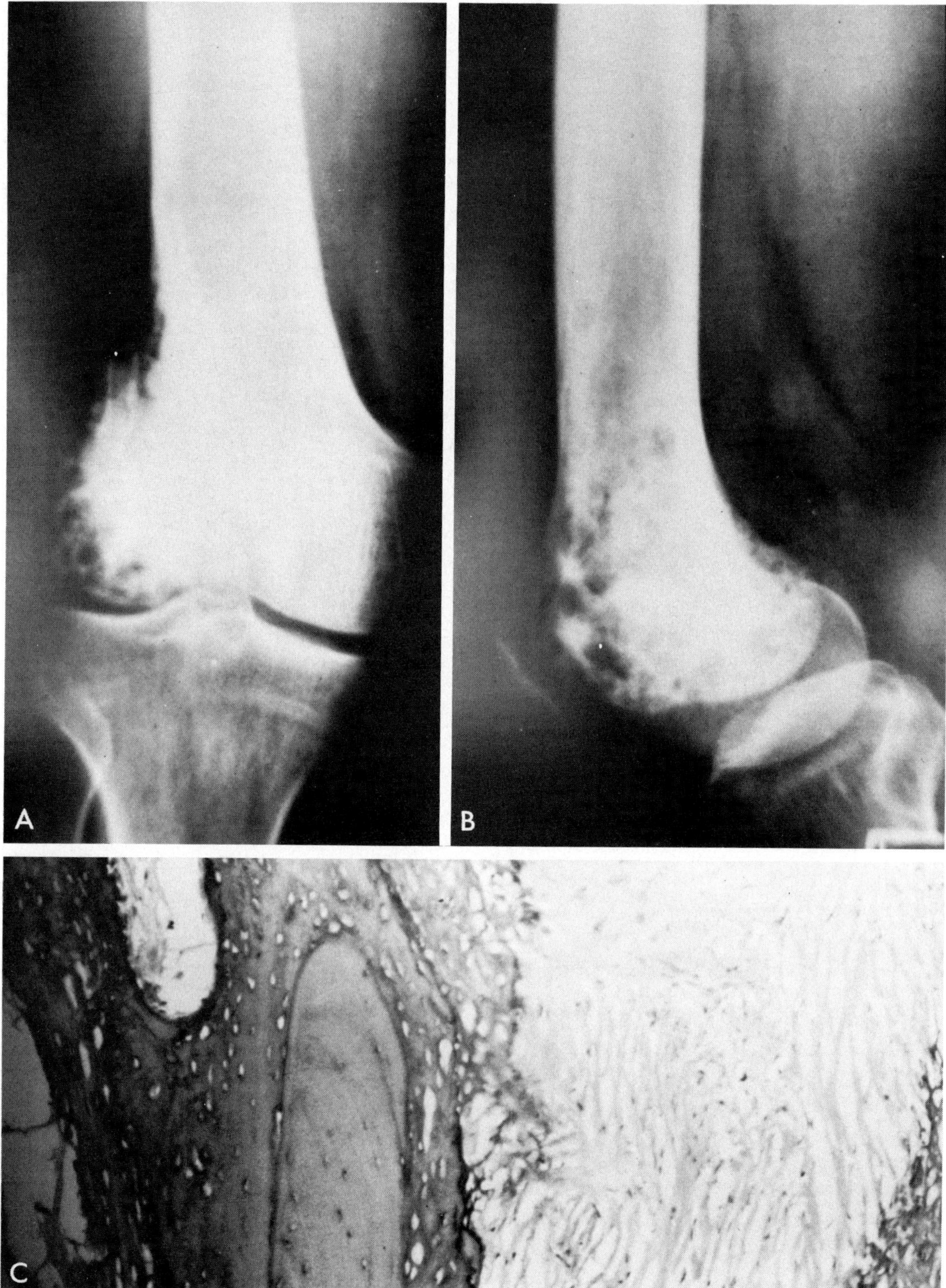

Figure 9–93. Anteroposterior (*A*) and lateral (*B*) radiographs of desmoplastic fibrous tumor. The lesion is poorly circumscribed, erodes through the cortical surface, and exhibits extensive calcification, but there is no evidence of osteoid-matrix production. The histologic picture (*C*) reveals dense collagen formation, a relatively acellular tumor, and extensive calcification.

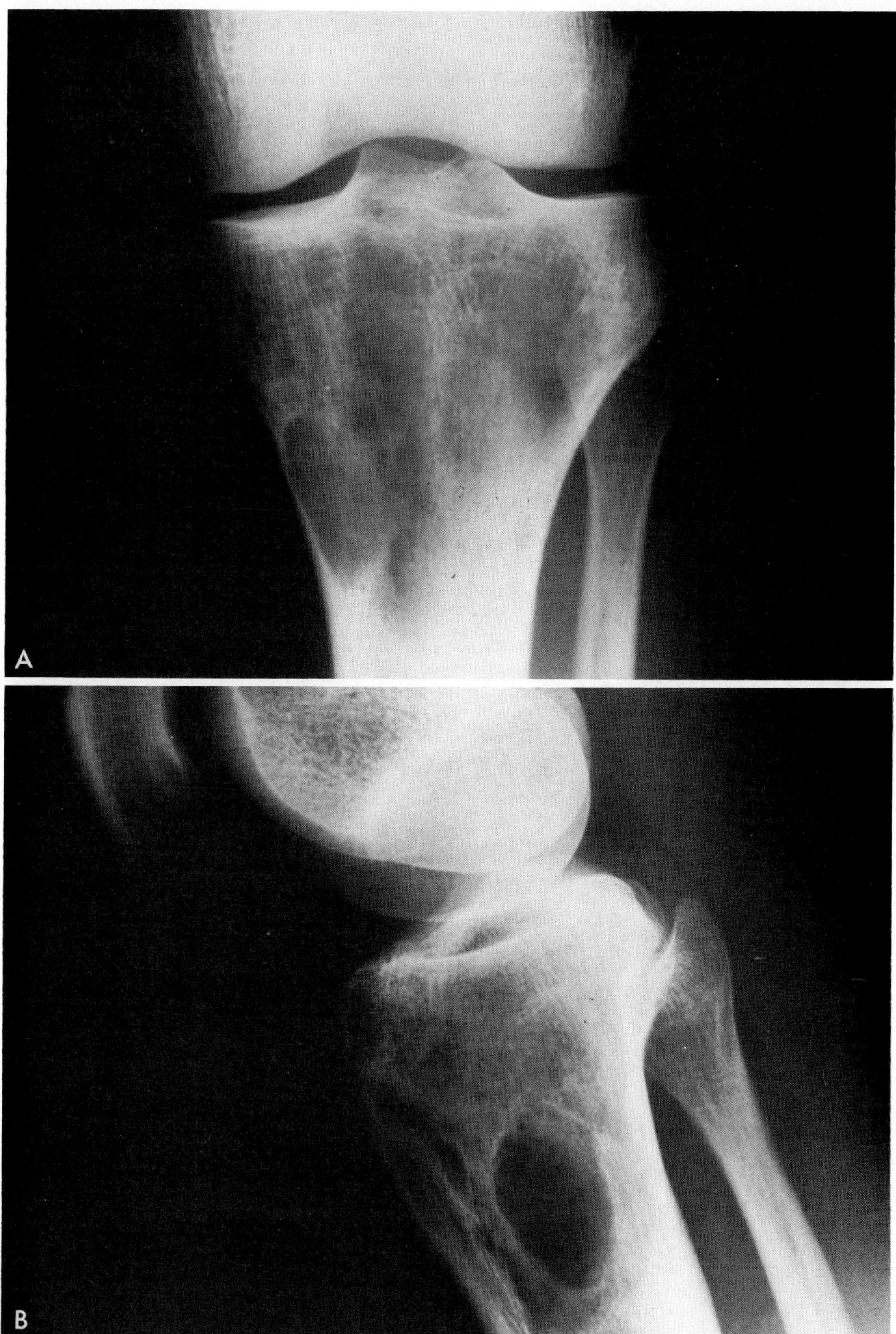

Figure 9–94. Fibrosarcoma. Anteroposterior (*A*) and lateral (*B*) radiographs of a fibrosarcoma in the epiphysis and metaphysis of the tibia. There is diffuse destruction of the entire epiphyseal portion of the tibia. A pre-existing benign-appearing defect is present in the metaphysis, indicating a previous nonossifying fibroma.

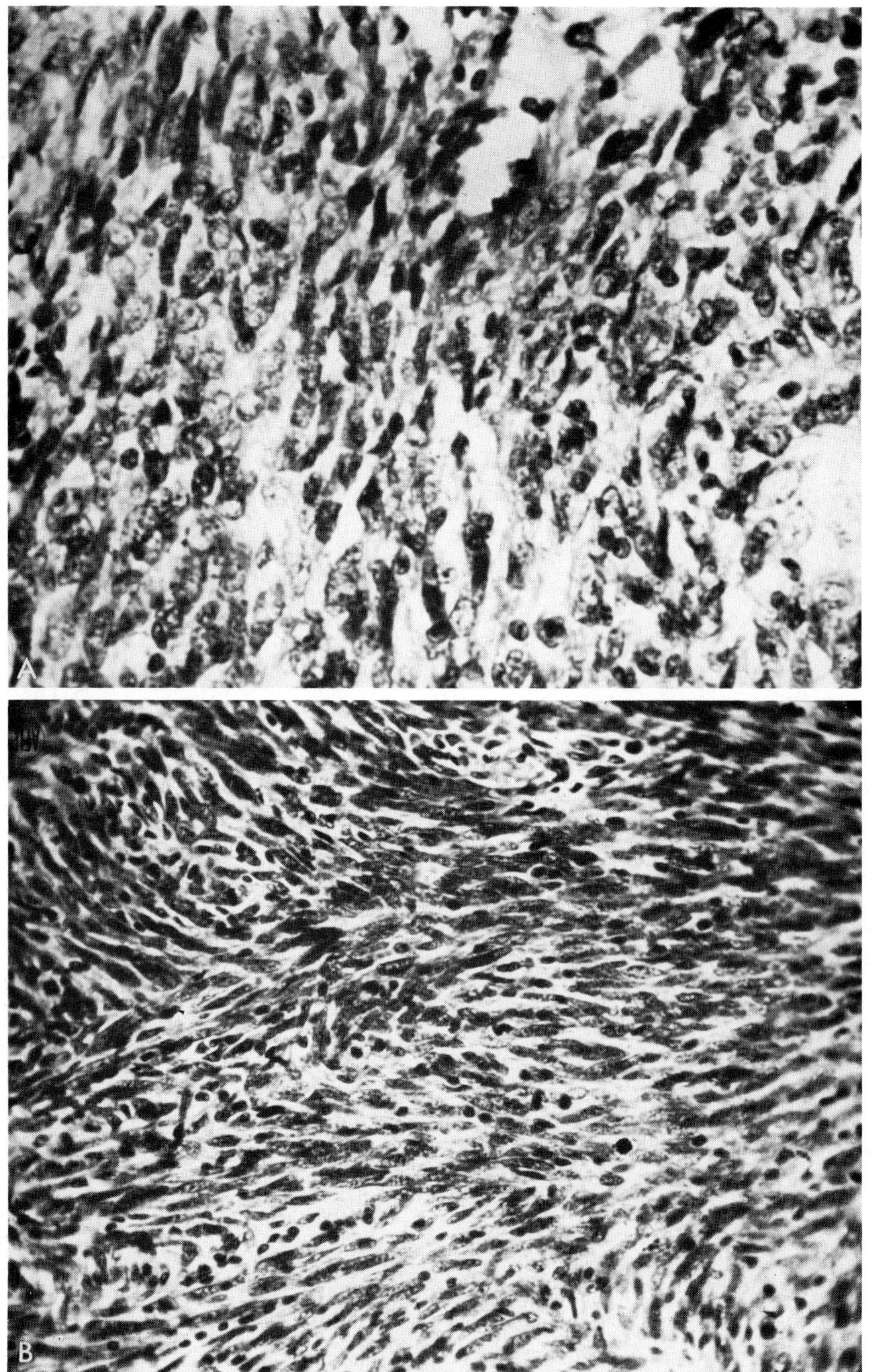

Figure 9–95. Fibrosarcoma. Histologic appearance of the fibrosarcoma illustrated in Figure 9–94. Portions of the lesion exhibit a benign-appearing pattern consistent with nonossifying fibroma (*C*). The remainder of the lesion consists of a moderate to markedly pleomorphic spindle cell tumor without identifiable matrix production (*A* and *B*).

Illustration continued on opposite page

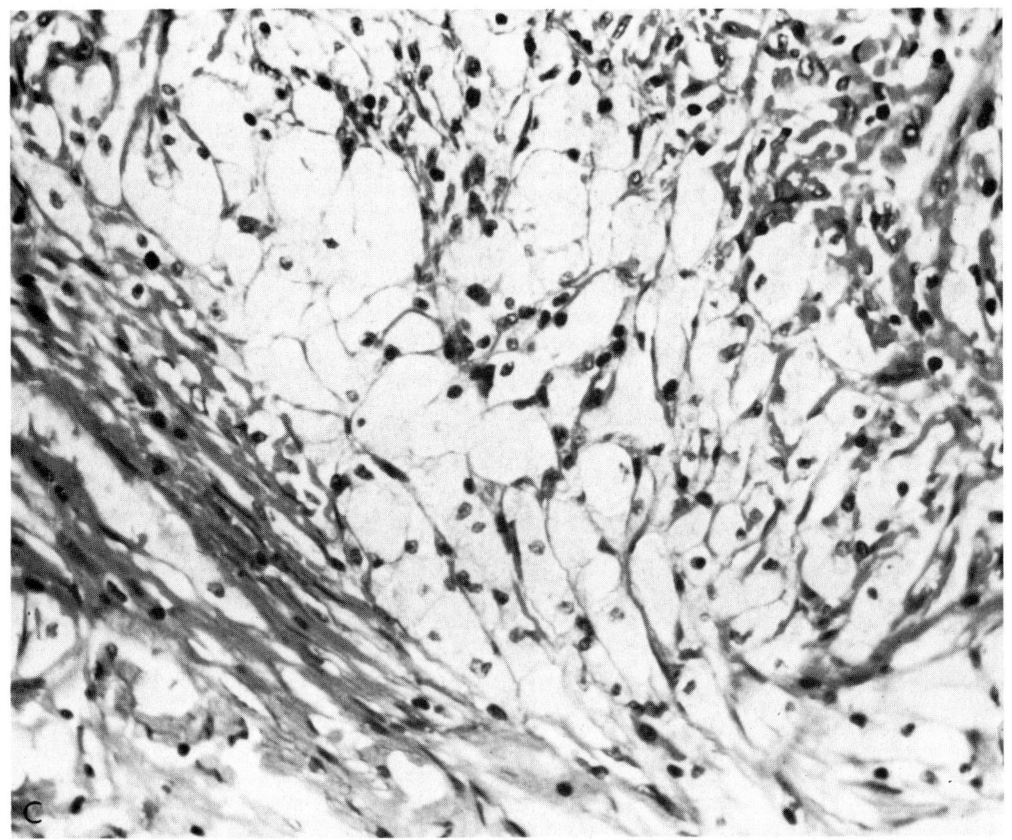

Figure 9–95 *Continued*

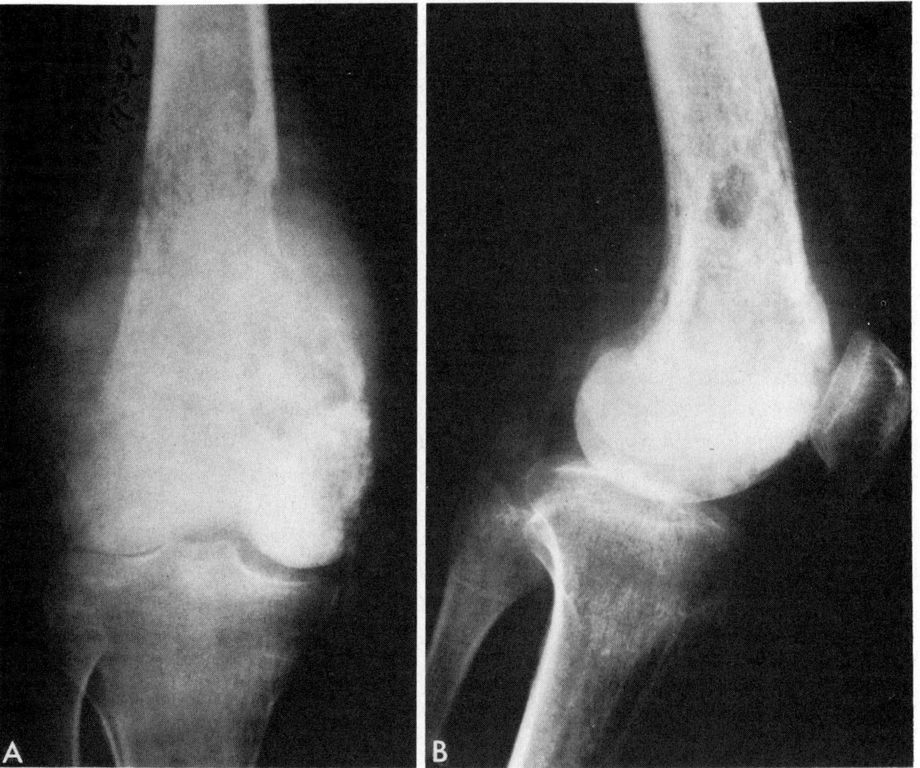

Figure 9–96. Fibrosarcoma. Anteroposterior (*A*) and lateral (*B*) radiographs of fibrosarcoma in lower femur. Note permeative destruction with poorly defined margins. A periosteal reaction is present at the site of cortical erosion. There is no identifiable calcification within the lesion.

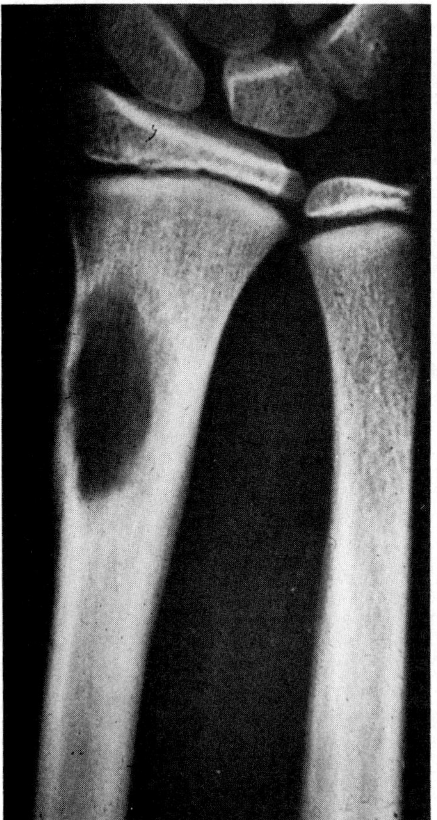

Figure 9–97

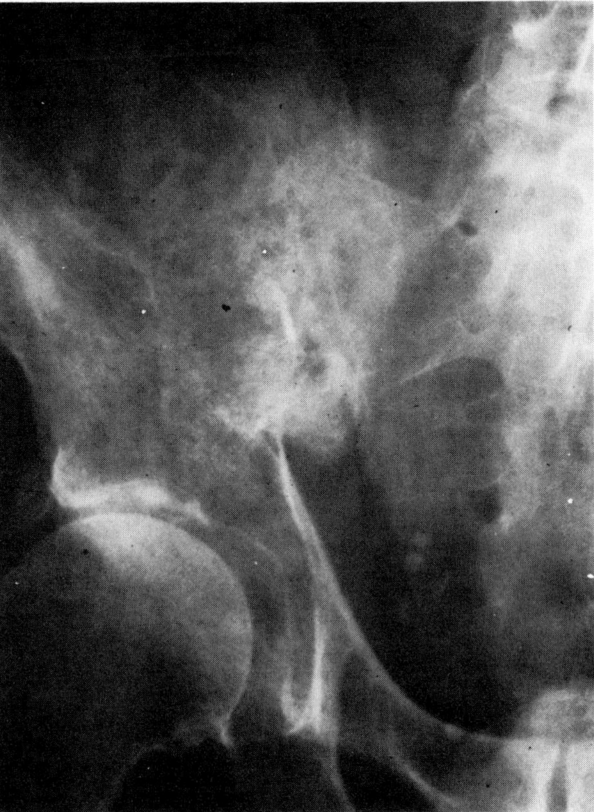

Figure 9–98

Figure 9–97. Fibrosarcoma. Radiograph of lytic destruction in the metaphysis of the distal radius. The lesion has a moth-eaten, destructive pattern with a poorly defined margin, but there is no permeative destruction and no identifiable periosteal reaction. This pattern is consistent with an intermediate rate of growth.

Figure 9–98. Fibrosarcoma. Radiograph of poorly defined lytic lesion in ilium. The margins are indistinct, and there is no identifiable calcification within the lesion.

FIBROSARCOMA OF BONE

Fibrosarcoma of bone is a primary malignant neoplasm, usually found in the metaphysis of long bone, exhibiting radiographic features of an aggressive growth pattern with indistinct margins. The lesion consists of fibrous connective tissue with variability of nuclear structure, pleomorphism, and mitotic activity. The matrix that is formed is purely collagenous. Occasionally, infarcted fragments of cortical bone are caught within the tumor. As a rule, there is no identifiable neoplastic bone formation by the tumor itself. It is a relatively rare tumor of bone, and in general the prognosis is better than that associated with osteosarcoma (Huvos, 1975).

Text continued on page 376

Figure 9–100. Fibrosarcoma. Note the moderate rate of growth with expansion of cortex and circumscribed margin in the medullary cavity. This moderate growth rate is characteristic of fibrosarcoma and allows for segmental resection in selected cases.

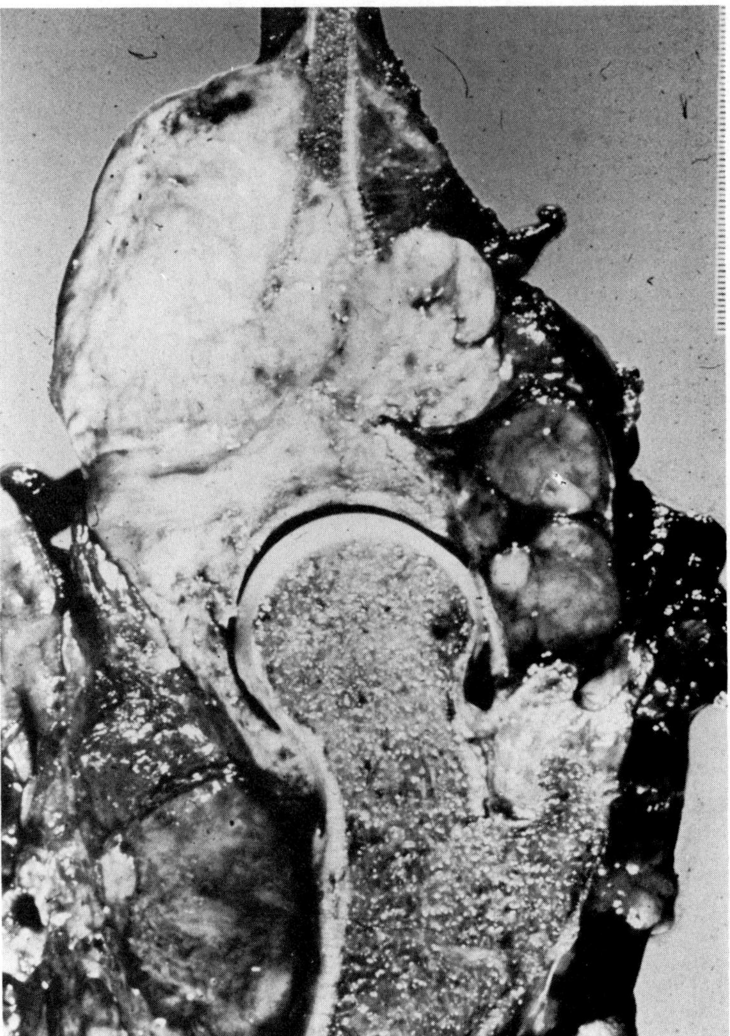

Figure 9–99. Fibrosarcoma. Gross specimen of the fibrosarcoma illustrated in Figure 9–98. Note extensive replacement of ilium and acetabulum by the white fibrous tumor. Erosion of the cortex on both surfaces is also evident.

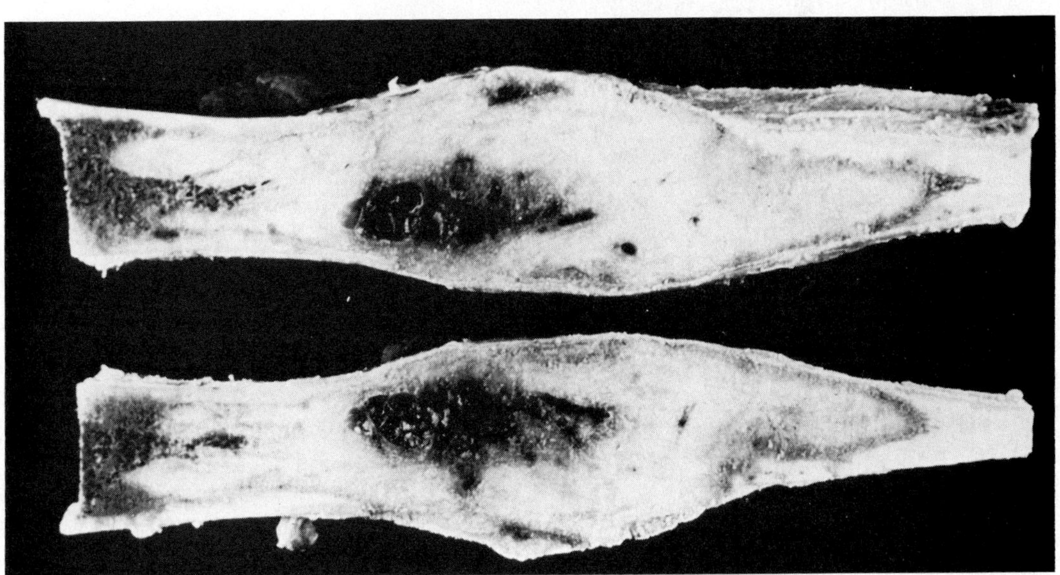

Figure 9–100. *See legend on opposite page*

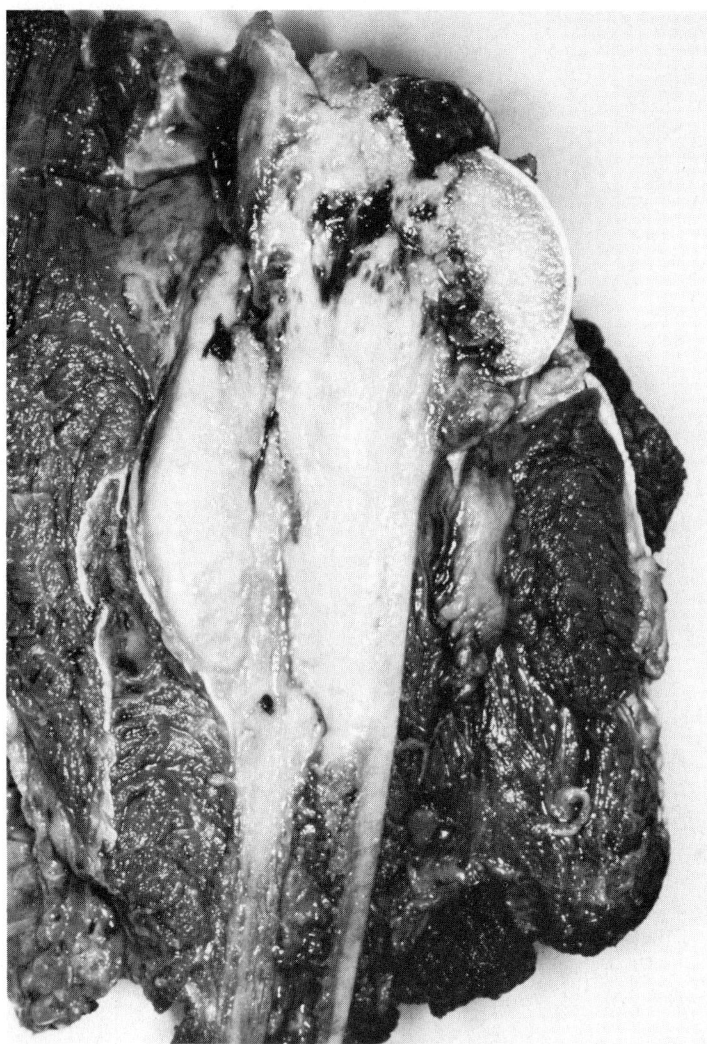

Figure 9–101. Fibrosarcoma. Gross specimen of fibrosarcoma with pathologic fracture, destruction of metaphysis and epiphysis, and erosion into adjacent soft tissue.

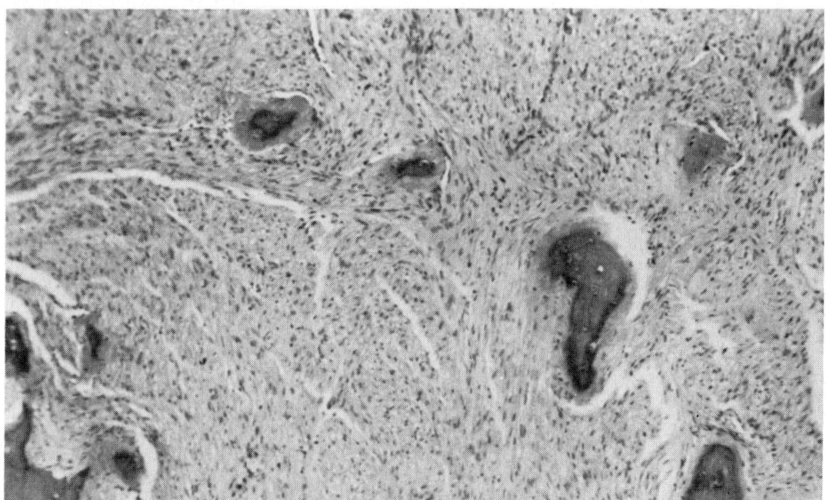

Figure 9–102. Fibrosarcoma. Fibrous tissue exhibiting moderate pleomorphism, even at this low magnification. There is no identifiable osteoid or chondroid-matrix formation.

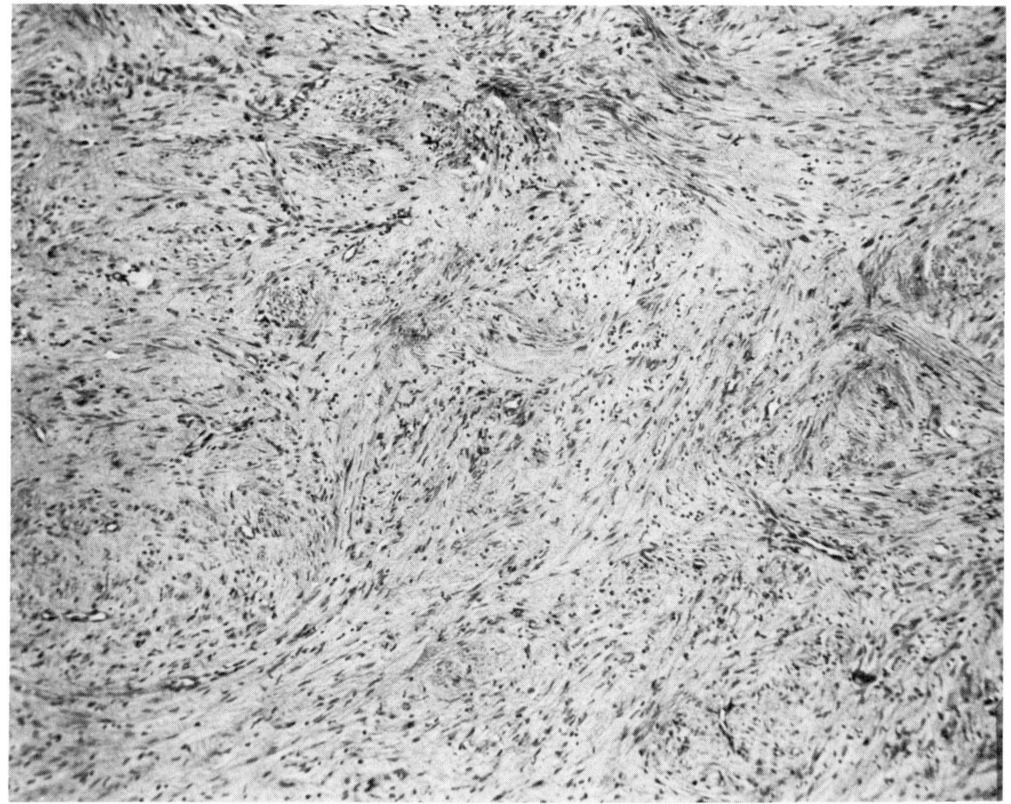

Figure 9–103. Fibrosarcoma. Mild to moderate pleomorphism of tumor. The tumor surrounds residual medullary trabeculae, and there may be some additional reactive bone formation. These residual trabeculae often infarct. There is no osteoid-matrix formation by the tumor.

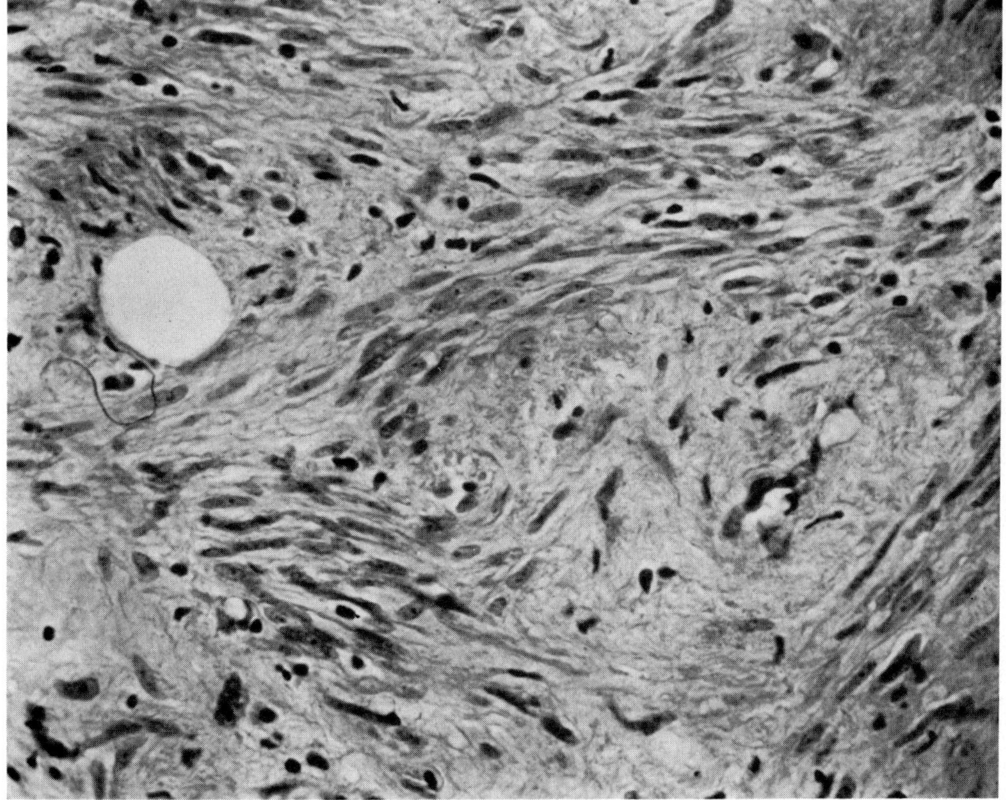

Figure 9–104. Fibrosarcoma. Moderate pleomorphism of fibroblasts and spindled collagen formation by the tumor.

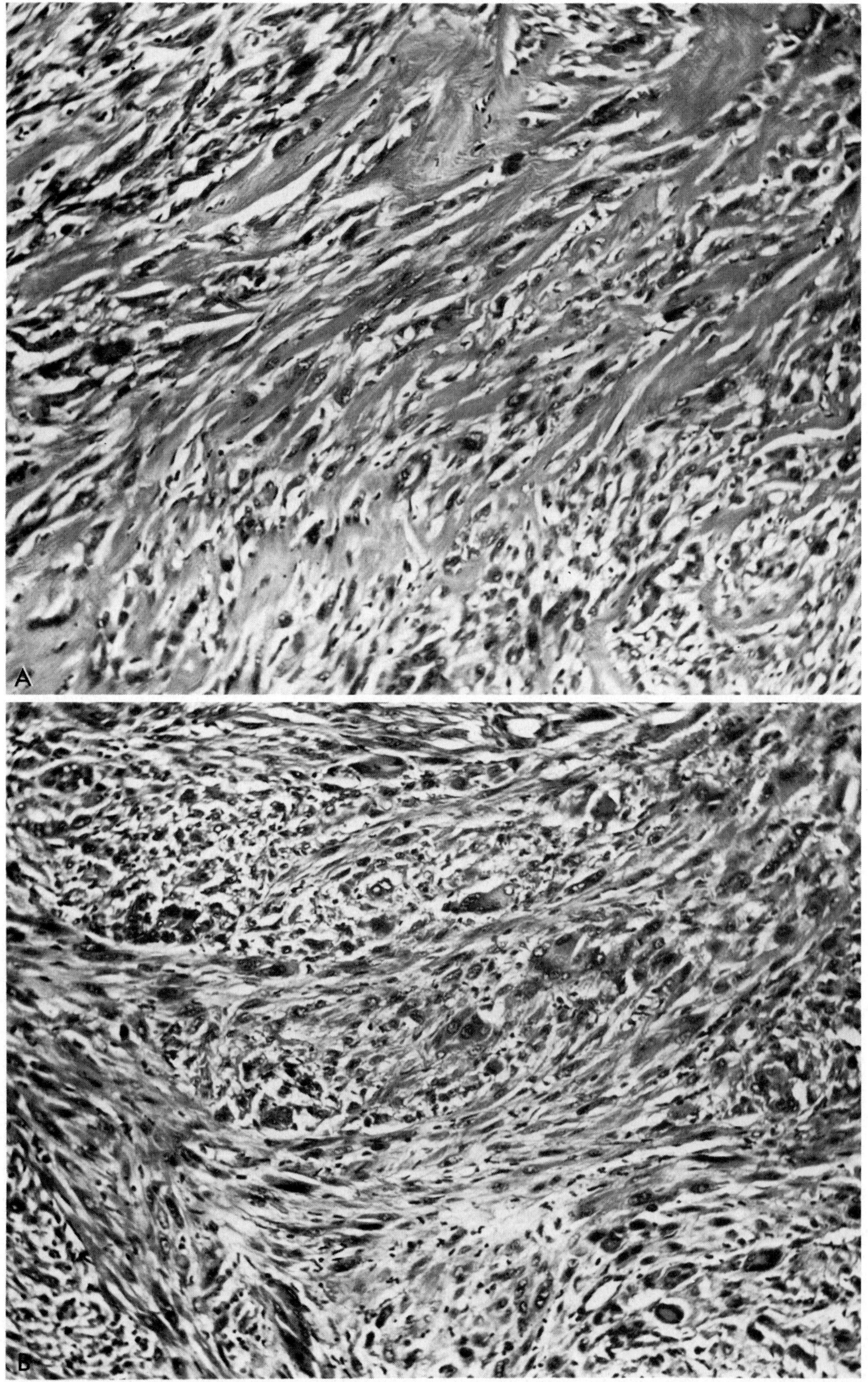

Figure 9–105. Fibrosarcoma. Moderate to severe pleomorphism and extensive mitotic activity in a relatively undifferentiated fibrosarcoma. Note the extensive collagen formed by the tumor.

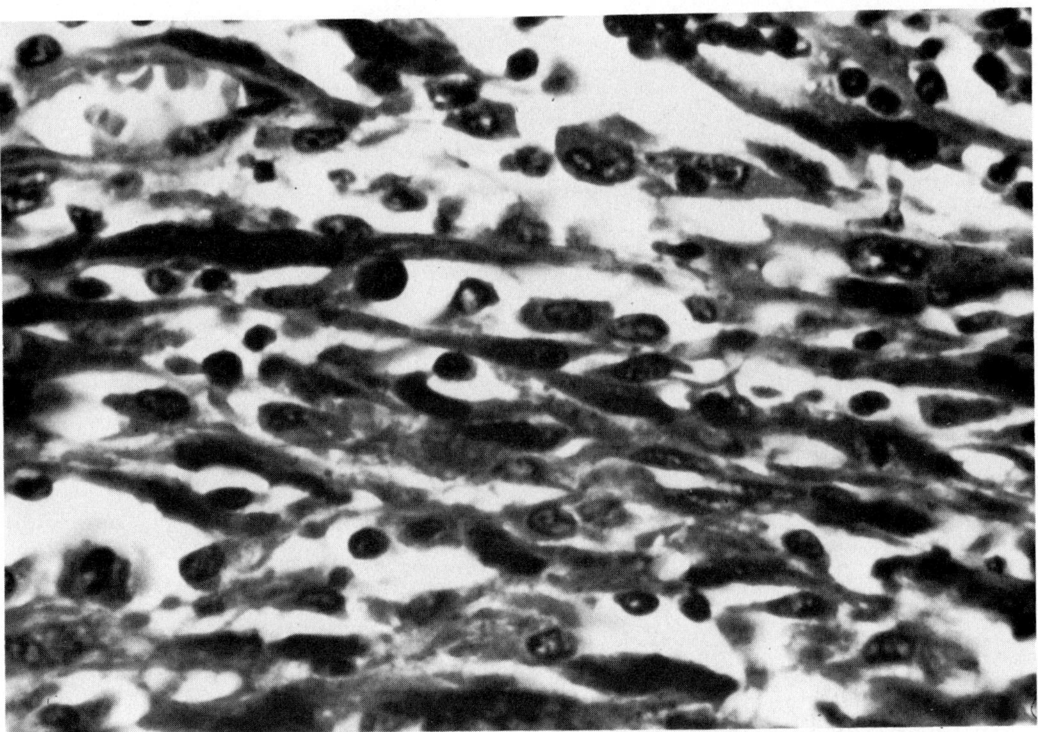

Figure 9–106. Fibrosarcoma. Spindled appearance with marked pleomorphism of the lesion. There is collagen-fiber formation, but no osteoid matrix is produced.

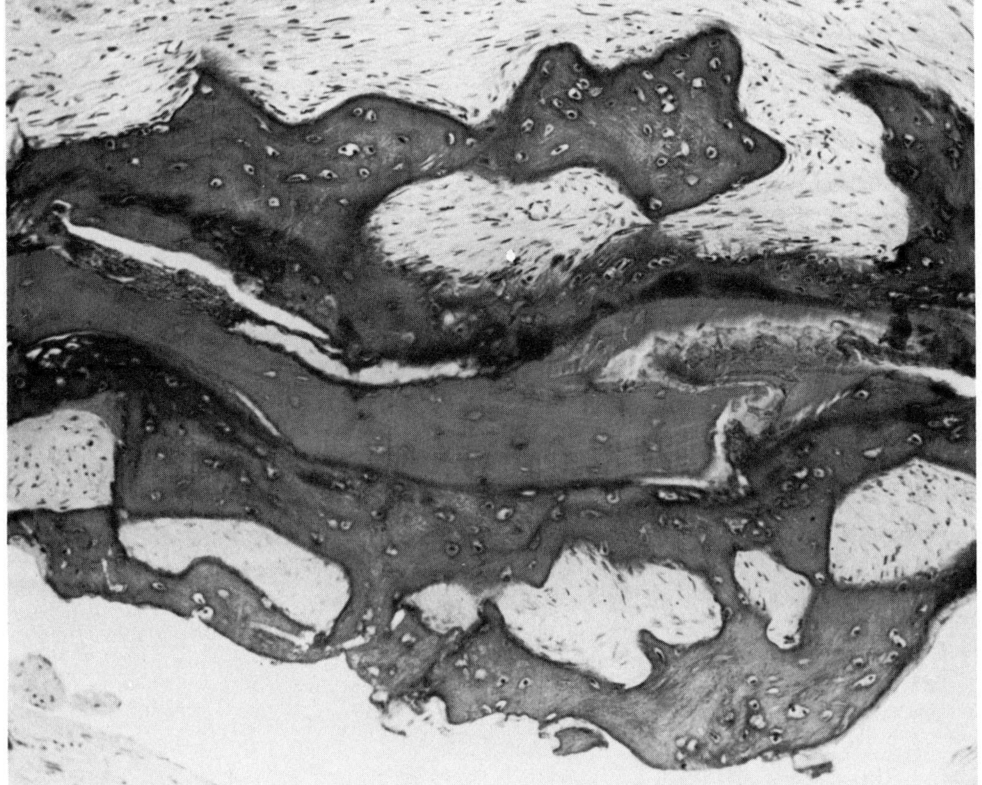

Figure 9–107. Fibrosarcoma. Sequestration of cortical bone fragments is a common occurrence in fibrosarcoma. A centrally located sequestered fragment is surrounded by reactive bone and fibroblastic tumor.

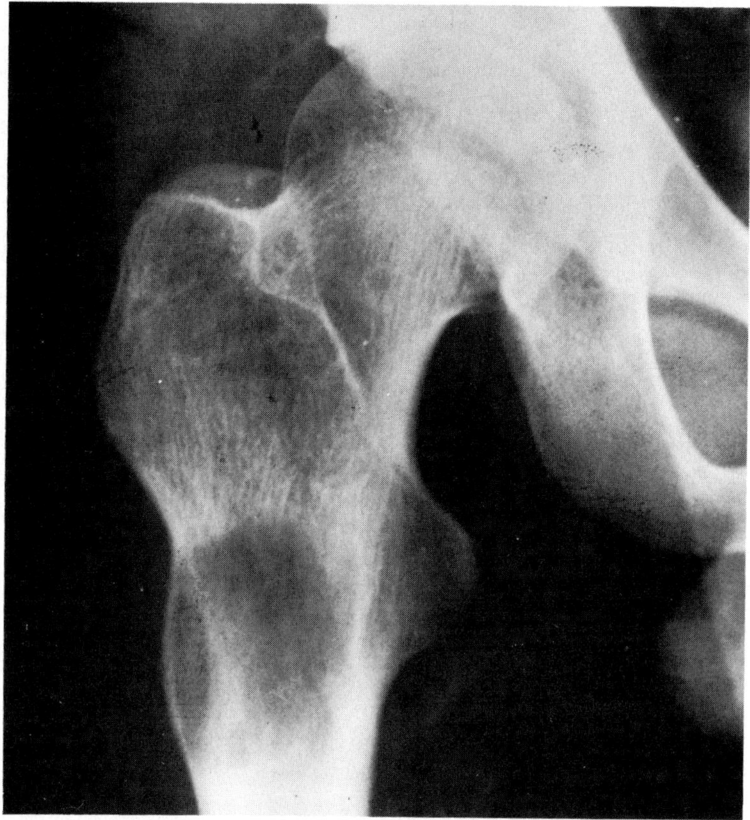

Figure 9–108. Malignant fibrous histiocytoma. Radiograph of circumscribed defect in the metaphysis of the femur. There is moth-eaten destruction at the margin but no identifiable periosteal reaction.

MALIGNANT FIBROUS HISTIOCYTOMA

The term "malignant fibrous histiocytoma" has been used to describe a separate group of tumors characterized by fibrous and histiocytic proliferation. These tumors are often secondary to pre-existing benign lesions, particularly infarcts, and were previously classified as osteosarcomas or fibrosarcomas. They should not show osteoid or chondroid matrix formation, should be composed of single or multinucleated histiocytes, and should contain xanthomatous material. The storiform pattern also seen in the benign nonossifying fibroma is a histologic feature.

Radiographic manifestations are those of a moderately aggressive malignant tumor, chiefly in the lower limb.

The prognosis of these tumors is essentially similar to osteosarcoma and fibrosarcoma of bone. Whether this entity represents a bona fide separate category of bone tumor has not been resolved to everyone's satisfaction.

Text continued on page 382

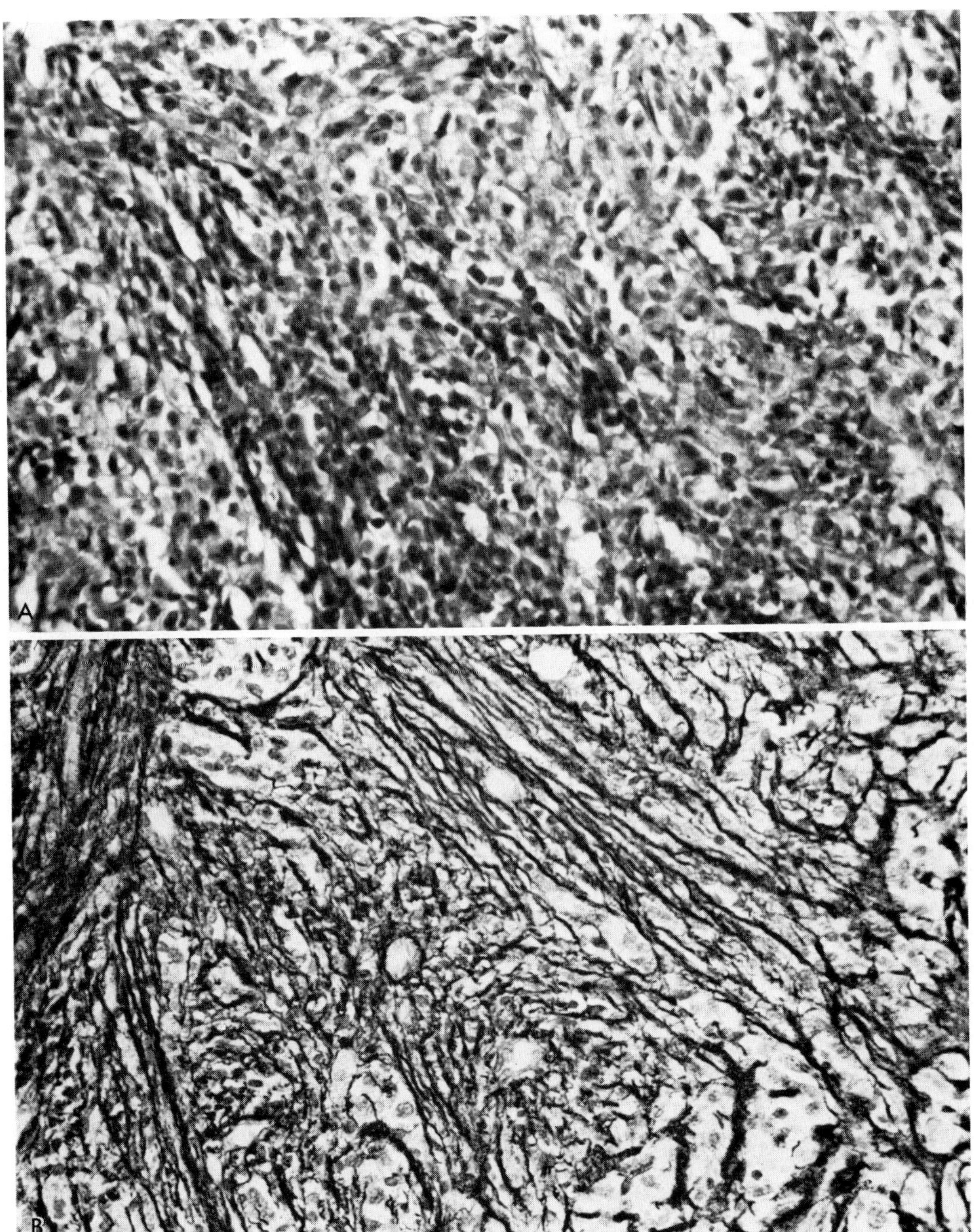

Figure 9–109. Malignant fibrous histiocytoma. Histologic pictures with hematoxylin and eosin (*A*) and reticulin stains (*B*) of lesion shown in Figure 9–108. Note the whorled fibrous pattern with numerous histiocytes and xanthomatous component. Other portions of the tumor exhibit a prominent round-cell component. There is no identifiable matrix production.

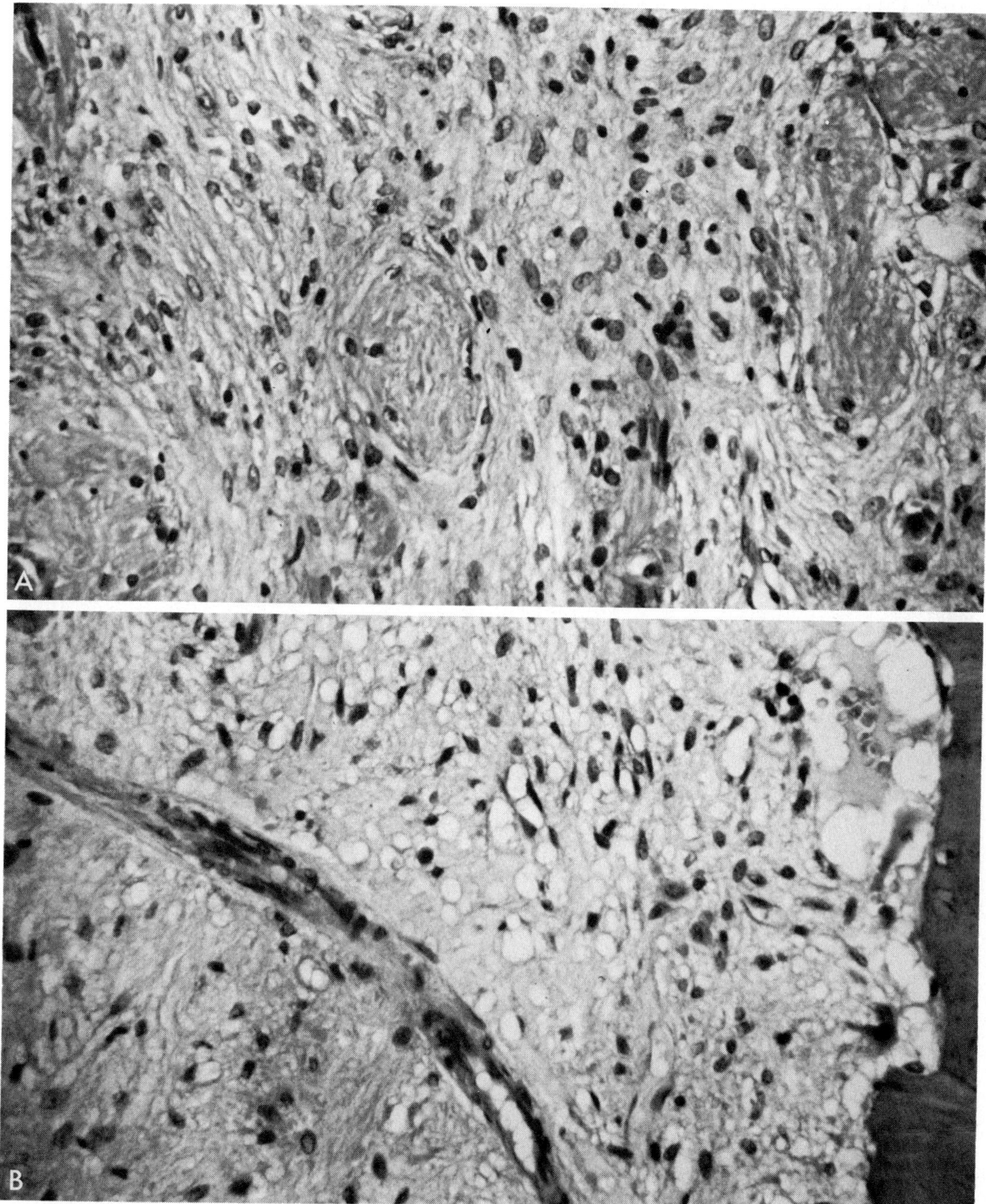

Figure 9–110. Histologic appearance of malignant fibrous histiocytoma characterized by spindled cellular component, xanthomatous deposits within the tumor, and moderate pleomorphism of the spindled cells.

Illustration continued on opposite page

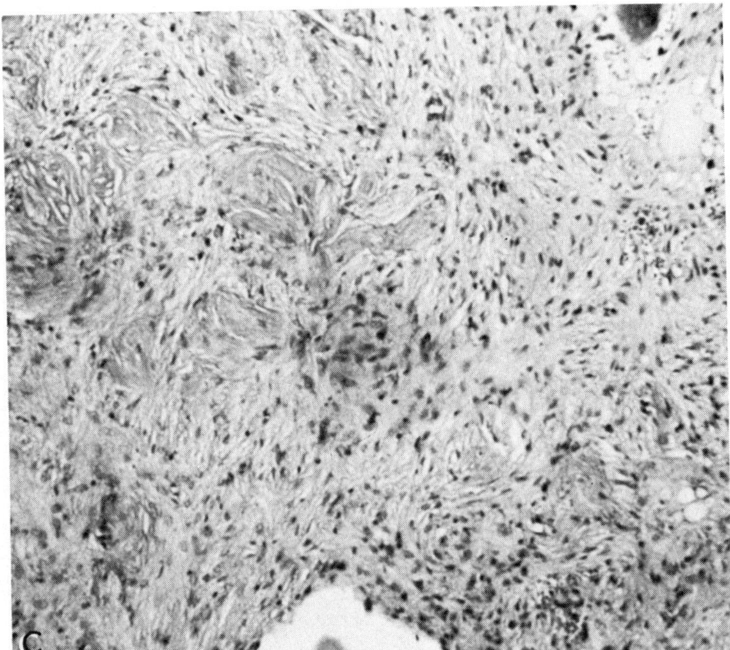

Figure 9–110 *Continued*

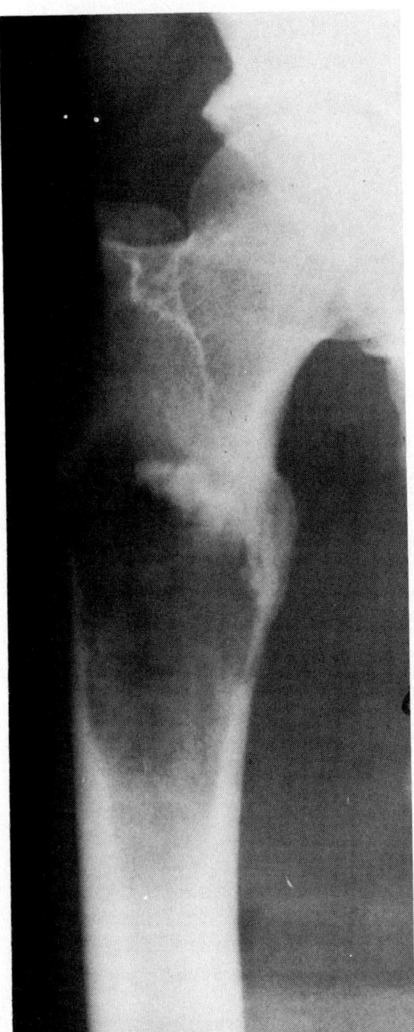

Figure 9–111. Malignant fibrous histiocytoma. Radiograph of poorly circumscribed lytic defect in the metaphyseal portion of the femur. A sclerotic calcified fragment is present in the upper portion of the lesion, suggesting either calcified cartilage or saponified fat. Malignant fibrous histiocytomas are often secondary to bone infarcts.

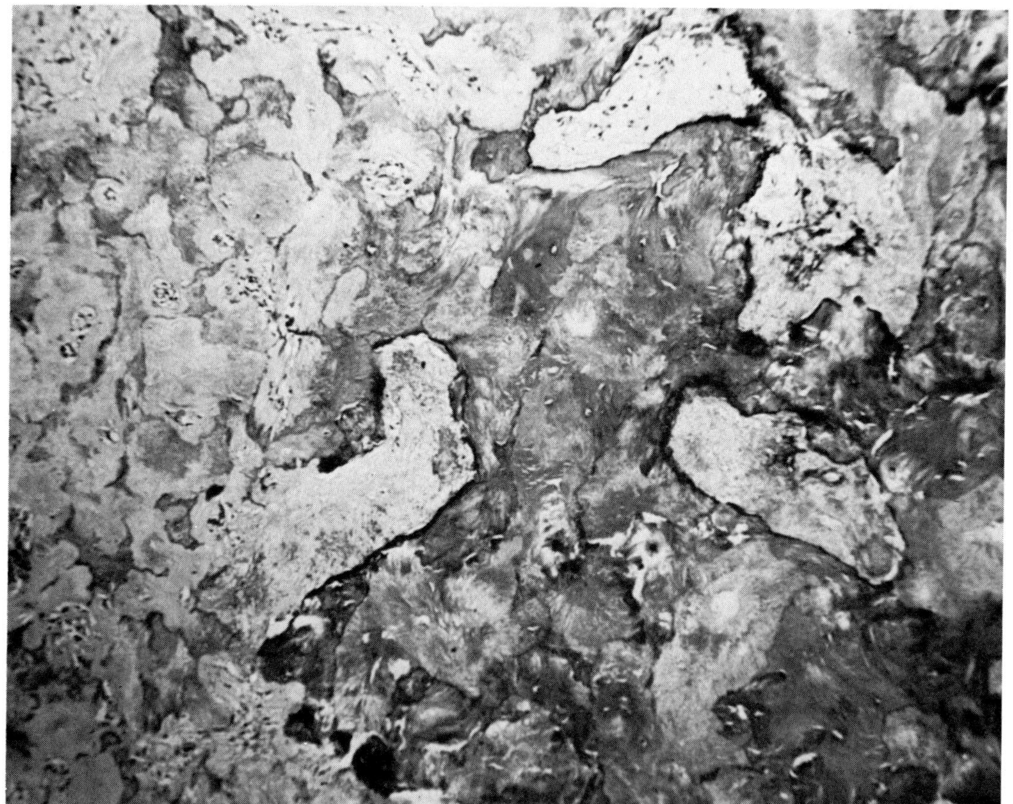

Figure 9–112. Malignant fibrous histiocytoma. Calcified ischemic bone removed from the lesion shown in Figure 9–111. This material indicates a previous infarct.

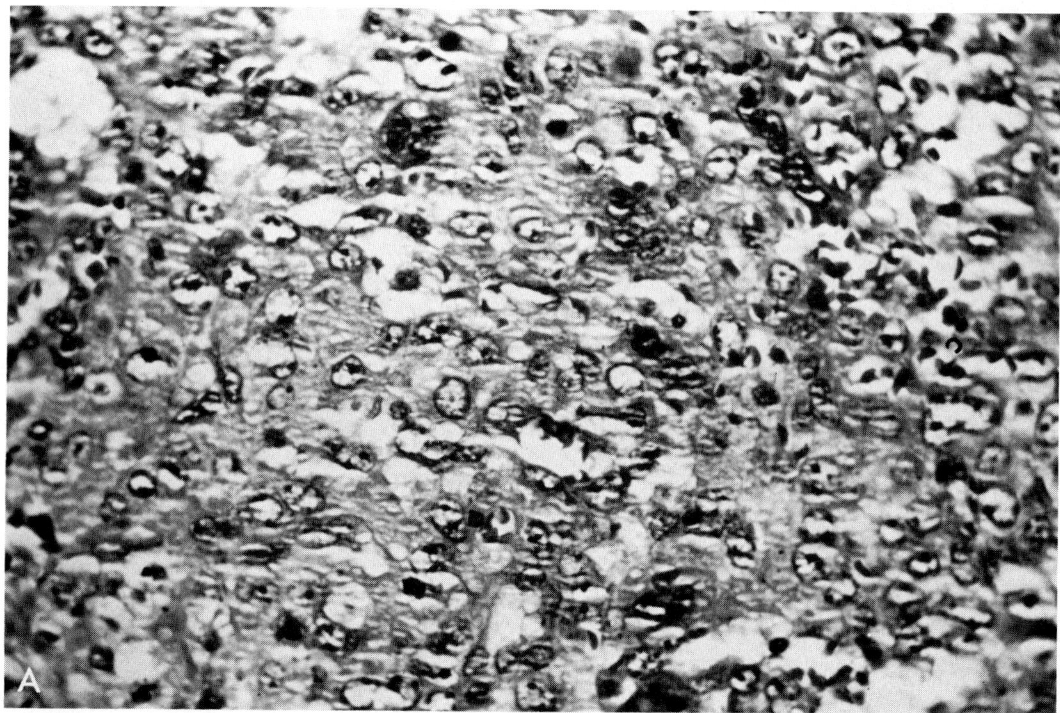

Figure 9–113. Histologic appearance of the malignant fibrous histiocytoma illustrated in Figures 9–111 and 9–112. There is marked variation in the histologic pattern, with extensive cellularity, fiber production, giant cells, and xanthoma cells. The tumor is clearly malignant. There is no identifiable osteoid- or chondroid-matrix production. The extreme variability leads some observers to doubt that the lesion represents a homogenous entity. These lesions were previously classified as malignant tumors arising in pre-existing infarcts, cysts, or lipomas; they have also been classified as osteosarcomas and fibrosarcomas.

Illustration continued on opposite page

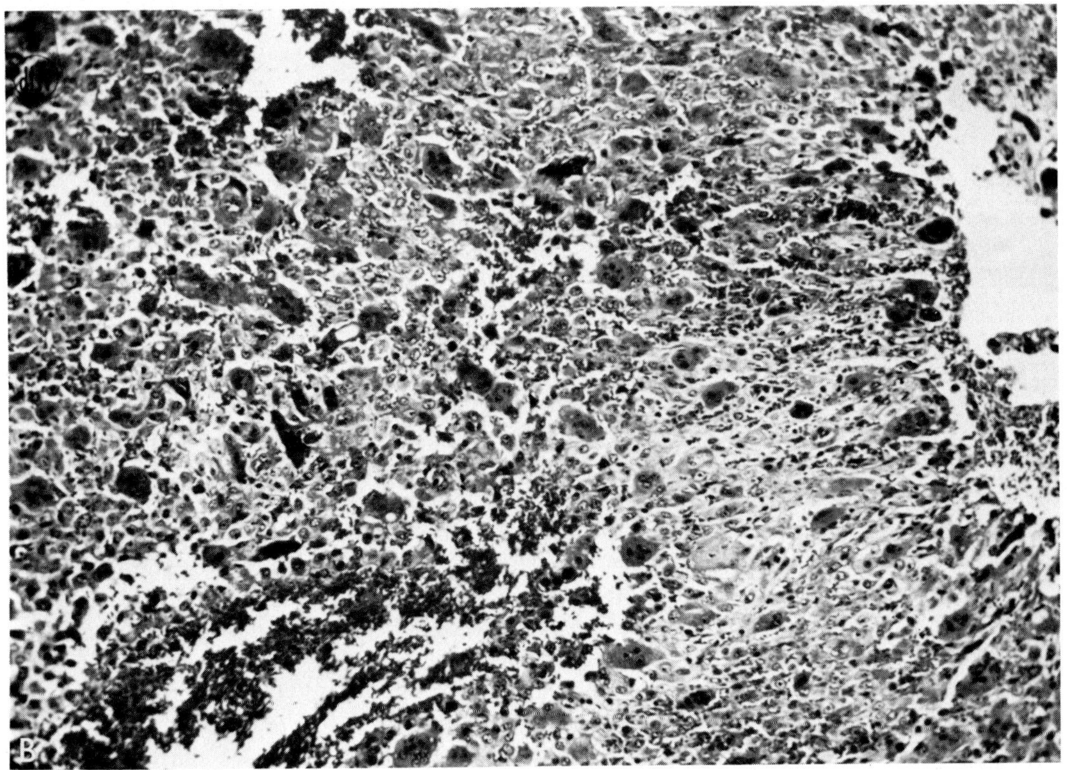

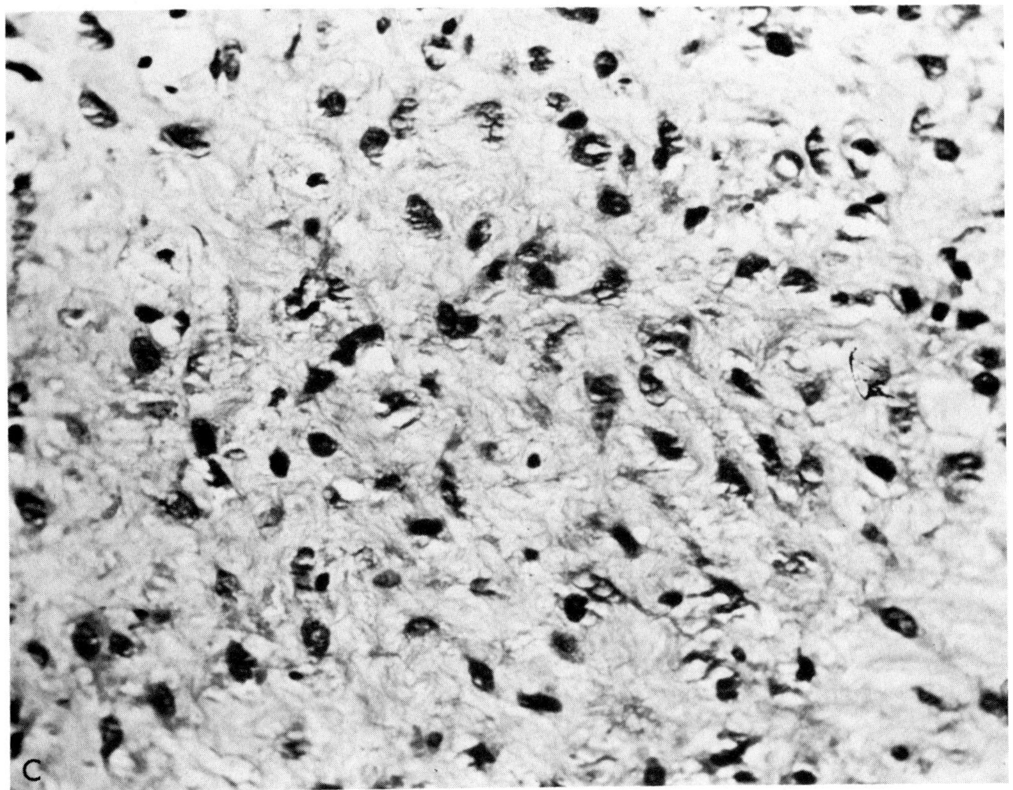

Figure 9–113 *Continued*

CARTILAGINOUS LESIONS

OSTEOCHONDROMA

The osteochondroma of bone is a common neoplasm that projects outward from the bone surface. It consists of a cartilage cap and an underlying bone stalk.

In normal growth and development, the ring of Ranvier is a thin, bony plate formed by the periosteum surrounding the proliferating cartilage cells of the growth plate (see pp. 4 to 6). A gap in this normal sleeve may be the origin of the osteochondroma. Whatever the precise origin, the lesion mimics a growth plate on the periosteal surface. It is a congenital anomaly leading to a "tumor"; cases of multiple osteochondromas are not infrequent but are probably genetically determined and not sporadic incidents in otherwise normal persons.

The histologic appearance of the lesion depends on the age of the patient. The cartilage cap reflects the growth phase of the individual. In children, actively proliferating cartilage may be seen; as the individual becomes older, the cartilage cap becomes less exuberant, and in individuals whose growth plates have fused there is a tendency for the cartilage cap to disappear and be replaced by bone through a process of endochondral ossification, similar to fusion of a growth plate.

Osteochondromas may be either pedunculated or sessile. Pedunculated lesions point away from the physis, and sessile lesions are seen at those sites at which muscle attachments are absent.

Malignant transformation of an osteochondroma is infrequent (Unni and Dahlin, 1979), but when it does occur, the cartilage portion becomes malignant, not the osseous portion. Rapid cartilage proliferation of an osteochondroma after growth-plate

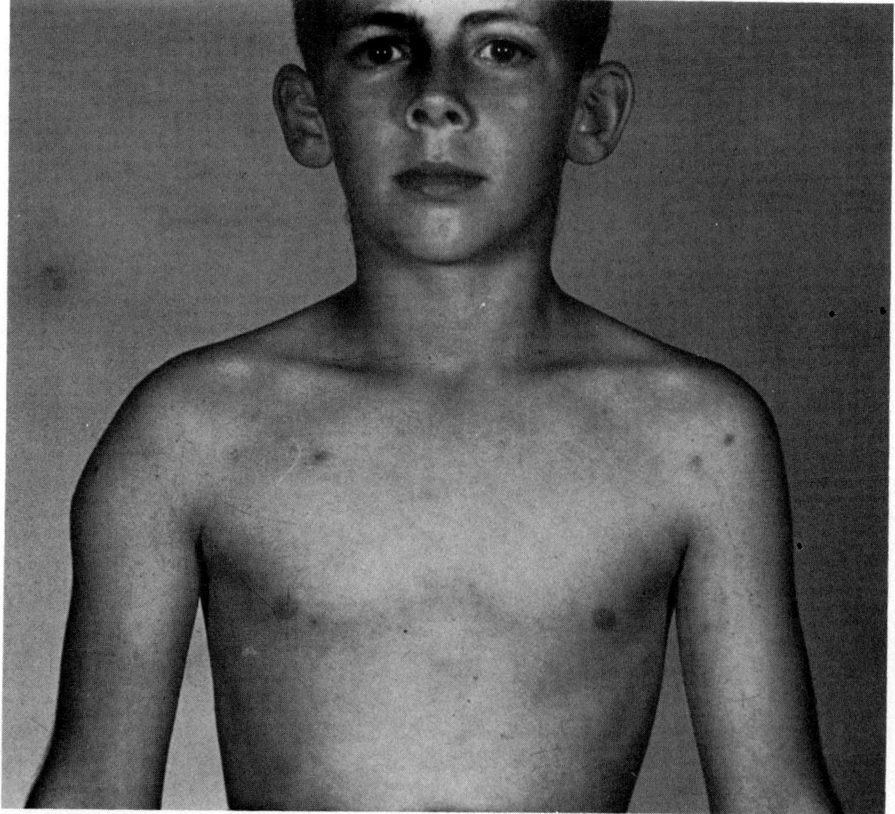

Figure 9–114. Osteochondroma. Shown here is a 12-year-old patient with tumor of shoulder. This tumor was asymptomatic and not noticed by parents.

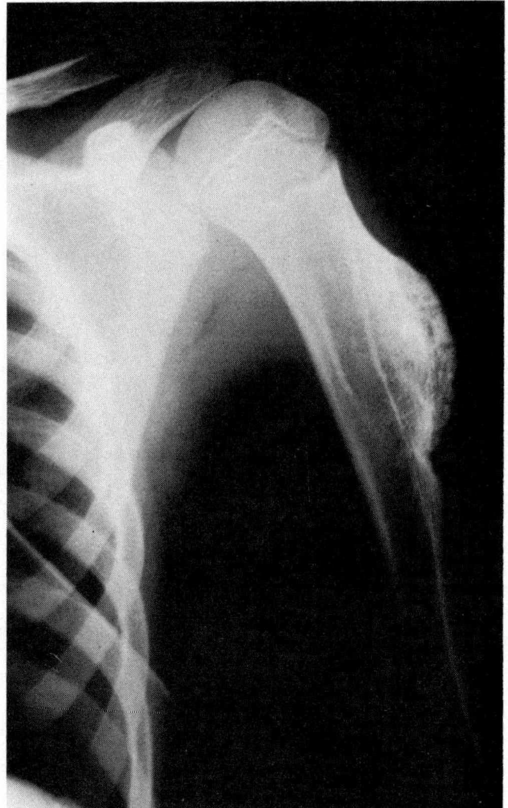

Figure 9–115. Osteochondroma. Radiograph of the patient shown in Figure 9–114 exhibiting a sessile lesion with a smooth contour, except in the distal portion of the lesion, where there is surface excavation.

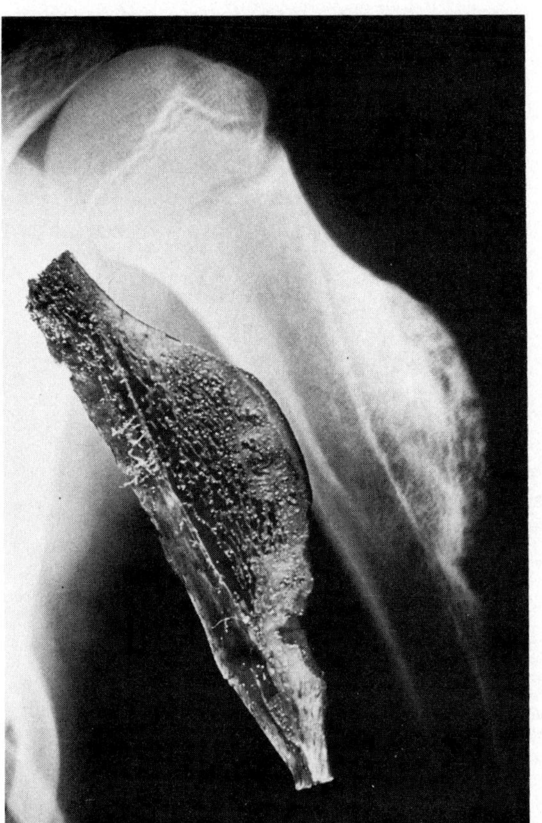

Figure 9–116. Osteochondroma. Radiograph and gross specimen of the sessile osteochondroma shown in Figure 9–115. Note the cartilaginous component causing the radiographic defect in the distal portion. Note incorporation of hematopoietic tissue into the base of the osteochondroma.

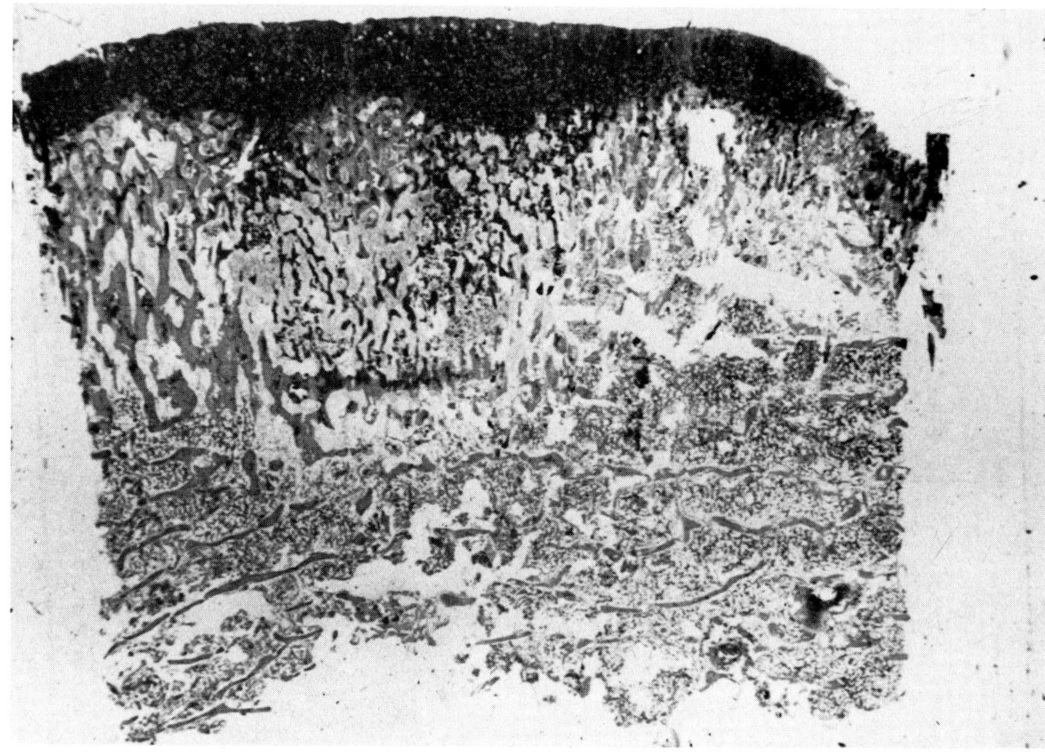

Figure 9–117. Osteochondroma. Macrosection of the osteochondroma shown in Figures 9–115 and 9–116. There is a prominent cartilaginous cap with transformation to bone, similar to what is seen in the normal growth plate. Note the incorporation of the hematopoietic marrow into the medullary spaces of the osteochondroma. The continuity of the marrow space from the parent bone into the osteochondroma is characteristic of the tumor and helps differentiate it from a parosteal osteosarcoma.

closure or invasion of the cartilage component into the bony portion should be regarded with suspicion.

An osteochondroma arising from an epiphysis and projecting from an articular surface will severely interfere with normal function of the joint. Such osteochondromas are also known as "dysplasia epiphysealis hemimelica," and they are similar in histologic appearance to the true osteochondroma.

Text continued on page 397

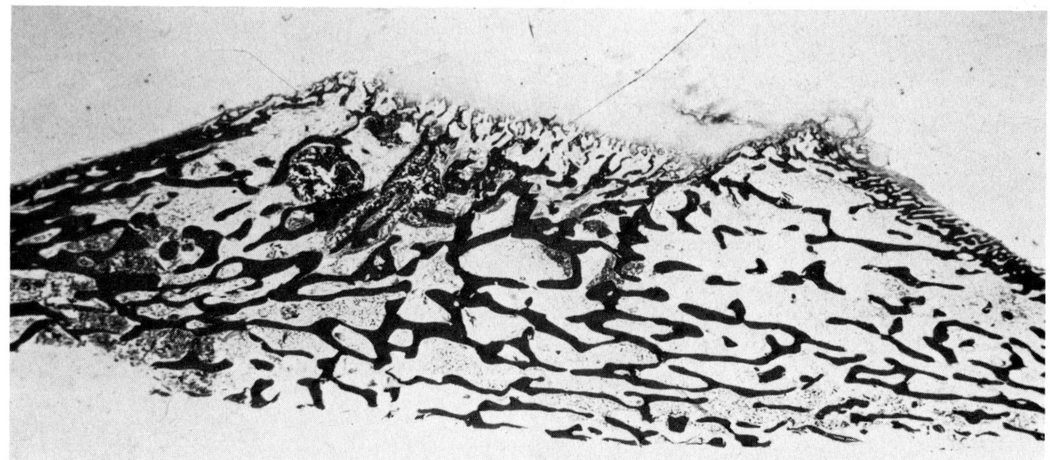

Figure 9–118. Osteochondroma. Macrospecimen of sessile osteochondroma. Note cartilage cap and conversion to bone with incorporation of marrow into the neoplastic bone.

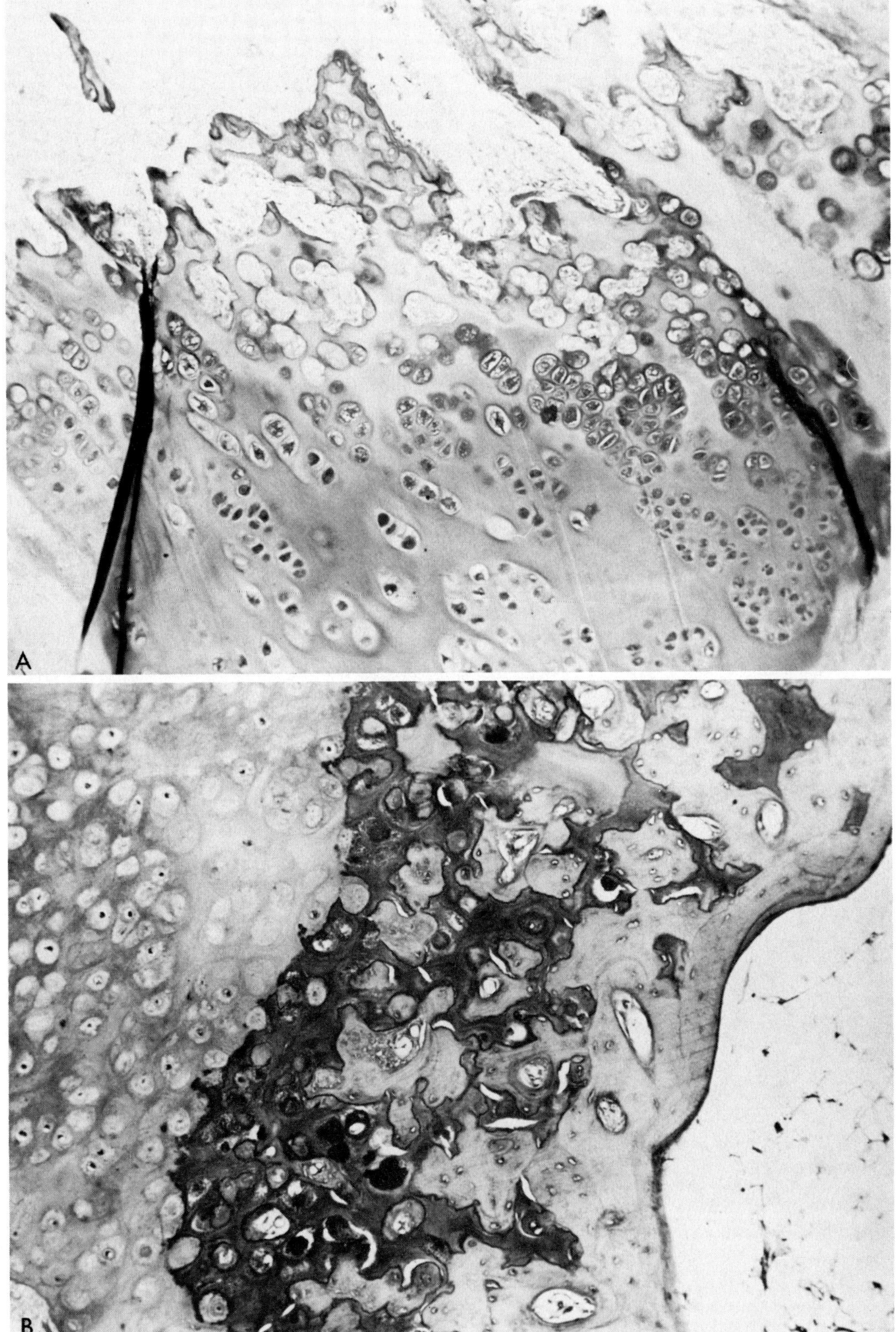

Figure 9–119. *A*, Osteochondroma in child. Conversion of cartilage to bone in a pattern similar to that occurring in the normal growth plate. Note column formation by cartilage cells and foci of calcification in the cartilage. *B*, Osteochondroma in adult. Note cessation of growth with abrupt transiton to bone.

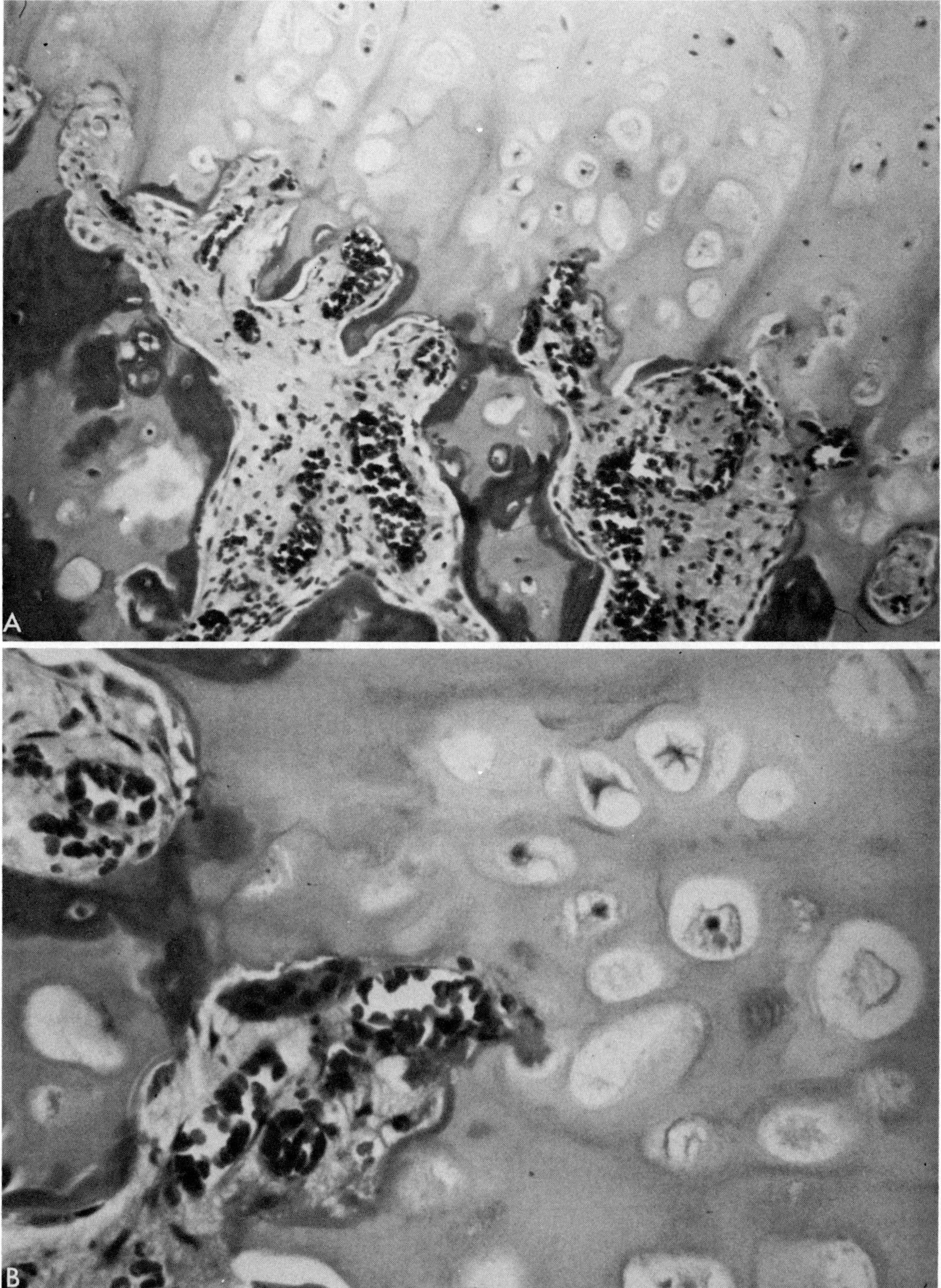

Figure 9–120. Osteochondroma. Conversion of cartilage to bone, mimicking normal growth plate activity.

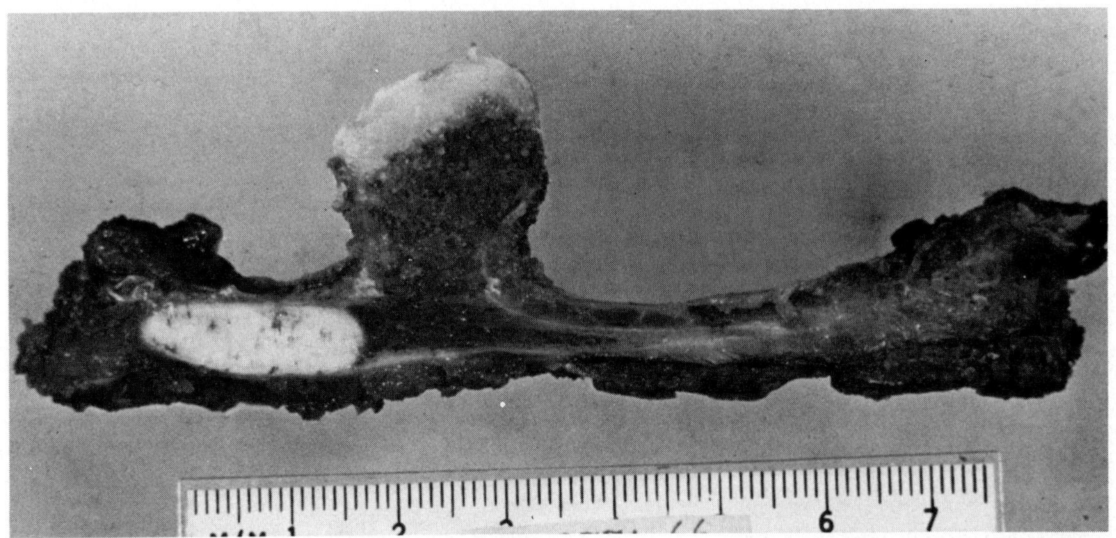

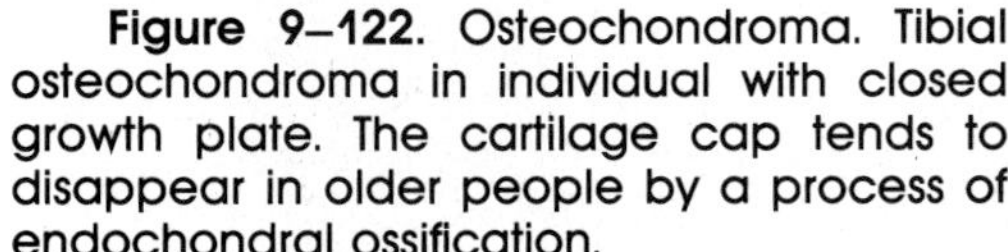

Figure 9–121. Osteochondroma. Gross photograph of an osteochondroma of a rib in a younger individual. Note the prominent cartilaginous cap. Compare with osteochondroma in an older individual (Fig. 9–122).

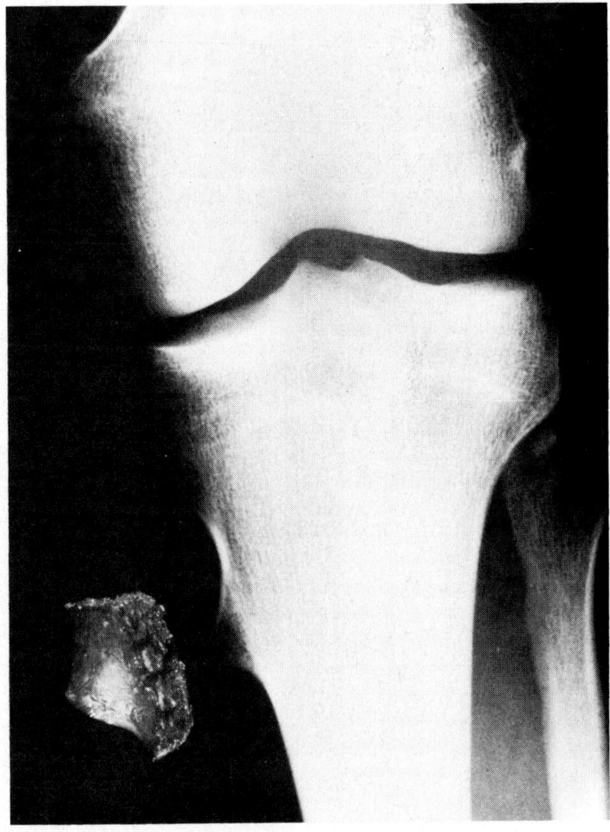

Figure 9–122. Osteochondroma. Tibial osteochondroma in individual with closed growth plate. The cartilage cap tends to disappear in older people by a process of endochondral ossification.

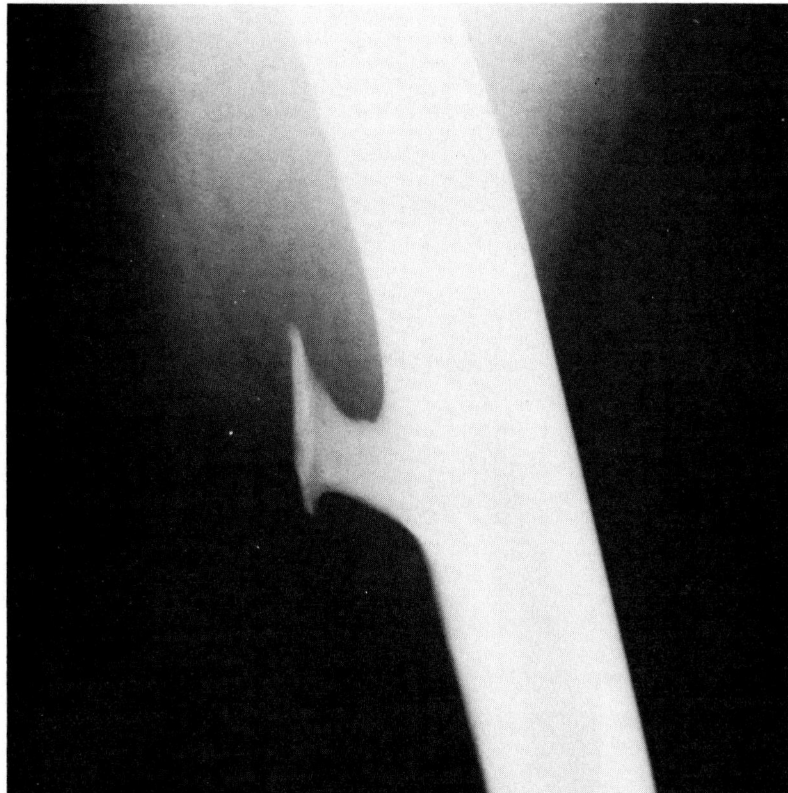

Figure 9–123. Osteochondroma. Radiograph of pedunculated osteochondroma in the diaphyseal portion of the bone. The lesion is contained within the intermuscular septum. It has a thin, blade-like stalk. The cartilage cap has been entirely replaced by bone.

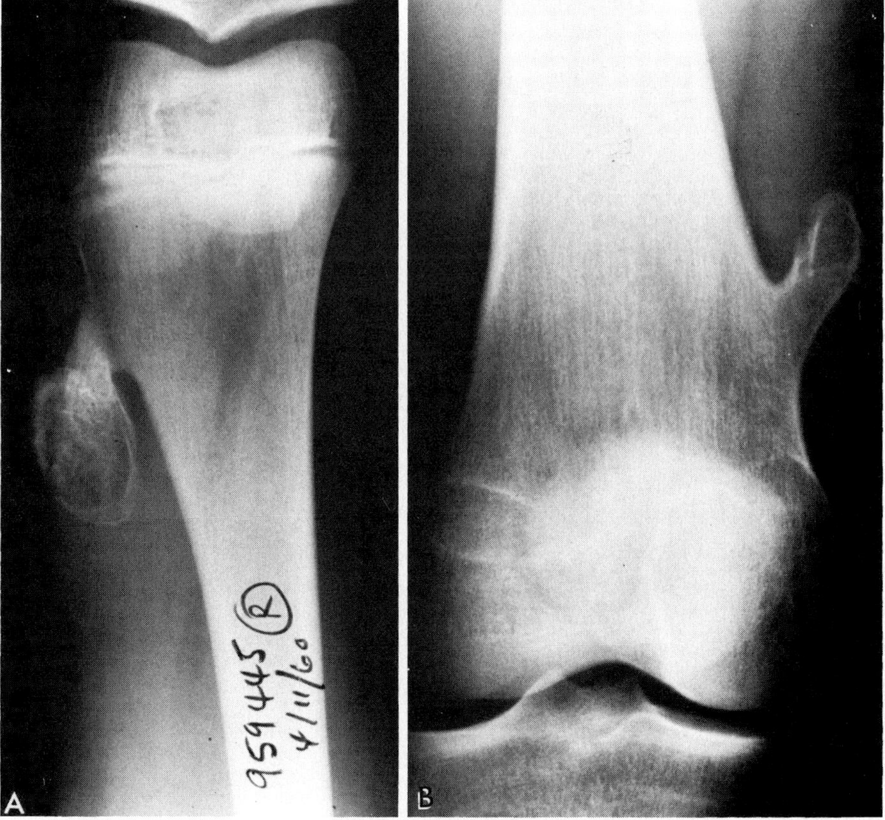

Figure 9–124. Osteochondroma. Two radiographs showing mature osteochondroma: stalked lesion pointing toward the diaphysis and away from the growth plate (Figs. 9–114 and 9–115).

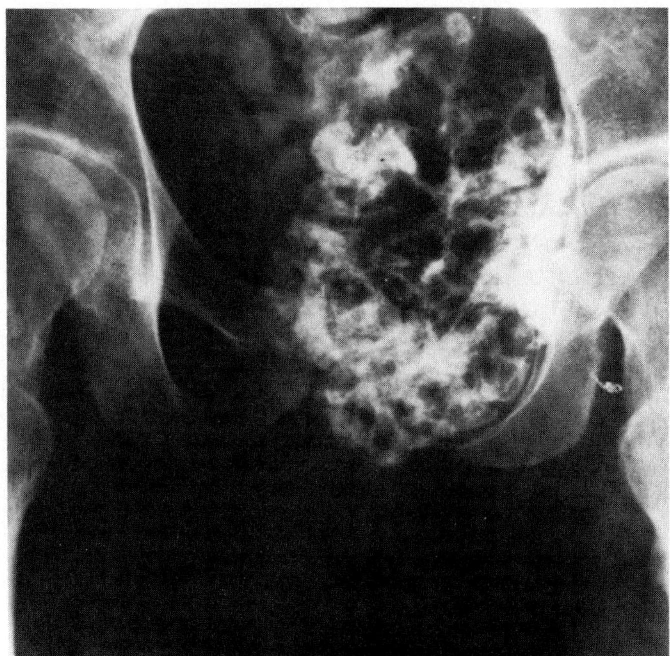

Figure 9–125. Radiograph of pelvic osteochondroma with large masses of cartilage. These lesions have high potential for malignant transformation. Most tumors of this size will exhibit malignant areas if sampled extensively.

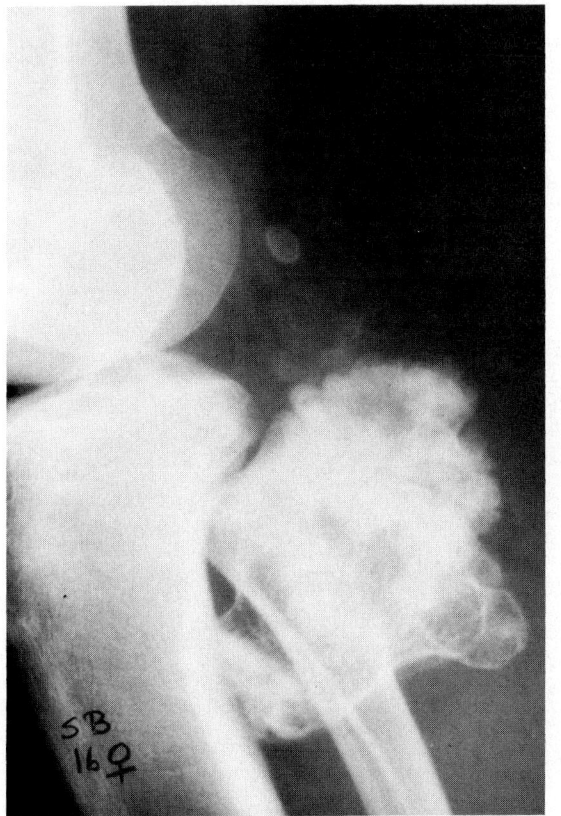

Figure 9–126. Osteochondroma. Radiograph of large lobulated osteochondroma in proximal fibula. The lesion must be differentiated from a parosteal osteosarcoma. The presence of normal marrow tissue within the trabeculae of neoplastic bone is histologic confirmation of osteochondroma rather than parosteal osteosarcoma.

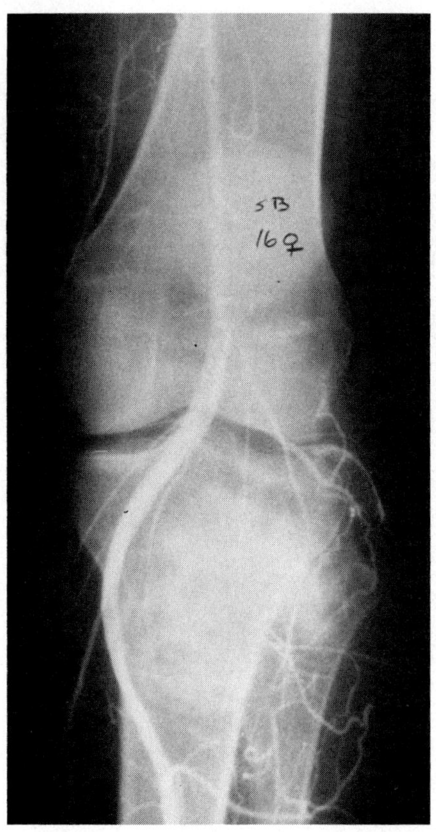

Figure 9–127. Osteochondroma. Angiogram of the large lobulated osteochondroma of the proximal fibula illustrated in Figure 9–126. The differential diagnosis includes a parosteal osteosarcoma. The distortion of the vessels around the tumor and the lack of tumor vascularity help the surgeon in establishing the diagnosis and determining the approach to the lesion.

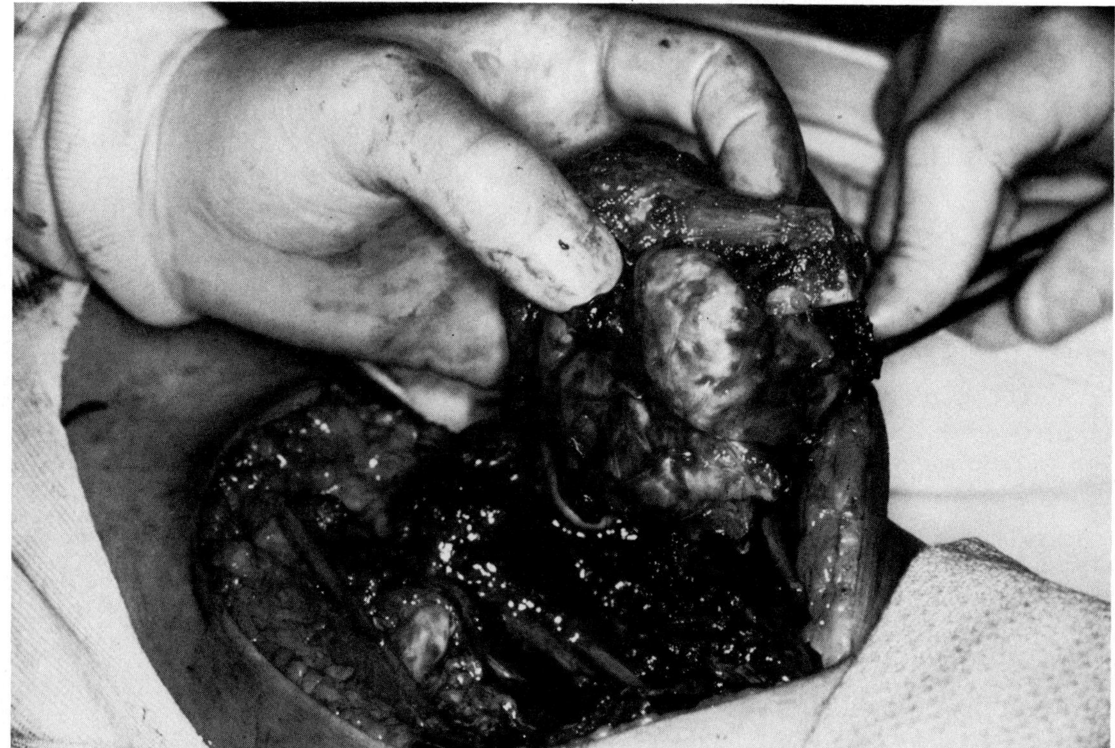

Figure 9–128. Osteochondroma. Surgical removal of the proximal fibula with the attached osteochondroma. Note the white, glistening appearance of the cartilage cap.

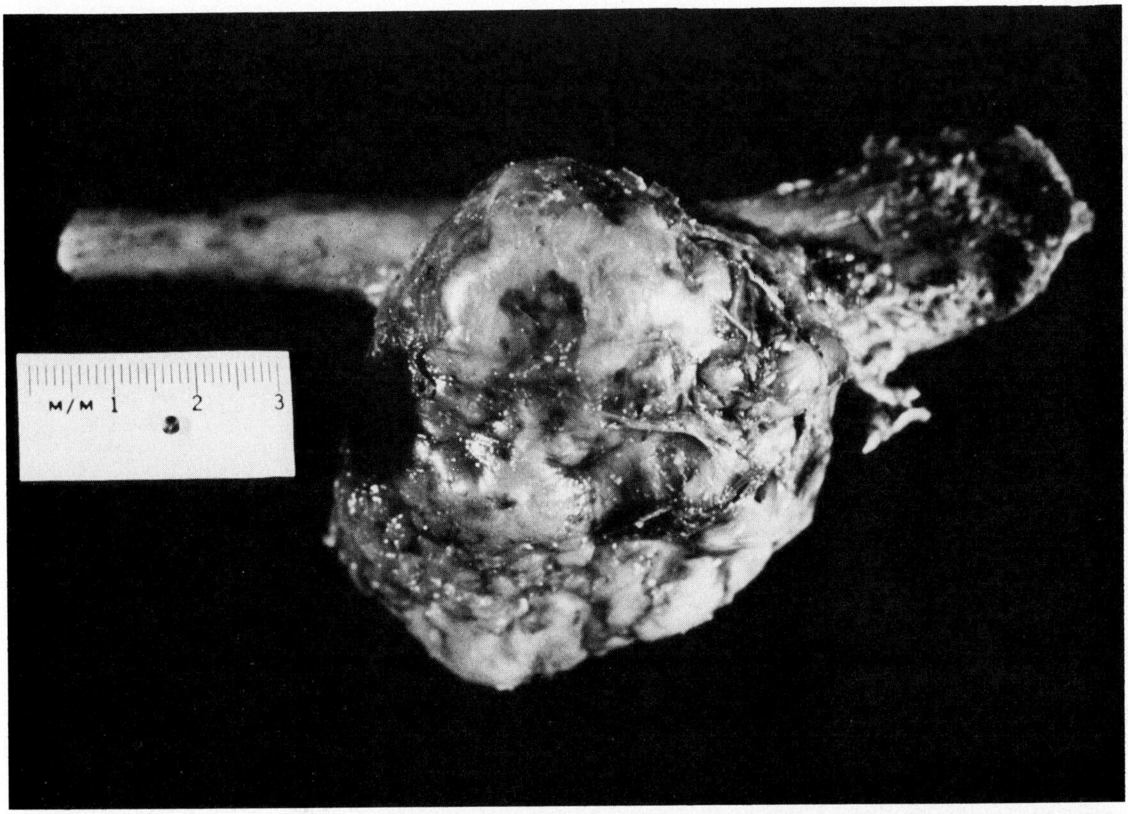

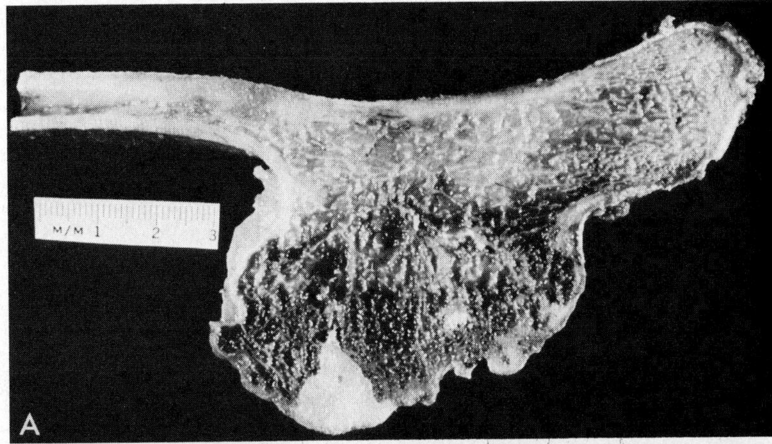

Figure 9–129. Osteochondroma. Gross specimen of the osteochondroma exhibiting a prominent cartilage cap.

Figure 9–130. Osteochondroma. Cut section (*A*) and specimen radiograph (*B*) of lesion exhibiting the cartilage cap. Portions of the cap have been completely replaced by bone. The neoplastic bone has been incorporated into the medullary cavity of the host bone, with formation of hematopoietic marrow within the neoplasm, a characteristic feature of osteochondroma.

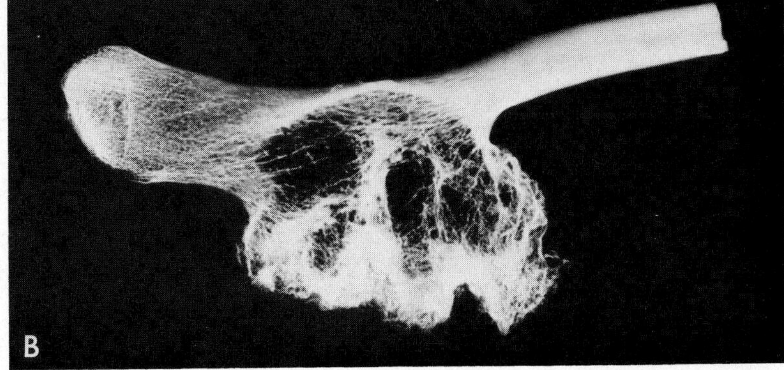

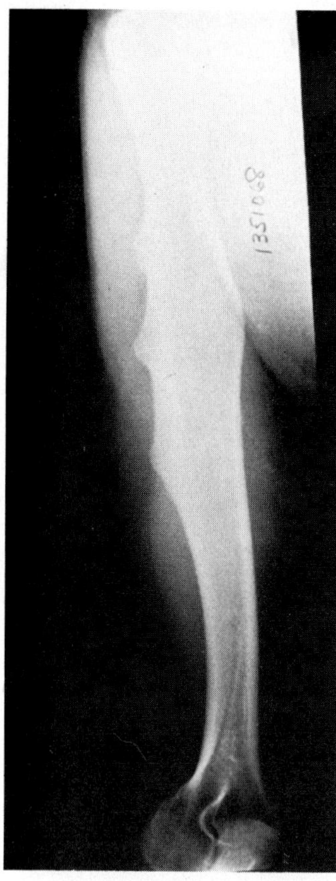

Figure 9–131. Osteochondromatosis. Osteochondromas are a congenital defect, and multiple osteochondromas as well as several osteochondromas in the same bone may occur.

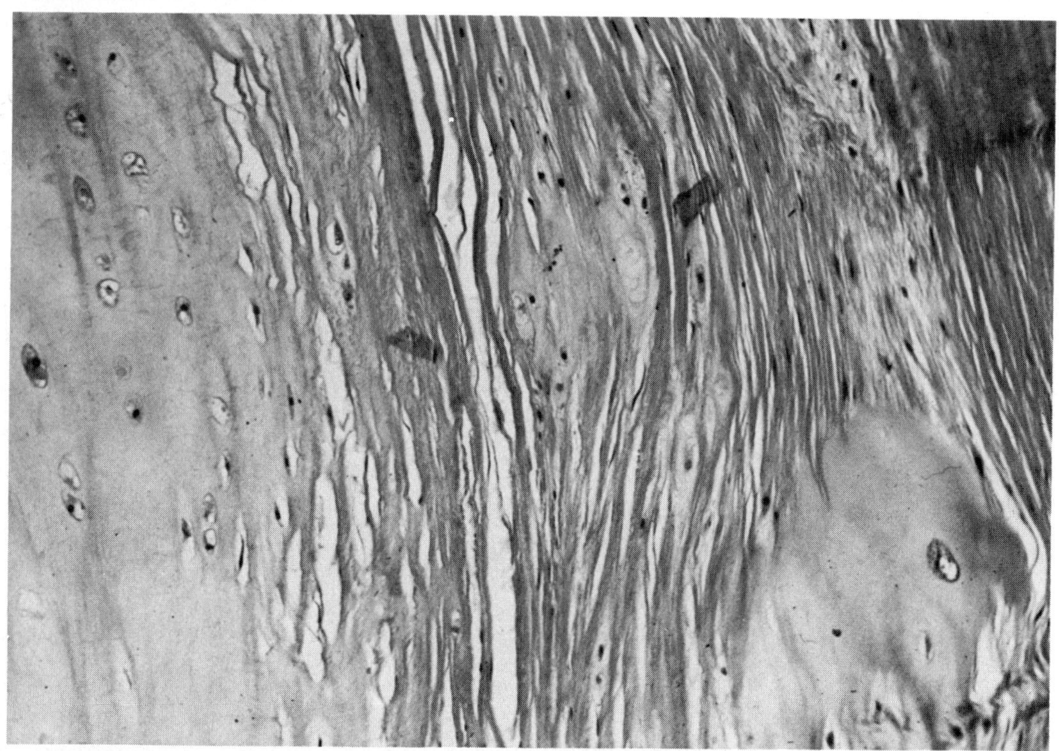

Figure 9–132. Osteochondroma. Formation of cartilage nodules in perichondrial membrane. This membrane must be removed to prevent local recurrence. Removing the osteochondroma through the apparent capsule (marginal excision) leaves the membrane and nodules behind, leading to recurrence.

Illustration continued on opposite page

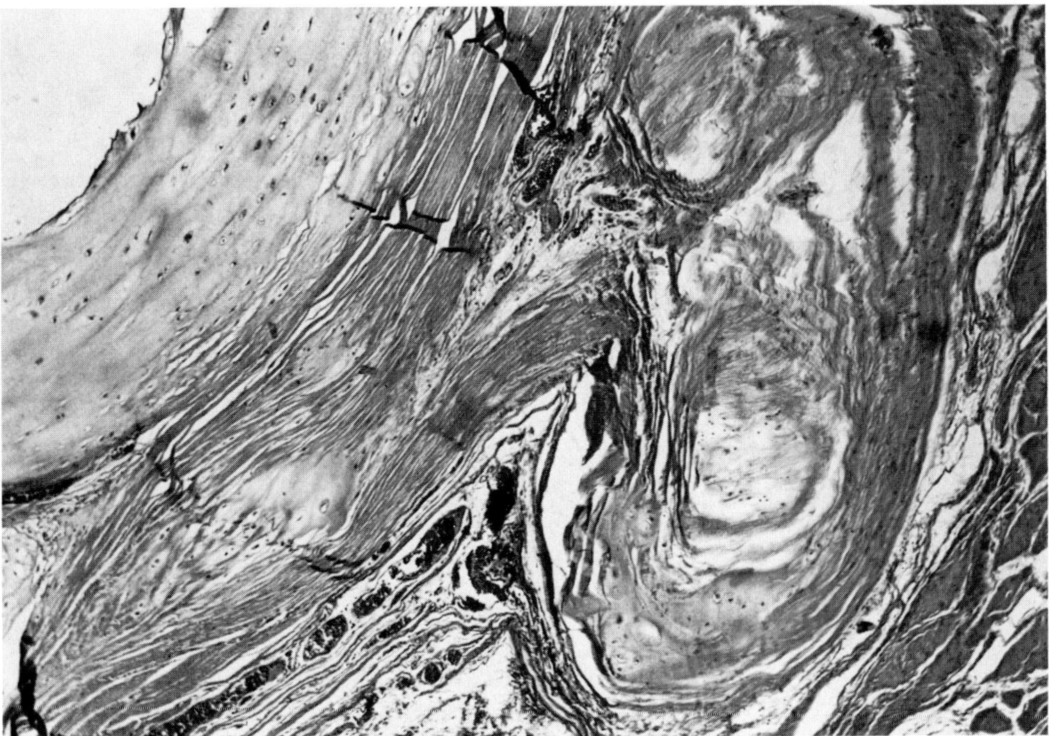

Figure 9–132 *Continued*

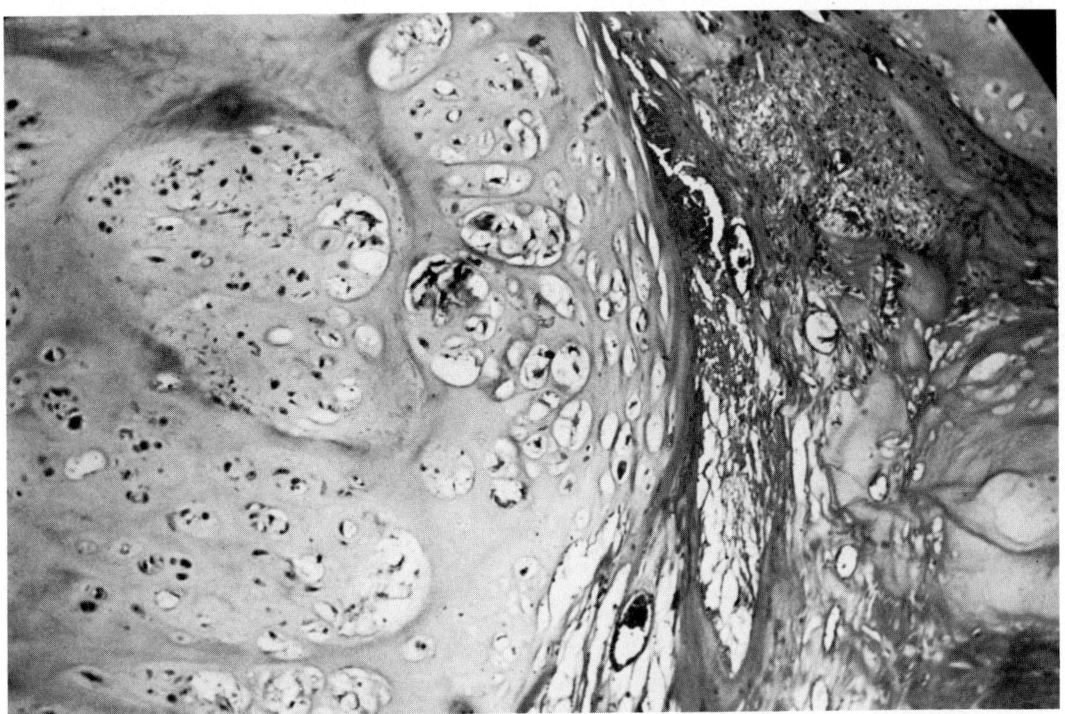

Figure 9–133. Osteochondroma. Histologic appearance of perichondrial membrane responsible for the formation of cartilage. Note the large clusters of cartilaginous cells as well as the newly formed cartilage within the connective tissue.

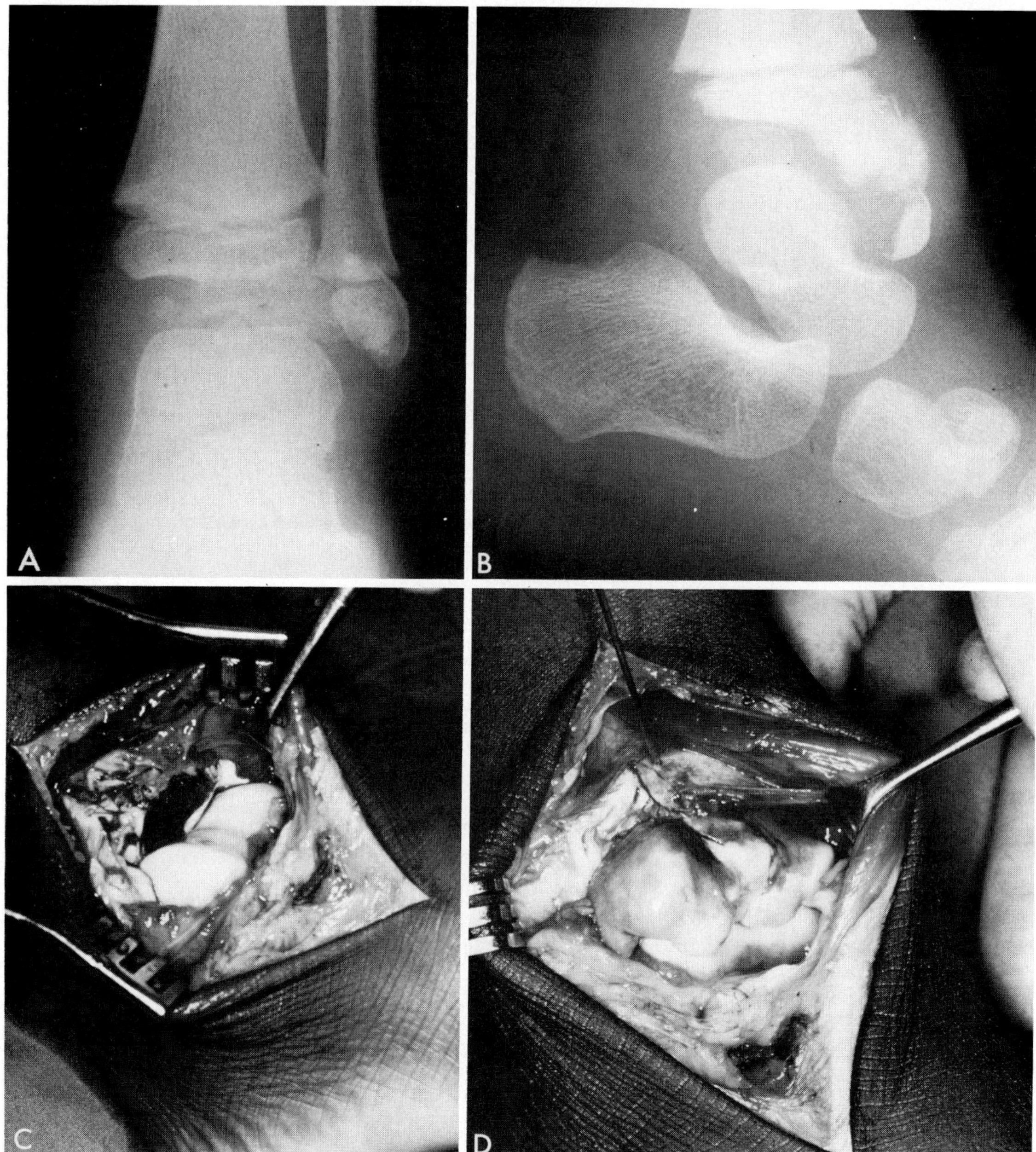

Figure 9–134. Radiographic (*A* and *B*) and gross (*C* and *D*) appearance of epiphyseal osteochondroma. A portion of the lesion has broken off into the joint space.

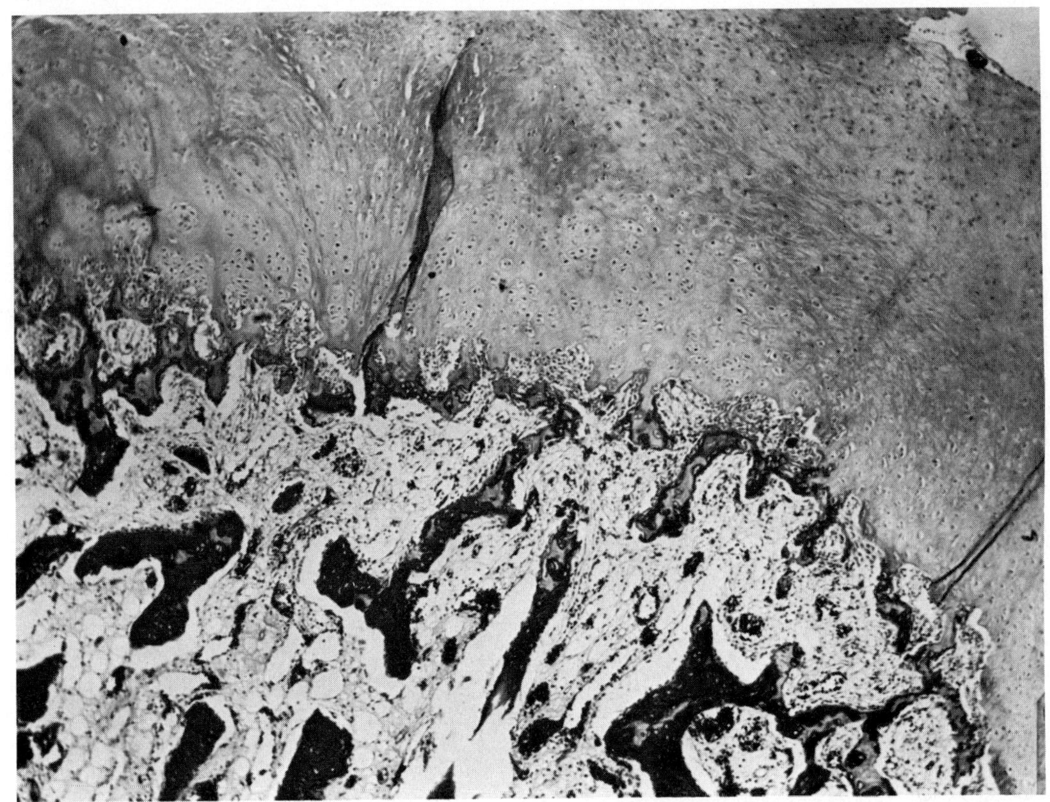

Figure 9–135. Epiphyseal osteochondroma. The histologic appearance of this lesion is identical with that of the usual osteochondroma. The difference lies only in the location of the lesion, and the surface cartilage is articular. The presence of the lesion at the joint causes major dysfunction.

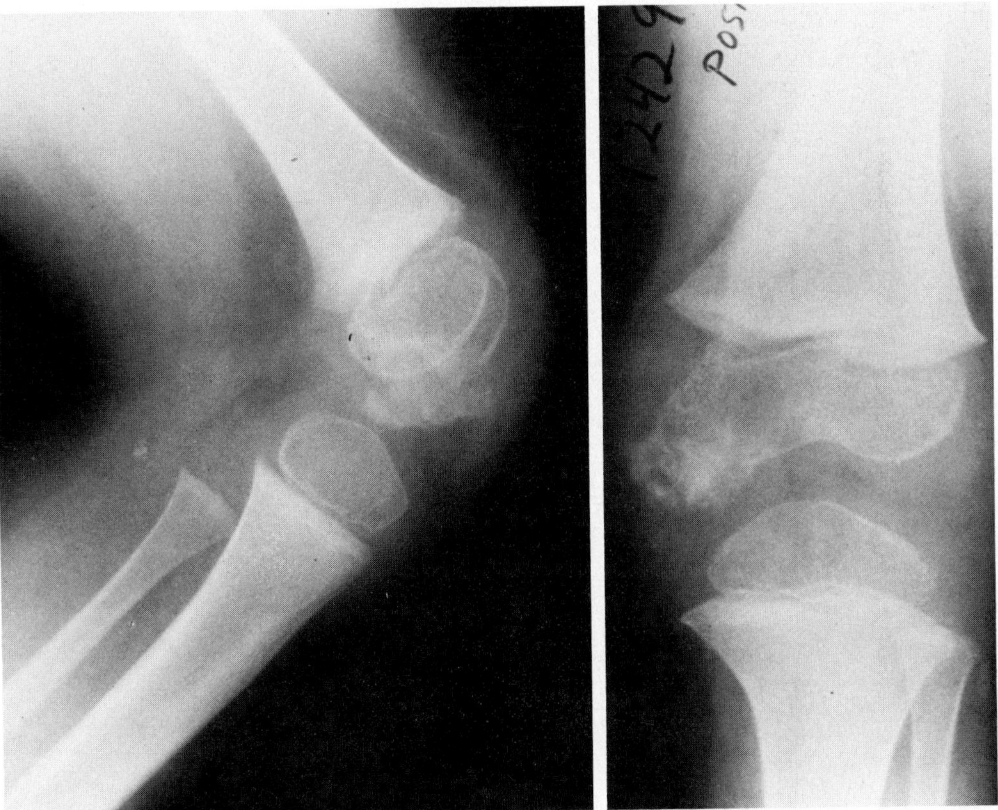

Figure 9–136. Epiphyseal osteochondroma. Lateral and anteroposterior radiographs of knee joint showing epiphyseal osteochondroma of lower femur.

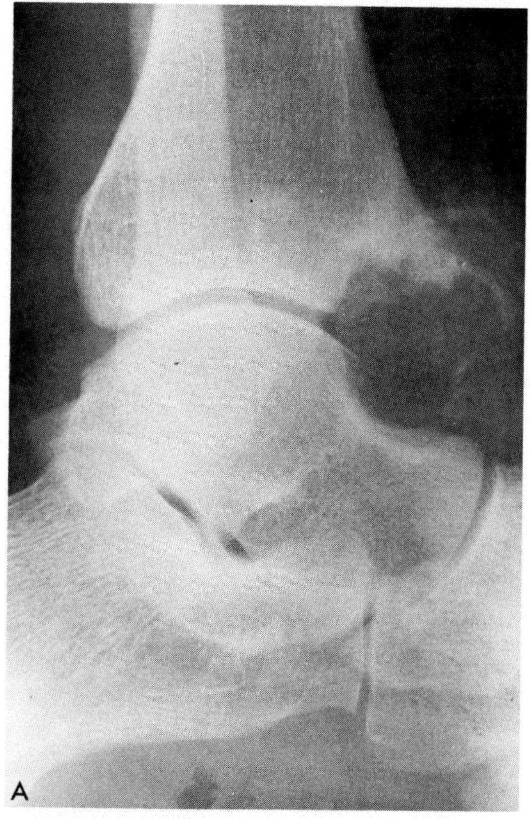

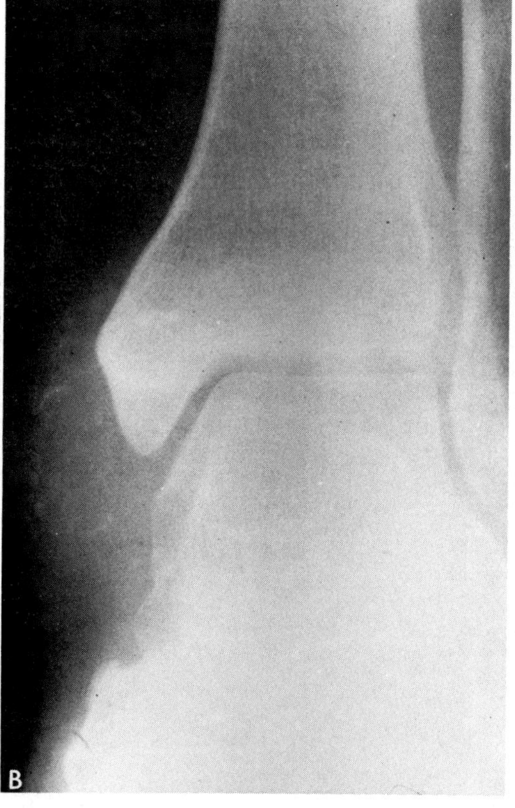

Figure 9-137. Epiphyseal osteochondroma. Lateral (*A*) and anteroposterior (*B*) radiographs showing epiphyseal osteochondroma of ankle joint in an adult.

SUBUNGUAL EXOSTOSIS

The subungual exostosis is a benign lesion of bone, arising from the terminal phalanx. Trauma may be an etiologic factor. It is different from the usual ostochondroma of bone, probably because of the difference in development of the terminal phalanx. A fibrous cap covers the distal primitive cartilage skeleton of the terminal phalanx, and osteochondromas arising at the site have the characteristics of fibrous cartilage, in addition to hyaline cartilage. The fibrous component is characterized by spindled stroma, with some hypercellularity and pleomorphism. Conversion to bone occurs at the base of the lesion, and despite the moderately ominous appearance of the spindled stroma, these lesions are uniformly benign. They are most commonly located at the distal tip of the phalanx of the great toe (Landon et al., 1972).

Text continued on page 404

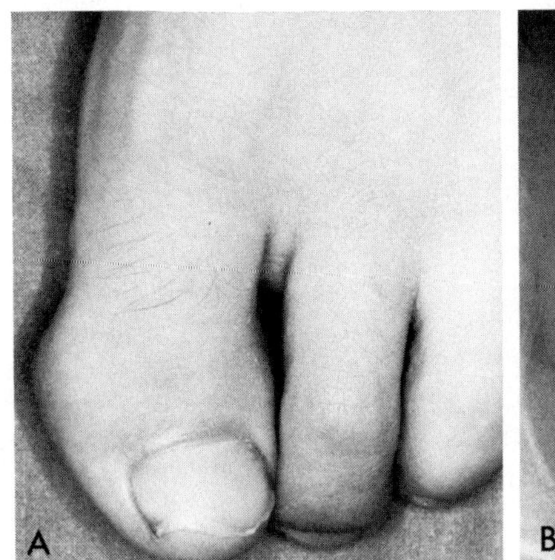
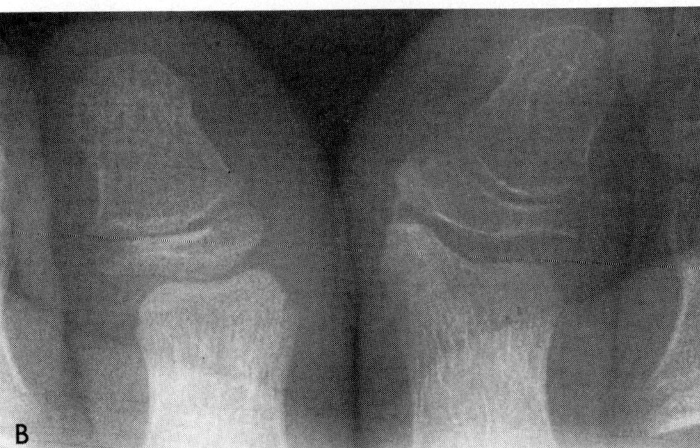
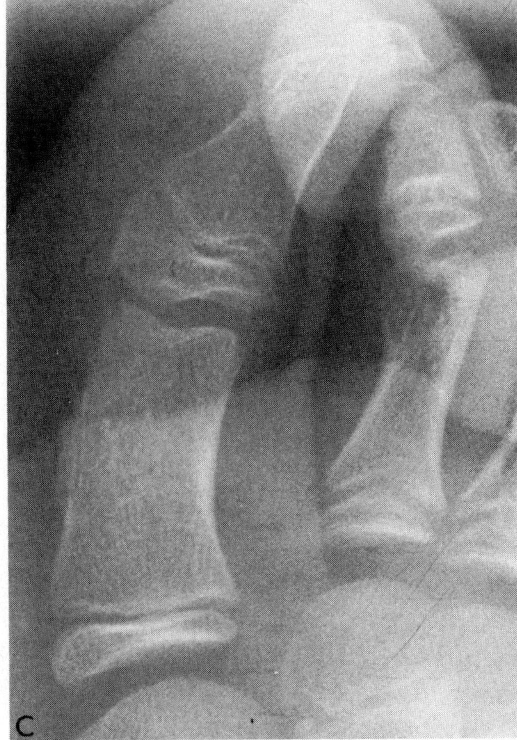

Figure 9–138. Epiphyseal osteochondroma. Clinical appearance (*A*), preoperative film (*B*), and postoperative (*C*) film of epiphyseal osteochondroma in the great toe.

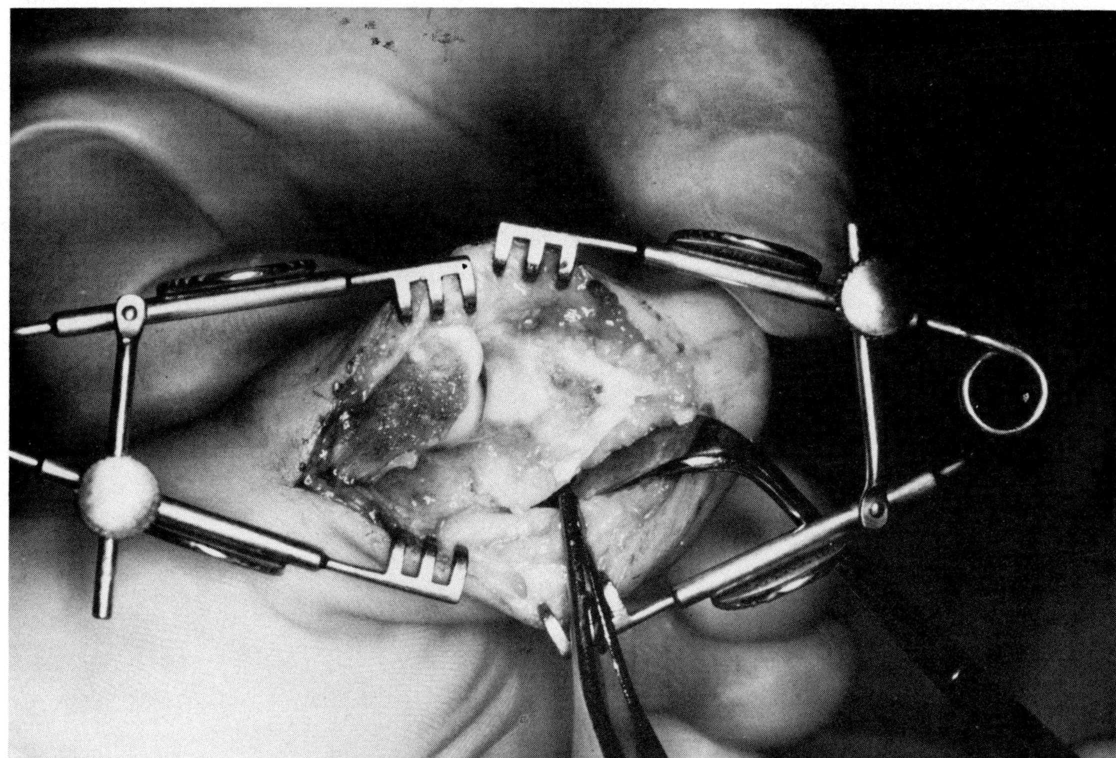

Figure 9–139. Epiphyseal osteochondroma. Intraoperative view of the lesion shown in Figures 9–138 and 9–140 after removal of the epiphyseal osteochondroma. Note that the remaining articular surface is normal.

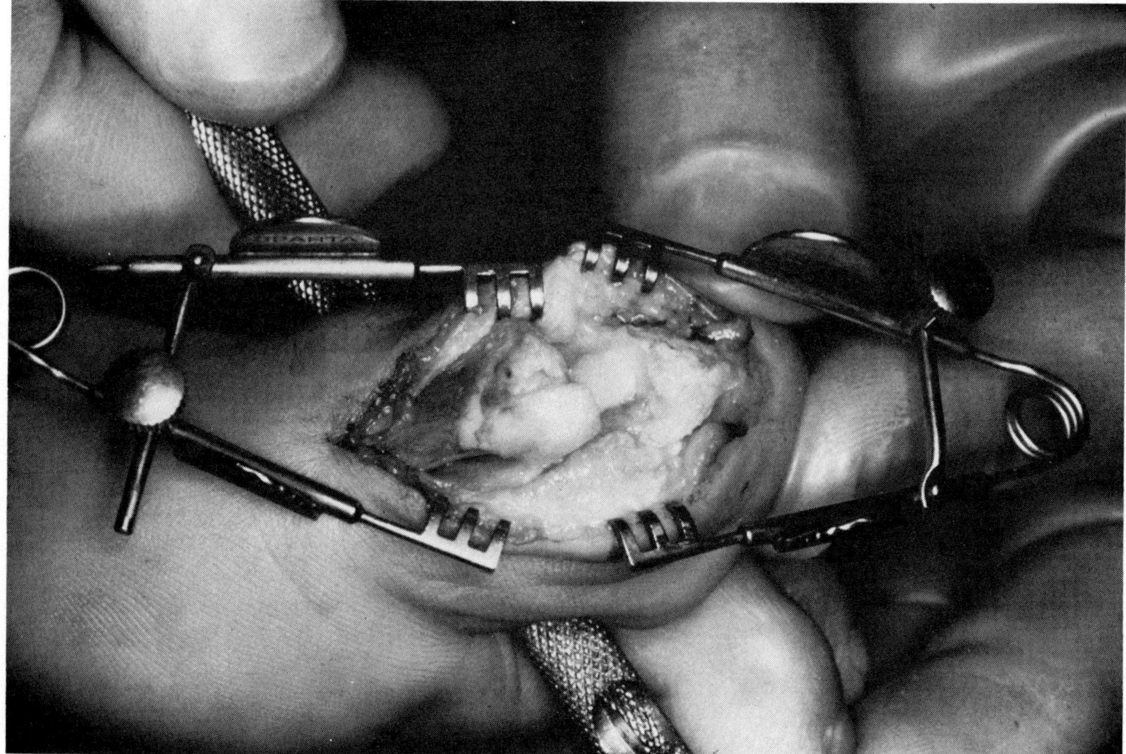

Figure 9–140. Epiphyseal osteochondroma. Intraoperative photograph of the lesion shown in Figures 9–138 and 9–139. Note the projection of the lesion into the joint.

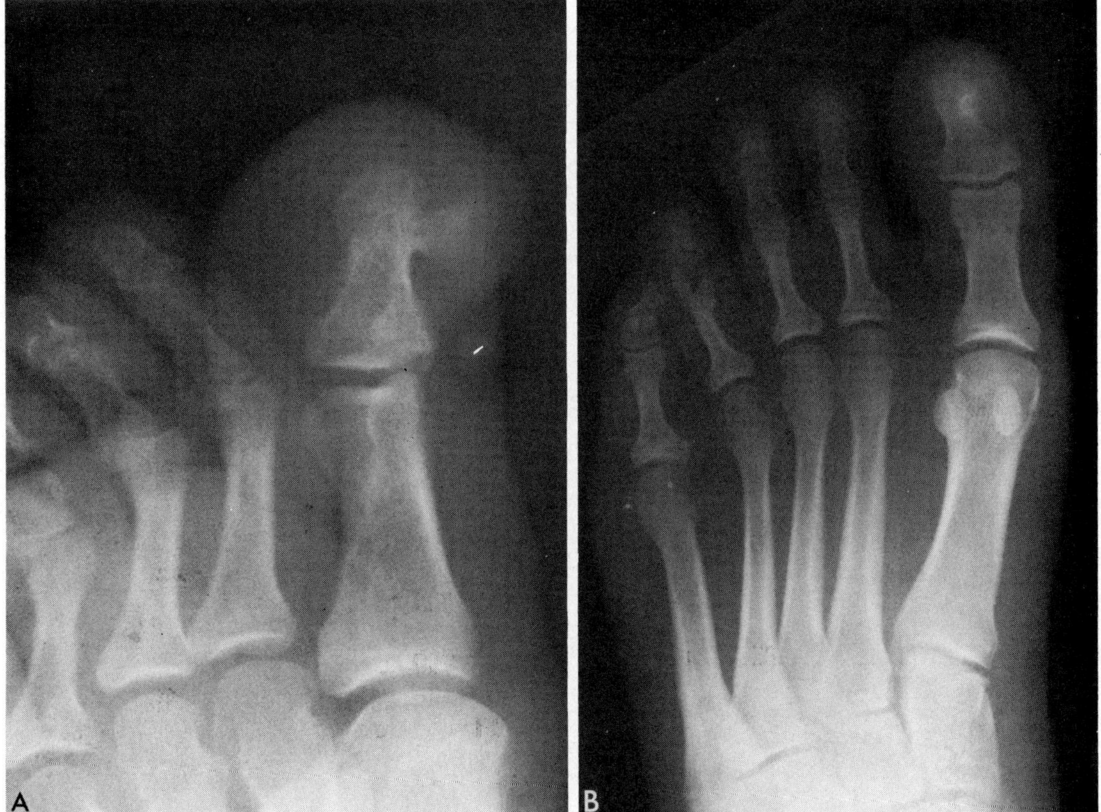

Figure 9–141. Subungual exostosis. Characteristic radiographic appearance of subungual exostosis. The lesion originates on the superior or lateral surface of the distal phalanx. It corresponds to the fibrous cap covering the cartilage anlage of the terminal phalanx.

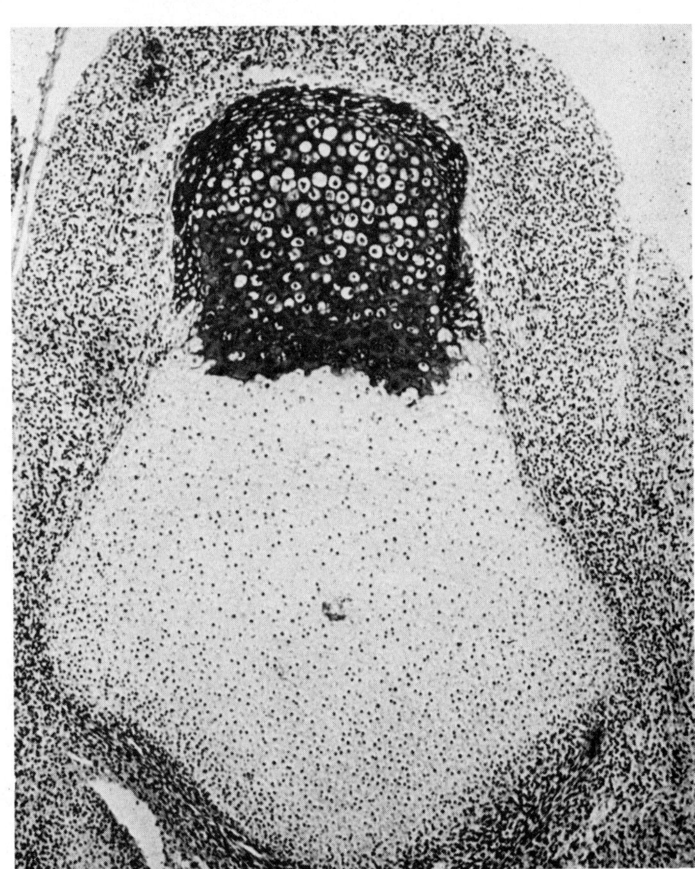

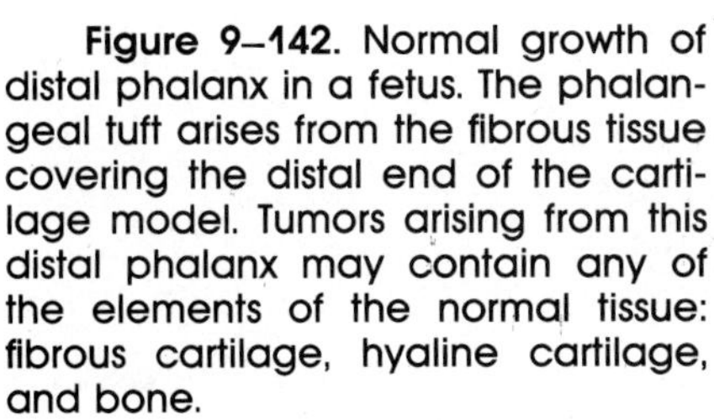

Figure 9–142. Normal growth of distal phalanx in a fetus. The phalangeal tuft arises from the fibrous tissue covering the distal end of the cartilage model. Tumors arising from this distal phalanx may contain any of the elements of the normal tissue: fibrous cartilage, hyaline cartilage, and bone.

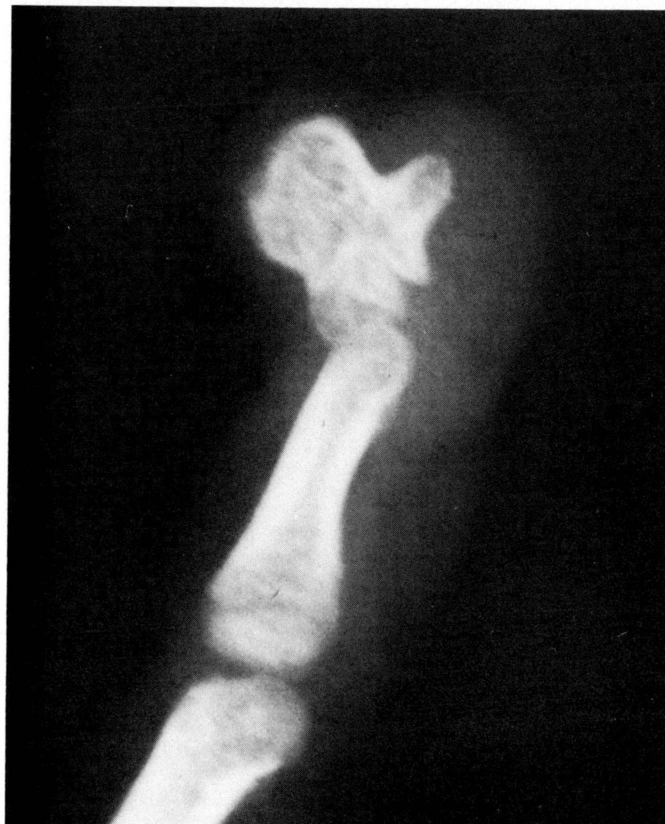

Figure 9–143. Subungual exostosis. Radiographic appearance of subungual exostosis in distal phalanx of digit.

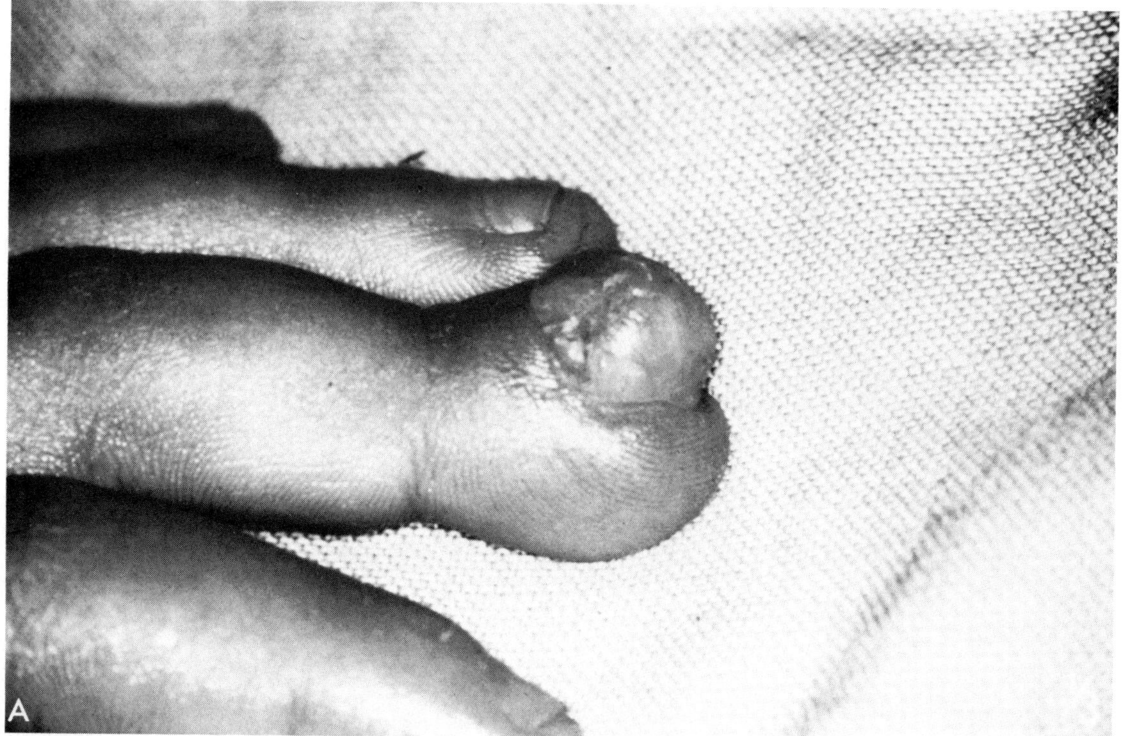

Figure 9–144. Subungual exostosis. Gross appearance of lesion (*A*) and appearance during surgical removal (*B*). The lesion exhibits a fibrocartilaginous surface.

Illustration continued on opposite page

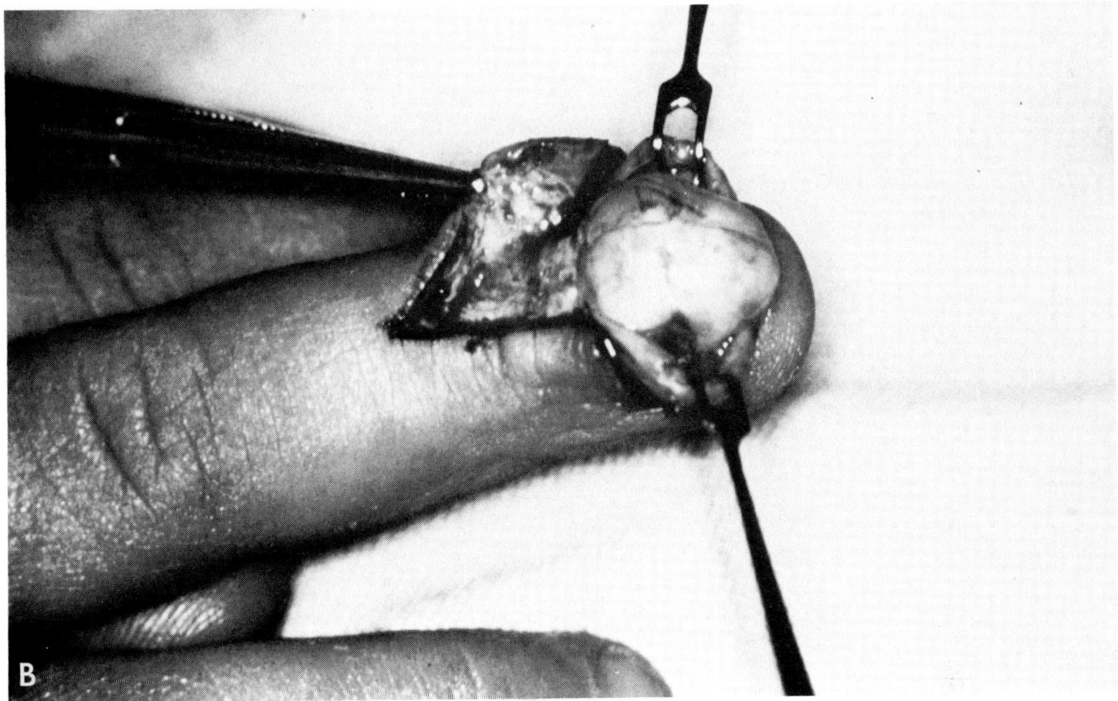

Figure 9–144 *Continued*

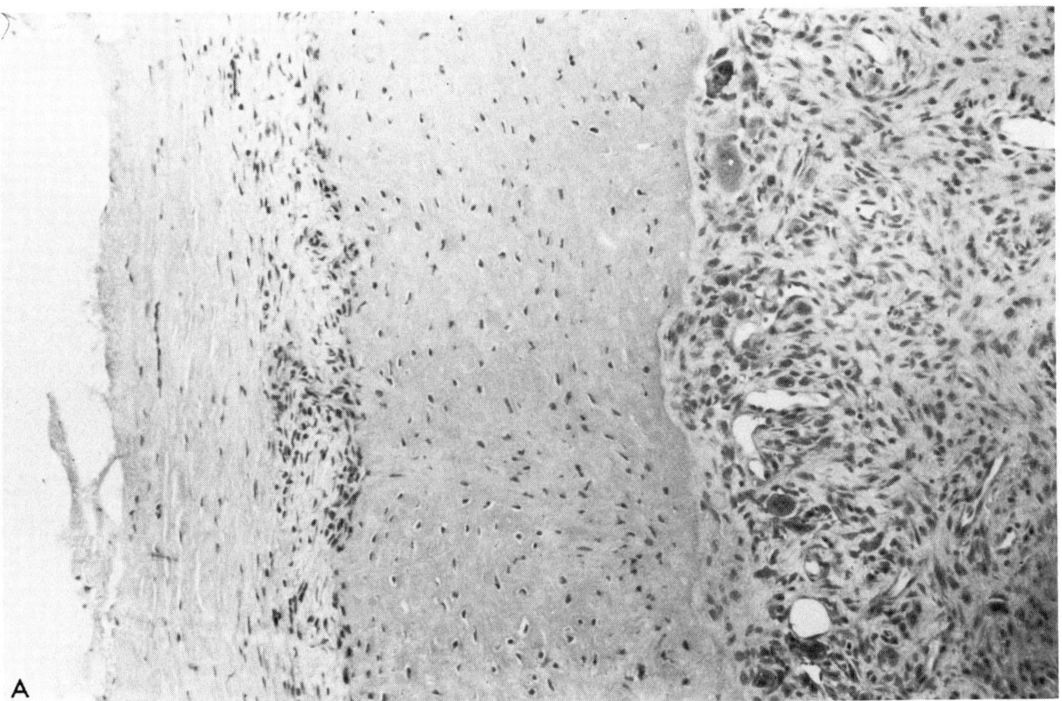

Figure 9–145. Subungual exostosis. Histologic appearance of subungual exostosis. Note the fibrous component, which may be prominent. These lesions have been erroneously diagnosed as parosteal sarcomas. There is a varying degree of cartilage formation and conversion to bone.

Illustration continued on following page

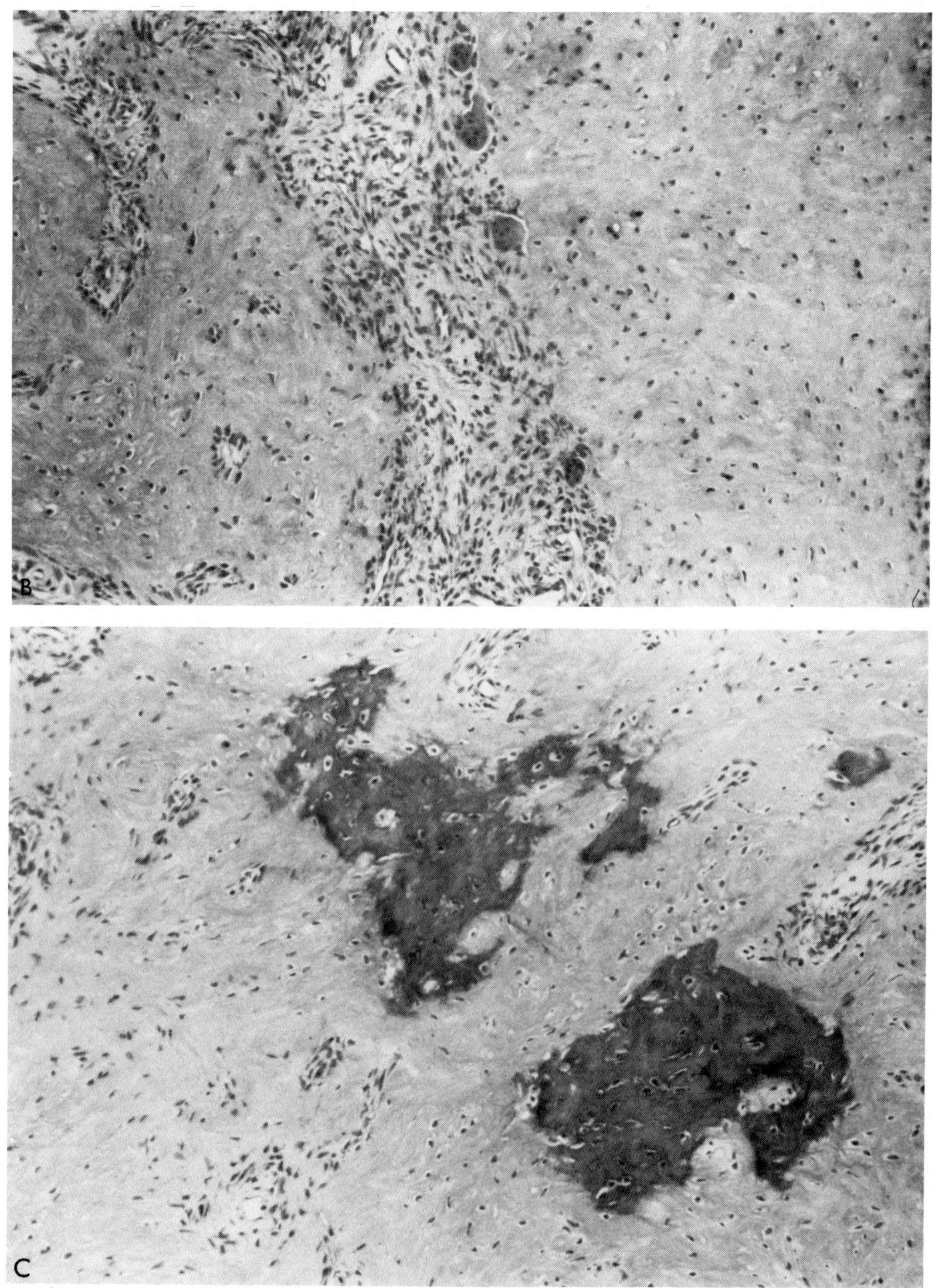

Figure 9–145 *Continued*

Illustration continued on opposite page

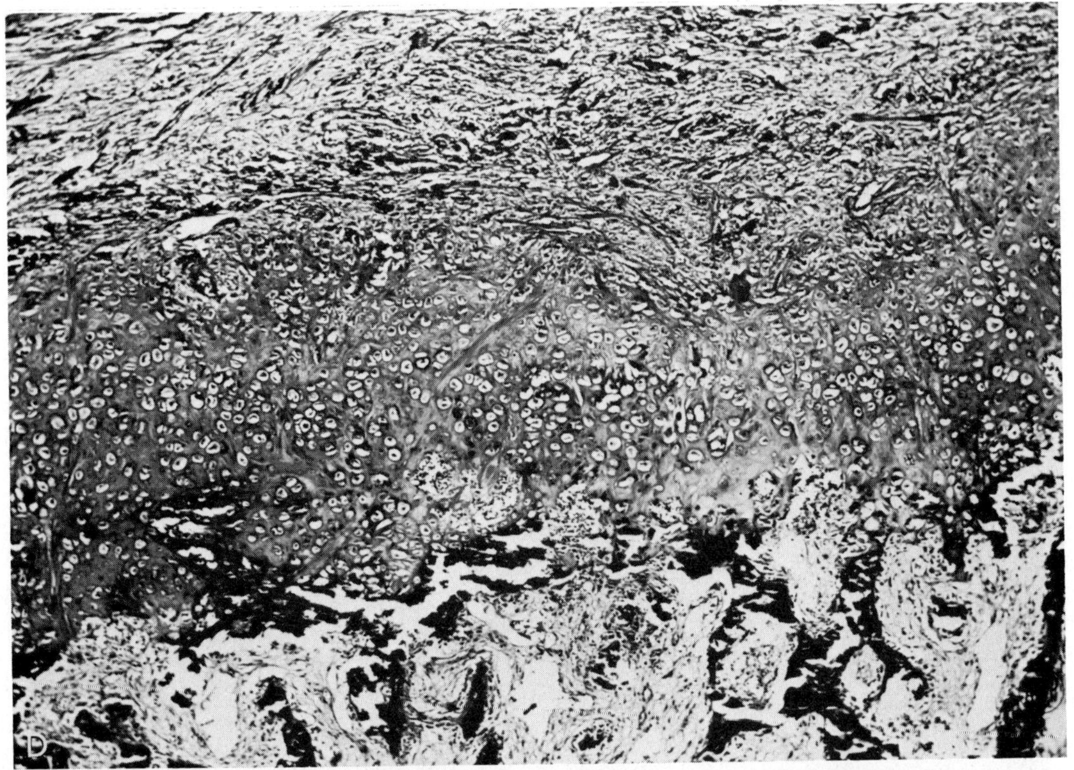

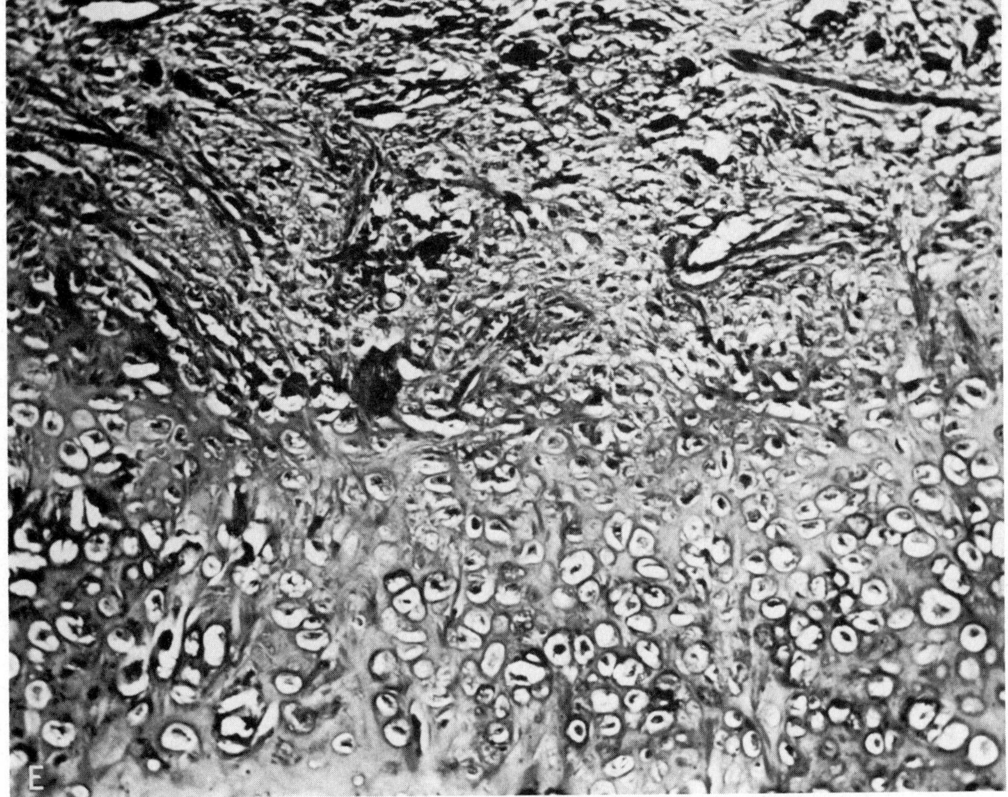

Figure 9–145 *Continued*

ENCHONDROMA

Enchondroma is a common anomaly of bone, arising in residual "islands" of cartilage left in the metaphysis as the physis grows away. These isolated cartilaginous areas existing within the metaphyseal portion of the bone continue their growth independently, expanding the bone, and occasionally break through the cortex into the adjacent soft tissue. Calcification of the cartilage is common. Enchondromas may be multiple (Ollier's disease, Maffucci's syndrome).

The histologic features of enchondroma are those of innocuous cartilage. The cartilage must be carefully studied for evidence of malignant transformation, especially in patients with Ollier's disease. Cartilage tends to reflect the age of the patient with the lesion. Thus, an individual in whom the skeletal growth phase is occurring will show relatively cellular cartilage, whereas the individual in whom the growth phase has ceased will exhibit more quiescent cartilage, and unusual growth activity in such

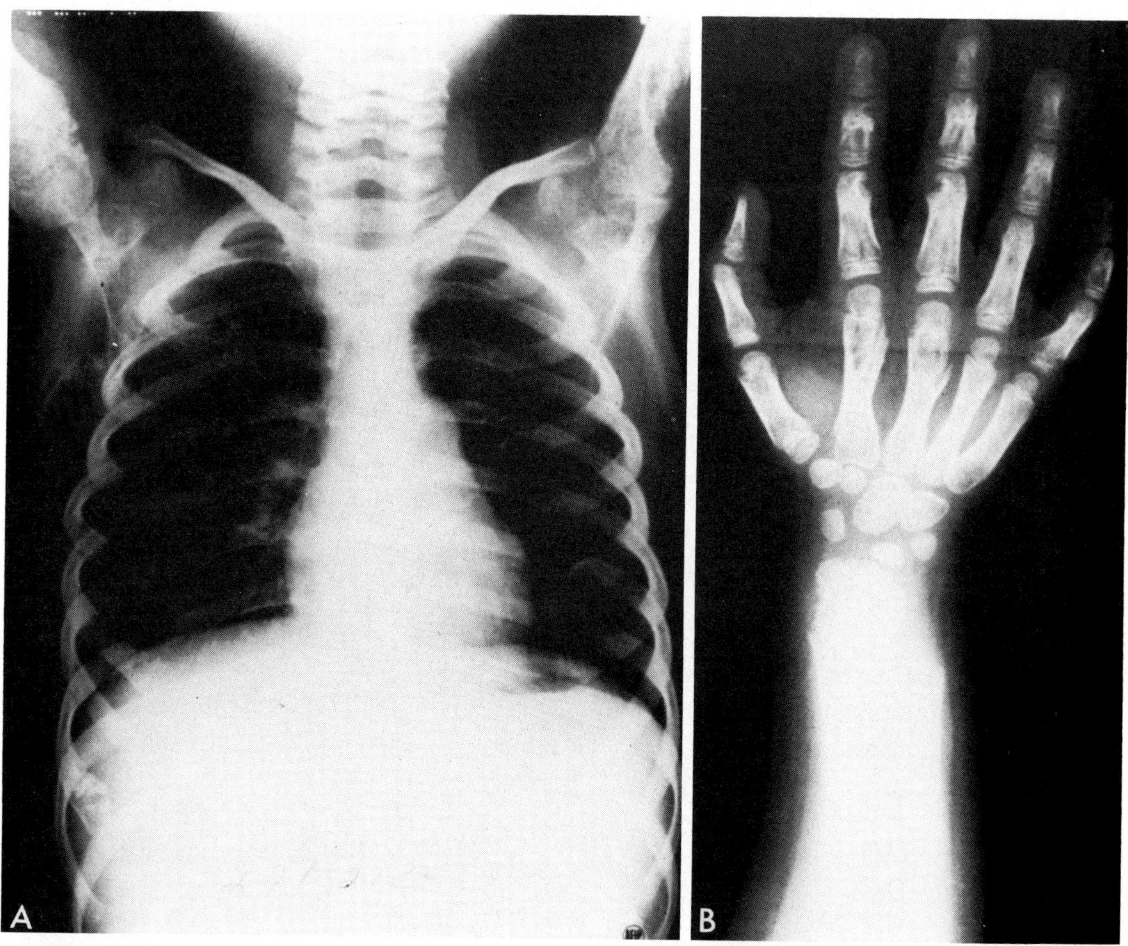

Figure 9–146. Enchondroma. Radiographs of chest (*A*) and hand (*B*) of a patient with Ollier's disease: multiple enchondromas in the skeleton of a child. These are characterized by irregular areas of radiolucency mixed with varied calcification and ossification. Expansion of bone and irregularities of growth in both length and diameter are common. The irregularities arise in the cartilage of the growth plate and are left behind within the metaphysis. As growth occurs, the radiolucencies tend to be longitudinally oriented in the metaphysis.

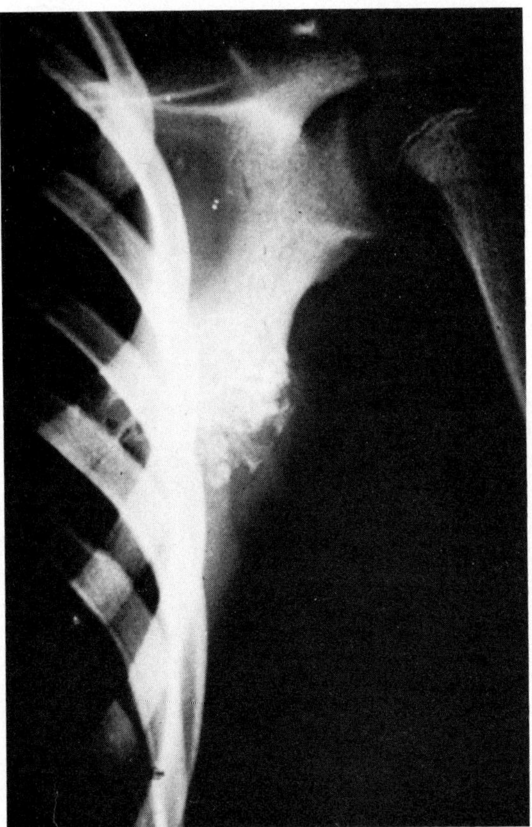

Figure 9–147. Enchondroma of scapula. Sharply circumscribed defect, with expansion of bone. Numerous punctate, or ring-shaped, calcifications are characteristic of the lobulations of cartilage matrix. The absence of periosteal reaction and expanded bone indicates a slow rate of growth.

an individual is a sign of malignant transformation. The normal characteristics of cartilage include uniform nuclei surrounded by relatively large lacunar spaces. Reduction of lacunar space or cellular proliferation without formation of normal lacunae indicates increased cellular growth and, very possibly, an aggressive or malignant cartilage tumor (i.e., chondrosarcoma). In larger bones, enchondromas do not erode the cortex. There should be no associated periosteal reaction, and deposits of cartilage are surrounded by lamellar bone.

Enchondromas may be seen in any bone preformed in cartilage. One should remember the possibility of malignant transformation when considering chondromas of the central skeleton (i.e., any bone proximal to the wrist and ankle). Chondromas of the distal skeleton, (i.e., hands and feet) very rarely become malignant (Dahlin and Salvador, 1974). Histologic transformation should not be confused with biologic behavior. Although some observers doubt the concept (Spjut et al., 1971; Unni and Dahlin, 1979), it is our opinion that the biologic malignant potential of a cartilage lesion of the central skeleton is somewhat ominous, regardless of its histology. Conversely, the malignant biologic potential of a lesion of the distal skeleton is virtually nonexistent. We therefore recommend prophylactic removal of easily accessible cartilaginous lesions of the central skeleton and close observation for those not removed.

Text continued on page 414

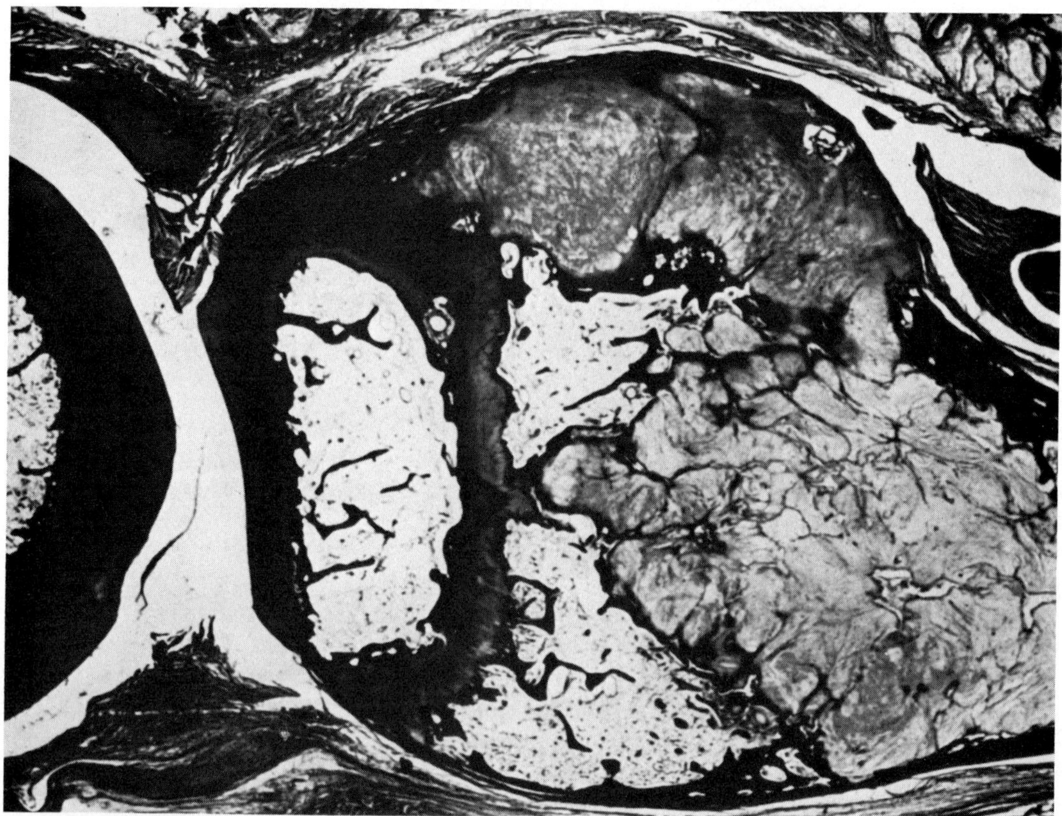

Figure 9–148. Enchondroma. Cartilaginous masses in the metaphyseal portion of bone. The shaft is expanded; the lesion is contained and surrounded by trabeculae of bone, indicating a slow rate of growth.

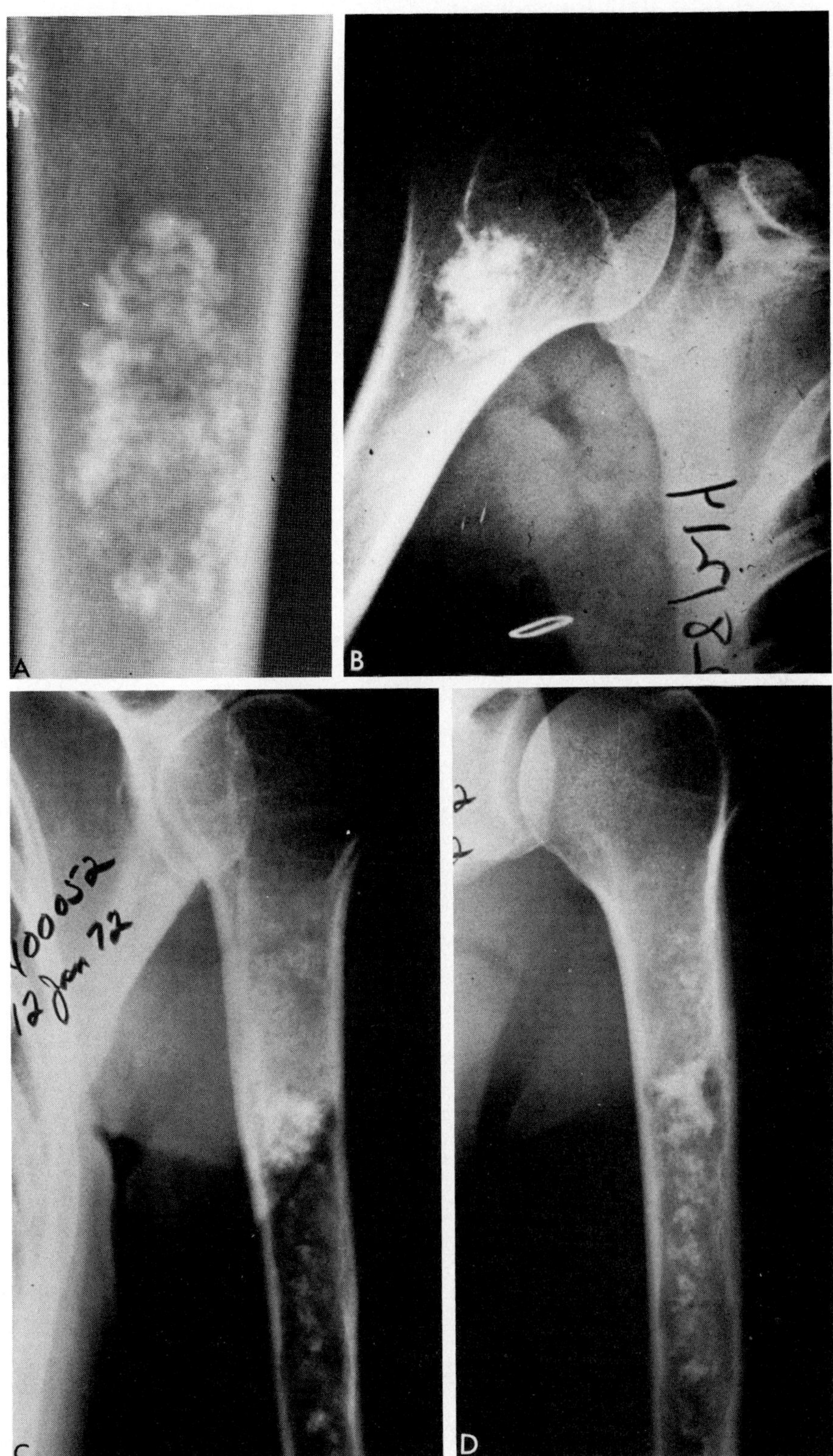

Figure 9–149. Enchondroma. Radiographic appearance of enchondromas in various portions of the skeleton. The lesions are sharply circumscribed and exhibit flocculent calcification.

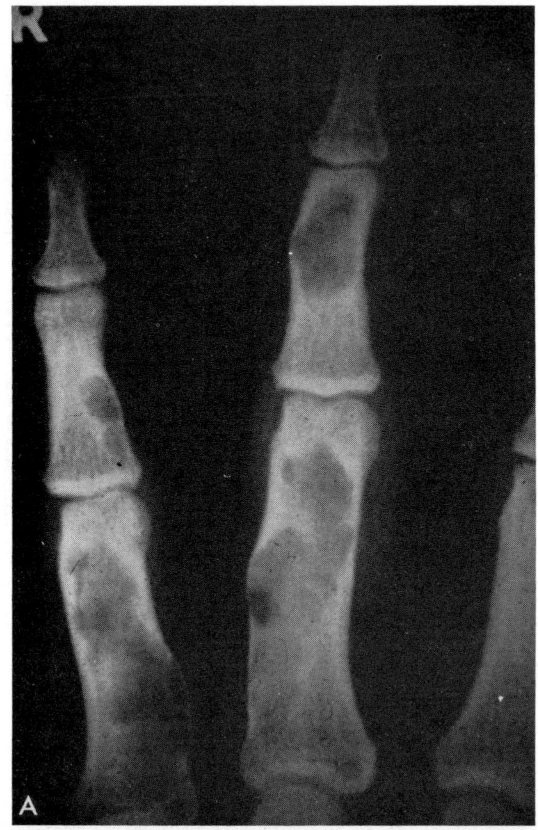

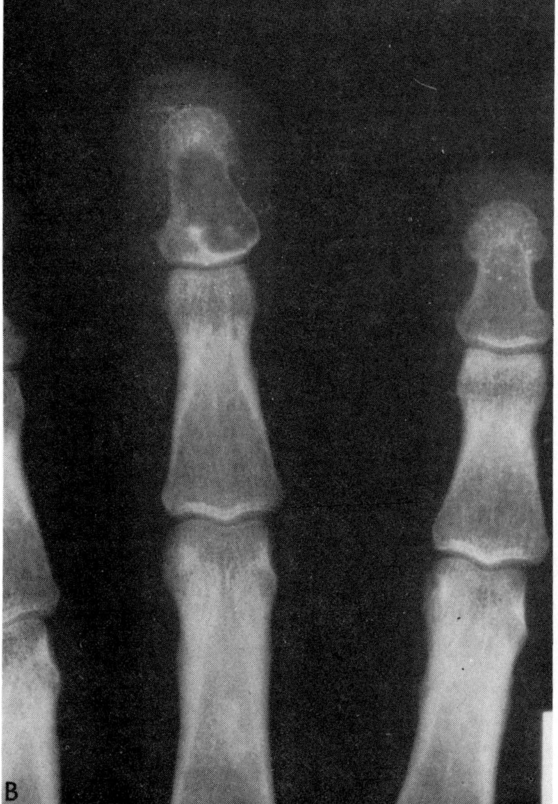

Figure 9–150. Enchondroma. Radiographic appearance of multiple enchondromas in the small bones of the hand. The lesions are lytic and sharply circumscribed, and they exhibit focal areas of flocculent calcification. Location in the peripheral bones of hand and foot is common.

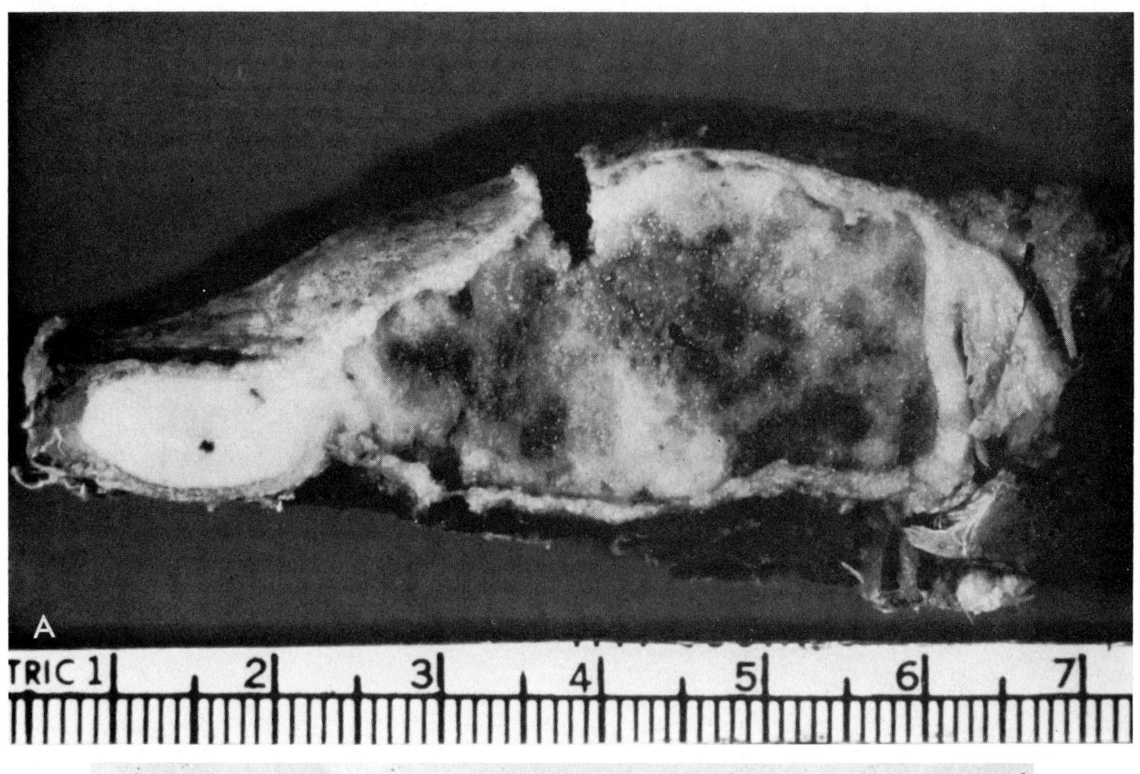

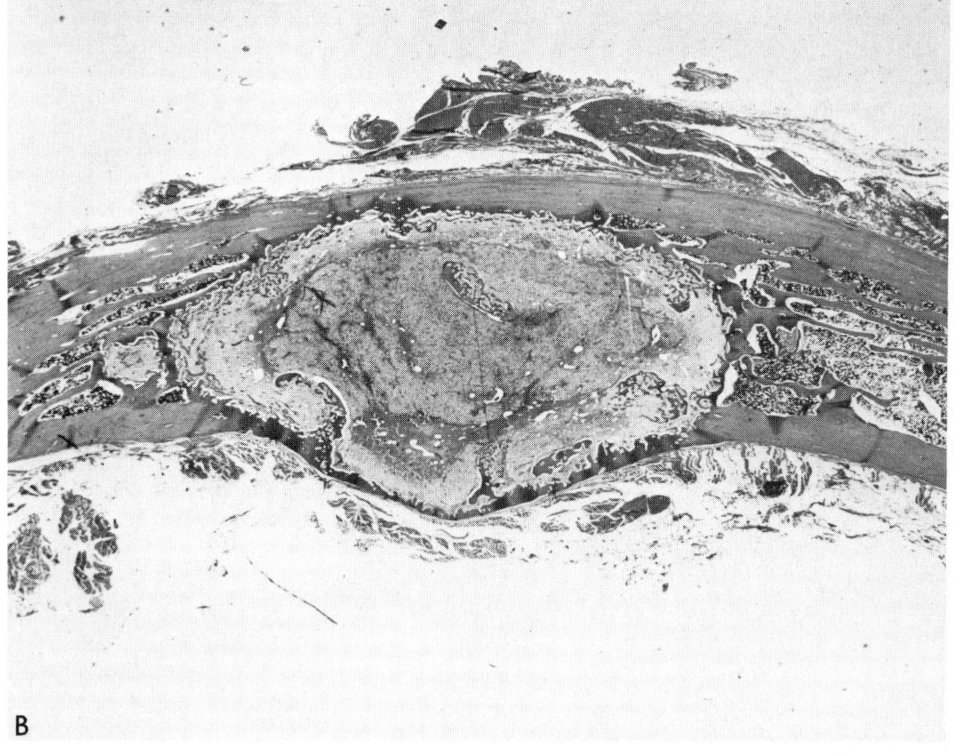

Figure 9–151. Enchondroma. Gross appearance *(A)* and macrospecimen *(B)* of enchondroma. Note the sharp circumscription and reactive bone formation around the margin of the tumor.

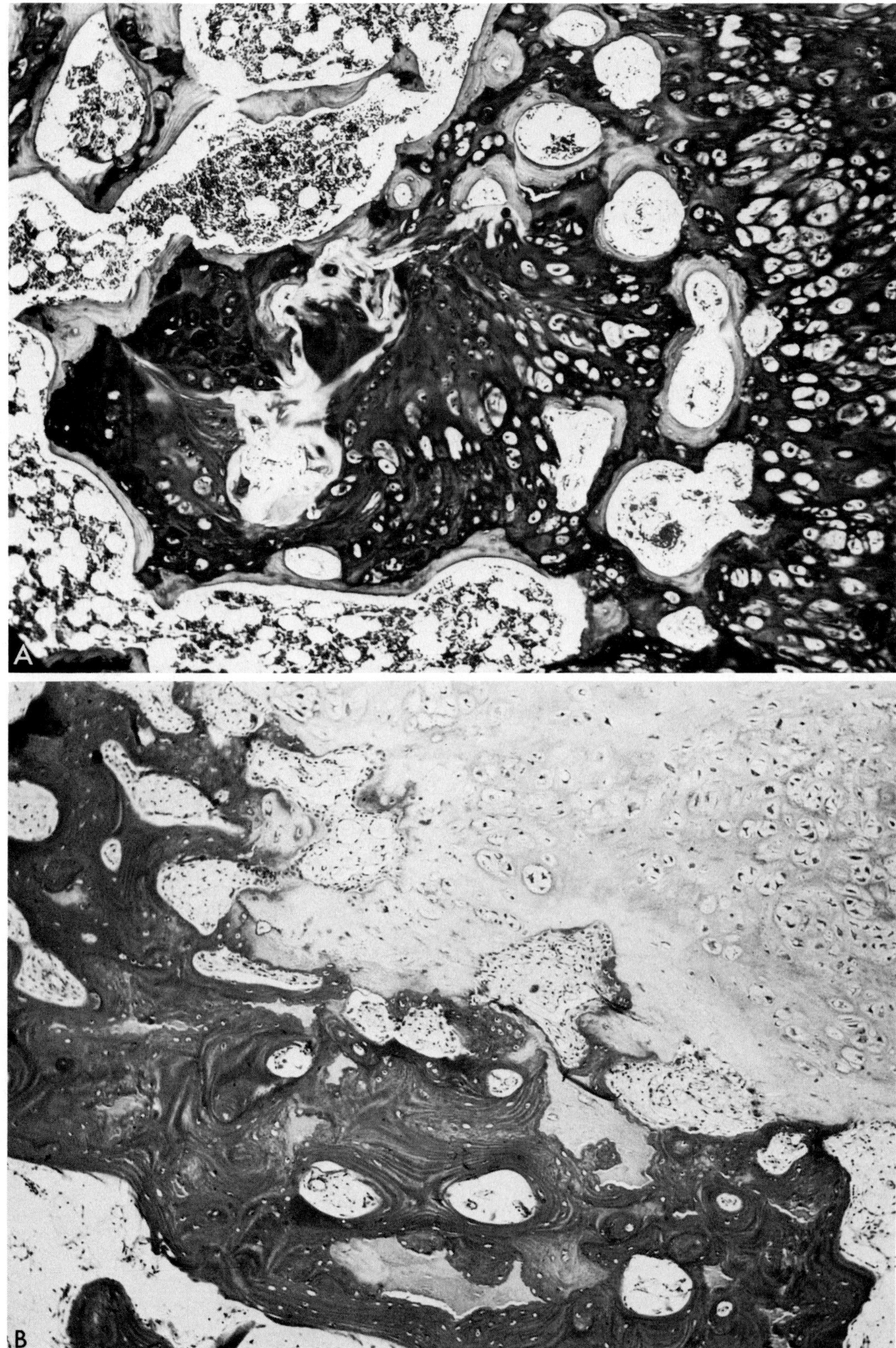

Figure 9–152

Illustration continued on opposite page

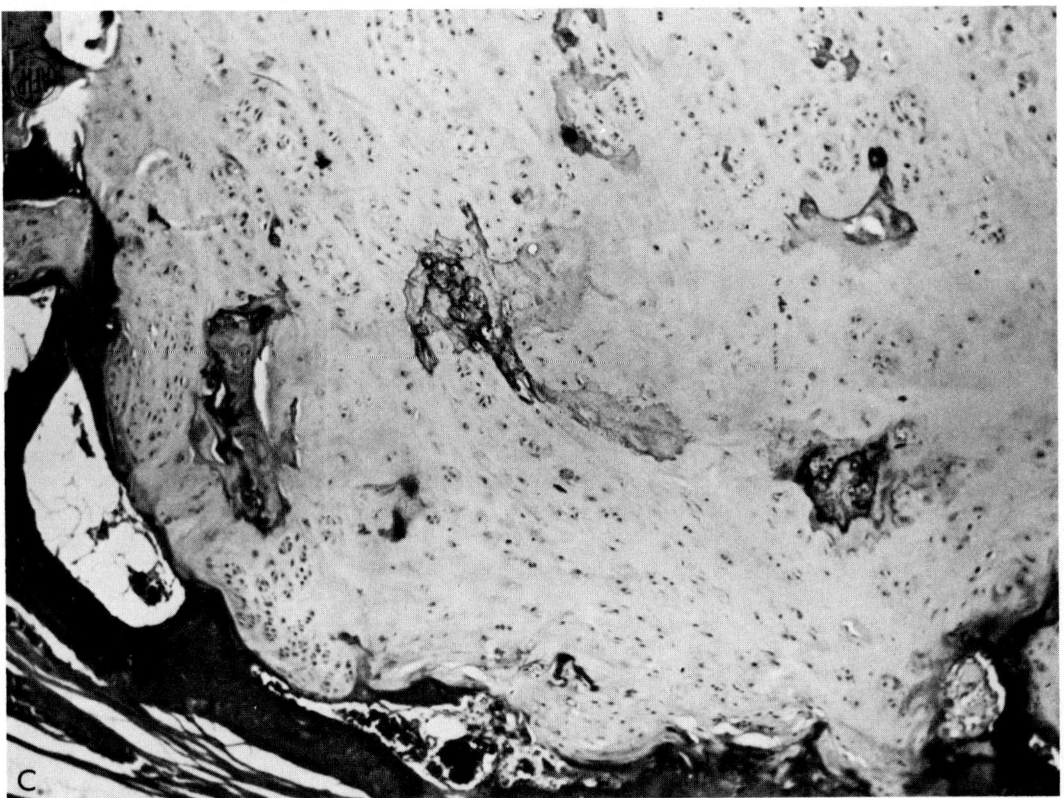

Figure 9–152. Enchondroma. Histologic appearance of benign enchondroma. There may be some variation in cellular size. The lacunar spaces may show variation, and a moderate degree of pleomorphism is present. Features identifying the lesion as benign include the small size of the nucleus within the lacunar space, the lack of mitotic activity, and the circumscribed nature of the cartilage deposits. Note the thin rim of bone surrounding the cartilage, a sign of benign enchondroma.

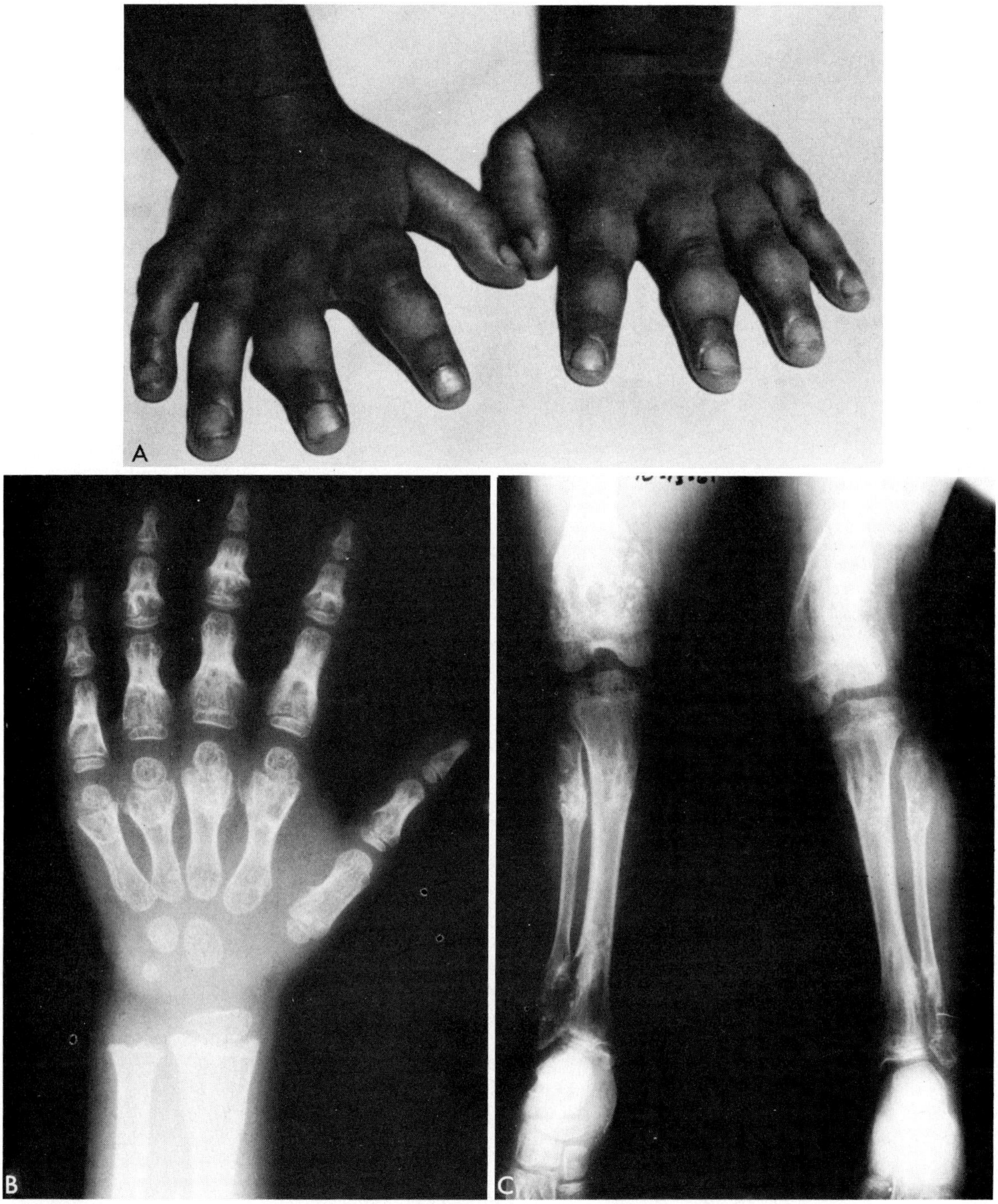

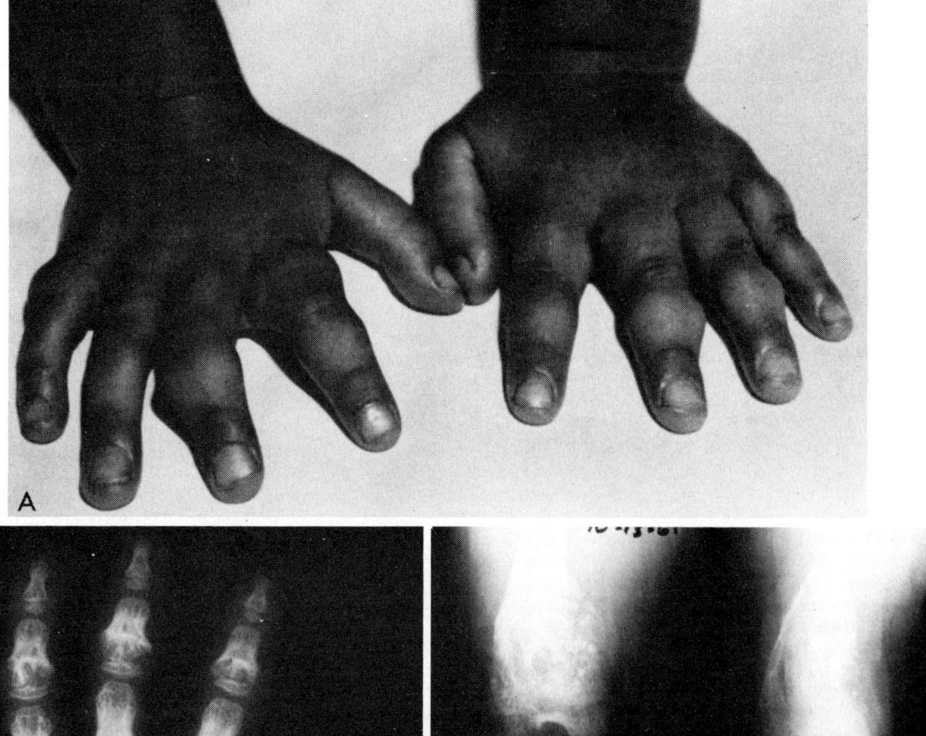

Figure 9–153. Gross appearance *(A)* and radiographs *(B* to *D)* of patients with Ollier's disease. Multiple enchondromas are evident throughout the skeleton. Surgical removal depends on symptomatology. *E,* Radiograph of a patient with Maffucci's syndrome exhibiting multiple angiomas with characteristic vascular calcification in addition to the multiple enchondromas.

Illustration continued on opposite page.

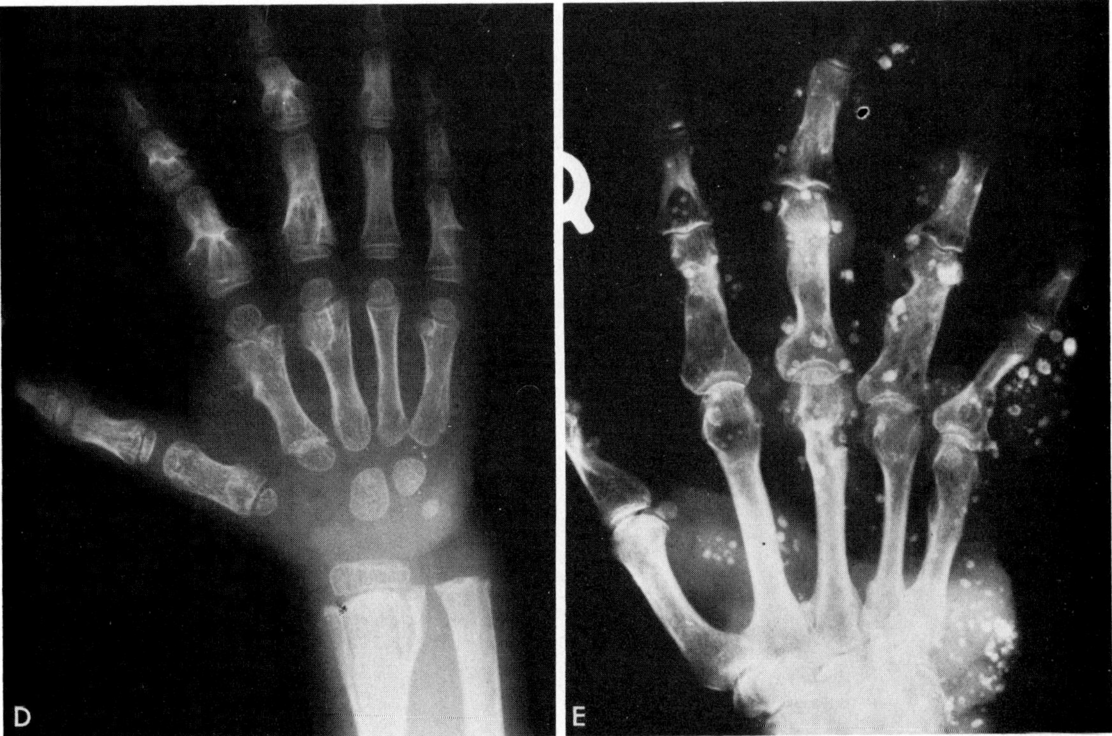

Figure 9–153 *Continued*

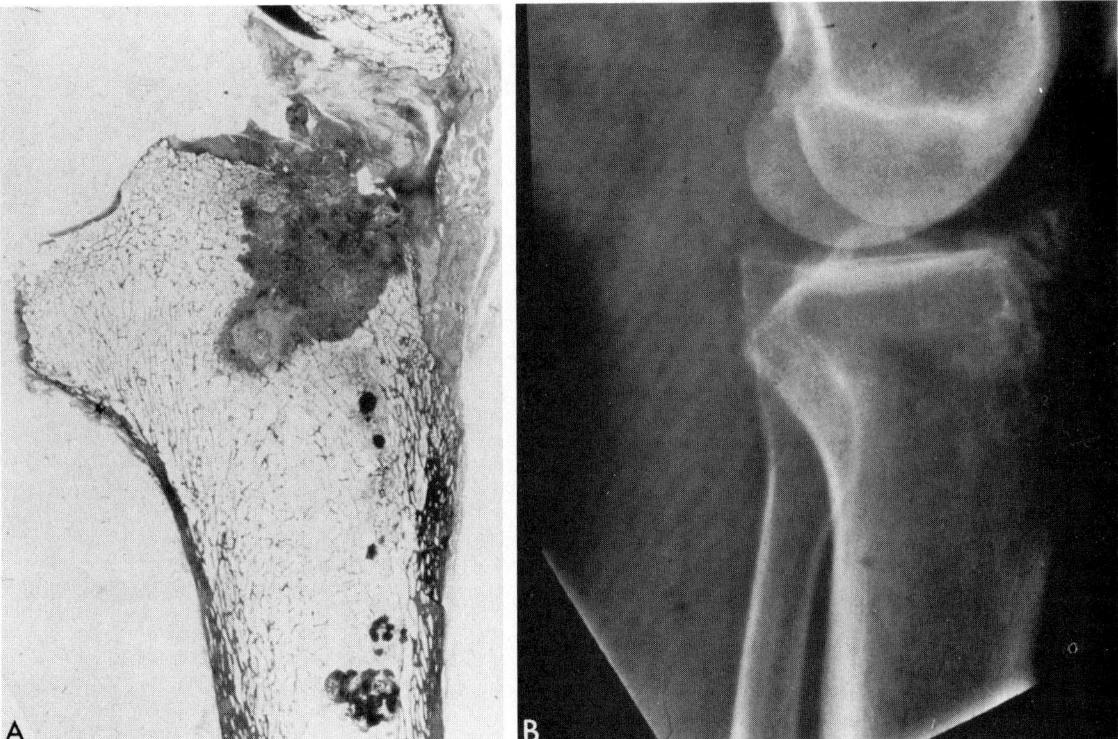

Figure 9–154. Enchondroma. Macrosection *(A)* and radiograph *(B)* of a tibia with a chondrosarcoma at the joint surface. Study of the amputated specimen reveals numerous smaller enchondromas within the medullary cavity that are not visible radiographically.

CHONDROSARCOMA

Histologic differentiation between benign and malignant cartilaginous neoplasms is difficult. The unequivocal enchondroma is a lesion in which there is no clinical, histologic, or radiologic suspicion of malignancy. It is a small, sharply circumscribed lesion, with a sharply defined radiographic margin, focal punctate calcification, no significant cortical erosion, and no periosteal reaction.

The presence of any symptom, such as pain, automatically makes the lesion suspicious. Evidence of recent activity, based on either clinical, histologic, or radiographic findings, is sufficient to warrant the suspicion of malignancy, and aggressive investigation must be instituted.

The clear-cut chondrosarcoma shows histologic changes of varying grades. The most subtle change is simply an increase in the number of cartilage cells per unit volume. The cartilaginous lacunae are maintained, and the nuclei exhibit slight hyperchromatism and some regenerative activity. More severe changes consist of loss of lacunar spaces, naked nuclei, spindling of nuclei, and myxoid changes in cartilaginous cells and stroma. Ultimately, undifferentiated tumor cells are present in which only a cartilaginous ground substance identifies the tumor as a chondrosarcoma.

One usually has no problem identifying the malignant characteristics of the grade 3 undifferentiated, spindled, or myxoid tumor. Difficulties abound in the differentiation between benign enchondroma and well-differentiated chondrosarcoma in which the cartilage nuclei and lacunae are maintained (Fig. 9–165A).

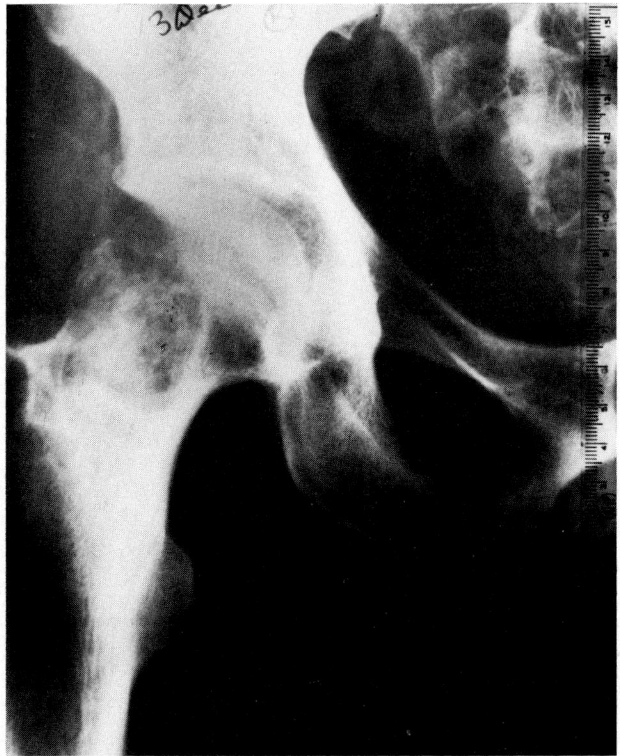

Figure 9–155. Chondrosarcoma. Poorly circumscribed lesion in the neck of the femur. The flocculent calcification is characteristic of cartilage matrix. The moth-eaten appearance of the lesion's margin indicates a moderately aggressive tumor. The lesion was not biopsied at this time, but 1 year later histologic study revealed well-differentiated chondrosarcoma.

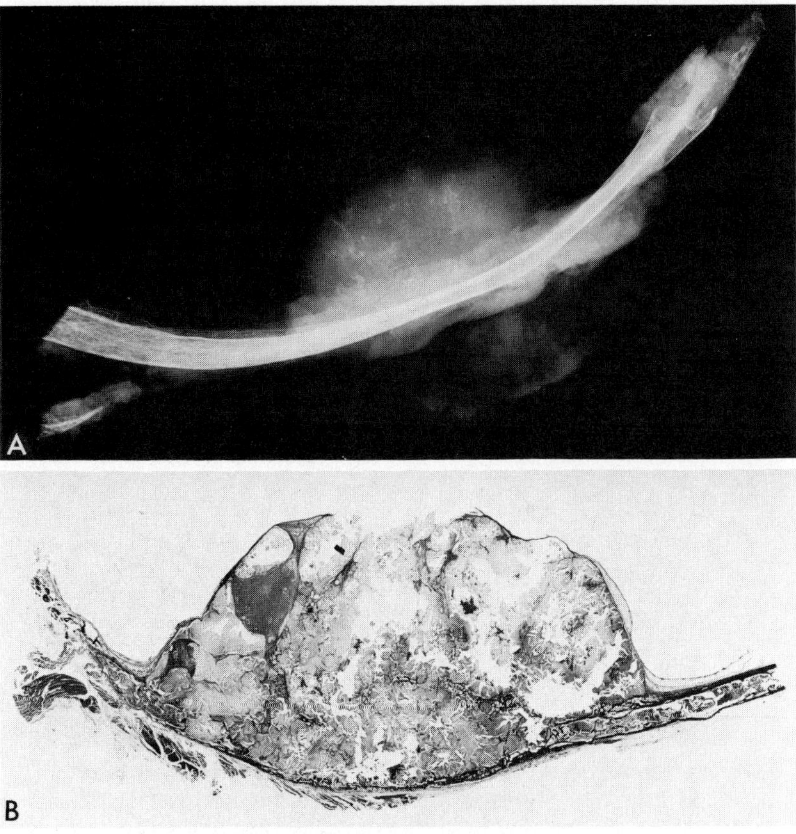

Figure 9–156. Chondrosarcoma. Specimen radiograph *(A)* and macrosection *(B)* of a rib containing a chondrosarcoma. Note the flocculent calcification characteristic of cartilage matrix. The lesion exhibits extensive myxoid component.

Radiographic features, such as loss of distinct margins, moth-eaten or permeative destruction, evidence of cortical erosion, and the presence of a periosteal reaction, all serve to make the physician suspect malignancy.

Numerous variants of chondrosarcoma exist. The clear cell variant (LeCharpentier et al., 1979) appears confined to the epiphysis; mesenchymal chondrosarcoma exhibits a compact highly cellular histologic appearance (Salvador et al., 1971). Survival studies for these variants of chondrosarcoma are not essentially different from those for chondrosarcoma as a whole, but depend upon histologic grade.

Differentiation is made between primary and secondary chondrosarcomas (Dahlin and Salvador, 1974). Primary sarcoma is a tumor arising de novo within the medullary cavity of a bone; secondary chondrosarcoma is a tumor arising in a pre-existing enchondroma. With the exception of the obviously different age group that will be affected by these two variants, prognosis is affected by the histologic grade rather than the mode of origin.

Chondrosarcomas are known to undergo "dedifferentiation" (Dahlin and Salvador, 1974; McCarthy and Dorfman, 1982). A relatively low-grade chondrosarcoma exhibits change to a poorly differentiated sarcomatous component. In some cases, the well-differentiated lesion may be benign pre-existing enchondroma with extensive calcification, and the secondary chondrosarcoma becomes a highly anaplastic sarcoma whose cartilaginous origin is difficult to discern. The poor prognosis of these tumors is a reflection of their undifferentiated histologic pattern.

Text continued on page 437

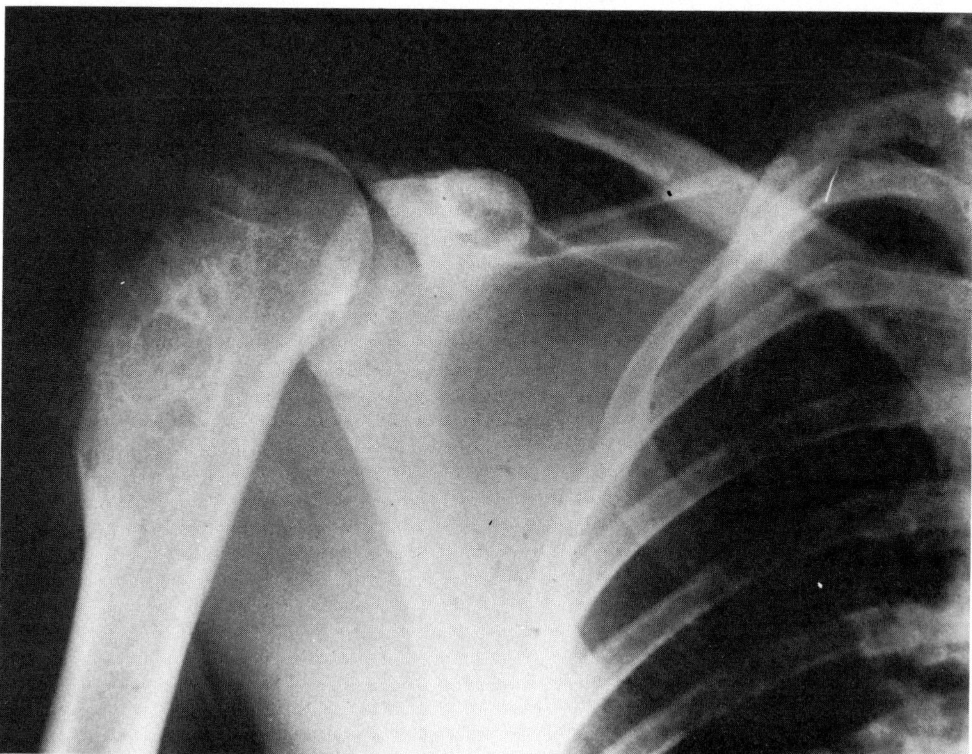

Figure 9–157. Chondrosarcoma. A well-defined lesion in the epiphyseal and metaphyseal portions of the upper humerus. There is expansion of the cortex but no active periosteal reaction. The matrix calcification is characteristic of cartilage but is not prominent in this lesion.

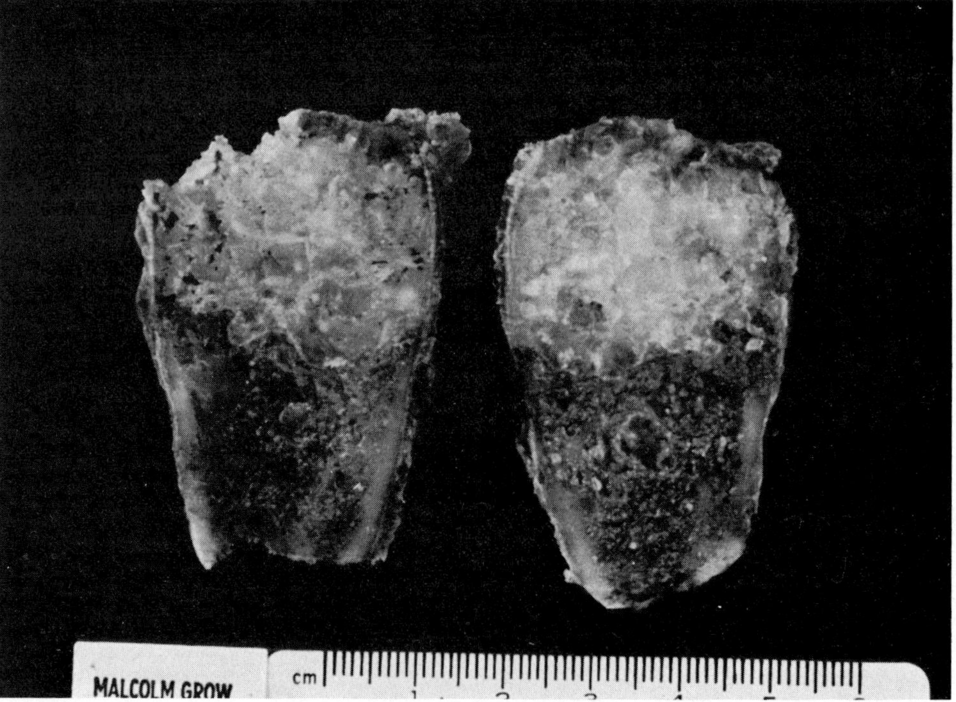

Figure 9–158. Gross specimen of the humerus illustrated in Figure 9–157 containing bluish-white cartilage mass replacing the medullary contents. Excision of the lesion reveals a small skip lesion located just beneath the primary tumor that is not evident on the preoperative radiograph.

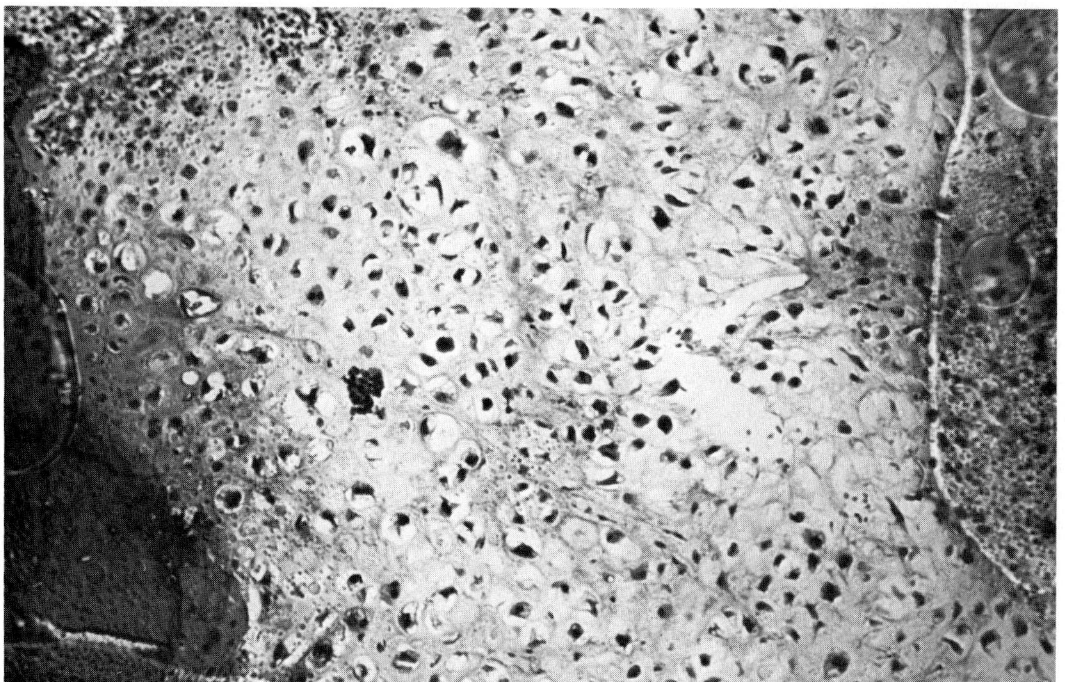

Figure 9–159. Chondrosarcoma. Histologic appearance of lesion illustrated in Figures 9–157 and 9–158. Note the plump chondroblasts, set in a myxoid stroma. There is moderate variation in size, shape, and staining quality of the cells in the presence of easily recognized chondroid matrix. This favors the diagnosis of a well-differentiated but malignant cartilage tumor.

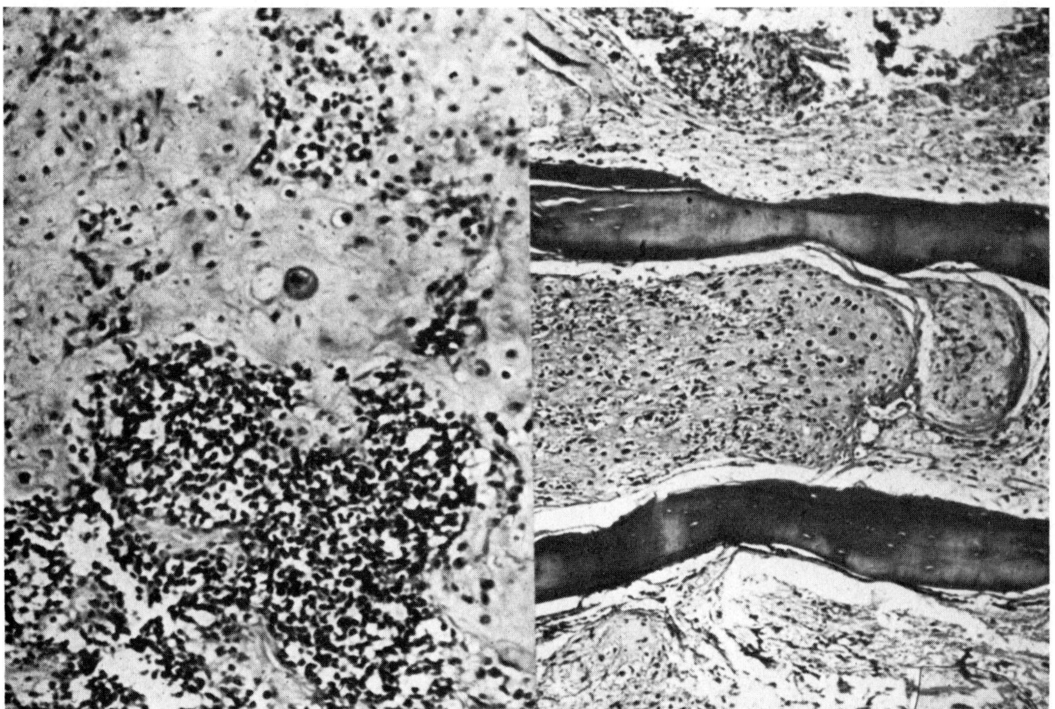

Figure 9–160. Chondrosarcoma. Spectrum of histologic changes seen in chondrosarcoma. On the left, clumps of chondroid matrix are intermingled with clusters of cells that are too undifferentiated to manufacture identifiable matrix. They consist of small, round nuclei with scanty cytoplasm. On the right, the tumor extends between trabeculae of bone and replaces the normal marrow. This rapidly growing advancing edge is not usually mineralized and thus cannot be seen radiographically. It presents a hazard to the surgeon who is planning a segmental resection for chondrosarcoma.

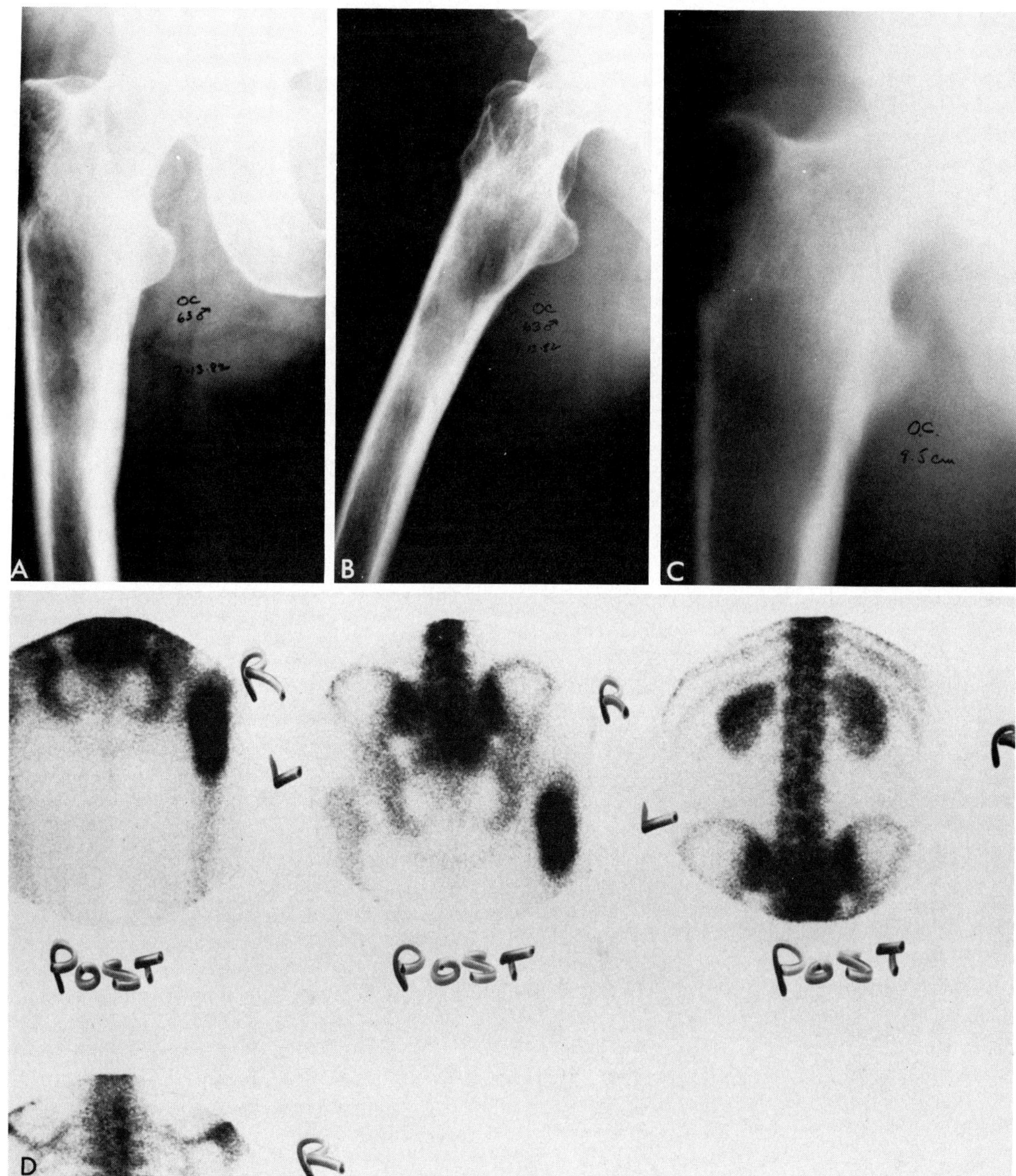

Figure 9–161. Anteroposterior *(A)* and frogleg *(B)* radiographs of proximal femur in a 63-year-old male patient with a 3-year history of pain. There is a large lytic defect that has eroded the cortex from within. Slight expansion and thickening of the medial cortex of the proximal femoral shaft are evident. There is no periosteal reaction. The bone scan *(D)* shows marked uptake in the proximal femur. The tomograms *(C)* demonstrate a purely lytic defect with water density and no matrix mineralization. The medial cortex is reinforced. The CT scan *(E* and *F)* through the lesion was interpreted as showing water density in the medullary cavity, leading to a radiographic impression of bone cyst.

Illustration continued on opposite page

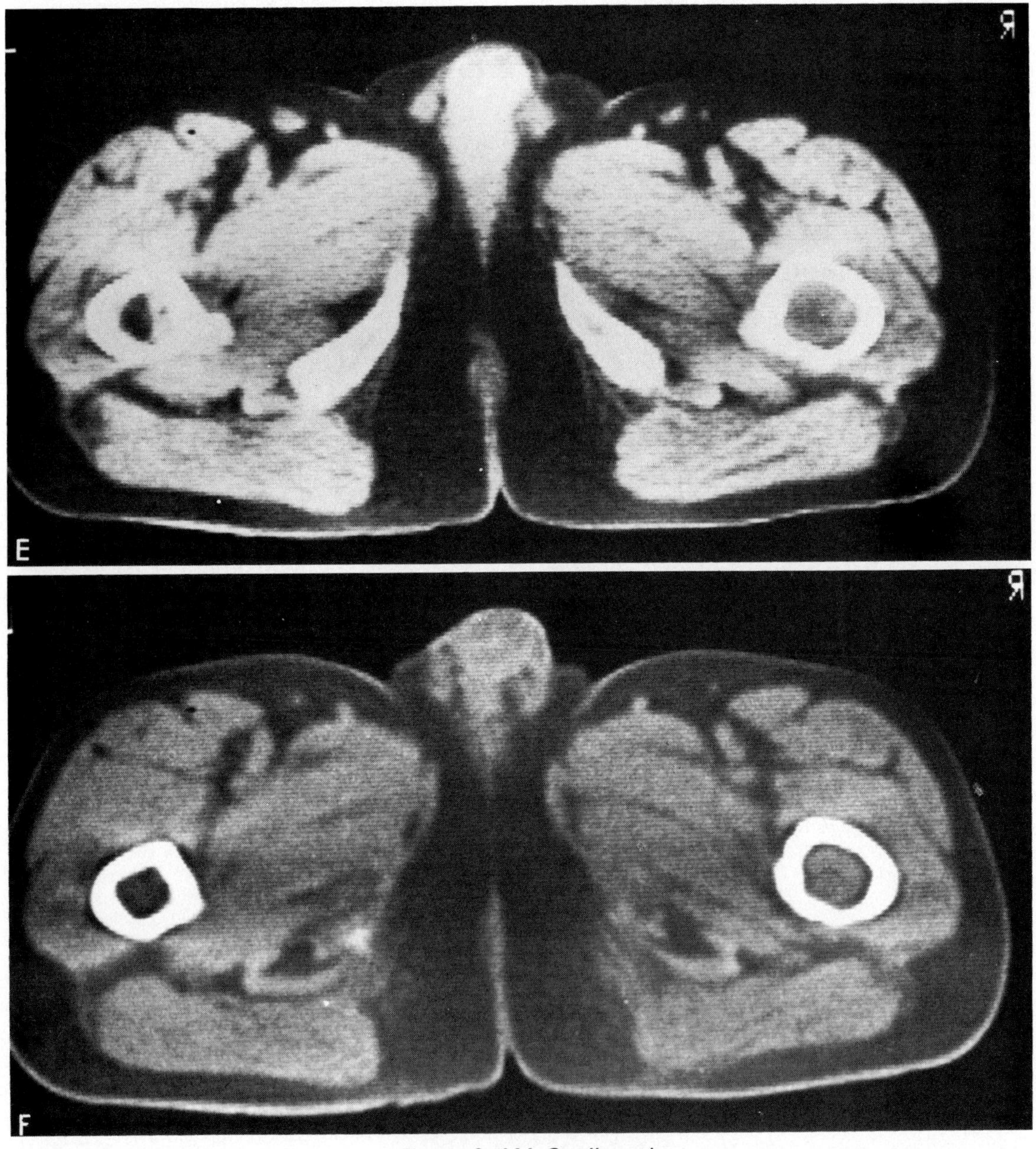

Figure 9–161 *Continued*

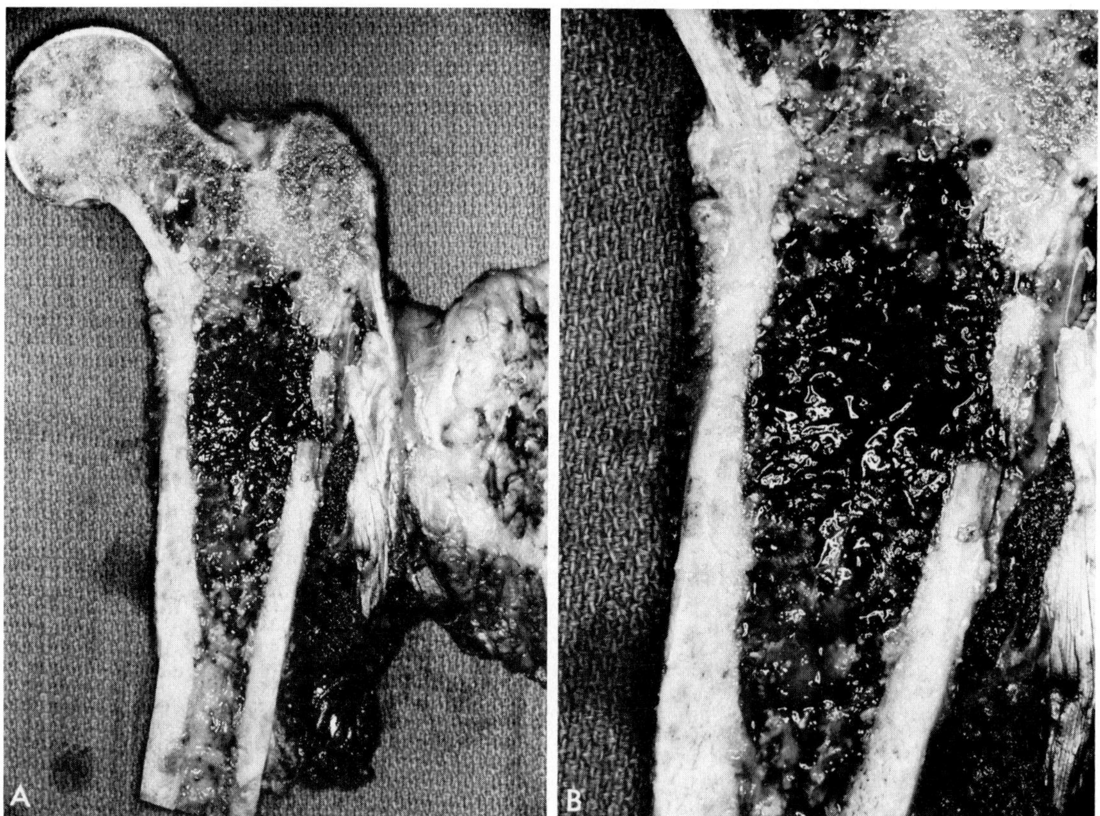

Figure 9–162. Low-power *(A)* and high-power *(B)* views of the surgical specimen illustrated in Figure 9–161 after resection. The extent of the lesion is evident at the distal margin but unclear at the proximal margin. The soft gelatinous consistency is evident.

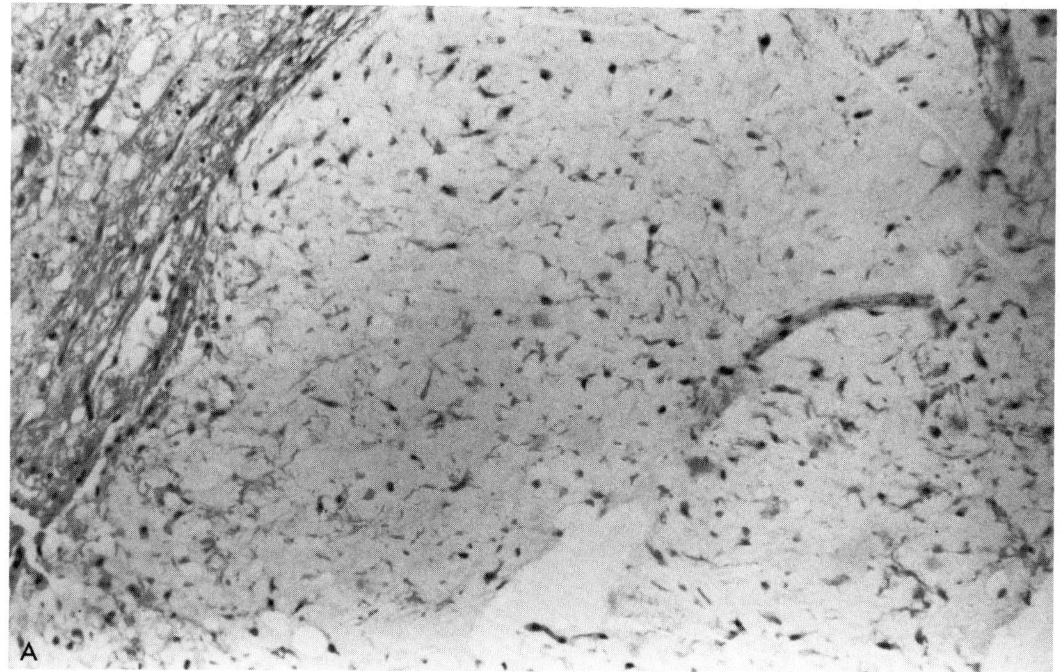

Figure 9–163. Chondrosarcoma. Histologic sections demonstrating a markedly myxoid tumor with isolated pleomorphic clusters of cells. The myxomatous nature of the chondrosarcoma may account for the water density evident on CT scan. Chondrosarcomas with extensive myxoid component are common.

Illustration continued on opposite page

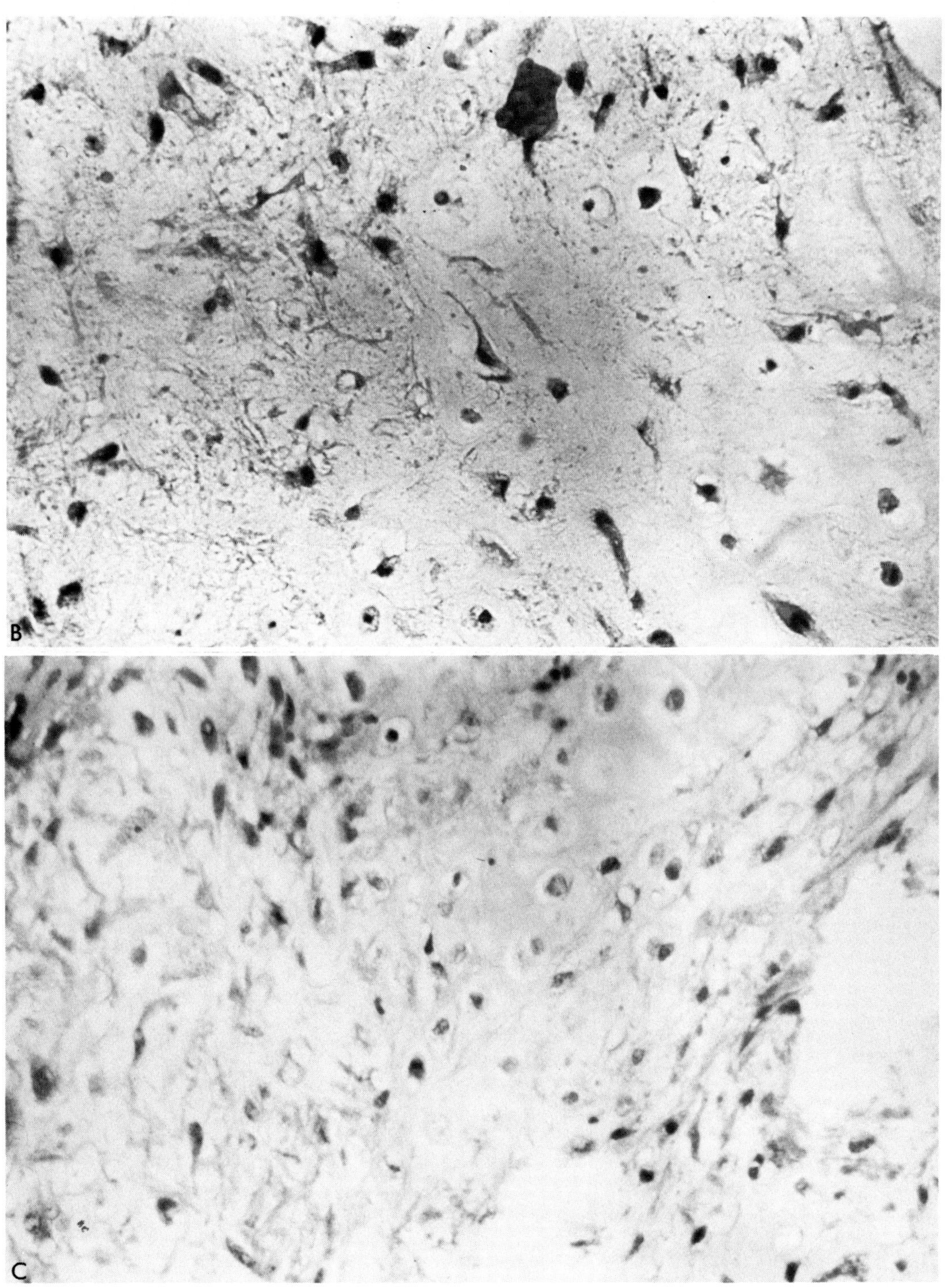

Figure 9–163 *Continued*

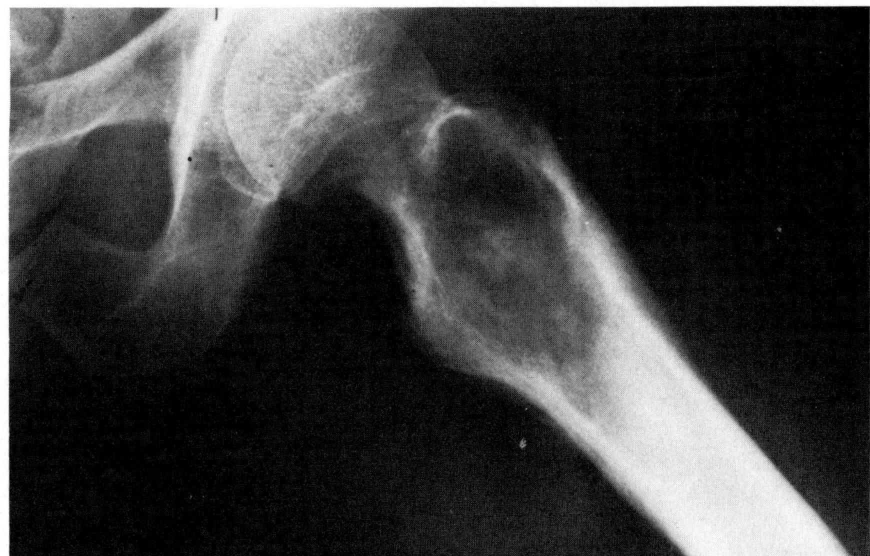

Figure 9–164. Chondrosarcoma. Lytic defect, metaphyseal portion of femoral neck; indistinct margin that fades into normal bone; focal irregular calcification within the defect. The poor definition of the lesion indicates intermediate aggressive growth; the calcification is consistent with cartilage.

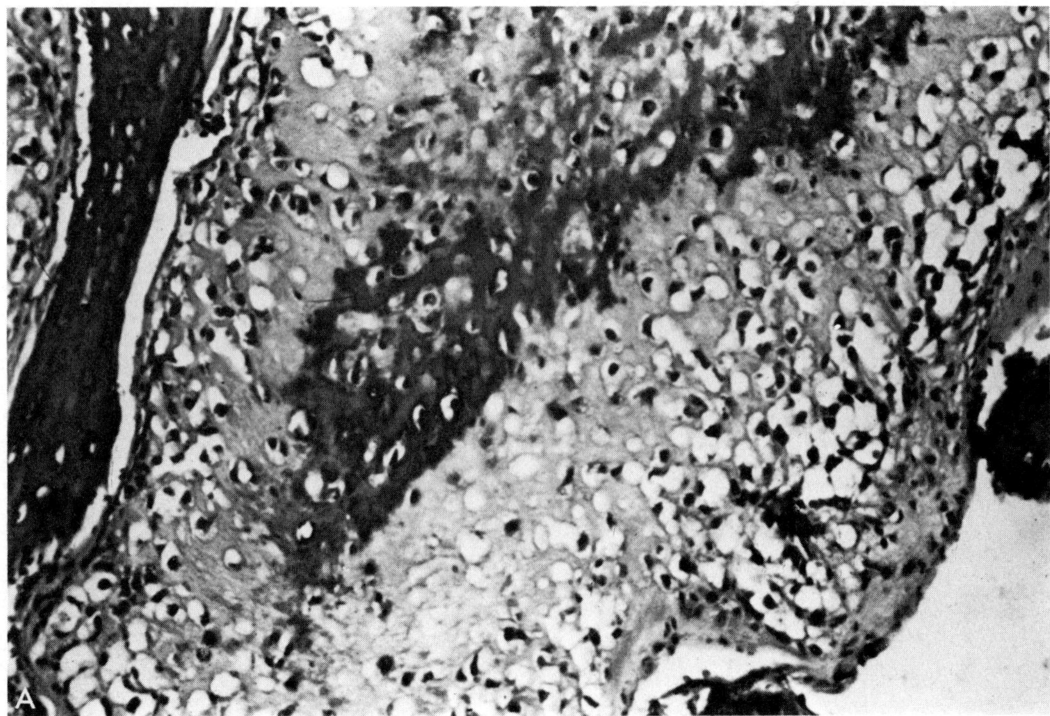

Figure 9–165. Spectrum of histologic changes seen in a single chondrosarcoma. In *A,* the lesion retains its basic cartilage nature, with foci of calcification. Lacunar spaces are large, and only the hypercellularity indicates a malignant tumor. In *B, C, D,* and *E,* there is progressive dedifferentiation of the neoplasm. Lacunar spaces are lost, the tumor is hypercellular, and stellate chondrocytes with marked pleomorphism and mitotic activity are evident. In *F,* the tumor is virtually unrecognizable as a chondrosarcoma.

Illustration continued on opposite page

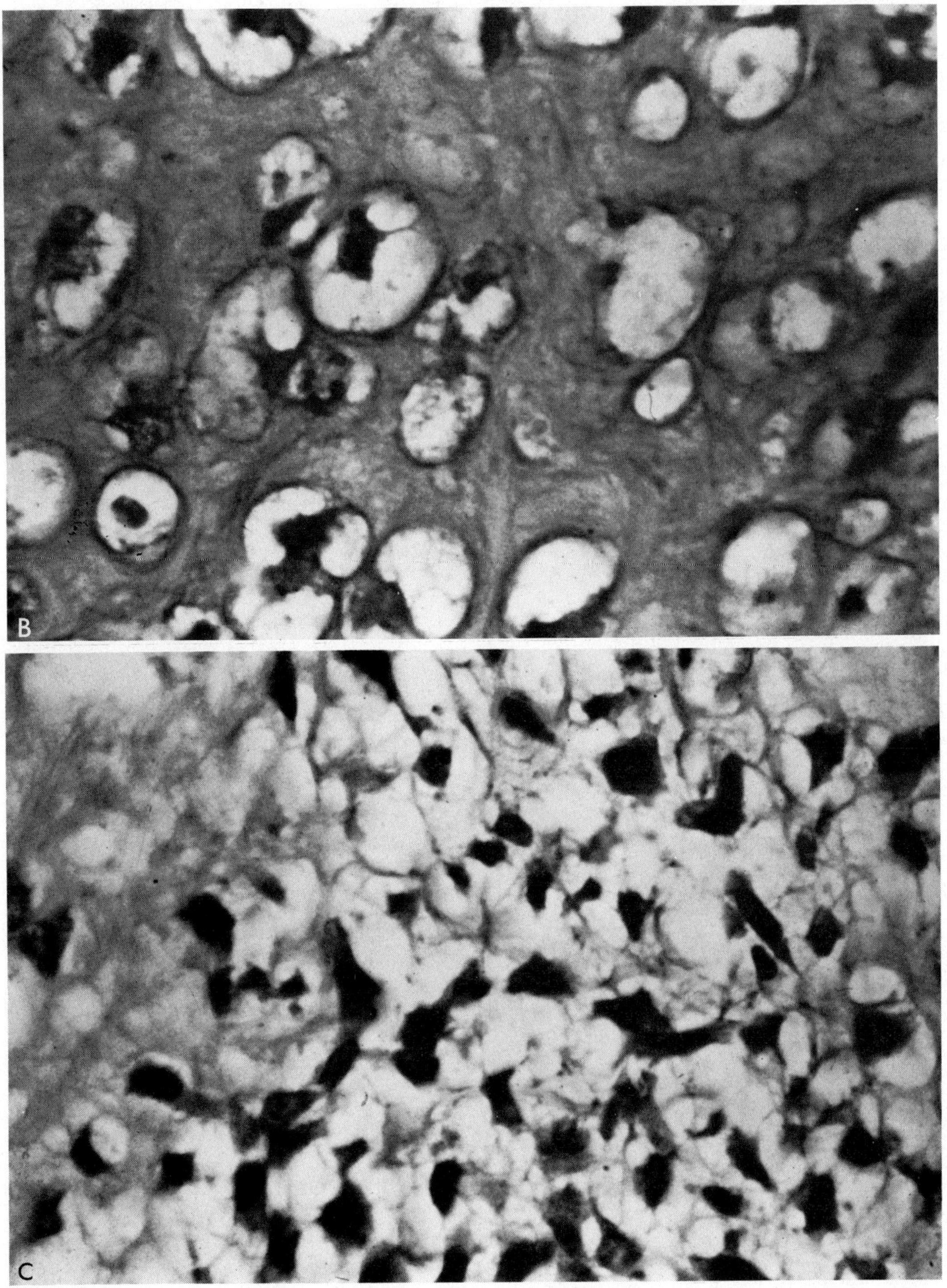

Figure 9–165 *Continued*

Illustration continued on following page

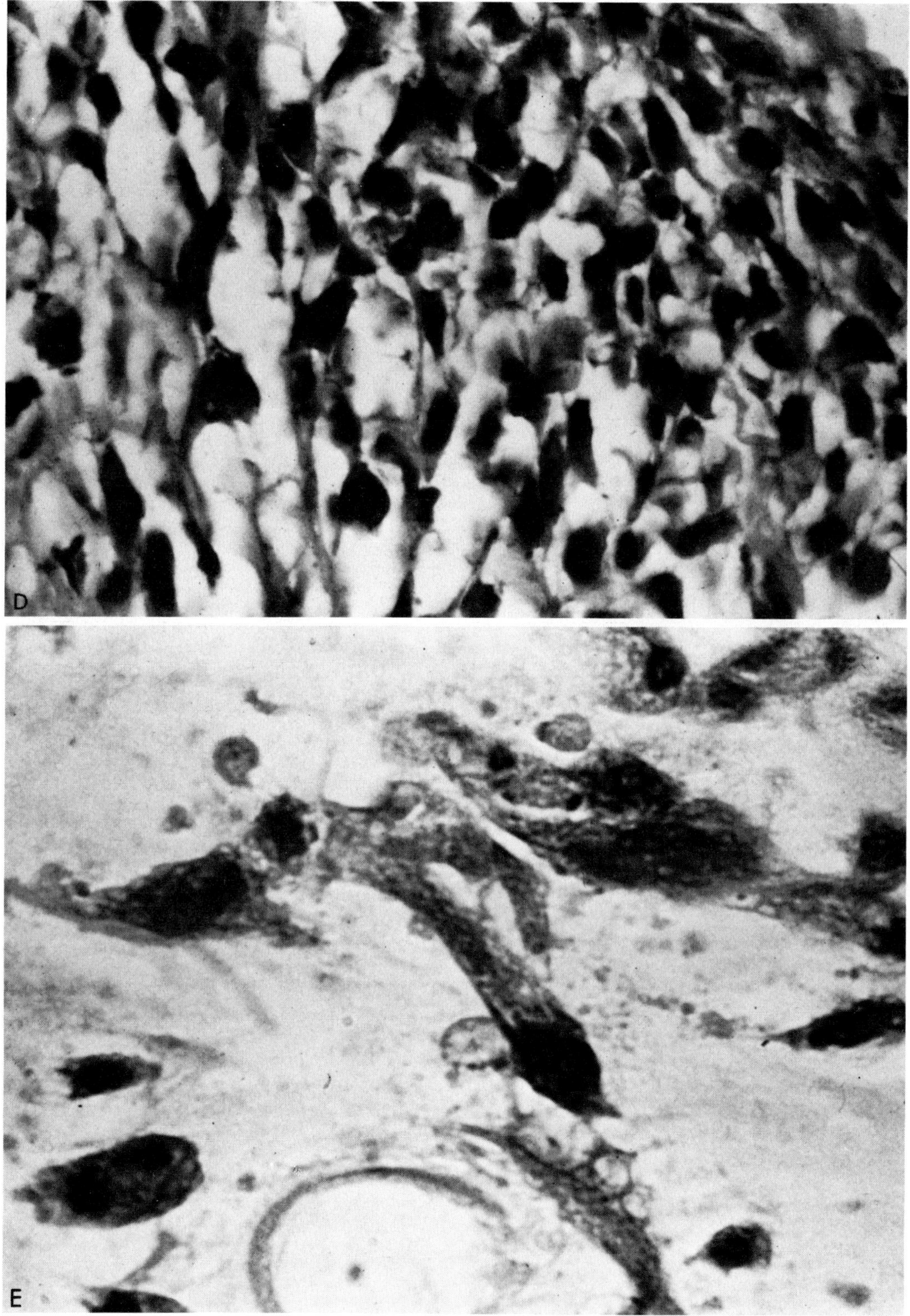

Figure 9–165 *Continued*

Illustration continued on opposite page

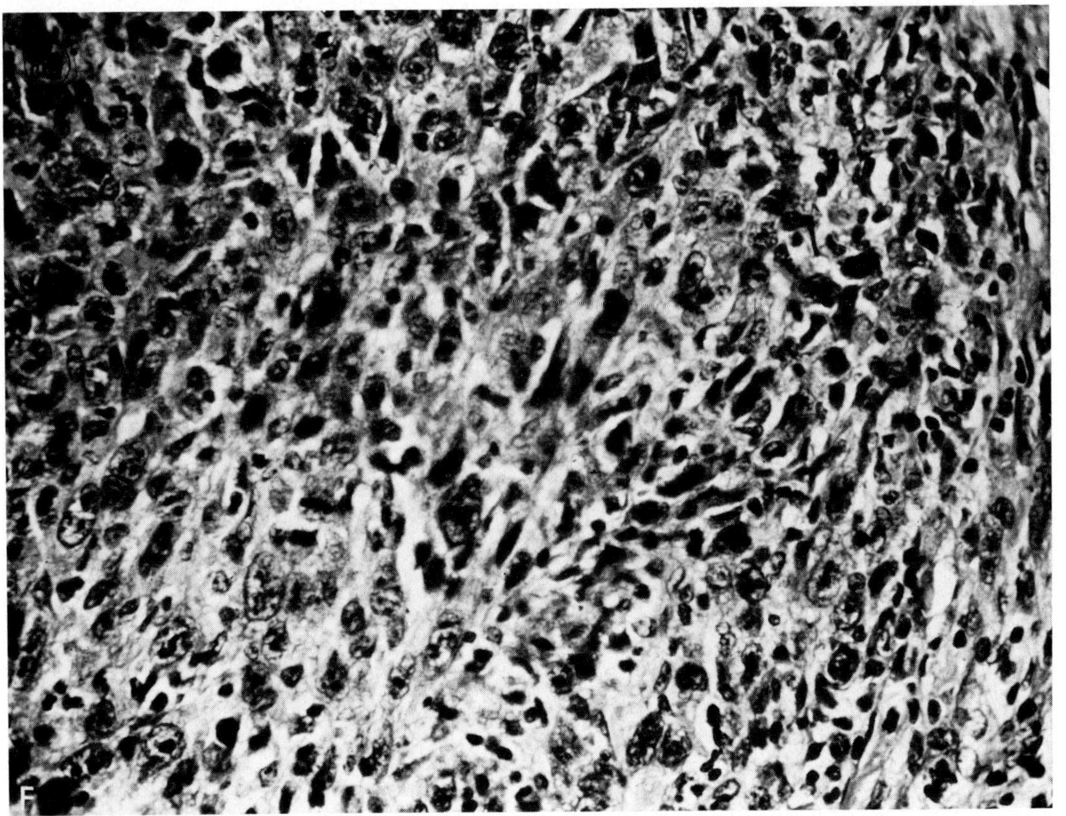

Figure 9–165 *Continued*

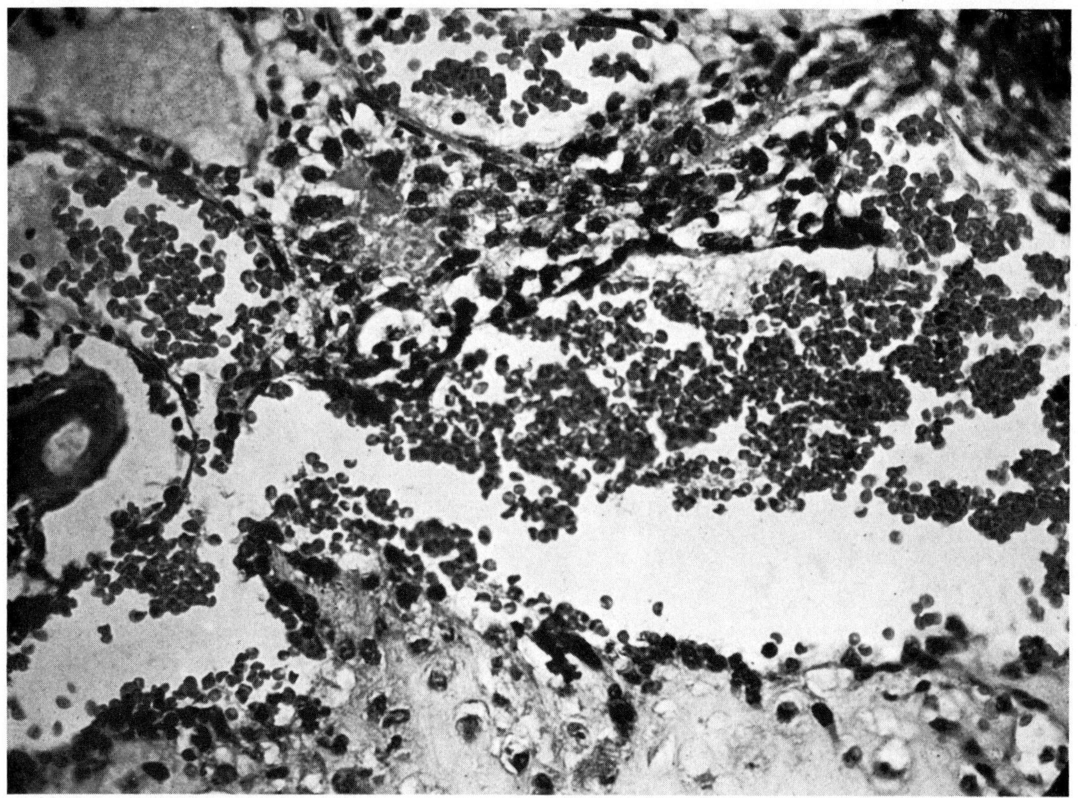

Figure 9–166. Chondrosarcoma. Focus of undifferentiated neoplastic cells in otherwise well-differentiated cartilage neoplasm. Foci of undifferentiated tumor must be sought in any cartilage lesion. Many cartilage lesions are large; the malignant focus may be quite small and easily missed unless the lesion is generously sampled and multiple sections made. The danger of missing a focus of this nature is potentiated by the use of the needle biopsy.

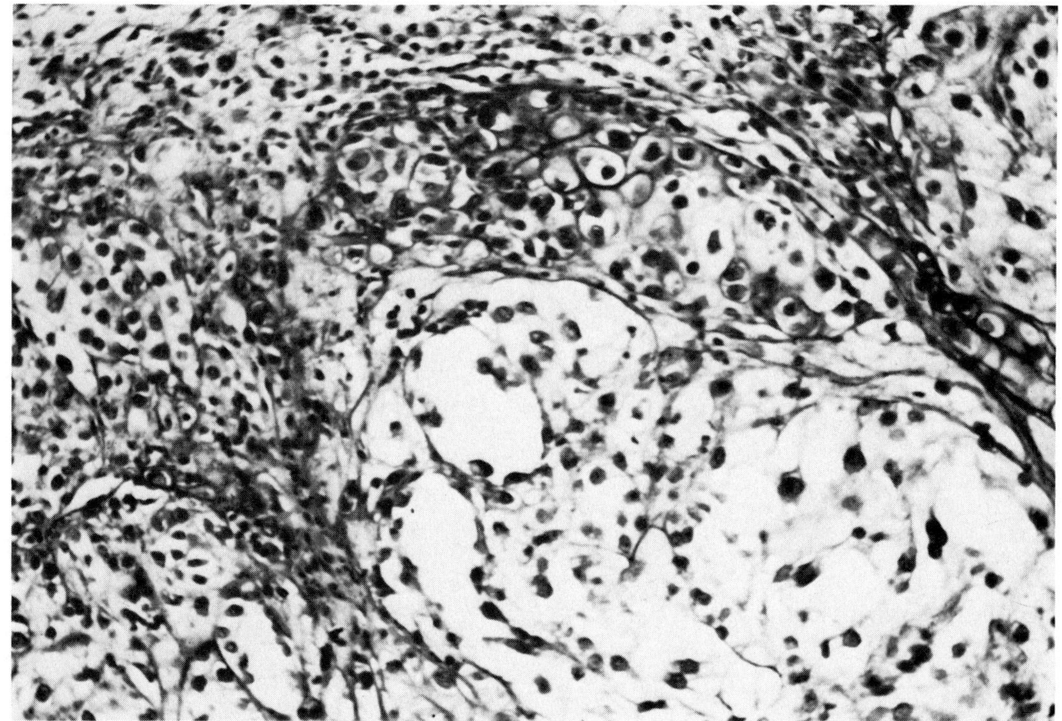

Figure 9–167. Chondrosarcoma. Myxoid matrix with cellular pleomorphism adjacent to other cell groups that are identifiable as cartilage. Such variability is common in chondrosarcoma.

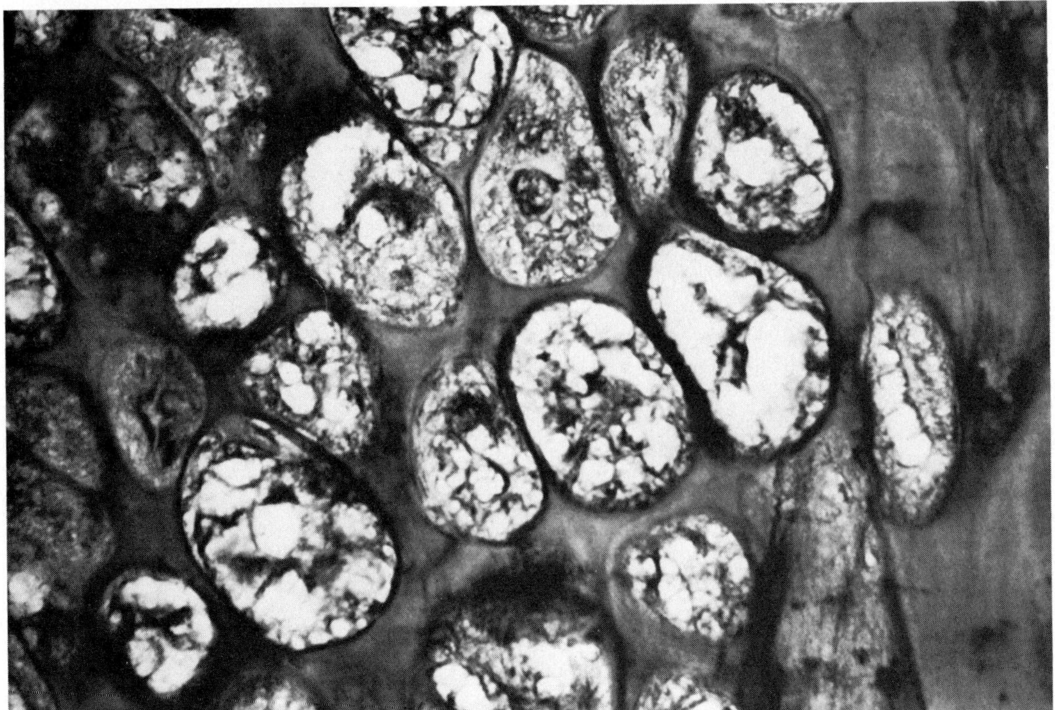

Figure 9–168. Chondrosarcoma. Large lacunar spaces, irregular pleomorphic chondrocytes. Cartilage cells are undergoing maturation process with hypertrophy, cell death, and matrix calcification. They are replaced by bone just as in the normal process of endochondral ossification, but their appearance is irregular because the neoplasm is disordered and the developmental process stops at any stage.

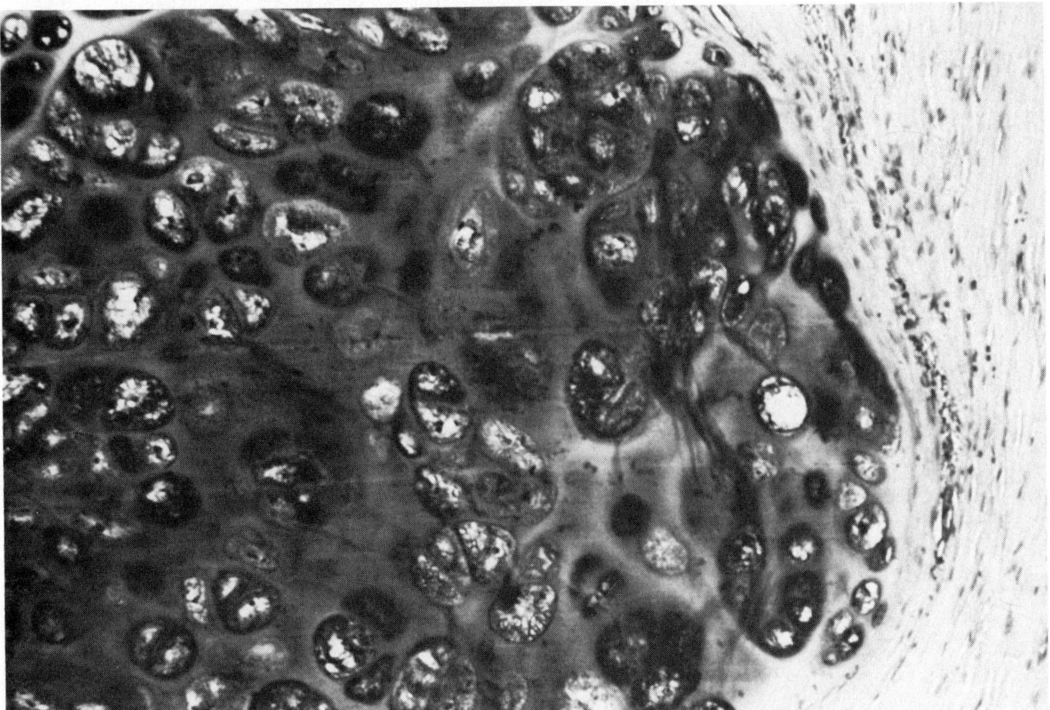

Figure 9–169. Chondrosarcoma. Hypercellular, moderately pleomorphic tumor arising from an osteochondroma. The junction with the surrounding tissue produces a pseudocapsule that strips readily from the lesion but that may contain tumor cells left behind as a focus for recurrent growth. The pseudocapsule must be removed to prevent recurrence.

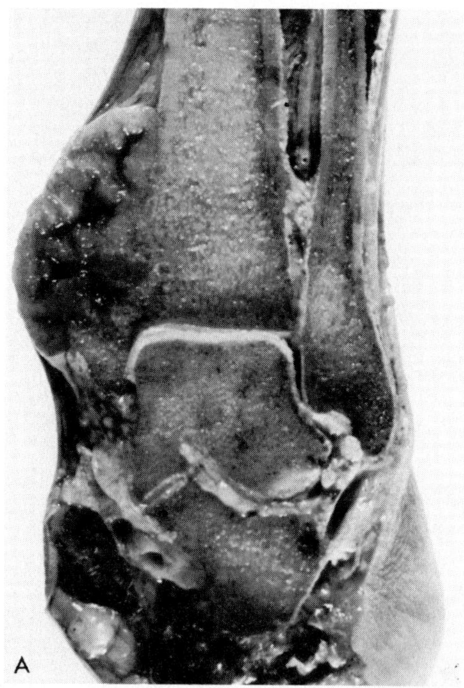

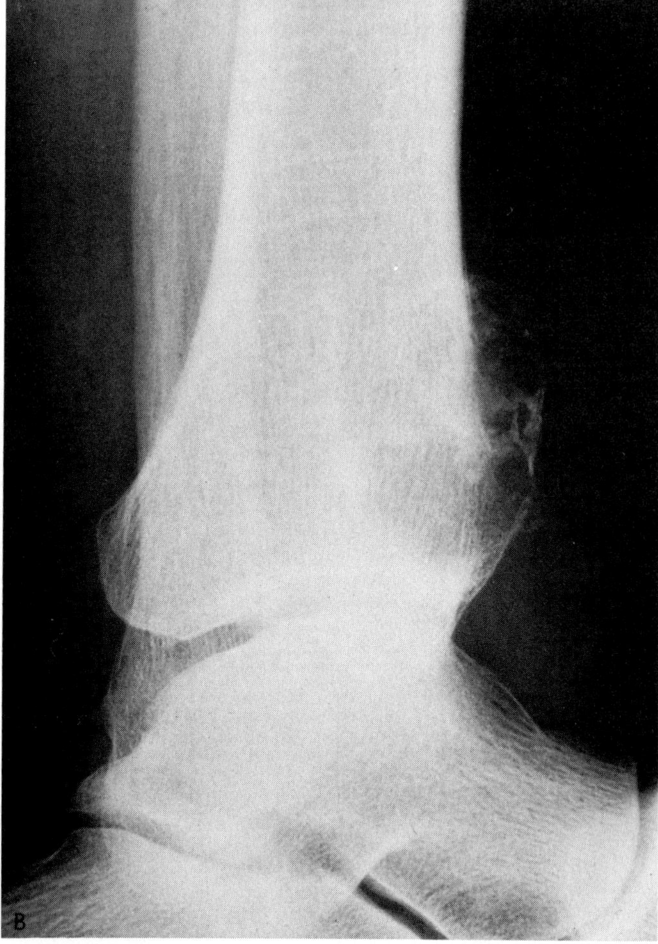

Figure 9–170. Gross appearance *(A)* and radiograph *(B)* of sharply defined expansile lesion in lower tibia in elderly male. The lesion had been locally excised but recurred within a year. Tumor is present within the medullary cavity of the tibia but also expands into the adjacent soft tissue. Cartilage tumors of the long bones above the ankle and wrist have a more ominous potential than lesions of the hands and feet.

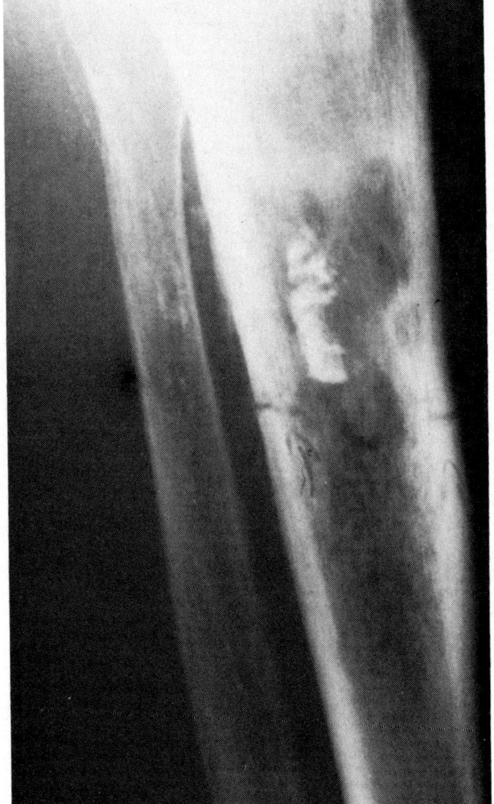

Figure 9–171. Chondrosarcoma. Radiograph of poorly circumscribed lytic defect in upper tibia with pathologic fracture. Calcification is present within the medullary cavity, indicating a previous enchondroma.

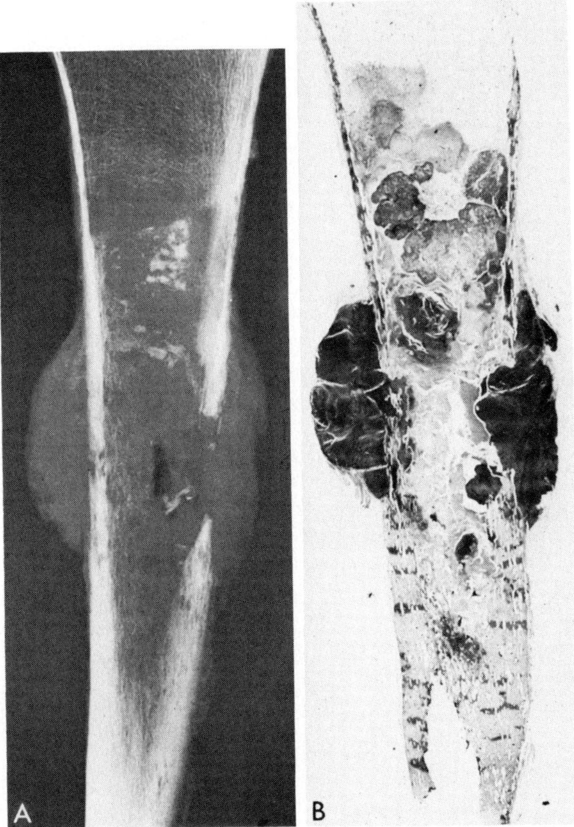

Figure 9–172. Chondrosarcoma. Specimen radiograph *(A)* and macrospecimen *(B)* of lesion illustrated in Figure 9–171 indicating focus of benign cartilage with extensive calcification, adjacent to undifferentiated tumor breaking out of the bone.

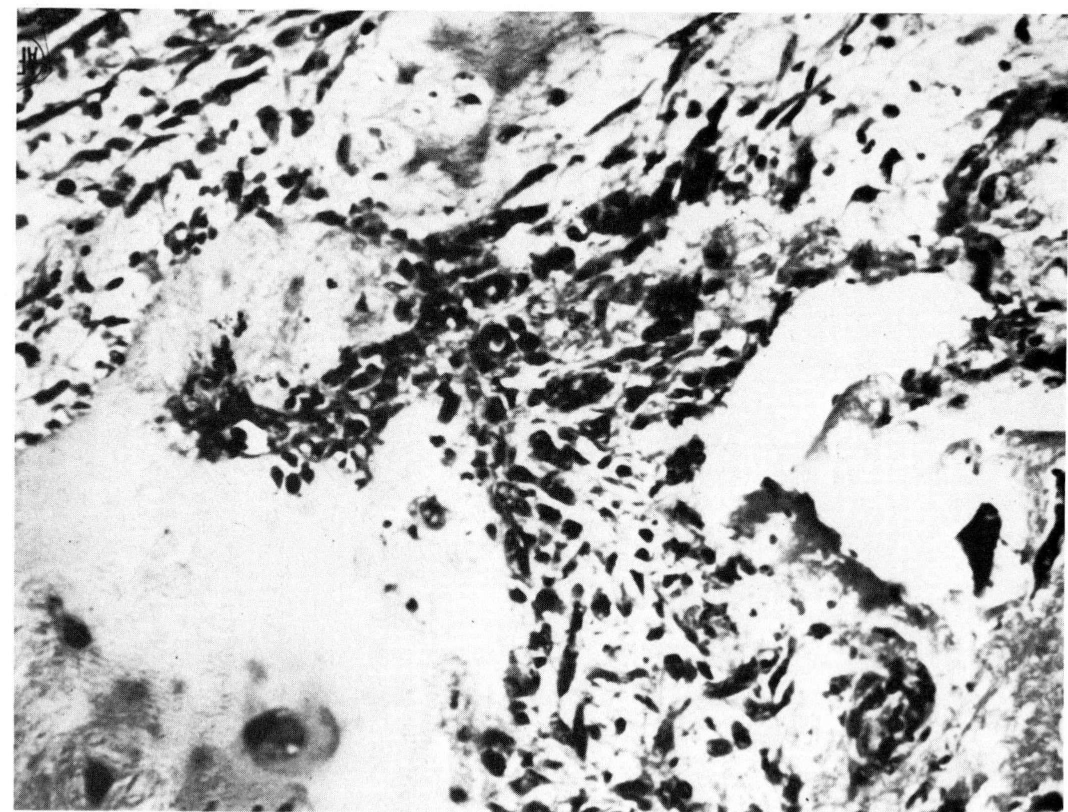

Figure 9–173. Chondrosarcoma. Histologic section of malignant tumor arising from pre-existing benign enchondroma. Foci of benign cartilage are present on the left of the photograph, and the undifferentiated tumor is evident on the superior surface and on the right.

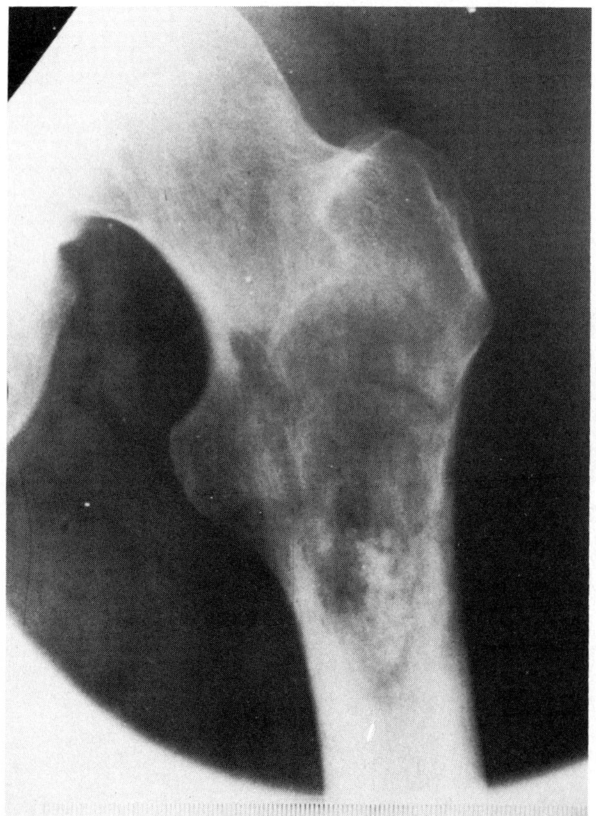

Figure 9–174. Chondrosarcoma. Radiograph of poorly circumscribed lesion in the neck of the femur, with focus of calcification in the inferior portion of the defect. Note the moth-eaten destruction, pathologic fracture, and flocculent calcification of pre-existing cartilage lesion.

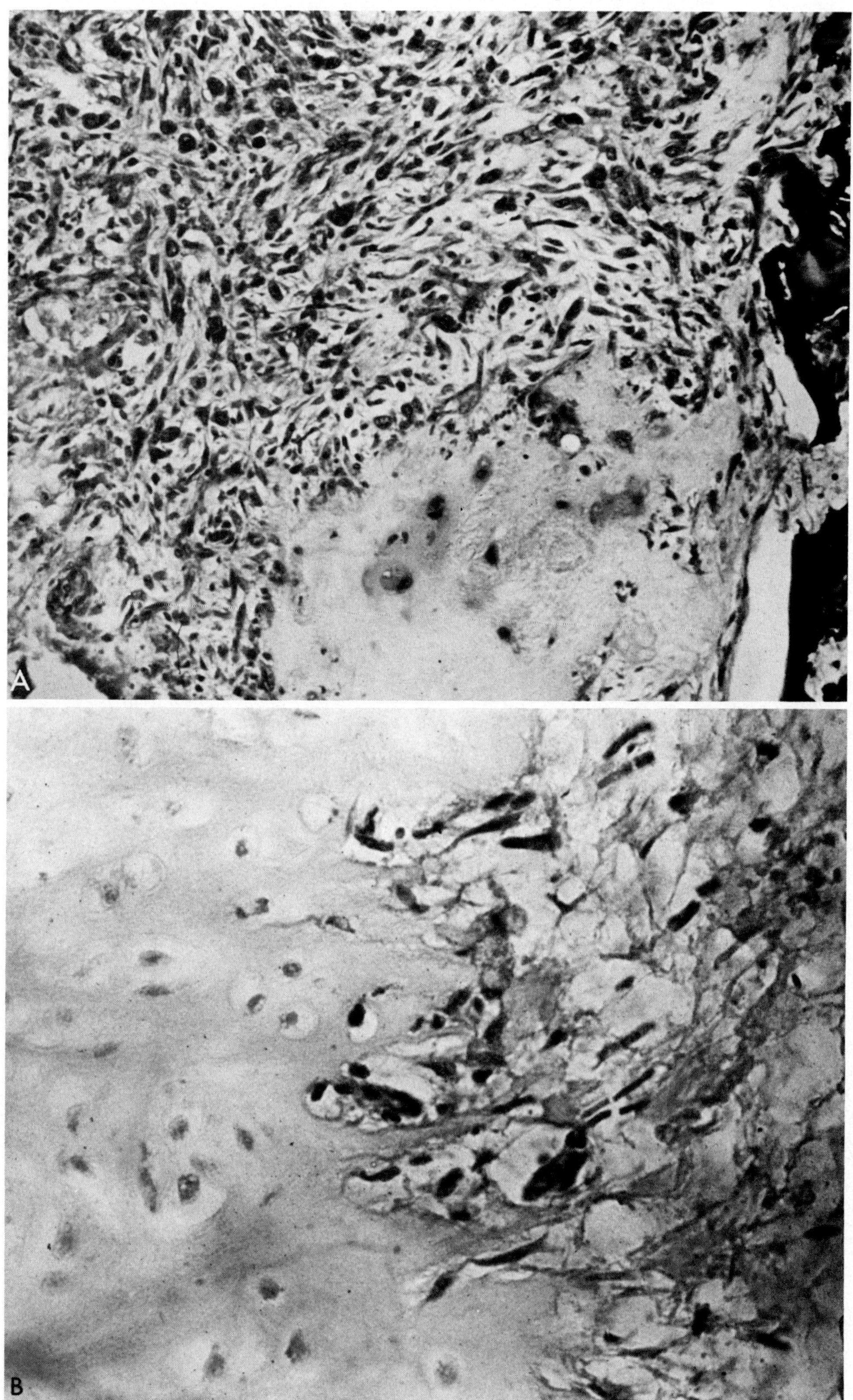

Figure 9–175. Chondrosarcoma. Histologic sections from lesion illustrated in Figure 9–174 exhibiting benign cartilage and direct transformation to markedly pleomorphic neoplasm.

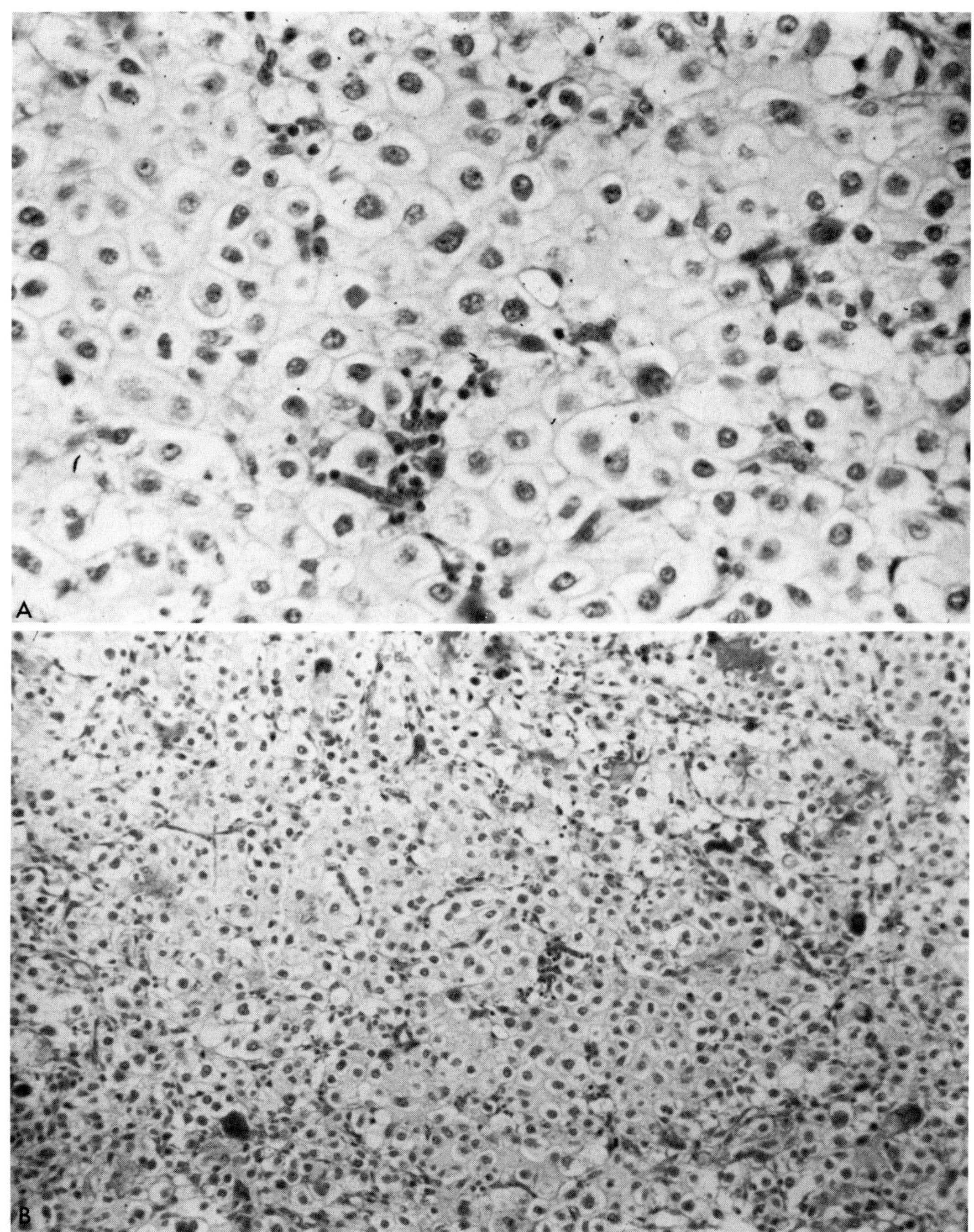

Figure 9–176. Chondrosarcoma. Histologic appearance of clear-cell chondrosarcoma. Polyhedral cells, distinct cell margins, a water-clear cytoplasm, and occasional giant cells are characteristic of this tumor.

Illustration continued on opposite page

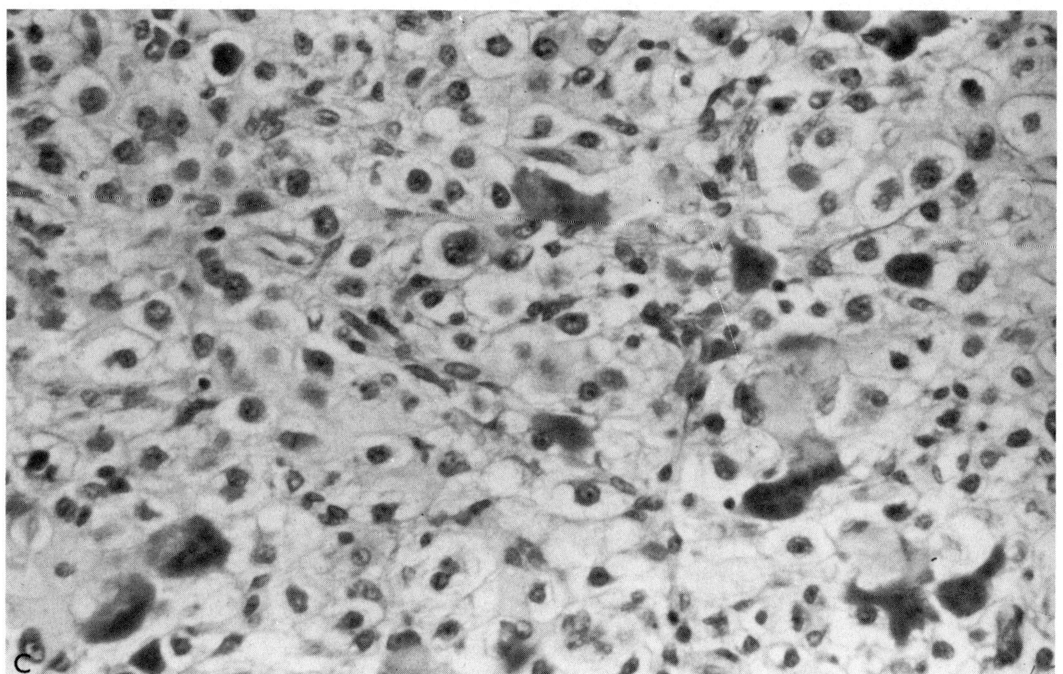

Figure 9–176 *Continued*

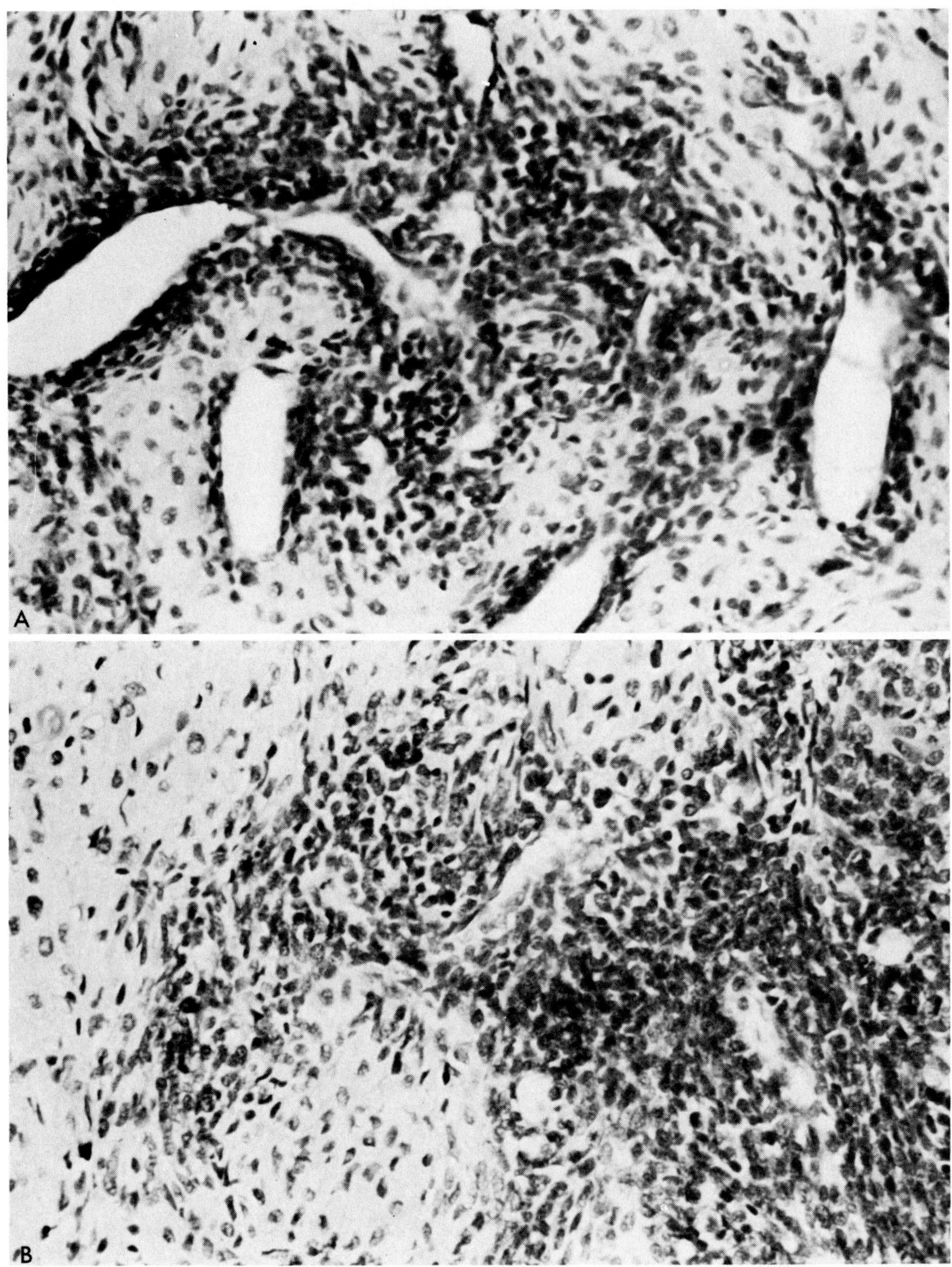

Figure 9–177. Chondrosarcoma. Histologic appearance of mesenchymal chondrosarcoma. The lesion consists of extremely cellular clusters mixed with chondroid matrix.

Illustration continued on opposite page

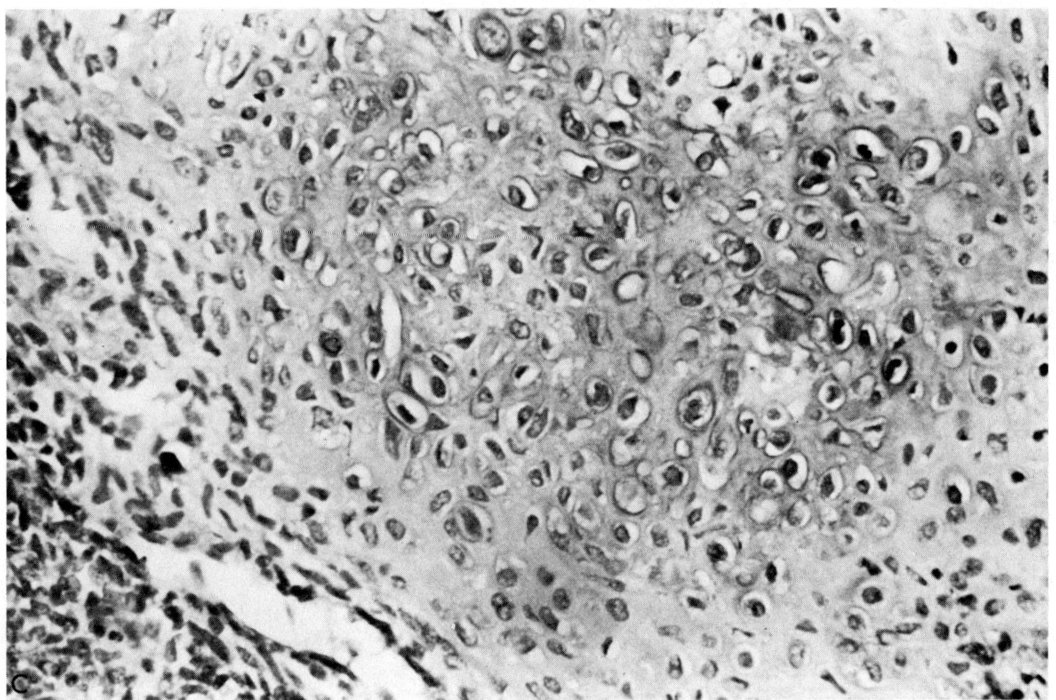

Figure 9–177 *Continued*

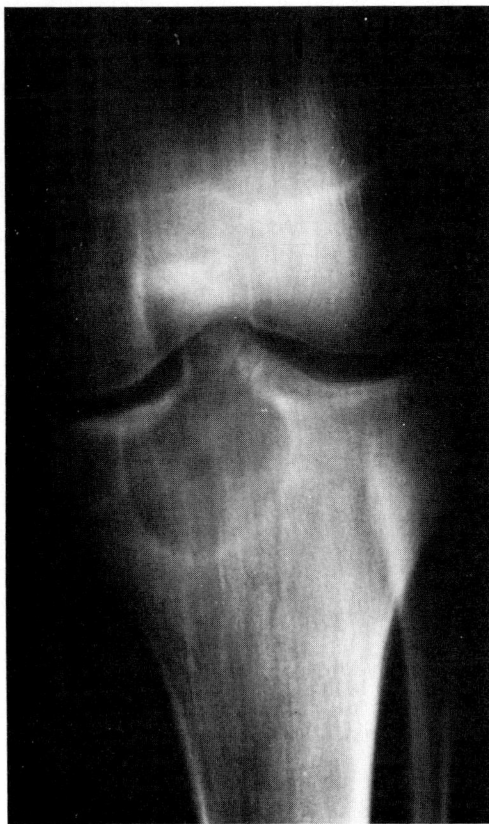

Figure 9–178. Chondroblastoma. Sharply circumscribed lytic defect located in the epiphysis of the upper tibia. The center of the lesion is located above the epiphyseal growth plate. After fusion of the growth plate, the lesion extends into the superficial metaphysis. Radiographically visible calcification is usually not present.

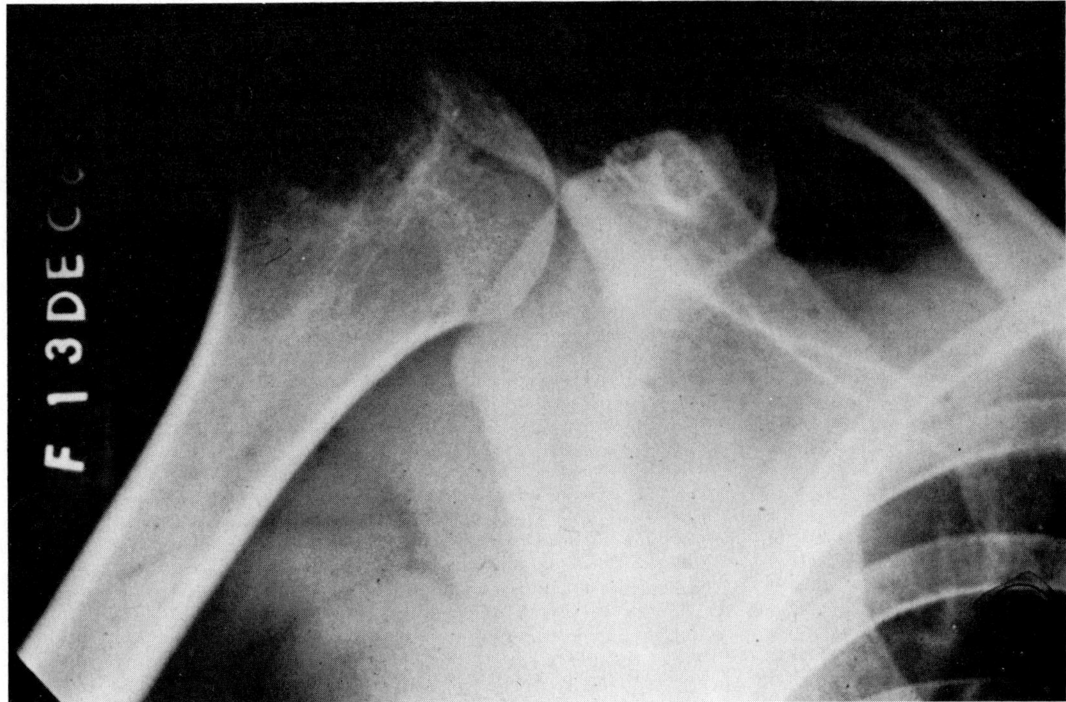

Figure 9–179. Chondroblastoma. Sharply circumscribed lytic defect located in the epiphyseal portion of the humerus, a classic location.

CHONDROBLASTOMA

The chondroblastoma (Codman's tumor, epiphyseal giant cell tumor) is an uncommon neoplasm. The typical lesion arises in the epiphysis; the radiographic appearance is one of a sharply circumscribed lytic lesion with a sclerotic rim and occasional punctate calcification.

The lesion consists of uniform small polyhedral cells with sharp cytoplasmic margins: It has been described as a "bird's-eye view of a cobblestone street." The lesion also includes giant cells, small amounts of chondroid material, and so-called "chicken-wire" calcification (Mirra, 1980). This "chicken-wire" calcification is associated with matrix secretion that stains positively with alcian blue, helping to differentiate it from the typical giant cell tumor of bone.

Chondroblastoma, as numerous other lesions, may alter its vascular bed and undergo transformation to an aneurysmal bone cyst. Occasional transformation into a malignant lesion has been described in the literature; all lesions of bone, be they benign neoplasms, anomalies, or inflammatory lesions, are capable of transformation into malignant neoplasms (Unni and Dahlin, 1979; Wirman et al., 1979).

The differential diagnosis of a sharply circumscribed solitary epiphyseal lesion must include the occasional enchondroma, chondrosarcoma, osteomyelitis, and bone cyst.

Text continued on page 447

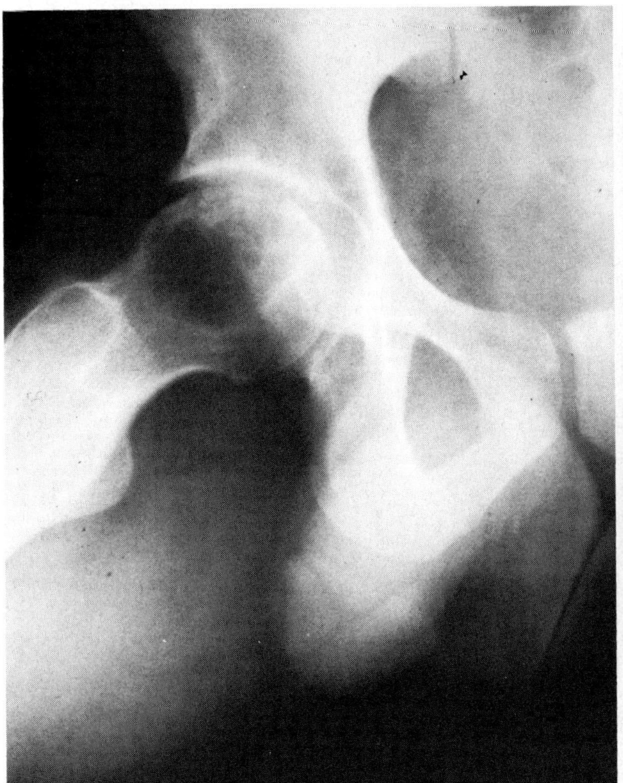

Figure 9–180

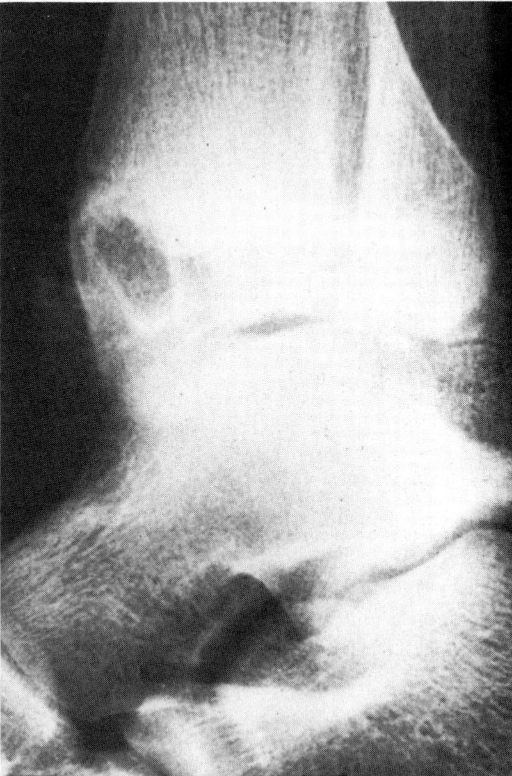

Figure 9–181

Figure 9–180. Chondroblastoma. Sharply circumscribed lytic defect located in the epiphyseal portion of the upper femur. Notice the uniform lytic appearance, with sclerotic rim and absence of extension into soft tissue.

Figure 9–181. Chondroblastoma. Lesion located in the distal portion of the tibia, extending beyond the fused growth plate and into the metaphyseal portion. There is a sharply circumscribed margin, with no evidence of calcification in the matrix.

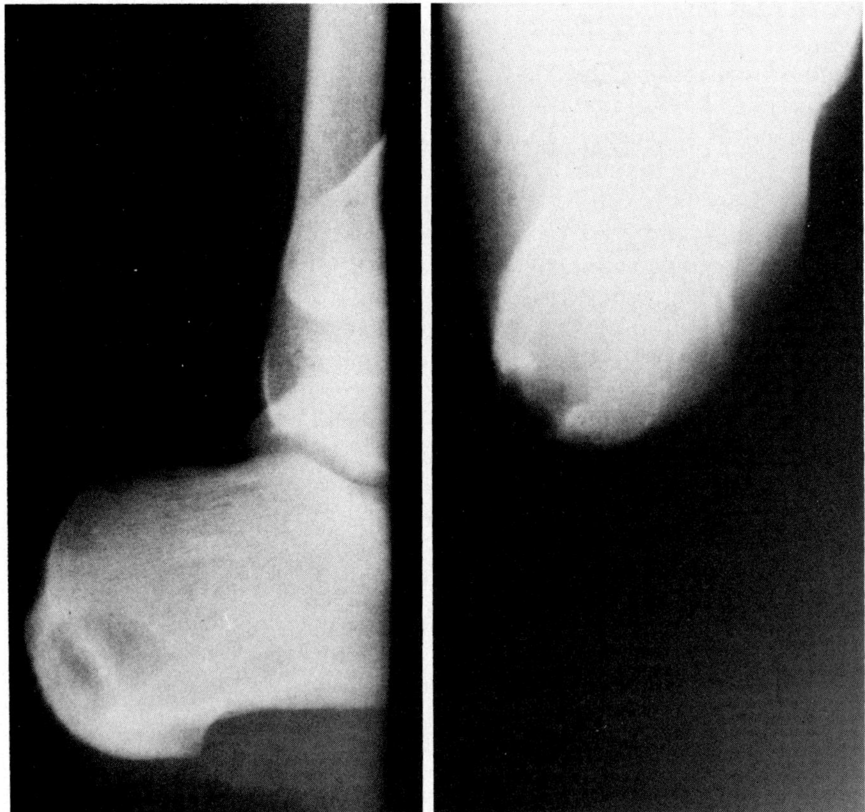

Figure 9–182. Chondroblastoma. Lesion located in the apophysis of the calcaneus. Lytic defect, sharply circumscribed. There is a narrow rim of bone outlining the lesion.

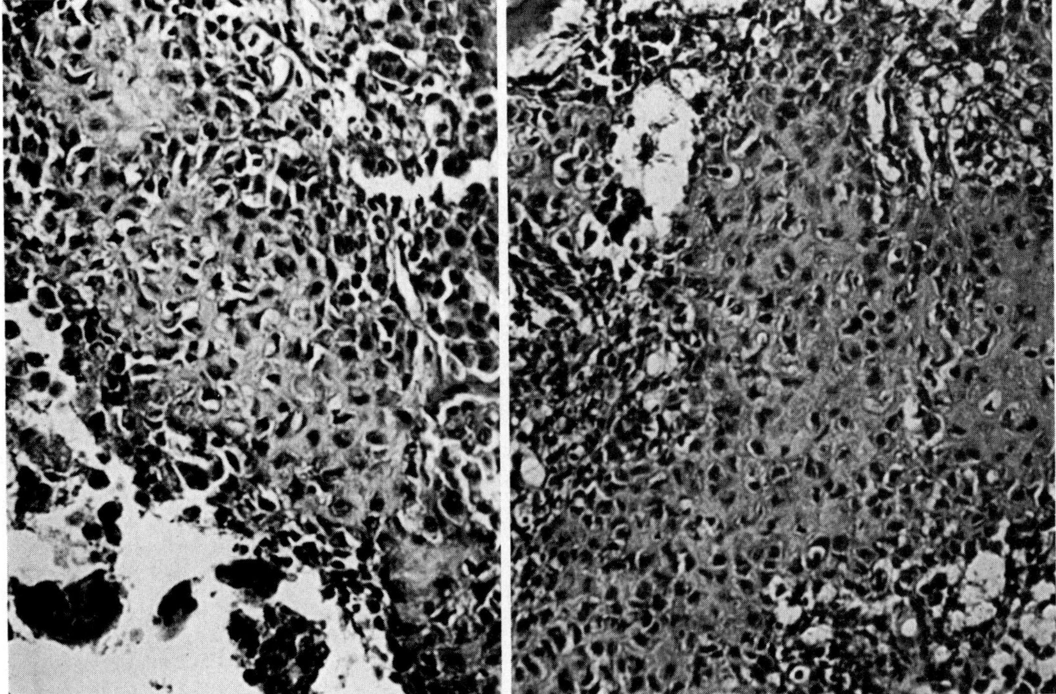

Figure 9–183. Histologic picture of chondroblastoma exhibiting the chondroid matrix formed by the tumor cells. The lesions are usually quite cellular but lack any significant pleomorphism.

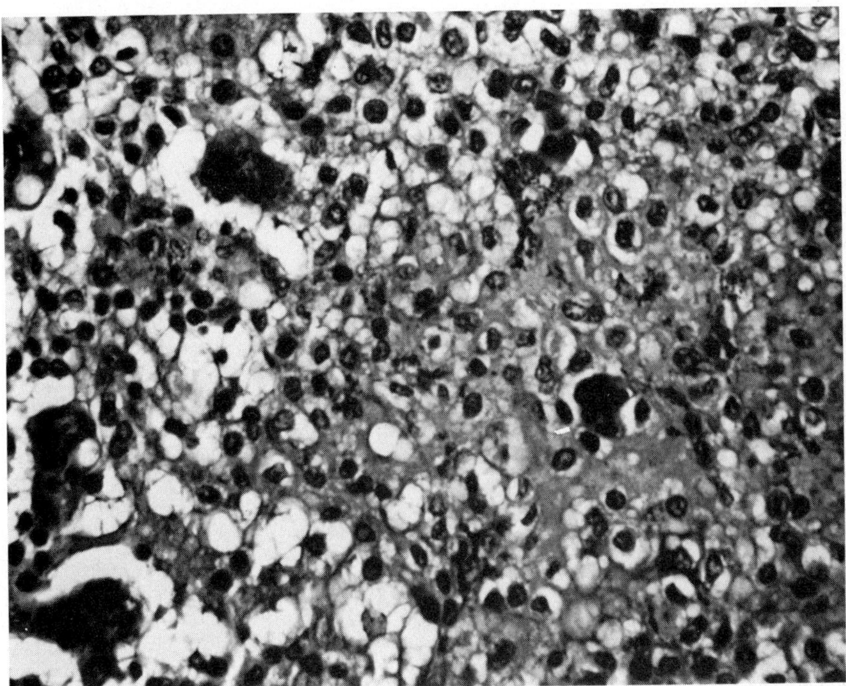

Figure 9–184. Chondroblastoma. Higher magnification of chondroid matrix production with occasional giant cells. Because of the uniformity of the small polyhedral cells, the histologic picture of chondroblastoma has been described as a "bird's-eye view of a cobblestone street."

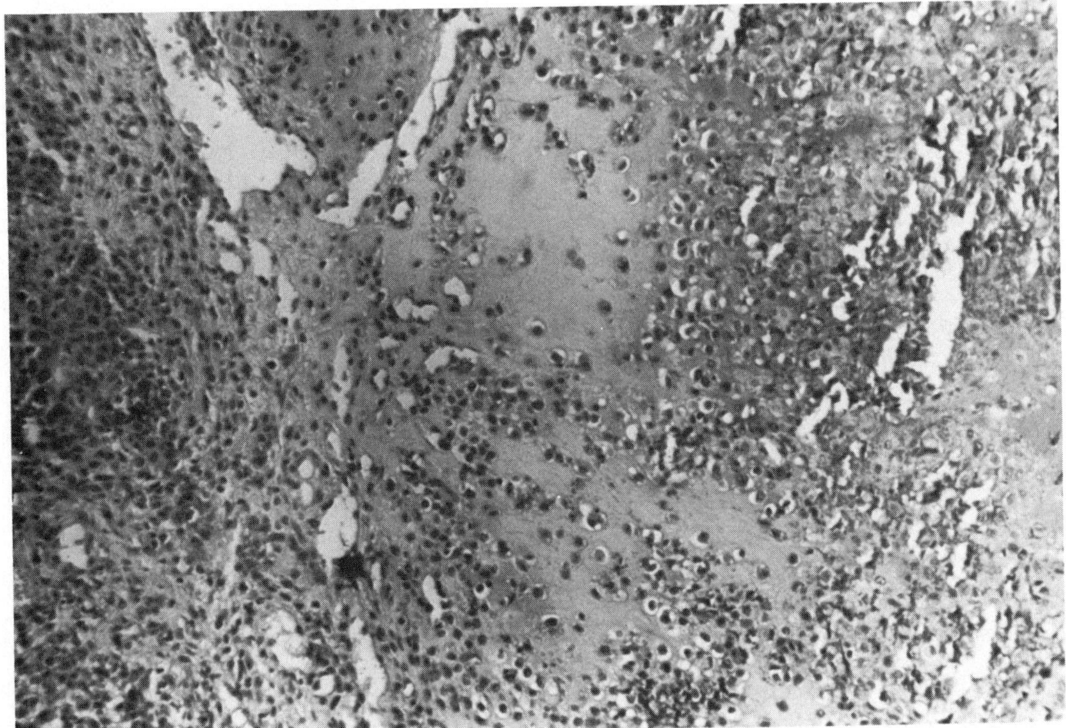

Figure 9–185. Chondroblastoma. Chondroid matrix production by tumor, with numerous chondroblasts in the midst of the matrix.

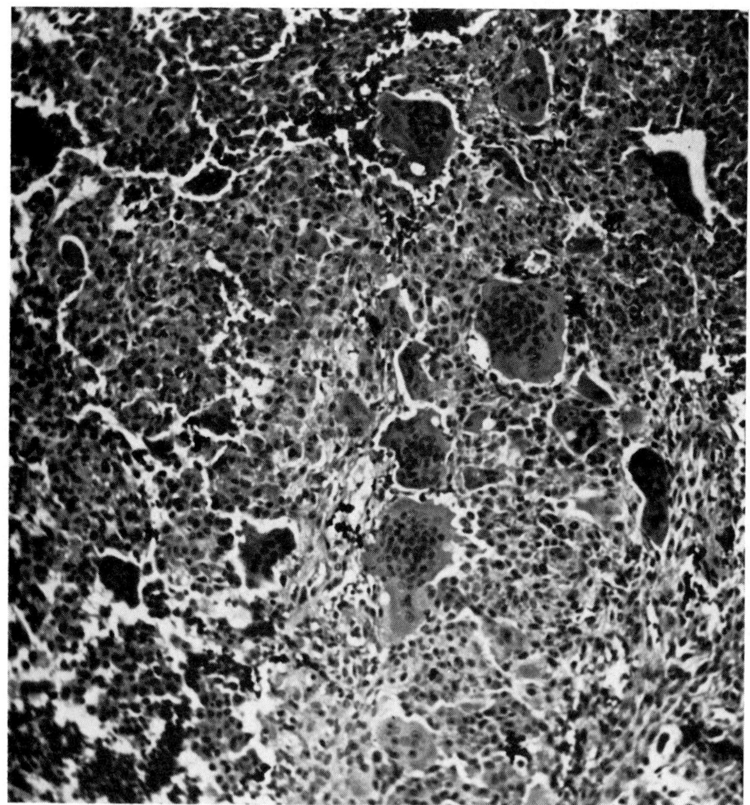

Figure 9–186. Chondroblastoma. A large number of giant cells may predominate in a chondroblastoma. Because of the presence of these giant cells, Codman named the lesion an "epiphyseal giant cell tumor." The predominance of these cells may often cause one to misdiagnose the lesion as a giant cell tumor of bone. The epiphyseal location without involvement of the metaphysis should suggest to the clinician that a chondroblastoma rather than giant cell tumor is present.

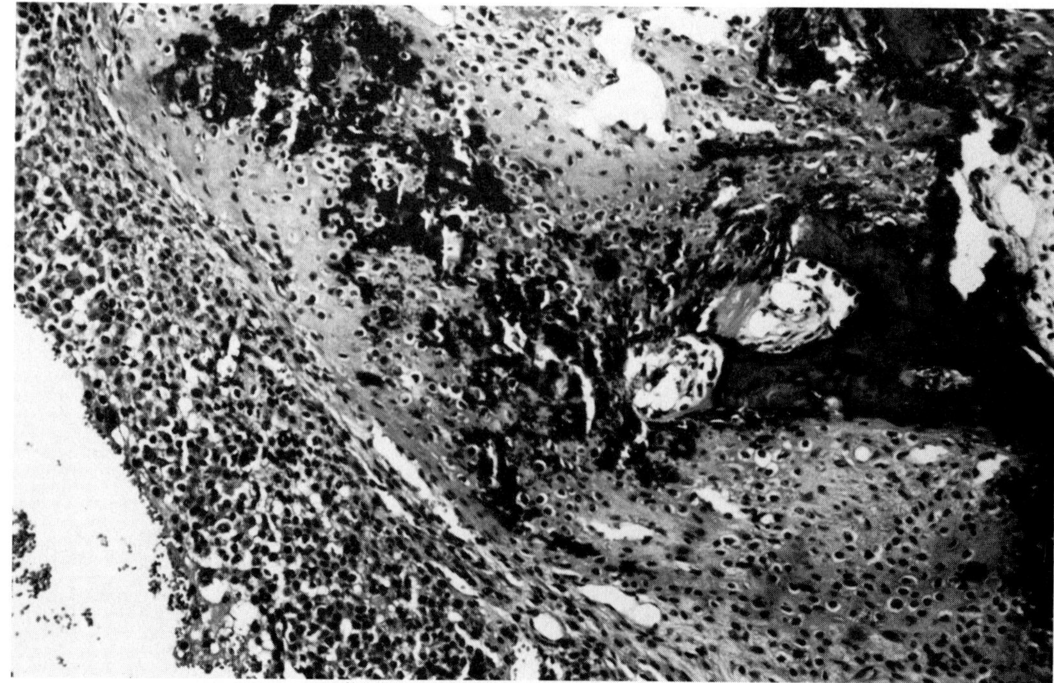

Figure 9–187. Chondroblastoma. Intense calcification within characteristic chondroblastoma.

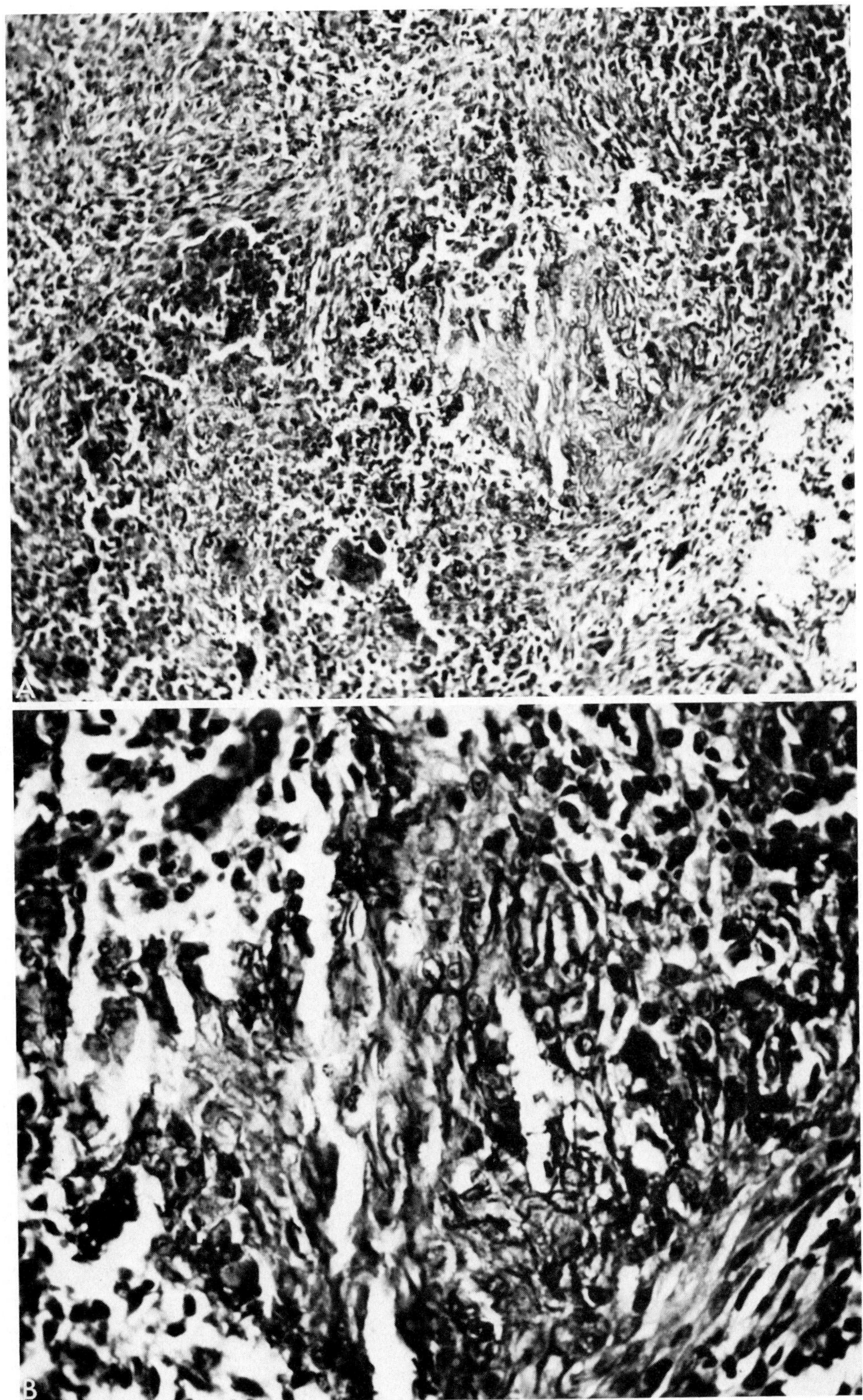

Figure 9–188. Chondroblastoma. Note the focus of minute calcification within the lesion. These small foci are always seen histologically, but only infrequently are they dense enough to become radiopaque.

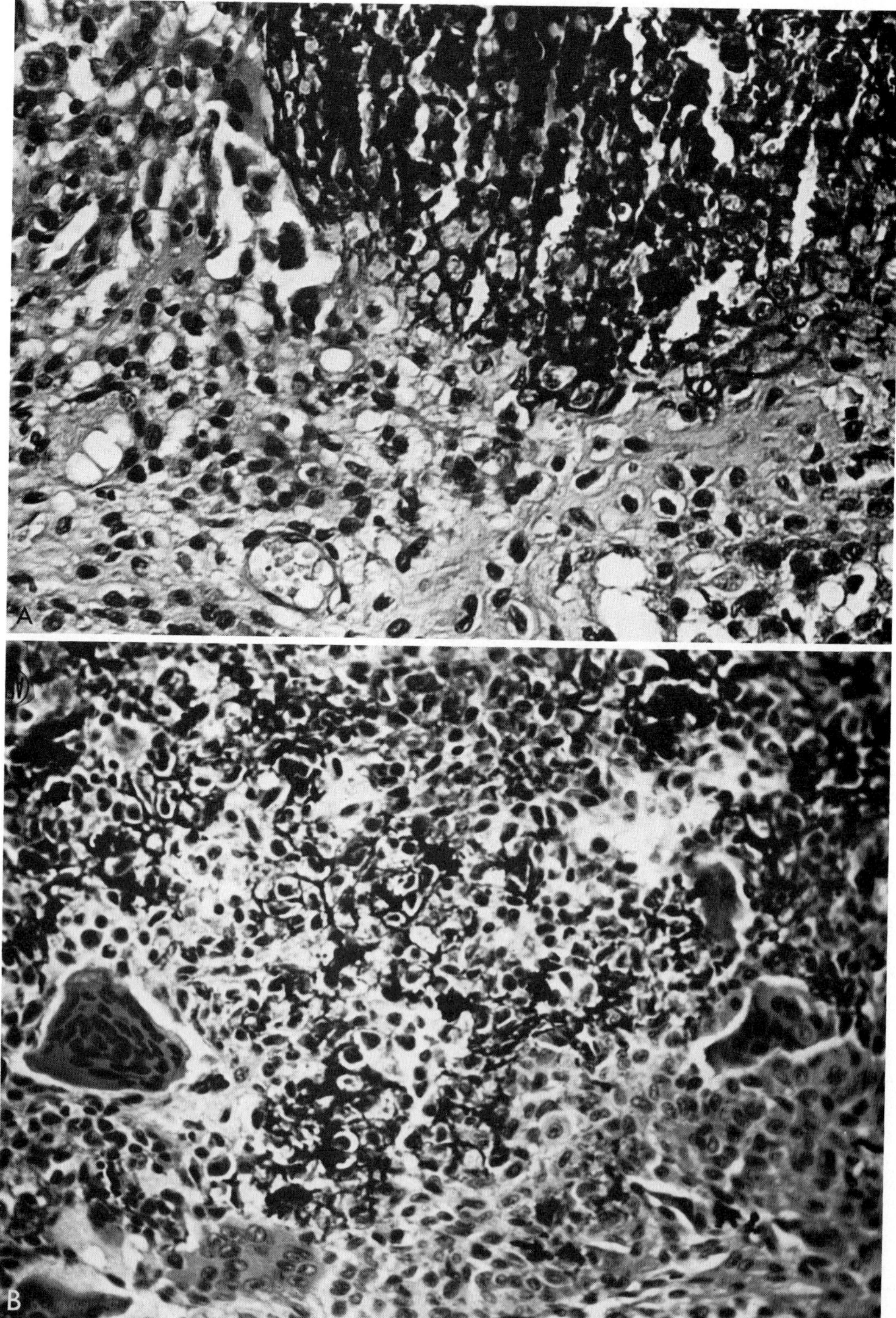

Figure 9–189. Chondroblastoma. Characteristic "chicken wire" calcification surrounding the individual cells.

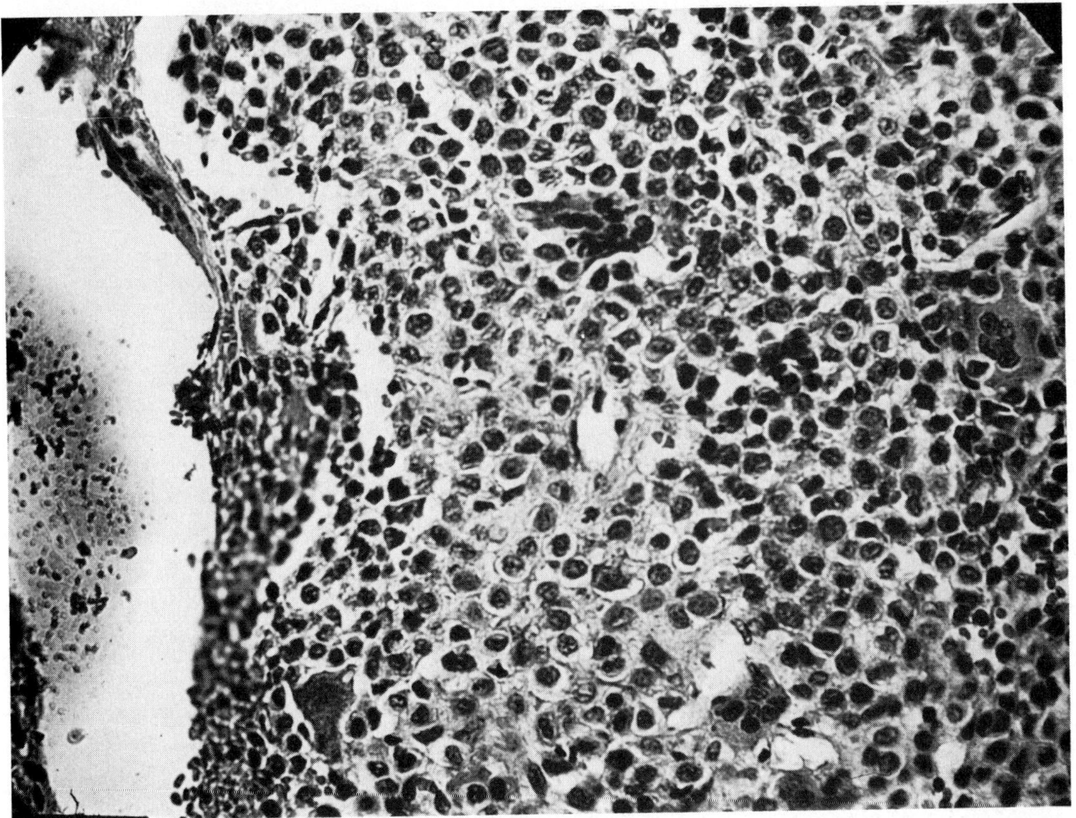

Figure 9-190. Chondroblastoma. Characteristic focus of the cellular matrix in chondroblastoma.

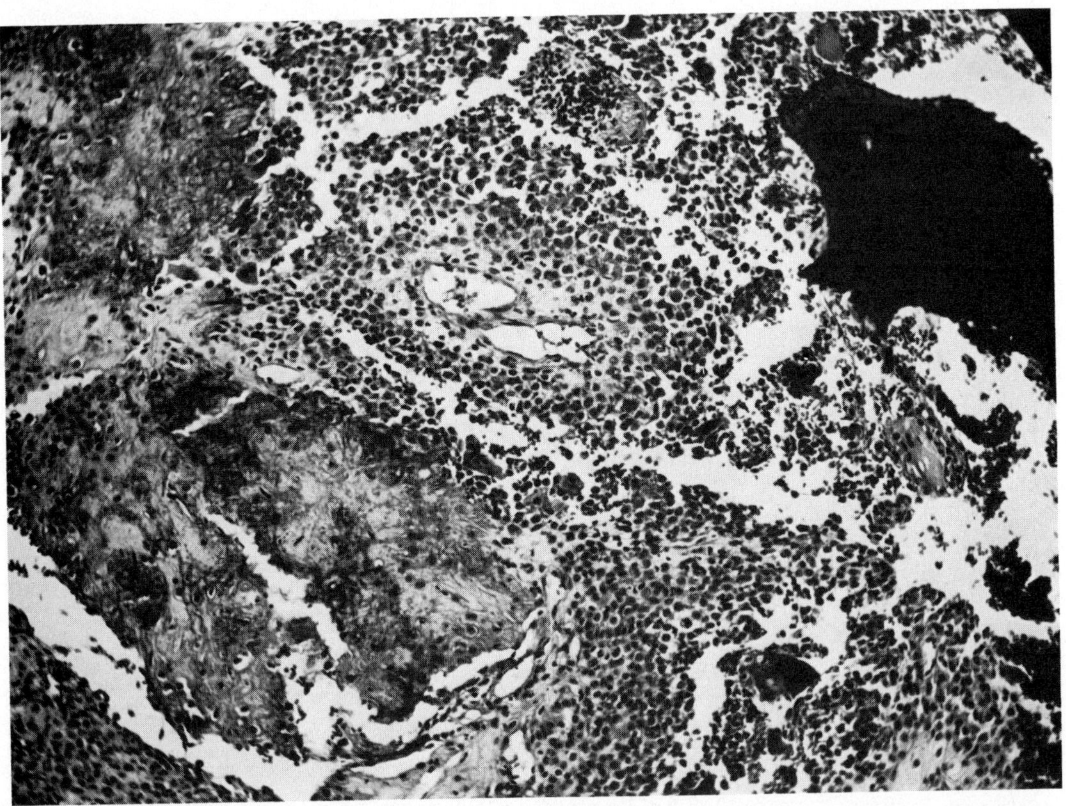

Figure 9-191. Chondroblastoma. Activation of the vascular network, especially after trauma, may cause a chondroblastoma to assume the clinical appearance of an aneurysmal bone cyst.

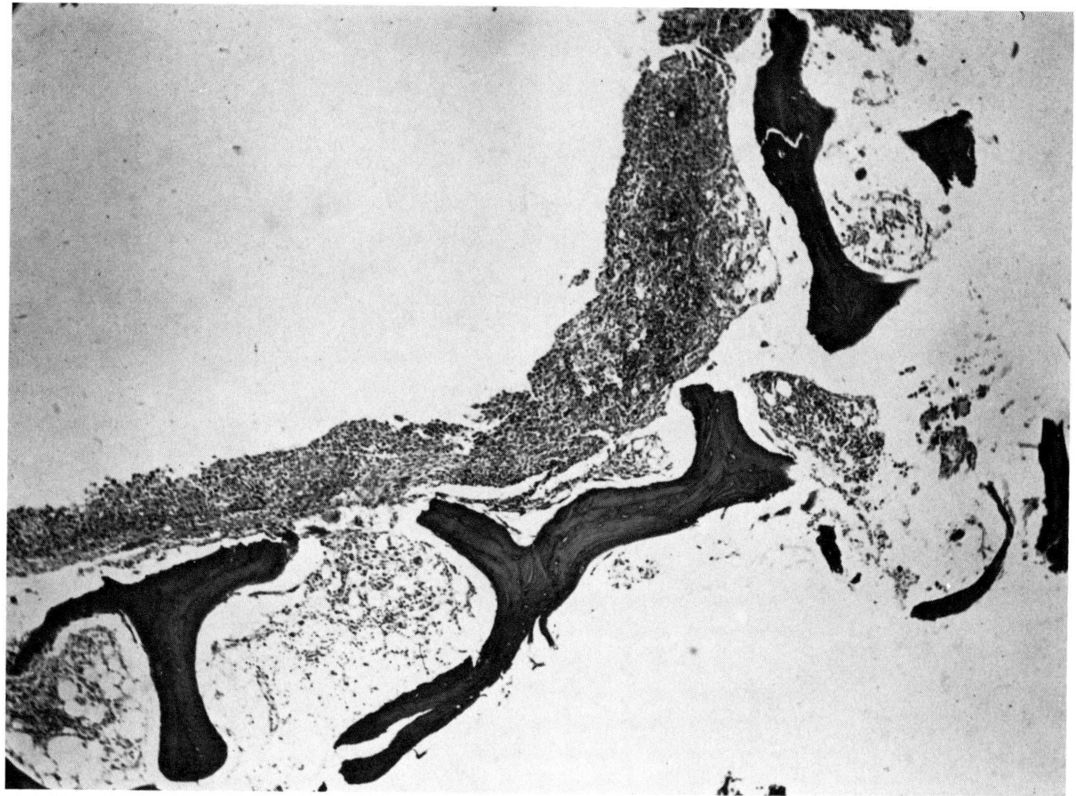

Figure 9–192. Chondroblastoma. Histologic view of the apophyseal chondroblastoma illustrated in Figure 9–182. Note cyst with lining surface composed of characteristic chondroblastic foci.

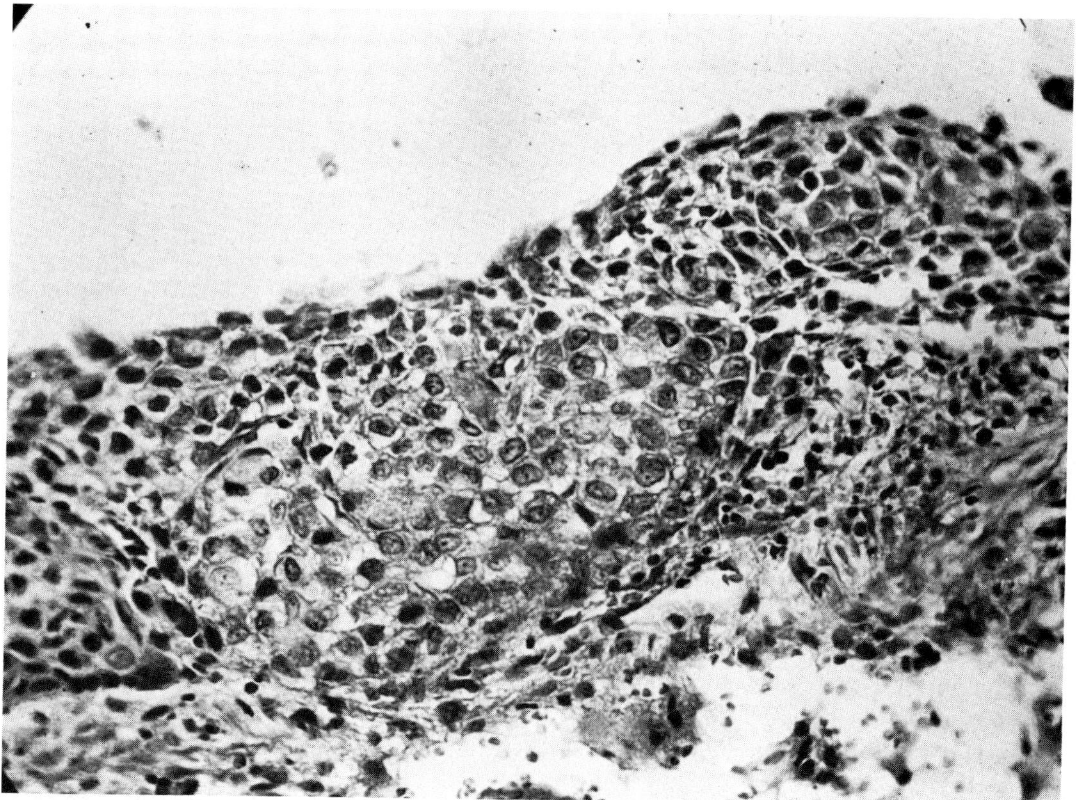

Figure 9–193. Chondroblastoma. Histologic view of the apophyseal chondroblastoma illustrated in Figures 9–182 and 9–192. Note the focus of characteristic chondroblastoma in the wall of the cyst.

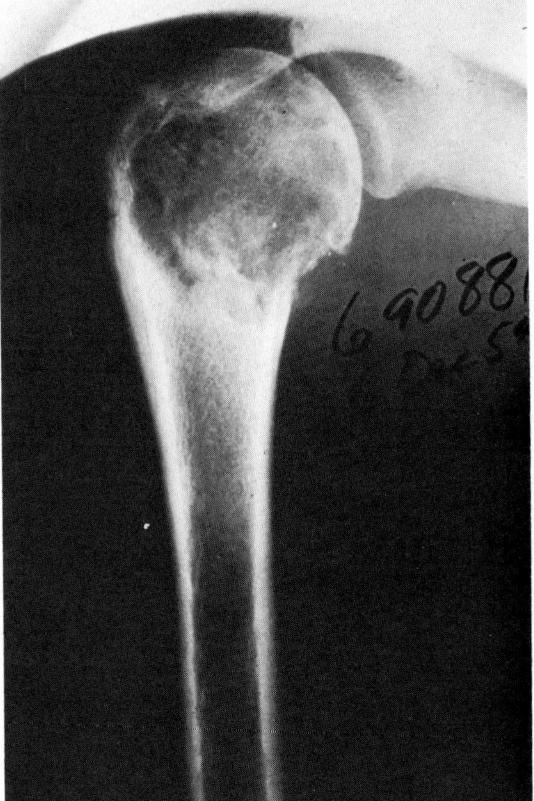

Figure 9–194. Chondroblastoma. Radiograph of a large lesion in the humeral head extending into the metaphysis. Note that even in this large lesion most of the tumor is epiphyseal, whereas in giant cell tumor of bone most of the lesion is metaphyseal. Pathologic fractures through such large tumors bring them to the clinician's attention.

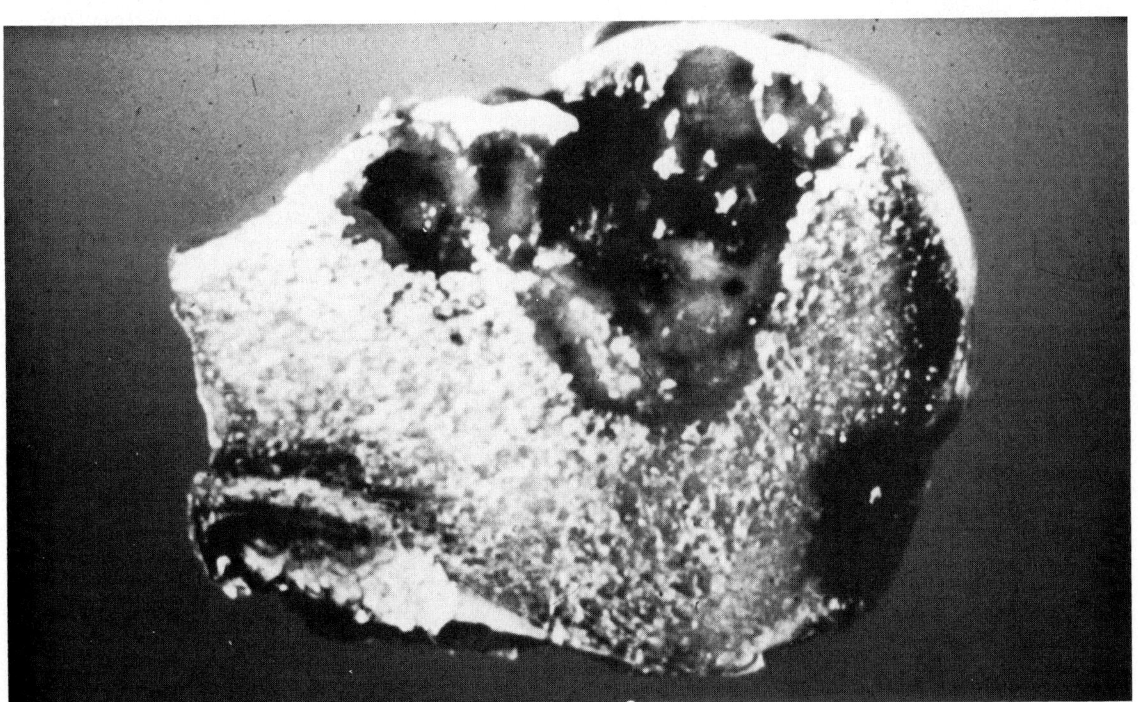

Figure 9–195. Chondroblastoma. Gross specimen of the humeral head with a blood-filled defect. The transformation to aneurysmal bone cyst is not uncommon in chondroblastoma.

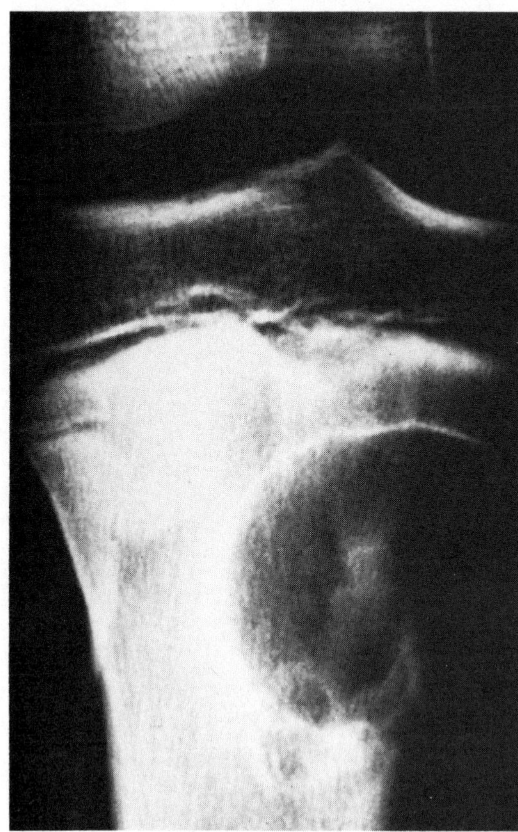

Figure 9–196. Chondromyxoid fibroma. The radiographic appearance of this lesion is similar to that of nonossifying fibroma. It is a sharply circumscribed metaphyseal defect, often with a sclerotic rim, and shows no evidence of calcification in the matrix. There is always a gap between the chondromyxoid fibroma and the epiphyseal growth plate.

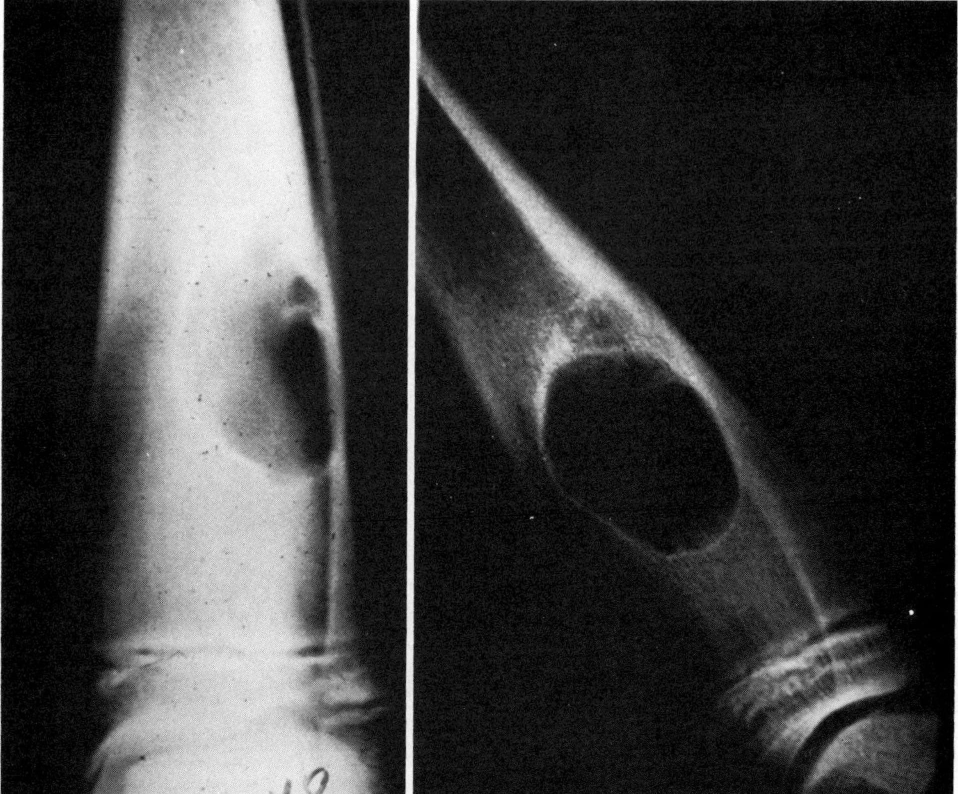

Figure 9–197. Chondromyxoid fibroma. Characteristic lytic metaphyseal eccentric defect at some distance from the epiphyseal growth plate.

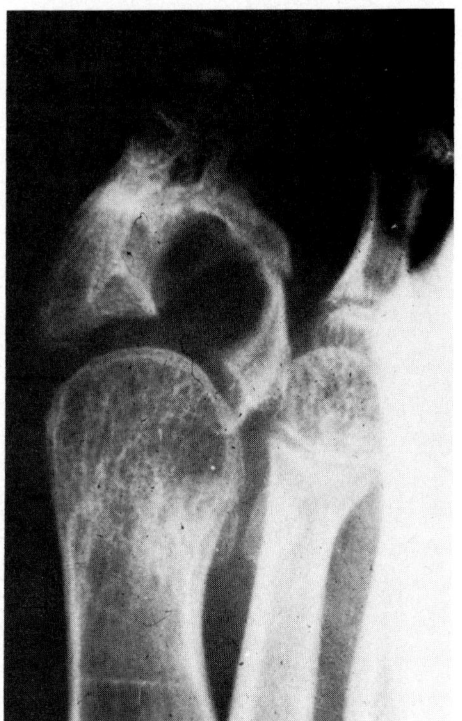

Figure 9–198. Chondromyxoid fibroma. This lesion has a tendency for localization in small bones of the hands and feet. A sharply circumscribed defect in the proximal phalanx of the great toe is shown here.

CHONDROMYXOID FIBROMA

The chondromyxoid fibroma is a metaphyseal lesion, typically located at some distance from the epiphyseal growth plate. It is a sharply circumscribed eccentric lesion with a sclerotic rim. The radiographic differential diagnosis includes the

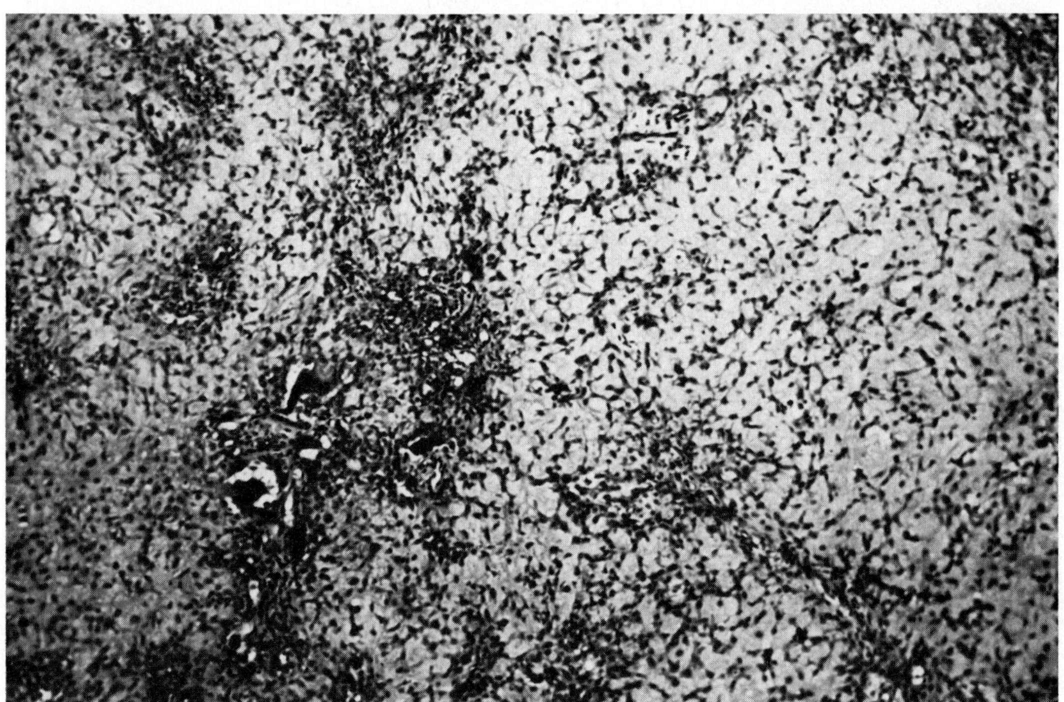

Figure 9–199. Chondromyxoid fibroma. Histologic appearance of characteristic chondromyxoid fibroma: spindled fibroblasts, occasional giant cells, and underlying chondroid matrix.

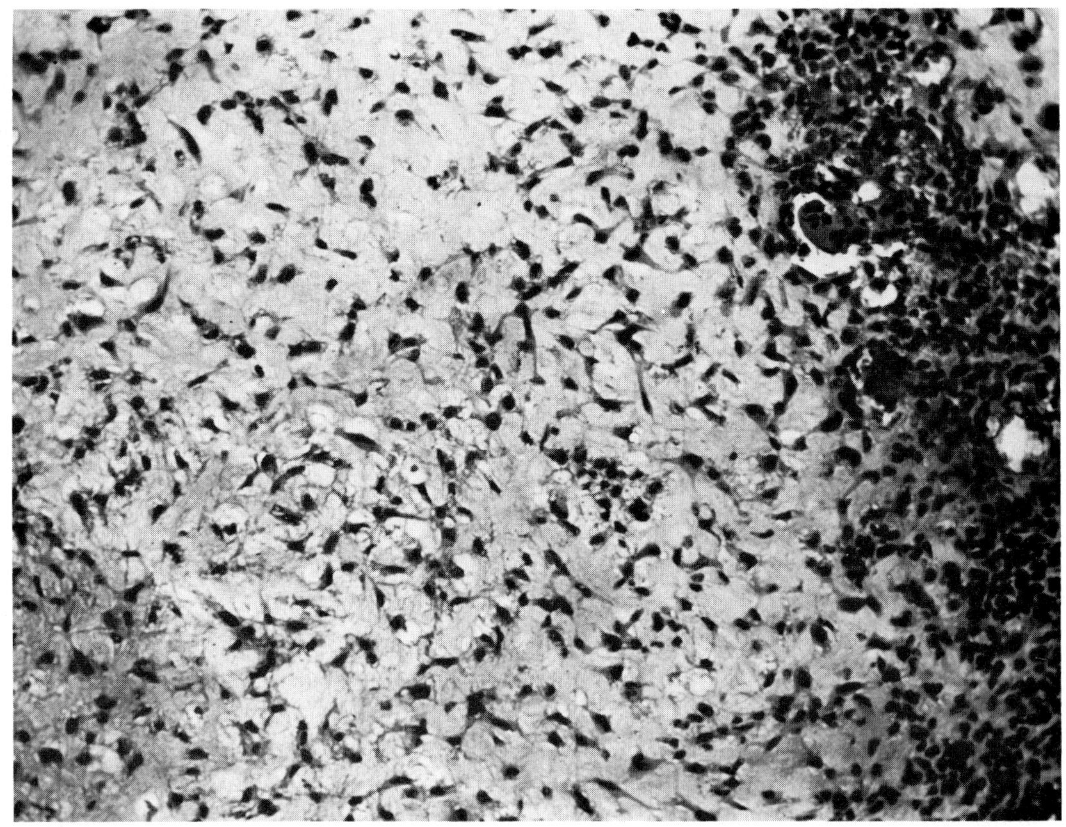

Figure 9–200. Chondromyxoid fibroma. Histologic picture of chondromyxoid fibroma showing spindled fibroblasts set in the chondroid stroma. Focal areas of increased cellularity are present, and giant cells may be identified.

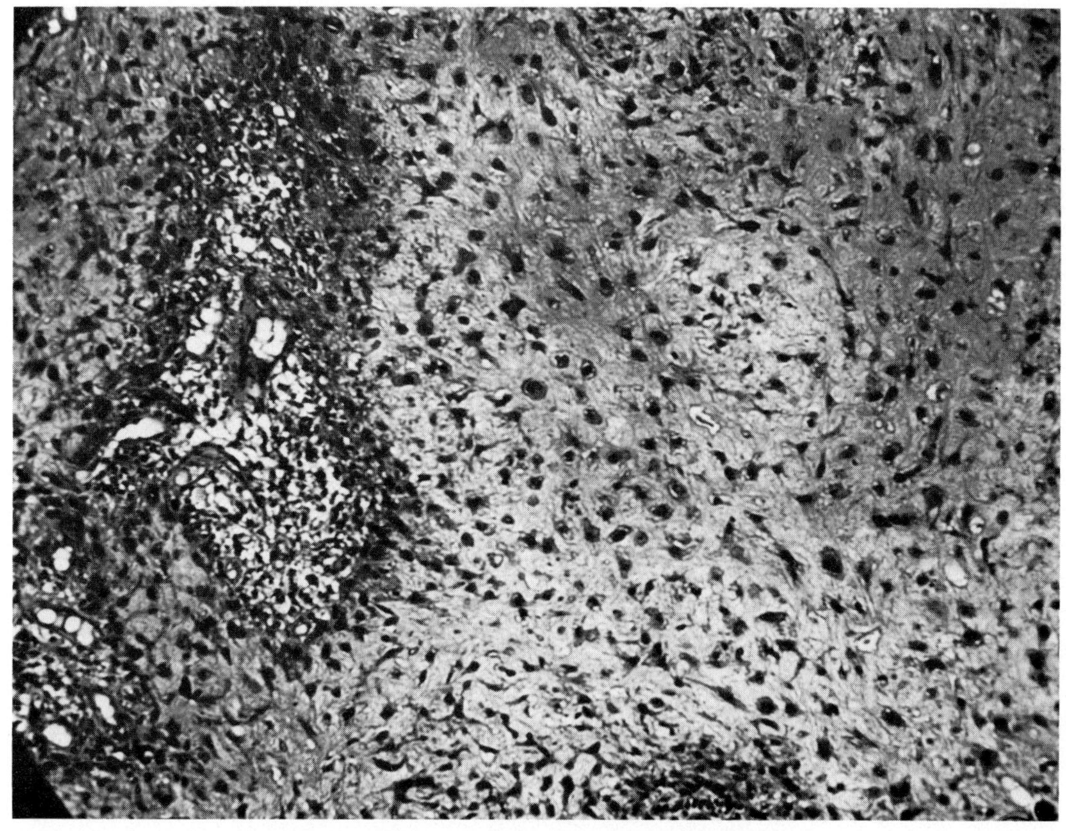

Figure 9–201. *See legend on opposite page*

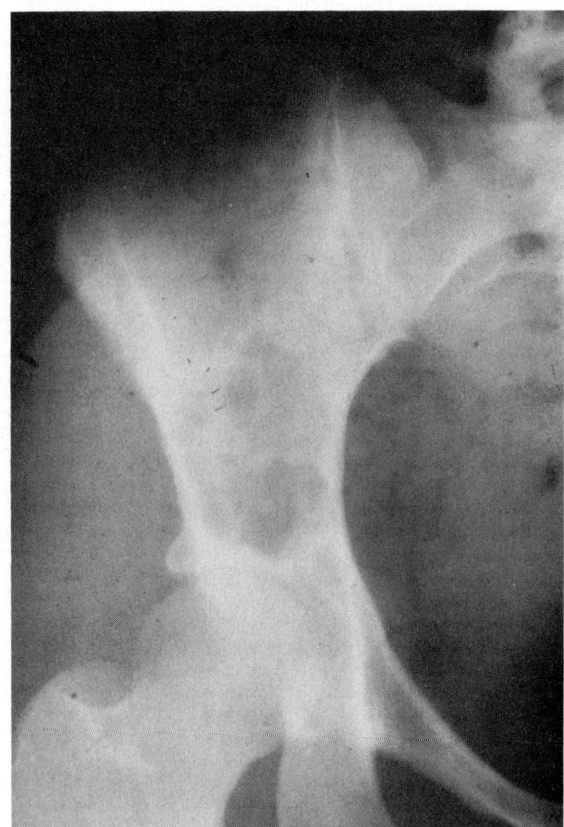

Figure 9–202. Chondromyxoid fibroma. Sharply circumscribed lytic defect located in the ilium, an unusual location. Apparent loculations are ridges on the cavity wall.

nonossifying fibroma of bone; the radiologist cannot differentiate the two, although there is a tendency for less septation in the chondromyxoid fibroma than in the nonossifying fibroma.

Histologically, the lesion consists of a varied mixture of elements, including a fibrous component, chondroid ground substance, and giant cells. There may be occasional bona fide cartilage cells, but the diagnosis of chondromyxoid fibroma does not depend on their presence. The extreme variability of chondroid, myxoid, and fibrous pattern associated with these lesions is characteristic, and giant cells may abound. The histologic features, although varied, are clearly benign and demonstrate minimal pleomorphism.

MISCELLANEOUS CARTILAGE LESIONS

In addition to the aforementioned clearly identifiable entities, numerous instances of bizarre or unusual cartilage lesions may be found in the literature (Lichtenstein and Bernstein, 1959). The physician should treat cartilaginous lesions with respect; their biologic potential in the proximal and axial skeletons may be ominous, and unless they are found as incidental lesions, the symptoms that prompt clinical investigation are suggestive of aggressive behavior.

Figure 9–201. Chondromyxoid fibroma. Histologic view demonstrating chondroid matrix, spindled, moderately pleomorphic fibroblasts, and more cellular elements with occasional giant cells.

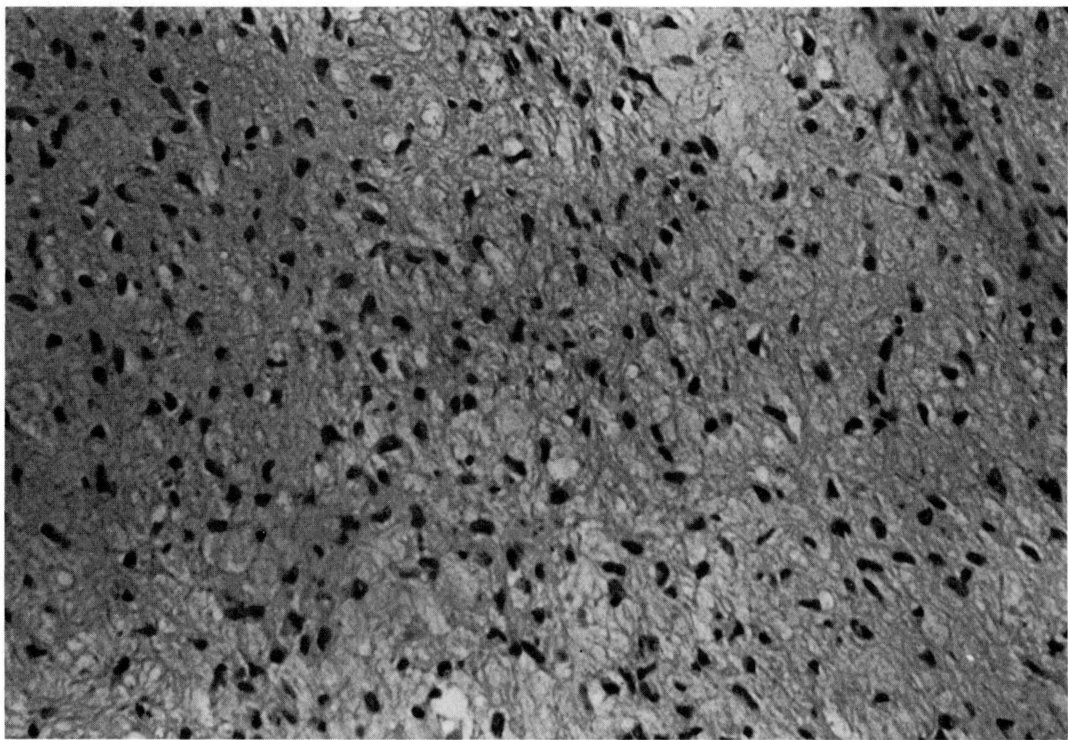

Figure 9–203. Chondromyxoid fibroma. Biopsied specimen of lesion illustrated in Figure 9–202. Note the characteristic histologic appearance of chondromyxoid fibroma, with spindled fibroblastic elements set in a chondroid stroma. Fibrous component predominates in this field.

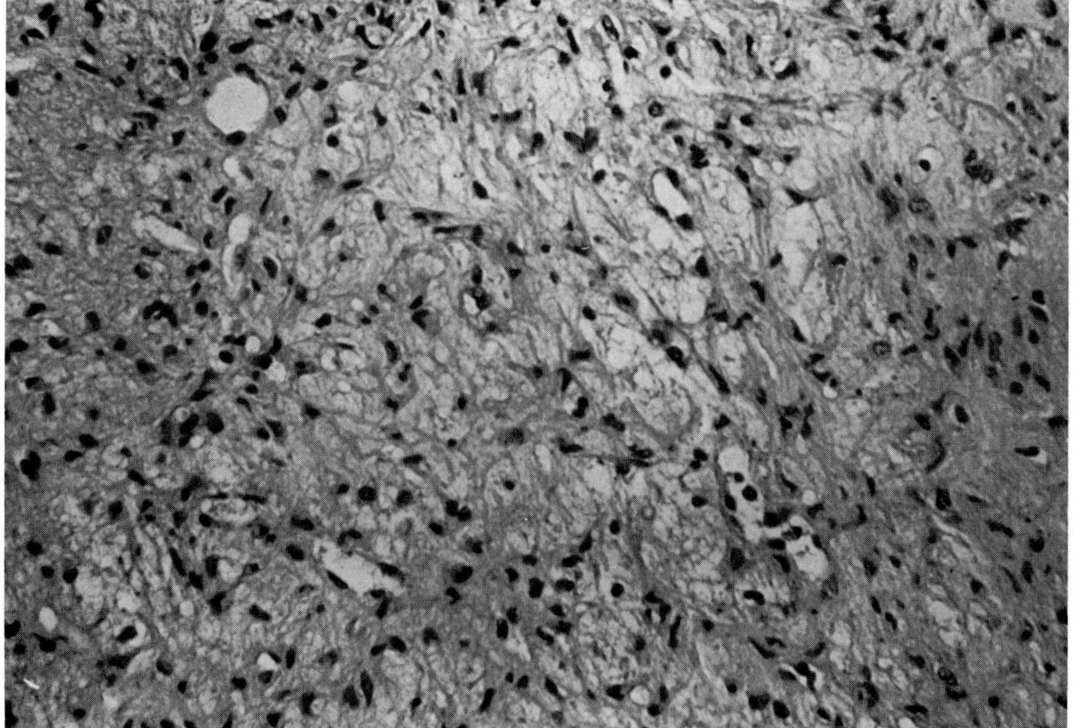

Figure 9–204. Chondromyxoid fibroma. Histologic picture similar to that shown in Figure 9–203, with stellate fibroblastic elements predominating.

CHORDOMA

Chordoma is a tumor arising from notochordal remnants. The tumor is therefore always found in the vertebral column and may often involve more than one vertebral body. Extensive tumor formation with involvement of soft tissue is common. The characteristic cell identifying the tumor is the physaliferous cell, which demonstrates a markedly vacuolated cytoplasm. The lesion exhibits a moderate degree of pleomorphism and, except in rare instances, shows no evidence of cartilage formation.

Text continued on page 457

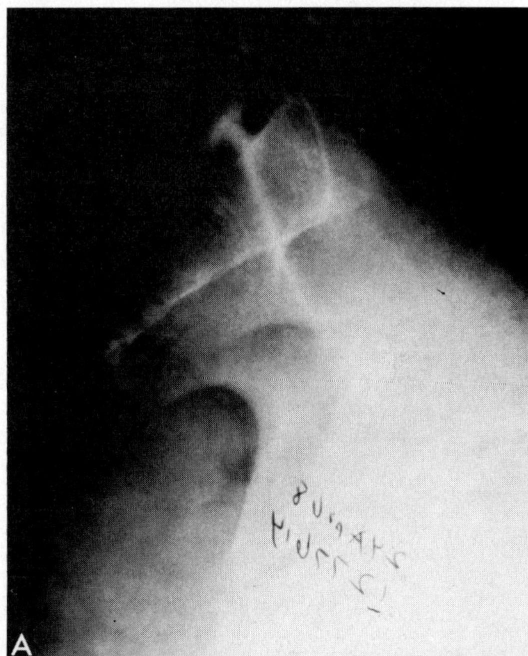

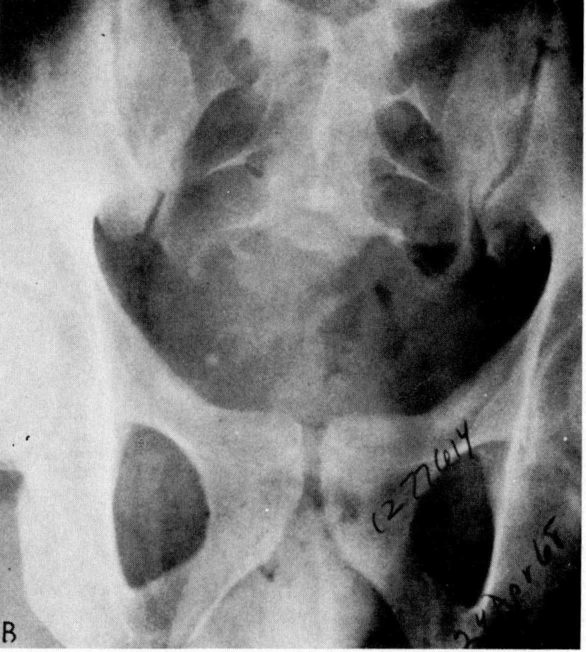

Figure 9–205. Lateral *(A)* and anteroposterior *(B)* radiographs of the pelvis of a 32-year-old male with a large chordoma of the sacrum. There is destruction of the distal portion of the sacrum beyond the S-3 level. The lateral view illustrates an abrupt cut off. The soft-tissue mass is not well-defined.

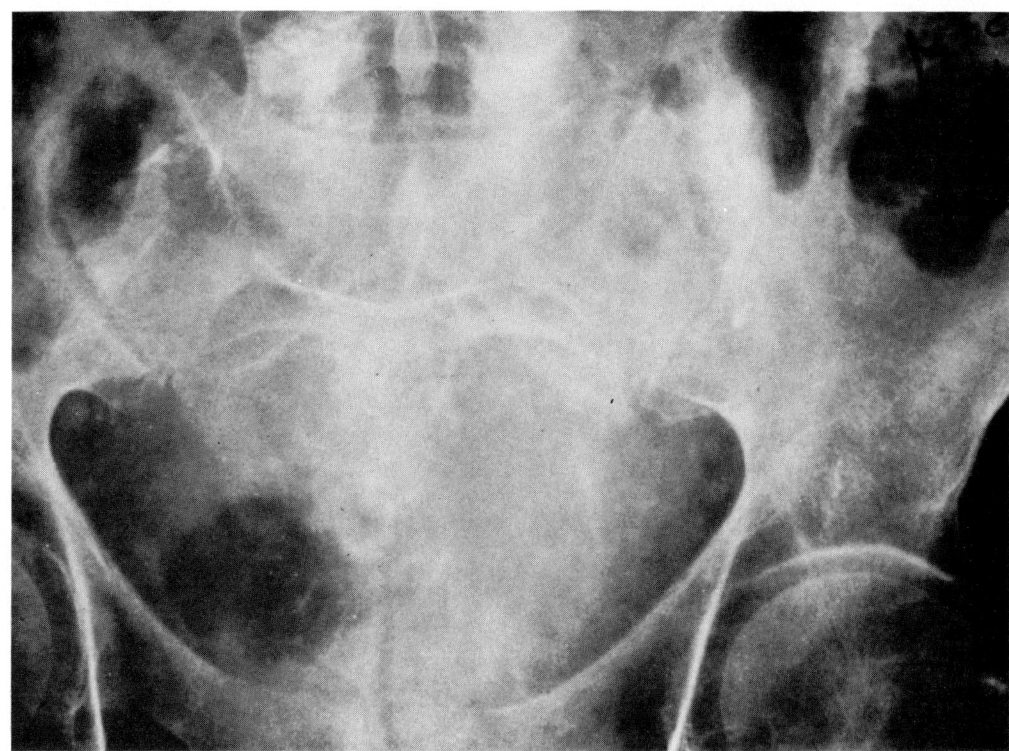

Figure 9–206. Chordoma. Anteroposterior radiograph of the pelvis of a 70-year-old male with a sacral chordoma. There is destruction of the terminal portion of the sacrum, and the lesion extends laterally to the midline in the proximal portion. There is an indistinct outline of the soft-tissue mass, with calcification scattered throughout the lesion.

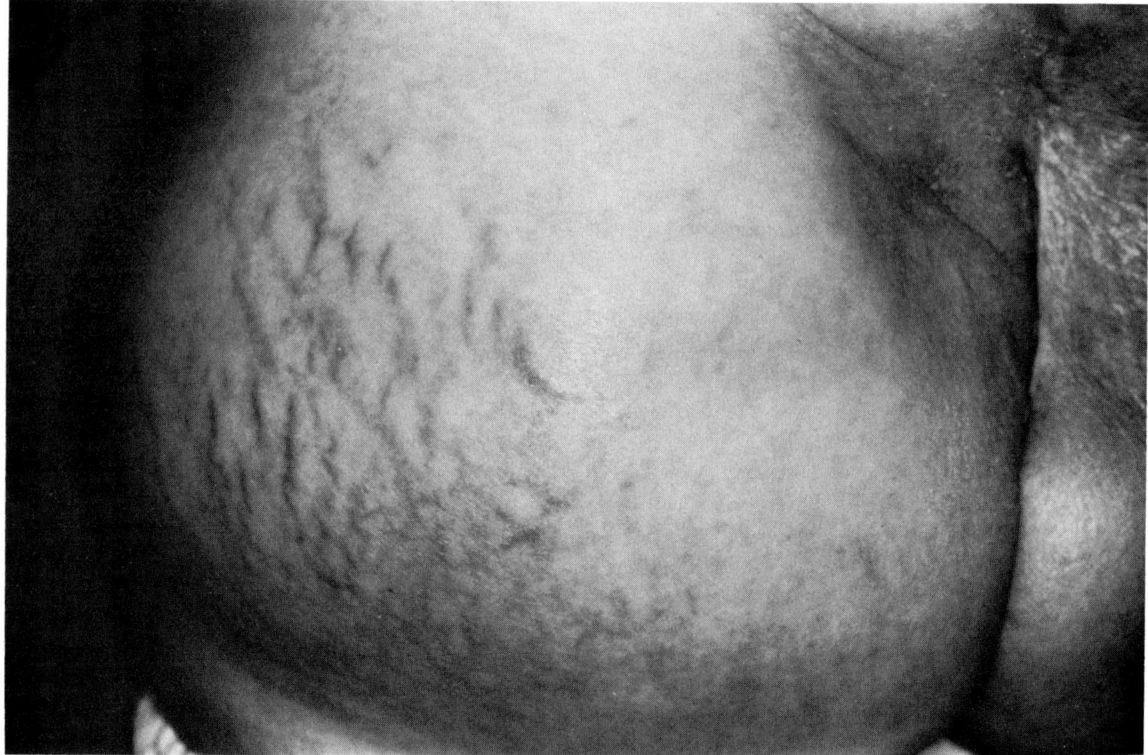

Figure 9–207. Chordoma. Clinical photograph of an extensive chordoma reaching bilaterally into the buttock of a 34-year-old female. She had previous surgical resection, but the tumor was never completely excised and has become increasingly painful. The lesion is very hard to palpation, and one can feel distinct lobulations through the skin of the buttock.

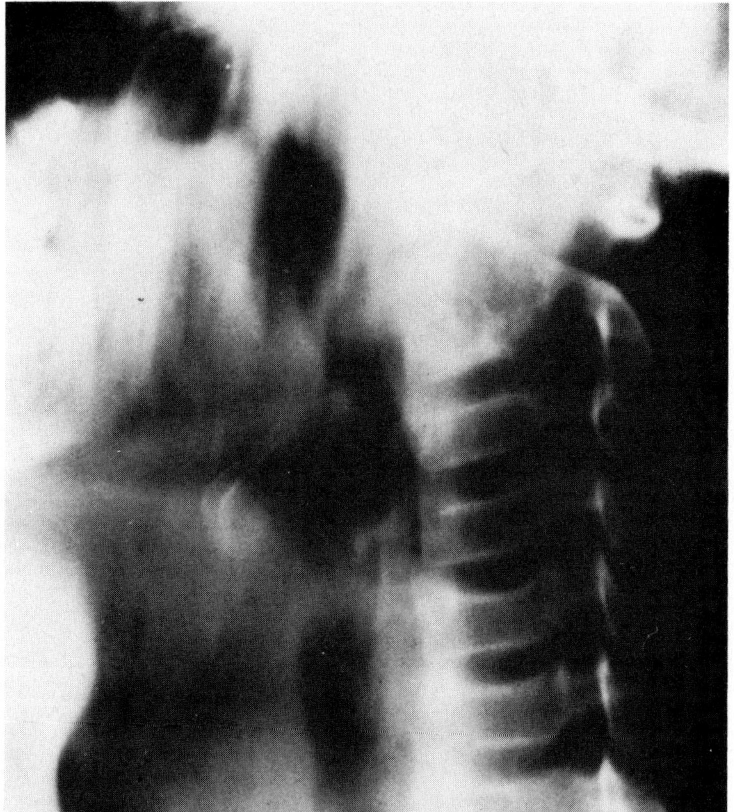

Figure 9–208. Chordoma. Lateral tomogram of the cervical spine in a 12-year-old male with a lytic lesion in the body of C-2. Approximately two thirds of chordomas originate in the sacrum; a large portion of the remainder originate in the base of the skull or the upper cervical spine. Remnants of notochordal cells are the source of these tumors.

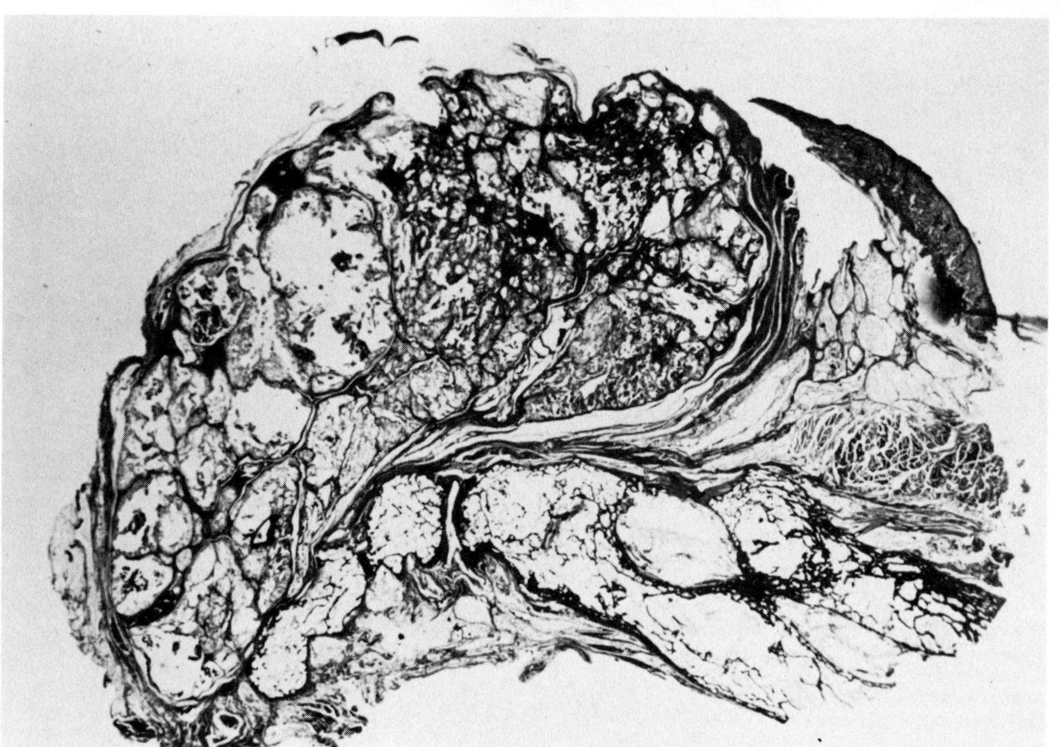

Figure 9–209. Chordoma. Macrosection of a chordoma illustrating the lobular nature of the basic lesion with the fibrous septa intervening between the lobules. These septa contain the vasculature for the tumor. There is frequent obliteration of these vessels by tumor, with resultant necrosis and cyst formation in the lesion.

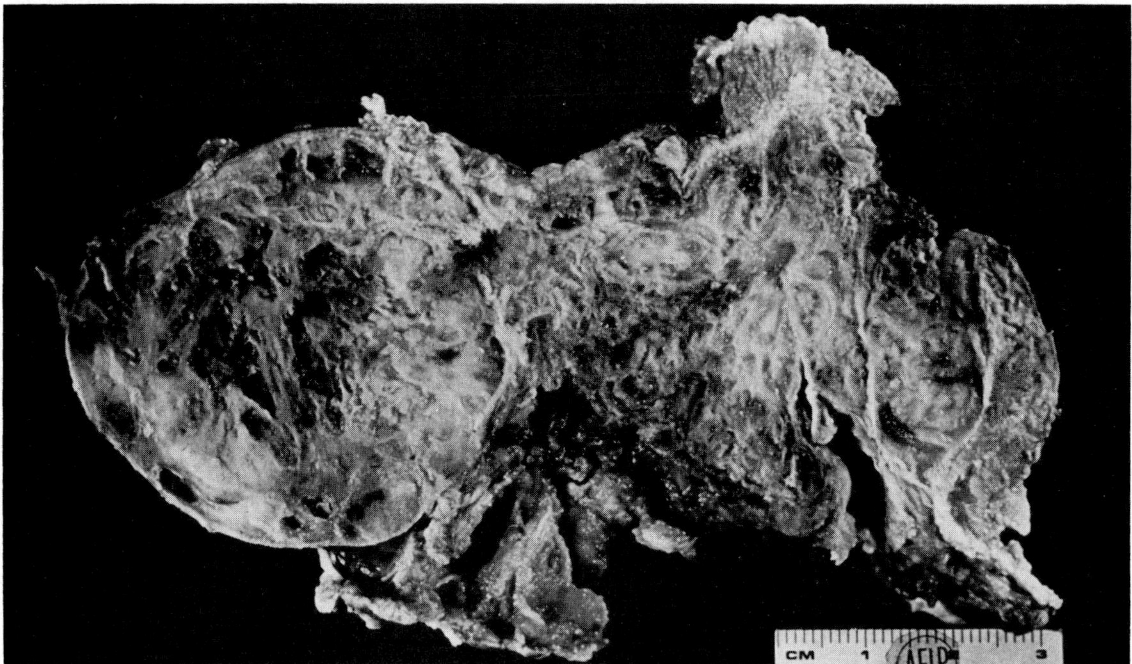

Figure 9–210. Chordoma. Hemisection of a chordoma. The lobular nature of the lesion is evident. The strands of fibrous connective tissue between the lobules are visible, and there are numerous areas of cystic degeneration.

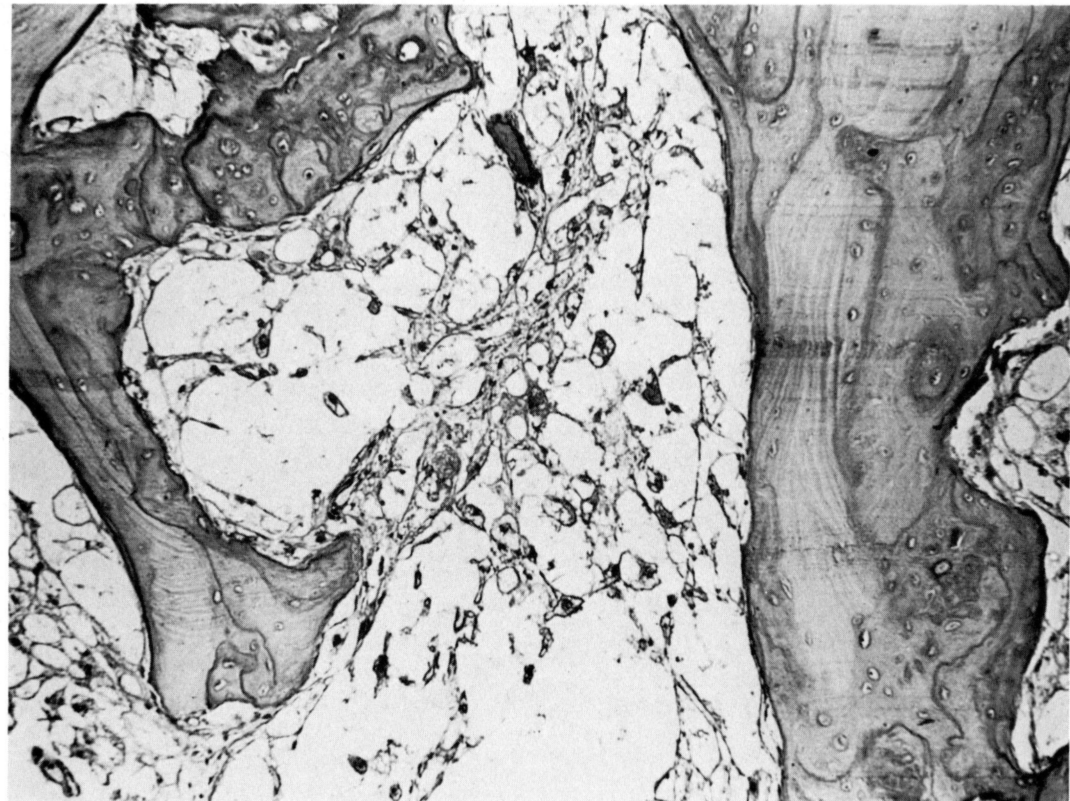

Figure 9–211. Chordoma invading bone. The bony structure appears relatively normal, although there is morphologic evidence of bone remodeling. The normal marrow has been replaced by tumor with vacuolated cytoplasm.

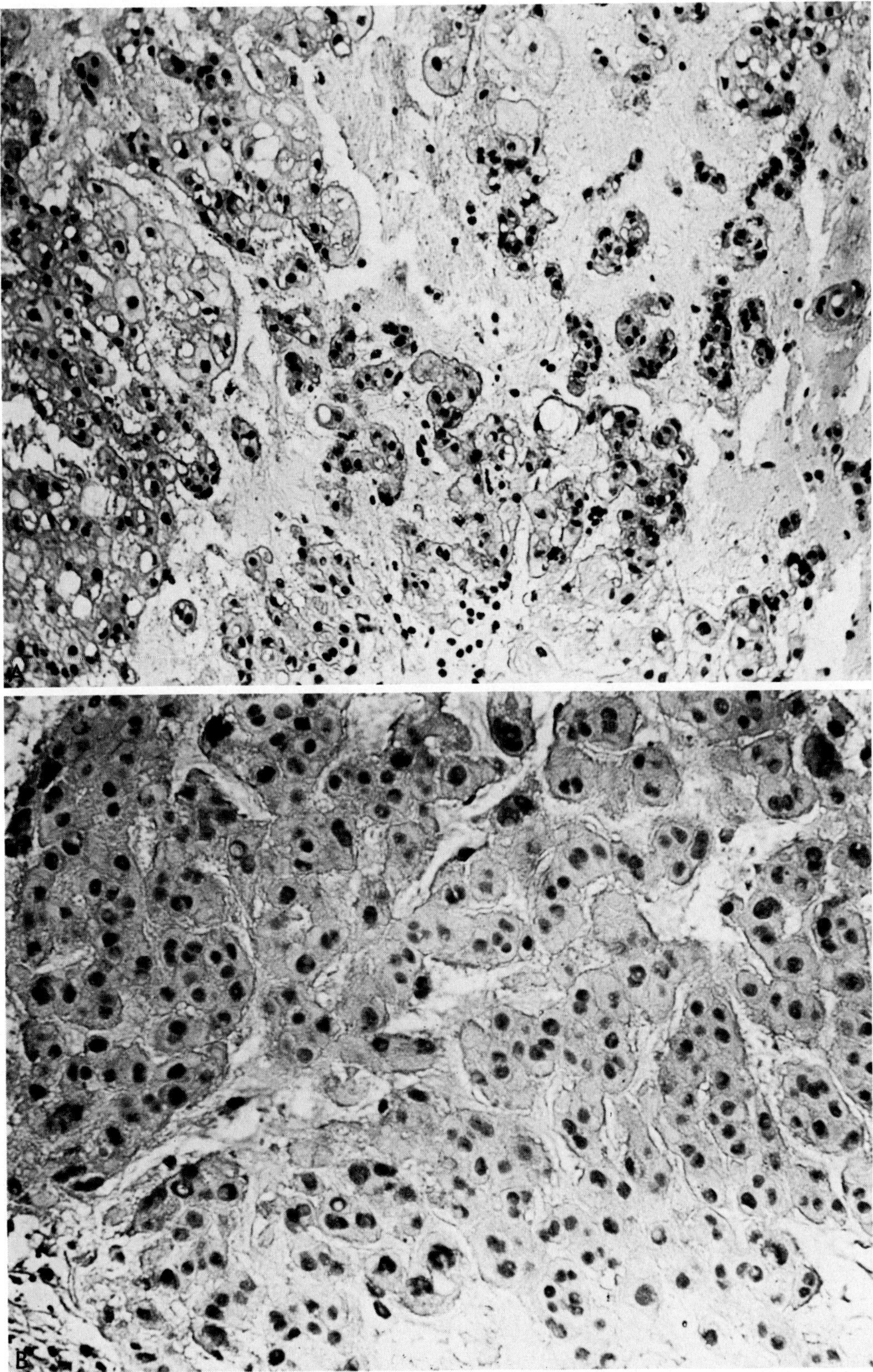

Figure 9–212. Chordoma. Cellular area of chordoma. The cells are large with a clearly visible central nucleus and numerous vacuoles in the cytoplasm. These vacuoles contain mucinous material.

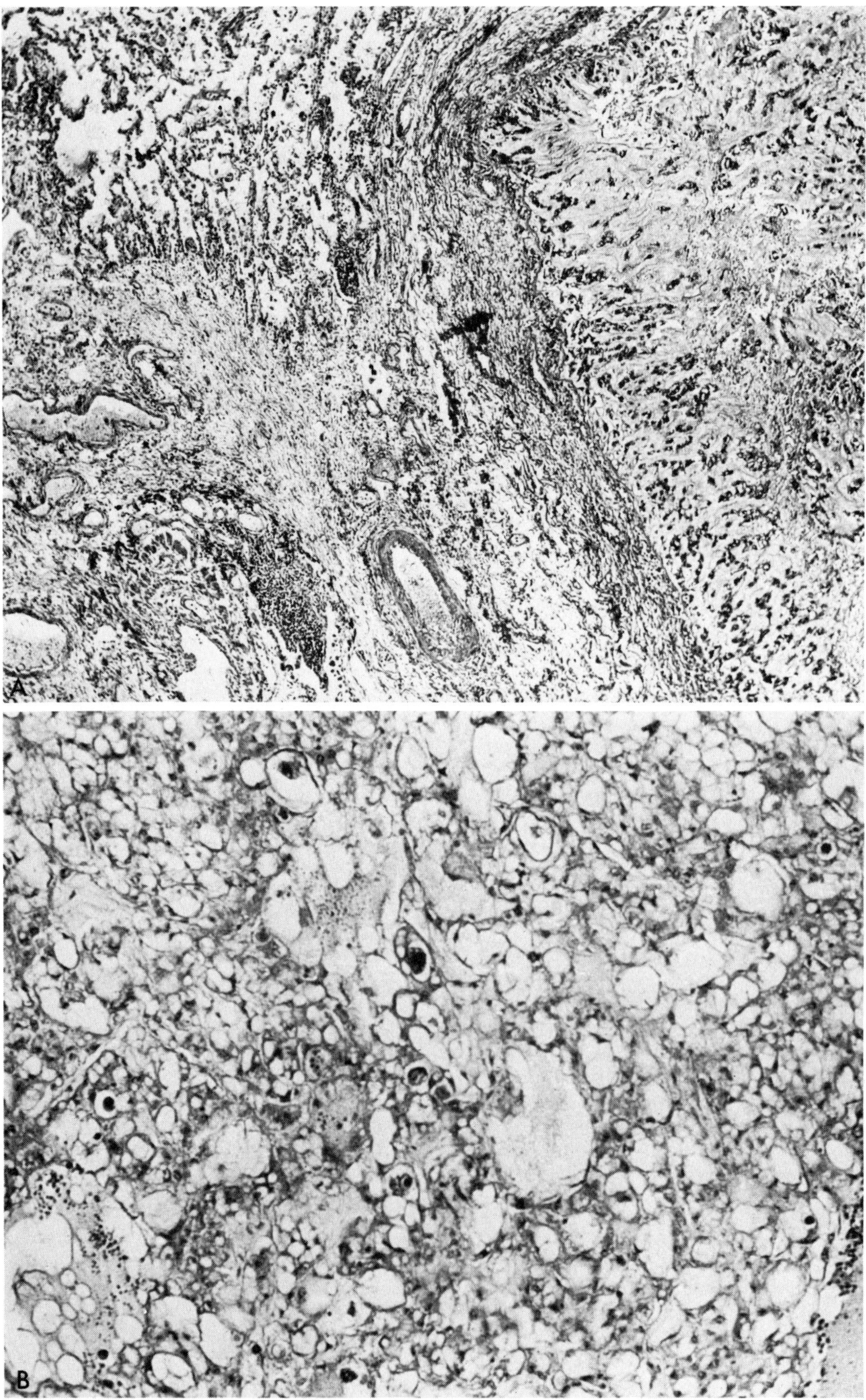

Figure 9–213. Chordoma. Varied histologic appearance of chordoma. The cells are large, and each has a central, clearly defined nucleus and homogeneous cytoplasm. Vacuoles are present in the cytoplasm of the cells. Fibrous septa surround distinct lobules of tumor.

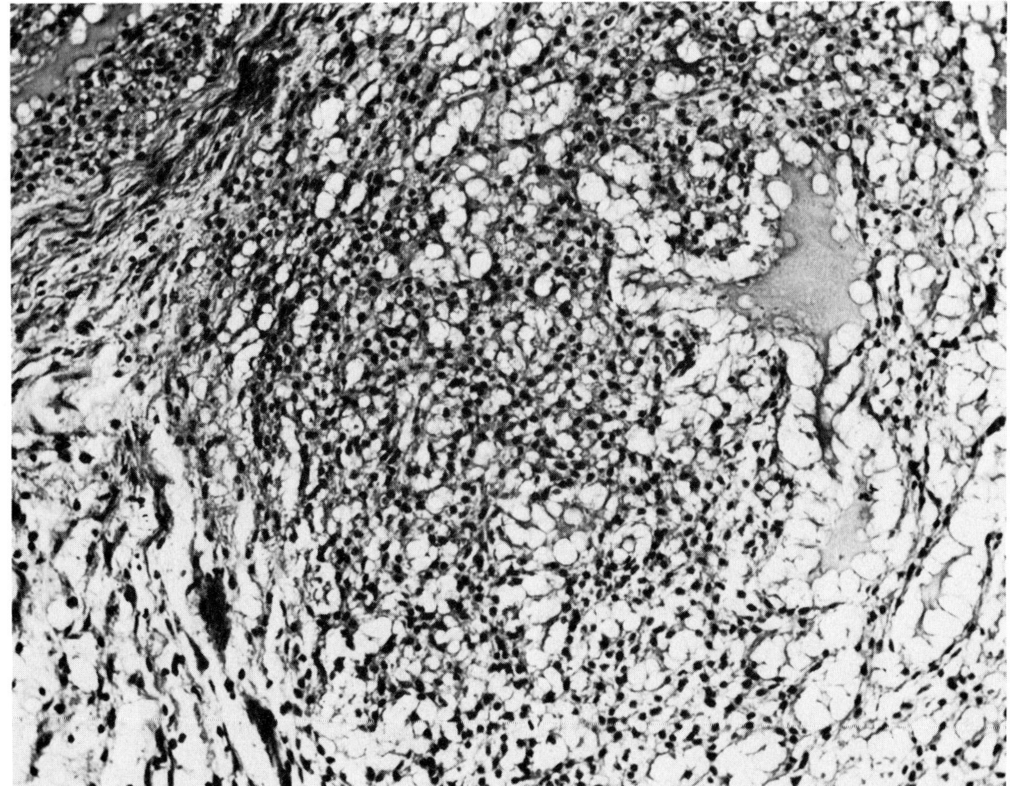

Figure 9–214. Chordoma. Histologic view of chordoma showing mucin-producing physaliferous cells. The lesion must be differentiated from chondrosarcoma and metastatic adenocarcinoma.

OSSEOUS LESIONS

The difficulties in the diagnosis of osteoid-producing neoplasms is not actually in differentiating among osteoid osteoma, osteoblastoma, and osteosarcoma, but rather in differentiating the lesions from benign traumatic, reactive, and inflammatory lesions. From the pathologist's view, the key is the purposeful and logical maturation of structure in the reactive process contrasted with the haphazard growth patterns of the neoplastic process.

OSTEOID OSTEOMA

Although not strictly speaking a neoplasm, osteoid osteoma demonstrates a histologic pattern that must be differentiated from that of a neoplasm. Osteoid osteoma consists of a sharply circumscribed lytic nidus surrounded by a variable rim of reactive sclerotic bone. The nidus should not be greater than 1.0 cm in diameter. The lesion consists of numerous osteoblasts and exhibits primitive bone formation and extensive vascularity. It produces pain, which is more pronounced at night (as opposed to stress fracture, which will respond favorably to rest). Aspirin provides some relief from the pain, which is possibly related to the extensive vascularity associated with the lesion. Radiographic differential diagnosis includes Brodie's abscess.

Osteoid osteomas may remain stable for many years, but pain usually requires operative intervention.

Text continued on page 463

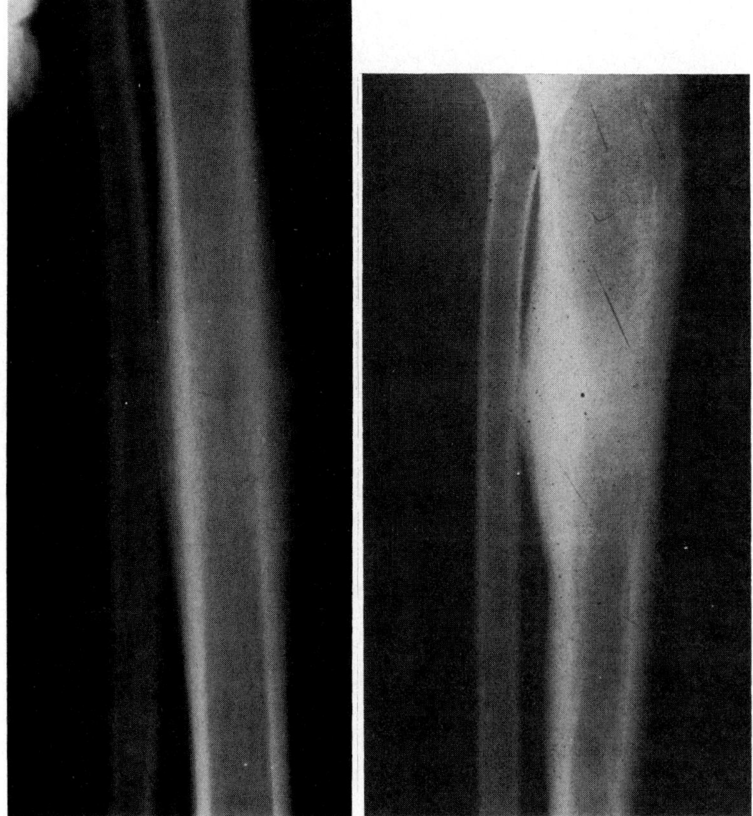

Figure 9–215   Figure 9–216

Figure 9–215. Osteoid osteoma. Radiograph of an osteoid osteoma of the tibia. The lesion is located in the anterior cortex. The periosteum has produced increased bone with expansion and thickening of the cortex, and there is a radiolucent region in the center of the thickened bone.

Figure 9–216. Osteoid osteoma. Radiograph of a tibia showing an osteoid osteoma characterized by an area of dense sclerosis that is disproportionate with the size of the lesion itself. The tumor appears in the periosteal cortical junction, and its nidus is less than 1.0 cm in diameter. Often, the nidus cannot be visualized radiographically.

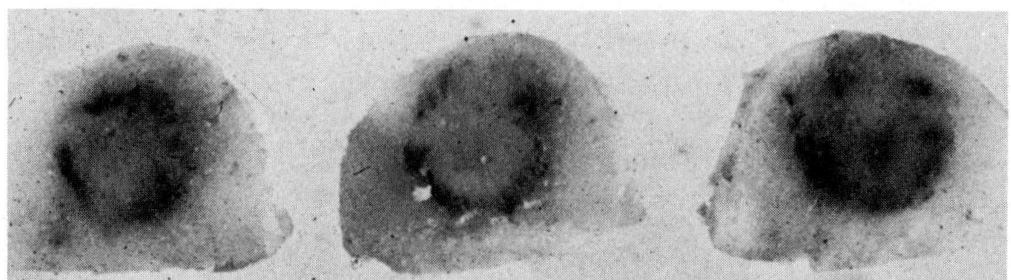

Figure 9–217. Osteoid osteoma. Gross sections of cortical bone containing an osteoid osteoma. Note the size of the nidus and the dark discoloration, features consistent with the increased vascularity of an osteoid osteoma.

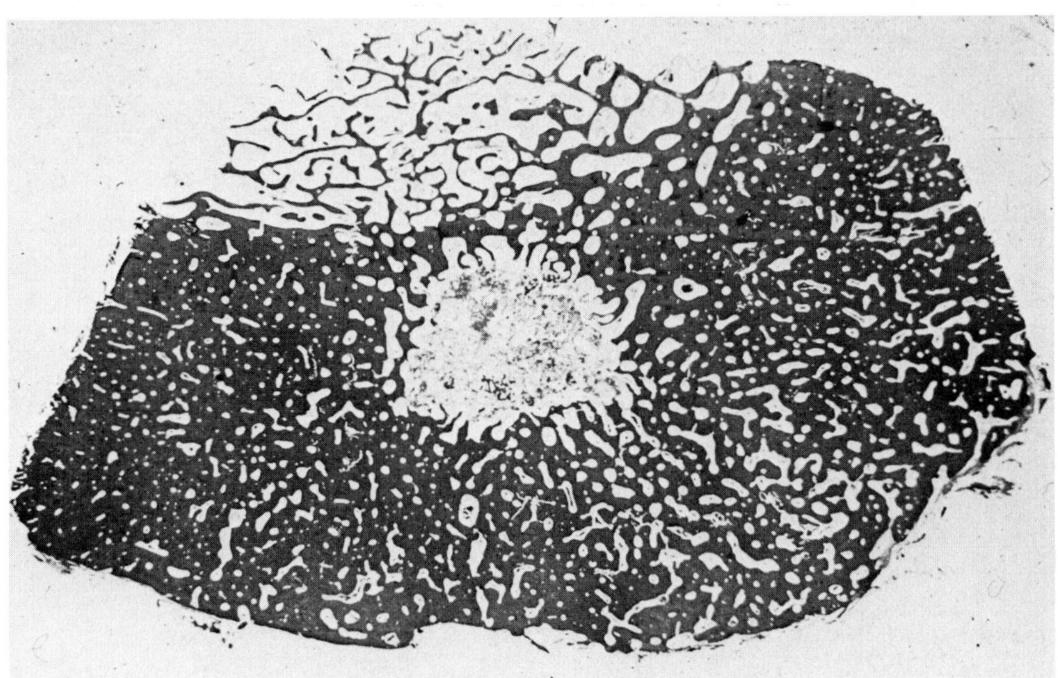

Figure 9–218. Osteoid osteoma. Macrosection of an osteoid osteoma exhibiting an extremely dense sclerotic margin with a central lytic nidus.

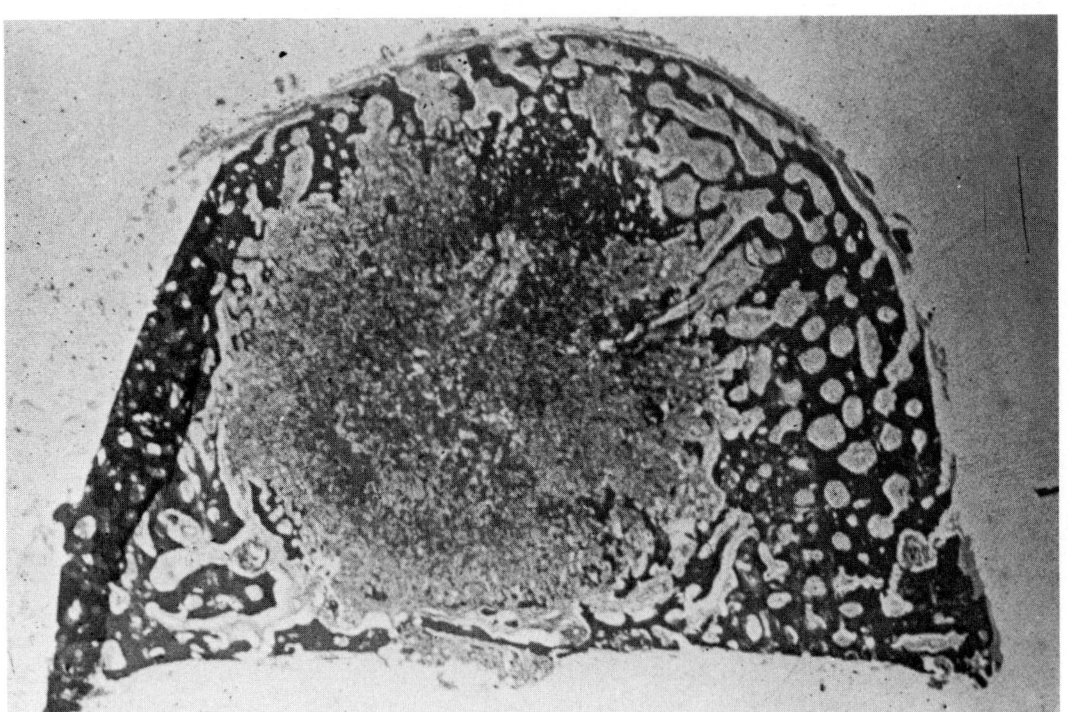

Figure 9–219. Osteoid osteoma. Macrosection of an osteoid osteoma exhibiting a nidus approximately 1 cm in diameter with sclerotic margin. There is somewhat less sclerosis in this specimen than in the one illustrated in Figure 9–218.

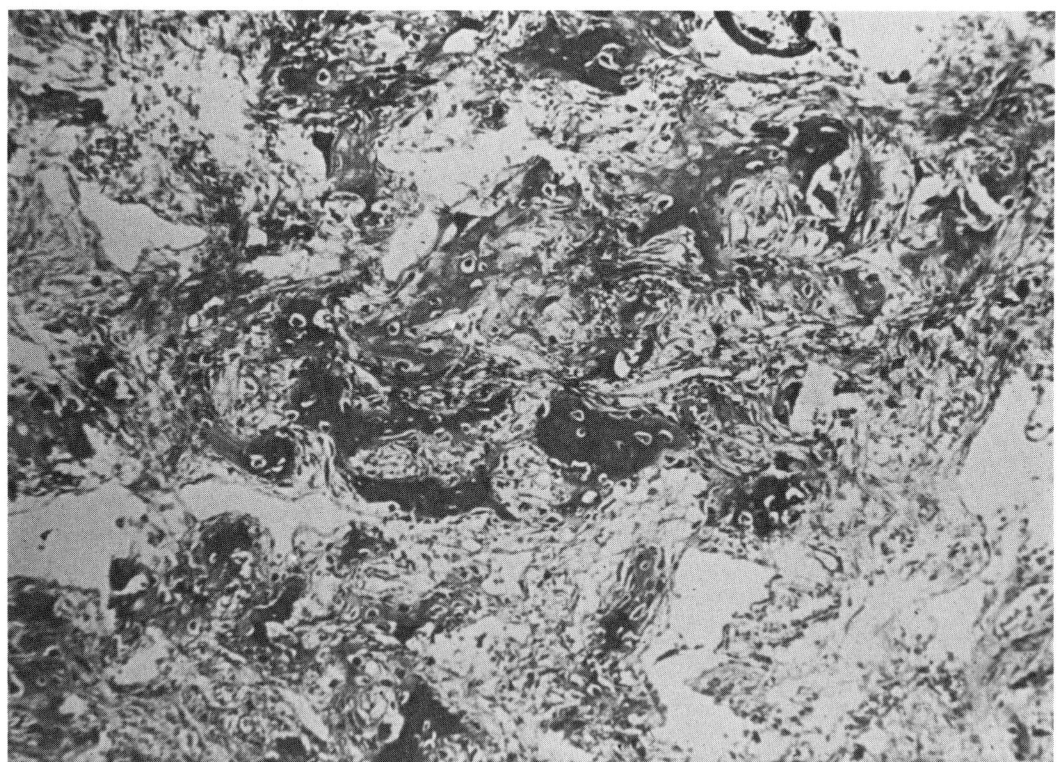

Figure 9–220. Osteoid osteoma. Histologic section from the nidus of an osteoid osteoma exhibiting neoplastic osteoid formation with extensive vascularity. The nidus alone suggests an osteoblastoma.

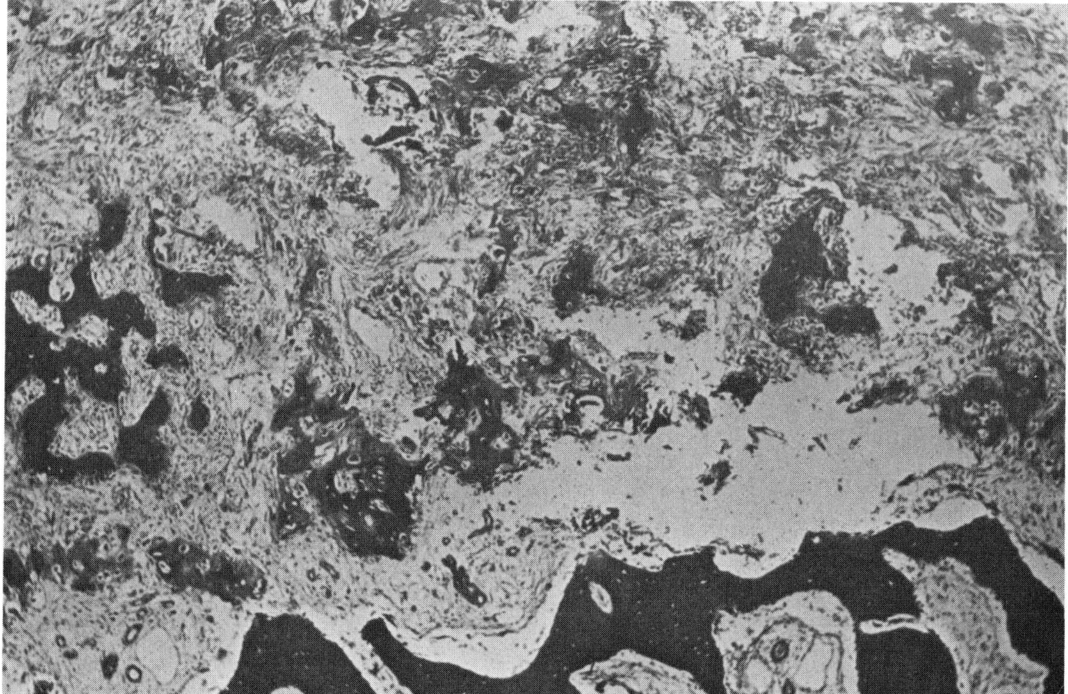

Figure 9–221. Osteoid osteoma. Histologic section from central area of osteoid osteoma exhibiting the neoplastic osteoid formation and increased vascularity as well as the dense sclerotic margin. The presence of a sclerotic margin confirms the slow-growing, benign nature of the process and serves to differentiate osteoid osteoma from osteoblastoma.

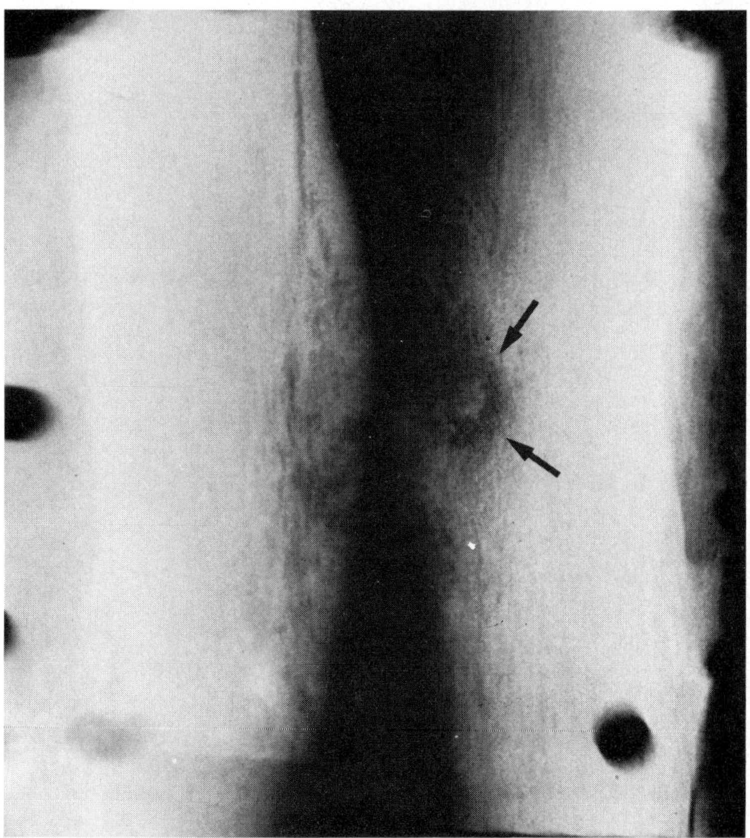

Figure 9–222. Specimen radiograph of the nidus (arrows) of an osteoid osteoma. There is thickened bone surrounding a lucent defect with a calcified center. The dark holes are surgical defects created during removal of the lesion.

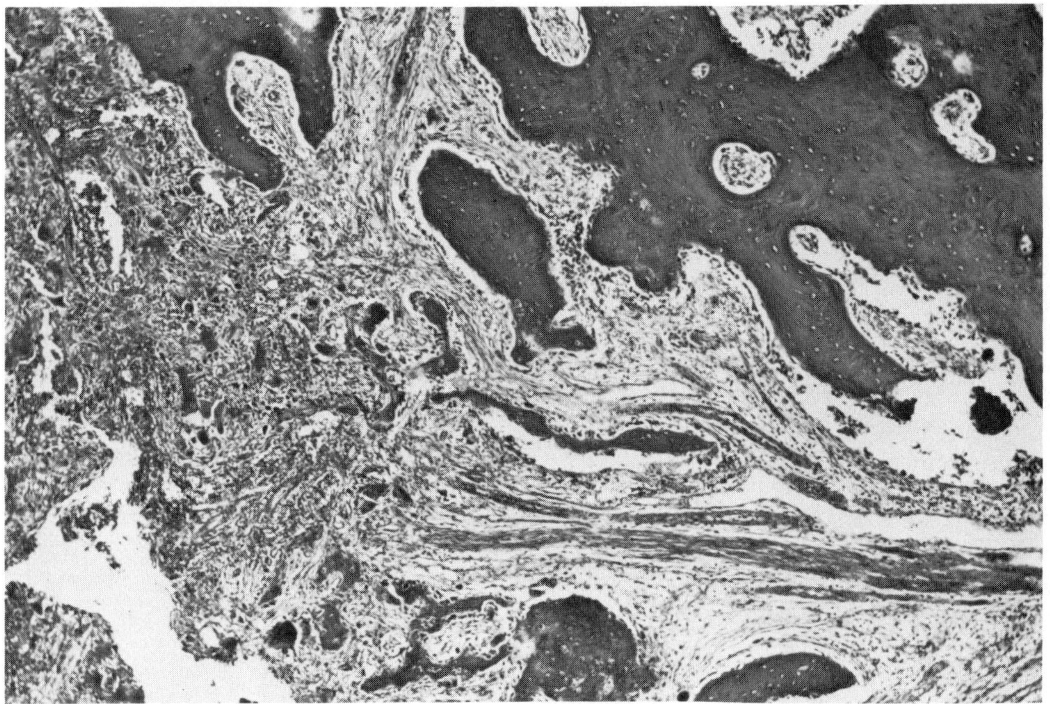

Figure 9–223. Osteoid osteoma. Margin of an osteoid osteoma showing a nerve fiber growing into the region.

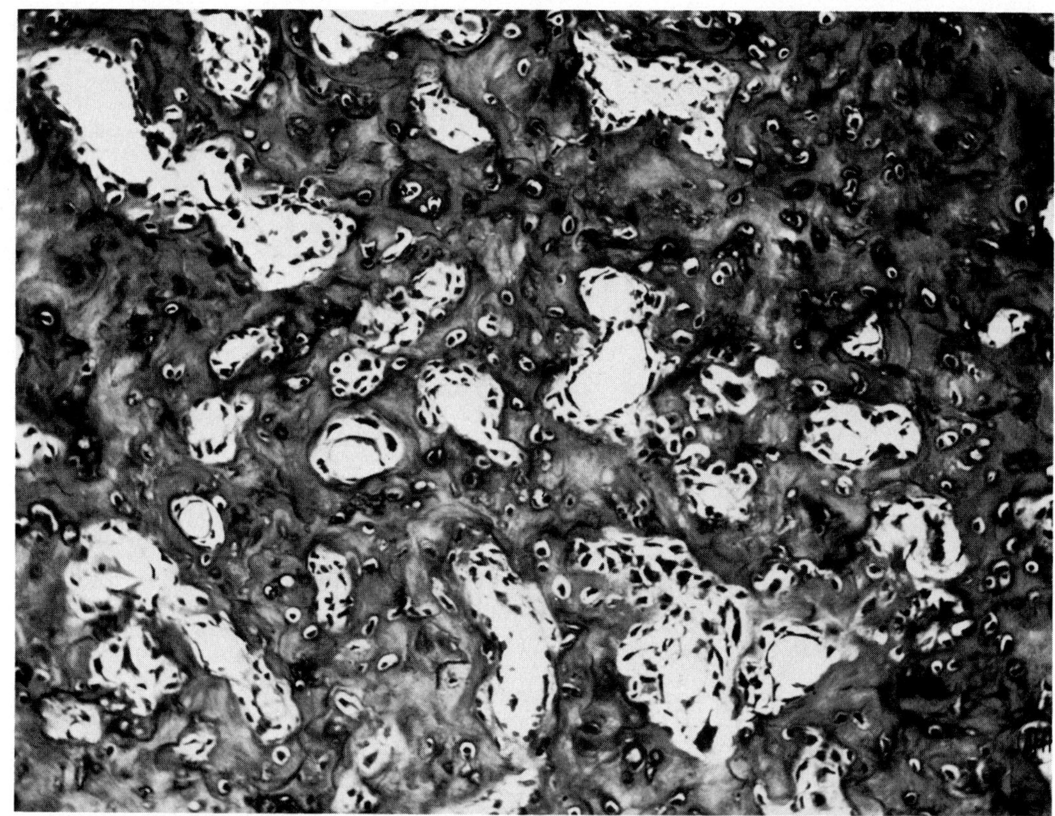

Figure 9–224. Osteoid osteoma. Older nidus of an osteoid osteoma with heavy mineralization and recognizable bone production. Radiographically, this nidus would appear fairly dense and sclerotic.

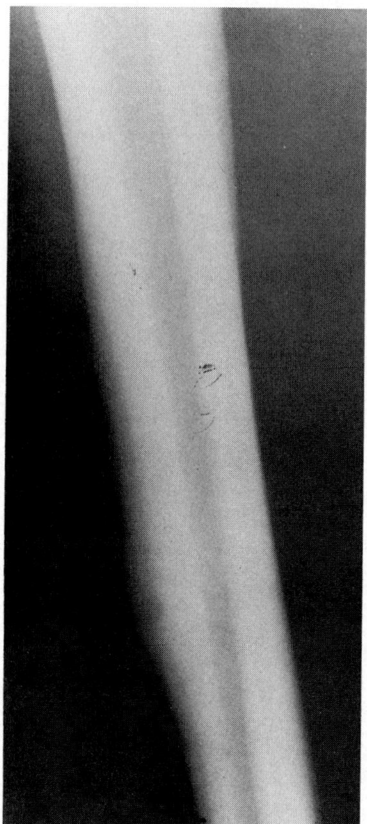

Figure 9–225. Osteoid osteoma. Radiograph of peripheral osteoid osteoma. The tumor may be present at any site in any bone. In this lesion, the nidus is located within the periosteum.

OSTEOBLASTOMA

The osteoblastoma is a rare neoplasm of bone, usually presenting in the vertebral column. It may also present in long bones, and then in the same location as the characteristic osteosarcoma. The lesion must have radiographically benign characteristics, or osteosarcoma must be considered. The typical osteoblastoma is sharply circumscribed, and it may be either lytic or sclerotic. Calcified lesions are usually seen in the vertebral bodies.

Histologically, the lesions exhibit a large number of bland, uniform osteoblasts with osteoid formation. The osteoid may or may not be calcified, and this will determine the radiographic appearance (lytic or sclerotic). Numerous vascular structures are often associated with the osteoblastoma, and transformation into an aneurysmal bone cyst is not uncommon. The benign nature of the lesion is determined by the uniform sheet-like proliferation of osteoblasts. Transition to clear-cut osteosarcoma has been documented (Unni and Dahlin, 1979).

A distinct group of neoplasms has emerged whose behavior is neither clearly benign nor outright malignant. These "aggressive osteoblastomas" are characterized by persistent growth, by extension into soft tissue, and, histologically, by the presence of "epithelioid" osteoblasts and sheet-like osteoid (Mirra et al., 1976; Case Records of the Massachusetts General Hospital [Case 40-1980]; Revell and Scholtz, 1979). Evidence of thin, lace-like osteoid or neoplastic cartilage suggests that a bona fide osteosarcoma rather than an aggressive osteoblastoma is present.

The classic osteoblastoma must be differentiated from the nidus of an osteoid osteoma. Histologically, the nidus of osteoid osteoma is similar to the osteoblastoma; radiographically, the osteoid osteoma is always surrounded by a sclerotic rim of bone. The osteoblastoma, however, is a neoplasm that expands slowly into the surrounding adjacent structures, and it elicits virtually no reactive bone formation.

Text continued on page 473

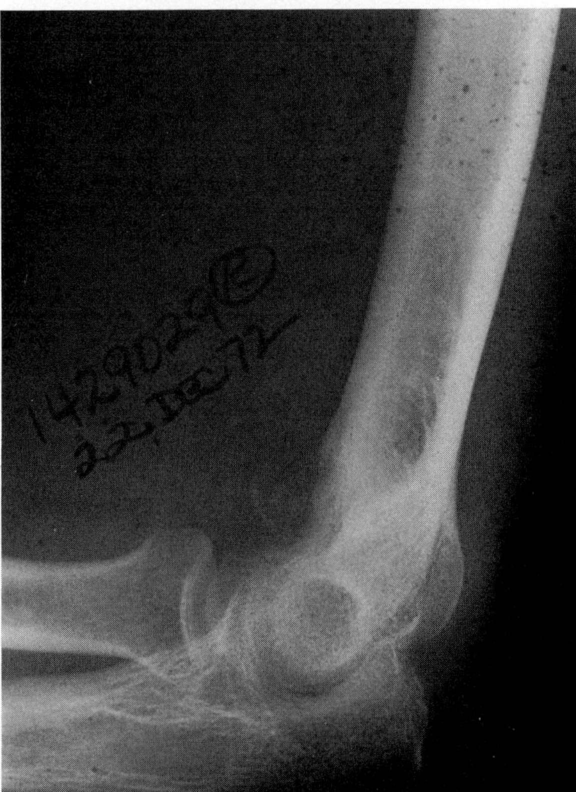

Figure 9–226. Osteoblastoma. Lateral radiograph of an elbow with an osteoblastoma in the distal humerus. Note the irregularity of the anterior cortex. There is apparent soft-tissue extension with calcification. Not much change is evident in the underlying bone.

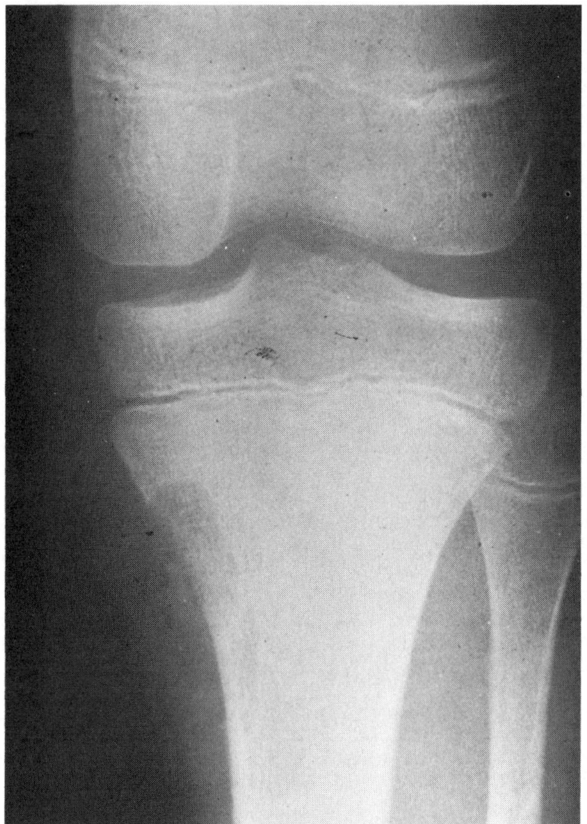

Figure 9–227. Osteoblastoma. Anteroposterior radiograph of the knee of a child who presented with local pain. An irregular lytic defect with bone production is evident in the proximal tibial metaphysis. Radiographic interpretation varied from osteosarcoma to fibrous dysplasia. Histologic study revealed an osteoblastoma.

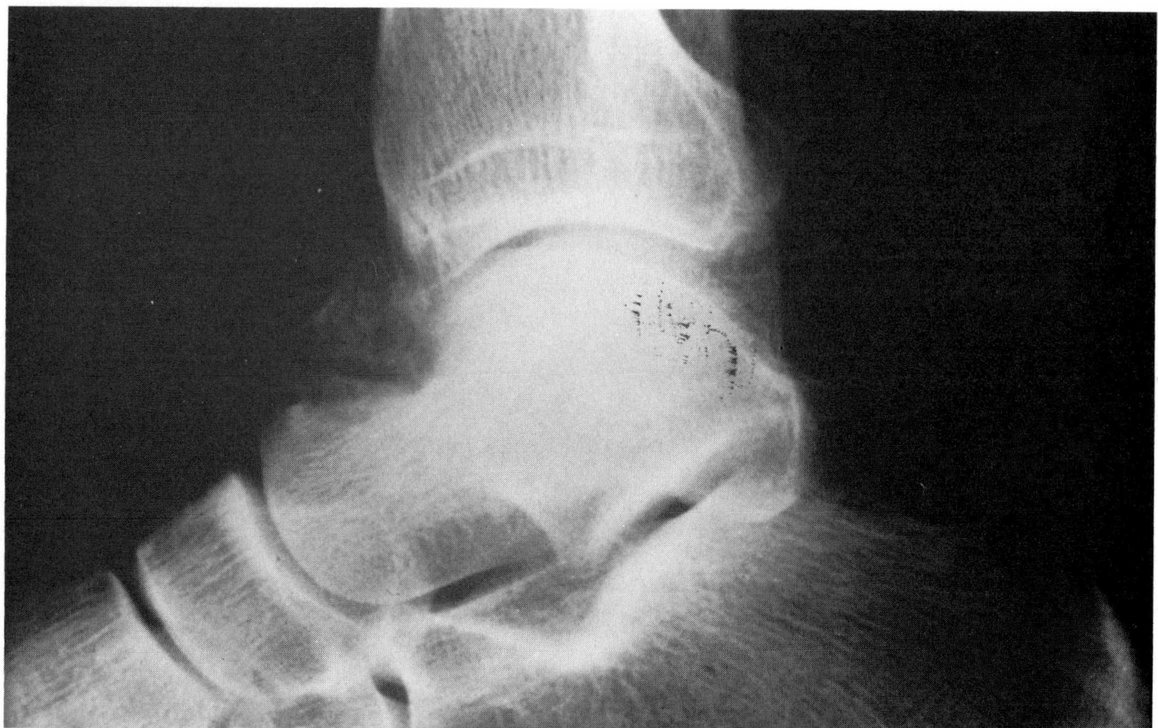

Figure 9–228. Osteoblastoma. Lateral radiograph of an ankle showing irregular soft-tissue density extending anteriorly from the body of the talus. There is irregular flocculent calcification within the soft tissue mass (often seen in synovial sarcoma), but the lesion proved to be an osteoblastoma.

Figure 9–229. Osteoblastoma. Lateral *(A)* and anteroposterior *(B)* radiographs of large osteoblastoma in sacrum. Note the sharp demarcation of the lesion. Osteoblastoma may or may not form radiographically visible matrix.

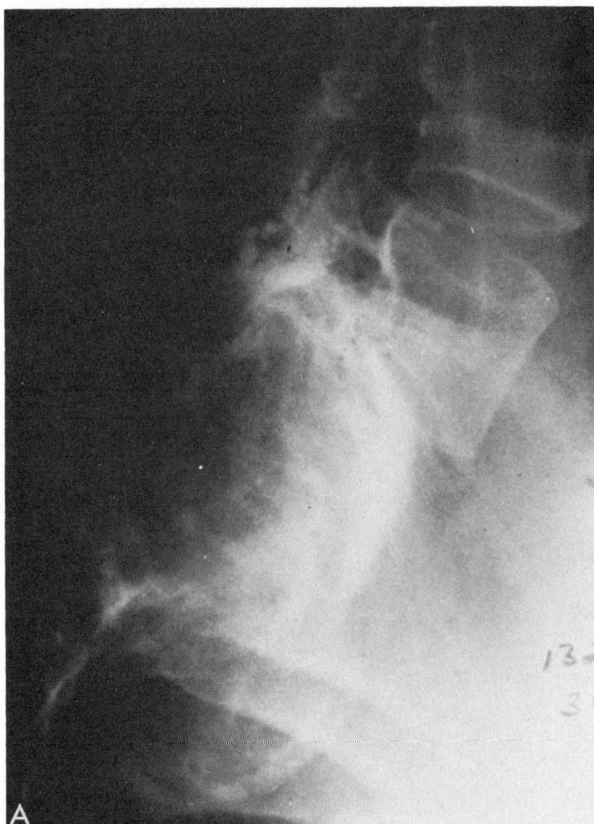
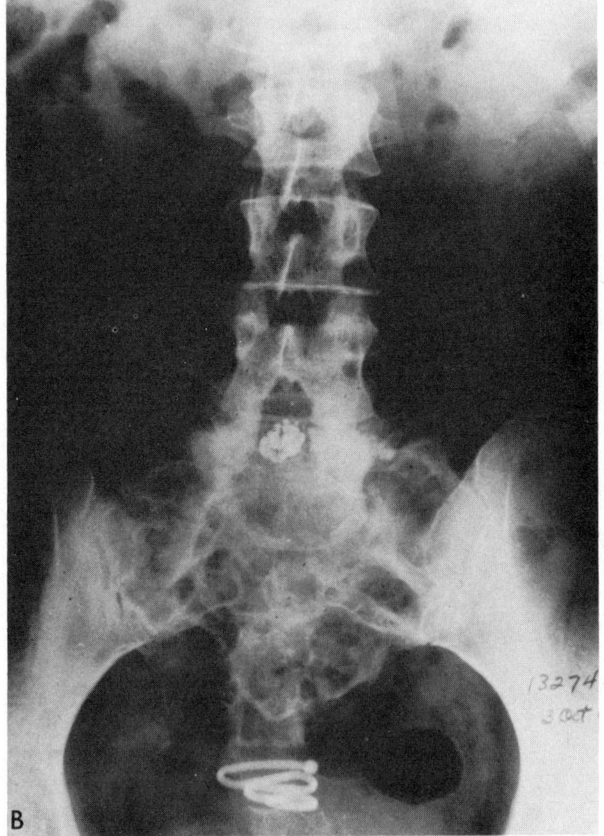

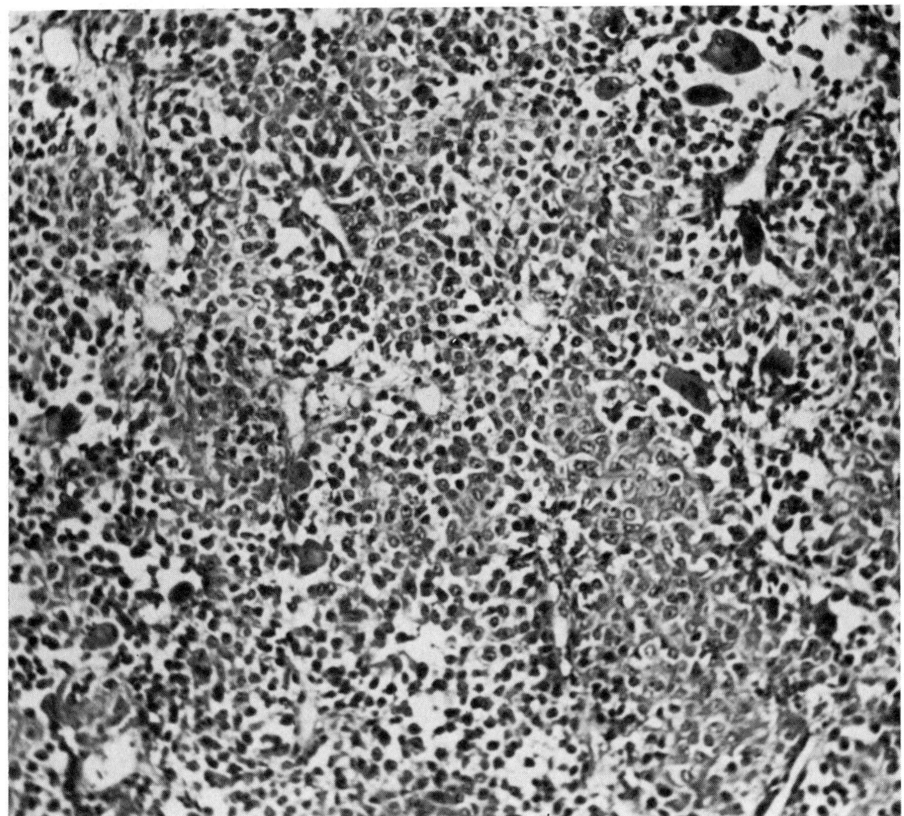

Figure 9–230. Osteoblastoma. Histologic picture of an osteoblastoma showing a cellular lesion with multiple giant cells and poorly mineralized osteoid matrix.

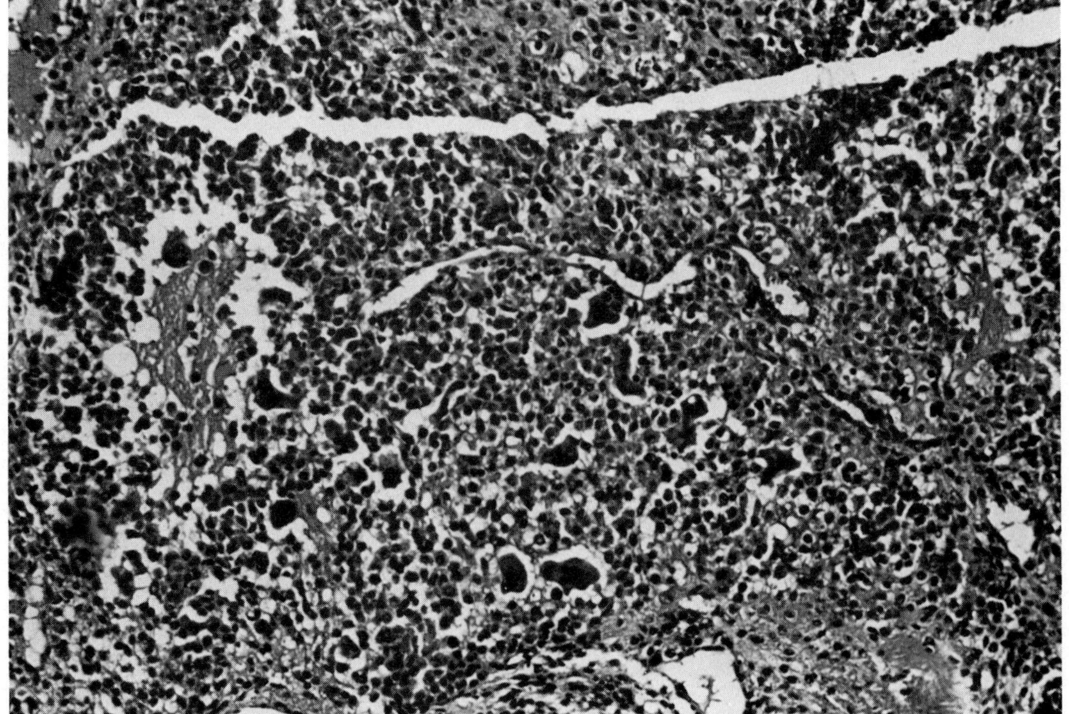

Figure 9–231. Osteoblastoma. Histologic view of osteoblastoma exhibiting numerous osteoblasts, primitive osteoid formation, and giant cells. The fairly uniform appearance of the osteoblasts indicates a benign process.

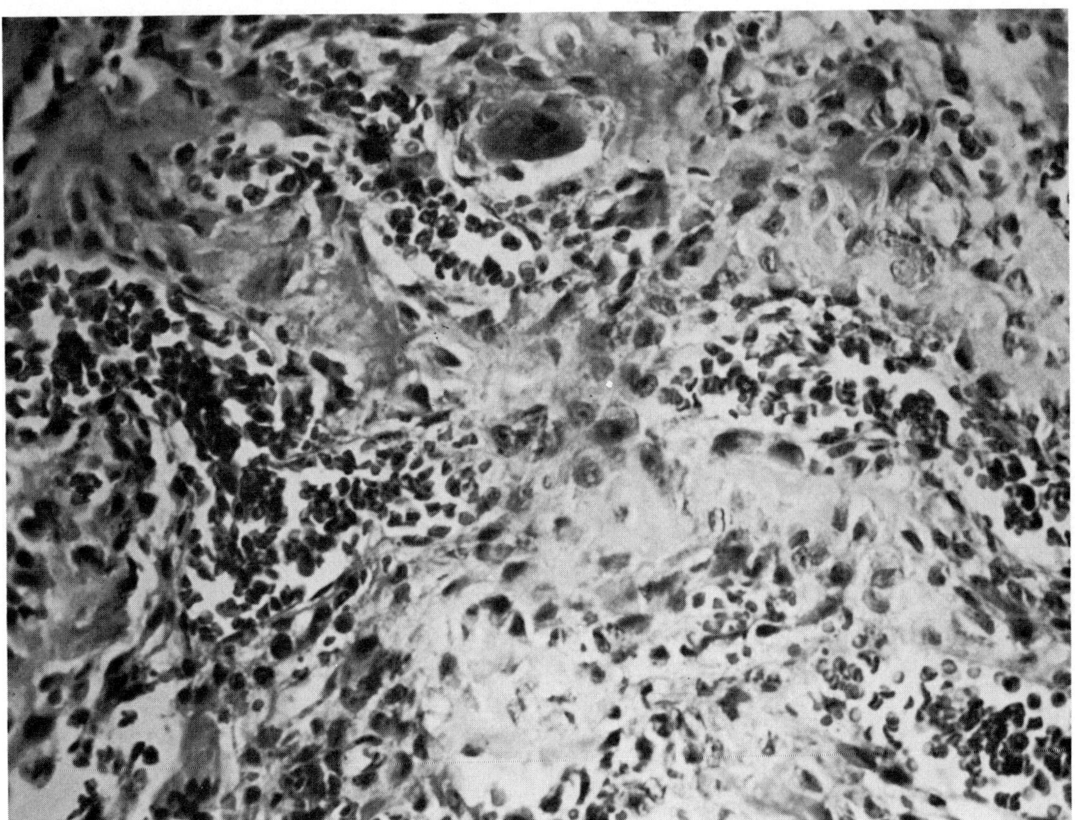

Figure 9–232. Osteoblastoma. A higher-power view of an osteoblastoma with numerous strands of irregular, poorly mineralized osteoid and cellular background. Giant cells are prominent. Note the numerous vessels.

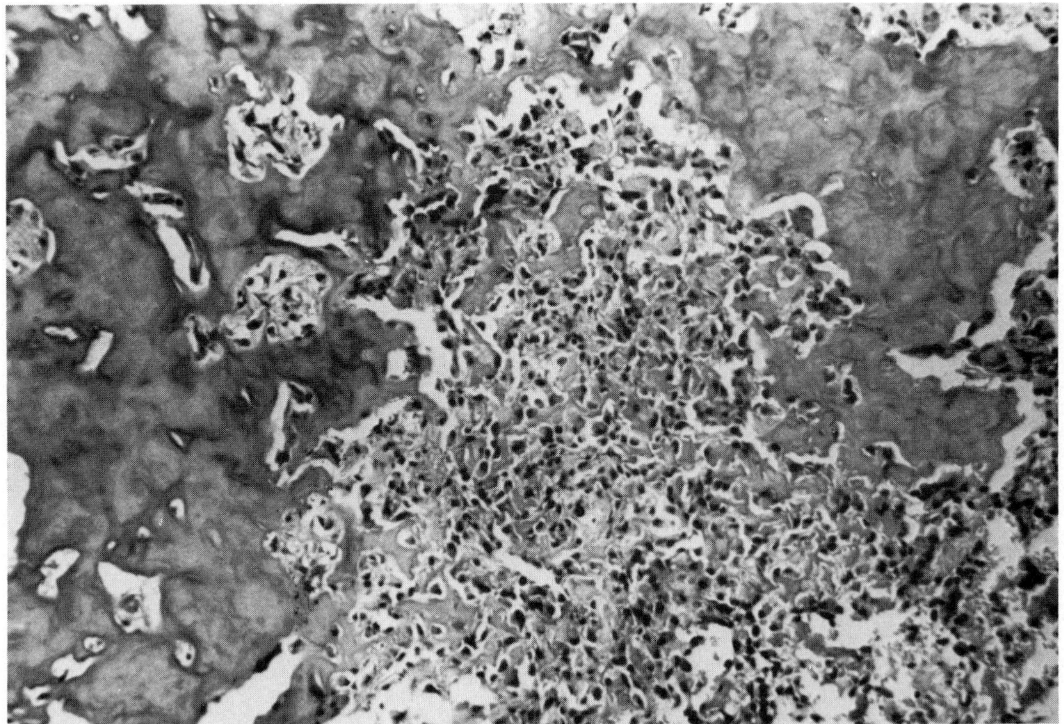

Figure 9–233. Osteoblastoma. Cellular lesion with more clearly defined trabeculae of osteoid and some mineralization.

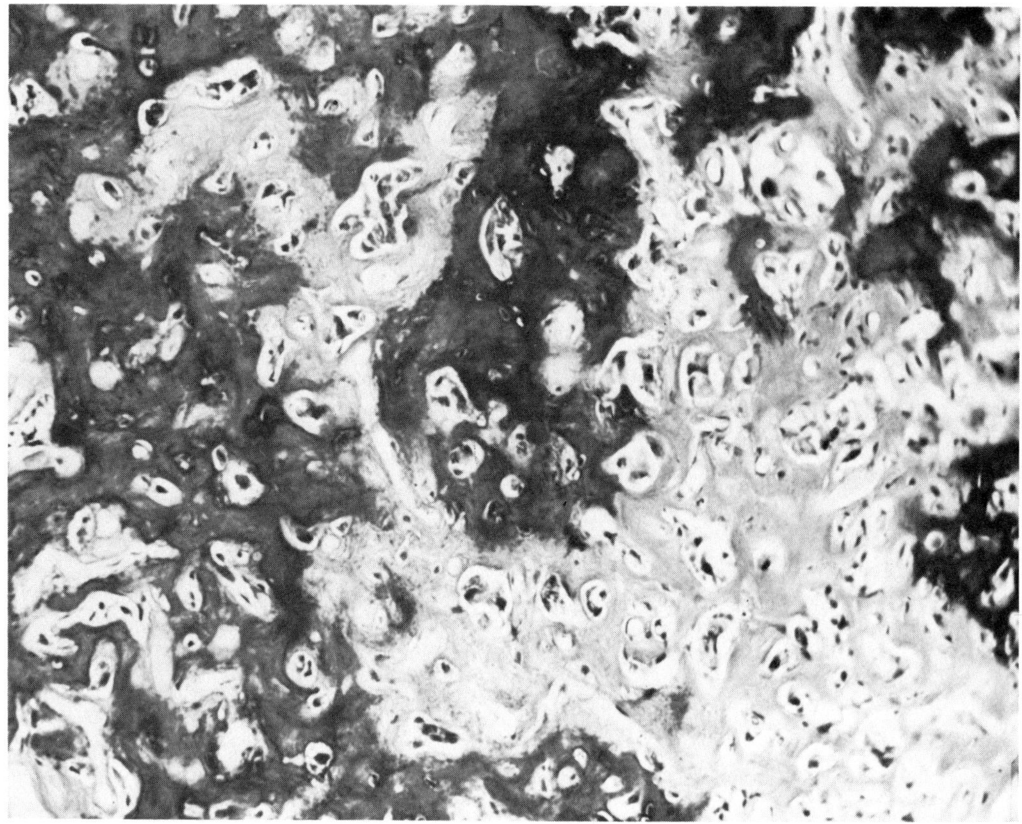

Figure 9–234. Osteoblastoma. Sclerotic focus in osteoblastoma. Extensive osteoid formation and mineralization reduce the cellular component. This represents a radiographically prominent older focus.

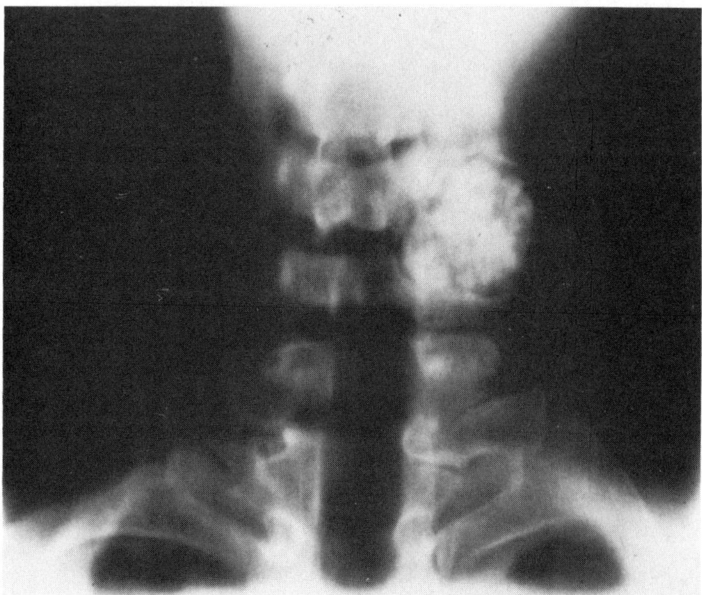

Figure 9–235. Osteoblastoma. Anteroposterior tomograph of cervical spine in a patient with a large osteoblastoma involving several contiguous vertebrae. The mineralized bone present makes the lesion clearly evident, and there is encroachment on the spinal canal.

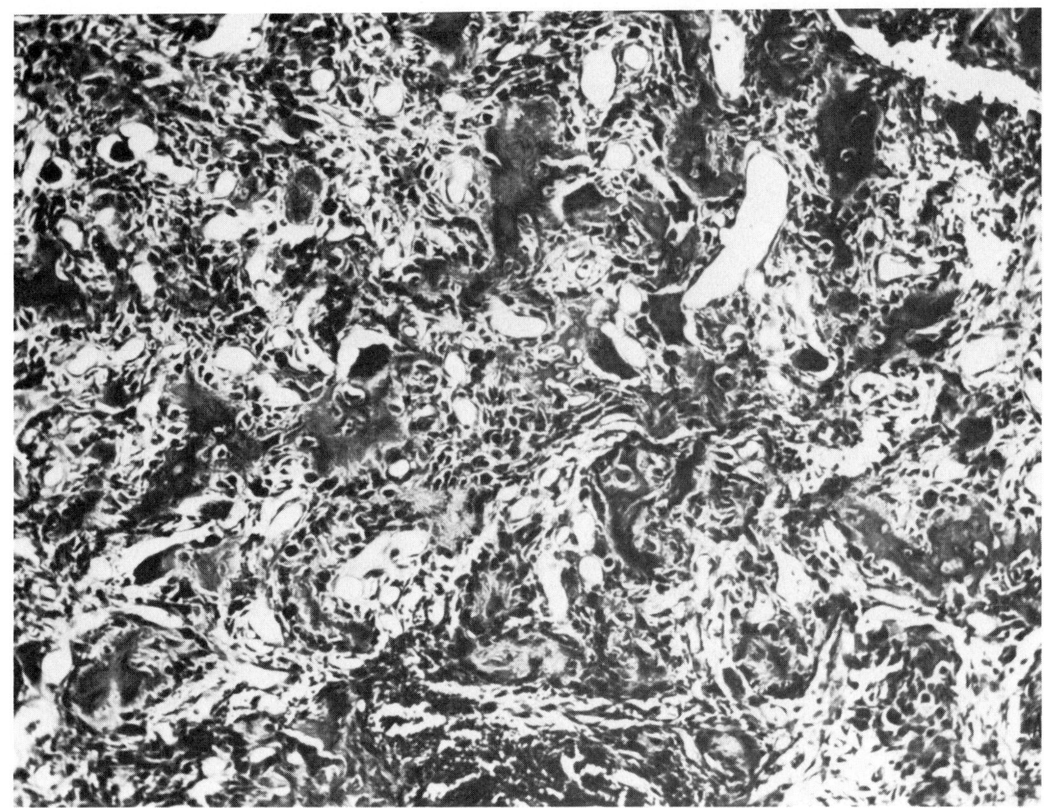

Figure 9–236. Osteoblastoma. Histologic appearance of a vascular focus in an osteoblastoma. Note the large, dilated vascular channels. If this area is activated by trauma or surgery, aneurysmal dilatation of the vessels can occur.

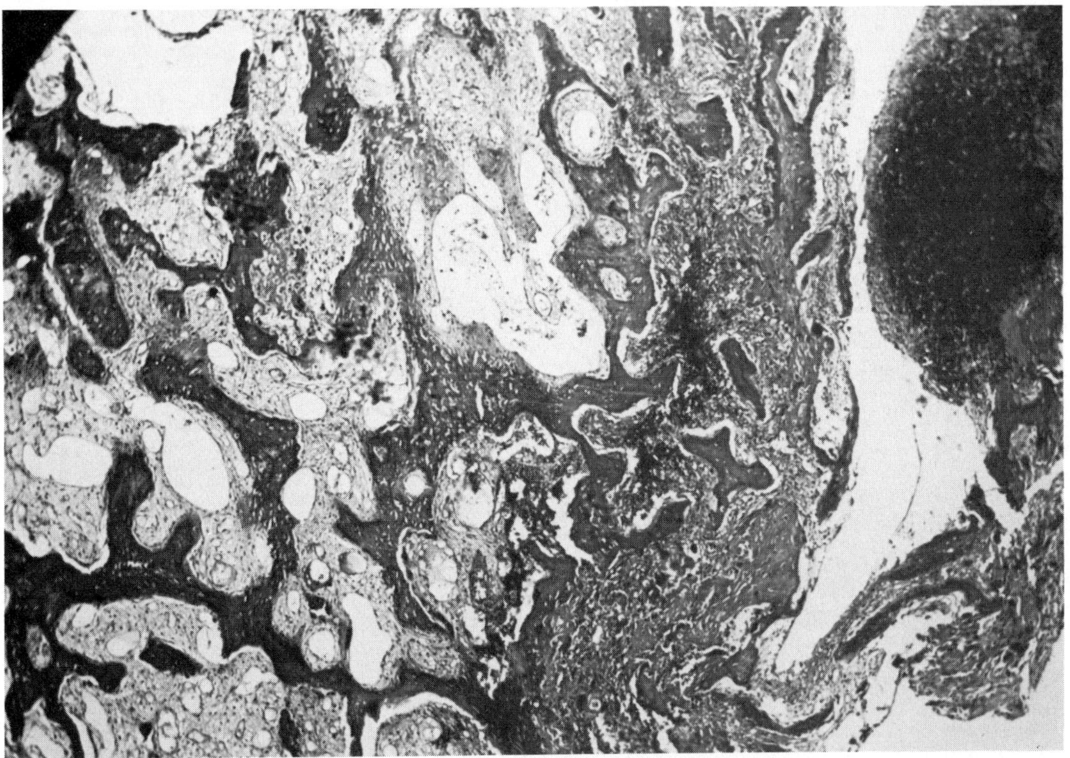

Figure 9–237. Osteoblastoma. Focus of aneurysmal cystic change in an area of osteoblastoma. Such change is a fairly common occurrence in osteoblastoma, presumably because of its frequent hypervascularity.

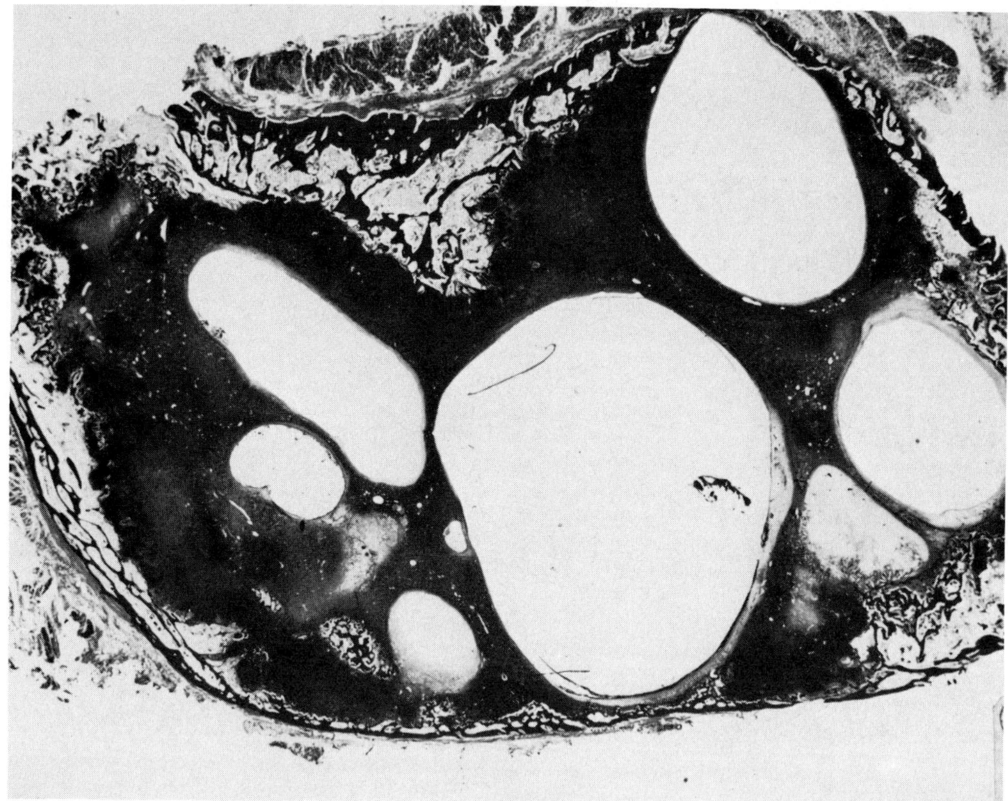

Figure 9–238. Osteoblastoma. Typical appearance of a lesion commonly diagnosed as aneurysmal bone cyst. The tissue evident between the cavities reveals an underlying osteoblastoma.

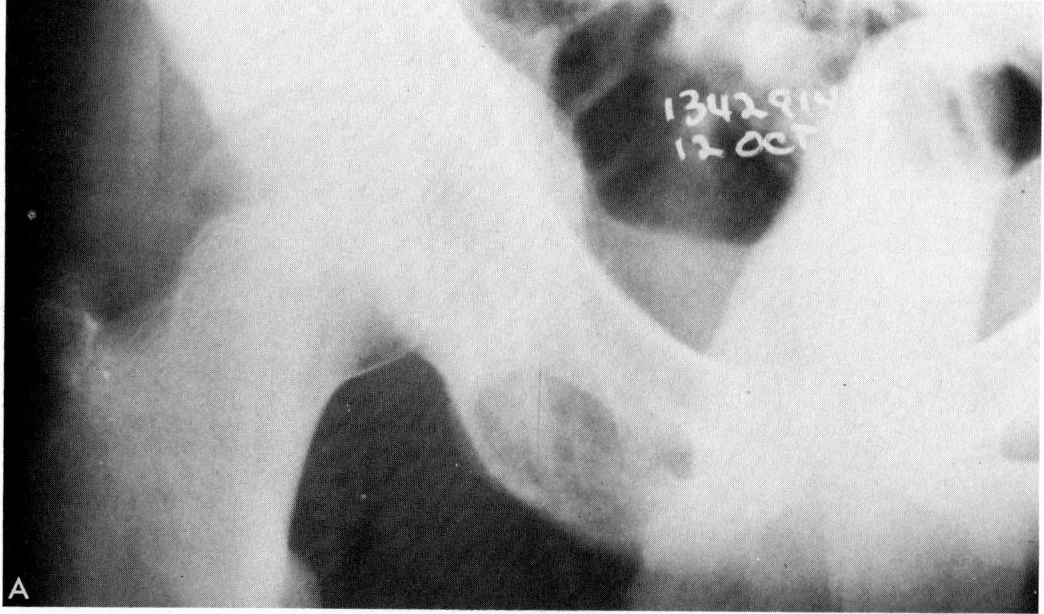

Figure 9–239. Osteoblastoma. Three-year progressive radiographic expansion of an osteoblastoma in the pubic ramus leading to aneurysmal bone cyst formation.

Illustration continued on opposite page

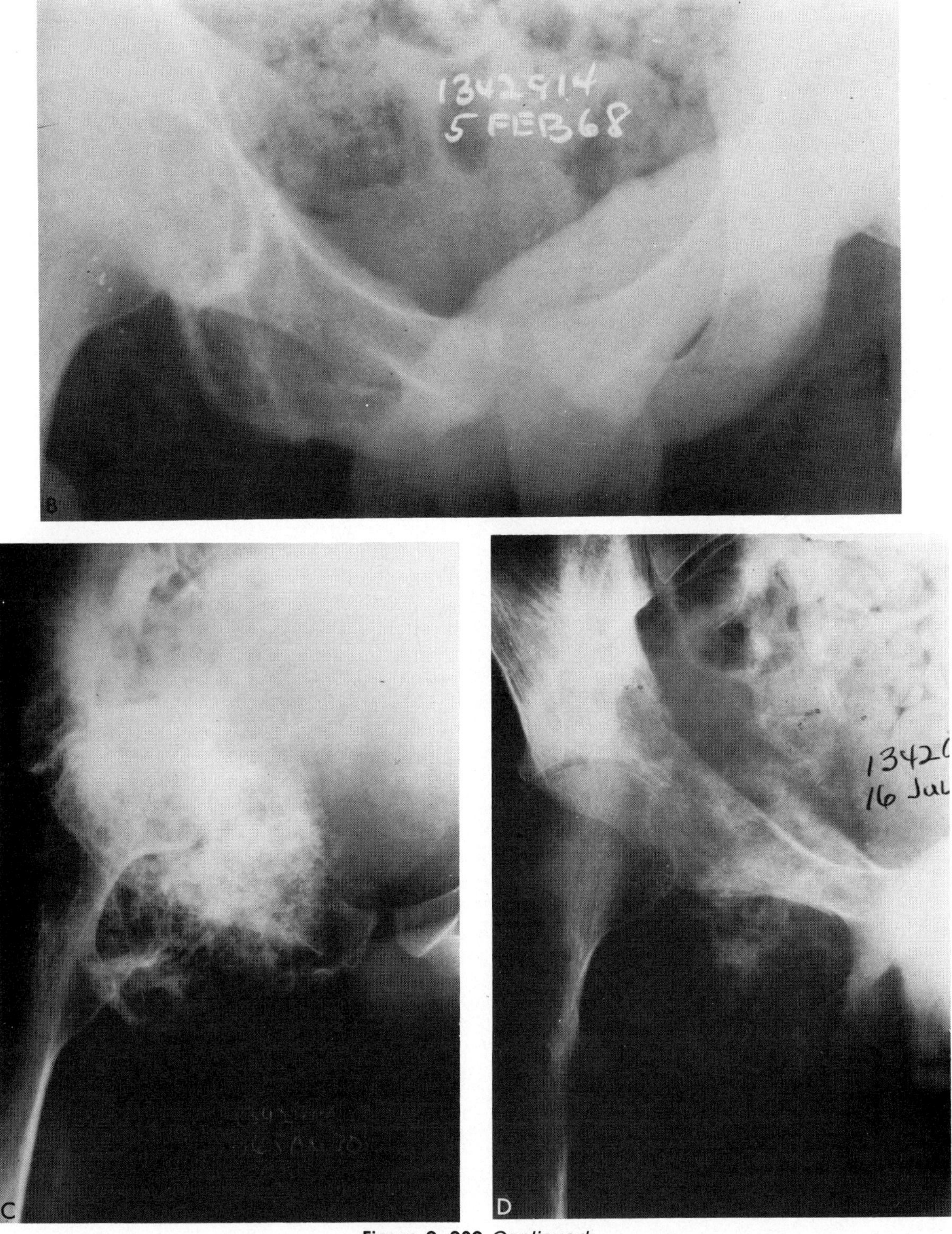

Figure 9–239 *Continued*

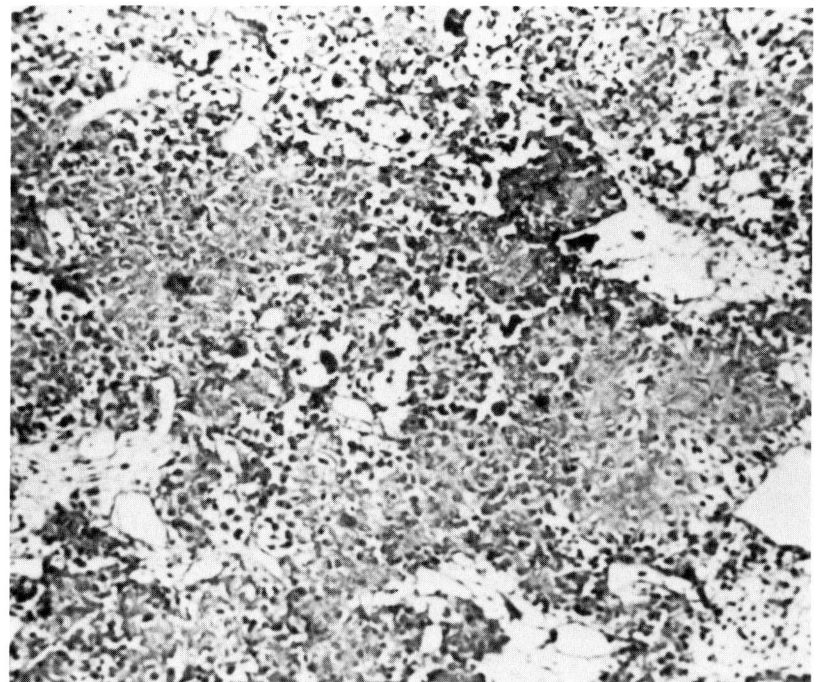

Figure 9–240. Osteoblastoma. Histologic appearance of initial biopsied specimen of the lesion illustrated in Figure 9–239A. Numerous osteoblasts, giant cells, primitive osteoid formation, and vascular spaces are present (see Fig. 9–230).

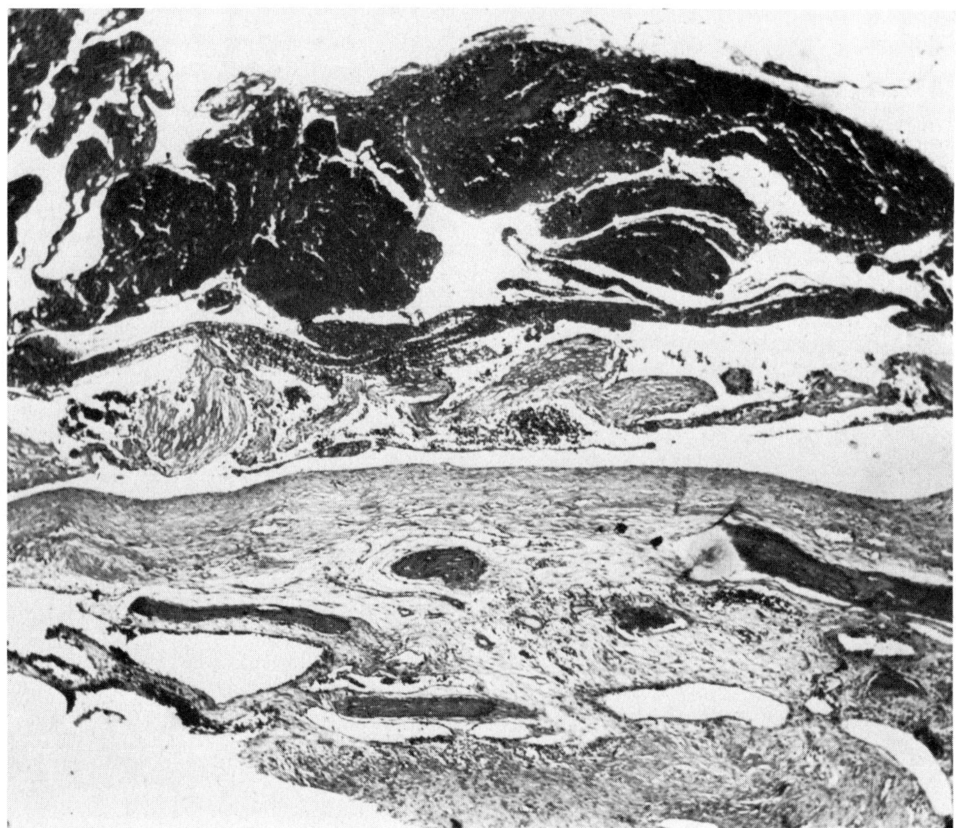

Figure 9–241. Osteoblastoma. Biopsied specimen of the lesion illustrated in the preceding two figures, obtained after progression to aneurysmal bone cyst. There are large vascular spaces present but no residual osteoblastic elements.

OSTEOSARCOMA

The osteosarcoma exhibits the radiographic features of a rapidly growing malignant process with poorly defined margins, permeative or moth-eaten destruction of bone, a classically metaphyseal or epiphyseal location, and evidence of neoplastic bone formation, although the latter feature may not always be present.

The histologic appearance of osteosarcoma varies extensively, but the diagnosis does not present difficulties. The lesion is usually an obvious malignant neoplasm, characterized by variation in size, shape, and staining characteristics of the osteoid-producing cells. Several types are identified, depending on the predominating histologic pattern. Categorization of separate tumor types is based on observation of such features as the degree of osteoid, cartilage, or fibrous matrix production and the presence of blood vessels, giant cells, or simple cellularity with little or no matrix production. There is no clear-cut relationship between cell type and survival (Scranton et al., 1975). Regardless of cell types, well-differentiated tumors are associated with a better prognosis than poorly differentiated tumors (Unni et al., 1977). Telangiectatic osteosarcomas are characterized by rapidly proliferating cells capable of removal of existing structures accompanied by numerous vascular channels. In these tumors, there is virtually no osteoid formation. Despite their unfavorable reputation, their prognosis is no worse than that associated with other histologic types (Huvos et al., 1982).

"Skip lesions" and multifocal lesions are described in the literature (Enneking and Kagan, 1975; Mahoney et al., 1979). Their significance is currently under debate. Although their possible presence would suggest the necessity for removing the entire bone when the osteosarcoma is being surgically treated, experience with only partial

Text continued on page 486

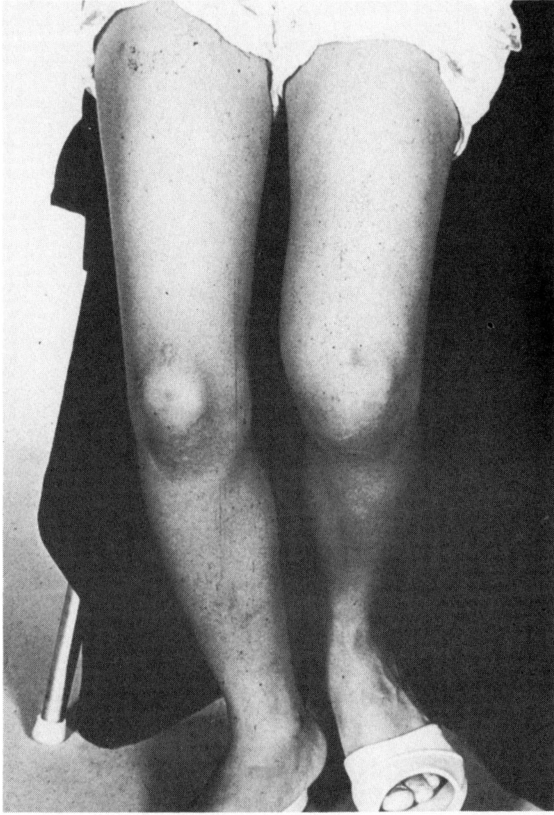

Figure 9–242. Osteosarcoma. Photograph of the lower limbs in a 13-year-old patient who fell and reported to the emergency room with a swollen knee. A history of trauma is a common presenting feature, but usually the trauma is minor and does not correspond to the severity of the physical or radiographic changes.

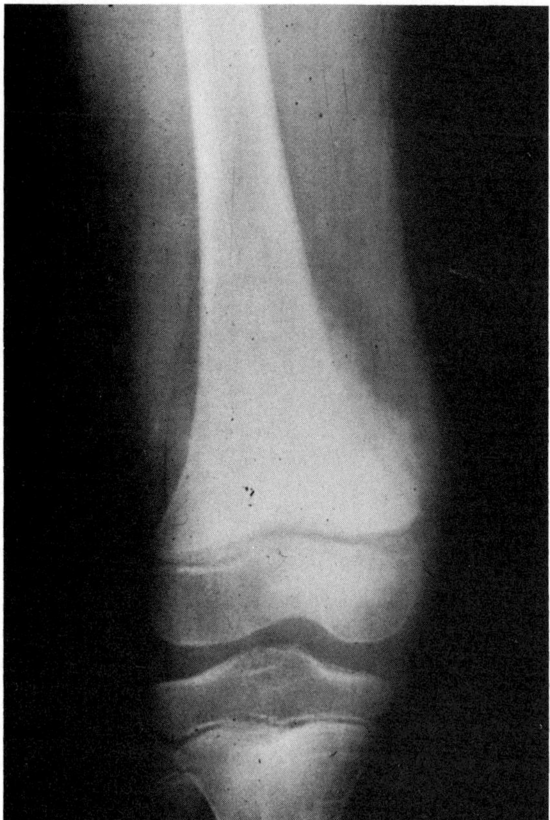

Figure 9–243. Osteosarcoma. Radiographic appearance of the left knee illustrated in Figure 9–242. The neoplasm is located in the metaphysis, expanding into the surrounding soft tissue with periosteal reaction and bony matrix formation. The increased density of the lesion is readily apparent.

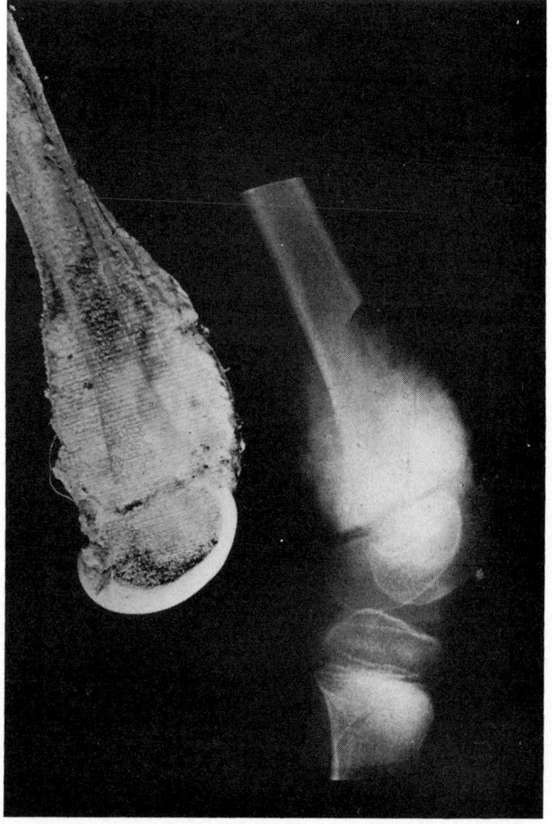

Figure 9–244. Osteosarcoma. Specimen radiograph and gross specimen exhibiting tumor involving the metaphysis and crossing the growth plate into the epiphysis. Note the presence of a characteristic Codman's triangle and extension of the tumor into soft tissue.

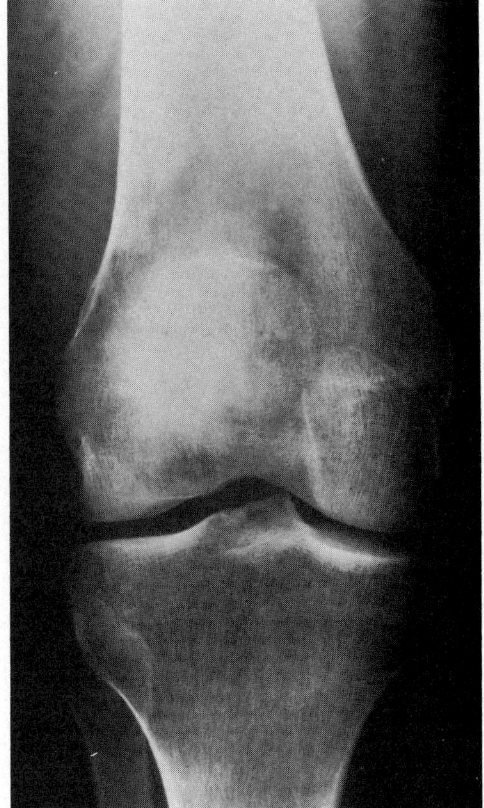

Figure 9–245. Osteosarcoma. Lytic defect in distal portion of femur with moth-eaten destruction of bone. There is no periosteal reaction, but the poor demarcation of the lesion indicates a malignant tumor.

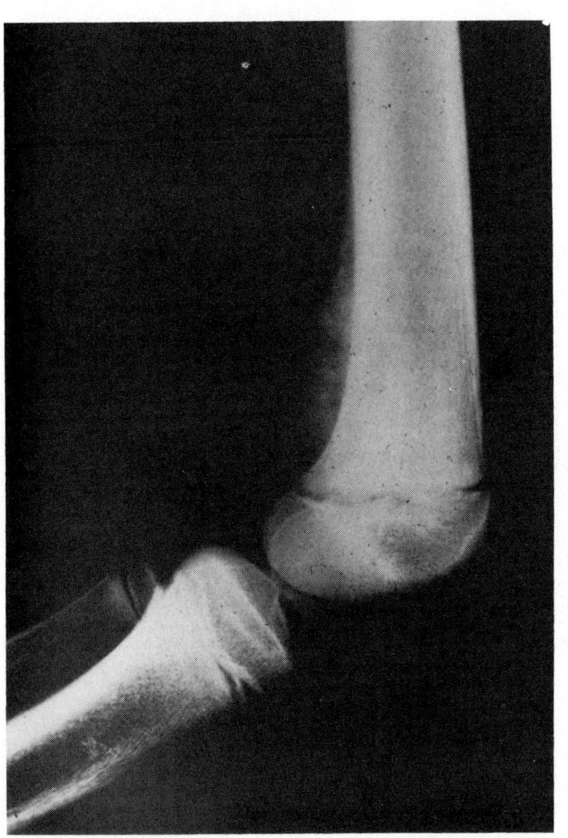

Figure 9–246. Osteosarcoma. Radiograph of an adolescent with osteosarcoma exhibiting periosteal reaction and permeative destruction of the lower distal femur.

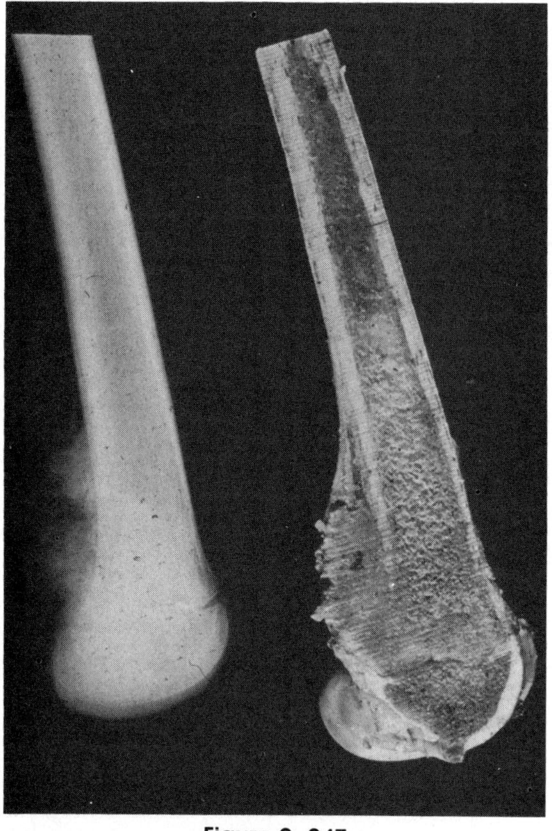

Figure 9–247

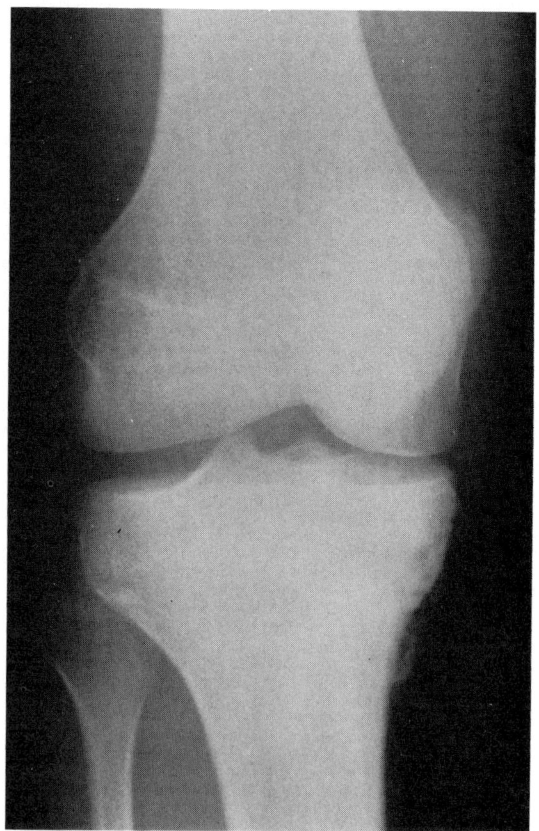

Figure 9–248

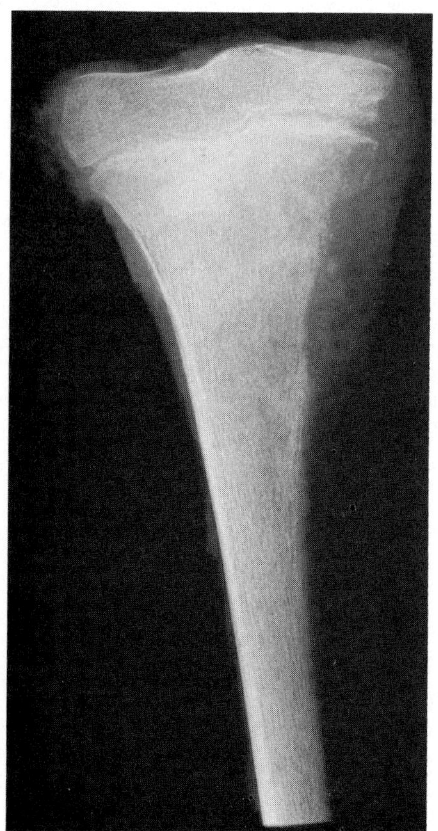

Figure 9–249

Figure 9–247. Osteosarcoma. Specimen radiograph and gross specimen exhibiting the extent of the tumor shown in Figure 9–246. Note crossing of the epiphyseal growth plate by the tumor and the characteristic Codman's triangle.

Figure 9–248. Osteosarcoma. Lesion located in the upper tibia demonstrating poorly circumscribed permeative destruction of the tibial bone and extension into the soft tissue.

Figure 9–249. Osteosarcoma. Specimen radiograph of lesion shown in Figure 9–248. Note the poorly defined permeative destructive pattern in the tibia and extension into the adjacent soft tissue.

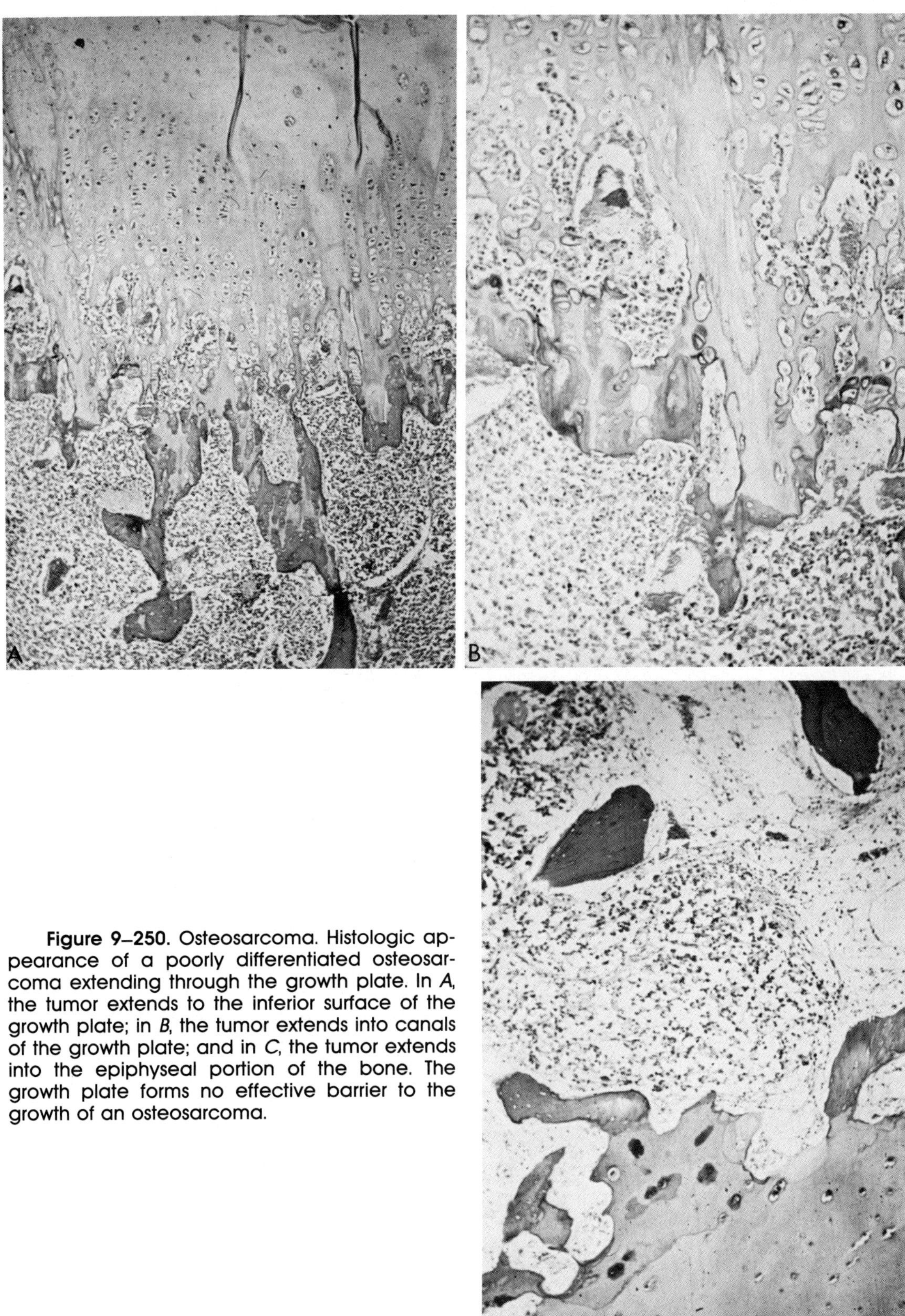

Figure 9–250. Osteosarcoma. Histologic appearance of a poorly differentiated osteosarcoma extending through the growth plate. In *A,* the tumor extends to the inferior surface of the growth plate; in *B,* the tumor extends into canals of the growth plate; and in *C,* the tumor extends into the epiphyseal portion of the bone. The growth plate forms no effective barrier to the growth of an osteosarcoma.

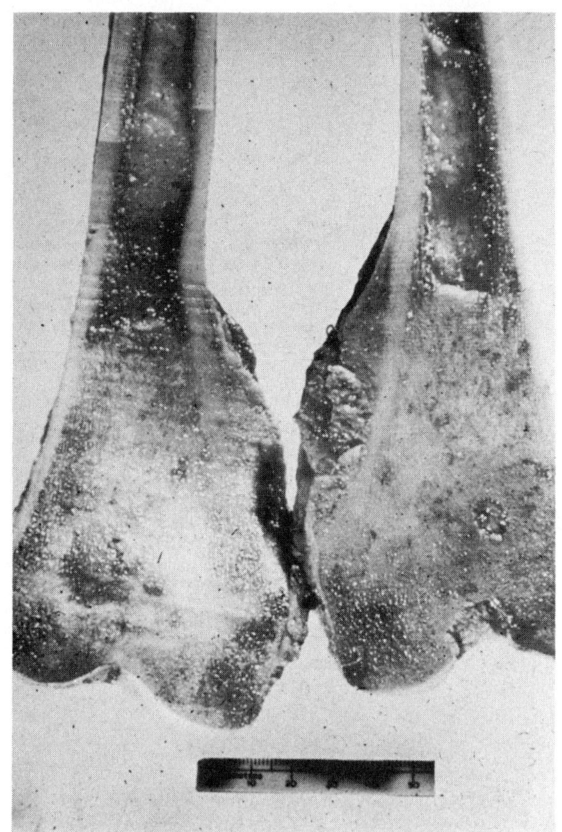

Figure 9–251. Osteosarcoma. Sclerotic osteosarcoma exhibiting dense sclerotic bone in the distal portion of the femur.

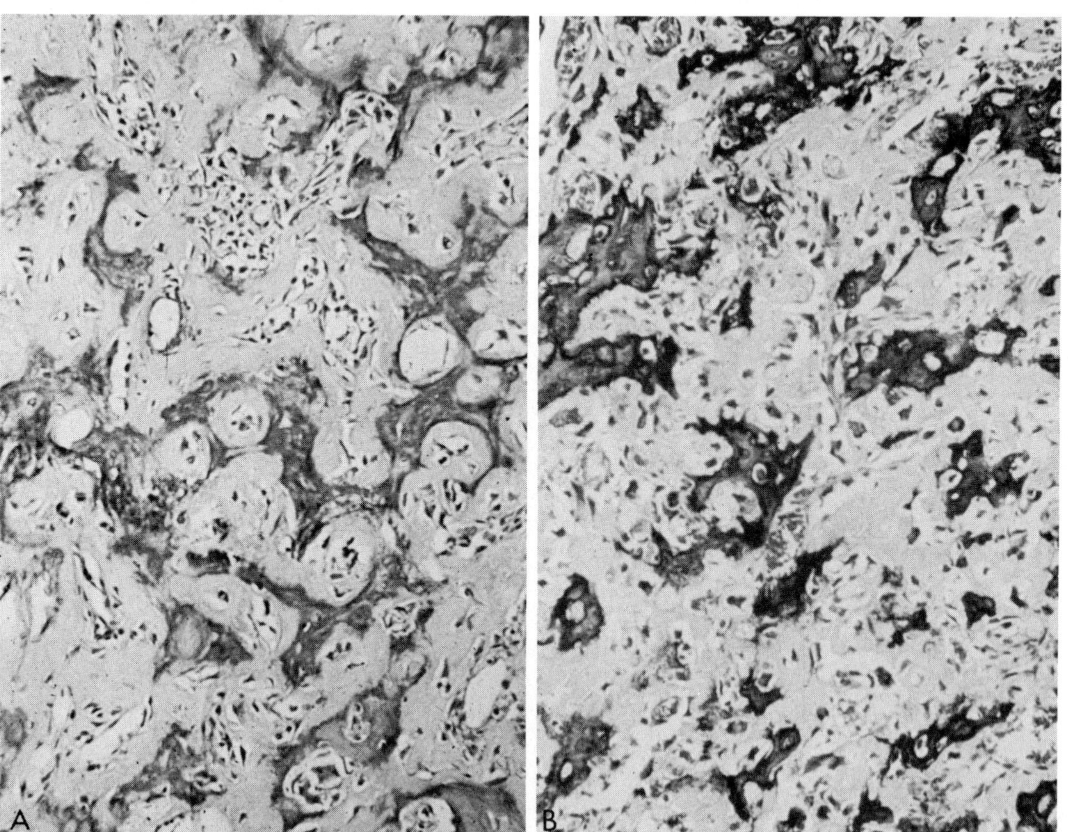

Figure 9–252. Osteosarcoma with extensive calcification of osteoid matrix. There is no convincing evidence that histologic type plays a role in survival. Grading of a tumor—any histologic subtype—is associated with survival.

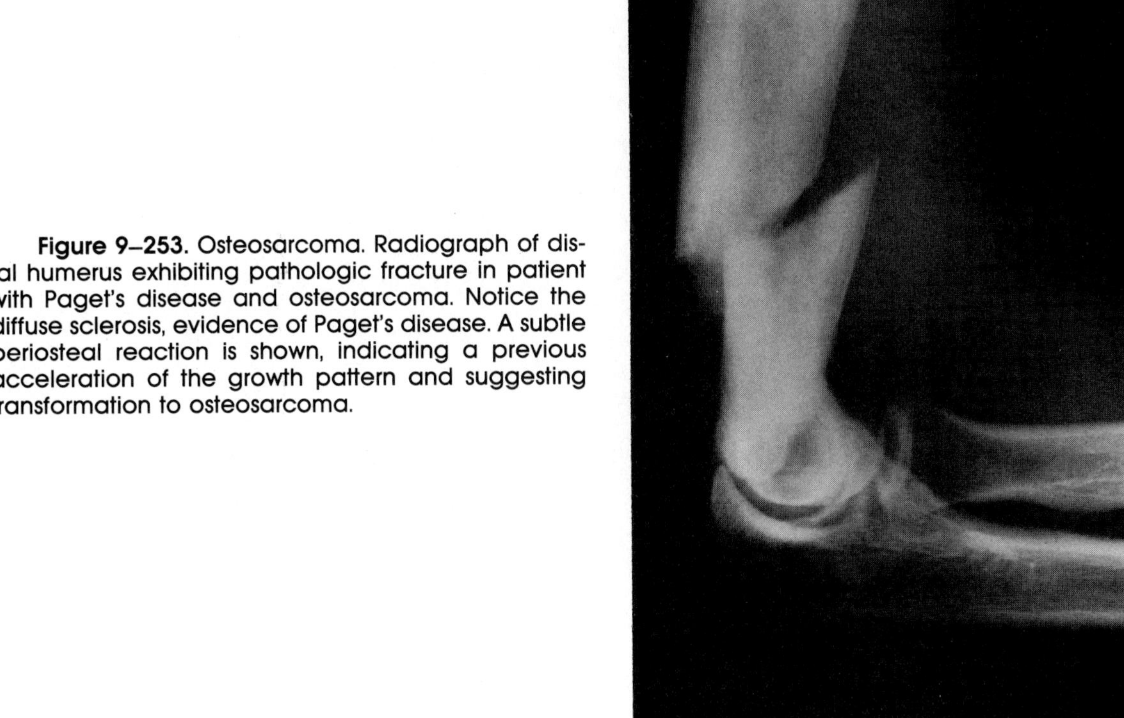

Figure 9–253. Osteosarcoma. Radiograph of distal humerus exhibiting pathologic fracture in patient with Paget's disease and osteosarcoma. Notice the diffuse sclerosis, evidence of Paget's disease. A subtle periosteal reaction is shown, indicating a previous acceleration of the growth pattern and suggesting transformation to osteosarcoma.

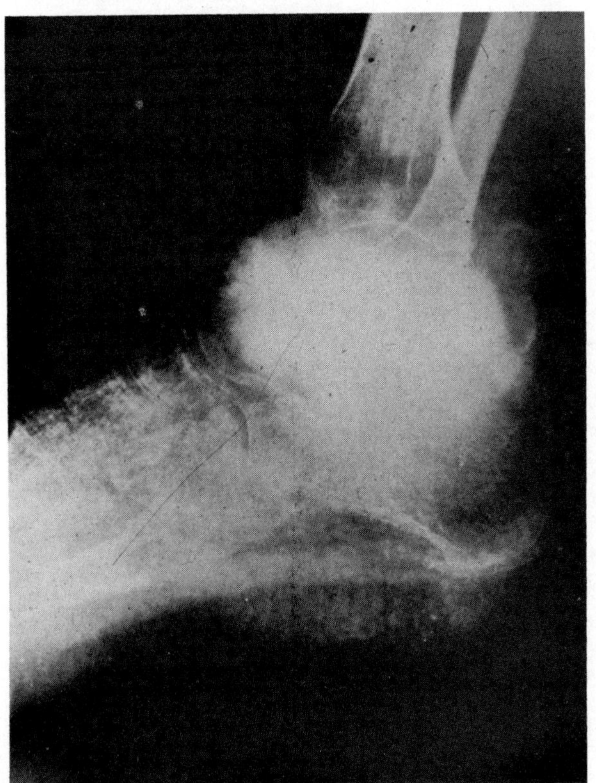

Figure 9–254. Osteosarcoma. Radiograph of osteosarcoma of the talus with expansion of the tumor beyond the confines of the bone.

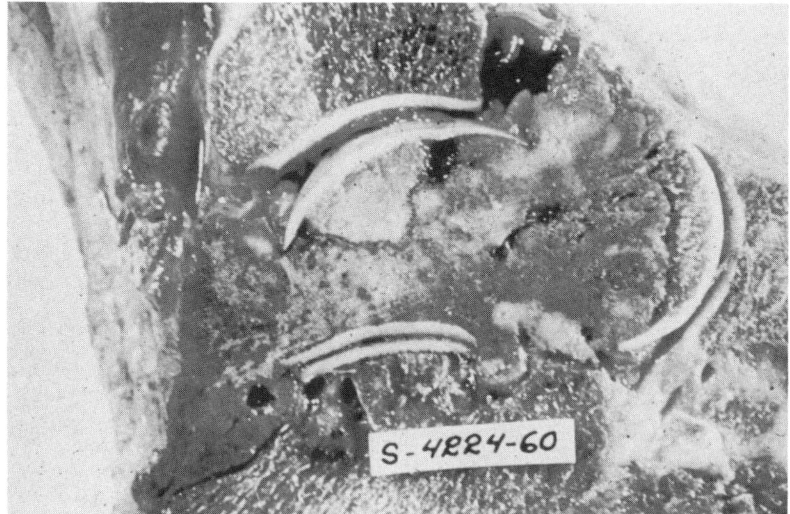

Figure 9–255. Osteosarcoma. Amputated specimen exhibiting the tumor expanding beyond the confines of the bone in all directions.

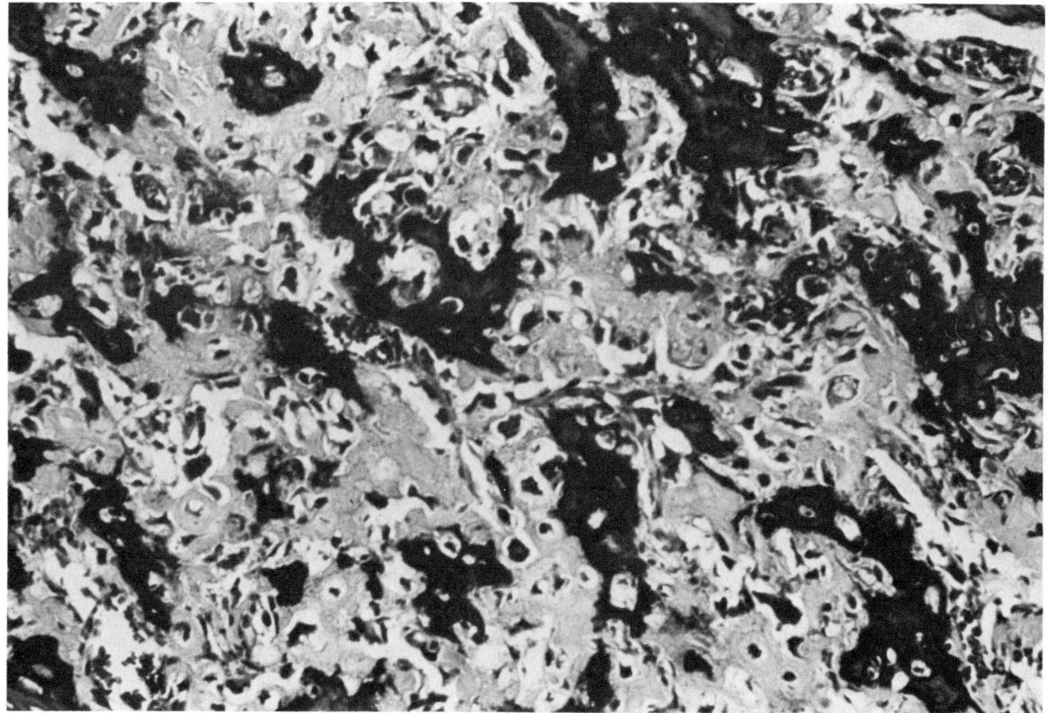

Figure 9–256. Osteosarcoma. Histologic pattern of osteosarcoma shown in Figures 9–254 and 9–255. Note the extensive sclerotic osteoid formation.

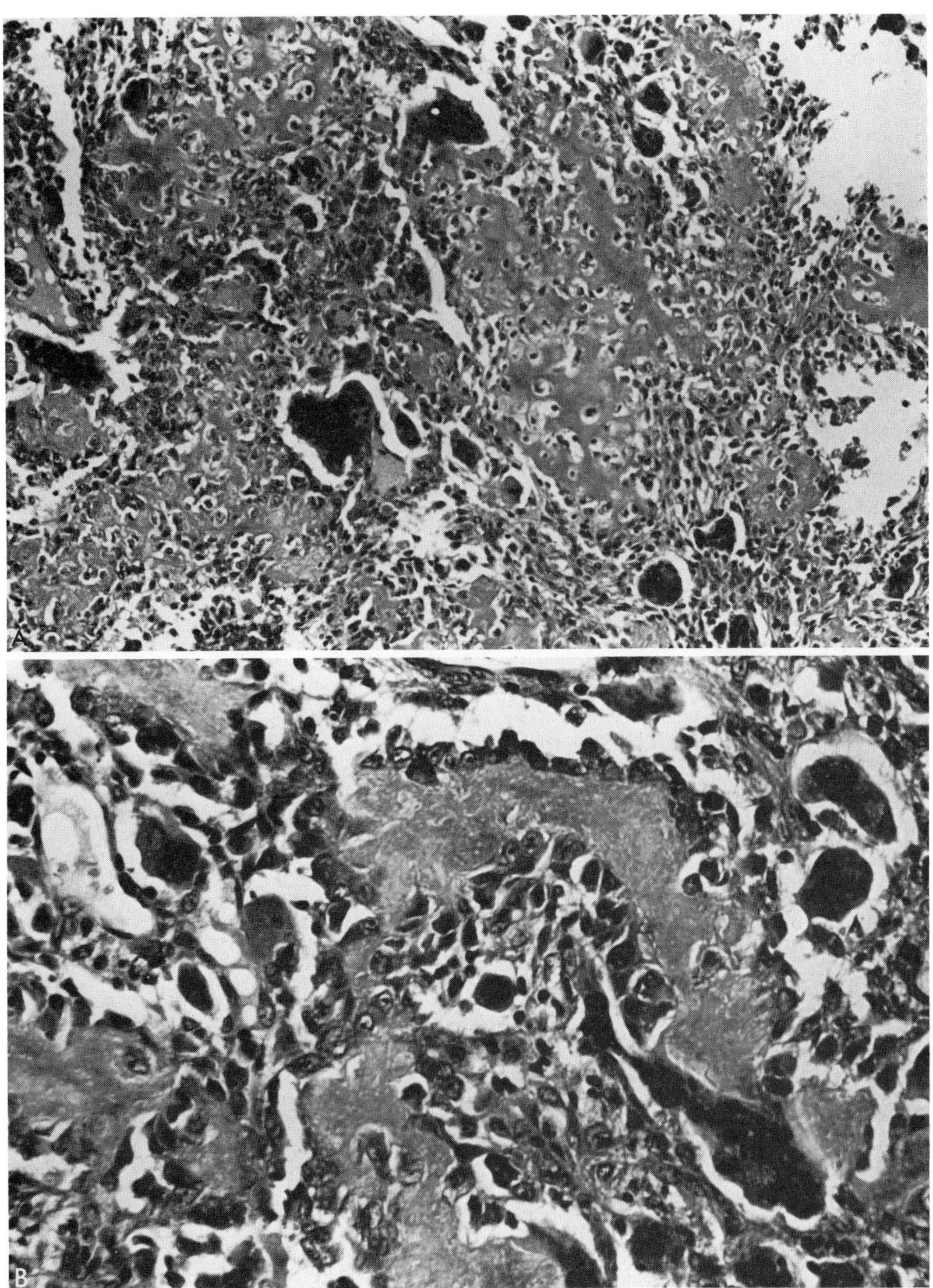

Figure 9–257. Osteosarcoma. Note the numerous giant cells. The tumor is characterized by marked pleomorphism, osteoid formation, and numerous large and pleomorphic giant cells.

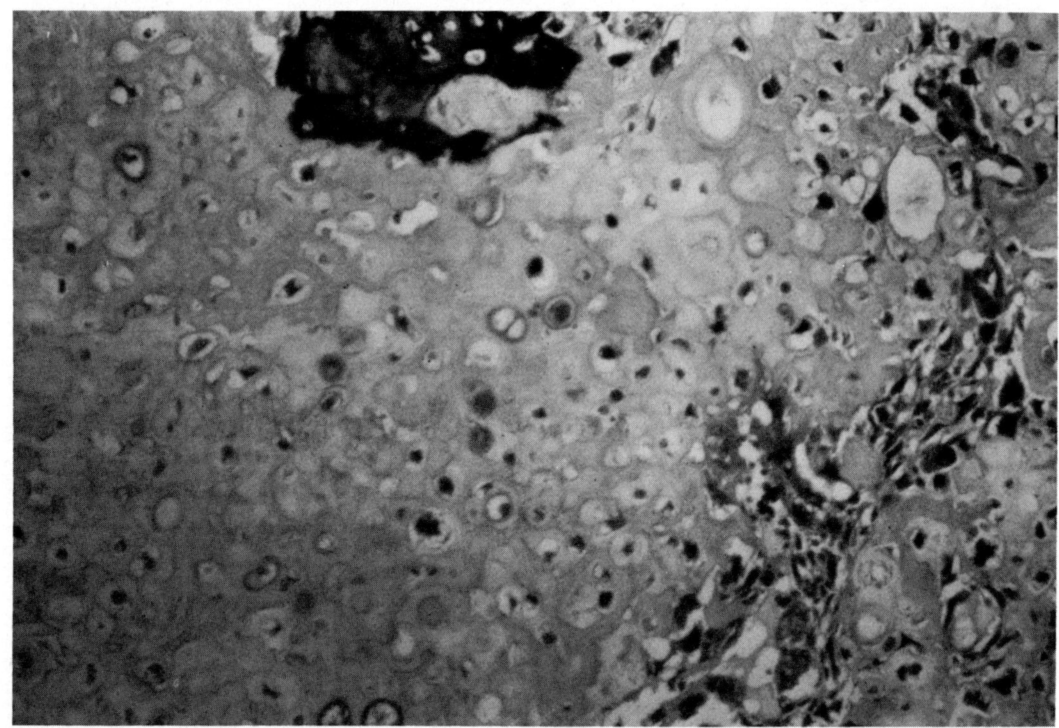

Figure 9–258. Osteosarcoma. A focus of malignant cartilage formation is evident. Clusters of pleomorphic cartilage cells may be present in any osteosarcoma.

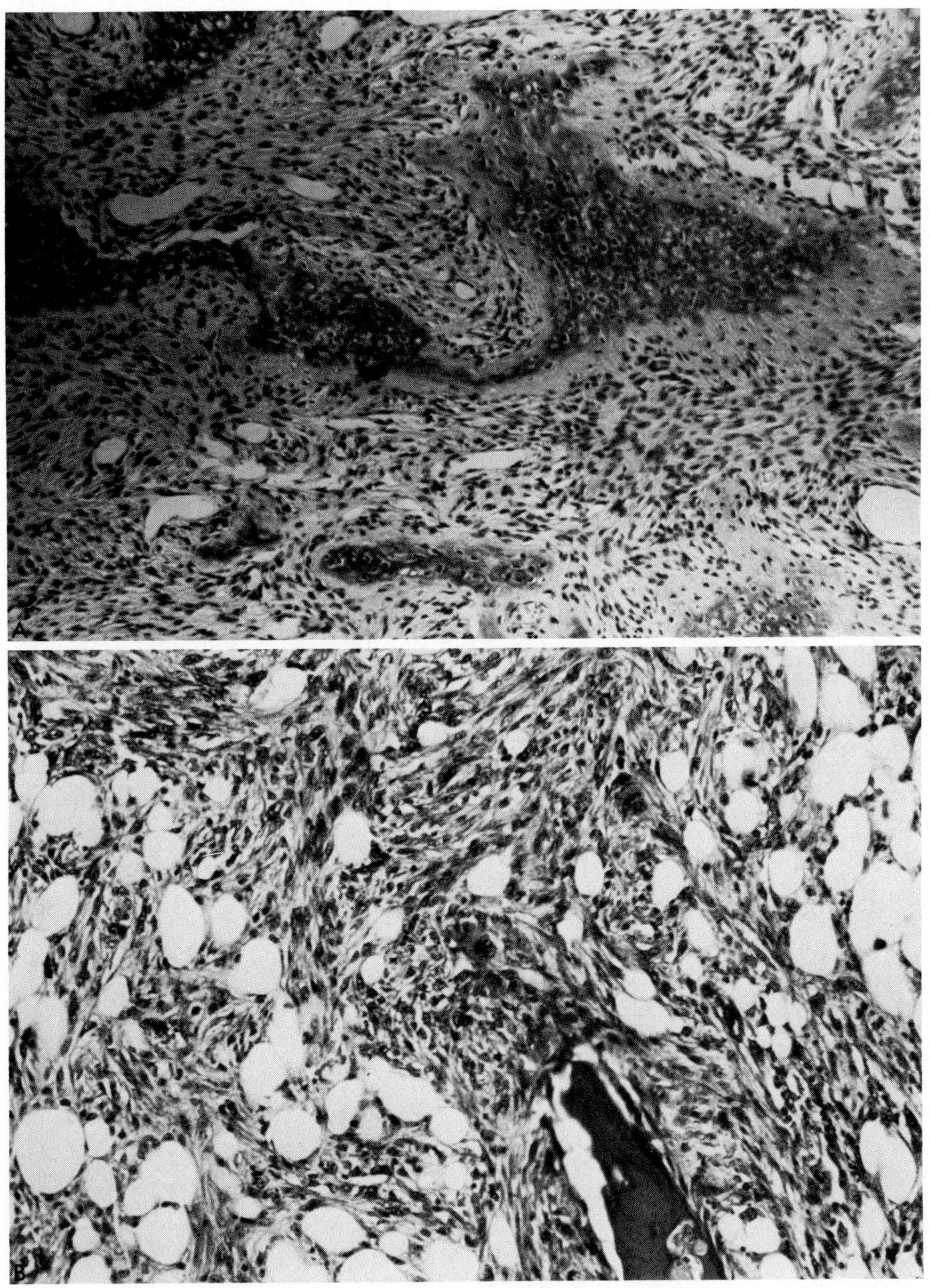

Figure 9–259. Osteosarcoma. Note the predominant fibrous pattern. The tumor is characterized by a spindled fibrous component with transformation to bone. There is some similarity to fibrous dysplasia, but the pleomorphism evident in this specimen indicates malignancy.

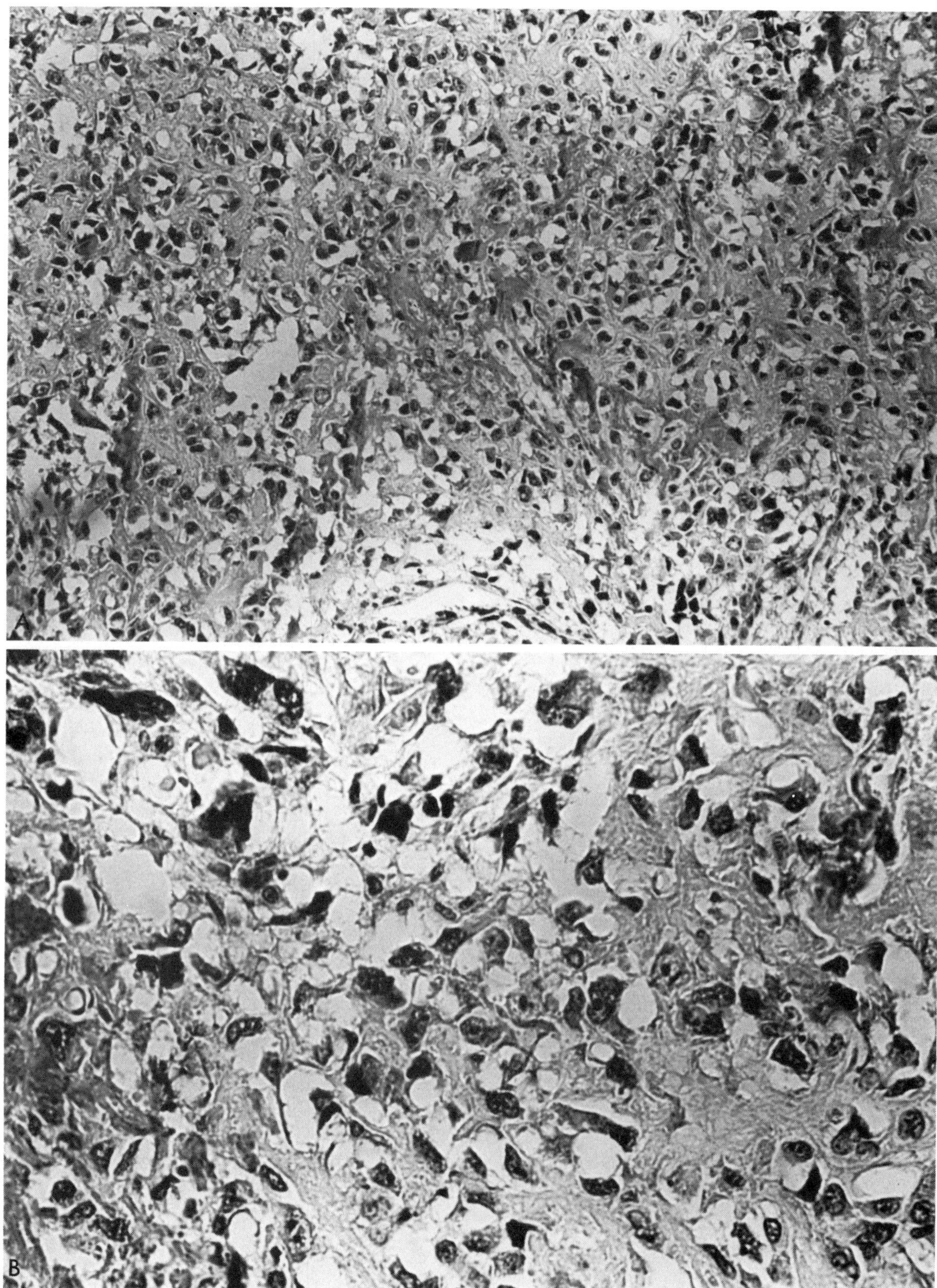

Figure 9–260. Osteosarcoma. Histologic appearance of a characteristic osteoid-producing osteosarcoma. The osteoblasts exhibit significant variation in cell size and shape, and osteoid formation is readily apparent. This lesion resembles osteoblastoma, but the pleomorphism indicates a malignant lesion.

Illustration continued on opposite page

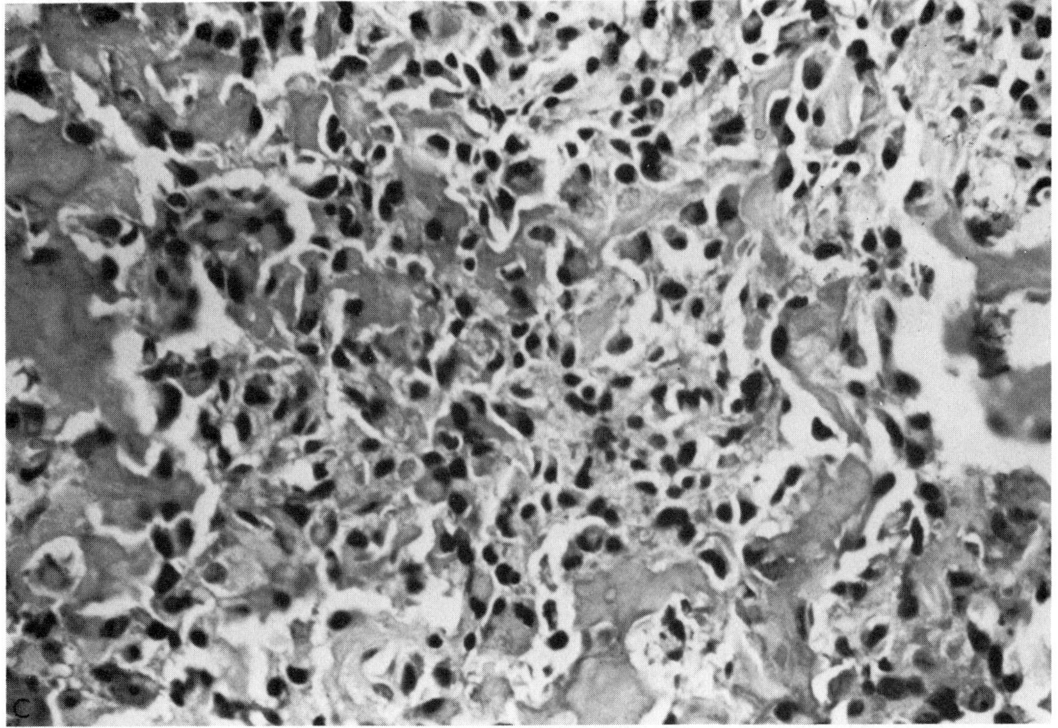

Figure 9–260 *Continued.*

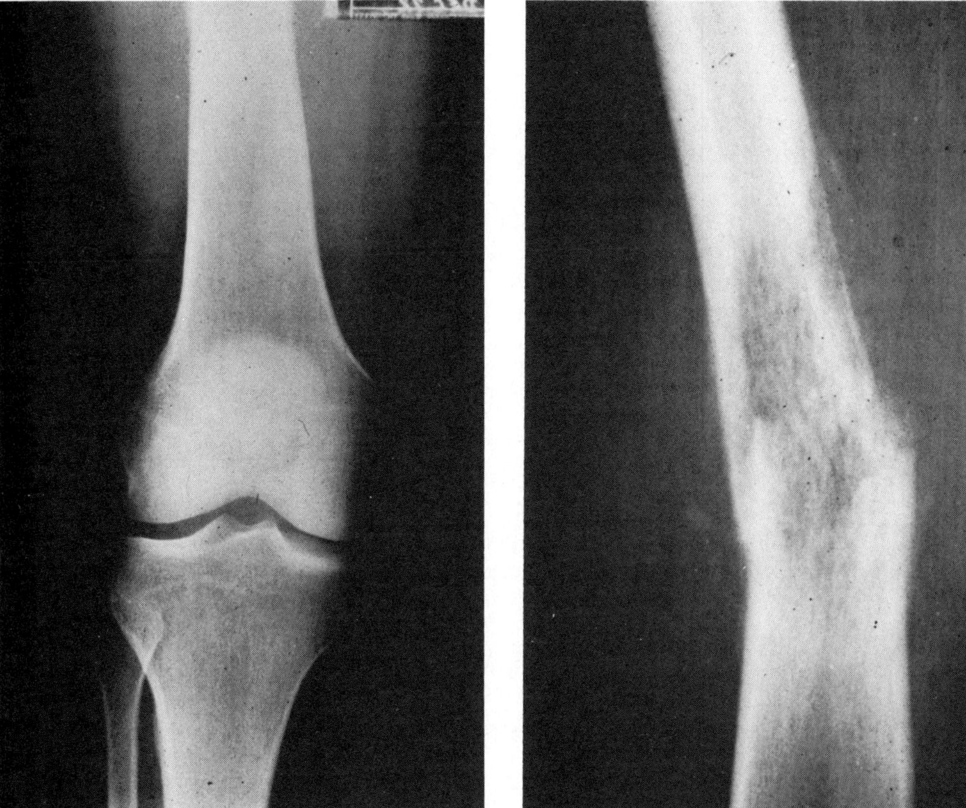

Figure 9–261. Osteosarcoma. Radiographic appearance of osteosarcoma in a 35-year-old female who complained of pain in the knee. Radiograph of the knee failed to reveal abnormality. During the radiographic examination, the patient suffered a pathologic fracture of the diaphysis. The lesion is obviously a malignant neoplasm, with permeative destruction and a Codman's triangle. The location and age are atypical for osteosarcoma but may reflect a long latent period before spurt in growth.

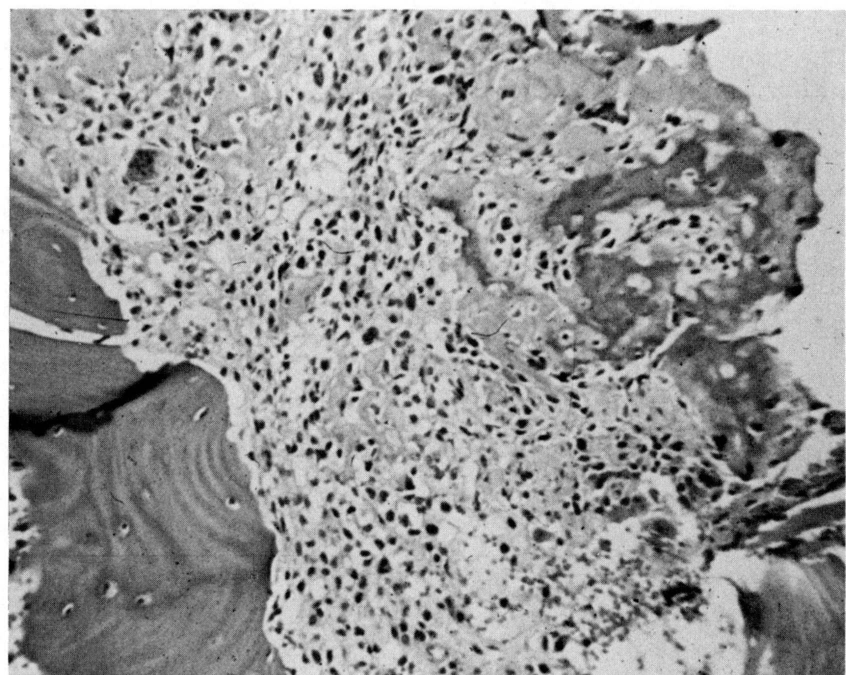

Figure 9–262. Osteosarcoma. Histologic appearance of osteoid-producing neoplasm shown in Figure 9–261. Note pleomorphic osteoblasts.

removal of the bone and the placement of a prosthesis does not appear to increase the risk of recurrence. Possibly, vigorous preoperative chemotherapy and radiation therapy are responsible for the ablation or control of skip lesions.

The incidence of osteosarcoma is highest in late adolescence and during the early 20s, coexisting with the cessation of skeletal growth and major internal remodeling. The second highest incidence is noticed in late adulthood, not only coexisting with the incidence of Paget's disease of bone but also indicating a true rise in incidence among the older adults who seem to have no evidence of Paget's disease.

Osteosarcoma is currently under aggressive investigation as a candidate for (1) new forms of therapy, including preoperative radiation and chemotherapy (Rosen et al., 1979), and (2) a valid prognostic reappraisal. The current prognostic view is more favorable than it was 20 or 30 years ago. Whether this optimism is justified (and preoperative therapy, selectivity of patient population, and/or more effective surgery really play a role in improved cure rates) or whether the biologic behavior of the tumor has changed has not yet been decided (Dahlin, 1979).

GIANT CELL TUMOR (OSTEOCLASTOMA)

The giant cell tumor of bone is a lesion that has aroused much controversy in the past with regard to etiology, site of origin, neoplastic vs. non-neoplastic state, therapy, and ultimate biologic potential. The opinions expressed in this syllabus are basically those taught by Dr. Lent Johnson of the Armed Forces Institute of Pathology; however, different viewpoints will be identified whenever possible to allow vital discussion whenever therapeutic implications are involved.

The giant cell tumor of bone is a tumor of osteoclasts and not a reactive process.

The lesion originates in the metaphysis (Bogumill et al., 1972). As opposed to chondroblastomas, all giant cell tumors of bone have the majority of their lesion on the metaphyseal side of the growth plate. When a giant cell tumor is seen in a patient whose growth plate has not fused it is always metaphyseal in location. On the basis of this fact, one must assume that the lesion originates in the metaphysis adjacent to the growth plate and expands into the epiphyseal portion of the bone once the growth plate has fused. Many observers deny the existence of a purely metaphyseal giant cell tumor. They claim that the tumor occurs in young adults and not in children. It appears illogical to us to assume that of all neoplasms of bone, only the giant cell tumor cannot be seen in the first 15 years of life, and yet as soon as the growth plate is fused, a significant number of large tumors suddenly appear, involving both metaphysis and epiphysis.

The early lesion is located eccentrically in the bone, but as it grows over time, the lesion will involve the full diameter of the bone, even when the tibia or femur is involved. It is sharply circumscribed expansile lesion, with a rather characteristic bubble pattern. These bubbles and delineating lines are really reactive trabeculae of bone formed by appositional bone growth. The giant cell tumor, removing numerous trabeculae by its neoplastic growth, prompts reinforcement of the remaining trabeculae, resulting in the "bubble" pattern.

As a rule, the giant cell tumor does not penetrate through the cortex, and there is usually no associated laminated or spiculed periosteal reaction. The tumor expands the cortex; that is, there is removal of cortex from the inside and deposition of periosteal new bone on the outer surface. If the tumor is aggressive, periosteal new bone formation may not be able to keep pace with the rate of bone destruction, and the tumor is contained solely by the fibrous periosteum. The periosteum itself is not often broached by the tumor, nor is the articular cartilage. The lesion is lytic, with no identifiable matrix production on radiographs.

Histologically, the lesion consists of giant cells and stromal cells with varying amounts of vascularity. The stromal cell is similar to the giant cell, and there should be no discernible difference between the nuclei of the giant cell and the stromal cell. Minimal amounts of osteoid may be seen, but large deposition of osteoid is not consistent with a giant cell tumor. The lesion can be graded on the basis of the degree of pleomorphism of the stromal and giant cell components. These grades are somewhat subjective and depend on the individual observer. Although it is possible to differentiate distinct grades of giant cell tumor, the purpose of this grading is to predict malignant behavior. However, regardless of the grade, occasional giant cell tumors have unpredictable malignant potential, and even grade 1 tumors have been known to metastasize (Unni and Dahlin, 1979).

Several giant cell tumors have been shown to be malignant from their inception. These tumors exhibit histologic changes consisting of variation in size, shape, staining characteristics, and mitotic activity that identify them as malignant tumors. Their radiographic appearance is malignant, with periosteal reaction and permeative to moth-eaten destruction of adjacent bone evident. They are to be differentiated from the usual giant cell tumor, which can be treated with more conservative methods.

It is important to ensure that the giant cell tumor is completely removed the first time surgical intervention is planned. The surgeon contemplating curettage should remember that giant cell tumors tend to invade adjacent structures slowly. The trabeculae that are permeated by the osteoclasts of the tumor will persist for some time after involvement; the tumor is therefore beyond the inner ridge of trabeculae. Curettage removes only the contents of the cavity. There is no removal of the contents of the area beyond the cavity that is formed by the reactive remnants of bone unless a conscious effort is made to curette the ridge of trabeculae forming the outer shell of the cavity. Failure to do so accounts for the extremely high recurrence rate documented in the literature. Recurrence is an expression of inadequate removal.

Much has been written about appropriate therapy for the giant cell tumor. Johnson and coworkers (1962) and Marcove and colleagues (1978) recommend sterilization of the cavity after curettage. Sterilization can be carried out by several methods, including cryosurgery as well as chemical cautery with phenol. The intent of both methods is the same: eradication of all cellular elements extending beyond the reach of the curette. The giant cell tumor, with its propensity to invade just beyond the limits of curettage, requires this type of sterilization in order to avoid recurrence. The 1978 data of Marcove, based on his observations gathered during performance of cryosurgery, indicate virtual elimination of recurrence. Likewise in our experience (G.P.B.), the rate of recurrence following appropriate surgery and phenolization has been virtually eliminated. Therapy remains controversial. There is general agreement that en-bloc resection of the tumor at the first operation is the procedure of choice in those bones that can be spared (ulna, clavicle, fibula) or in those in which fusion can provide good function (ankle, wrist, finger). At the knee, resection creates major reconstructive problems. Curettage with phenol or liquid nitrogen is the preferred therapy.

Differential Diagnosis. Hyperparathyroidism may produce lytic defects in bone with numerous giant cells. A brown tumor usually exhibits a much more cellular, spindled stroma, and there is a pronounced difference between the appearance of the giant cell and that of the stromal cell.

Codman described the chondroblastoma as an "epiphyseal giant cell tumor." The majority of the lesion is located within the epiphysis. Occasionally, borderline lesions make differential diagnosis between giant cell tumors and chondroblastoma difficult, but the center of the lesion will be either above or below the epiphyseal growth plate, and the lesion will therefore give a clue to its site of origin. Histologic analysis reveals chondroid substance and "chicken-wire" calcification, classic for chondroblastoma and not seen in the giant cell tumor of bone.

The osteoblastoma may contain a large number of giant cells, but extensive osteoid formation and numerous osteoblasts are not features of a giant cell tumor of bone.

An osteosarcoma with a prominent giant cell component can be confused with a giant cell tumor of bone. The more malignant radiographic appearance and the poorly differentiated neoplastic osteoid formation should serve to differentiate the osteosarcoma from a giant cell tumor.

The nonossifying fibroma of bone is eccentric and metaphyseal, almost always at some distance from the growth plate. As a rule, the radiographic appearance creates no difficulty in differentiating it from the giant cell tumor of bone. In atypical locations, however, the spindled fibrous stroma and occasional giant cells should serve to distinguish it from the uniform giant and stromal cell found in the giant cell tumor.

Fibrosarcoma may have numerous giant cells, but location, malignant radiographic appearance, the presence of malignant fibrous stroma should serve to alert the histologist that he is not dealing with a bona fide osteoclastoma.

The giant cell tumor of tendon sheath (nodular synovitis) may invade and replace bone. Although giant cells are plentiful in these lesions, the stroma contains numerous xanthomatous and fibrous components, not present in giant cell tumor.

Giant cells are ubiquitous; they may be present in any lesion of bone, benign, malignant, or reactive. Their presence must be gauged in the context of other associated findings. The mere presence of occasional or even numerous giant cells does not signify a diagnostic entity.

Text continued on page 523

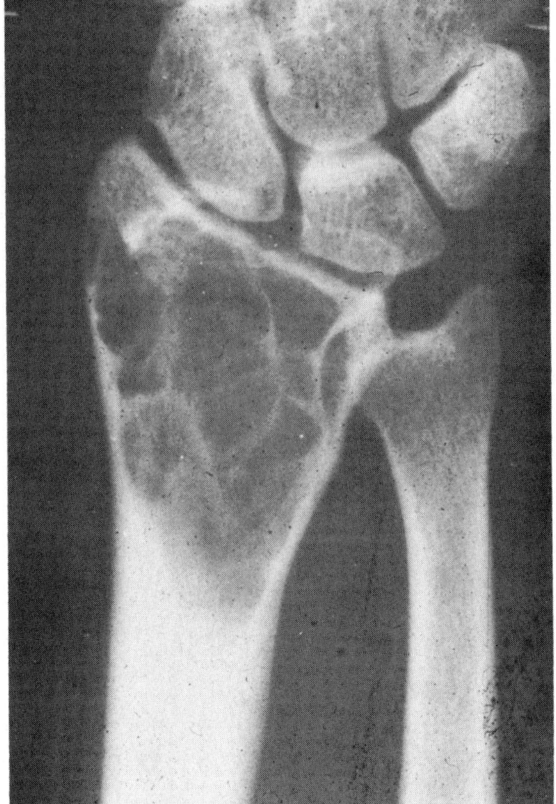

Figure 9–263. Giant cell tumor. Radiograph of the wrist demonstrating an expansible bubbly defect in the distal portion of the radius. There is involvement of metaphyseal and epiphyseal portions of the bone. Note the absence of a periosteal reaction.

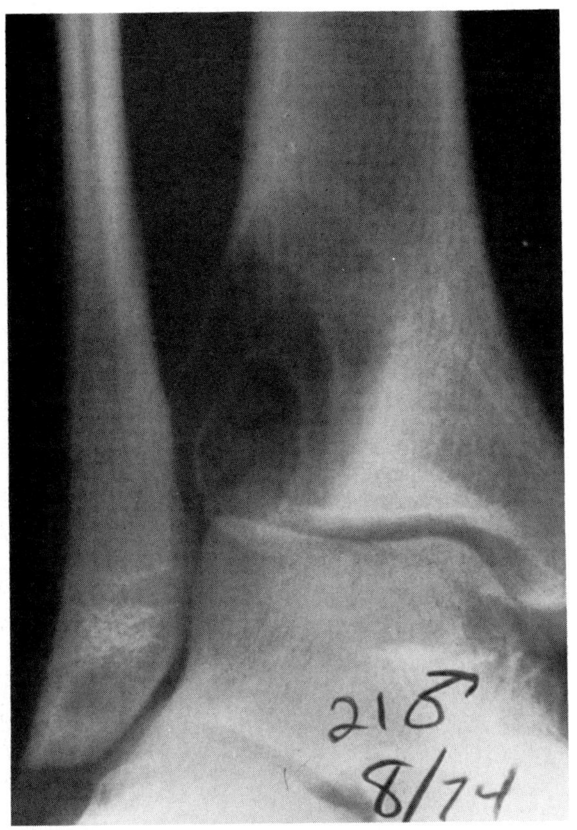

Figure 9–264. Giant cell tumor. Radiograph of distal tibia showing an eccentric radiolucent defect in the metaphysis and epiphysis extending to the articular surface. There are rings suggesting cortical "windows" of various size that are due to bone removal by tumor cells.

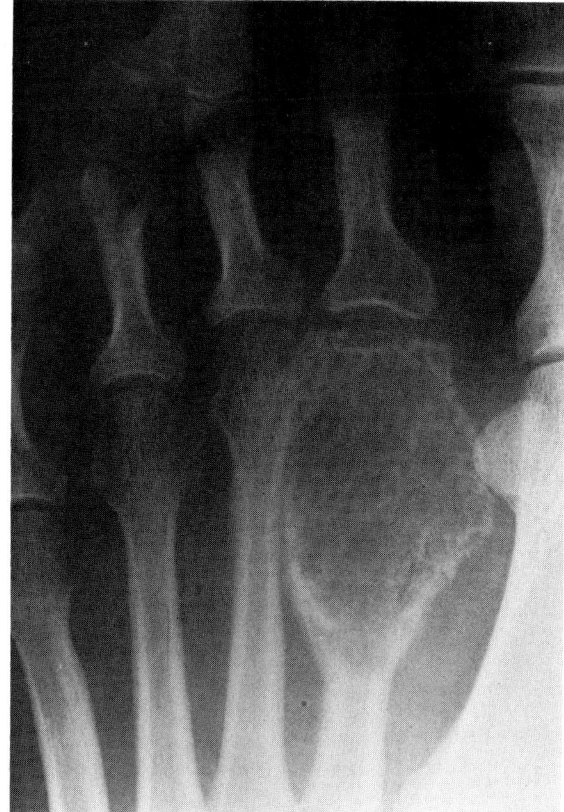

Figure 9–265. Giant cell tumor. Radiograph of foot with an expanded "soap-bubble" defect in the second metatarsal. When the lesion involves small tubular bones, it immediately becomes central rather than eccentric. Growth of the tumor and erosion of the endosteal surface are slow enough to allow periosteal new bone formation to keep pace, so the cortex is not markedly thinned.

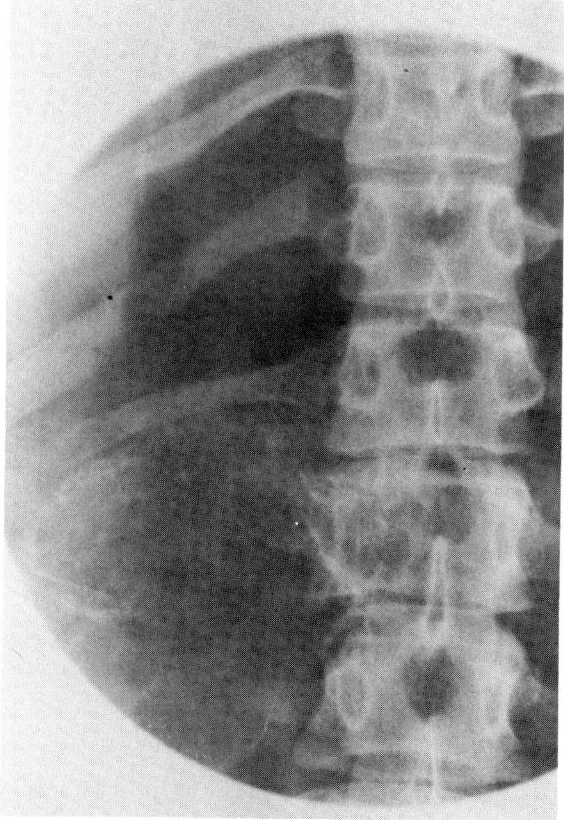

Figure 9–266. Giant cell tumor. Expansile "soap-bubble" lesion with poorly defined peripheral markings of a giant cell tumor in the transverse process of the first lumbar vertebra. Note encroachment into the body of the vertebra.

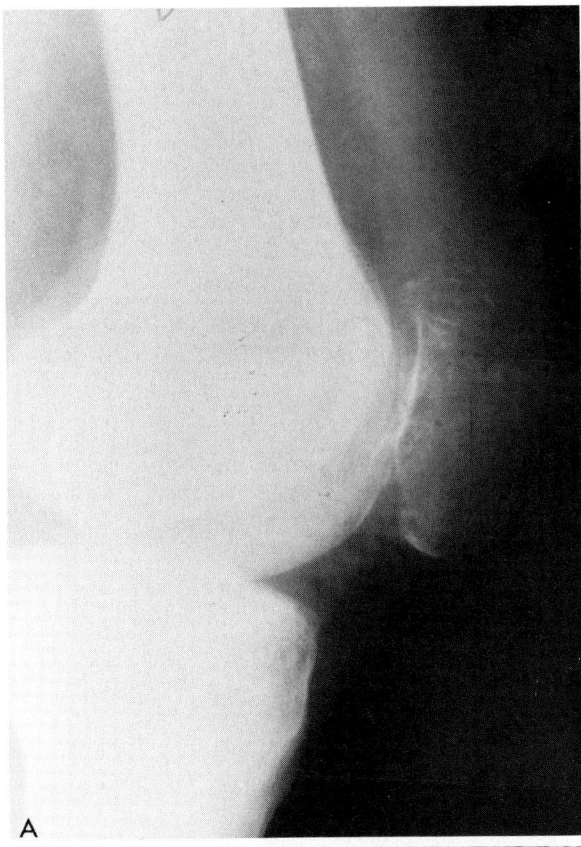

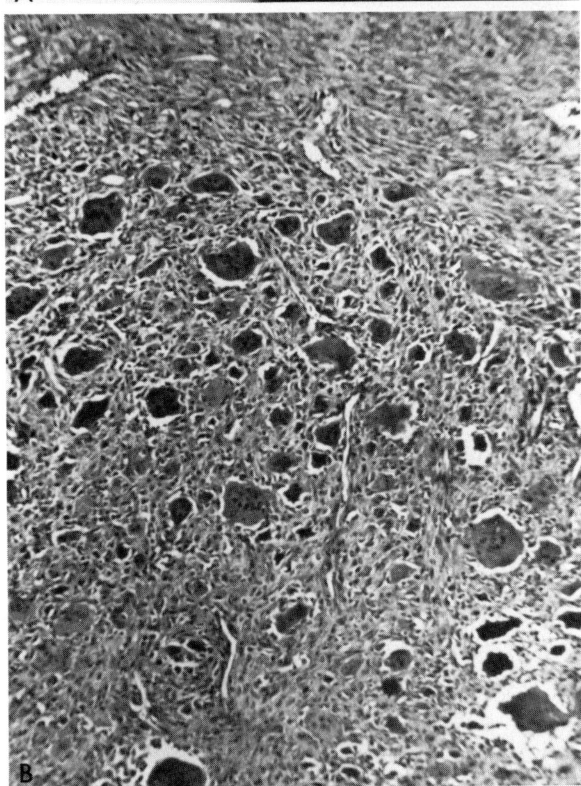

Figure 9–267. Lateral radiograph (*A*) and histologic appearance (*B*) of a lesion involving the patella. Giant cell tumor has been found in almost every bone of the body, although it usually occurs in the ends of long bones.

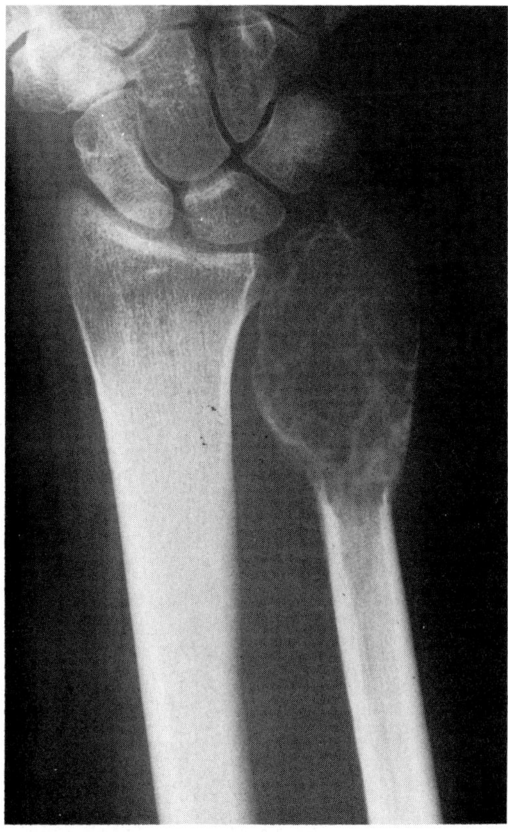

Figure 9–268

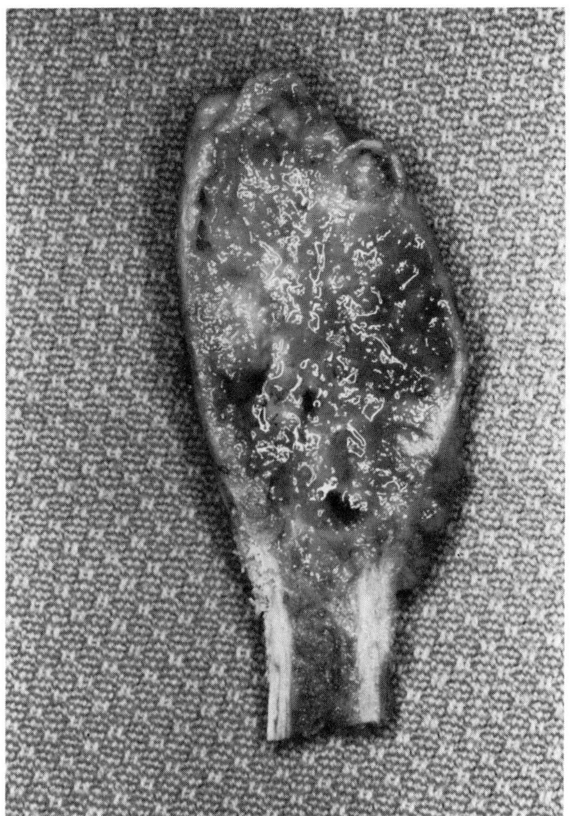

Figure 9–269

Figure 9–268. Giant cell tumor. Radiograph of wrist with typical appearance of giant cell tumor of the distal ulna. Periosteal new bone formation is unable to keep pace with the rapid tumor growth in all portions of the lesion, and there are defects in the peripheral shell of bone. The radiographs were interpreted as aneurysmal bone cyst.

Figure 9–269. Giant cell tumor. Gross specimen of the lesion shown in Figure 9–268. Note that the lesion is solid and completely fills the expanded area of the bone. The lesion is predominantly yellow and brown. The periosteal new bone is eggshell thin. There is sharp demarcation of the proximal margin in the medullary cavity.

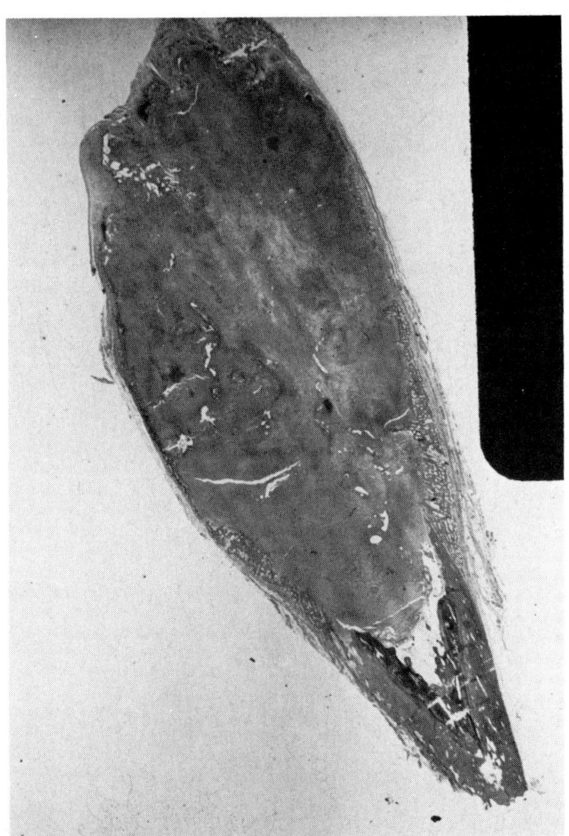

Figure 9–270. Giant cell tumor. Macrosection of the distal ulna containing giant cell tumor. Note the expansion of the bone with a thin, incomplete, bony shell around the lesion. The distal portion of the shell is irregular and partially covered with articular cartilage of the distal radioulnar joint.

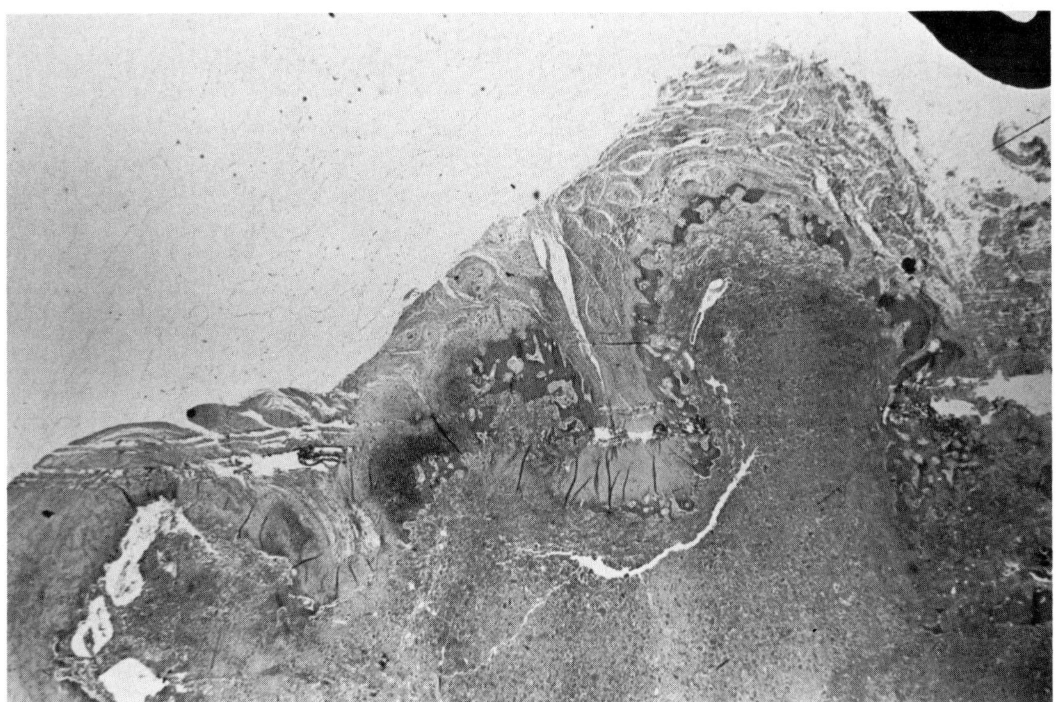

Figure 9–271. Giant cell tumor. Distal end of macrosection shown in Figure 9–270 illustrating the extension of giant cell tumor to the edge of the incompletely contained periosteal shell. Note the dark area of cartilage callus. The thin periosteal shell frequently fractures with muscle pull.

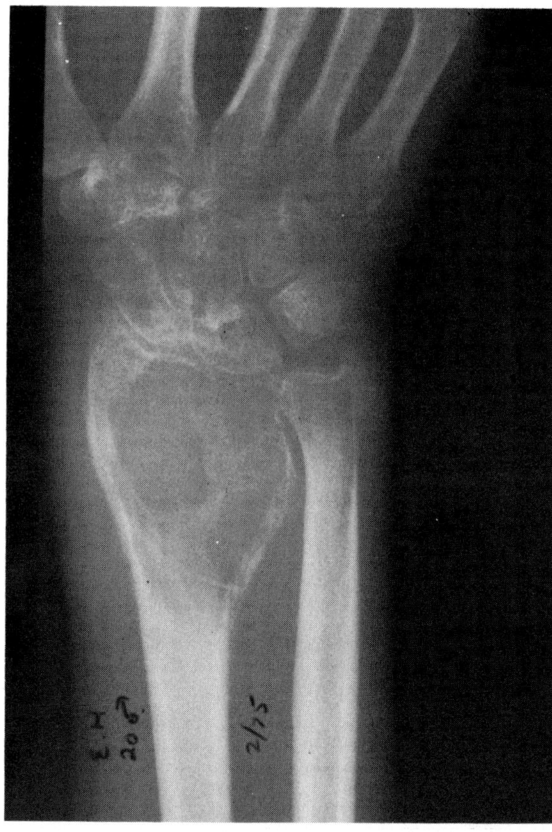

Figure 9–272

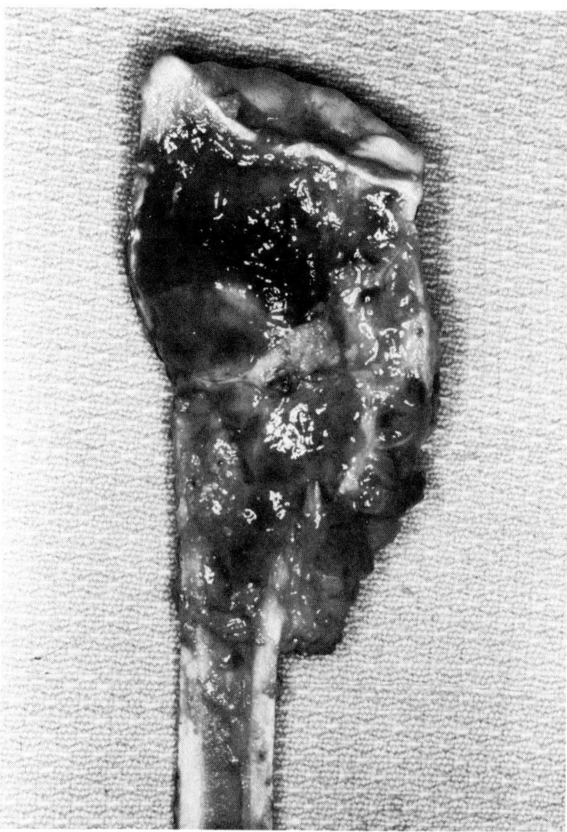

Figure 9–273

Figure 9–272. Giant cell tumor. Expansile lytic lesion of distal radius. Note the osteoporosis of the wrist due to hyperemia induced by the tumor and by disuse of the joint because of pain. The subchondral articular bone is thinned, and the proximal portion of the lesion is not sharply outlined but fades into the trabecular bone.

Figure 9–273. Giant cell tumor. Gross specimen of the lesion illustrated in Figure 9–272. Note the thinning of the articular surface and the subchondral bone with a small crack in the center that allows extrusion of tumor into the joint space. This did not create a problem for the patient. There is erosion of the cortex on the volar aspect of the bone (right) with soft tissue extension. En-bloc excision of the lesion and the adjacent pronator teres muscle was performed. The patient is free of recurrence 8 years after surgery.

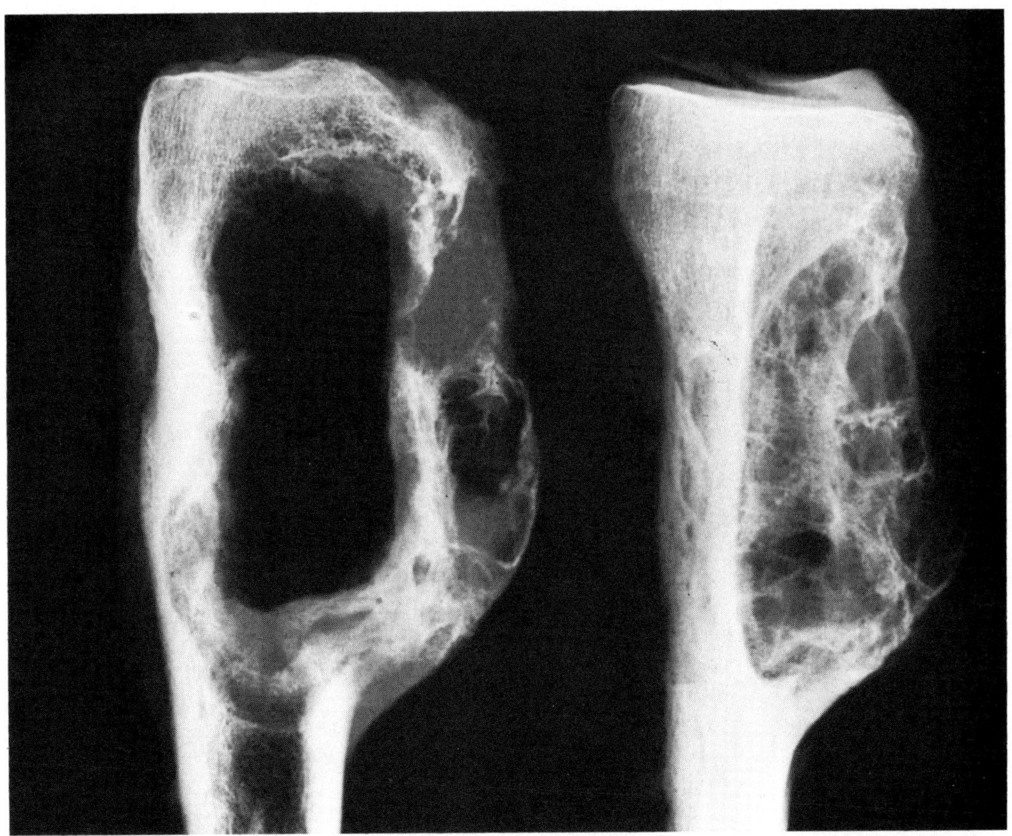

Figure 9–274. Giant cell tumor. Specimen radiograph of a recurrent giant cell tumor.

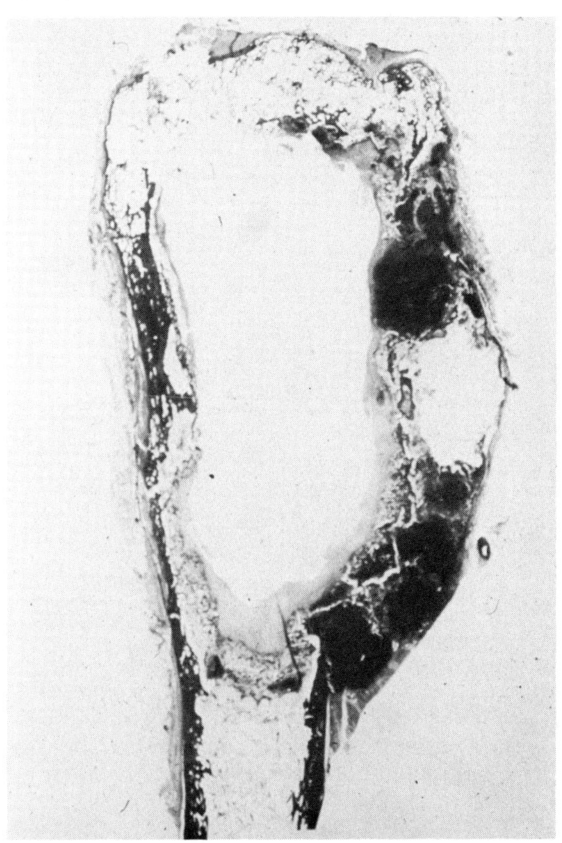

Figure 9–275. Giant cell tumor. Macrosection of the recurrent giant cell tumor shown in Figure 9–274. The curetted cavity is present in the center of the lesion, but "recurrent" (residual) tumor is present in several areas around the margin.

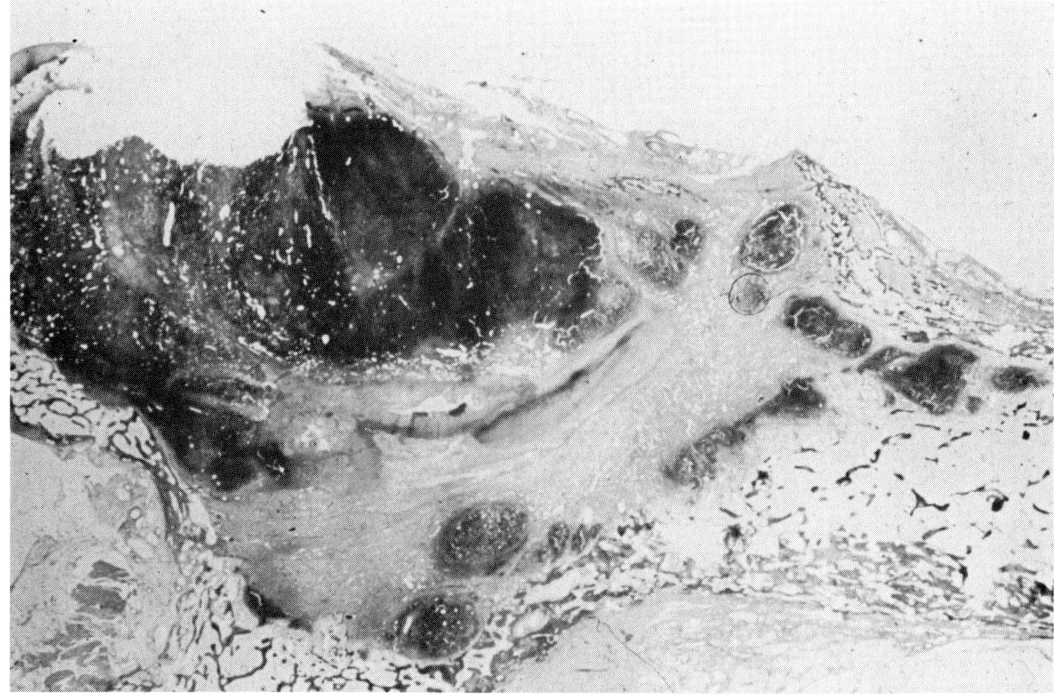

Figure 9–276. Giant cell tumor. Recurrent giant cell tumor with clusters of tumor both within and beyond the margins of the fibrous wall of the curetted cavity.

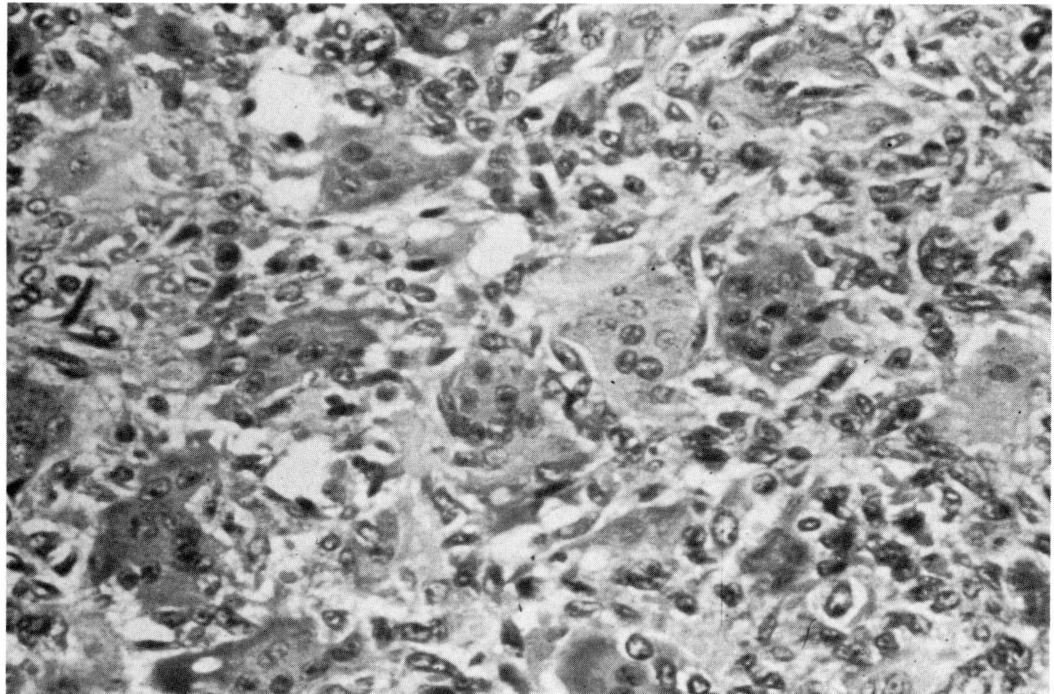

Figure 9–277. Giant cell tumor. Characteristic giant cells and stromal cells of a grade 1 giant cell tumor. Note the similarity of the nuclei within the giant cells to those of the stromal cells.

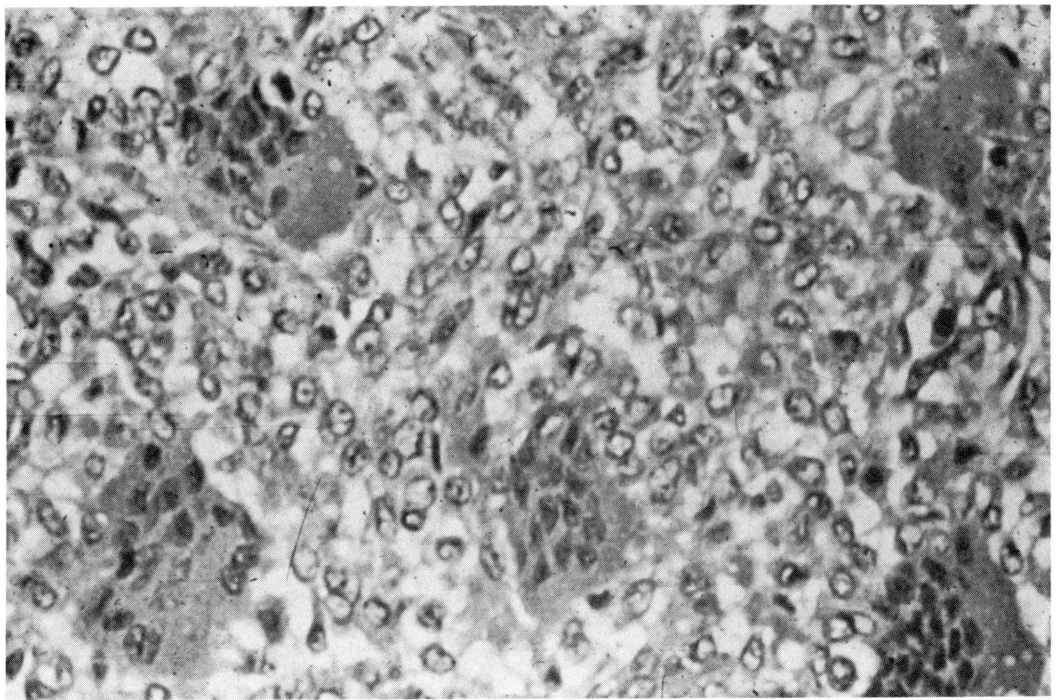

Figure 9–278. Giant cell tumor (grade 1). Appearance of lesion after re-excision.

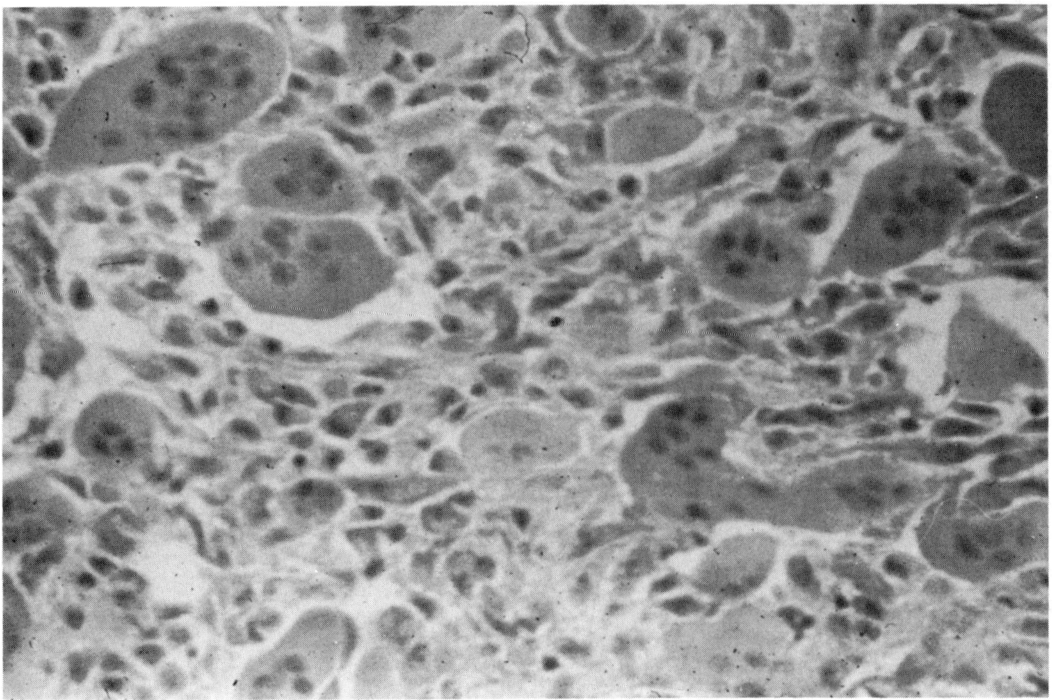

Figure 9–279. Giant cell tumor (grade 2). Note the variation and pleomorphism of the stromal cells.

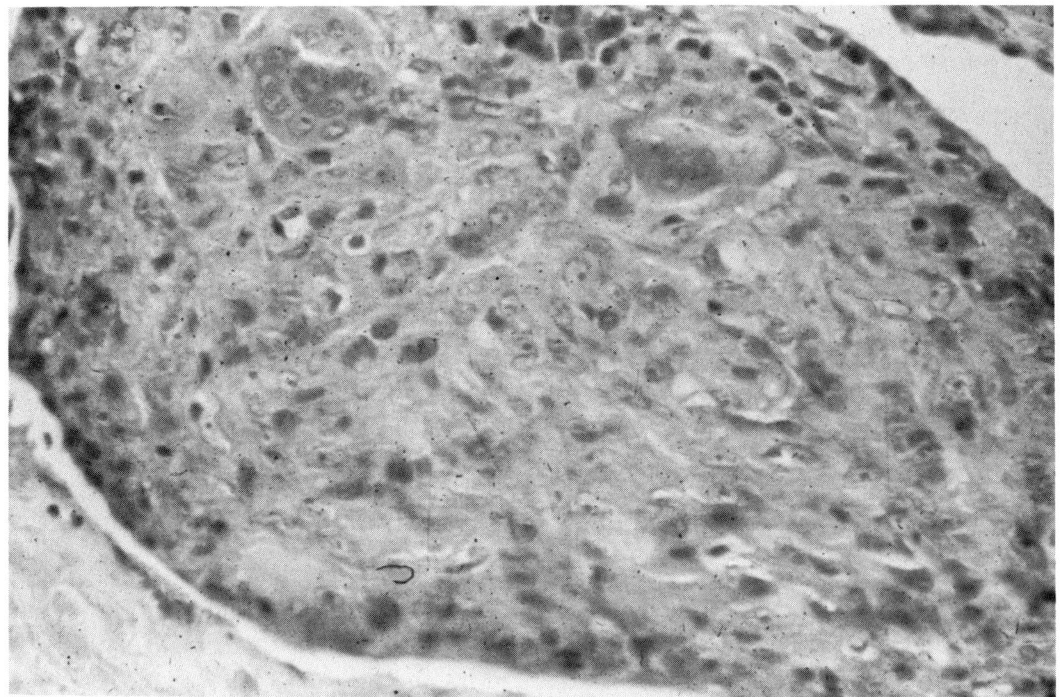

Figure 9–280. Giant cell tumor. Histologic picture of grade 2 giant cell tumor showing extension of a tumor nidus into a vessel (note the vessel lining at the corners of the photograph). Despite the vascular invasion, the tumor did not metastasize.

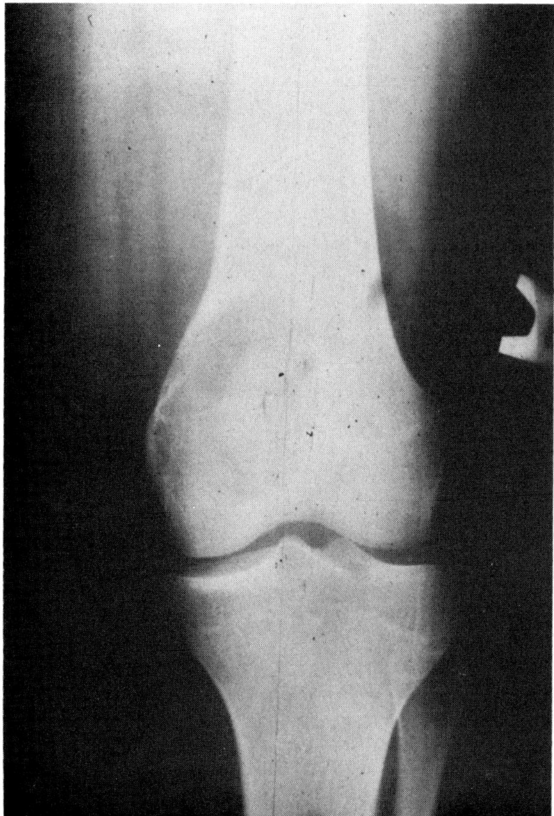

Figure 9–281. Giant cell tumor. Anteroposterior radiograph of the knee showing a giant cell tumor of the distal femur in a pregnant patient. The lesion is well circumscribed.

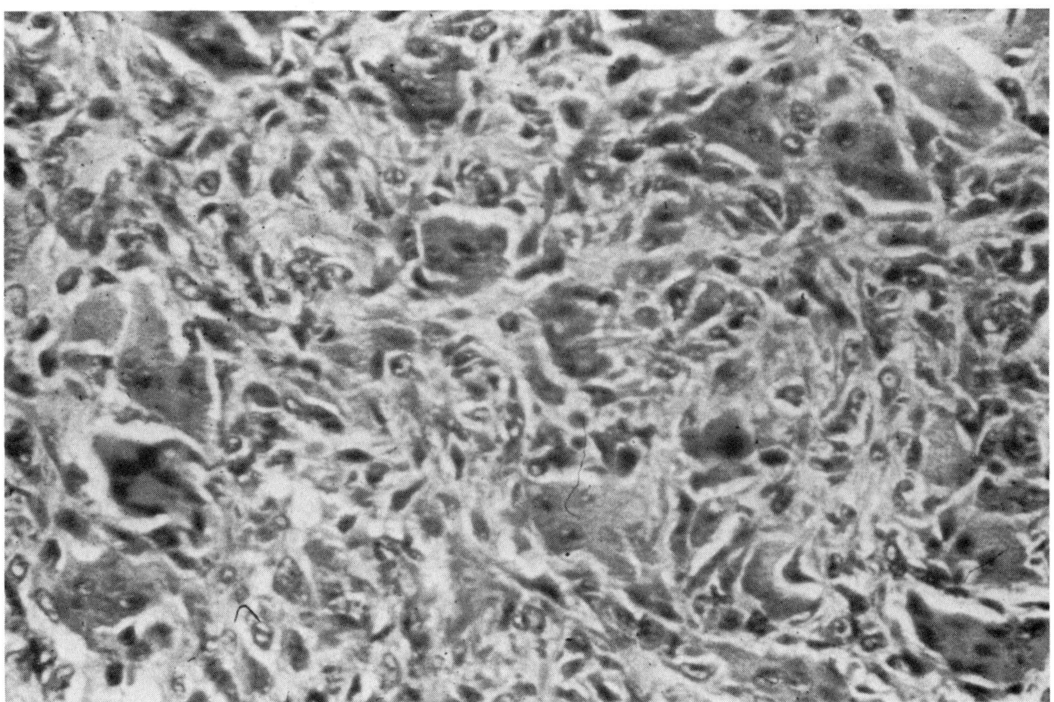

Figure 9–282. Giant cell tumor. Histologic appearance of lesion shown in Figure 9–281. There is moderate pleomorphism of the stromal component, suggesting a high-grade tumor. Despite the ominous histologic appearance, these lesions seldom metastasize in gravid patients but rather revert to a more benign appearance after the conclusion of the pregnancy.

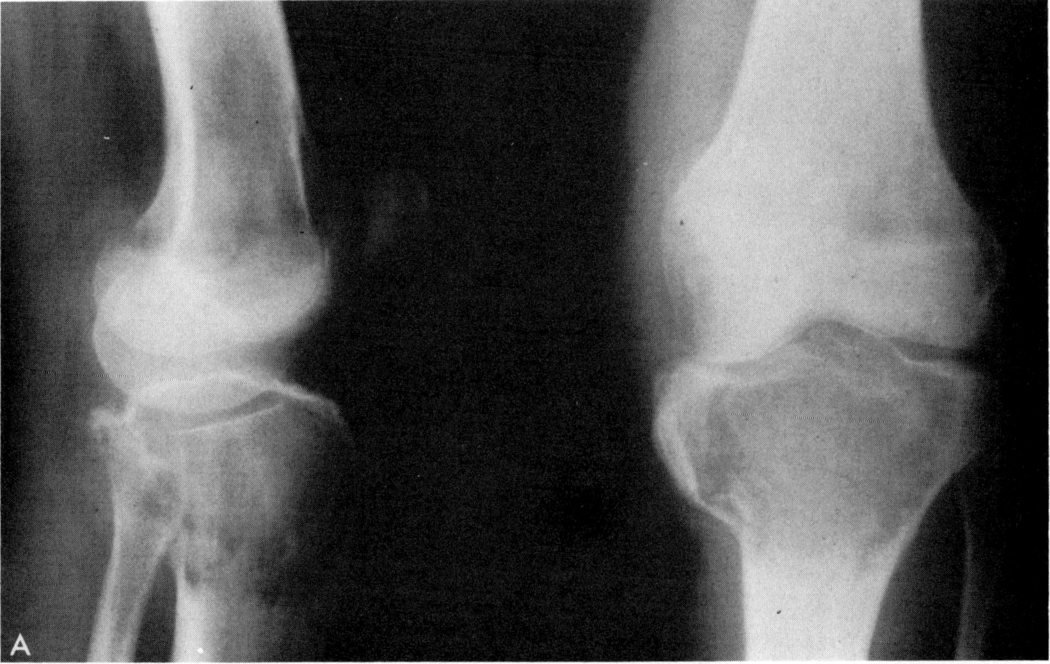

Figure 9–283. Giant cell tumor. Anteroposterior (A) and lateral (B) radiographs show giant cell tumor of the knee in a 26-year-old pregnant patient. She experienced pain for many months, but no radiographs were taken until she sustained a pathologic fracture while getting out of a bathtub. The lesion was partially curetted several days after delivery of a normal baby. Histologic sections (C to E) reveal a markedly pleomorphic giant cell tumor with prominent spindle-cell component within the stroma and extensive mitotic activity.

Illustration continued on following page

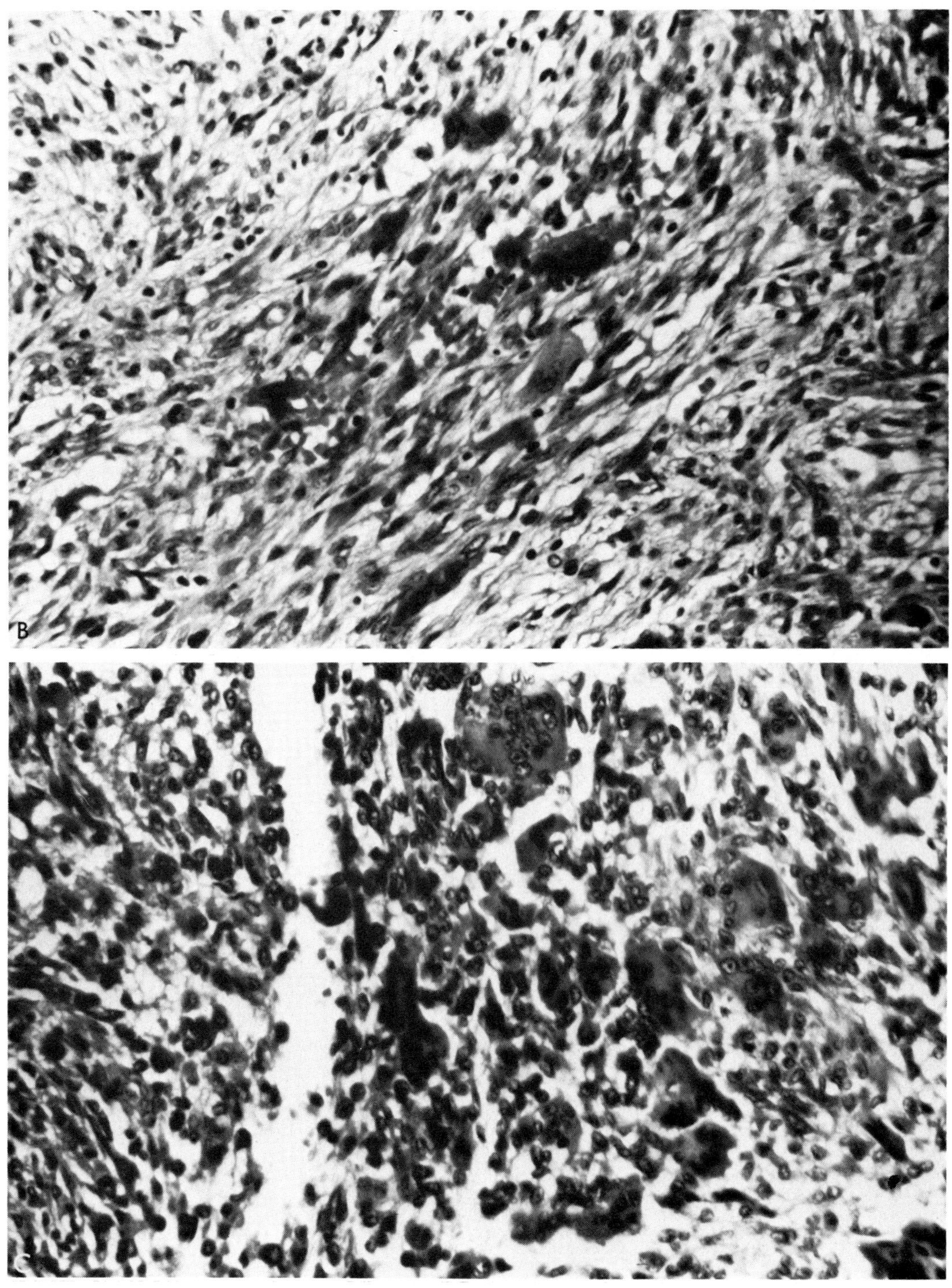

Figure 9–283 *Continued.*

Illustration continued on opposite page

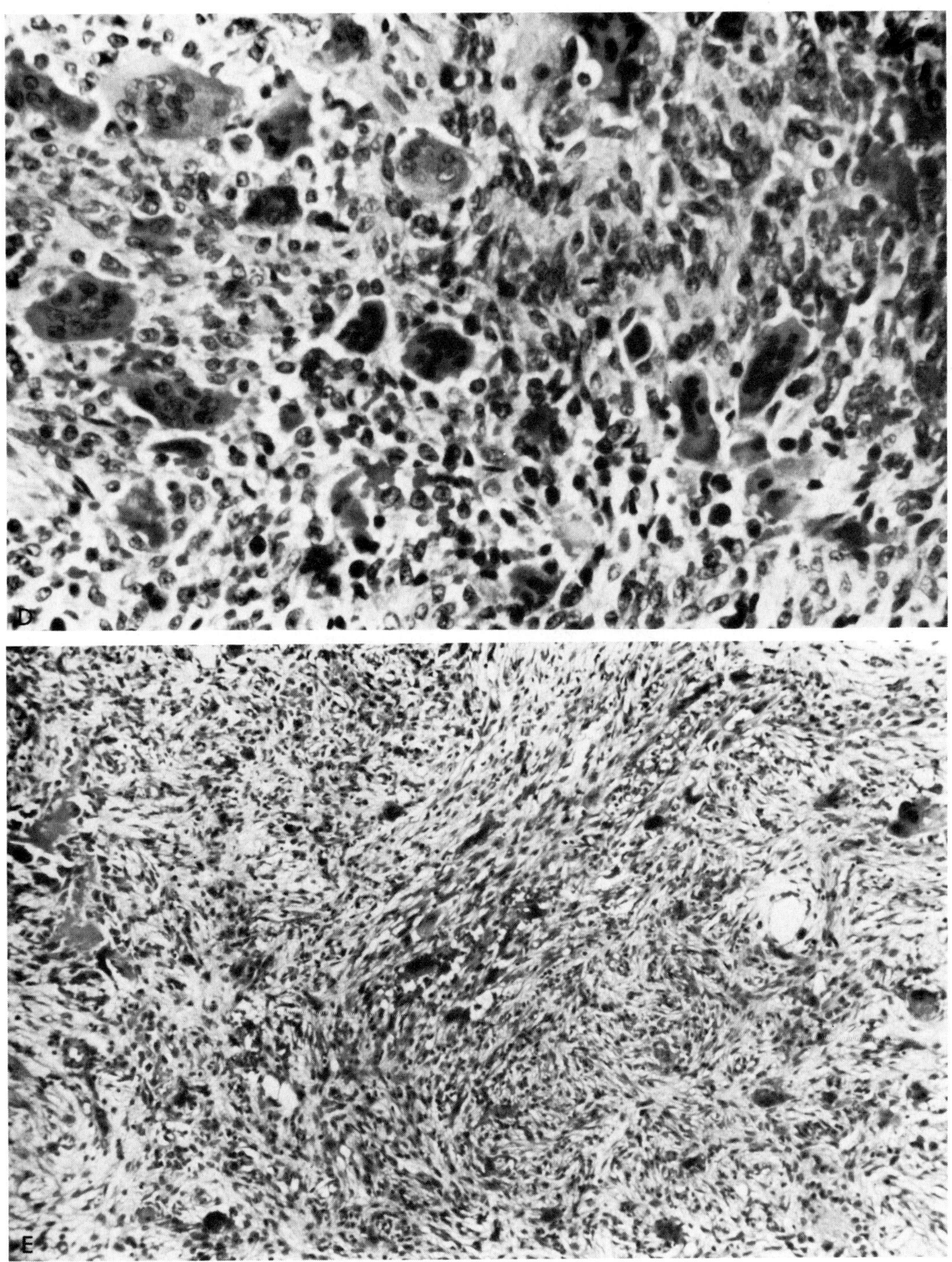

Figure 9–283 *Continued.*

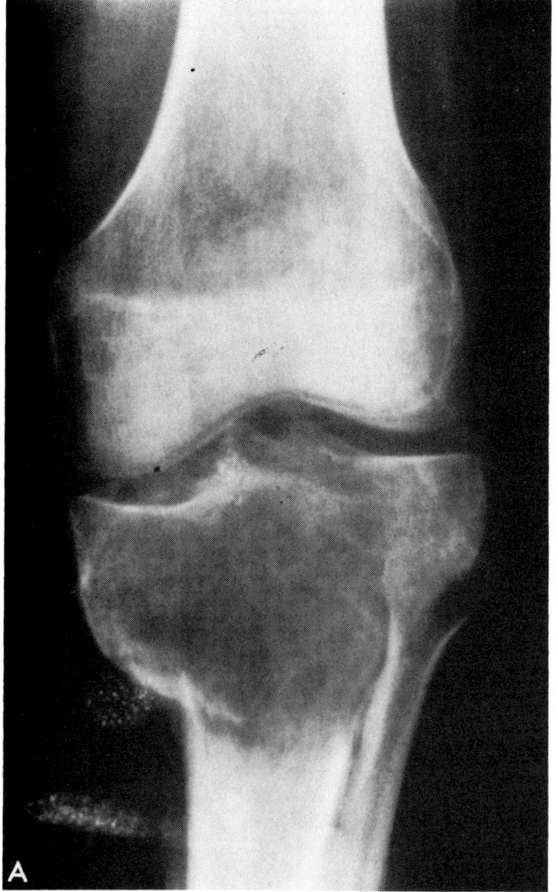

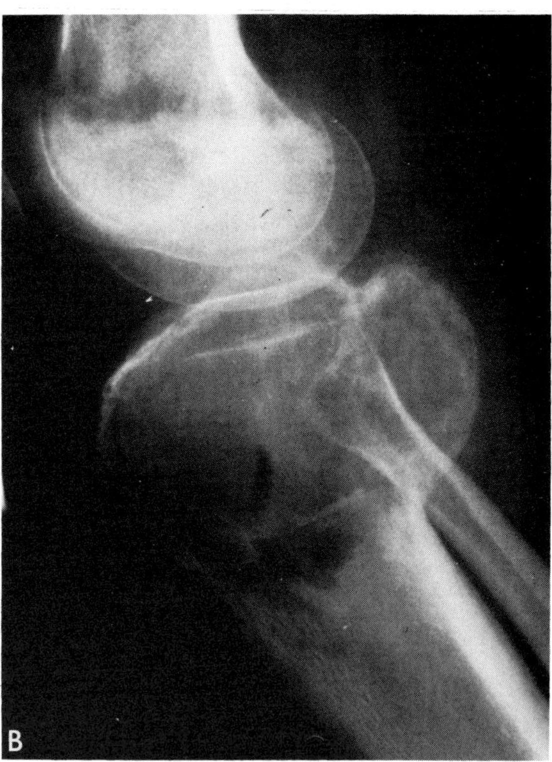

Figure 9–284. Giant cell tumor. Anteroposterior (*A*) and lateral (*B*) radiographs of the knee of the patient illustrated in Figure 9–283, 6 weeks after delivery. There has been healing of the posterior extension of the tumor and of the fractured tibial plateau. The patient no longer experiences night pain. Note the marked subchondral and metaphyseal resorption bands due to hyperemia from the tumor, fracture, and biopsy.

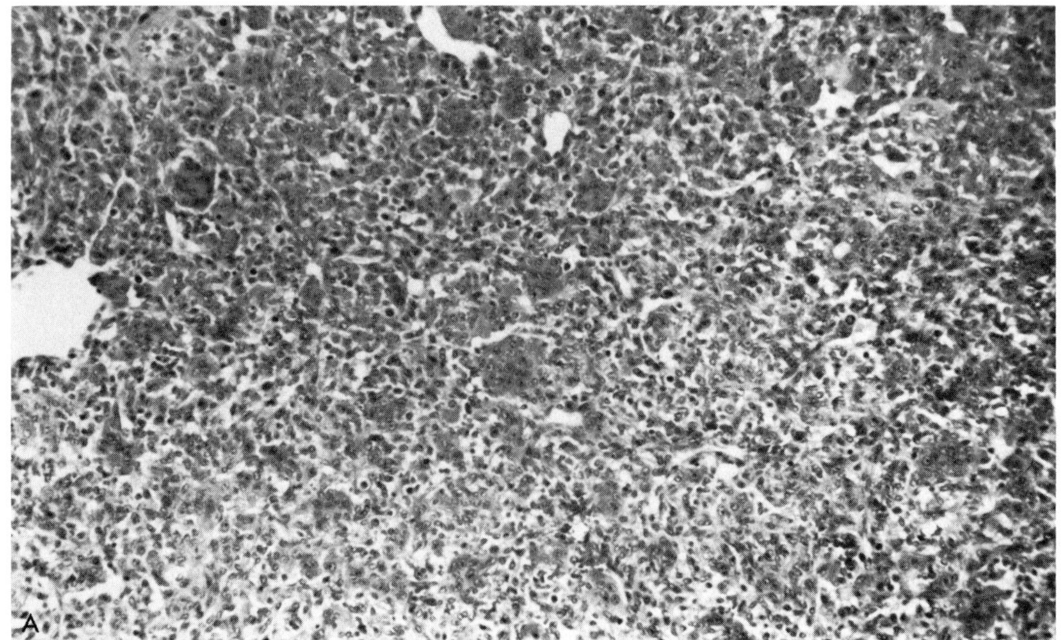

Figure 9–285. Giant cell tumor. Histologic appearance of giant cell tumor shown in Figure 9–284, after curettage. The lesion exhibits a grade 1 giant cell tumor with little pleomorphism, no significant mitotic activity, and no evidence of a spindled stromal component. Note the significant change that has occurred in the 6 weeks since the original biopsy was done (Fig. 9–283).

Illustration continued on opposite page.

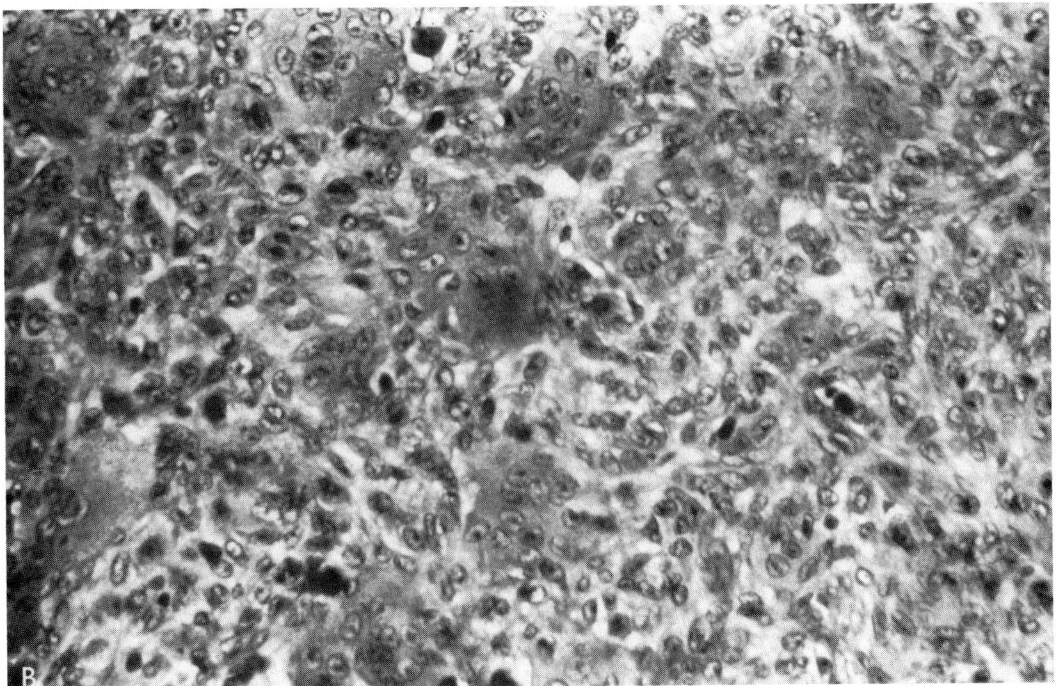

Figure 9–285 *Continued.*

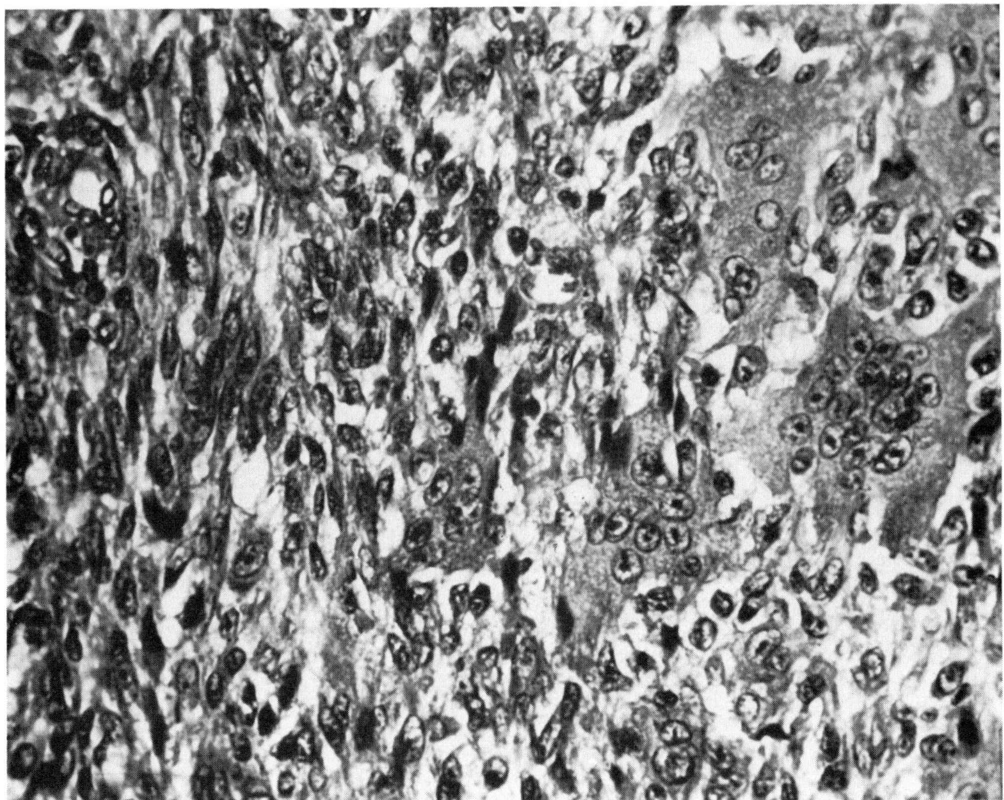

Figure 9–286. Giant cell tumor (grade 2). The pleomorphism in the stroma and the numerous mitoses throughout the specimen indicate a fairly aggressive, but not malignant, tumor.

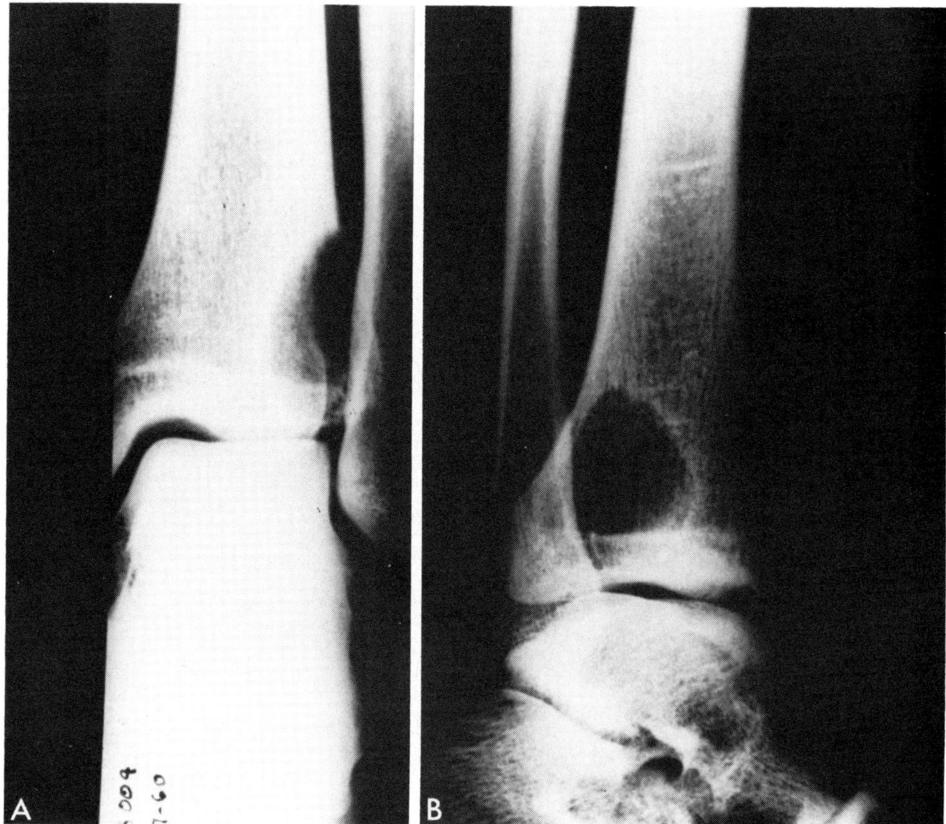

Figure 9–287. Giant cell tumor. Anteroposterior (A) and lateral (B) radiographs of the distal tibia of a patient whose growth plate has recently closed. There is an eccentric lytic lesion. Biopsy revealed giant cell tumor. Note that the center of the lesion is well within the metaphysis. Although the tumor extends into the epiphysis, it has not yet reached the joint line.

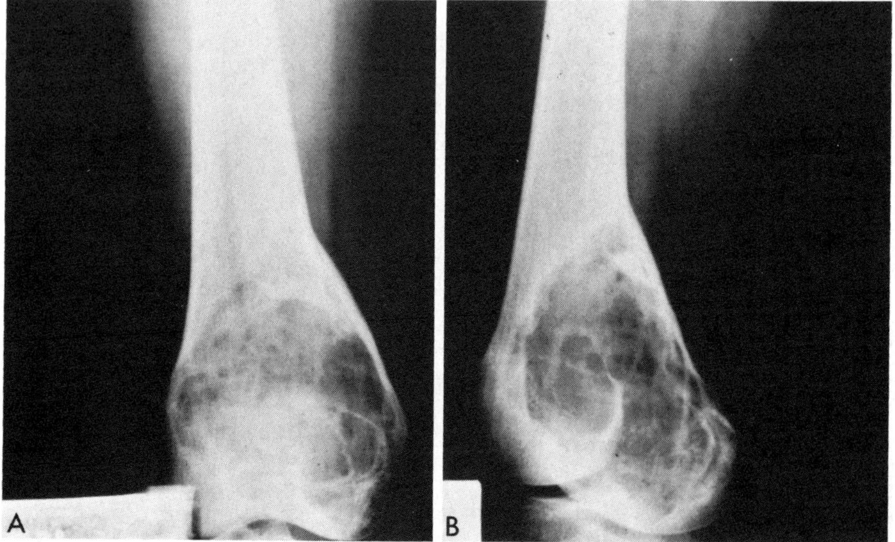

Figure 9–288. Giant cell tumor. Anteroposterior (A) and lateral (B) radiographs of a distal femur that contains a giant cell tumor. As in the lesion shown in Figure 9–287, the center of this tumor is on the metaphyseal side of the growth-plate scar, although it has extended far enough into the epiphysis to approach the articular surface.

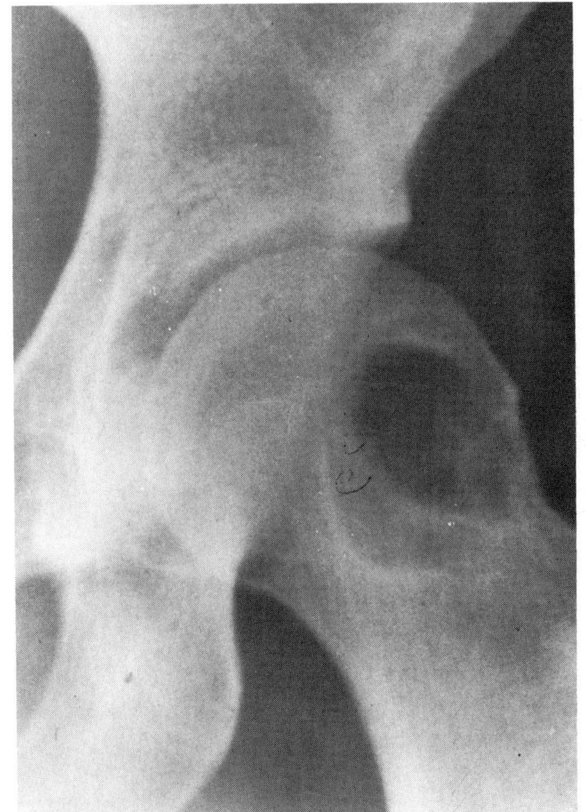

Figure 9–289. Giant cell tumor. Anteroposterior hip radiograph of a patient with a giant cell tumor of the femoral neck. This lesion is clearly within the metaphysis and has not yet encroached on the epiphysis.

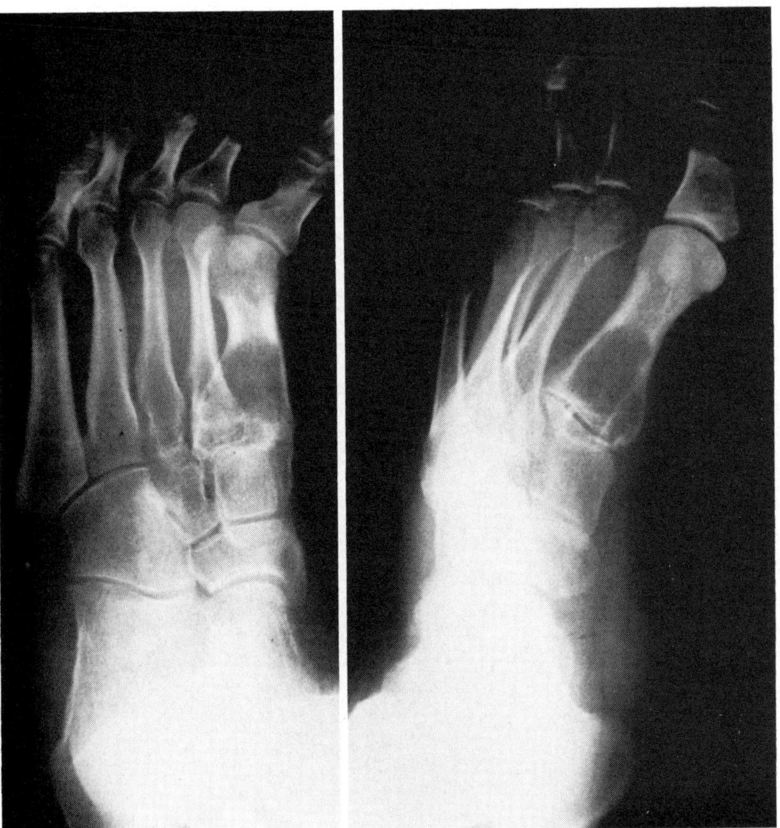

Figure 9–290. Giant cell tumor. Radiographs of the foot of a patient with a giant cell tumor in the proximal end of his first metatarsal. There has been minimal expansion of the bone. The lesion is purely resorptive in nature and is well outlined. When a giant cell tumor occurs in a bone that has only one physis, the lesion is present at the end of the bone containing that physis.

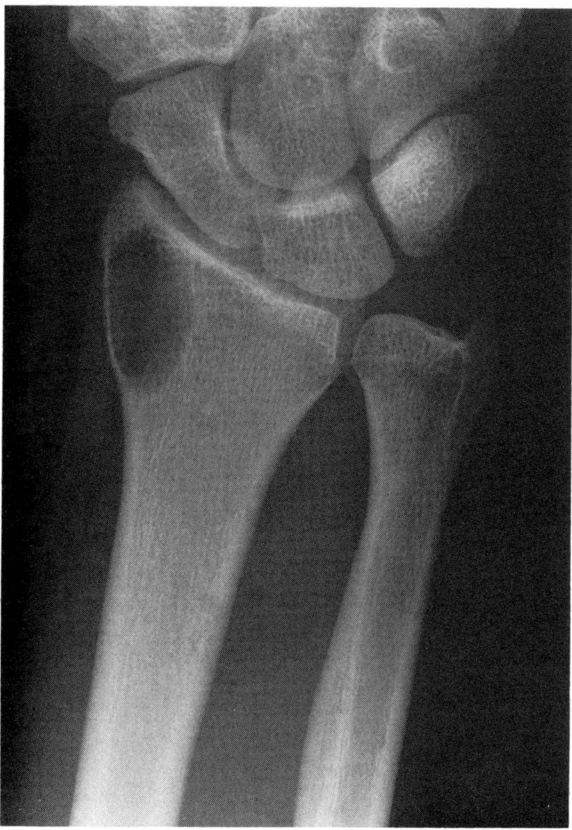

Figure 9–291. Giant cell tumor. Early giant cell tumor of distal radius. The small size of the tumor does not require reinforcement of remaining trabeculae, and therefore the "soap-bubble" pattern is not yet apparent. The center of the lesion is on the metaphyseal side of the old growth plate. Although it has extended into the epiphysis, it has not yet reached the subchondral bony plate.

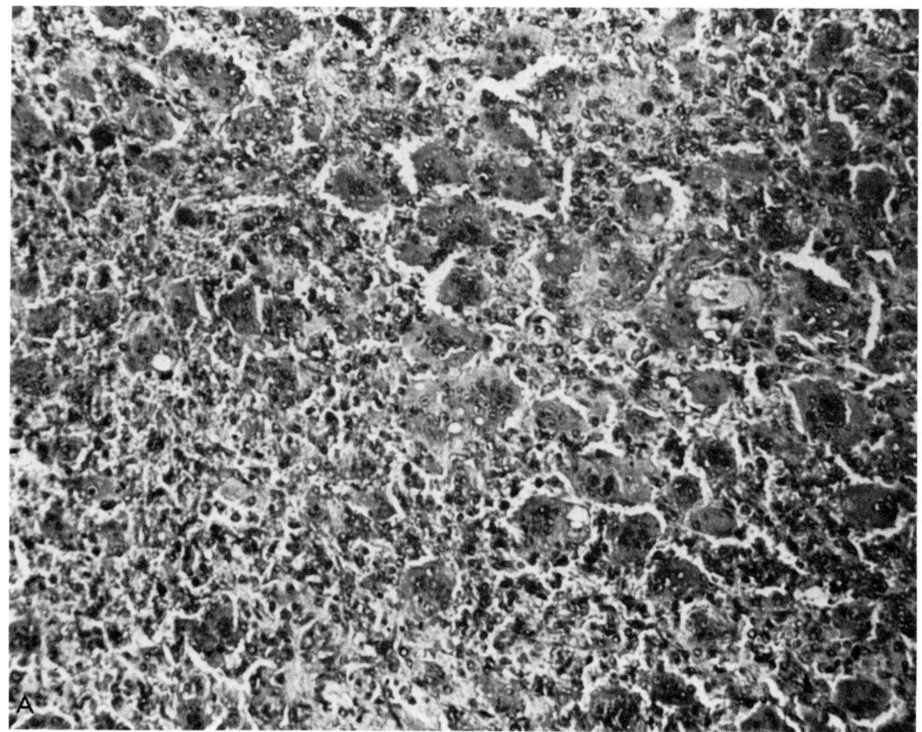

Figure 9–292. Giant cell tumor. Histologic appearance of a grade 1 giant cell tumor demonstrating uniform stromal and giant cell nuclei.

Illustration continued on opposite page

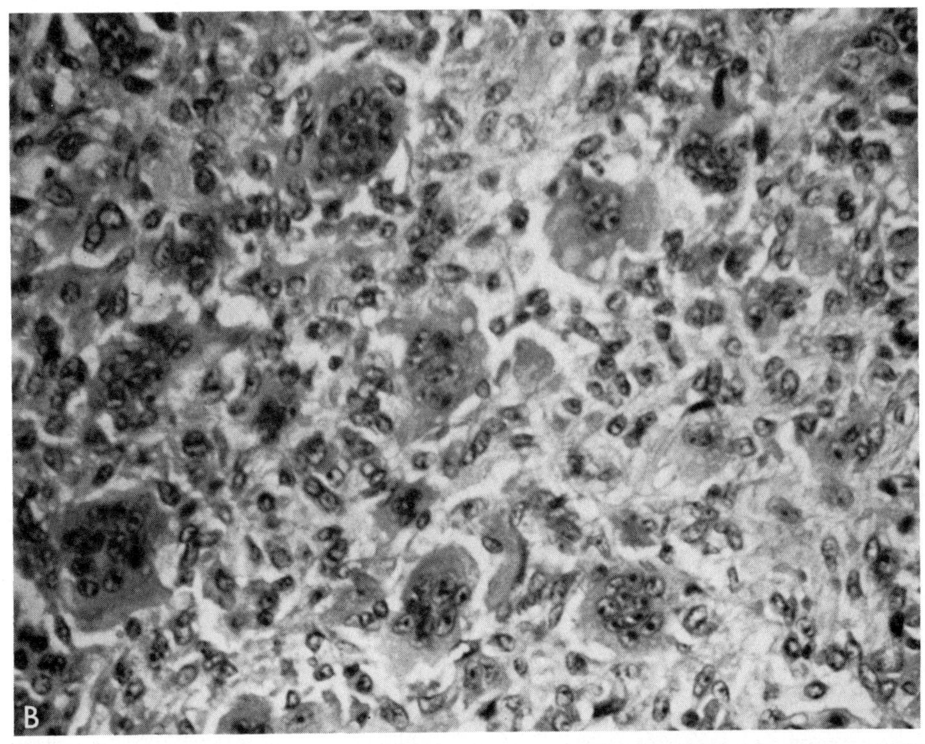

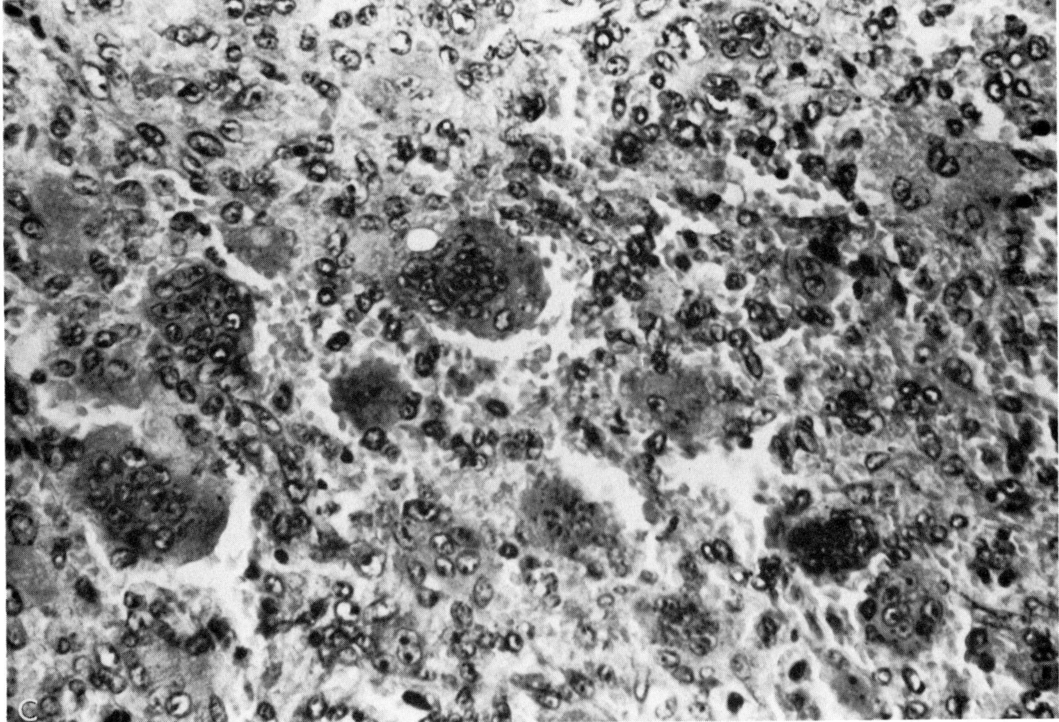

Figure 9–292 *Continued.*

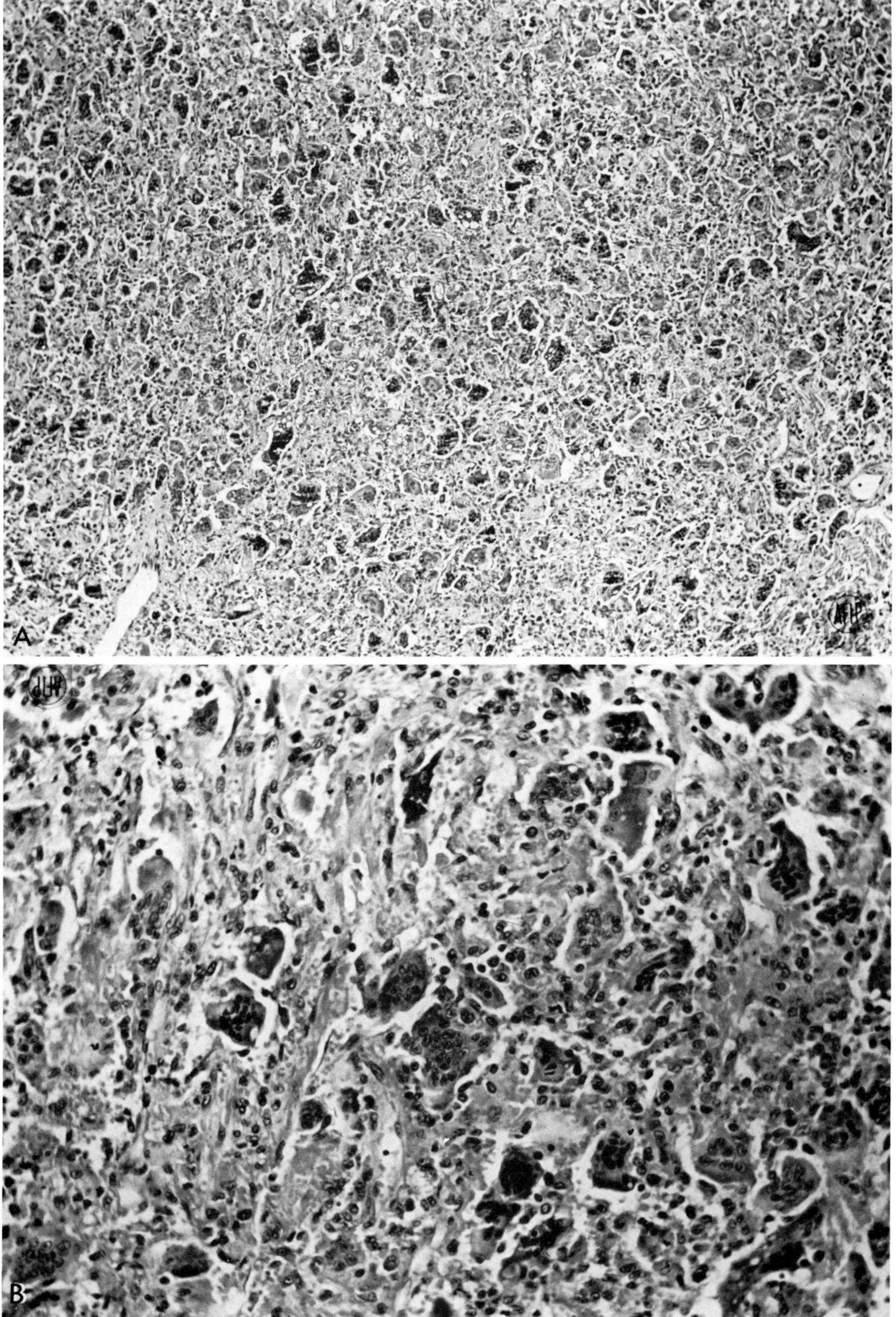

Figure 9–293. Histologic appearance of grade 2 giant cell tumor. Note the slight variation in the appearance of giant cells and stromal cells and the tendency for spindled stromal transformation.

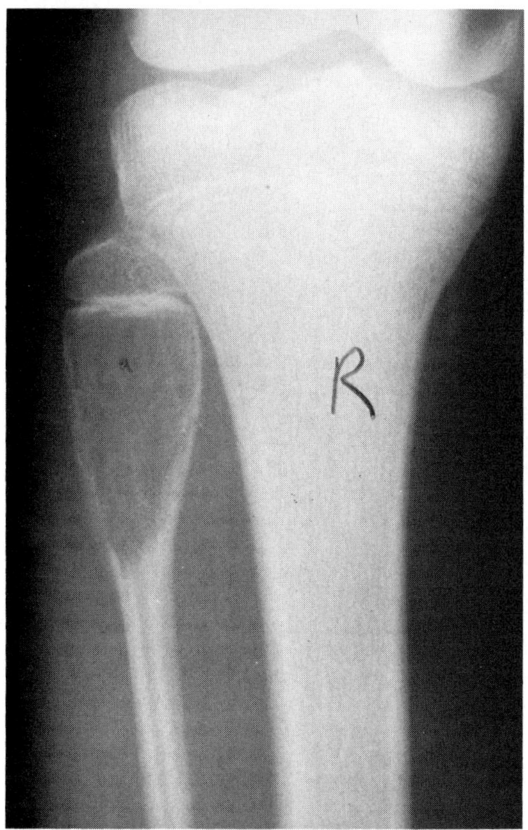

Figure 9–294

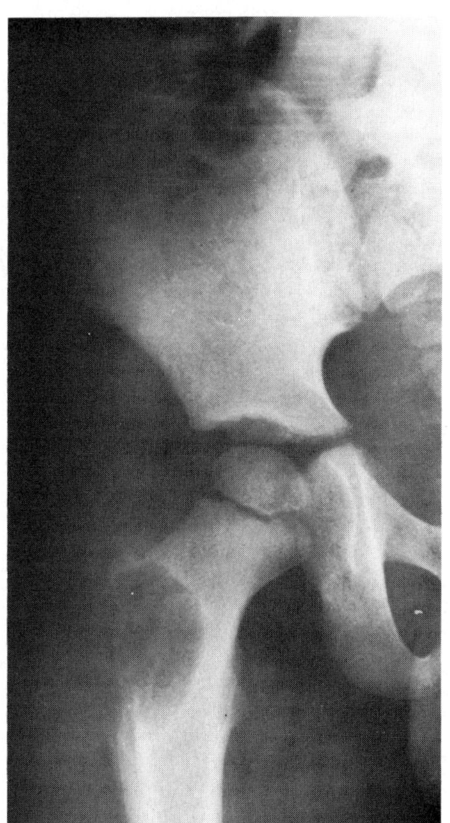

Figure 9–295

Figure 9–294. Giant cell tumor. The lesion is present in the proximal fibula in a 12-year-old female. The lesion is solid and has characteristic histology.

Figure 9–295. Giant cell tumor. Anteroposterior radiograph of the hip in a child with a giant cell tumor in proximity to the greater tuberosity of the femur.

Figure 9–296. Giant cell tumor. The lesion is present in the proximal tibial metaphysis in an 8-year-old male. In children, there is a higher tendency for tumors to undergo vascular malformation, tumor necrosis, and cystic change.

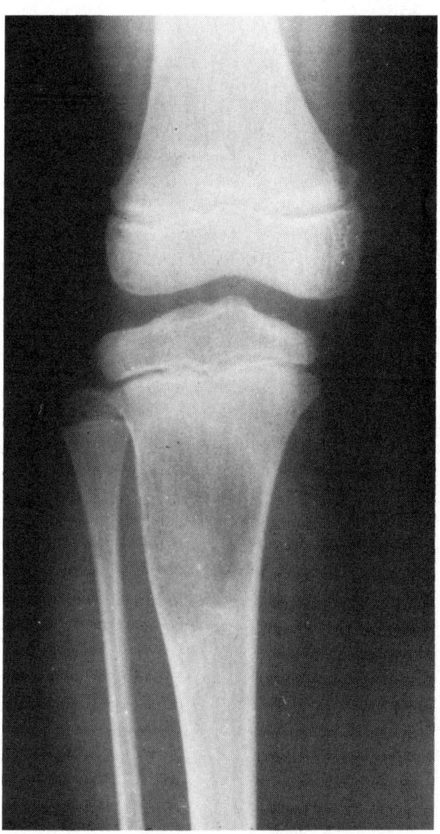

Figure 9–296

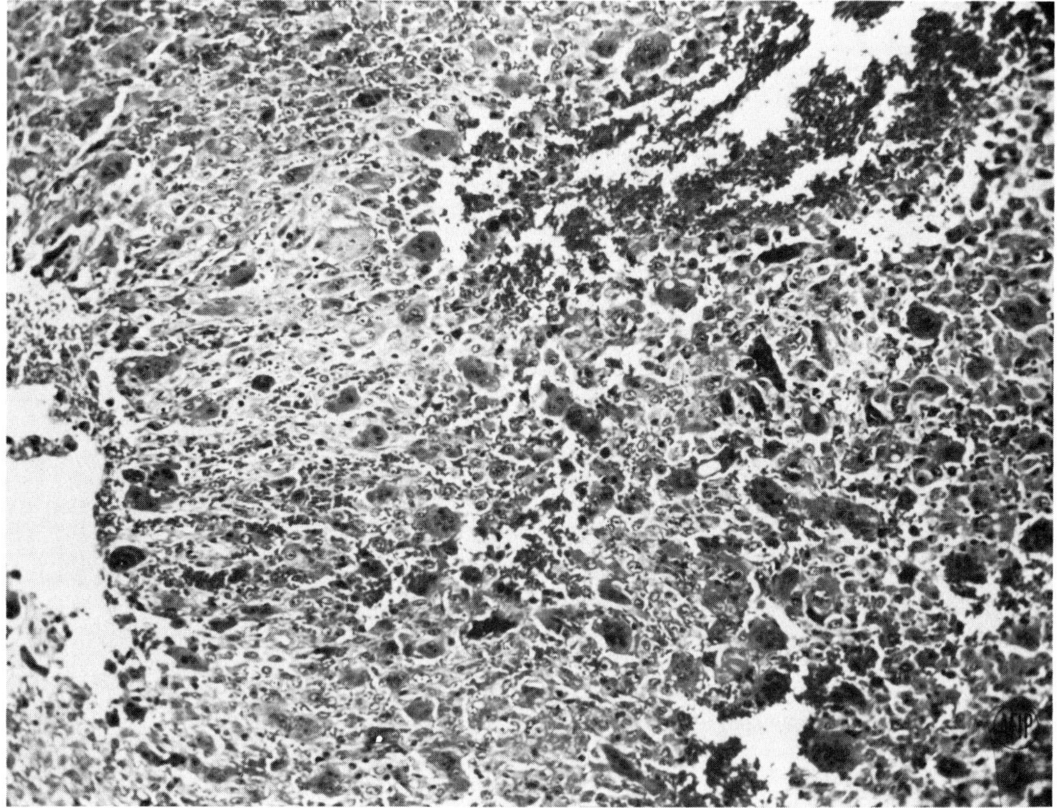

Figure 9–297. Giant cell tumor. Histologic picture of a giant cell tumor in a child showing areas of necrosis, hemorrhage, and early formation of blood-filled spaces. This lesion may be a precursor of aneurysmal cystic change.

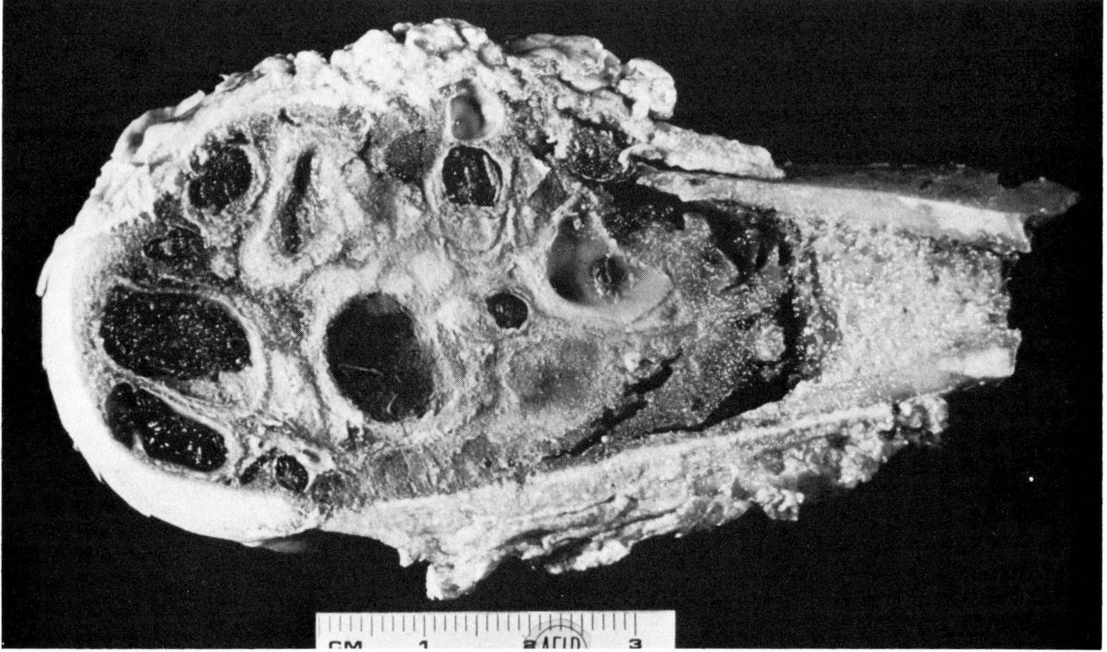

Figure 9–298. Giant cell tumor. Note the numerous areas of cystic degeneration. Although the cysts are fairly numerous and some of them may have been blood-filled, most of the lesion is solid.

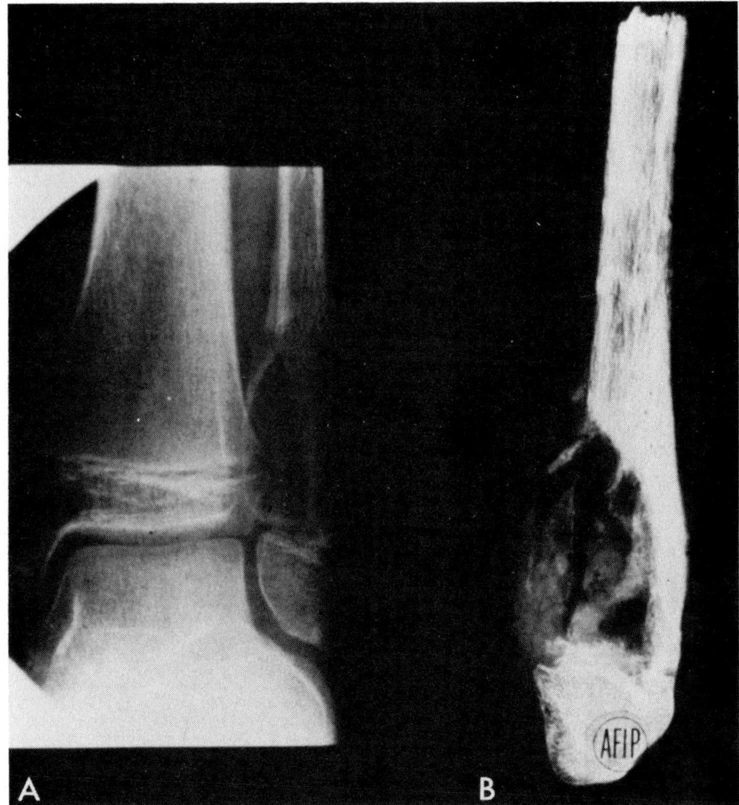

Figure 9–299. Giant cell tumor. Clinical (*A*) and specimen (*B*) radiographs of a distal fibula with an expansile lytic defect in the fibular metaphysis.

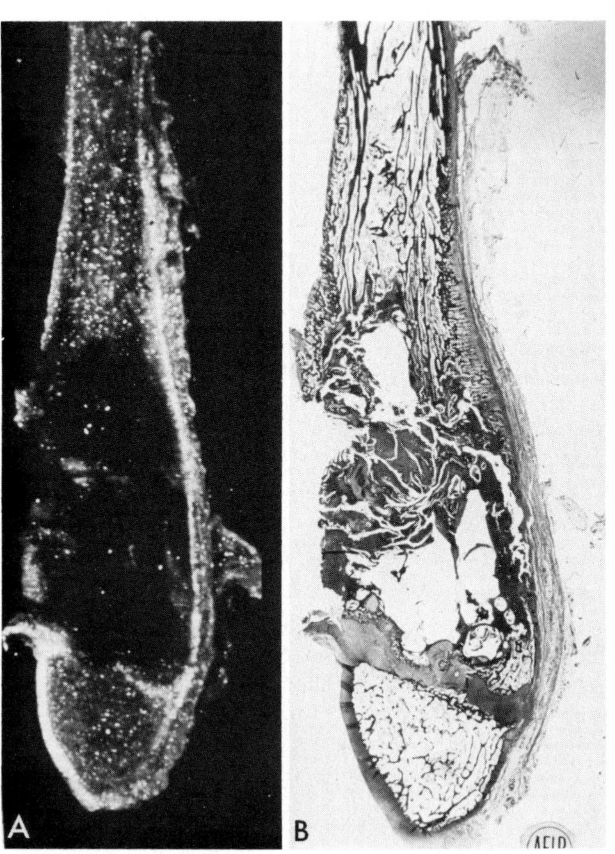

Figure 9–300. Giant cell tumor. Gross specimen (*A*) and macrosection (*B*) of the lesion shown in Figure 9–299. Note the partially solid, partially cystic, somewhat hemorrhagic lesion, confined to the fibular metaphysis.

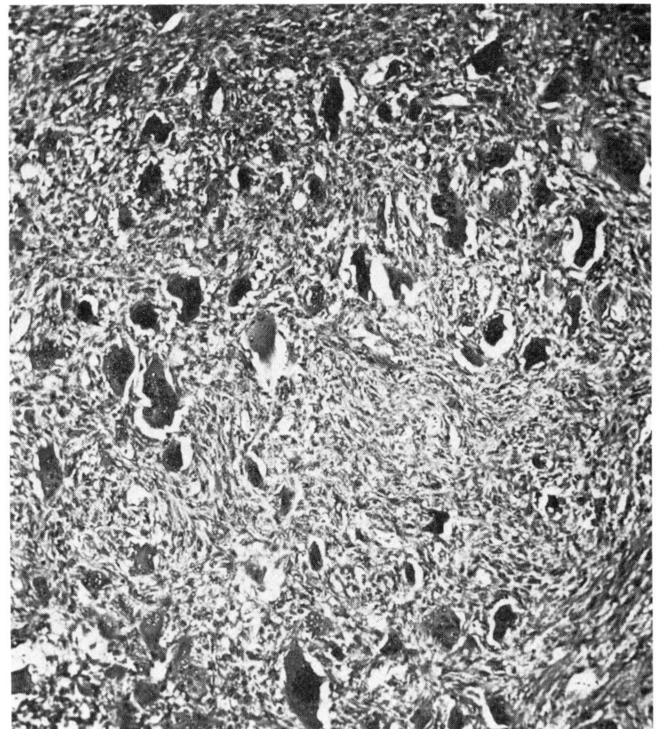

Figure 9–301. Giant cell tumor. Histologic specimen from the tumor shown in Figures 9–299 and 9–300. The appearance is typical of that of a giant cell tumor. The stroma is moderately fibrotic, and giant cells are fairly numerous. There are no areas of hemorrhage or hemosiderin deposits.

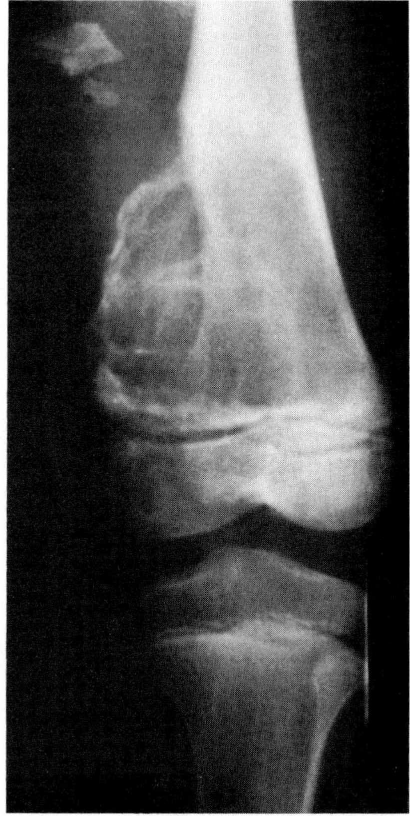

Figure 9–302. Giant cell tumor. In younger children, such as the 5-year-old male whose radiograph is shown here, the lesions may be predominantly cystic, with varying amounts of unclotted blood in the cystic cavity. This anteroposterior radiograph of the knee illustrates an expansile trabeculated defect in the distal femur and expansion of the metaphysis. There is an associated radiolucency in the medial aspect of the femoral epiphysis.

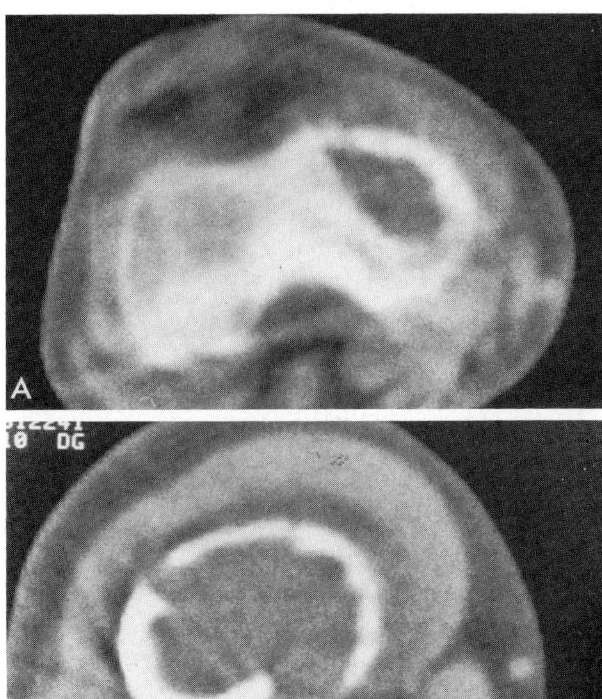

Figure 9–303. Giant cell tumor. CT scans of the epiphysis and diaphysis of a distal femur showing rarefaction in both areas, consistent with loss of trabecular bone. There is a soft-tissue density within the bone cavity that suggests a solid lesion. The posterior cortex of the femur is markedly thinned.

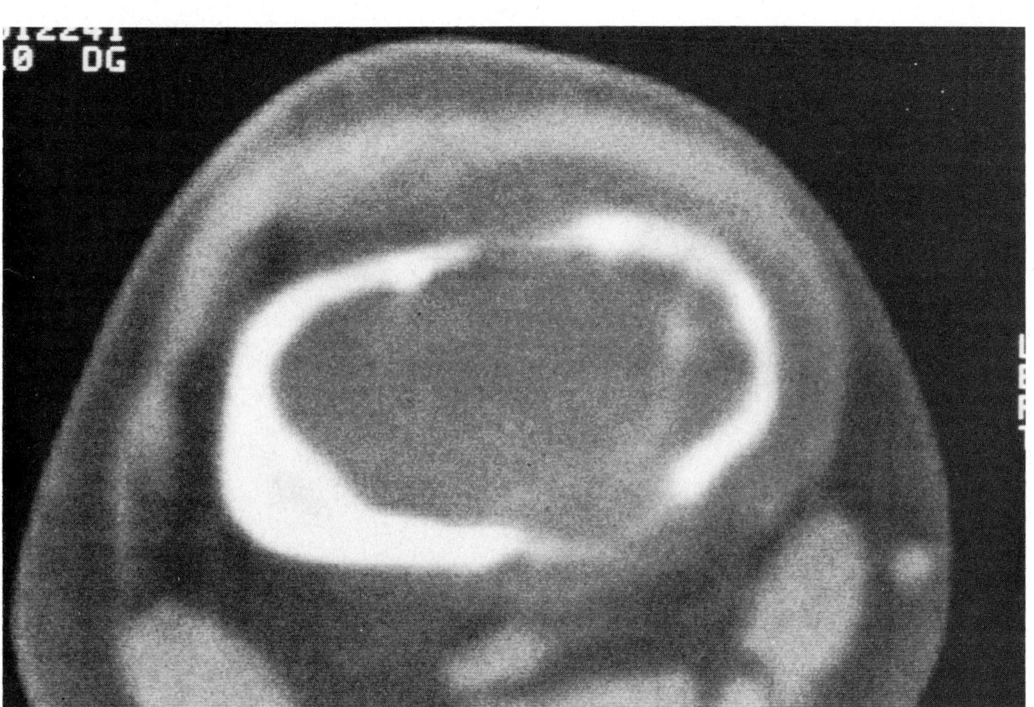

Figure 9–304. Giant cell tumor. CT scan through the femoral metaphysis showing expansion of the bone and marked thinning of the cortex anteriorly and posteriorly. Periosteal new bone is present without extension into soft tissue.

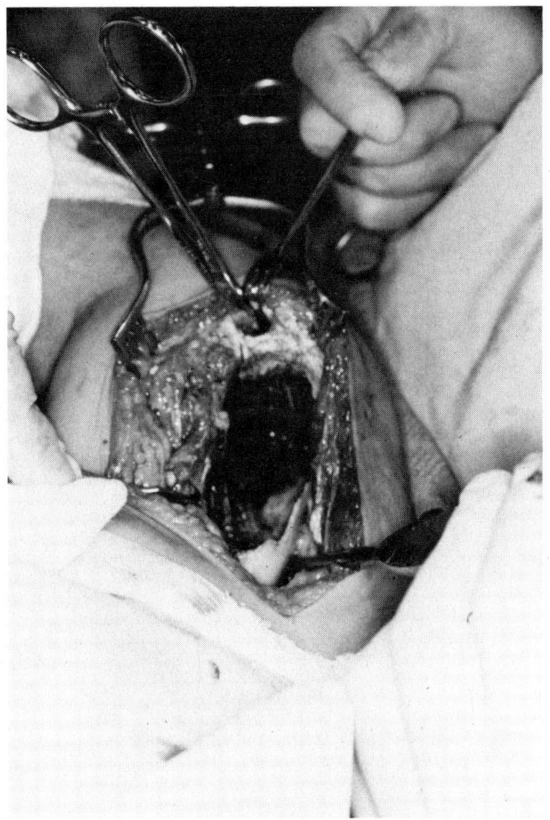

Figure 9–305. Operative photograph of the lesion shown in Figure 9–304. Note the large cavity that remained following thorough curettage of the lesion. There is also a cavity in the epiphysis, with a 1 cm defect in the growth plate causing communication of both cavities. This did not cause problems in the postoperative period. The wall of the cyst was 1 cm thick in some areas, but only 1 mm thick in others. All areas of the wall showed the typical histologic appearance of a giant cell tumor.

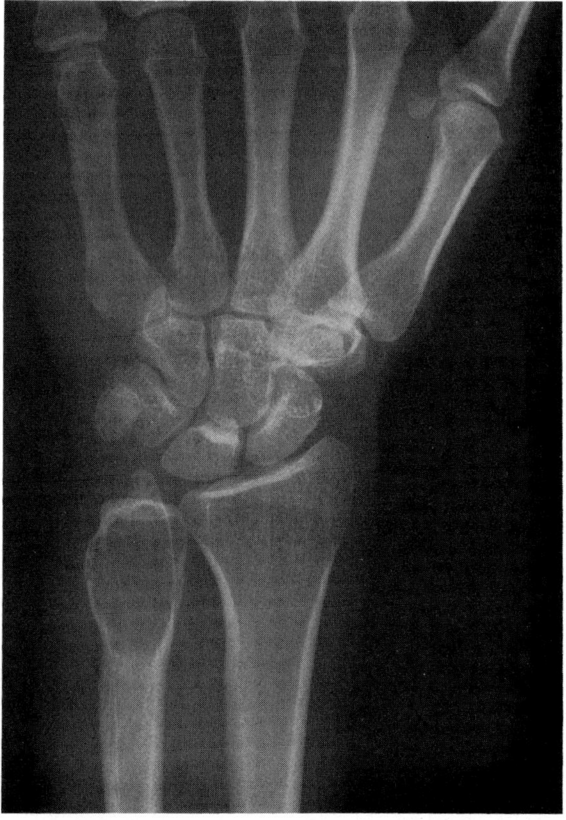

Figure 9–306. Giant cell tumor. Radiograph of wrist of an adult patient with an expansile lesion in the distal ulna. At surgery, this proved to be a cystic giant cell tumor. At the patient's request, the lesion was curetted but the bone was not resected; however, the tumor recurred, and the distal ulna was resected 1 year after curettage. This case illustrates the major problem in the management of giant cell tumors: frequent recurrence following curettage.

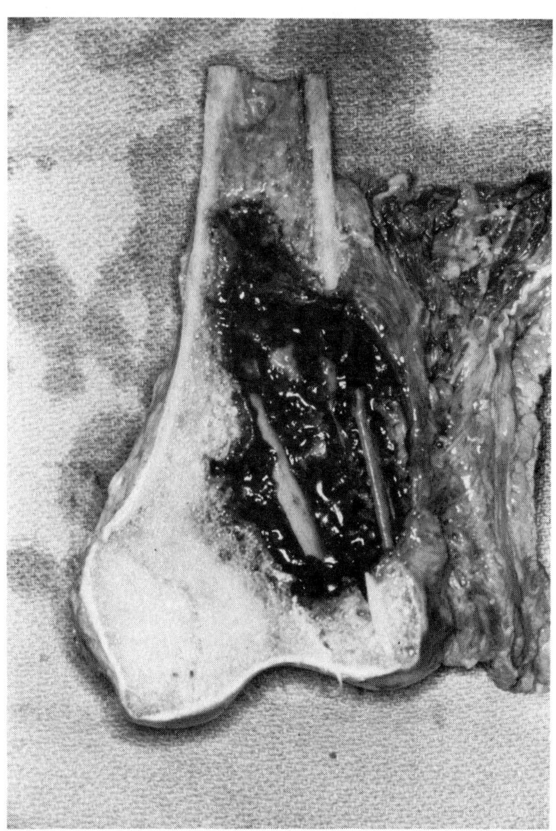

Figure 9–307. Giant cell tumor. Gross specimen of a distal femur with a recurrent giant cell tumor that appeared in a 37-year-old patient. Curettage and bone graft were attempted twice, most recently 10 months before resection. Note the persistent presence of the struts of bone graft. There has been incorporation of the grafts distally near the articular surface; however, there is a satellite area of tumor extending into the trabecular bone of the metaphysis and diaphysis around the edge of the tumor. It is very difficult to curette this region adequately, and therefore enlargment of the preoperative cavity created by the tumor is necessary. Unless some form of chemical cautery or cryosurgery is used to eliminate cells in the trabecular interstices, the recurrence rate is unacceptably high.

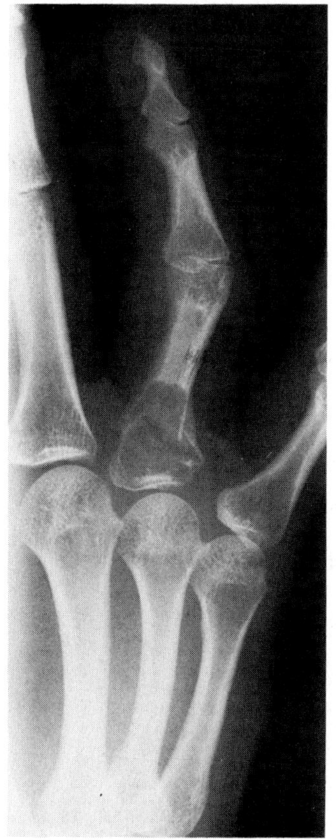

Figure 9–308. Giant cell tumor. Radiograph of hand demonstrating a pathologic fracture through a giant cell tumor in the proximal phalanx. Because of the marked weakening of bones produced by this osteoclastic tumor, pathologic fractures are very common. It is thought by some that curettage of lesions in the phalanges and metacarpals is always followed by recurrence, and the primary treatment should be some form of resection.

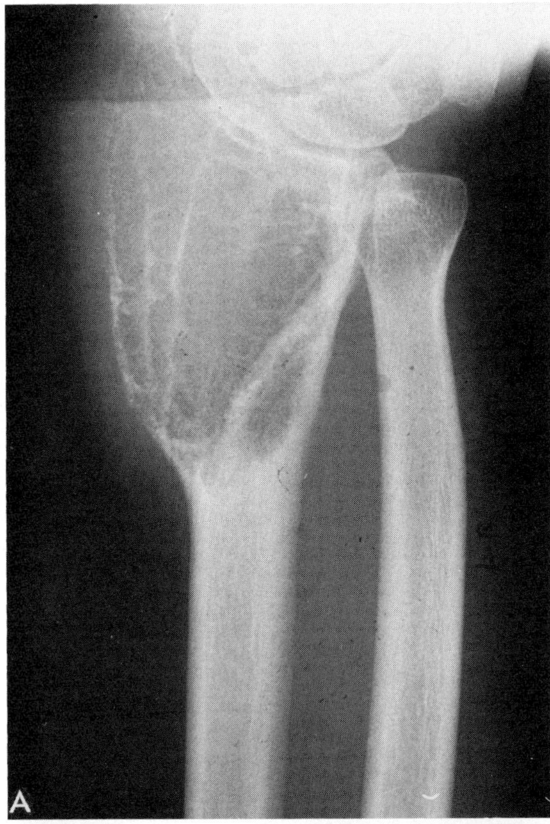

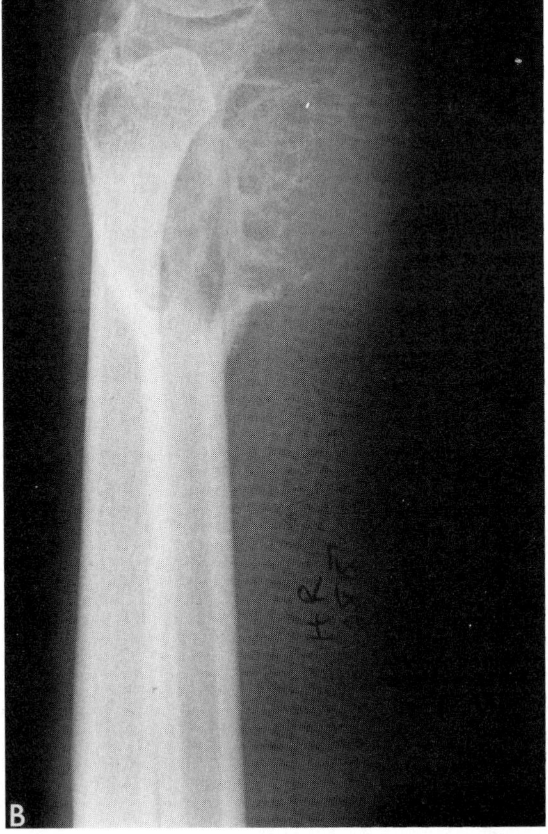

Figure 9–309. Anteroposterior (*A*) and lateral (*B*) radiographs of giant cell tumor of the distal radius. There has been marked expansion, with thinning and virtual absence of the subchondral bone and the subperiosteal bone on the volar aspect. Such growth that exceeds the ability of the body to maintain periosteal containment indicates fairly aggressive behavior and probable grade 2, if not actually malignant, histologic features.

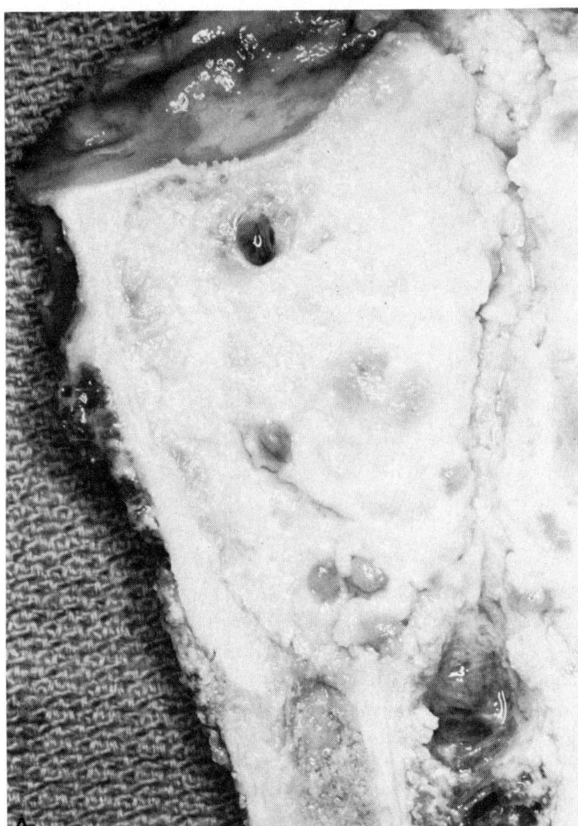

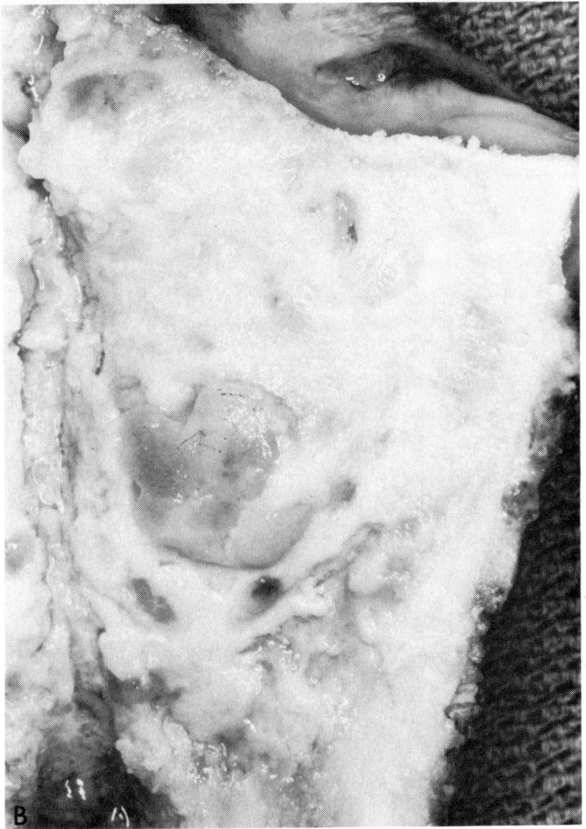

Figure 9–310. Gross specimens of distal radius showing two distinct patterns of tissue. In the bone closer to the dorsal cortex and extending proximally is a yellowish, granular tissue. This proved to be a low-grade spindle-cell component that was thought to be malignant. The central portion of the tumor exhibits myxomatous changes, numerous giant cells, and a pattern typical of benign giant cell tumor. The patient has done well during the 5 years following resection.

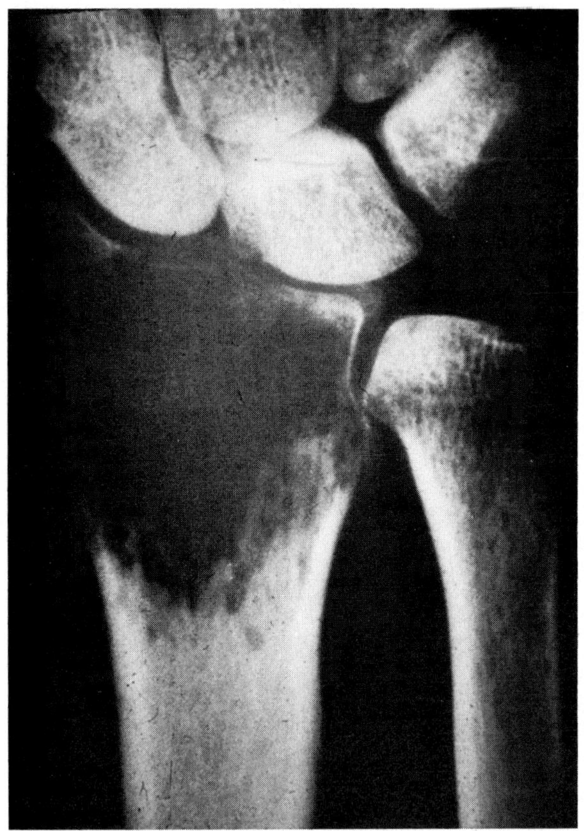

Figure 9–311

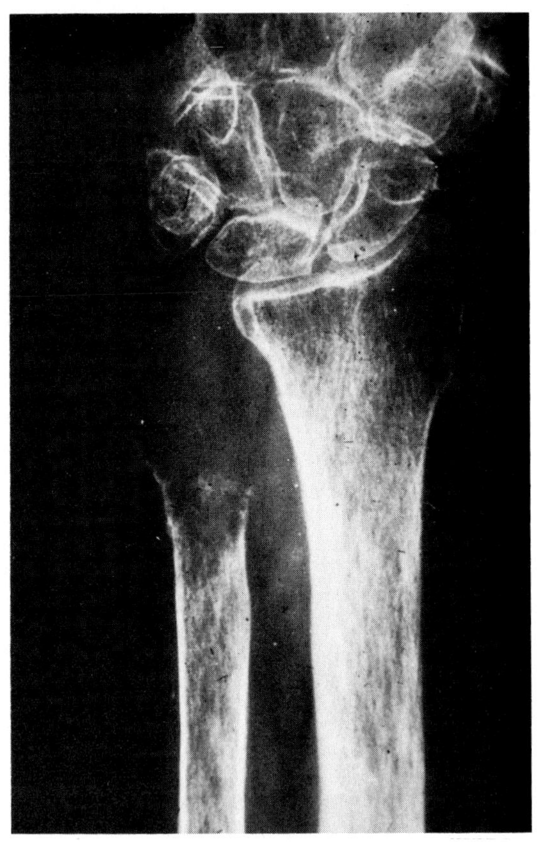

Figure 9–312

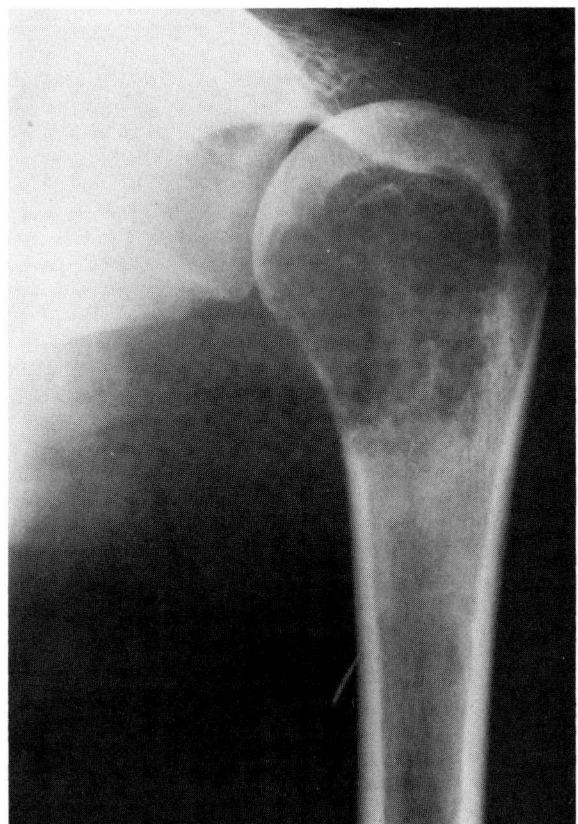

Figure 9–313

Figure 9–311. Giant cell tumor. Lytic defect in distal radius in a 30-year-old female. The irregular absorptive margin extending proximally into the metaphysis and the lack of periosteal new bone on the surface indicate that this is a very rapidly growing, possibly malignant, tumor. However, the histologic appearance was consistent with that of a benign lesion.

Figure 9–312. Giant cell tumor. Anteroposterior radiograph of the wrist with a malignant giant cell tumor of the distal ulna. There has been extensive resorption of bone of the ulna, with irregular, poorly defined margins extending proximally. The cortex of the distal ulna is completely eroded, and there is no periosteal new bone formation visible. Note the marked osteoporosis of the adjacent radius, the remainder of the ulna, and the carpal bones.

Figure 9–313. Giant cell tumor. Malignant giant cell tumor of the proximal humerus. Although the histologic findings in this case clearly indicated malignancy, the radiographic features are consistent with those of a benign lesion. Even the malignant lesion has its epicenter in the metaphysis.

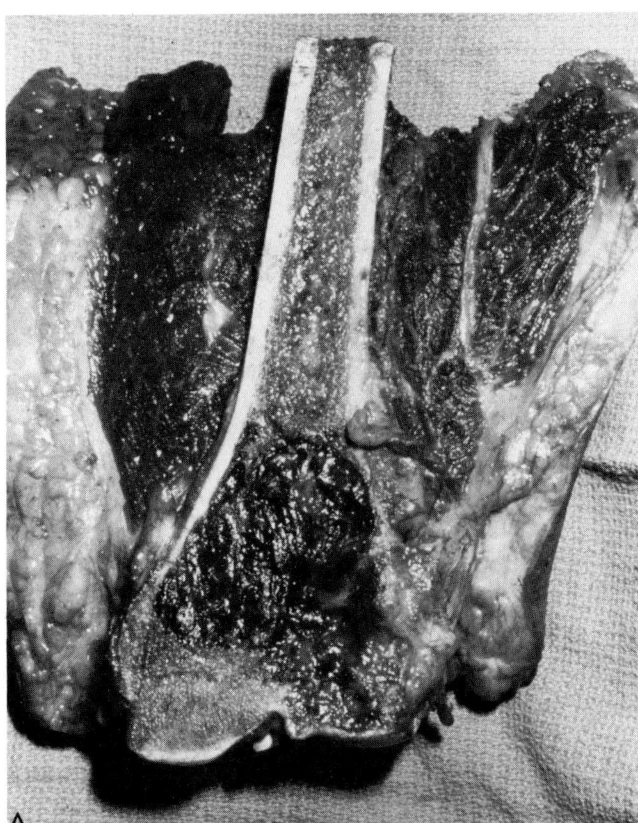

Figure 9–314. Giant cell tumor. Gross specimens of the distal femur in a patient with a malignant giant cell tumor that was curetted once. There was a soft-tissue recurrence within a few months, and within 1 year there were pulmonary metastases. Following amputation of the bone, the pulmonary metastases were resected. Limited and less than optimal chemotherapy was given, and the patient has remained well since that time, although he has bilateral pulmonary metastases that have not grown in more than 3 years. He refuses further therapy.

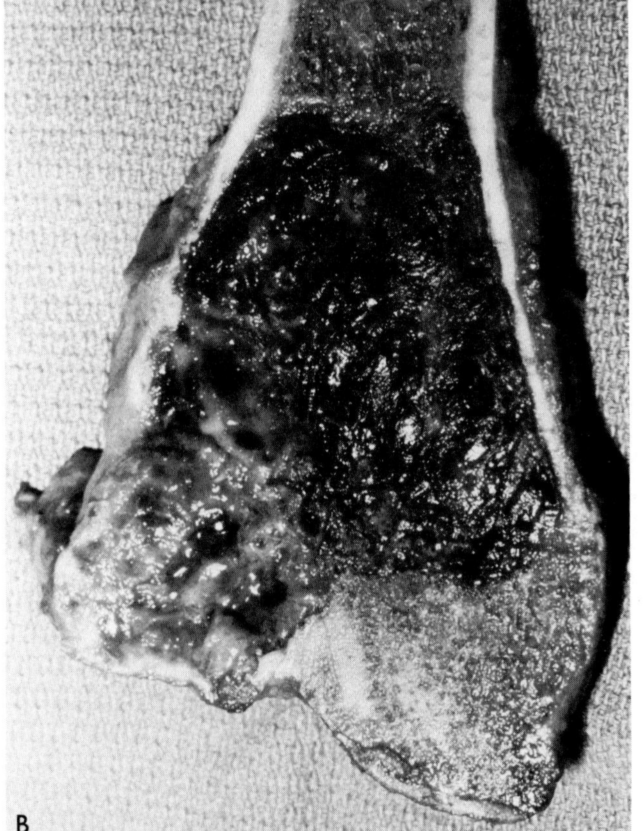

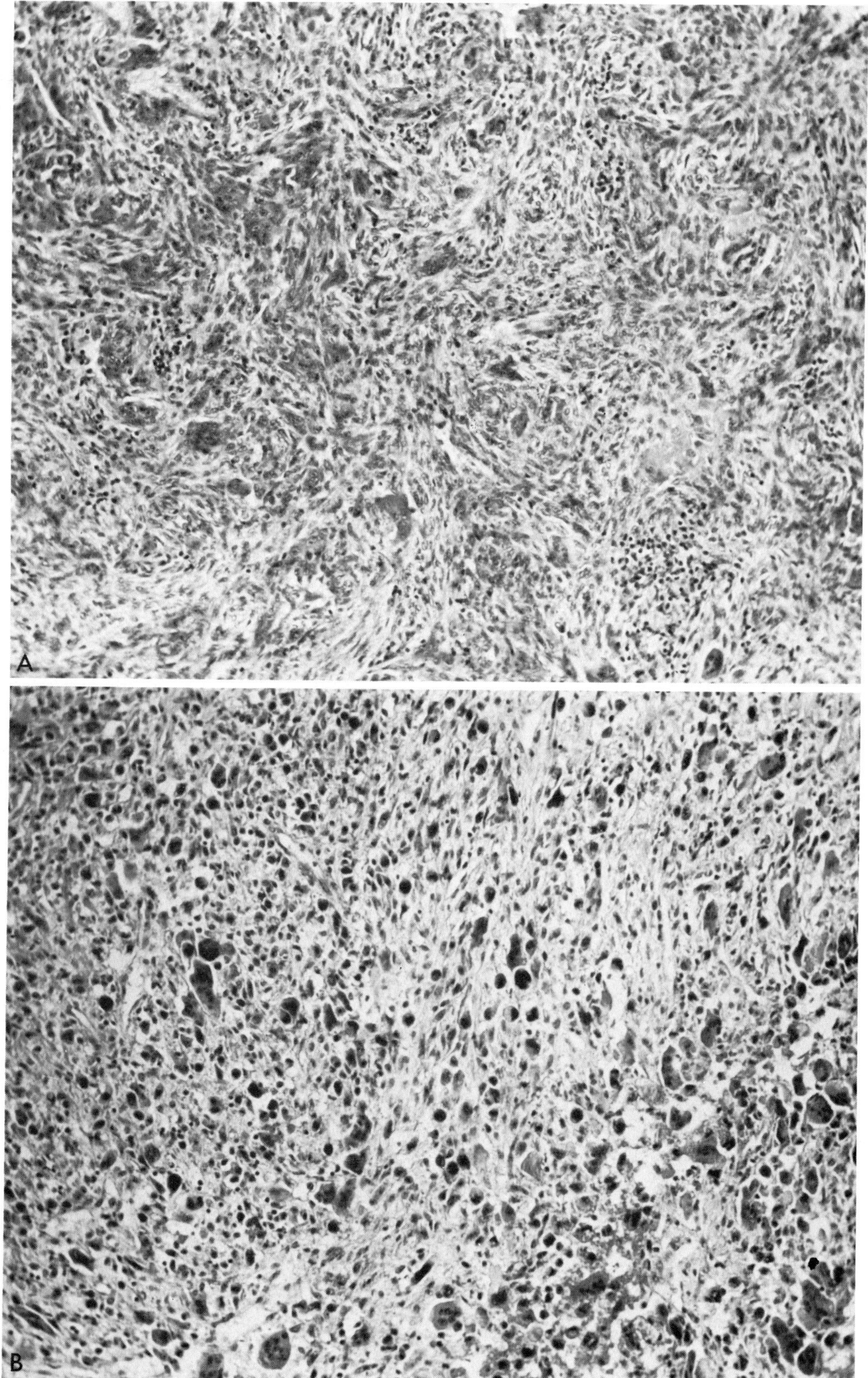

Figure 9–315. Giant cell tumor. Histologic appearance of malignant giant cell tumor of bone. The marked pelomorphism of the stromal cells and the small, irregular giant cells indicate a grade 3 tumor in *A* and *B* but outright malignant tumor in *C* to *F*.

Illustration continued on opposite page

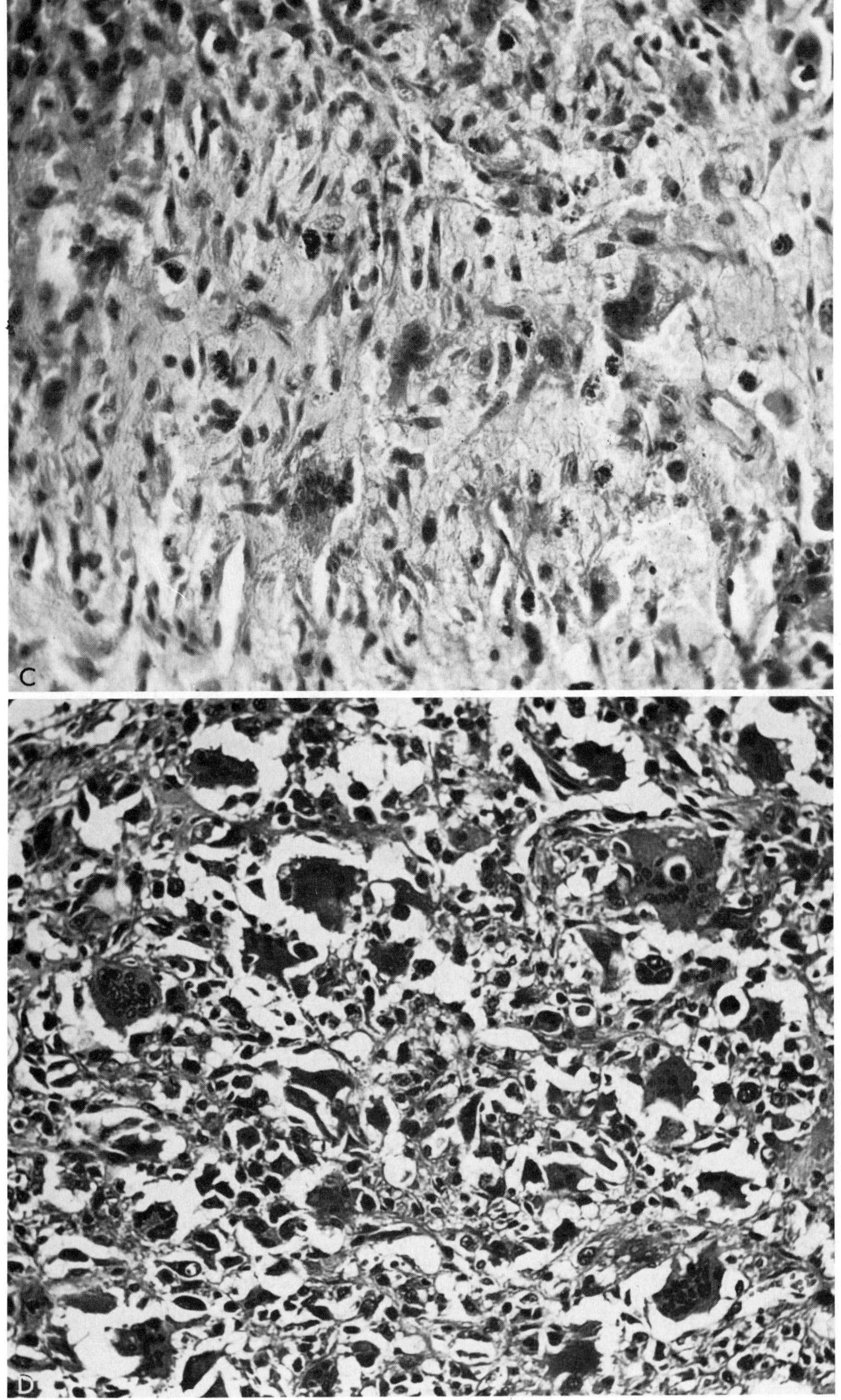

Figure 9–315 *Continued.*

Illustration continued on following page

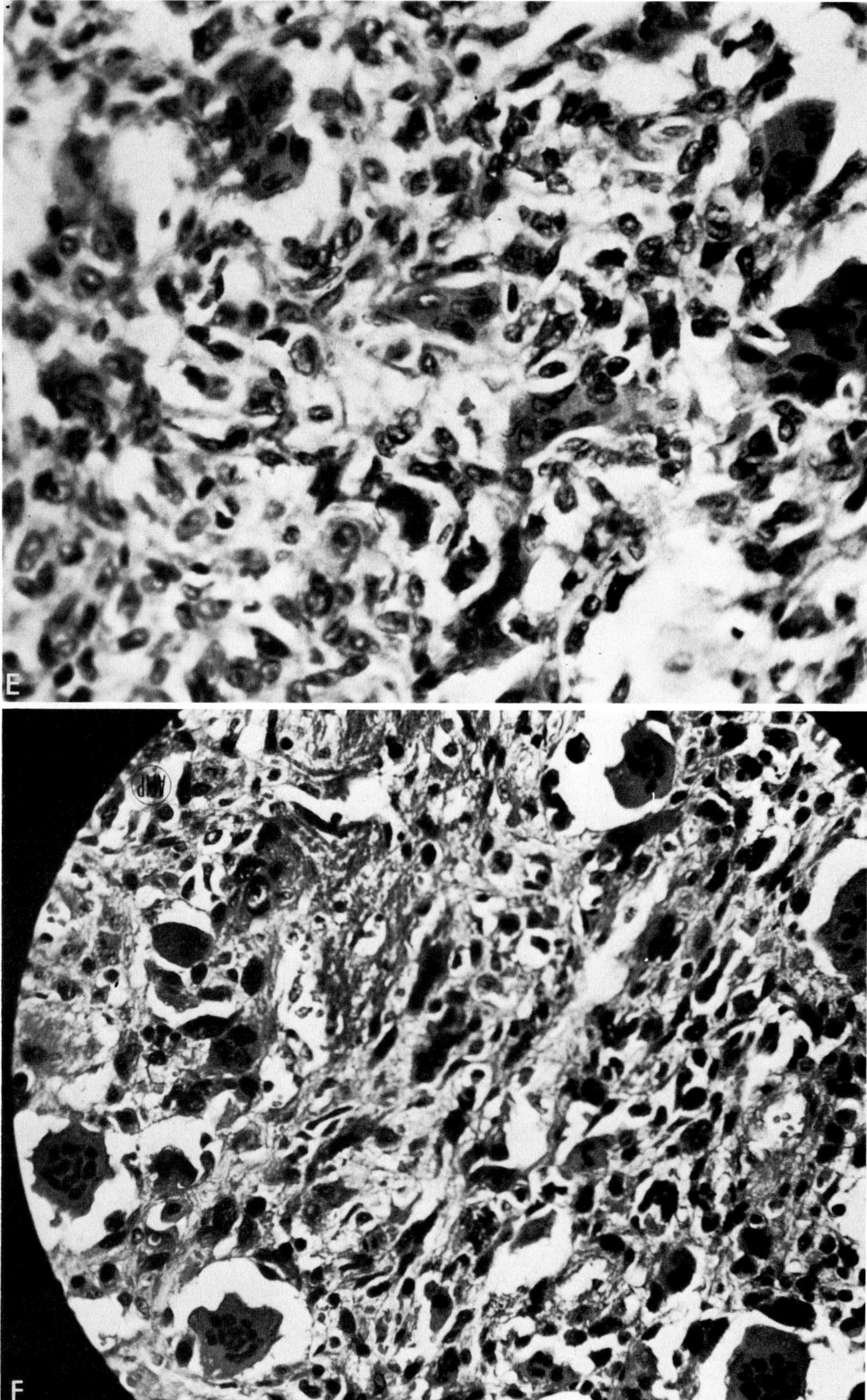

Figure 9–315 *Continued.*

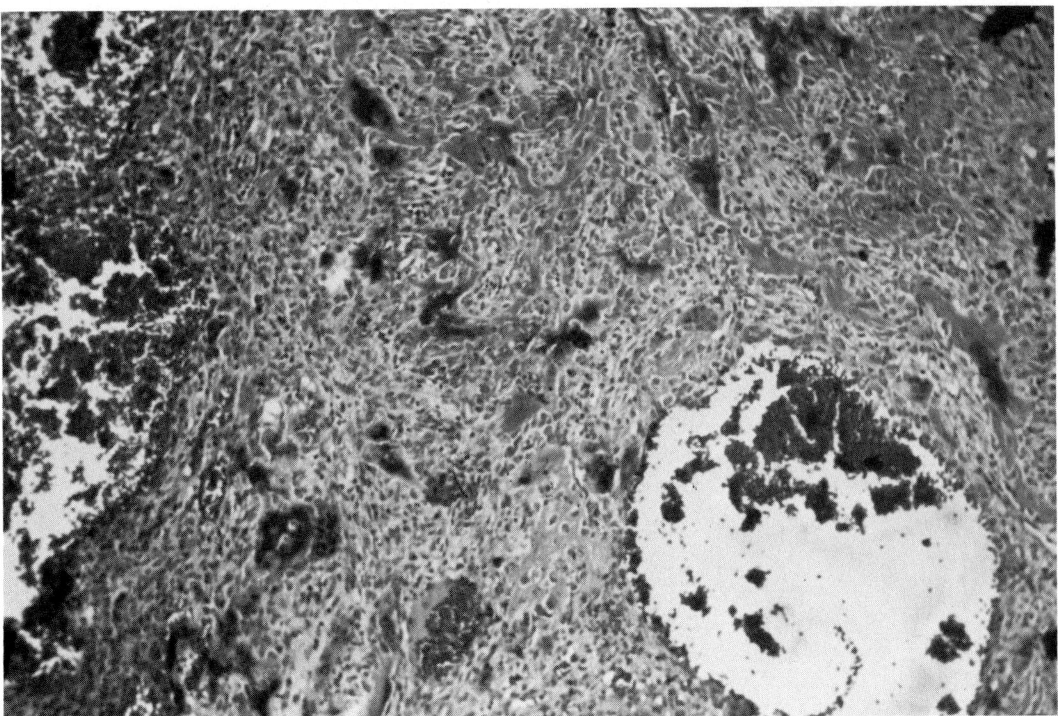

Figure 9–316. Giant cell tumor. Malignant giant cell tumor showing aneurysmal vascular changes in the stroma. Such vascular changes can occur in any lesion of bone and is quite common in giant cell tumor.

ROUND CELL TUMORS

Round cell tumors of the bone can be classified into three different groups: (1) Ewing's sarcoma, (2) primary lymphoma (reticulum cell sarcoma of bone), and (3) multiple myeloma.

EWING'S SARCOMA

Ewing's sarcoma and the primary lymphoma of bone consist of sheets of uniform small cells. These tumors grow fairly rapidly, with variable reactive processes within the bone. In the classic Ewing's sarcoma, the lesion grows so quickly that there is virtually no reaction whatsoever. A permeative destructive pattern is noted radiographically, and the characteristic periosteal "onion-peel" reaction is evident. Histologically, the tumor consists of sheets of uniform small cells with virtually no cytoplasm, forming no organoid pattern. Differential staining utilizing glycogen has been used to distinguish Ewing's sarcoma from primary lymphoma, but this is not always reliable. Electron microscopic differentiation can be carried out as well. The differential diagnosis must include secondary neoplasms, particularly neuroblastoma, which has a tendency for bone involvement.

The prognosis associated with Ewing's sarcoma used to be uniformly dismal, and indeed survival was considered nonexistent in the early 1960s. The advent of aggressive chemotherapy and radiation therapy has dramatically changed survival statistics associated with Ewing's sarcoma, and patients should be treated quickly and aggressively in order to maintain the current 50 per cent survival rate (Maurer, 1978).

Text continued on page 533

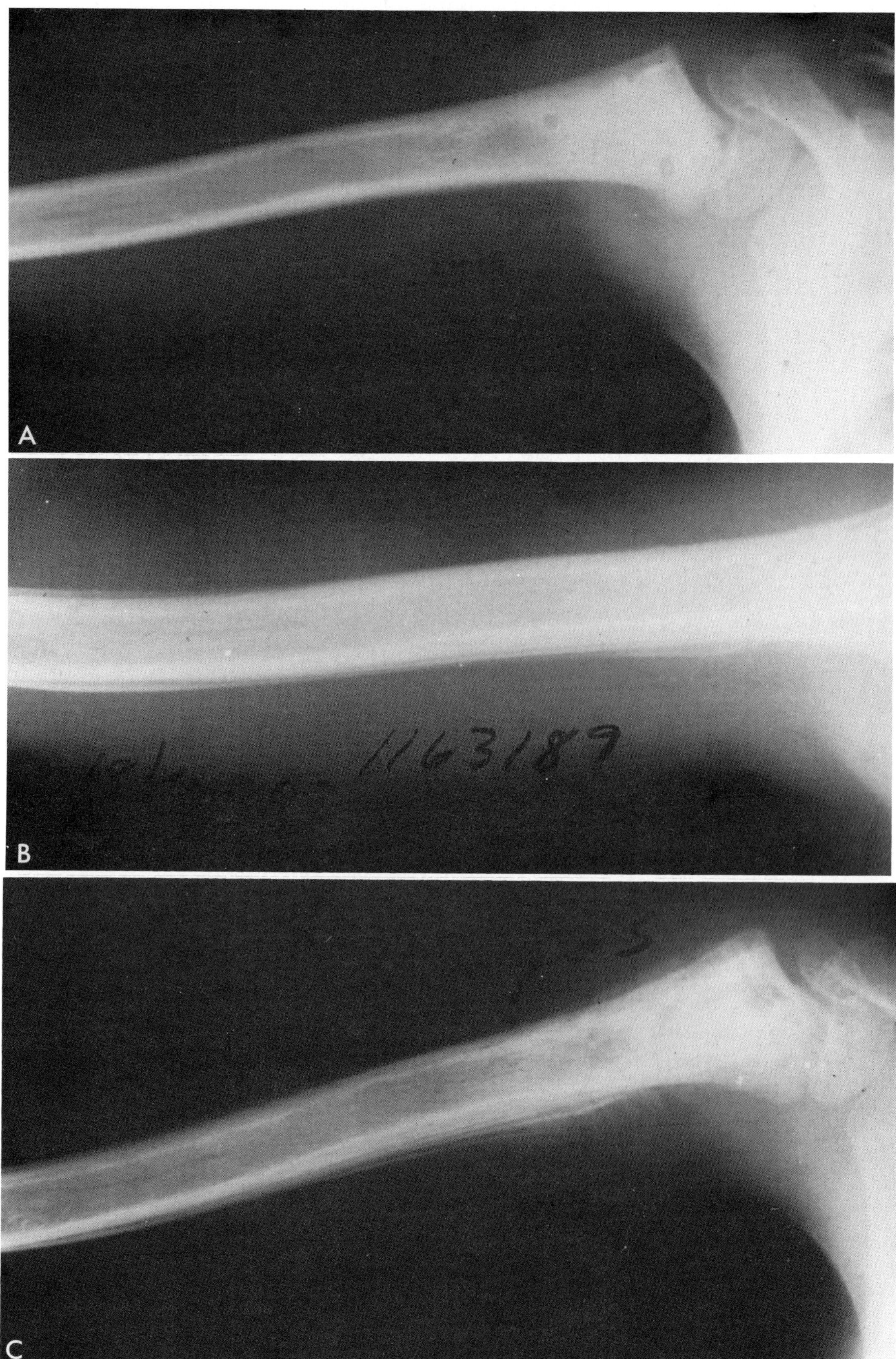

Figure 9–317. *See legend on opposite page.*

Illustration continued on opposite page

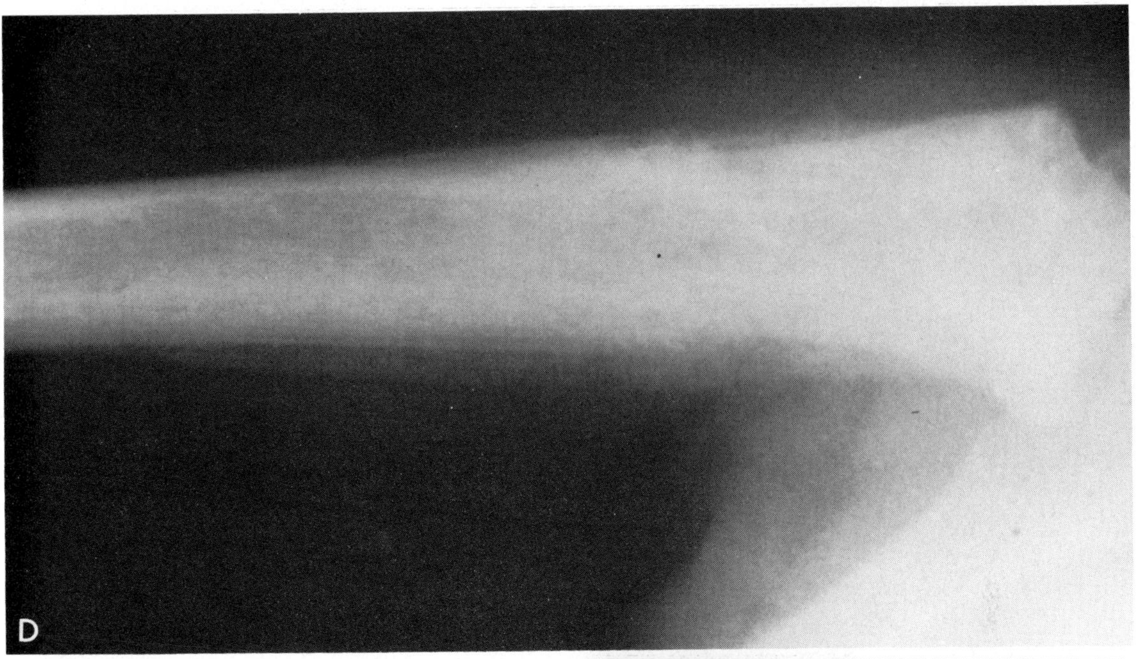

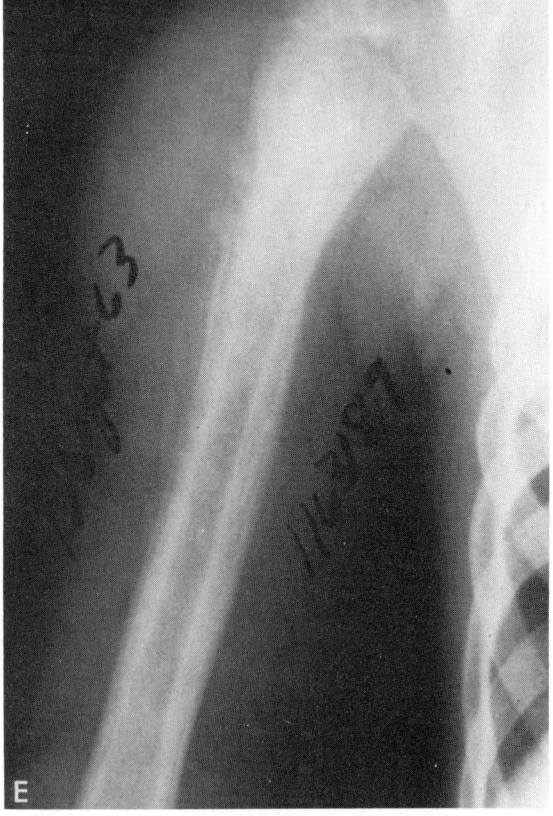

Figure 9–317. Ewing's sarcoma. Series of radiographs of humerus of a 6-year-old child with a 9-month history of pain in the arm, fever, chills, and elevated white-blood count. *A* shows lucencies in the proximal metaphysis without much periosteal reaction. The patient clinically responded to antibiotics until 4 months later (*B*), when a new wave of activity caused formation of periosteal reactive bone, with lytic and productive areas in metaphysis and diaphysis. Further activity produced several layers of periosteal laminar reaction and a sunburst pattern, visible 2 months later (*C*). One month later (*D*), there is more fill-back, followed by further "blow-out" (*E*) with large soft tissue mass under deltoid areas in which the periosteal reaction is unable to contain the tumor.

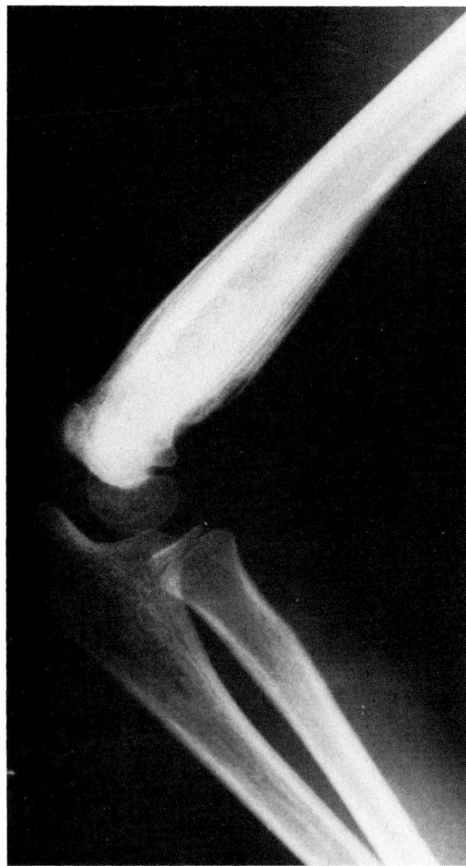

Figure 9–318. Ewing's sarcoma. Radiograph of Ewing's sarcoma with the characteristic "onion-peel" feature, consisting of concentric layers of periosteal elevation. There is permeative destruction of the lower humerus. Multiple layers of periosteal reactive bone indicate episodes of increased lesional activity (i.e., expansion) interspersed with pauses during which the periosteum can deposit bone in its new position before another wave of activity pushes it outward again.

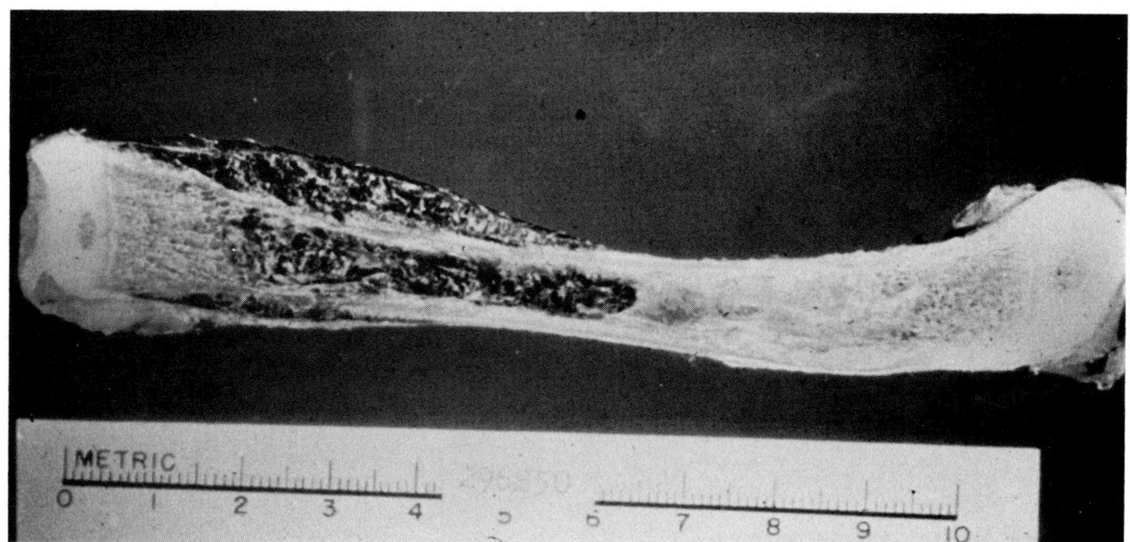

Figure 9–319. Ewing's sarcoma. Hemisection of bone containing Ewing's sarcoma. Note that periosteal reaction matches intraosseous extent of tumor.

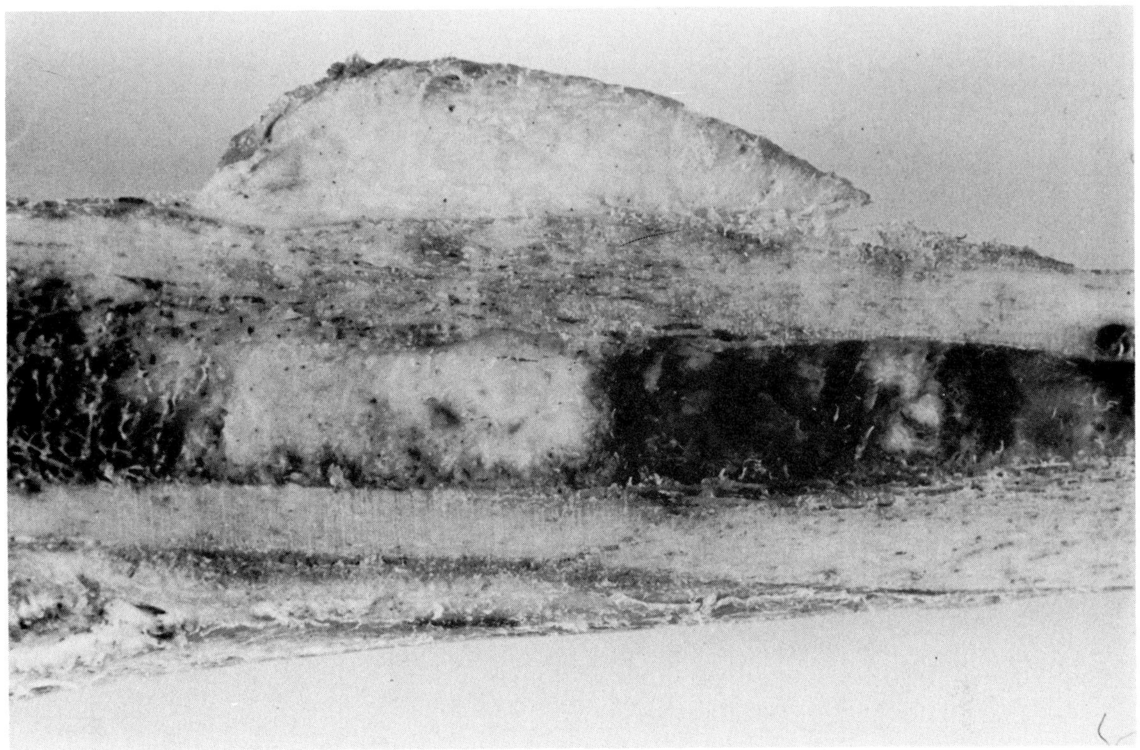

Figure 9–320. Ewing's sarcoma. Gross specimen of Ewing's sarcoma. The hemorrhagic component within the medullary cavity is secondary to biopsy. Note the extensive permeative destruction of the cortex and extension of tumor into soft tissue.

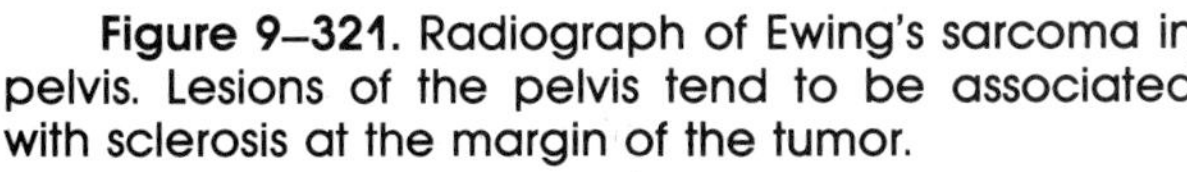

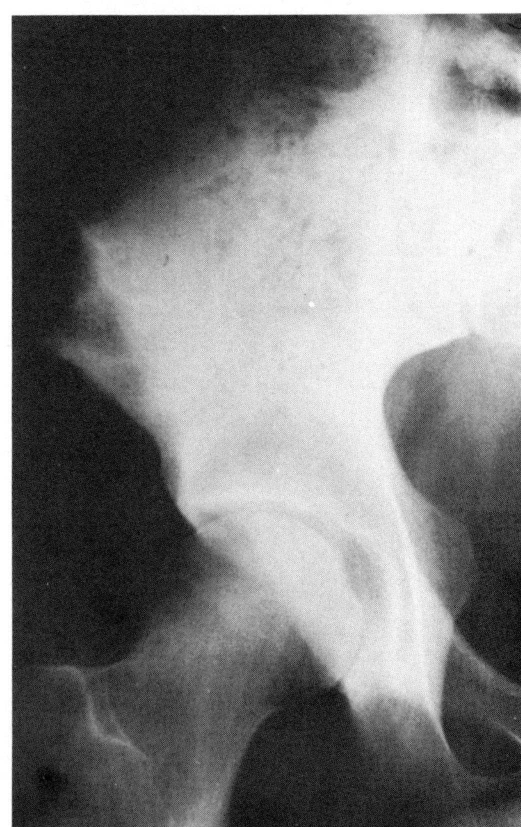

Figure 9–321. Radiograph of Ewing's sarcoma in pelvis. Lesions of the pelvis tend to be associated with sclerosis at the margin of the tumor.

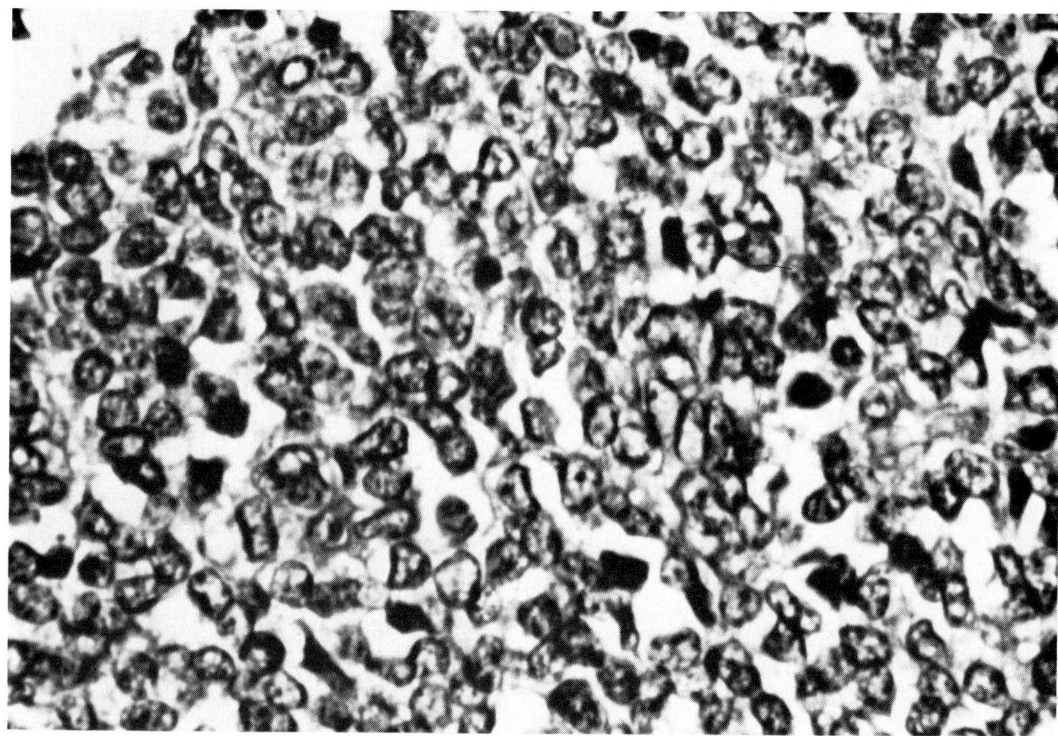

Figure 9–322. Ewing's sarcoma. High-power view of Ewing's sarcoma. More or less uniform cells with minimal cytoplasm are characteristic. Mitoses are frequent. No matrix is produced. Vessel formation is seldom conspicuous, and their absence may lead to areas of infarction with liquefactive necrosis of portions of the tumor. Absorption of breakdown products of the tumor will produce systemic signs of infection.

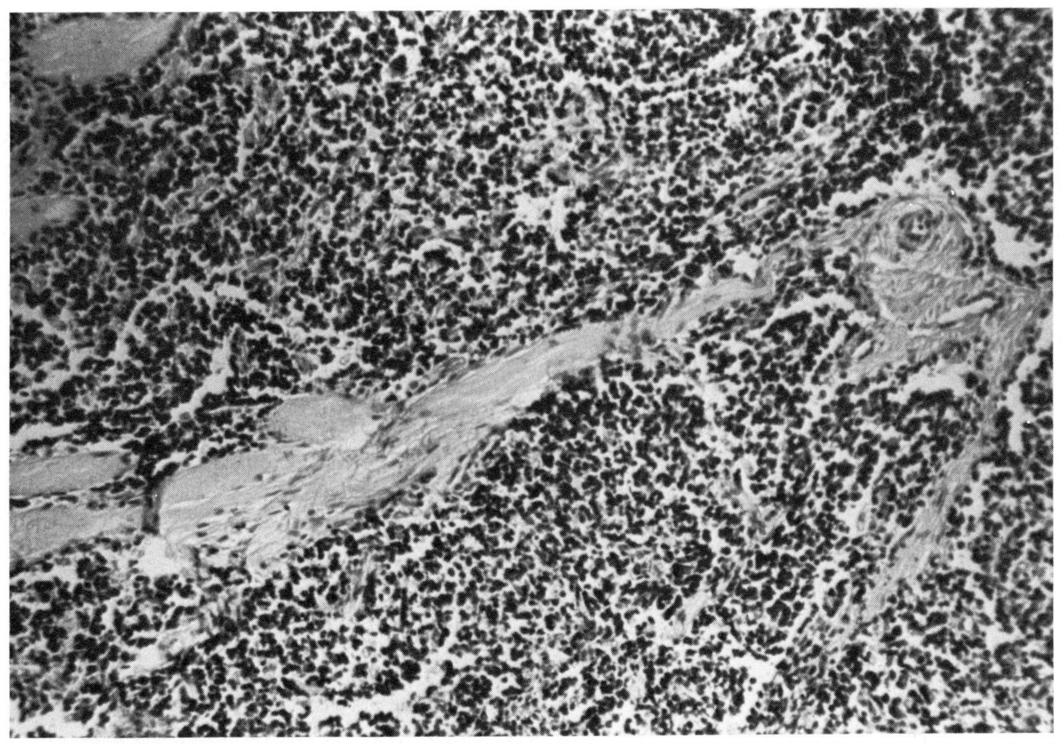

Figure 9–323. Ewing's sarcoma. The tumor consists of a sheet-like infiltrate of round cells invading between muscle fibers. No well-defined stroma is produced by the cells.

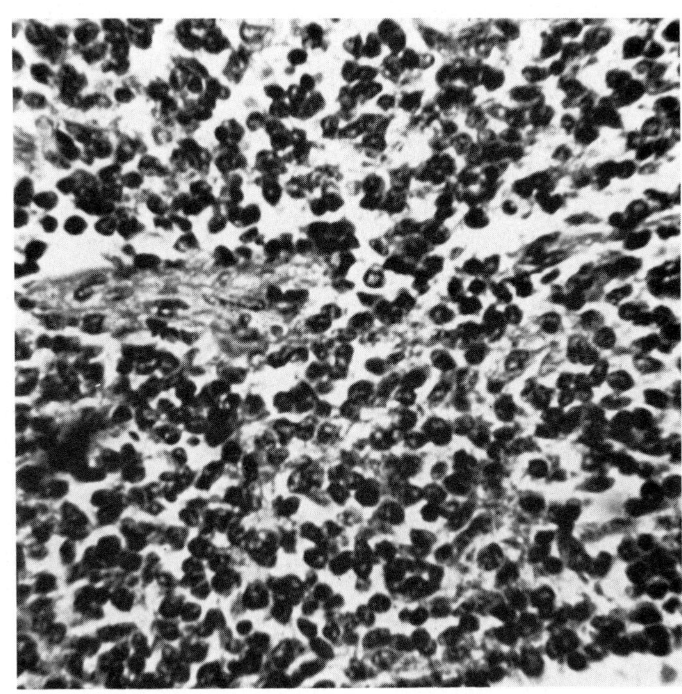

Figure 9–324. Ewing's sarcoma. High power view of lesion illustrated in Figure 9–323. Note the uniform round-cell nuclei with minimal cytoplasm, characteristic features of Ewing's sarcoma.

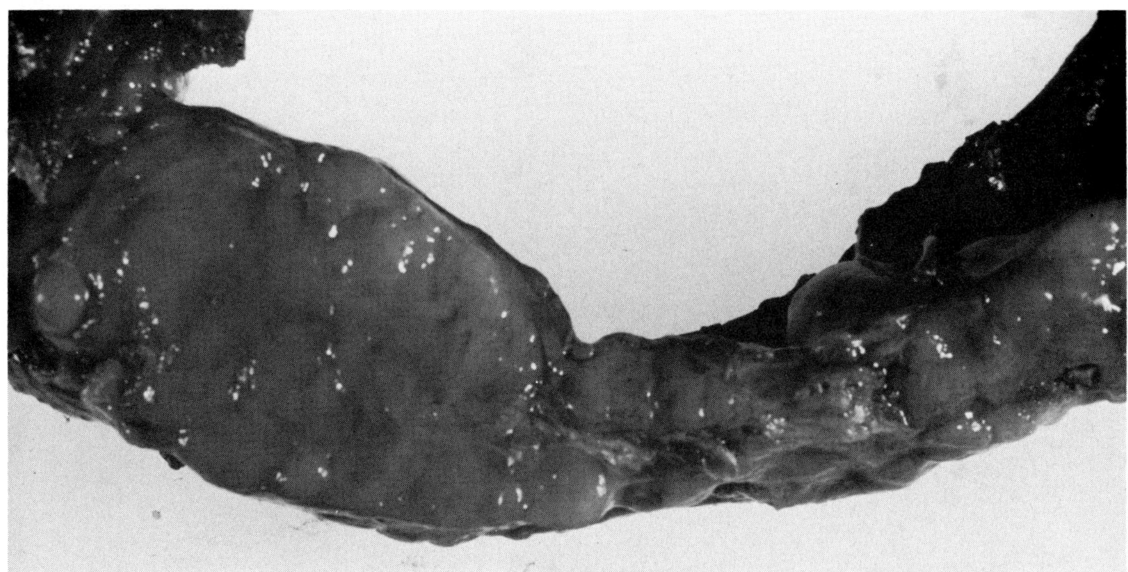

Figure 9–325. Primary lymphoma. Gross photograph of rib with primary lymphoma (reticulum cell sarcoma). The tumor replaces bone with relatively little reaction. It exhibits a "fish-flesh" consistency.

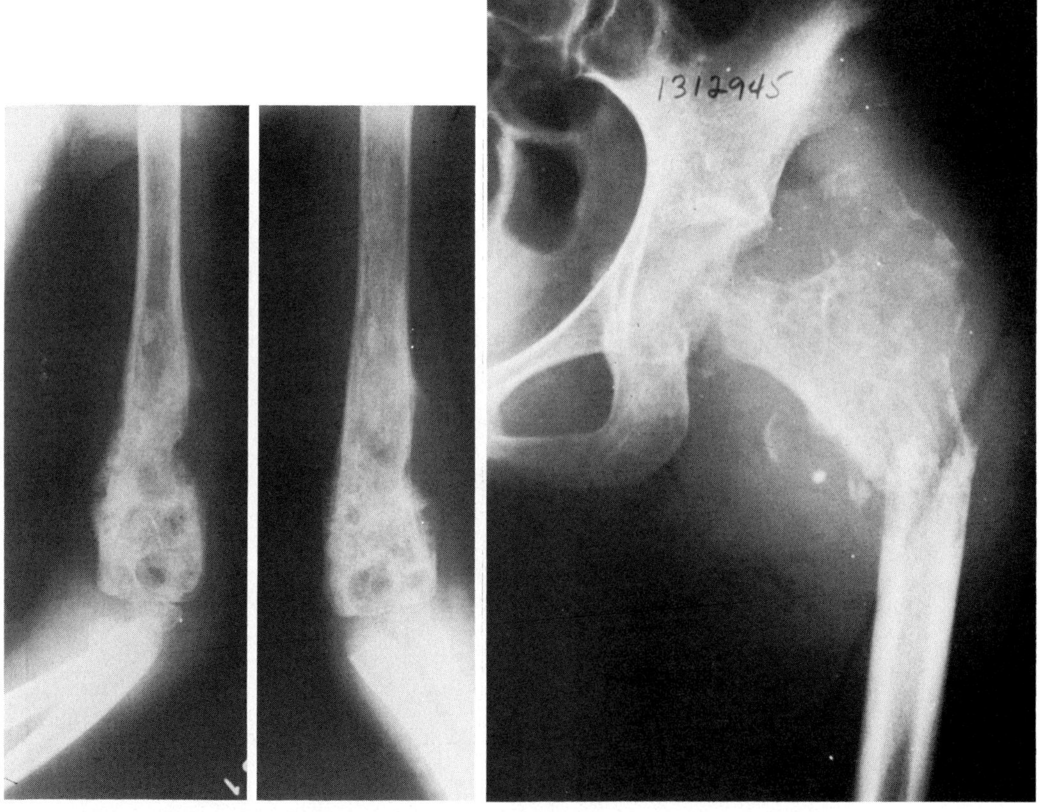

Figure 9–326   **Figure 9–327**

Figure 9–326. Primary lymphoma. Radiographs of lower humerus with primary lymphoma of bone. The permeative destruction of the cortex with periosteal reaction indicates a malignant process.

Figure 9–327. Primary lymphoma. Radiograph of irregular, extensive, destructive process in the femoral head and trochanter.

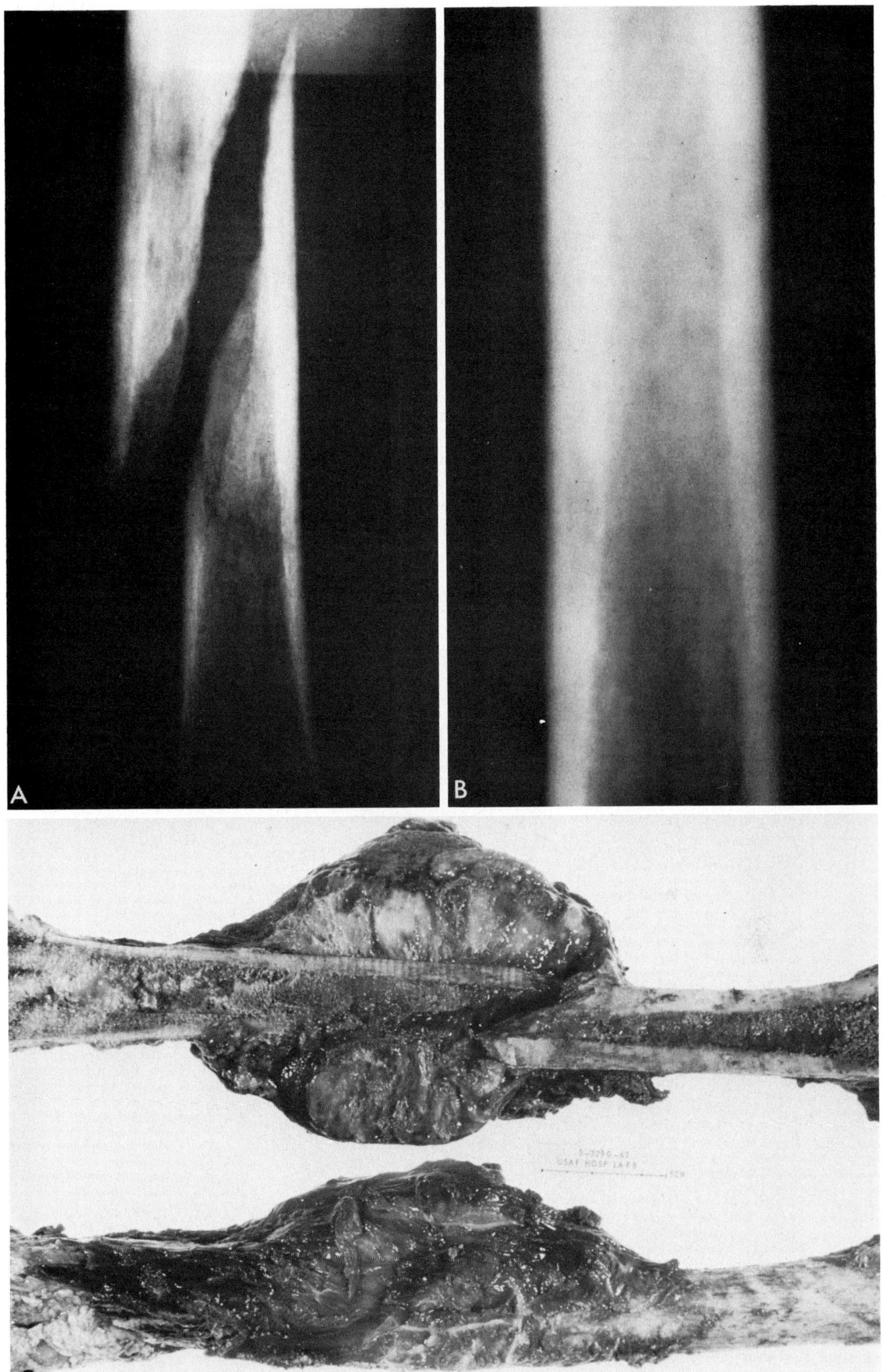

Figure 9–328. Primary lymphoma. Radiographs (*A* and *B*) and gross specimen (*C*) of femur with primary lymphoma. Radiograph of the femur shows subtle permeative destruction not easily visualized. The tumor involves bone and soft tissue more extensively than indicated by the radiograph. The massive involvement with minimal reaction is characteristic of primary lymphoma in long bones.

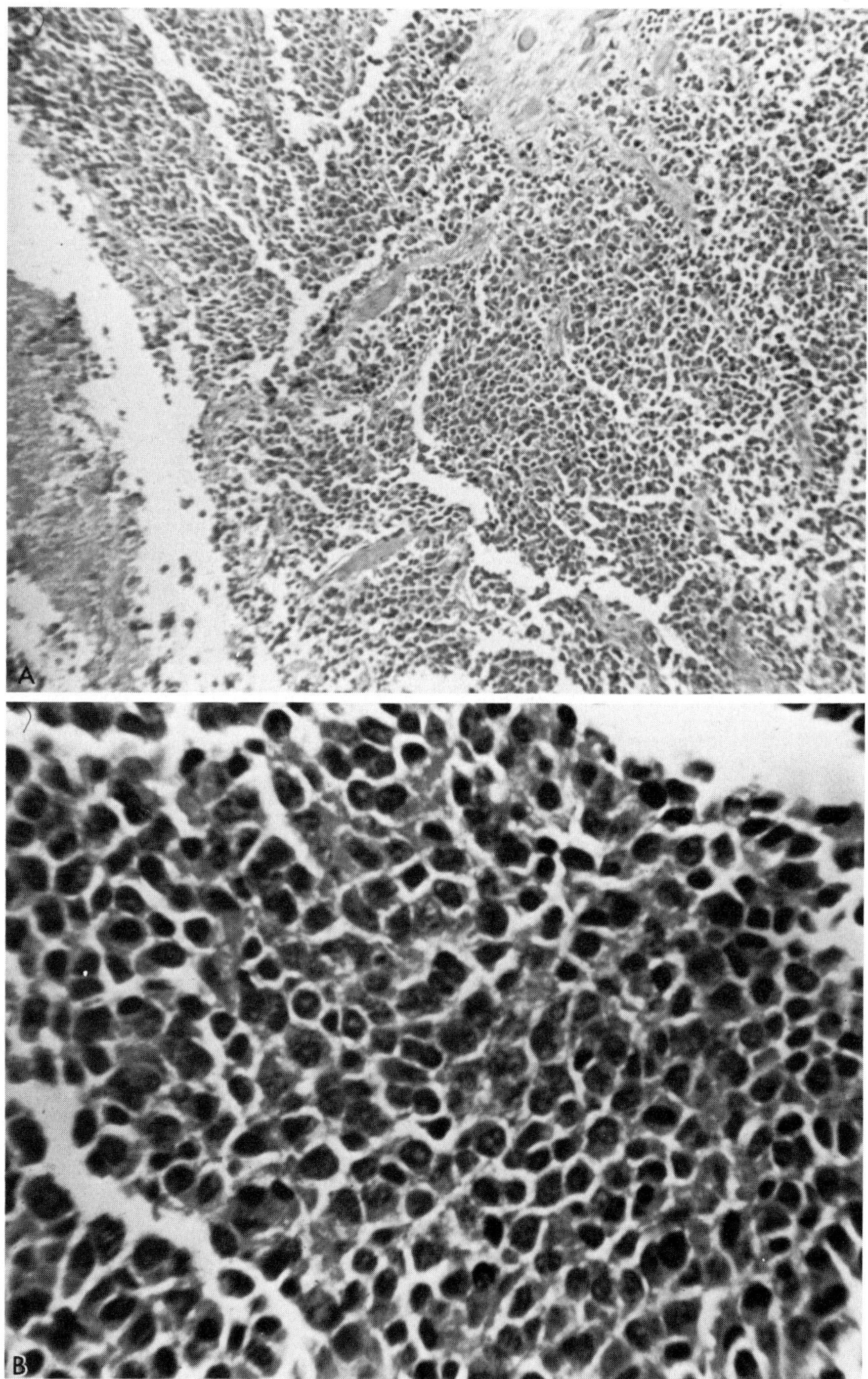

Figure 9–329. Primary lymphoma. Histologic sections of primary lymphoma. Compared with the cells in Ewing's sarcoma, the cells in this tumor are large and pleomorphic, with identifiable cytoplasmic content and margins. The monomorphous, sheet-like infiltrate is characteristic of both Ewing's sarcoma and primary lymphoma.

PRIMARY LYMPHOMA

Primary lymphoma of bone exhibits a histologic appearance that is similar to that of Ewing's sarcoma, and differentiation between the two lesions may be difficult. Classically, it is a slower growing tumor, and it involves an older age group. In view of the slightly slower growth rate, reactive processes are more pronounced. The cells of the lymphoma tend to be somewhat larger, with more prominent cytoplasm; a reticular meshwork appears, but the undifferentiated sheet-like infiltration is the same in both lesions, and the absence of glycogen has been used as a histochemical identifier (Boston et al., 1974). Aggressive radiation and chemotherapy have markedly improved the outlook for these patients.

MULTIPLE MYELOMA

Multiple myeloma is an infiltration of the marrow by plasma cells. The general appearance of the lesion is that of a circumscribed lytic defect without any significant osteoblastic reaction. The extremely rare case of multiple myeloma associated with osteosclerosis is the oddity; in principle, myeloma is always lytic (Kyle, 1975; Rogers et al., 1977, Rodriguez et al., 1976). Myeloma may present without identifiable osseous lesions and simply exhibit diffuse osteoporosis. Histologically, the plasma cell infiltrate is generalized and demonstrates no reactive bone formation (unless the patient has been treated). On closer examination the immaturity and variability of the plasma cells can be identified. The lesion must be differentiated from a plasma cell osteomyelitis, which may lead to a solitary or multiple osseous defects mimicking myeloma. A diagnosis should never be made without confirmatory laboratory data.

Text continued on page 545

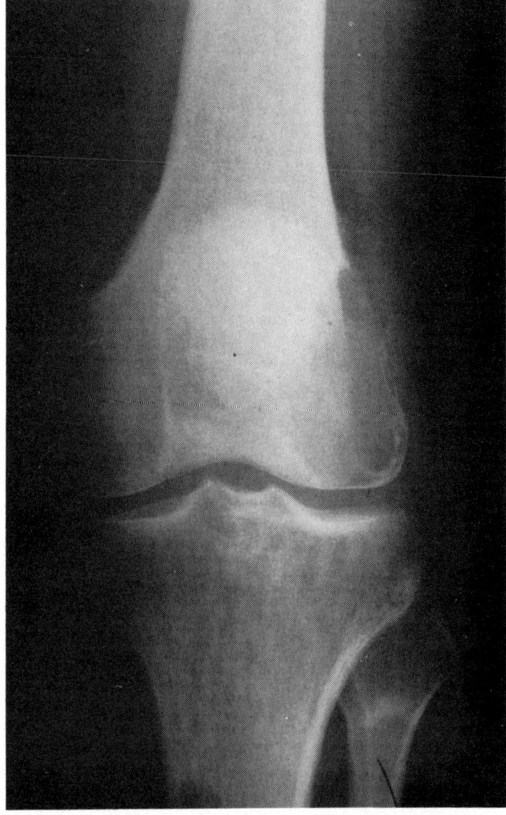

Figure 9–330. Multiple myeloma. Radiograph of a knee exhibiting a large lytic defect in the lateral femoral condyle. There is minimal reaction on the surface of the bone, even though a large portion of the surface has been removed by the tumor. Solitary myeloma is a very uncommon lesion. A focus of plasma cell myeloma may appear to be the only lesion, but the disease almost always becomes disseminated within 2 years.

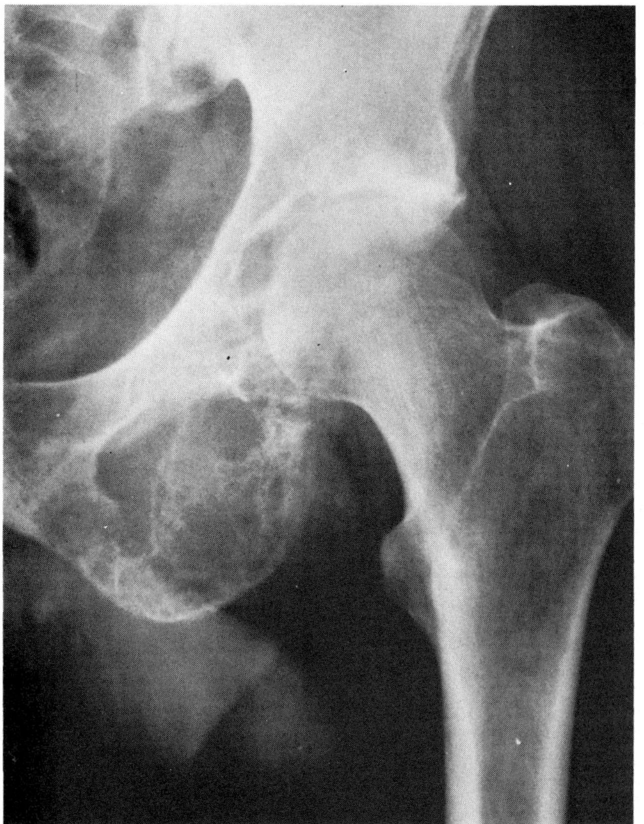

Figure 9–331. Multiple myeloma. Anteroposterior radiograph of left hip in a 39-year-old male who stumbled and developed hip pain. The radiograph shows a large lytic defect in the ischium and inferior pubic ramus. Plasma proteins reveal a monoclonal "spike," and iliac marrow biopsy reveals infiltrates of myeloma cells.

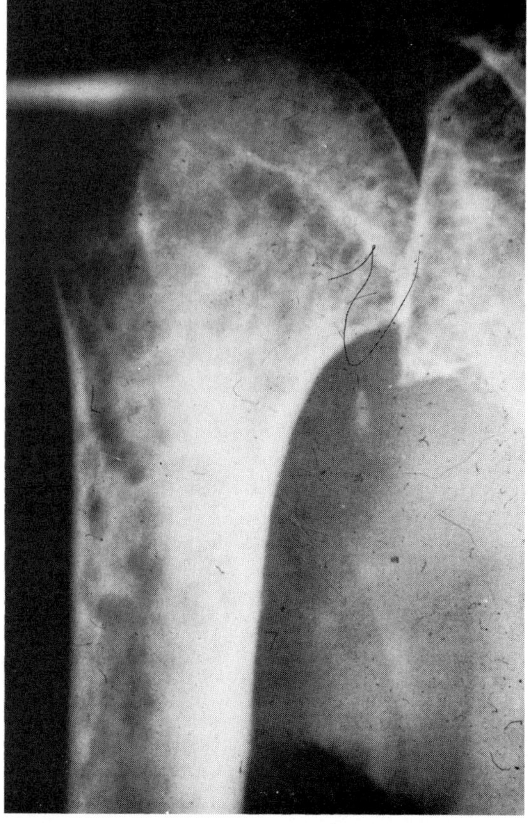

Figure 9–332. Multiple myeloma. Anteroposterior radiograph of shoulder exhibiting diffuse lytic changes in the humerus and glenoid. There is no periosteal reaction. The lesion could be misconstrued as osteoporosis of disuse in a painful shoulder.

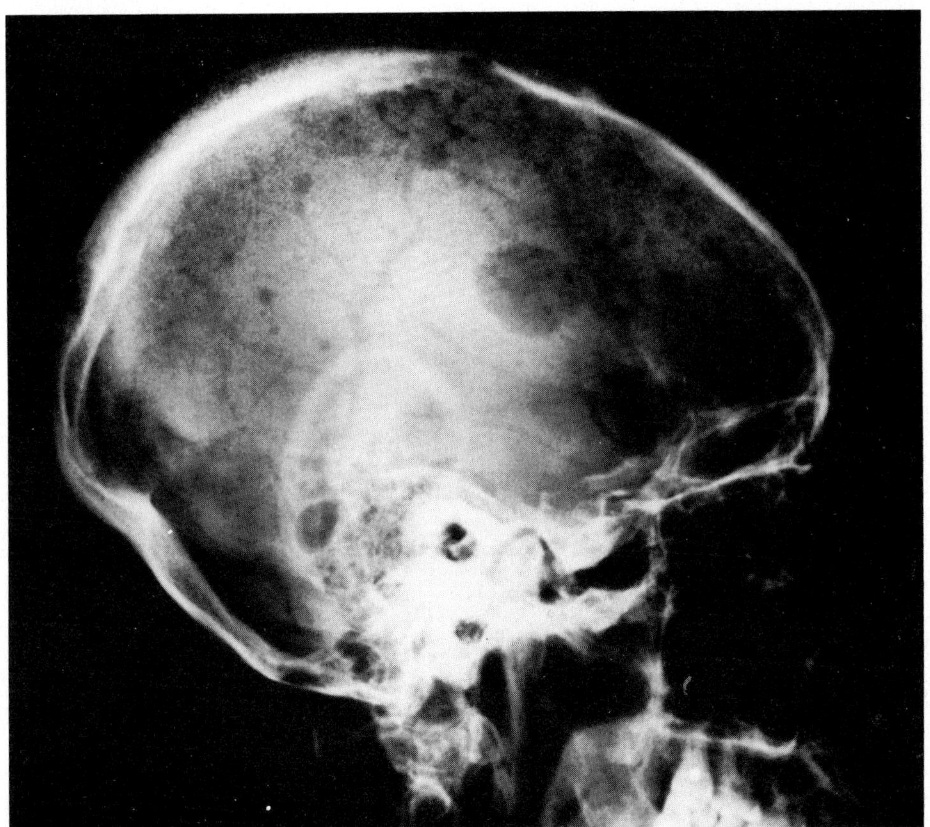

Figure 9–333. Multiple myeloma. Lateral radiograph of skull exhibiting discrete defects in the calvarium. There is minimal sclerotic reaction around these lytic foci. This is more pronounced around the larger, presumably older, focus. The smaller foci have almost no reaction.

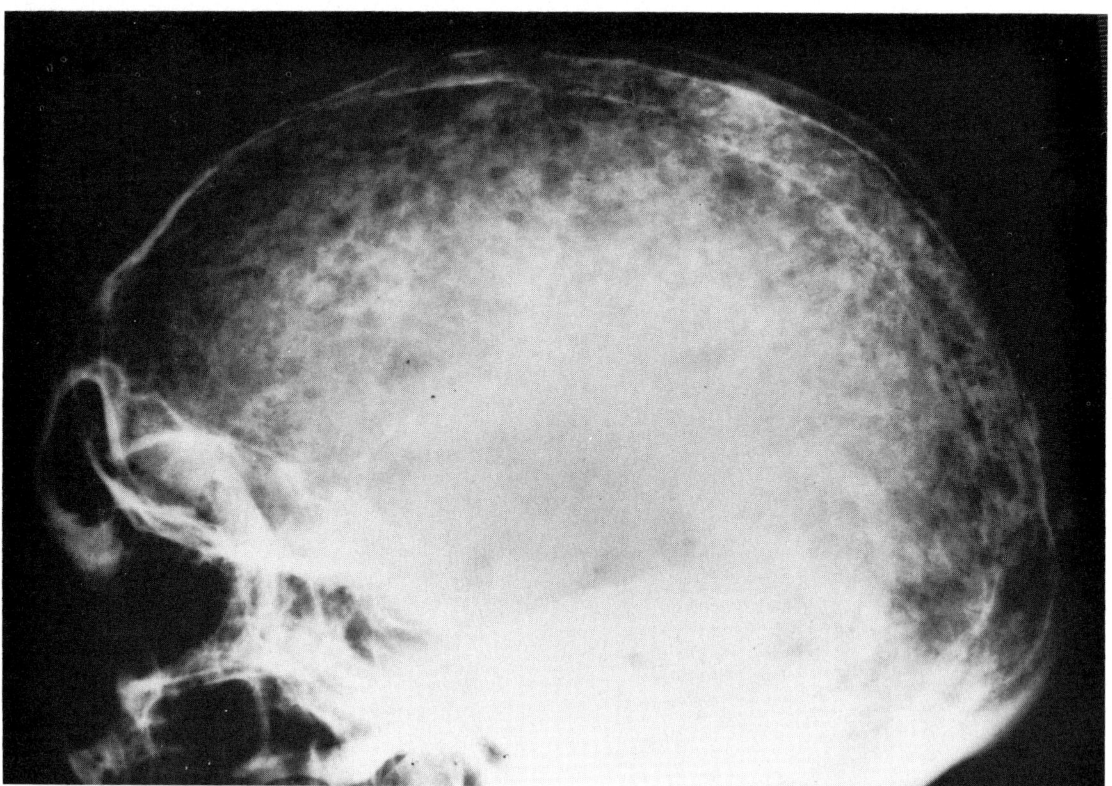

Figure 9–334. Multiple myeloma. Lateral radiograph of skull exhibiting more diffuse involvement with multiple small lytic defects.

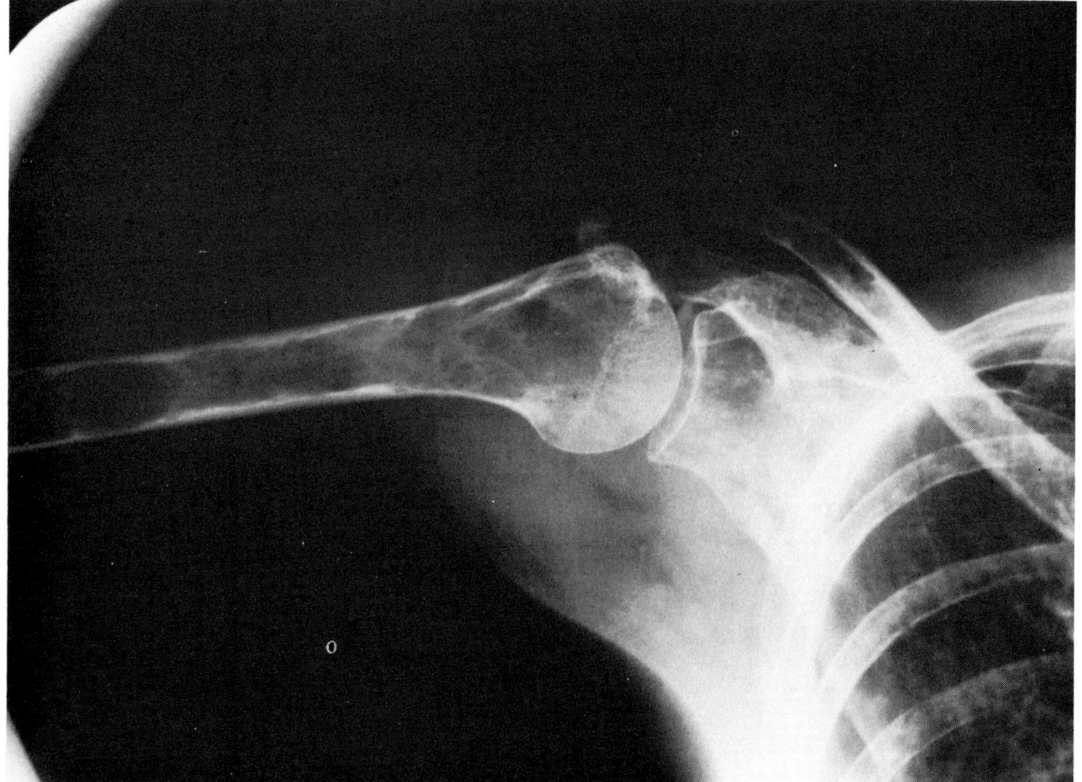

Figure 9–335. Multiple myeloma. Anteroposterior radiograph of shoulder joint with discrete punched-out lesions in the medullary cavity of the humerus. These remove cortical bone from within, but there is no periosteal reaction. Frequently, lesions of multiple myeloma are "cold" on bone scan because bone reaction is minimal.

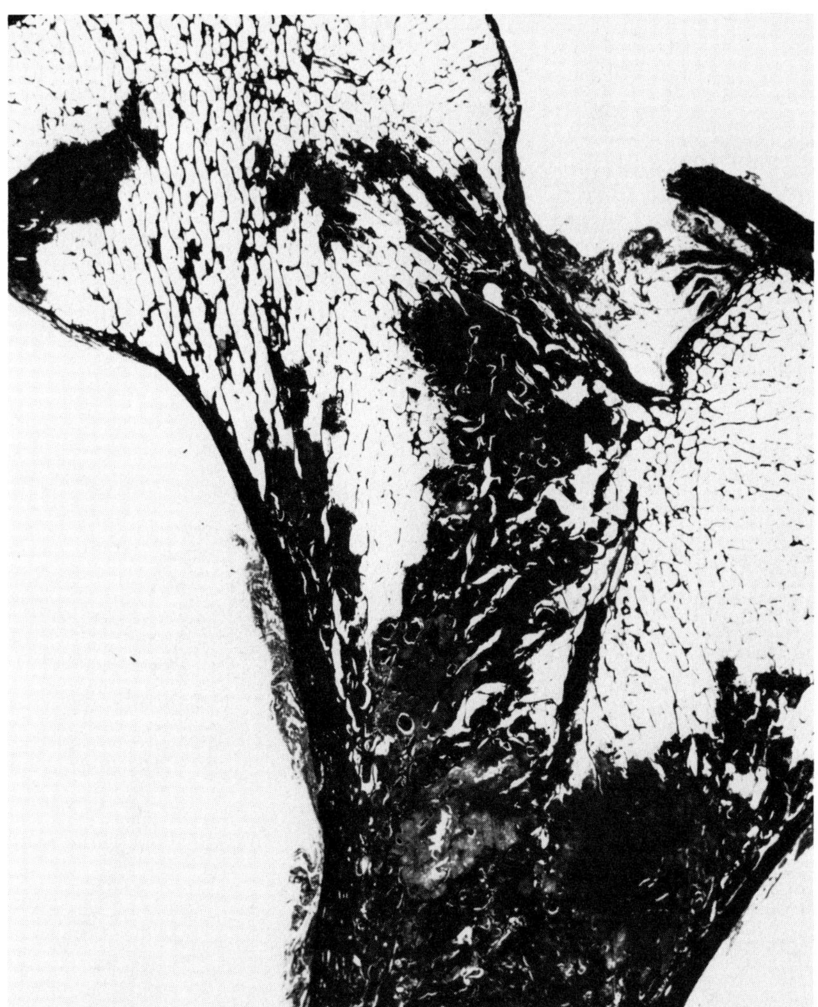

Figure 9–336. Multiple myeloma. Macrosection of proximal femur with extensive deposits of myelomatous tissue scattered throughout the bone. Unlike many other lesions, myeloma can produce multiple deposits of abnormal cells without becoming confluent.

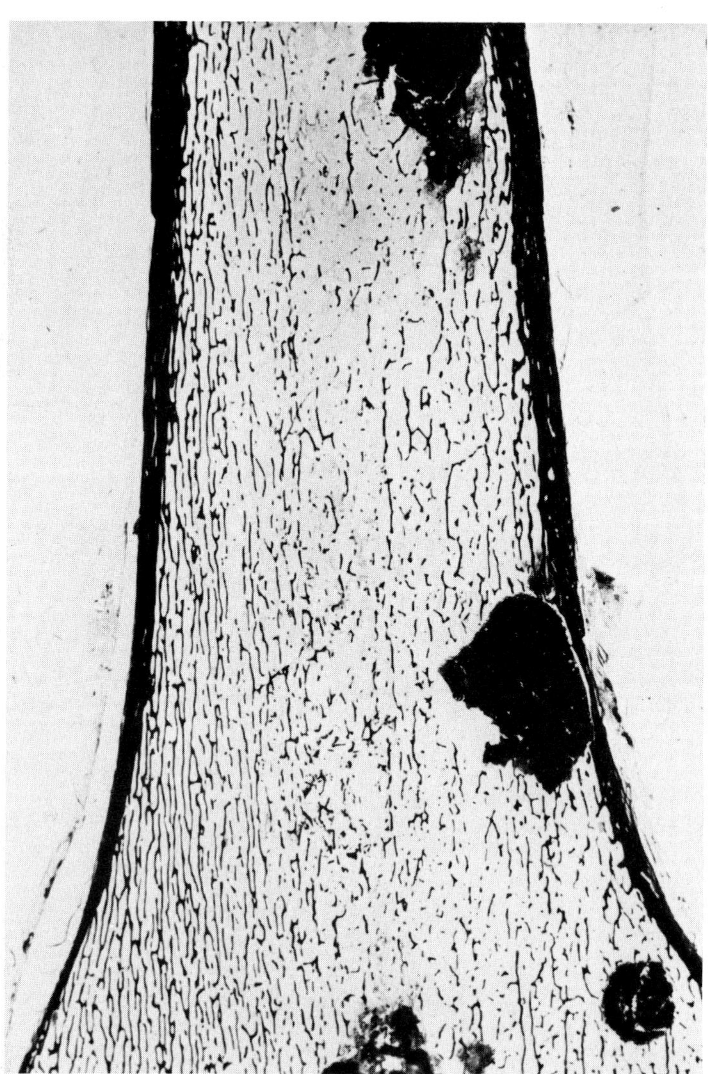

Figure 9–337. Multiple myeloma. Macrosection of distal femur with several large myeloma deposits. Note the moderate osteoporosis evident throughout the specimen.

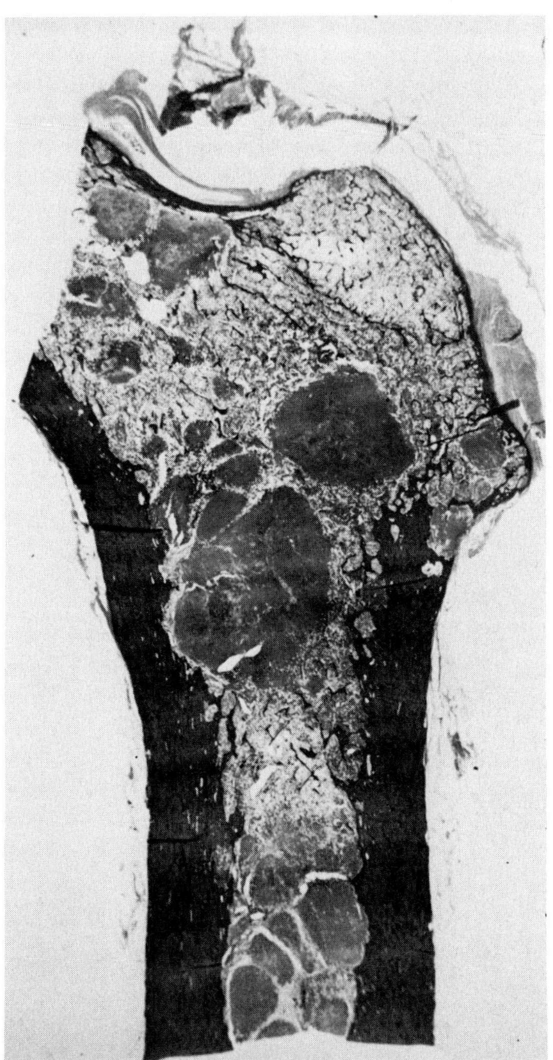

Figure 9–338. Multiple myeloma. Macrosection of proximal femur with a number of myeloma lesions. There is erosion of the cortex from within the medullary cavity, with absence of periosteal reaction.

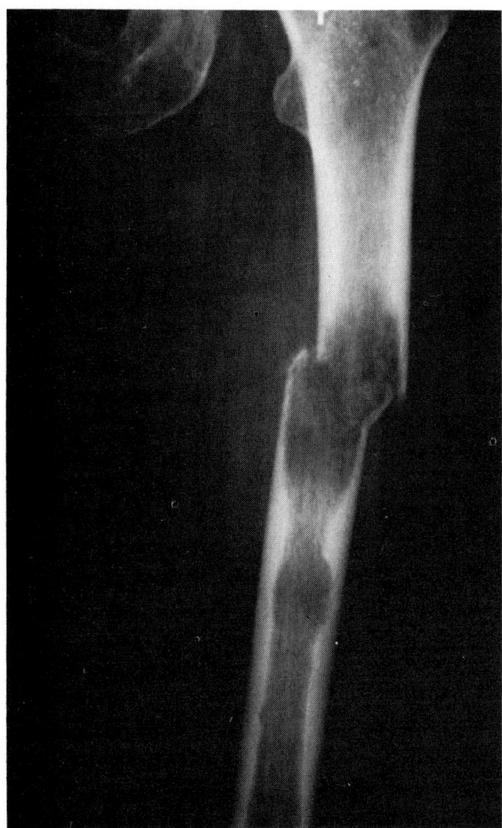

Figure 9–339. Multiple myeloma. Radiograph of femur with pathologic fracture through a focus of myeloma. Note the striking osteoporosis and the lack of periosteal reaction.

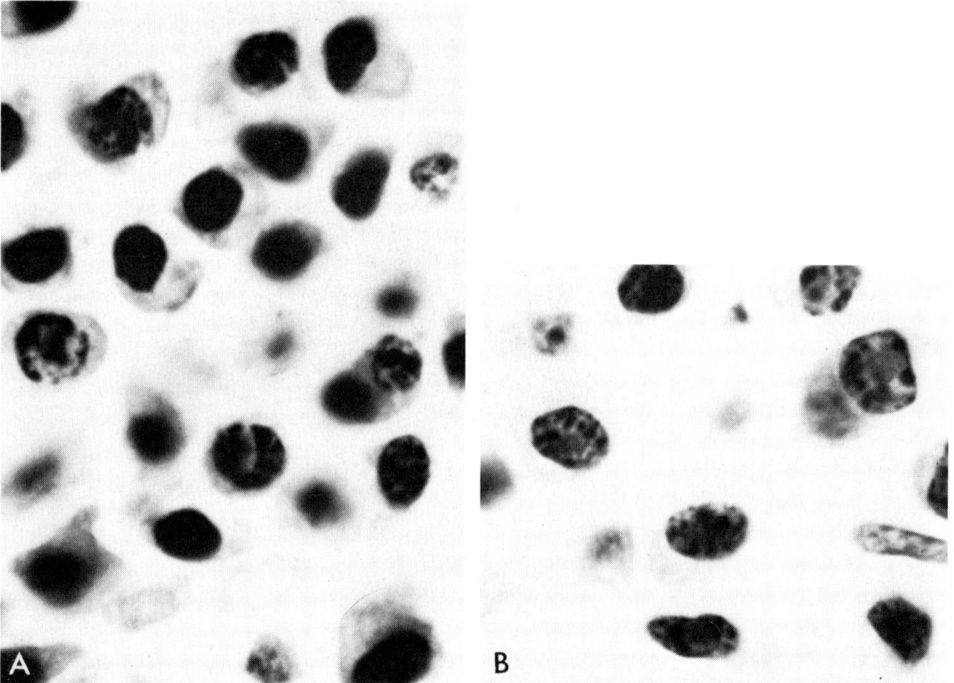

Figure 9–340. Histologic appearance of multiple myeloma. The cells are readily recognized as plasma cells with moderate variability. In some cells, chromatin is clumped around the periphery of the nucleus. Other cells exhibit the more characteristic dense nuclei, eccentrically located. Cytoplasm usually stains darkly with hematoxylin-eosin, owing to large numbers of protein-producing ribosomes.

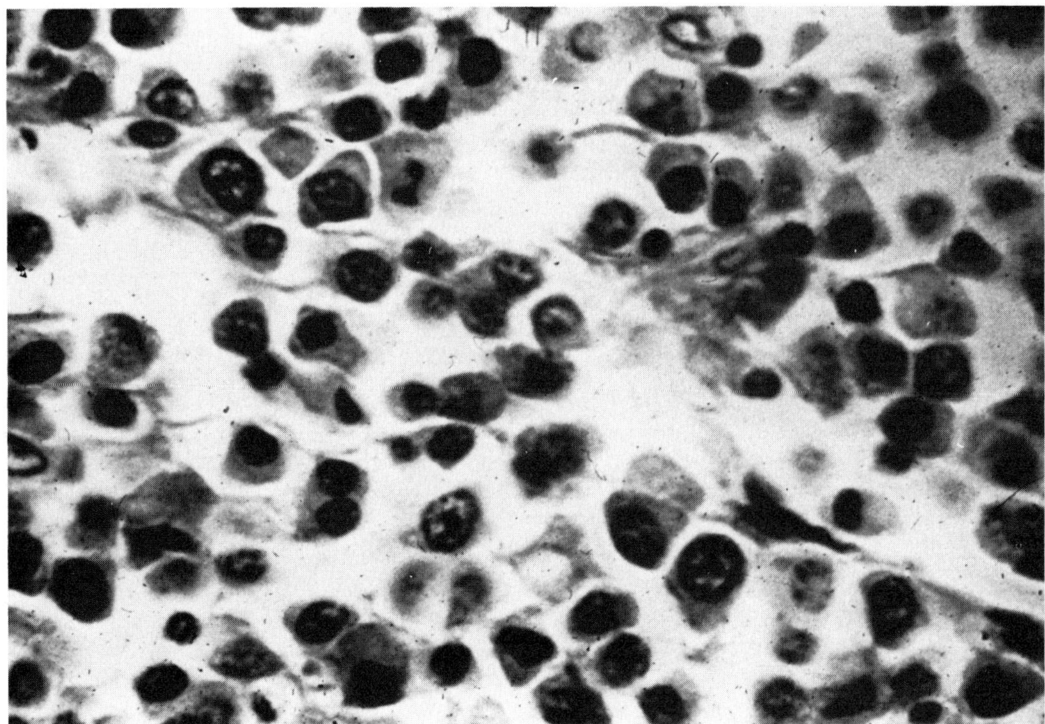

Figure 9–341. Multiple myeloma. Histologic appearance of multiple myeloma. Note the variability in nuclear characteristics and in size, shape, and staining quality of cells.

Figure 9–342. Multiple myeloma. Lateral radiograph of lumbosacral spine of a patient with myeloma. Occasionally, patients will have diffuse disease without discrete lesions, and severe osteoporosis will be the only radiographic finding. This radiograph illustrates severe osteoporosis with regressive remodeling of the vertebral bodies and "codfish" vertebrae. Pathologic fractures are very common in these porotic vertebrae.

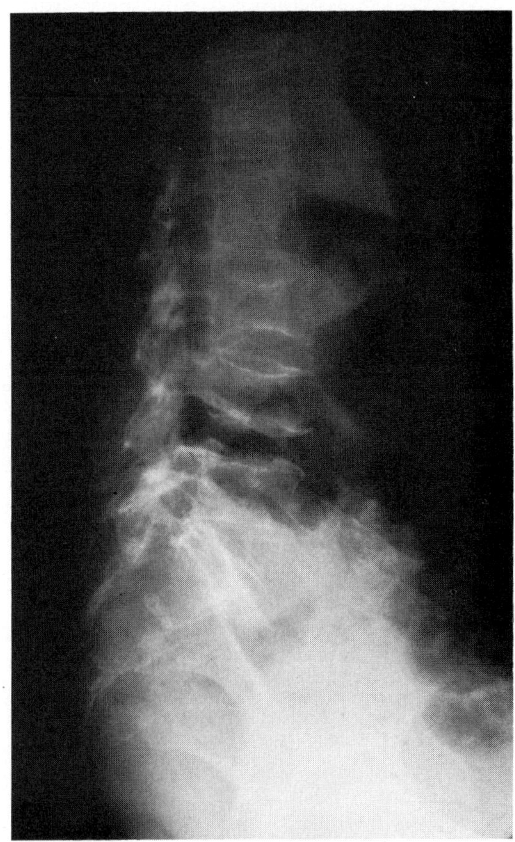

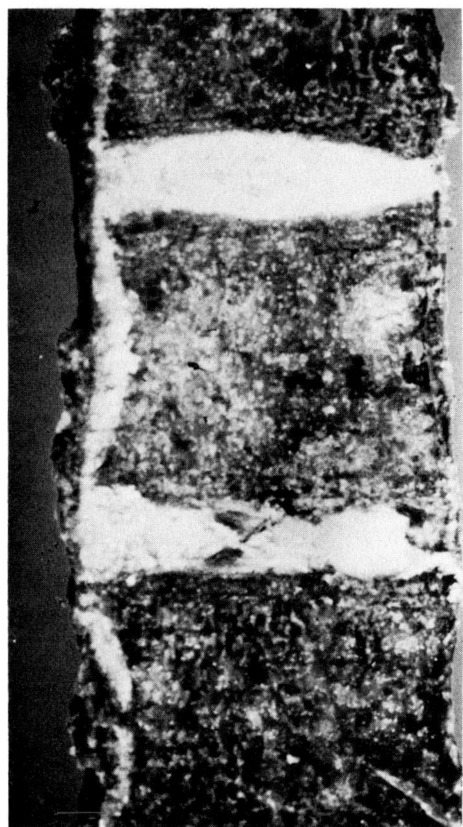

Figure 9–343. Multiple myeloma. Gross specimen of a vertebral body containing large deposits of myeloma. The myeloma cells will infiltrate between the existing trabeculae and can involve the body extensively before any radiographic changes are visible. Only after trabeculae are removed does the focus become apparent.

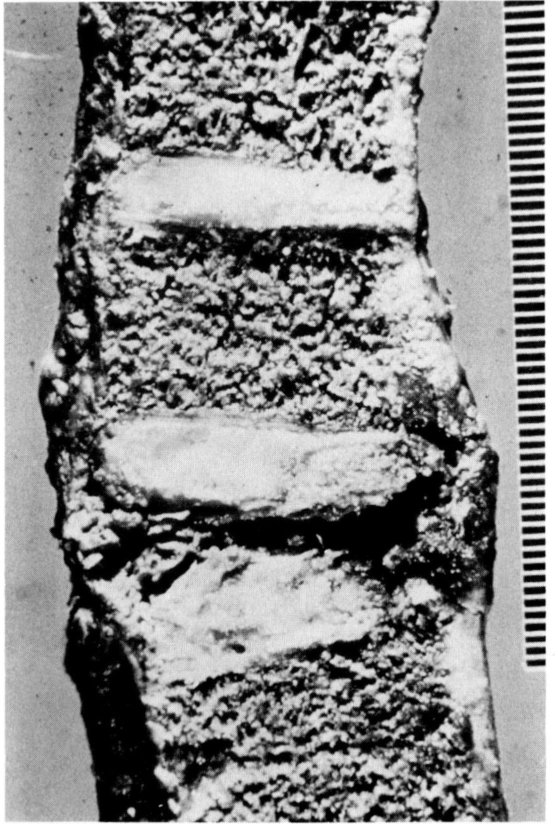

Figure 9–344. Multiple myeloma. Gross specimen of vertebral bodies in multiple myeloma. There is almost complete collapse of one vertebral body, with only a small portion of bone remaining anteriorly and posteriorly.

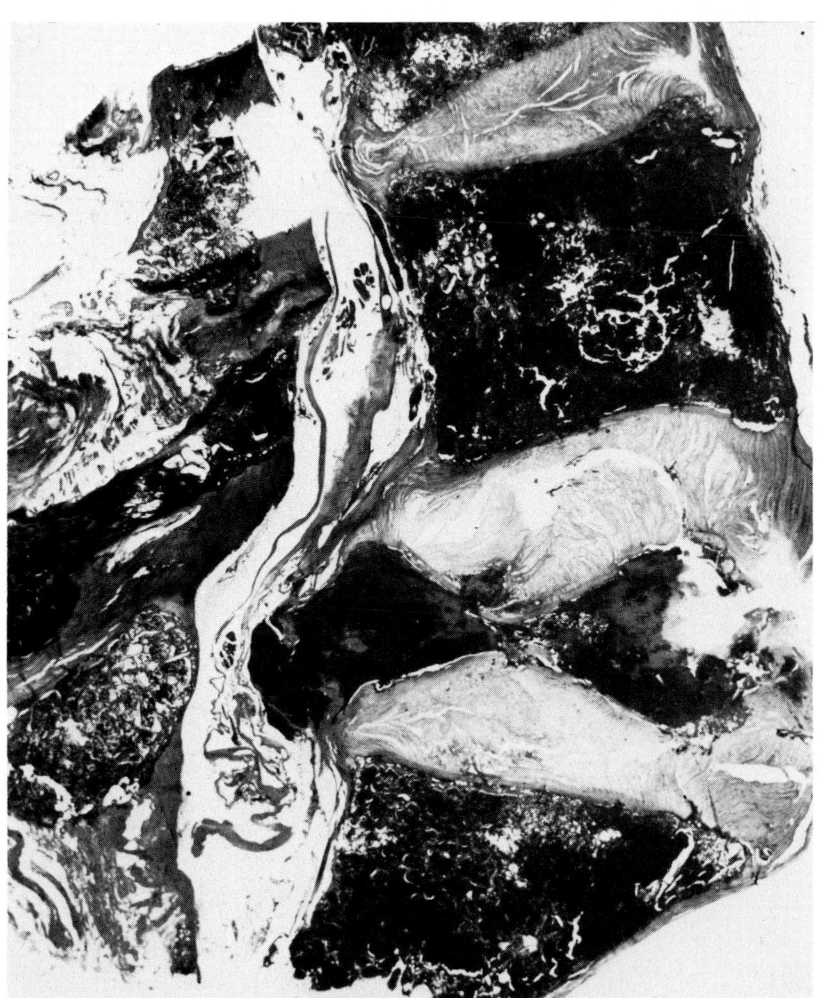

Figure 9–345. Multiple myeloma. Macrosection of vertebrae with collapse of a vertebral body extensively involved with myeloma.

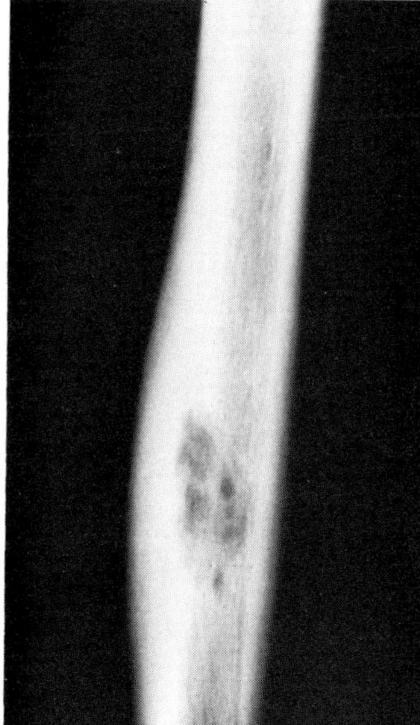

Figure 9–346. Eosinophilic granuloma. Sharply circumscribed lytic defect in the diaphysis of long bone. There has been periosteal thickening of the bone outside the lesion. Eosinophilic granuloma may appear in any bone, commonly in the diaphysis.

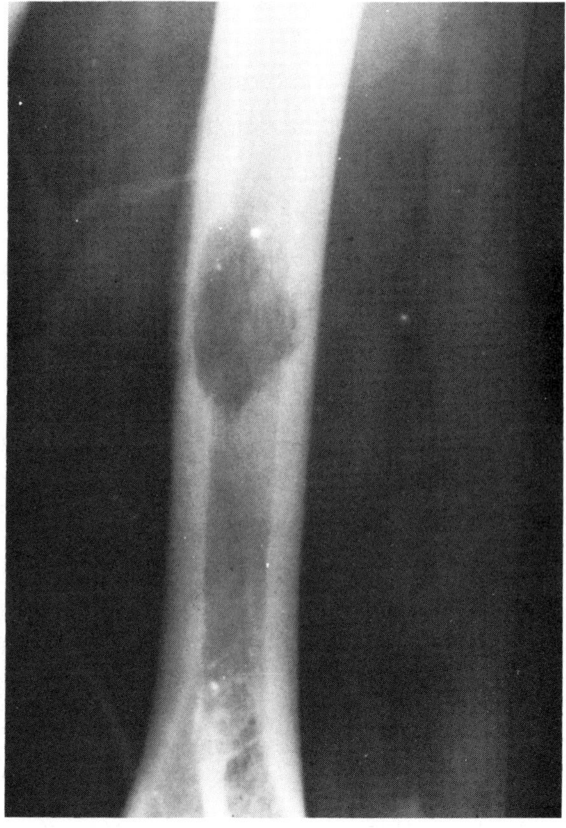

Figure 9–347. Eosinophilic granuloma. Radiograph of humerus with an irregularly shaped, sharply circumscribed lytic defect in the diaphysis. The cortex has been eroded from within. There is minimal periosteal reaction. There is no evidence of matrix mineralization.

Figure 9–348. Eosinophilic granuloma. Lateral radiograph of the cervical spine in a 12-year-old girl having a history of chronic upper respiratory infections and experiencing a stiff neck for 5 to 6 months. The film illustrates almost total collapse of the body of C-5, with intact posterior elements remaining.

Figure 9–349. Eosinophilic granuloma. Anteroposterior radiograph of the femur in a child with a large lytic defect in the medullary cavity and inner cortex. There has been a marked expansion of the bone with periosteal new bone production. This massive reaction is more typical in a young child.

HISTIOCYTIC LESIONS (HISTIOCYTOSIS X)

EOSINOPHILIC GRANULOMA OF BONE

The eosinophilic granuloma of bone is considered one of the histiocytoses, but despite the classic description of Lichtenstein and recent electron microscopic evidence of a uniform organelle in all three entities, the association of eosinophilic granuloma, Hand-Schüller-Christian disease, and Letterer-Siwe disease has been questioned persistently. By far, the most common of these manifestations is the eosinophilic granuloma of bone, which exists as a lytic lesion with a polymorphus infiltrate replacing bone. As opposed to the aforementioned round cell tumors, the eosinophilic granuloma is a *polymorphous* infiltrate (more than one cell type). The basic cellular component underlying the process consists of normal, mature histiocytes. These are usually accompanied by numerous eosinophiles and may occasionally be accompanied by lymphocytes, neutrophils, and plasma cells. However, these lesions always contain a generous histiocytic component, regardless of what other cells are present.

Radiographically, eosinophilic granuloma is a sharply circumscribed lytic defect demonstrating variable reaction. It may exist in monostotic or polyostotic form and may involve all parts of the skeleton (Case Records of the Massachusetts General Hospital [Case 7-1980]; Hartman, 1980). The lesion is self-limited; curettage or biopsy is the only procedure necessary, and even after incomplete removal the lesion will often disappear without further treatment.

Text continued on page 550

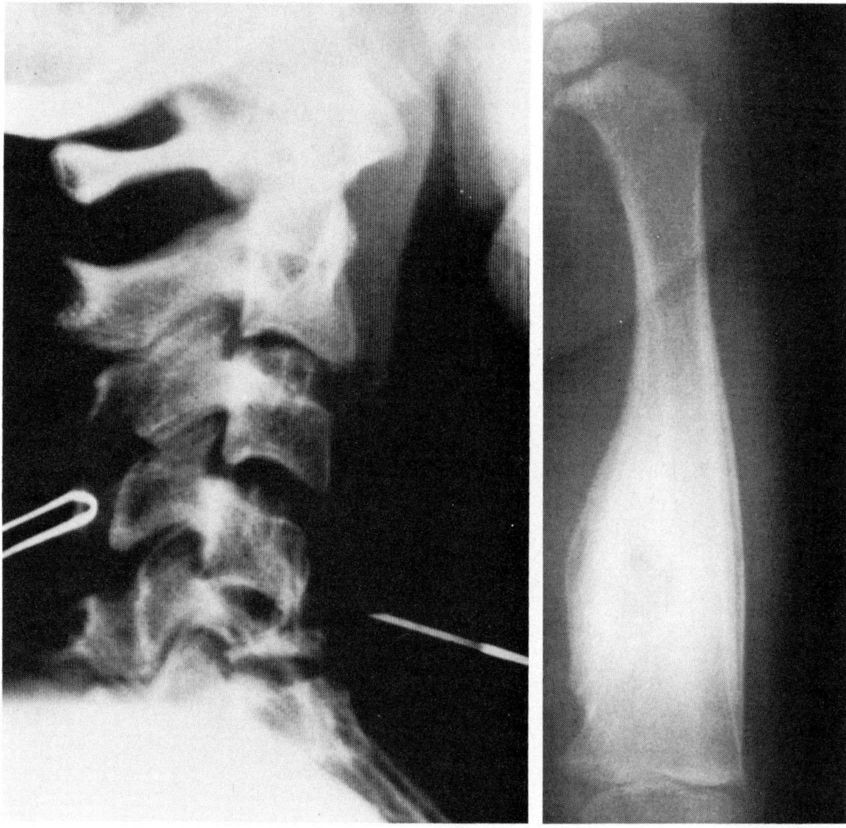

Figure 9–348   Figure 9–349

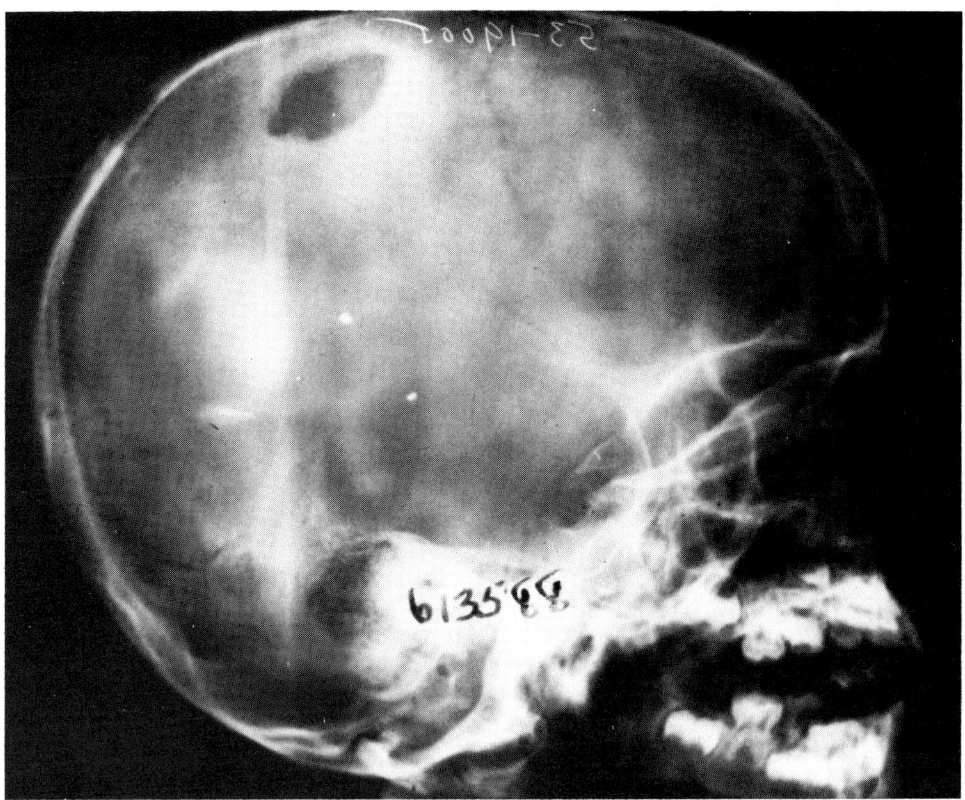

Figure 9–350. Eosinophilic granuloma. Lateral radiograph of the skull of a patient with an eosinophilic granuloma. Note the large, sharply marginated defect in the calvarium. There is no mineralized matrix in the defect. Sclerotic bony margins indicate that the process is long-standing.

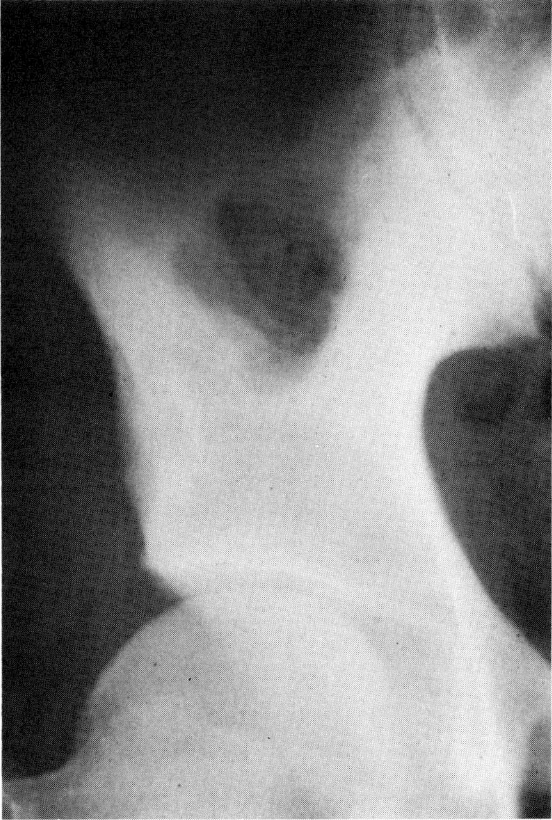

Figure 9–351. Eosinophilic granuloma. Radiograph of sharply circumscribed defect in the wing of the ilium. There is no significant sclerotic reaction and no periosteal reaction.

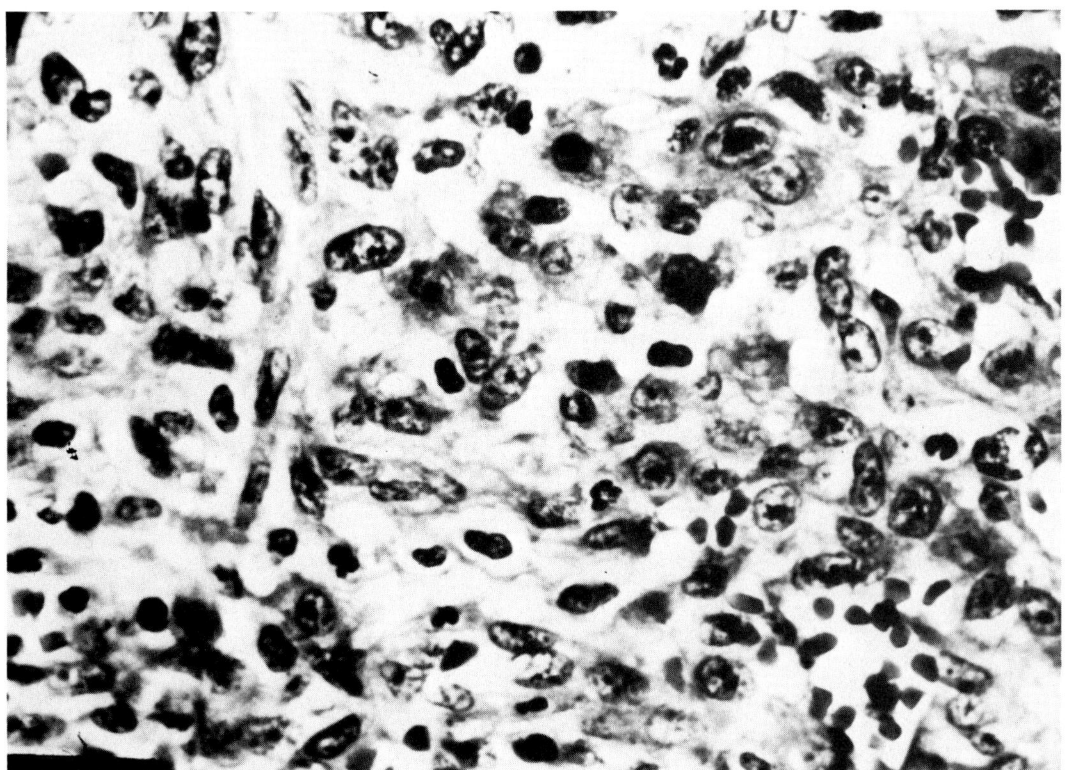

Figure 9–352. Eosinophilic granuloma. Histologic appearance of eosinophilic granuloma. The characteristic cell of the lesion is the histiocyte, which has a large vesicular nucleus, prominent nucleolus, and a moderate amount of cytoplasm. Other types of inflammatory cells are frequently present. The histiocyte is difficult to distinguish from immature fibroblasts and endothelial cells in granulation tissue.

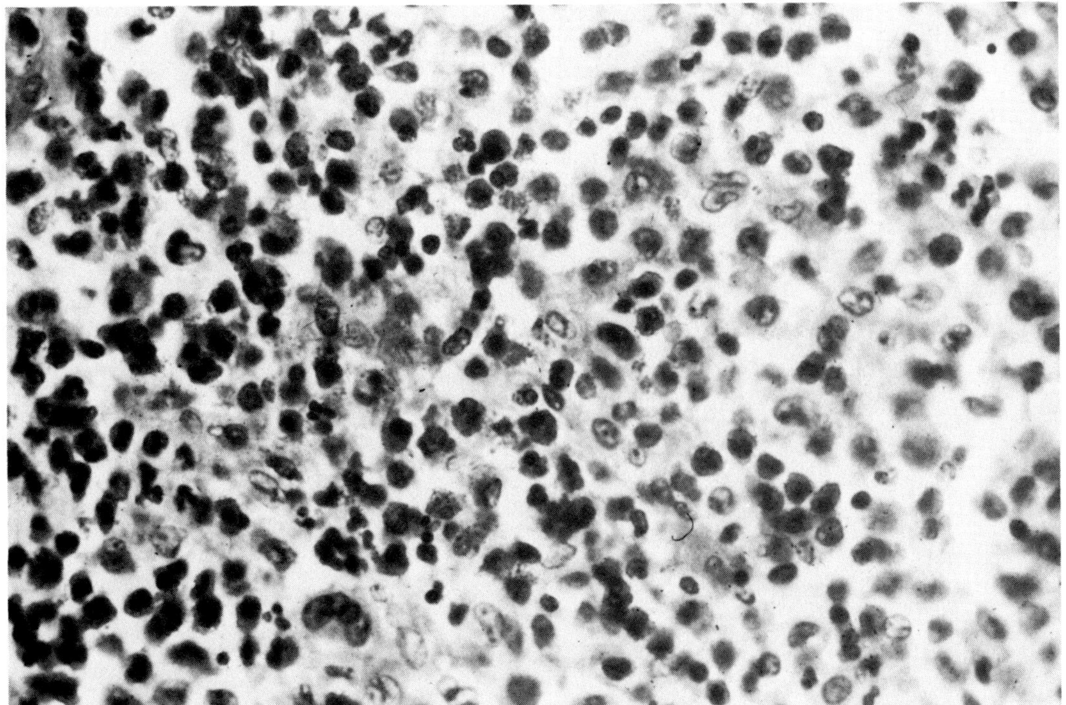

Figure 9–353. Eosinophilic granuloma. Section of an eosinophilic granuloma with an admixture of eosinophiles and histiocytes. The histiocytes constitute the basic cellular component of the lesion, but the eosinophiles are commonly present. Compared with histiocytes, they have a darker-staining cytoplasm with smaller, bilobed nuclei.

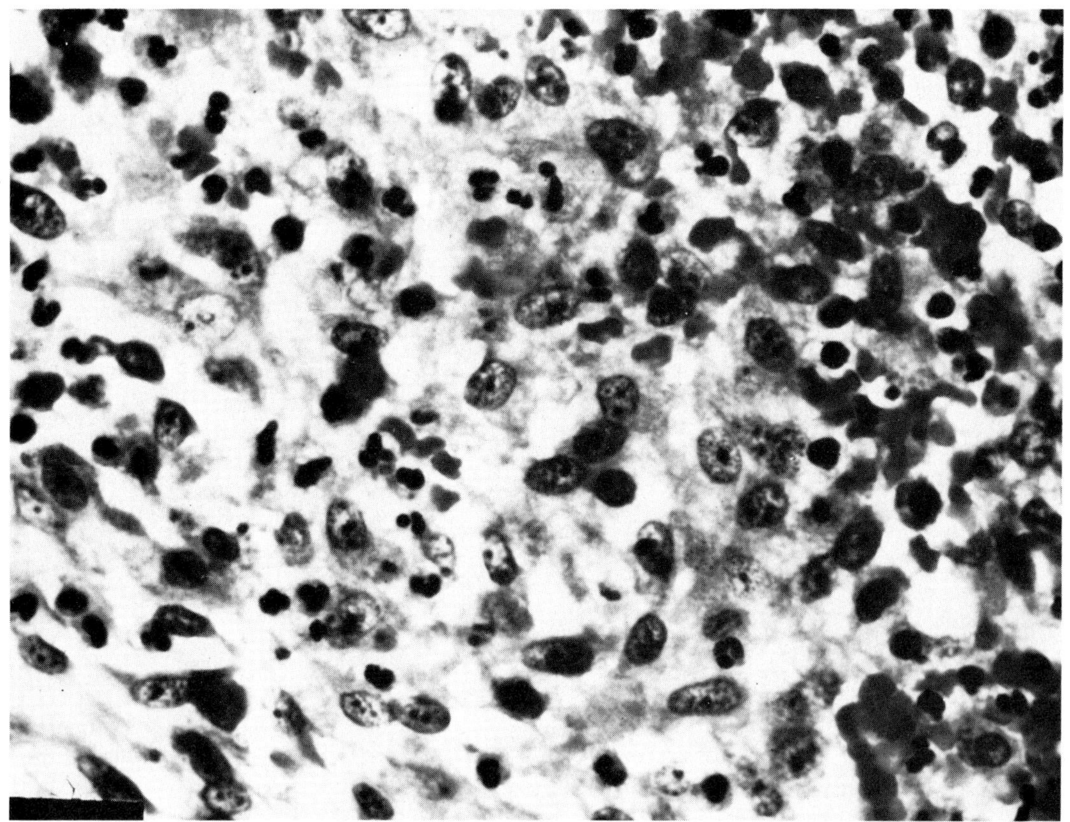

Figure 9–354. Higher-power view of a focus of eosinophilic granuloma. Well-defined histiocytes, a few scattered polymorphonuclear leukocytes, and eosinophils are present.

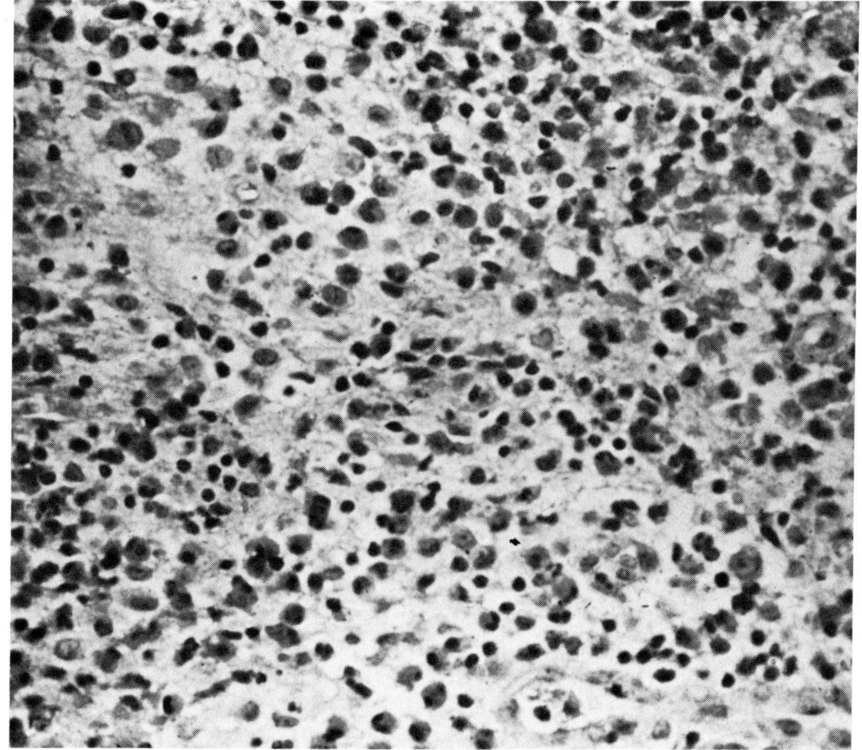

Figure 9–355. Eosinophilic granuloma. Polymorphous infiltrate composed of histiocytes, eosinophilic granulocytes, and occasional lymphocytes. The essential cell is the histiocyte, and the other components may vary in amount.

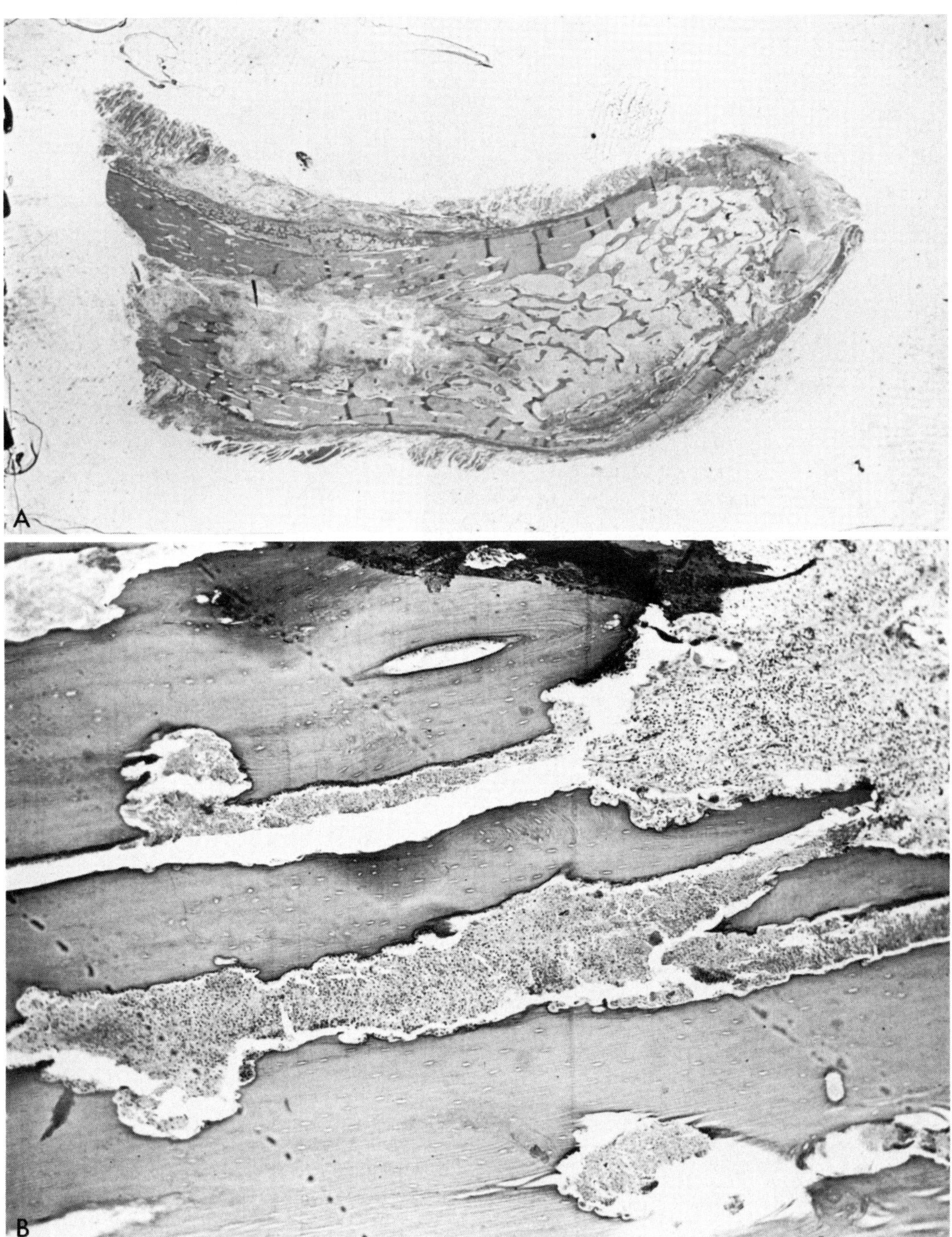

Figure 9–356. Eosinophilic granuloma. Macrosection *(A)* and histologic section *(B)* of eosinophilic granuloma invading the cortical bone of the clavicle. Note the large resorption cavities, filled with lesional tissue.

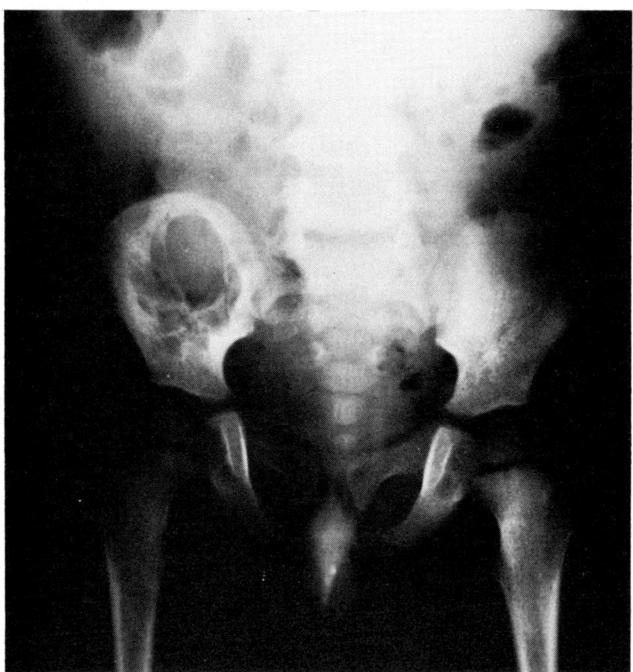

Figure 9–357. Hand-Schüller-Christian disease. Anteroposterior radiograph of the pelvis in a 2-year-old male with a large, purely lytic defect in the ilium. There is minimal reactive bone and no expansion of the iliac wing itself.

HAND-SCHÜLLER-CHRISTIAN DISEASE AND LETTERER-SIWE DISEASE

Whereas the eosinophilic granuloma may be a unifocal or multifocal lesion, Hand-Schüller-Christian disease involves bone and also viscera. Letterer-Siwe disease is also a disseminated disease. The unifying component of all three entities is the

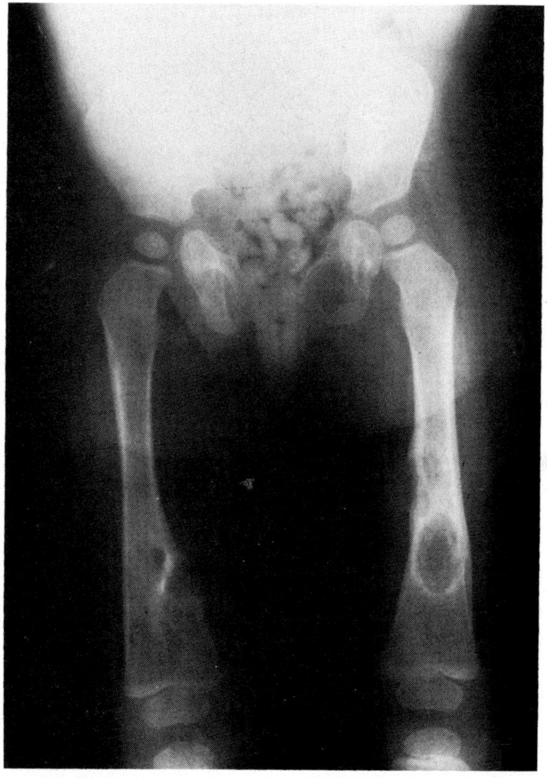

Figure 9–358. Hand-Schüller-Christian disease. Pelvis and femurs of a 15-month-old female with Hand-Schüller-Christian disease. Note the large, well-circumscribed defects. Some are outlined by sclerotic bone, but others erode through the cortex and have no significant reaction.

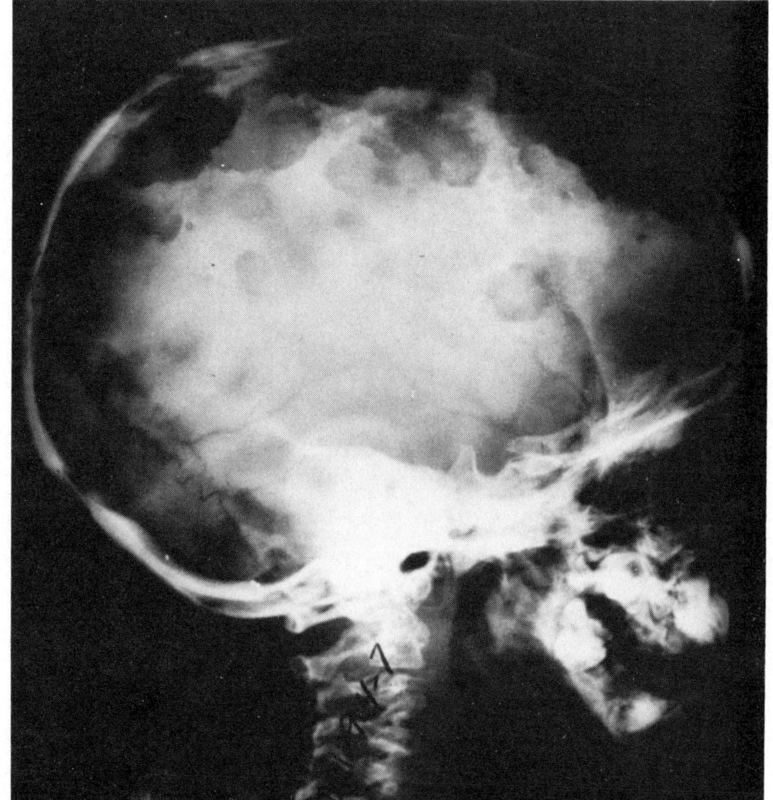

Figure 9–359. Hand-Schüller-Christian disease. Lateral radiograph of the skull in a 7-year-old male with multiple calvarial defects. Most of them have minimal reaction around the periphery and show apparent mineralization in the defect itself.

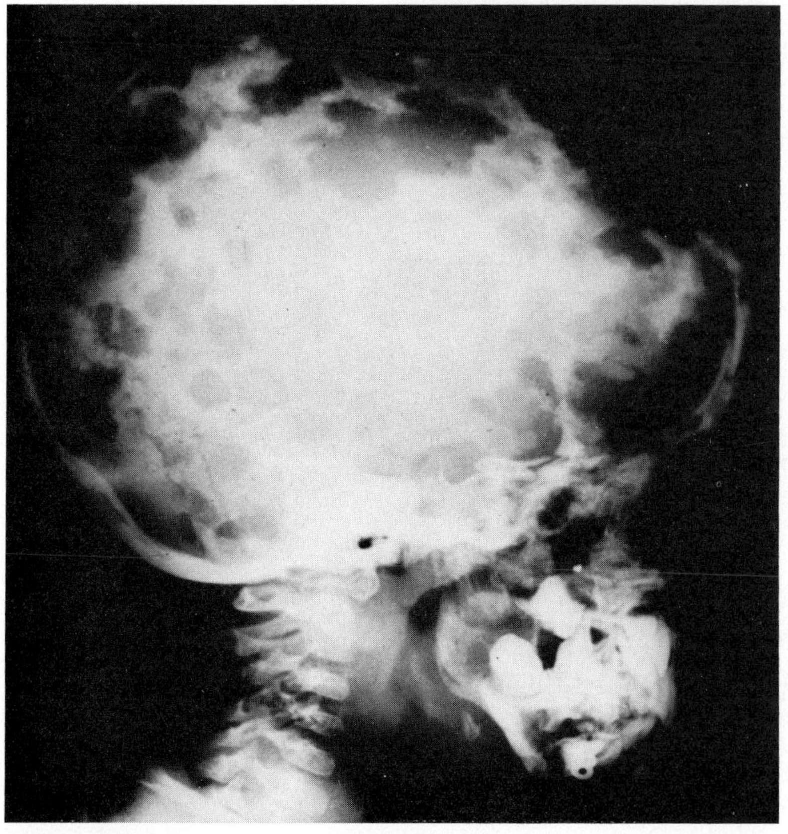

Figure 9–360. Hand-Schüller-Christian disease. Lateral radiograph of skull in a 4-year-old male with extensive involvement. Such extensive involvement often includes the viscera.

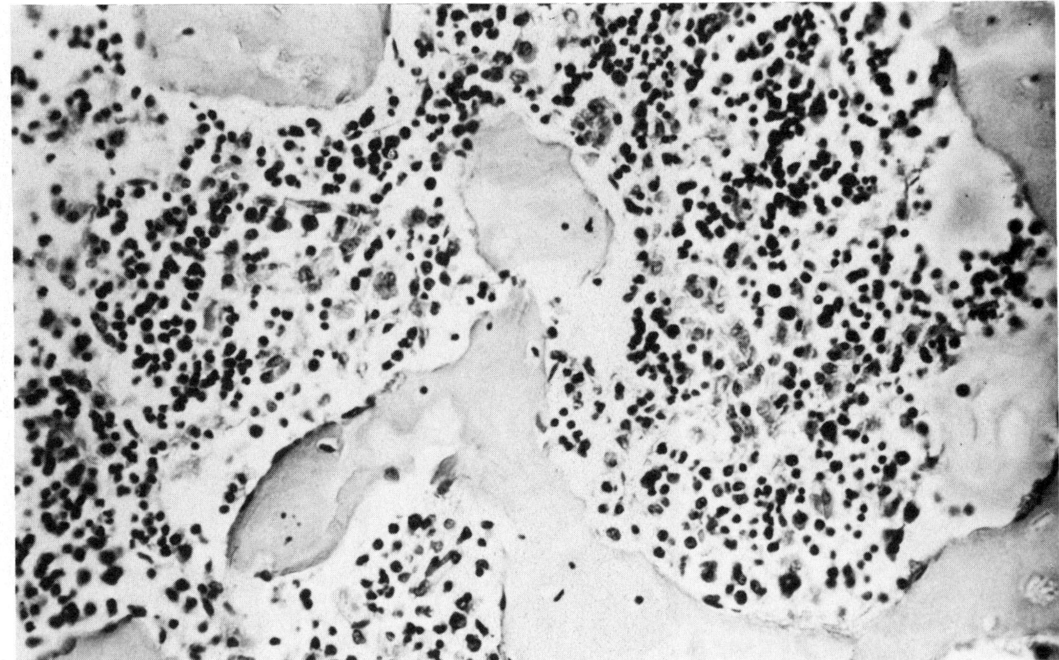

Figure 9–361. Hand-Schüller-Christian disease. Biopsied specimen of a lesion in the bone of a child with Hand-Schüller-Christian disease. The marrow has been extensively replaced with chronic inflammatory cells and numerous histiocytes.

proliferation of an abnormal histiocyte. The histologic appearance of Hand-Schüller-Christian disease is similar to that of eosinophilic granuloma; the more serious involvement in Hand-Schüller-Christian disease is due to the greater extent of the lesion rather than to any histologic difference (Mickelson and Bonfiglio, 1977).

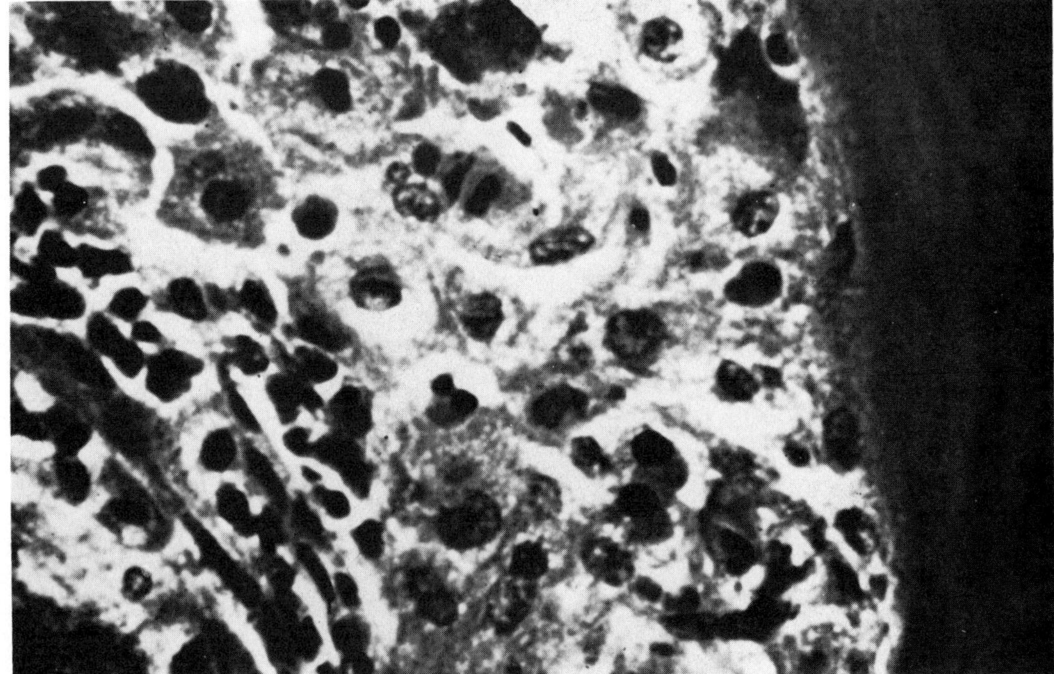

Figure 9–362. Hand-Schüller-Christian disease. Shown here is a section through the lesion. Note the large cells with central nuclei and fairly prominent cytoplasm, some of which is fairly light-staining. Note that the lesion extends to the surface of the bone.

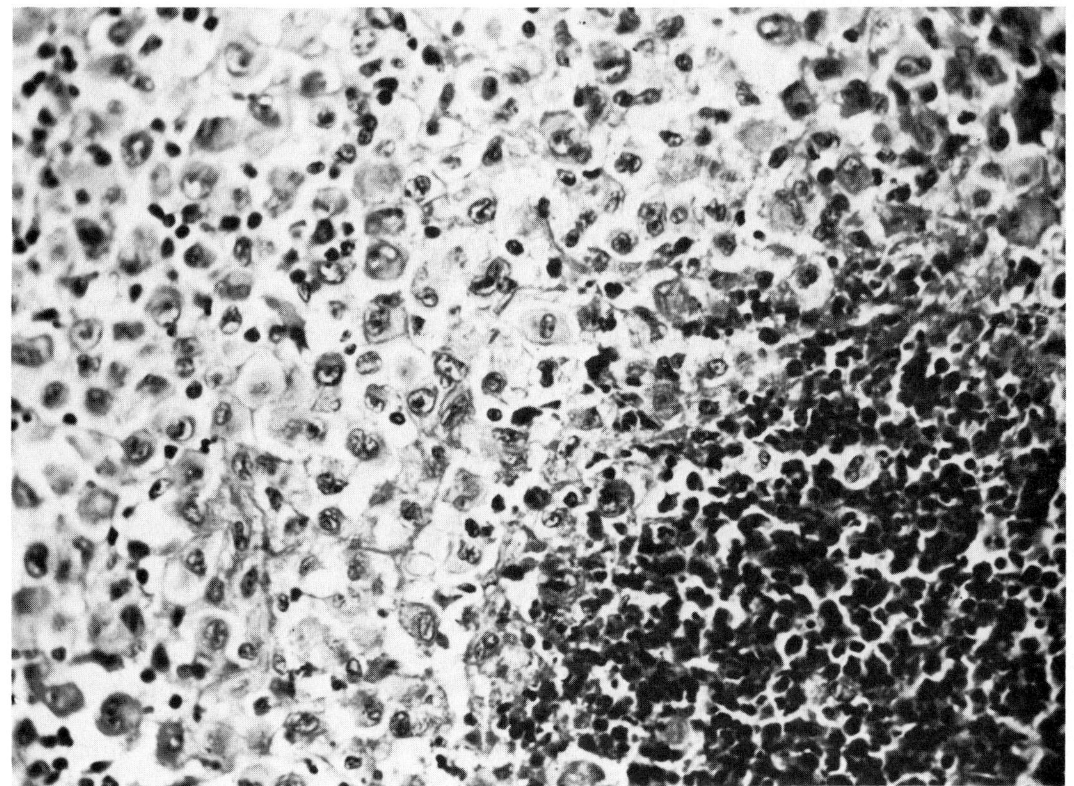

Figure 9–363. Hand-Schüller-Christian disease. Biopsied specimen of a cervical lymph node in a patient with this disease. Note the extensive replacement of the node by sheets of hystiocytes. The eosinophiles are not a prominent feature in this field.

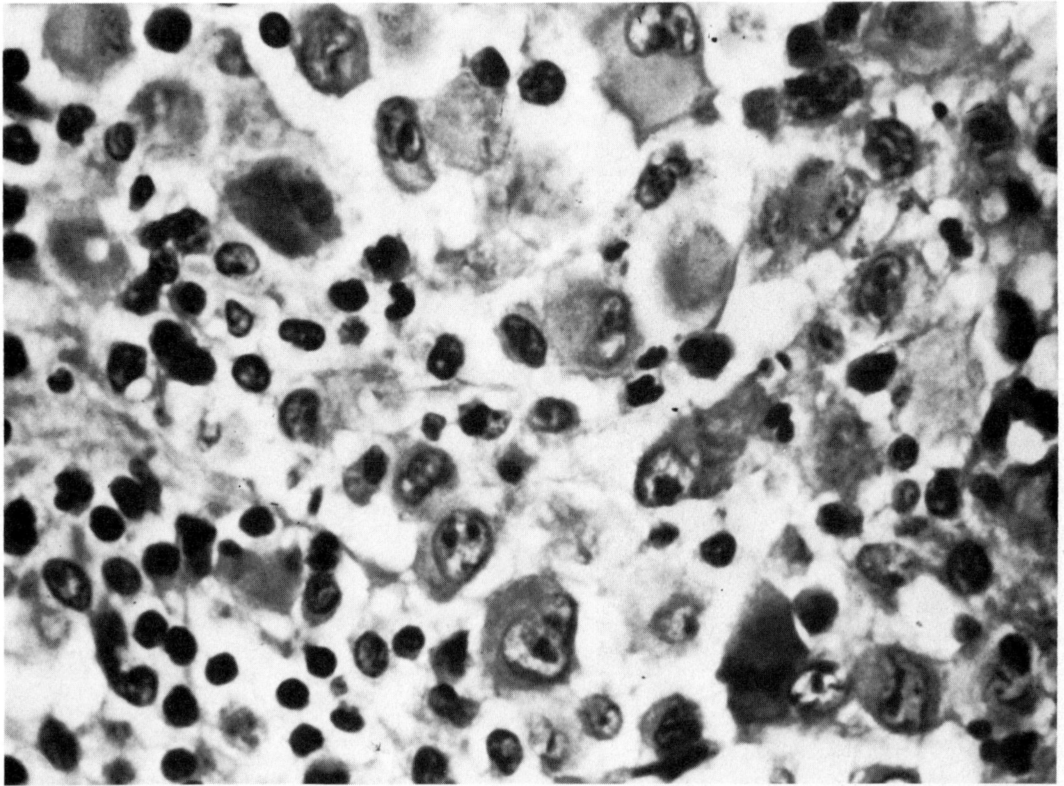

Figure 9–364. Hand-Schüller-Christian disease. Higher-power view of a biopsied specimen of a cervical nodé clearly demonstrating histiocytes and other inflammatory cells. Eosinophiles are present but not in large numbers.

TUMORS ARISING FROM PERIOSTEUM

PAROSTEAL TUMORS

Neoplasms arising within the medullary cavity of bone may have their counterpart in lesions that arise on the surface of the bone: parosteal osteosarcomas, chondrosarcomas, and fibrosarcomas. These lesions, as a group, are of lesser malignant biologic potential than are their counterparts within the medullary cavity (Unni, 1976). However, once a tumor of parosteal origin penetrates into the medullary cavity, it assumes the same biologic potential as a primary intramedullary lesion.

As a group, the parosteal sarcomas tend to have a much more benign appearance than their intramedullary counterparts. Thus, the differential diagnosis between a parosteal osteosarcoma and a benign reactive process is difficult. In particular, the tumor must not be confused with myositis ossificans secondarily attached to bone or with a sessile osteochondroma. The rude awakening comes 5 to 10 years later, when metastases are apparent.

The histologic appearance of a parosteal osteosarcoma has features not compatible with a reactive process. One must pay particular attention to the differentiation pattern of the bone, which is most mature in the center of the lesion and least mature at the periphery; in addition, the connective tissue between trabeculae of bone will exhibit cellularity with cytologic abnormalities instead of fatty or hematopoietic marrow. Myositis ossificans, maturing to form trabeculae of bone, will be accompanied by sinusoidal vascular channels in the adjacent connective tissue. Parosteal sarcoma, forming radiating bands of bone, will be accompanied by cellular connective tissue. On close inspection, the spindled-cell nuclei will exhibit pleomorphism, variation in size and staining characteristics, and mitotic activity. Although these changes may be

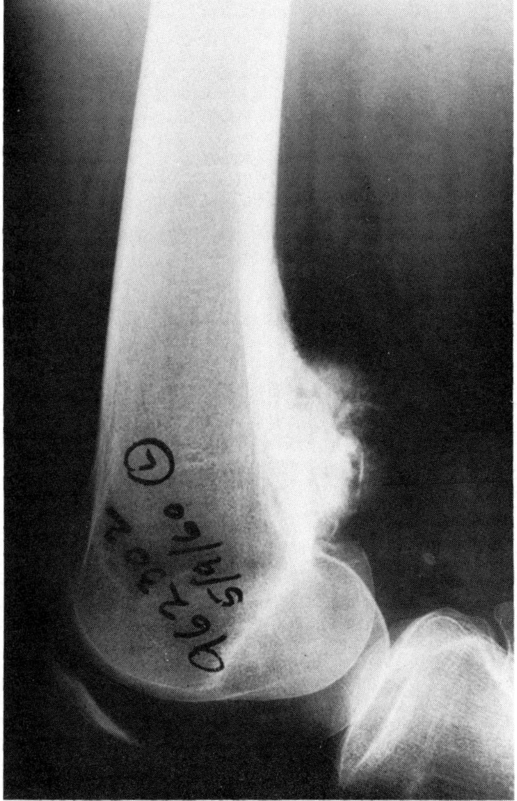

Figure 9–365. Parosteal sarcoma. Lateral radiograph of distal femur with a parosteal sarcoma on the popliteal surface of the metaphysis. The lesion does not involve the medullary cavity. It projects from the surface of the bone with irregular contour and mineralization, particularly on the periphery.

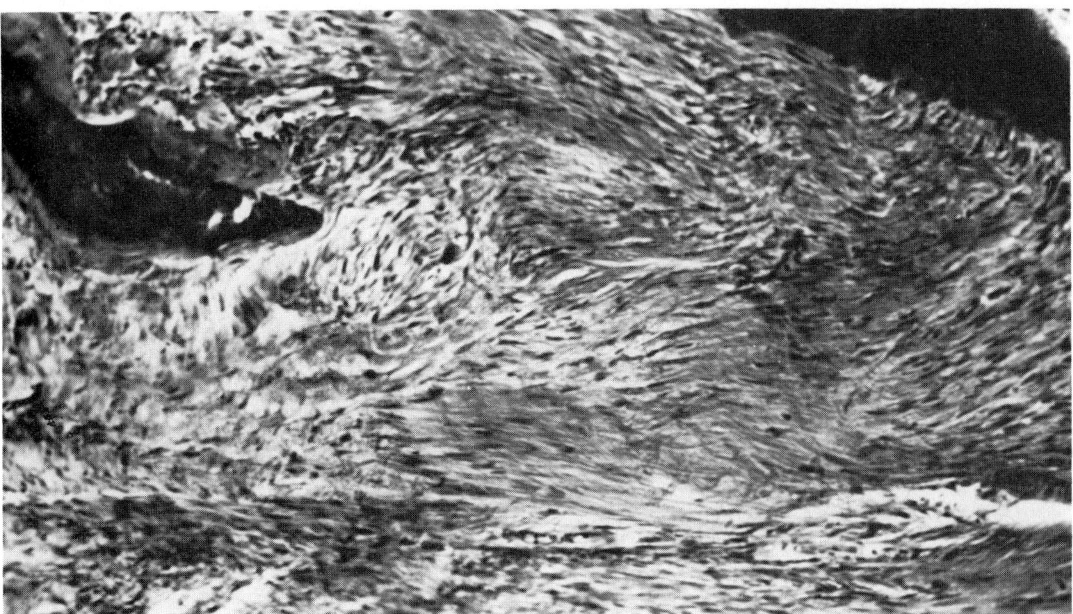

Figure 9–366. Parosteal sarcoma. Histologic appearance of the lesion shown in Figure 9–365. The base of the lesion contains a relatively benign-looking fibrous stroma with scanty to profuse bony trabeculae. The benign appearance is quite deceptive and frequently misleads the pathologist into diagnosing osteochondroma. However, the fibrous stroma is totally atypical for an osteochondroma, which should have normal marrow. Compare with Figure 9–117.

minimal, they contrast with the uniformly benign appearance of the cellular component accompanying bone formation in myositis ossificans or any other reactive process.

Radiographically, parosteal osteosarcoma exhibits the most mature bone formation in the area closest to the cortex, and the periphery of the lesion will be least differentiated. In this respect, the tumor contrasts sharply with a myositis ossificans,

Text continued on page 581

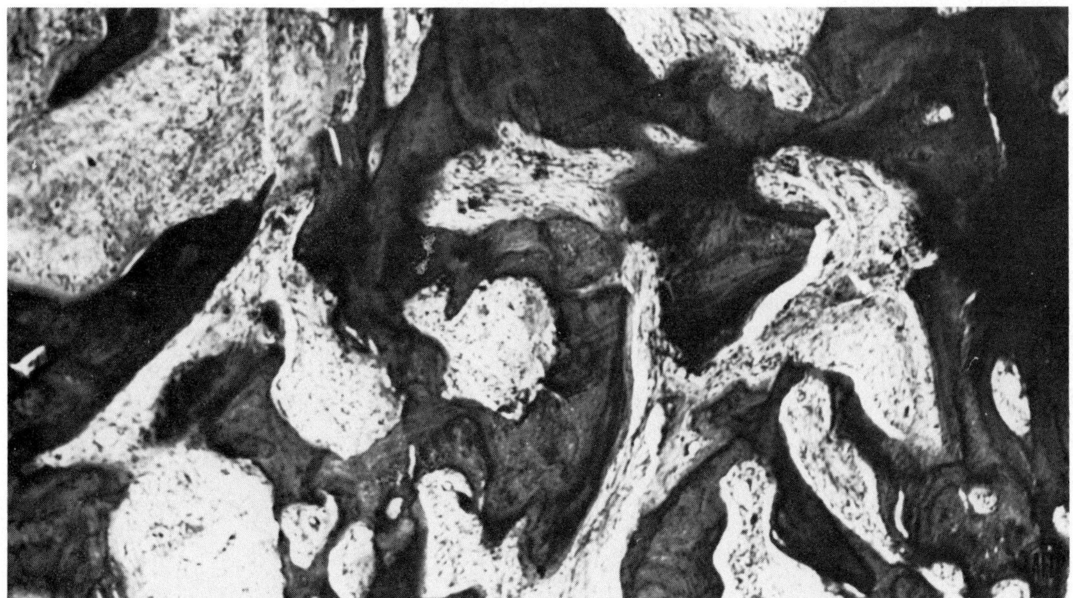

Figure 9–367. Parosteal sarcoma. Another region of the stalk of the parosteal sarcoma shown in Figures 9–365 and 9–366. Although more bone is evident, all the spicules are abnormal, and the intervening stroma indicates a low-grade sarcoma.

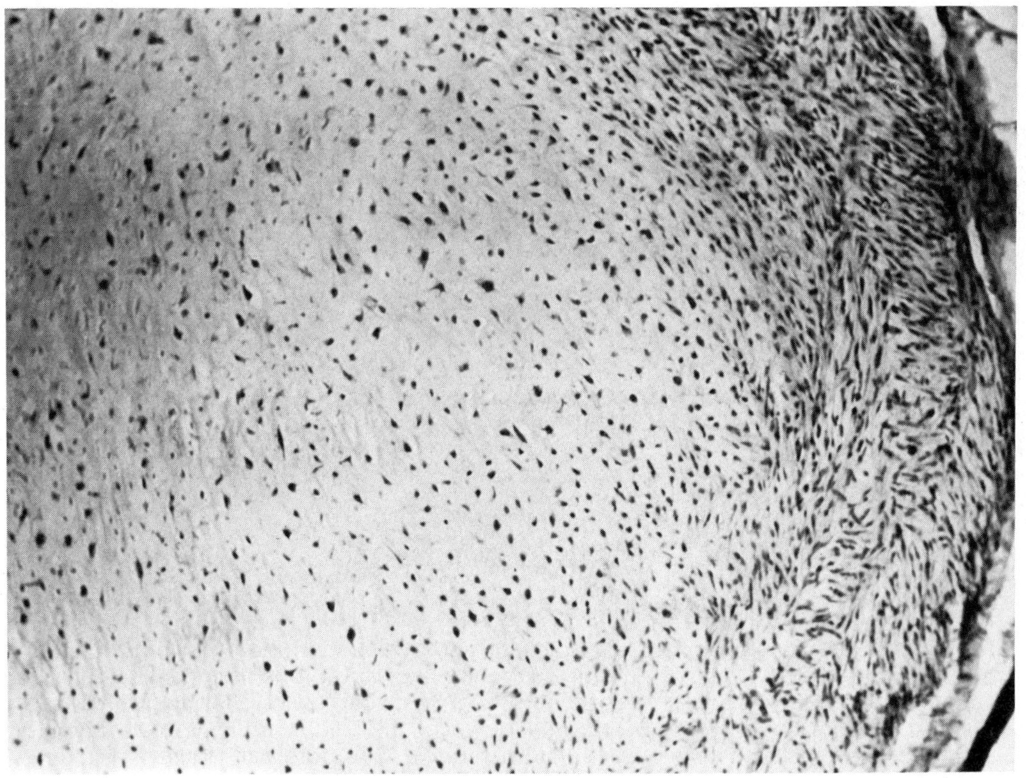

Figure 9–368. Parosteal sarcoma. Section through the surface of the osseous projection, with a cartilaginous cap similar to that seen in osteochondroma.

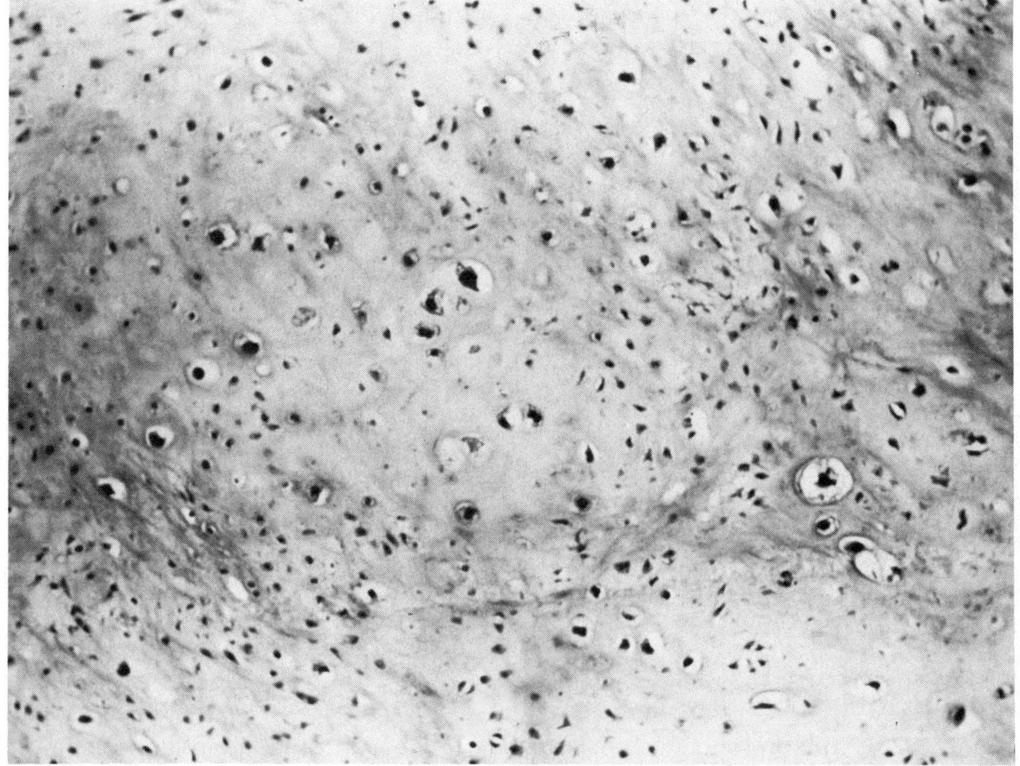

Figure 9–369. Parosteal sarcoma. Higher-power view of the cartilage cap of the parosteal sarcoma shown in Figure 9–368. The cellularity is greater than that demonstrated by benign osteochondroma.

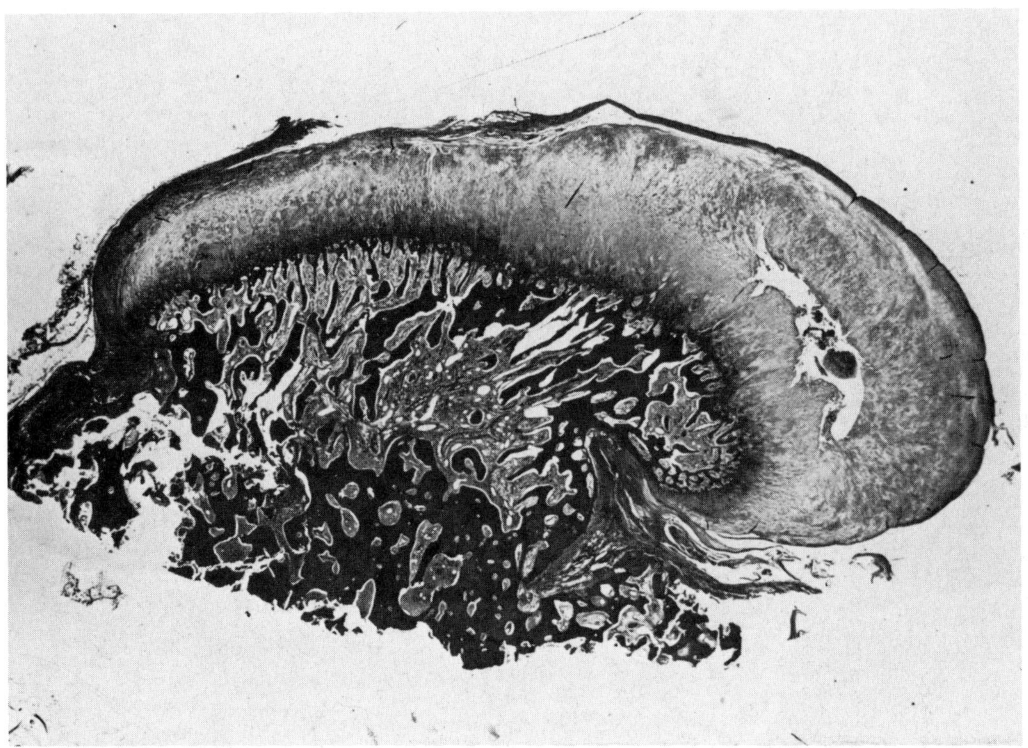

Figure 9–370. Parosteal sarcoma. Note the fairly thick cartilage cap. The stroma between the spicules of bone is fibrous rather than fatty.

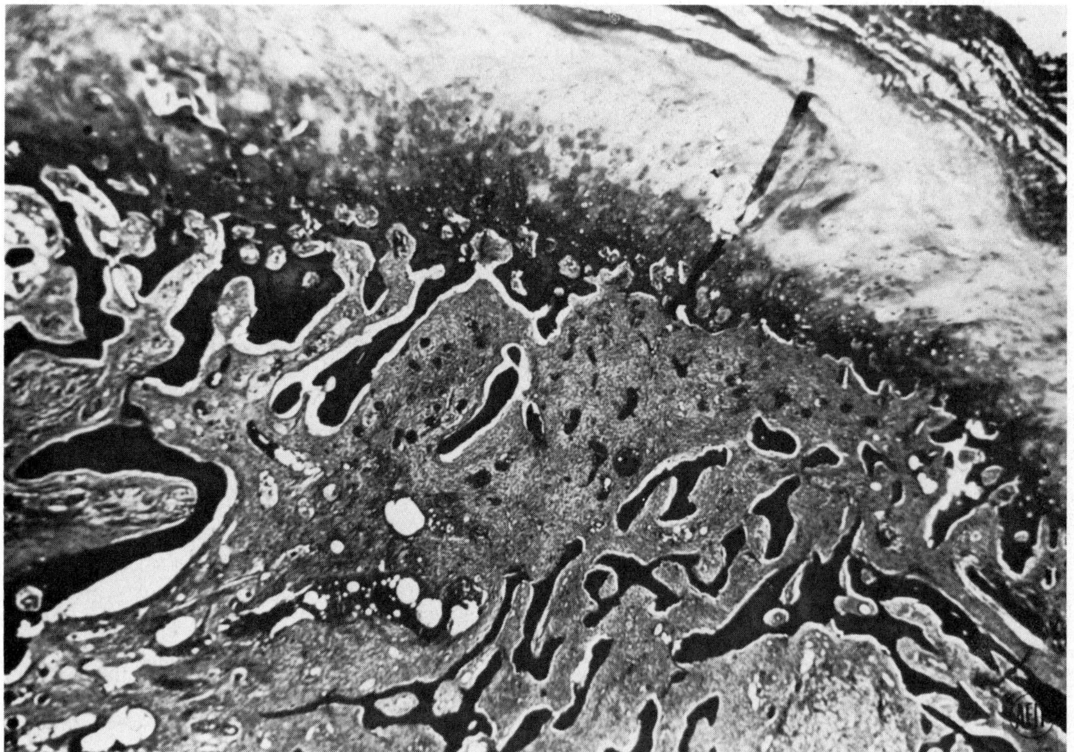

Figure 9–371. Parosteal sarcoma. Higher-power view of the parosteal sarcoma shown in Figure 9–370 demonstrating the area between the cartilage cap and the stalk of the parosteal sarcoma. The medullary cavity is filled with a fibrous stroma rather than normal marrow, which helps differentiate the lesion from an osteochondroma (Figs. 9–117 and 9–118).

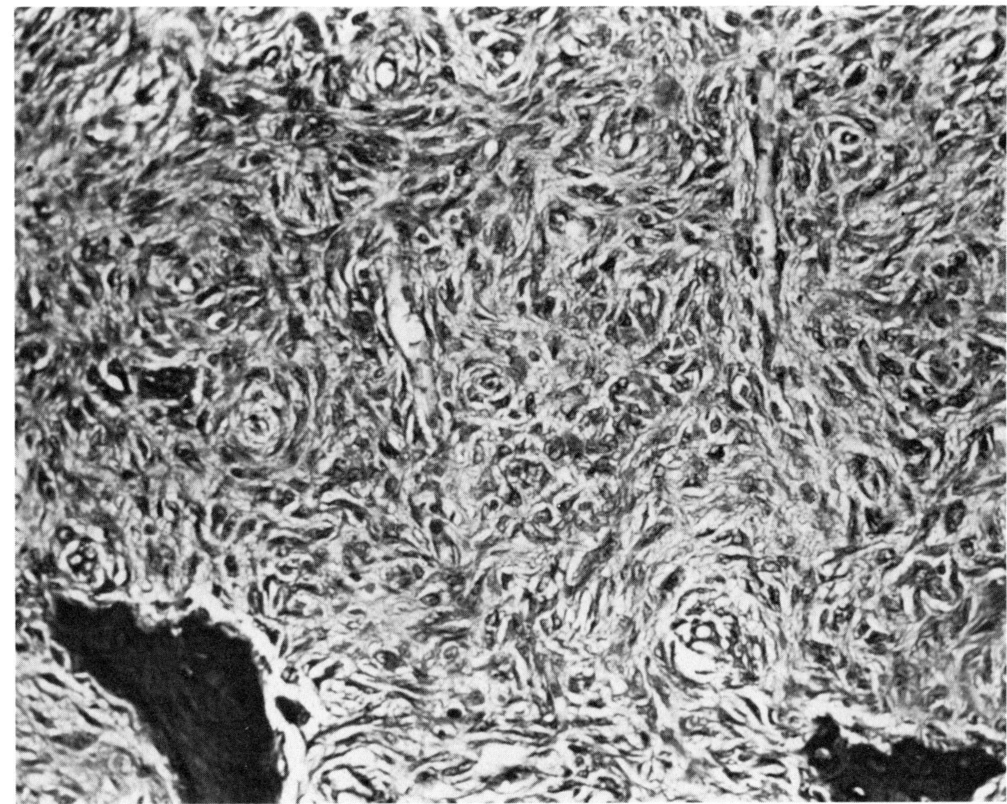

Figure 9–372. Parosteal sarcoma. Still higher-power view of the parosteal sarcoma. There is sarcomatous stroma in the medullary spaces of the lesion.

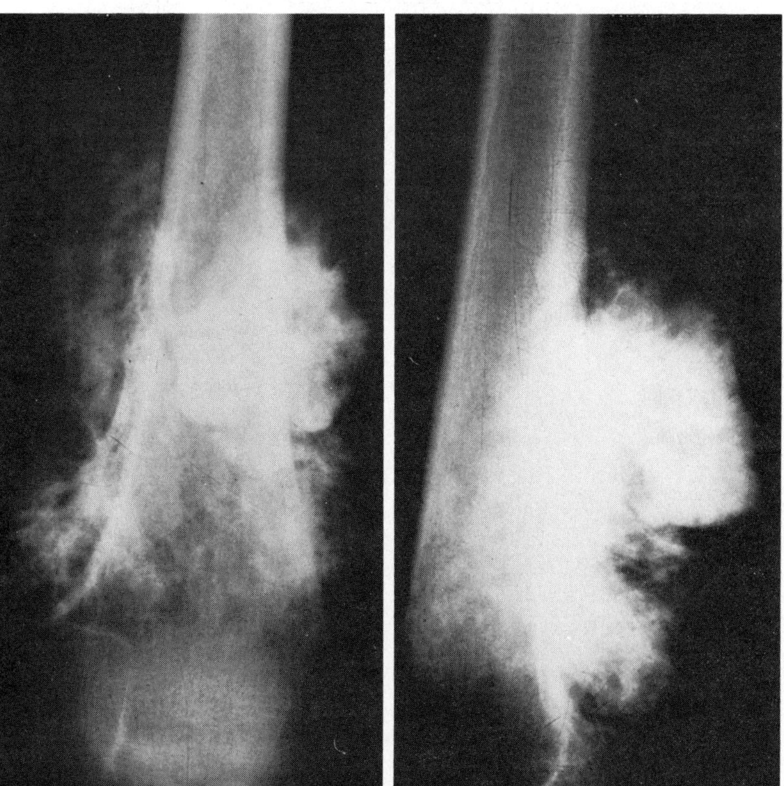

Figure 9–373. Parosteal sarcoma. Anteroposterior *(A)* and lateral *(B)* radiographs of lesion in distal femur of a 22-year-old male. The lesion extends around the circumference of the bone. In most parosteal lesions, there is a projection that will show a relatively clear area between the lesion and the cortical surface. This area is due to origin of the tumor at one portion of the surface. As it expands, it leaves a periosteal fibrous zone between the lesion and the cortex.

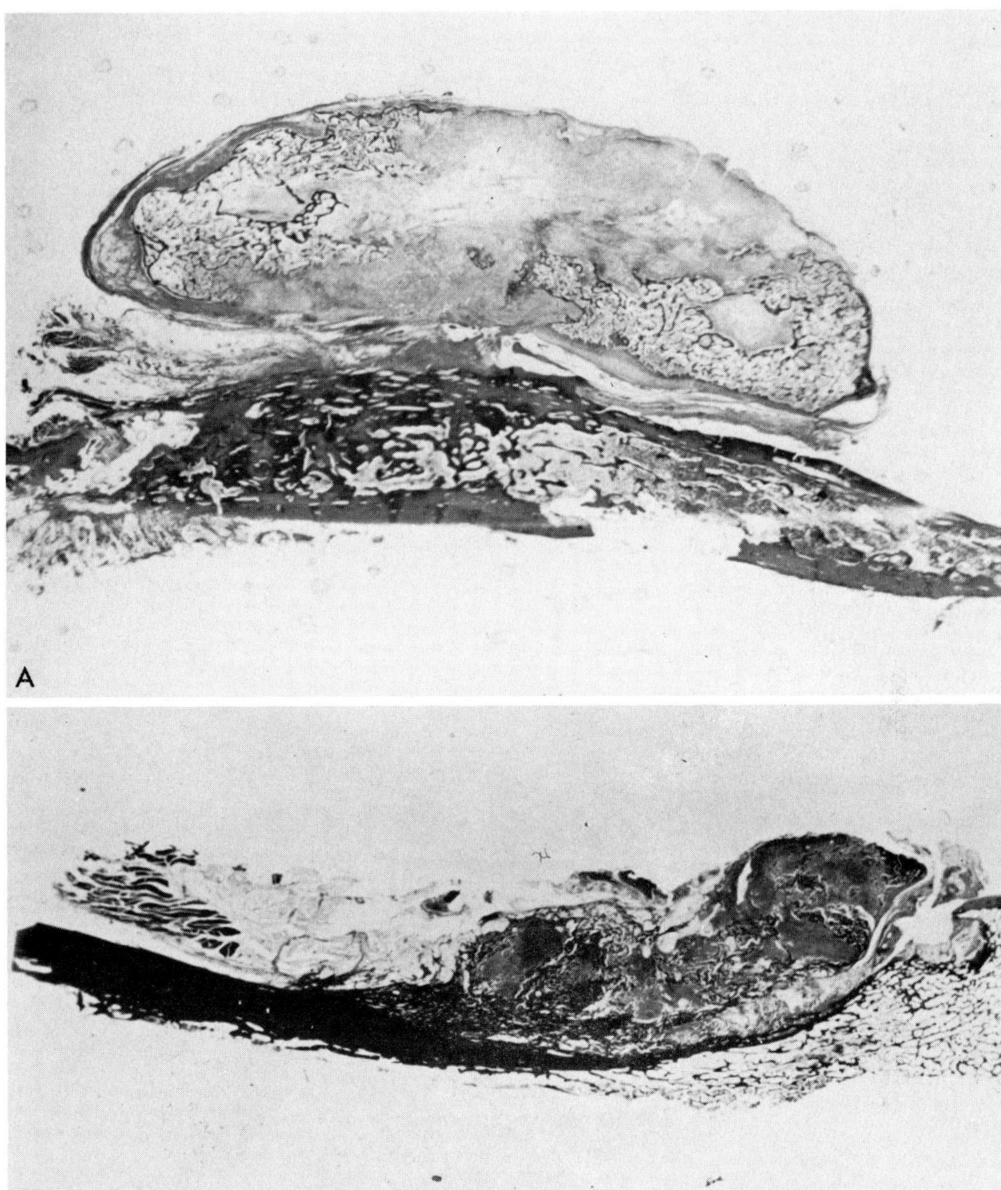

Figure 9–374. Parosteal sarcoma. Macrosections of two parosteal sarcomas illustrating the clear periosteal space between the lesion and the underlying cortex. In both lesions, there is an area in which the tumor originates from the cortex and is intimately associated with it. The bulk of the lesion, however, is clearly separate. It is very tempting for the surgeon to utilize this cleavage plane and simply cut throught the stalk of the lesion in removing it. However, this procedure is very dangerous and almost guarantees that tumor will be left behind in the cortex. It results in an unacceptably high rate of recurrence (approaching 100 per cent).

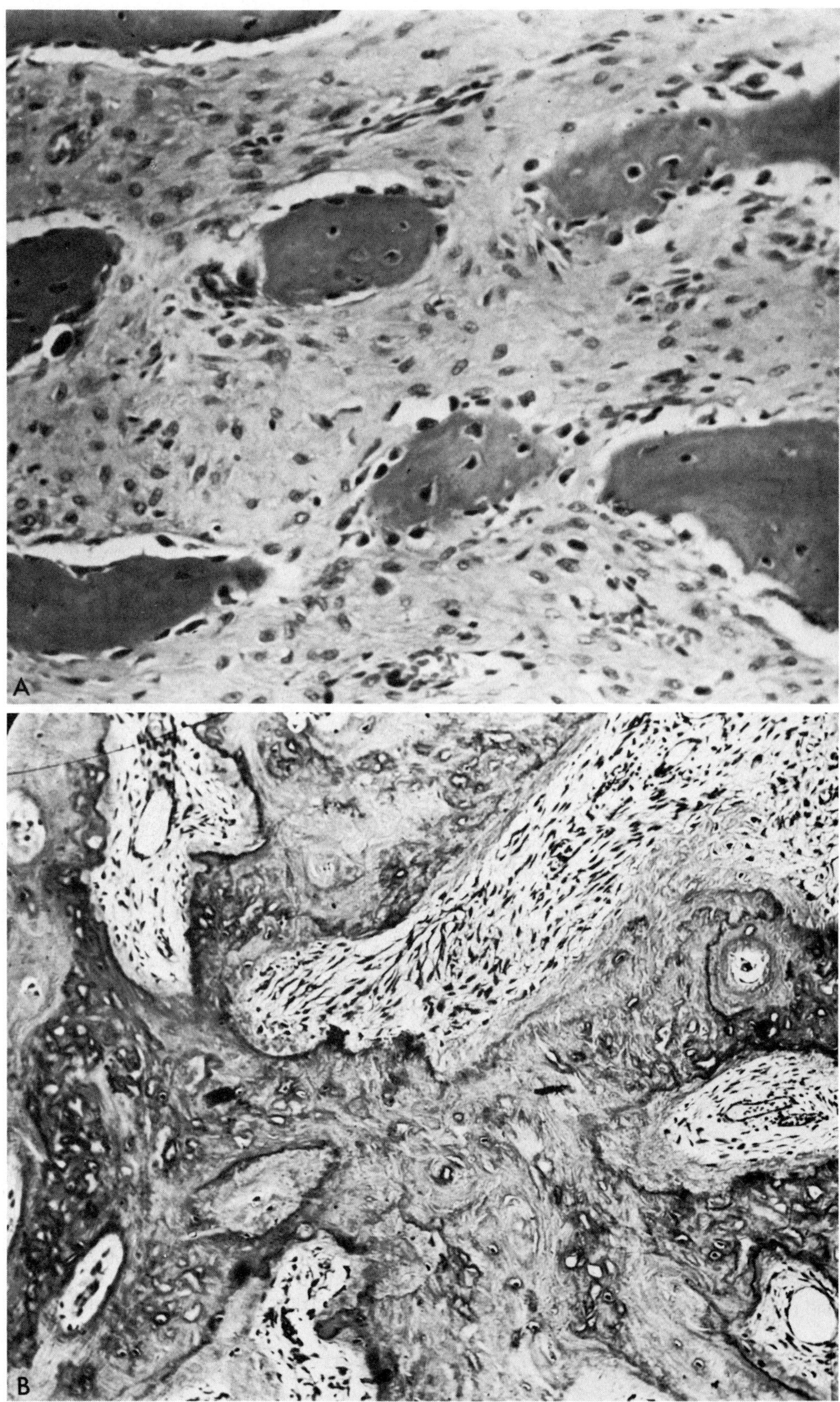

Figure 9–375. Parosteal sarcoma. Histologic variation seen in the osseous portion of parosteal sarcoma. *A,* Benign-appearing fibrous stroma is present between normal-appearing trabeculae of bone. It would be very difficult to characterize this type of tissue as a malignant lesion when taken out of context of the entire histologic picture. *B,* Highly cellular lesion with numerous cement lines and an irregular osseous pattern. The intervening fibrous stroma is cellular.

Illustration continued on opposite page

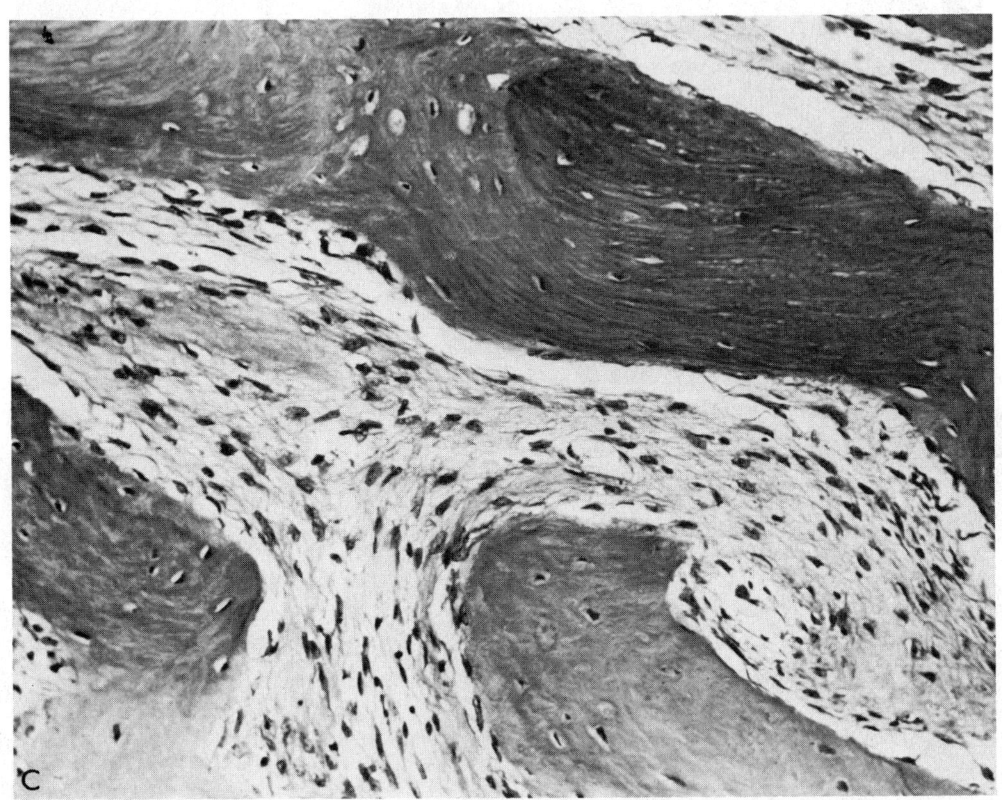

Figure 9–375 *(Continued). C,* Similar lesion, with benign-appearing fibrous stroma and trabeculae of relatively normal lamellar bone.

Illustration continued on following page

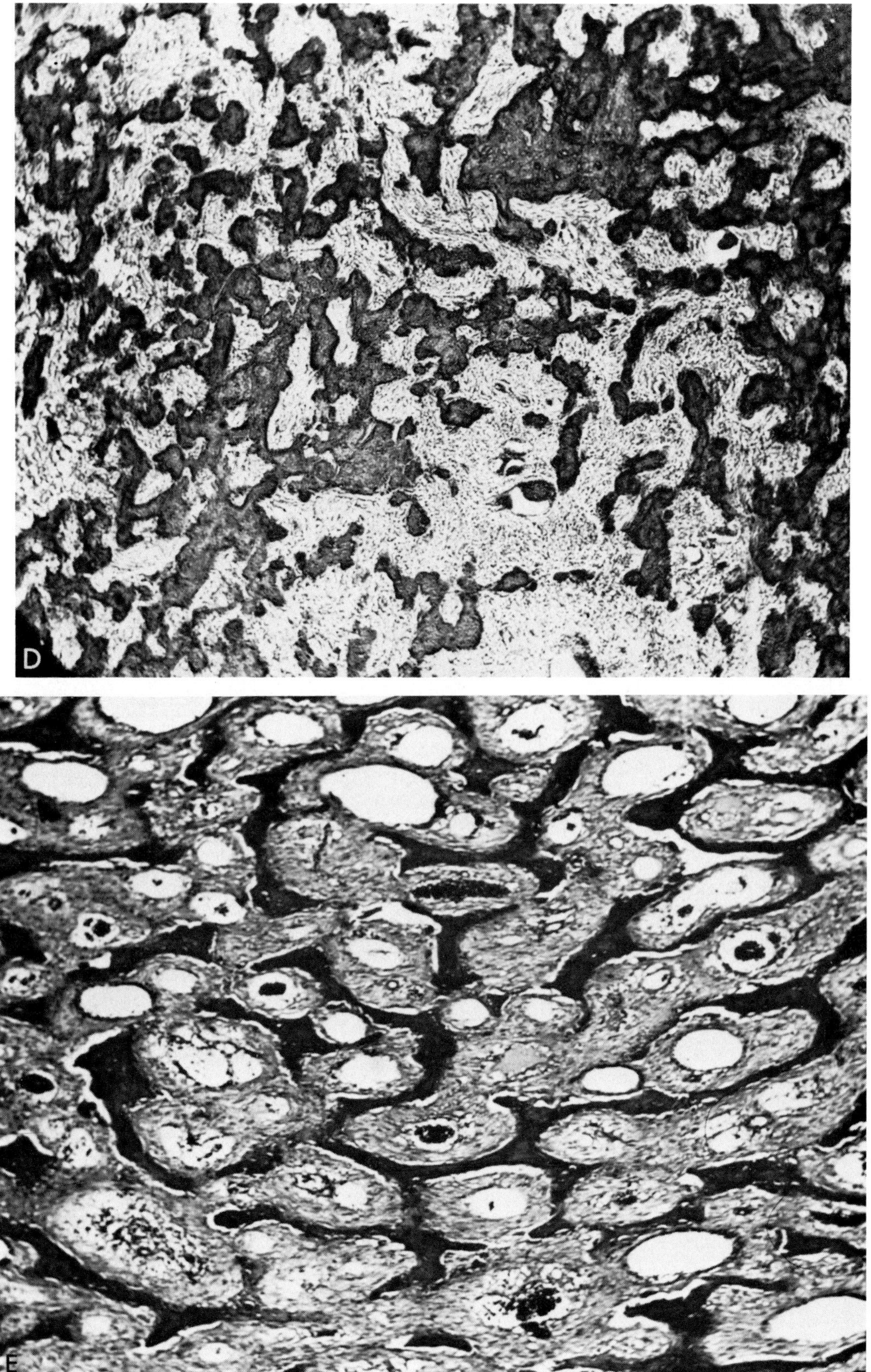

Figure 9–375 *(Continued). D*, Relatively dense, quite abnormal acellular bone. The fibrous stroma suggests the correct diagnosis. *E*, Vascular field in parosteal tumor.

Illustration continued on opposite page

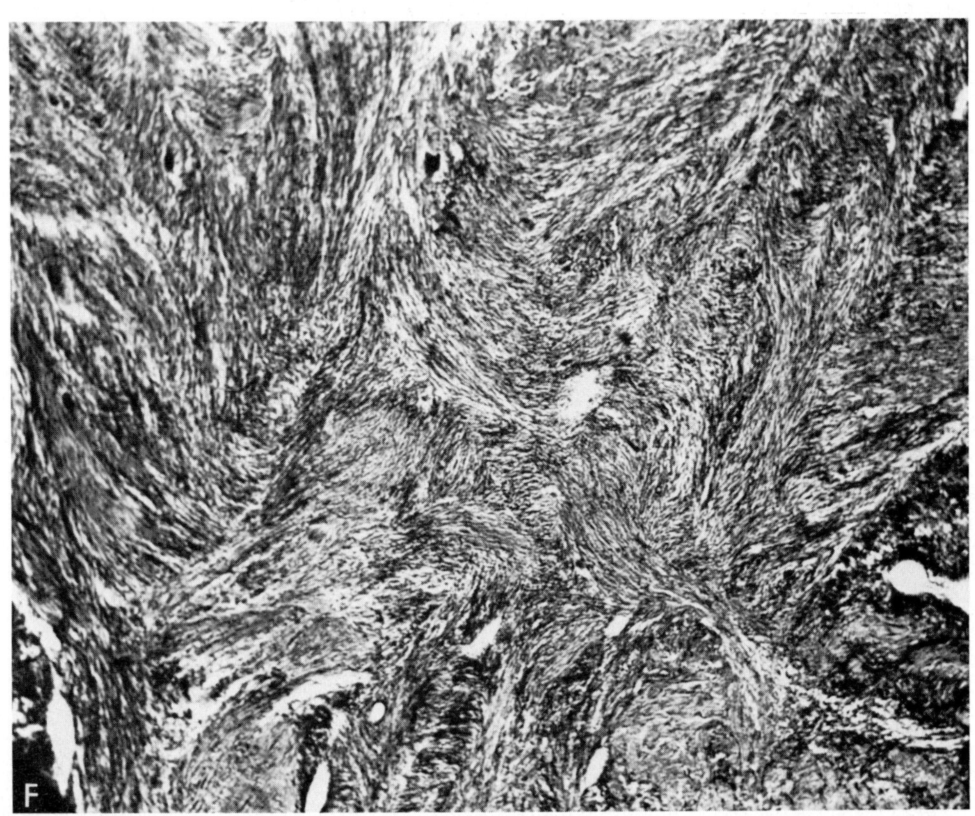

Figure 9–375 *(Continued). F,* Heavily collagenized focus of malignant fibrous stroma. Cells are not prominent; the lack of mitoses makes one reluctant to call this a malignant tumor.

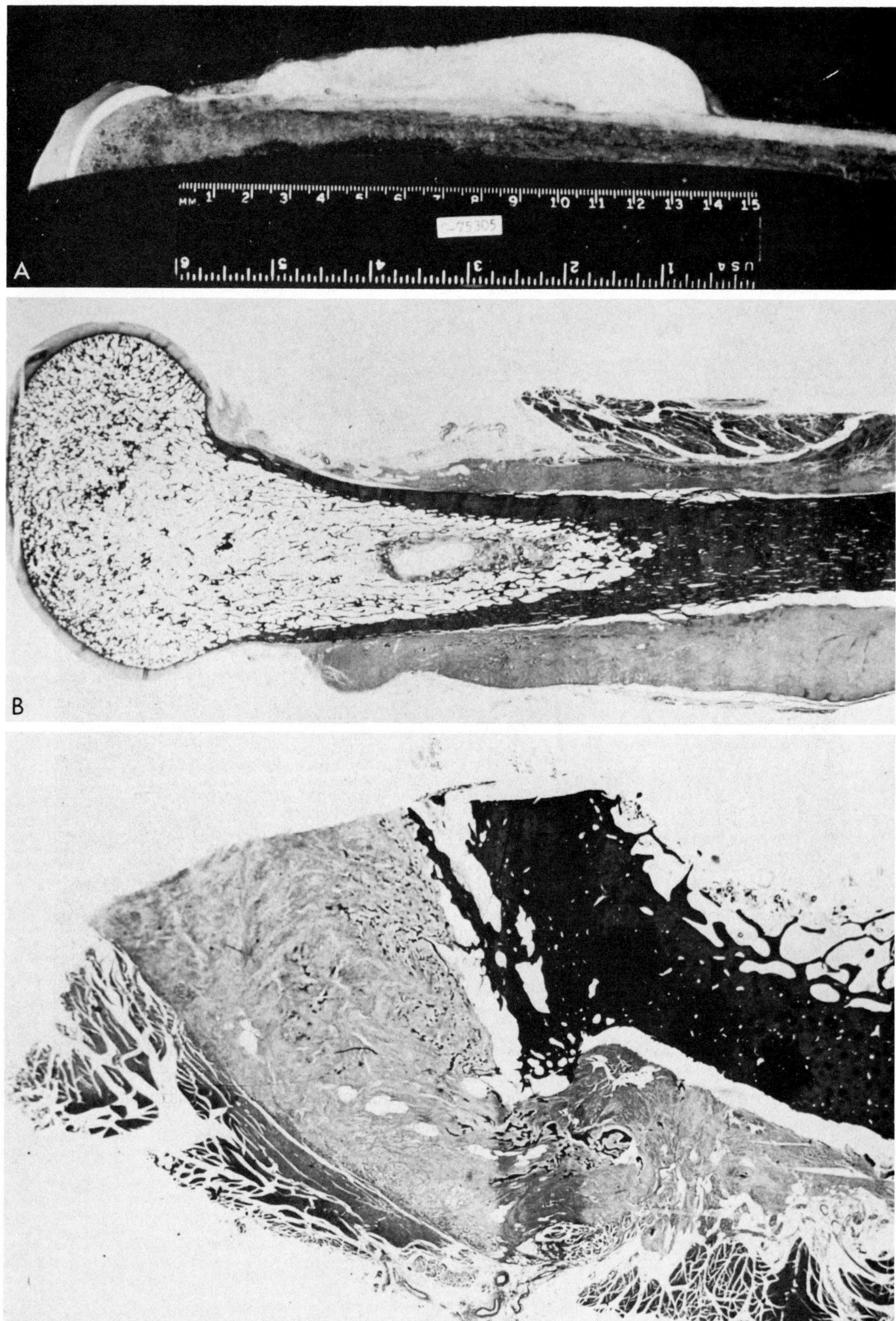

Figure 9–376. *A*, Parosteal fibrosarcoma on the surface of the distal femur. *B*, Macrospecimen of the same lesion, showing that it is entirely on the surface, with no intramedullary involvement. *C*, Cross section of an area through the tumor. Note the lack of medullary penetration.

Illustration continued on opposite page

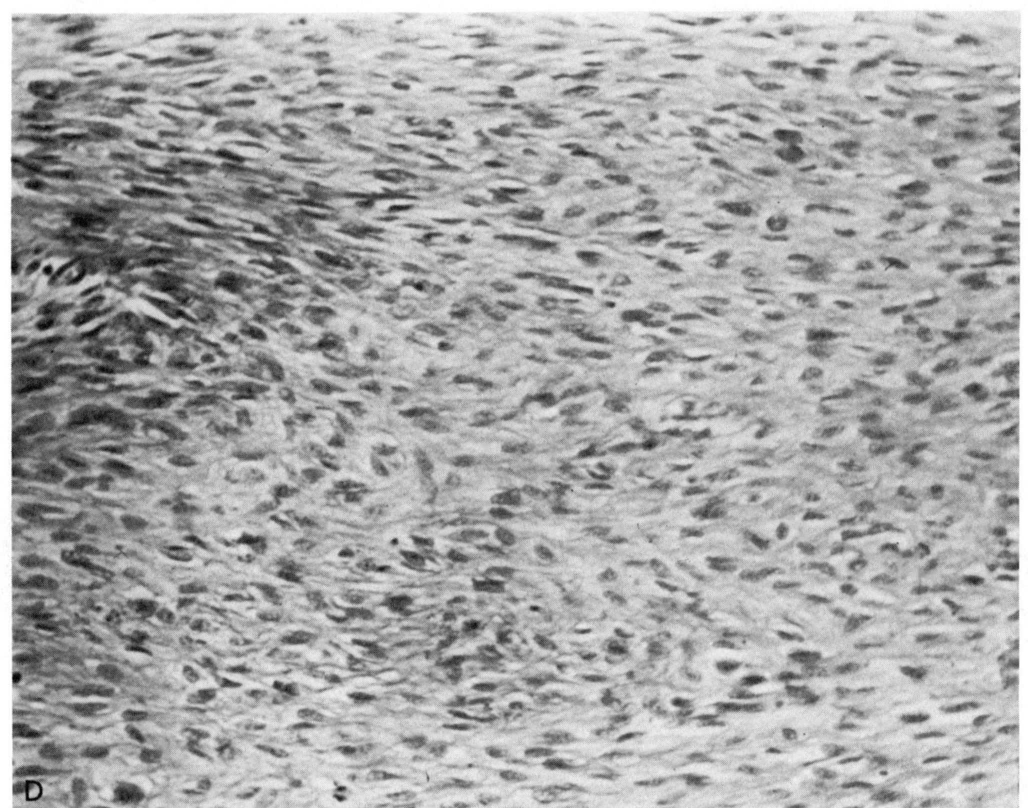

Figure 9–376 *(Continued). D,* Low-grade fibrous stroma without significant mitotic activity or cellular pleomorphism. The lesion shows soft-tissue density radiographically.

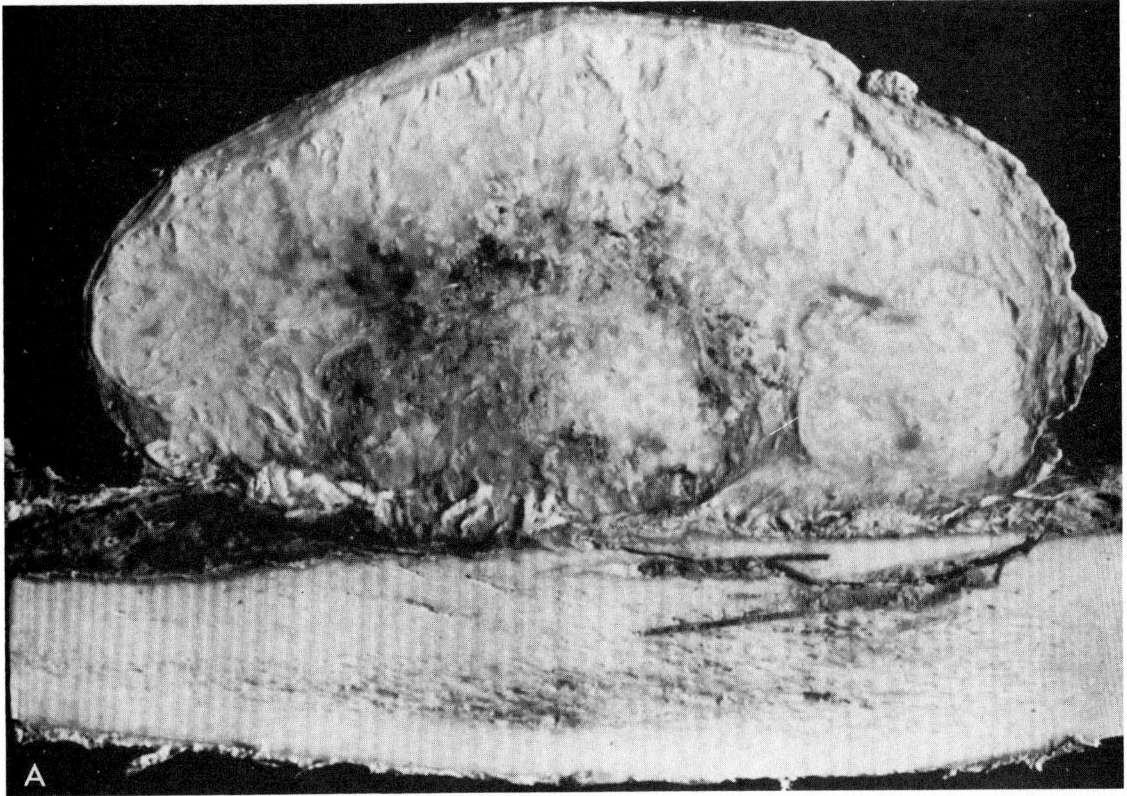

Figure 9–377. Parosteal chondrosarcoma. *A,* Gross specimen on the surface of the cortex of the humerus.

Illustration continued on following page

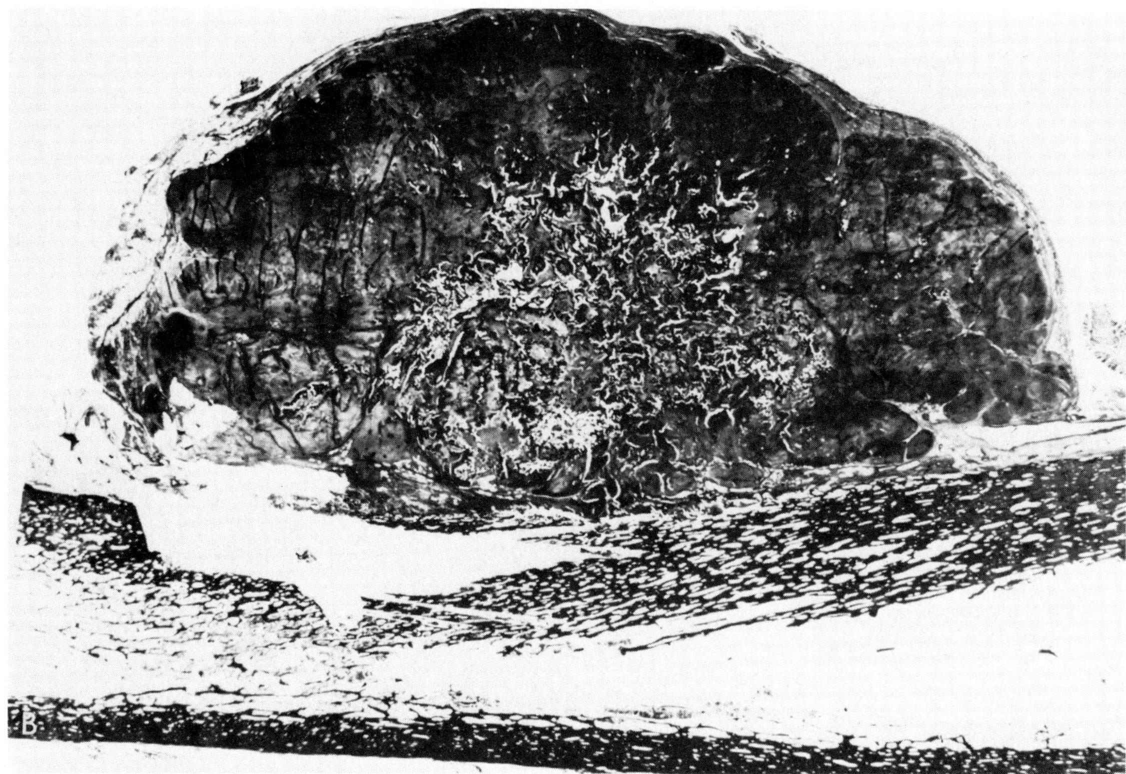

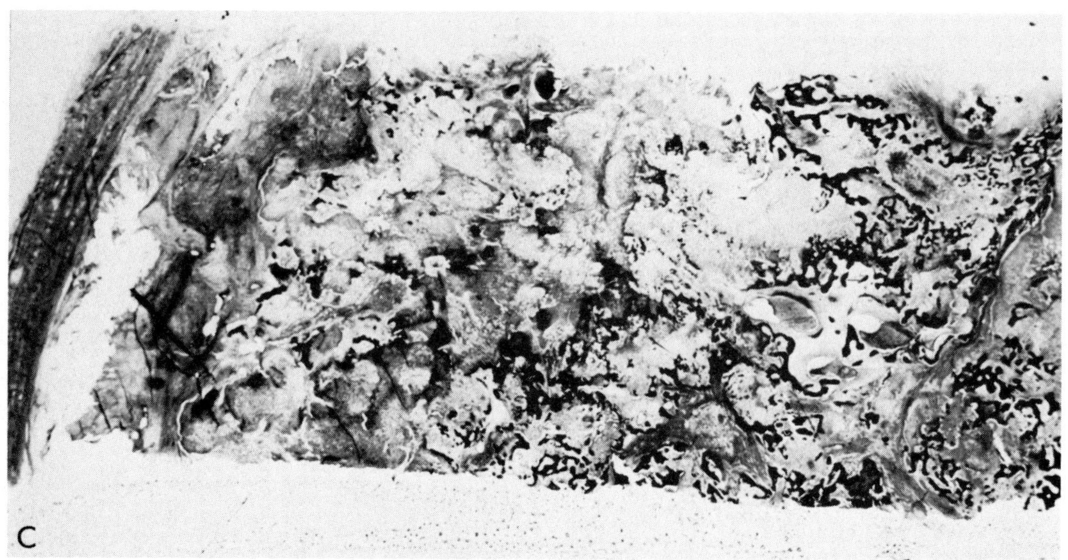

Figure 9–377 *(Continued). B*, Macrosection of the same lesion, showing the central ossified core with a large peripheral chondromatous surface. *C*, Section through the entire extent of the lesion from cortex to surface of the lesion (left).

Illustration continued on opposite page

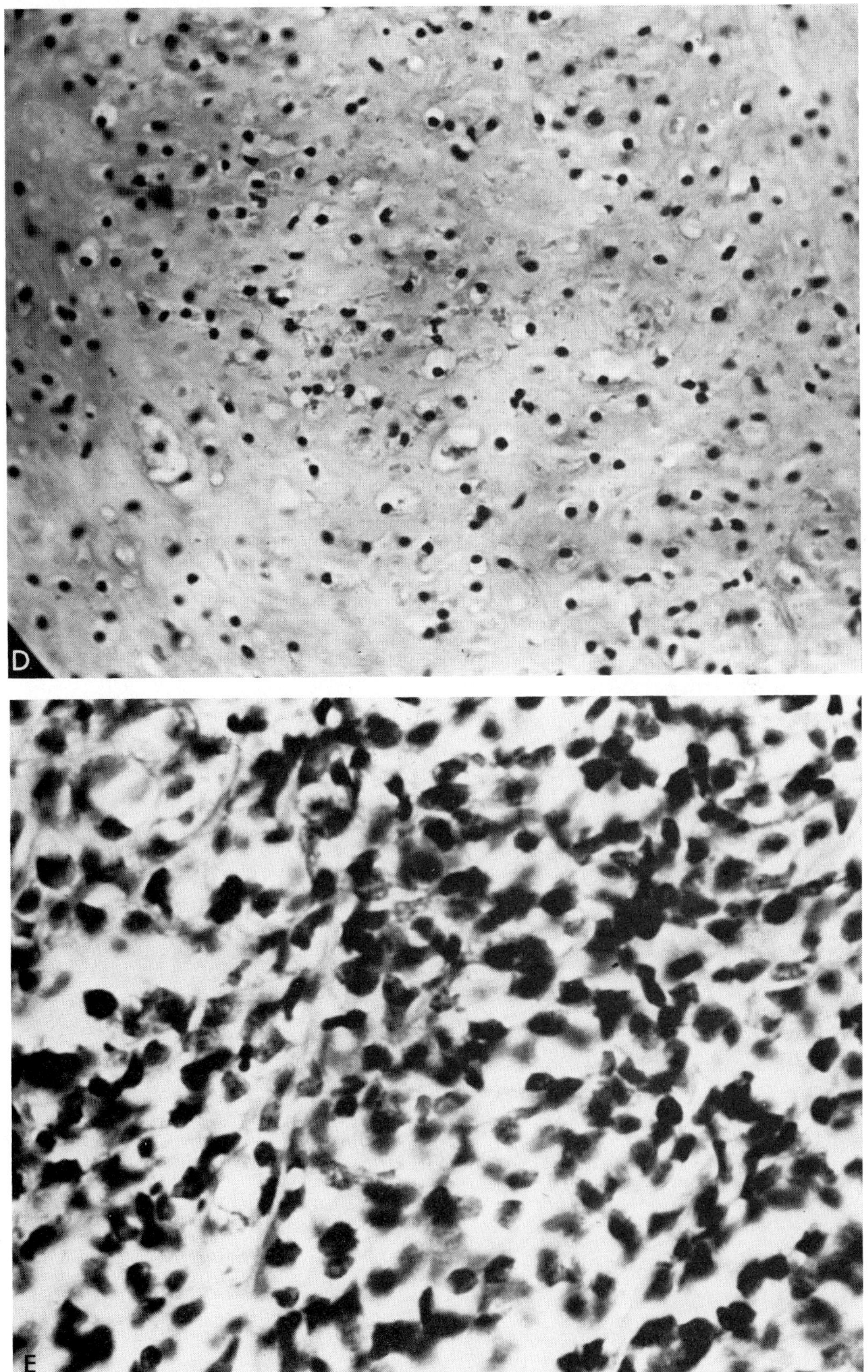

Figure 9–377 *(Continued). D,* Representative section of the tumor, with relatively benign-appearing cartilage. *E,* Representative section of the periphery of the lesion, consisting of sheets of undifferentiated small round cells, a histologic picture similar to that of Ewing's sarcoma. Sampling only a small portion of this large tumor could result in an inaccurate diagnosis and inappropriate therapy.

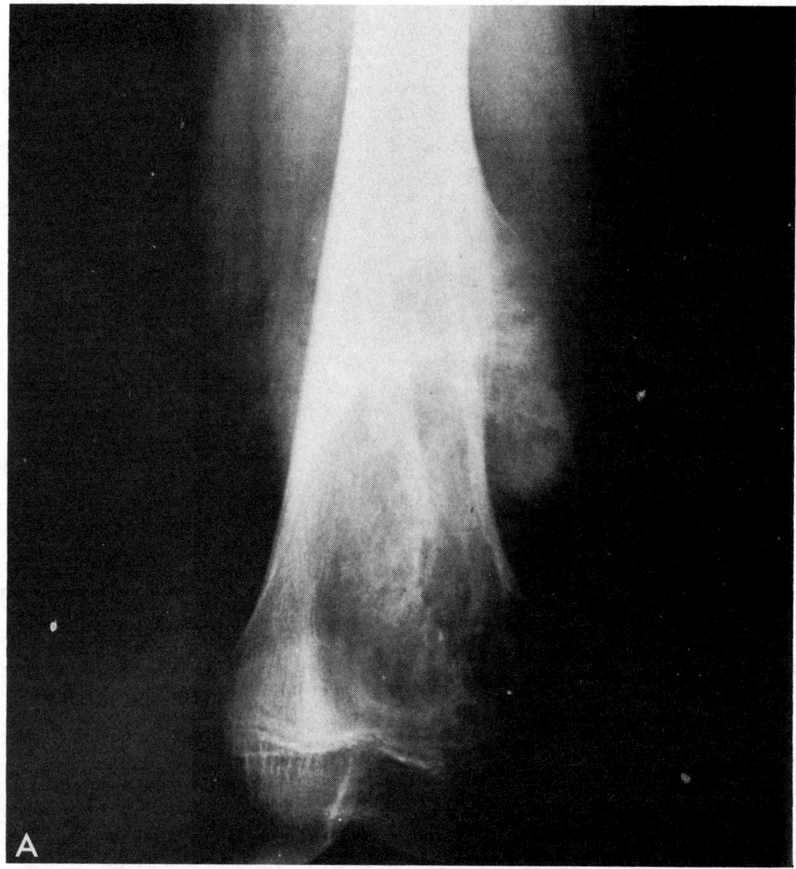

Figure 9–378. Parosteal sarcoma. Radiograph *(A)* and histologic sections *(B* and *C)* of parosteal tumor in a 15-year-old girl. Histologic study reveals an innocuous fibrous lesion with minimal pleomorphism. An occasional bone spicule is formed by the tumor. Amputation was performed at midthigh. Eleven years later, the lesion recurred in the soft tissue of the thigh.

Illustration continued on opposite page

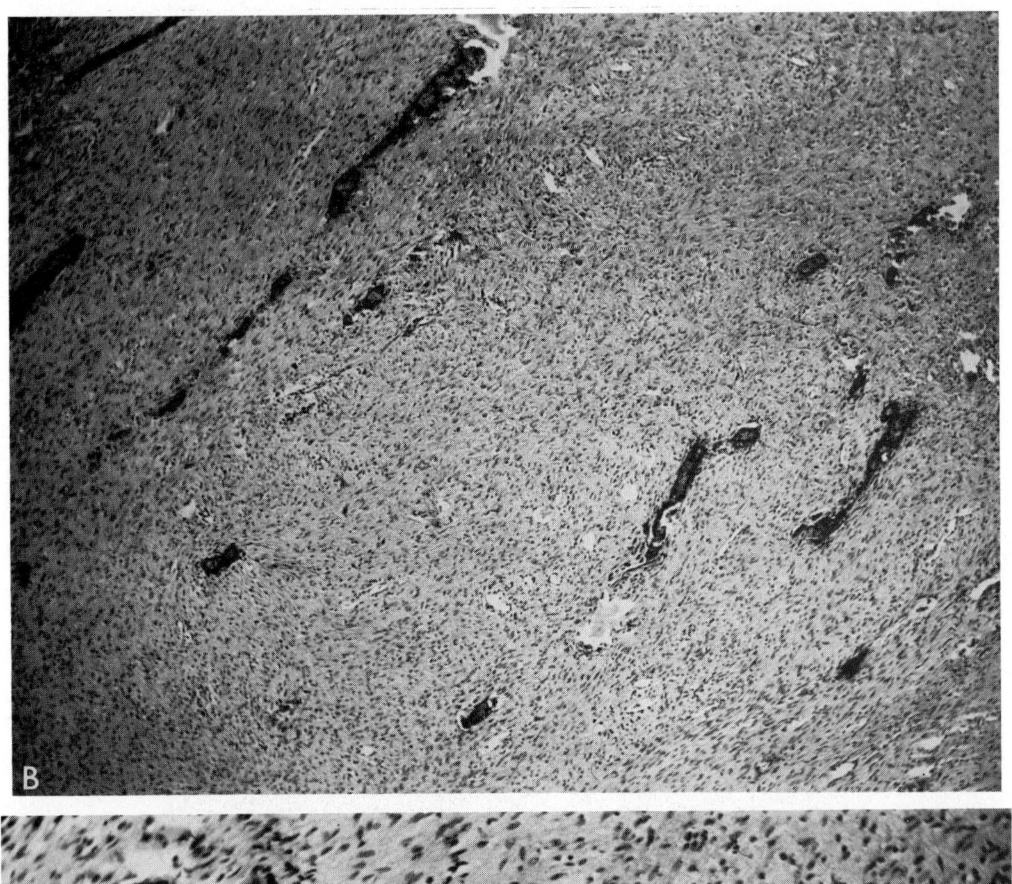

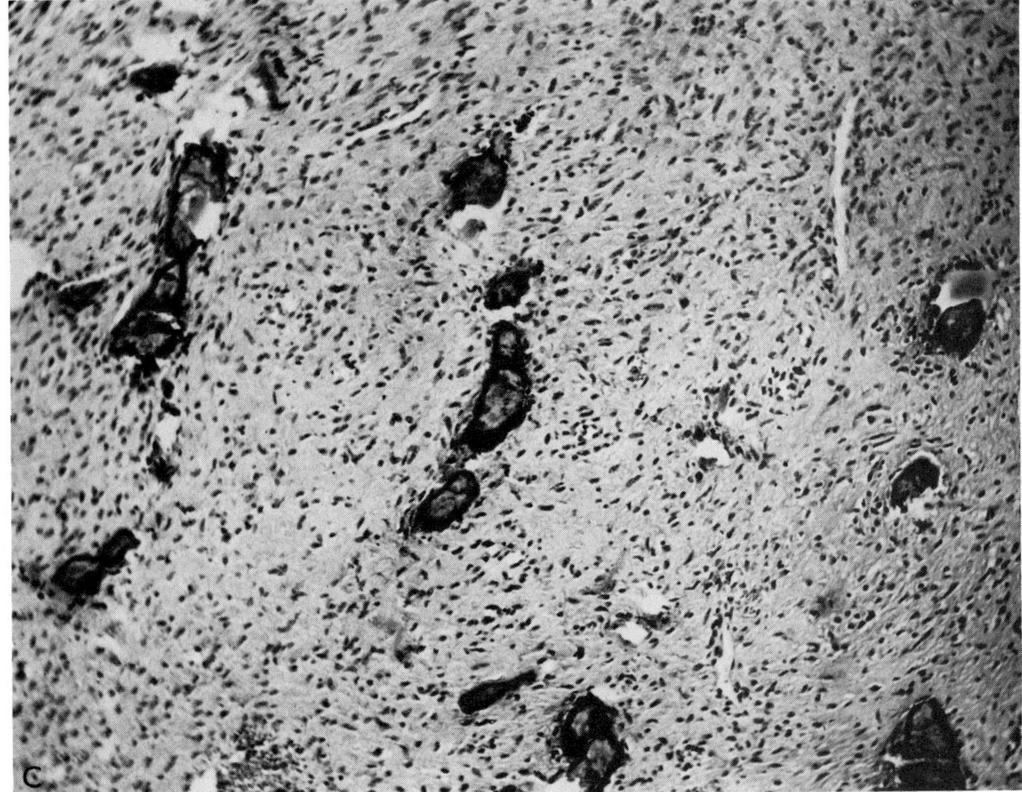

Figure 9–378 *Continued.*

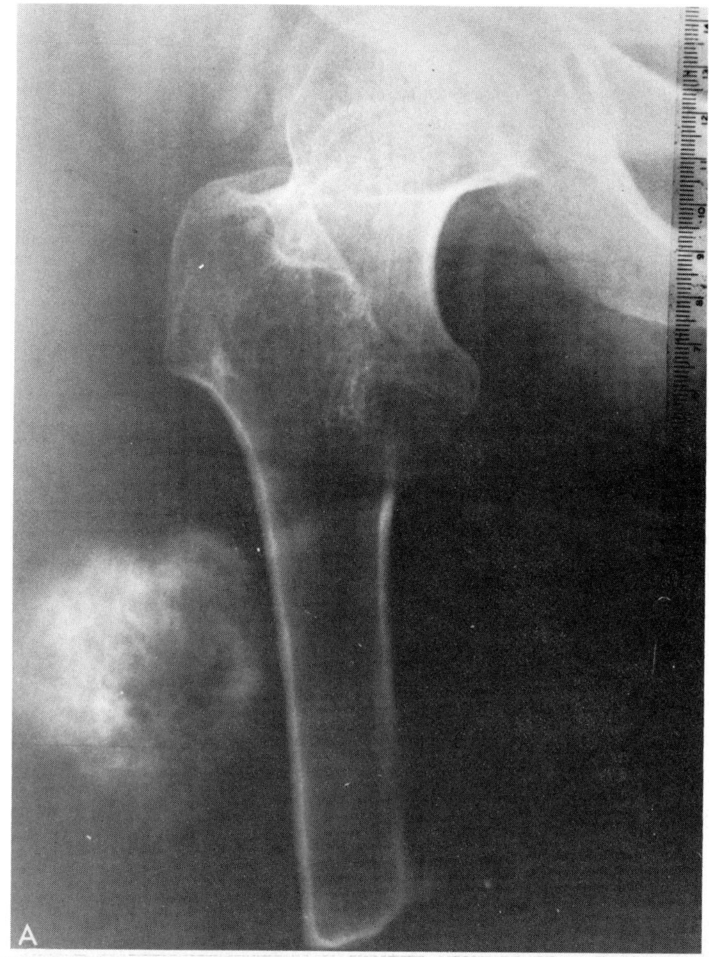

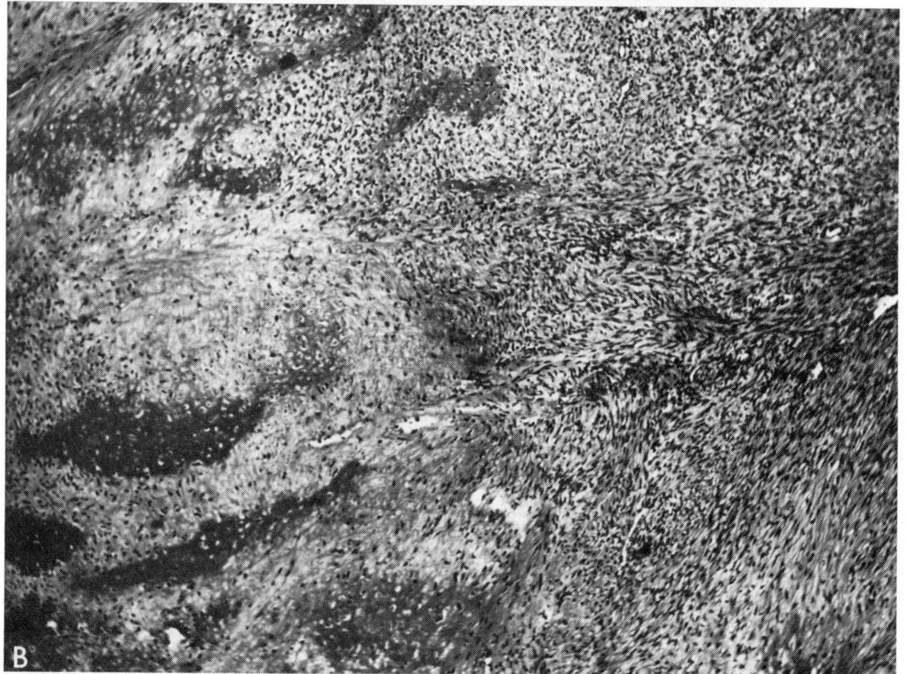

Figure 9–379. *A*, Radiograph of hip showing recurrence in the soft tissue of the thigh of the parosteal sarcoma shown in Figure 9–378. The large soft-tissue mass is heavily calcified, and the margin is indistinct. *B* to *D*, Representative fields from this tumor exhibit its fibrous and chondromatous nature, blending into more actively cellular, less differentiated regions with significant pleomorphism. Note the histologic transformation of the lesion over the 11 year period.

Illustration continued on opposite page

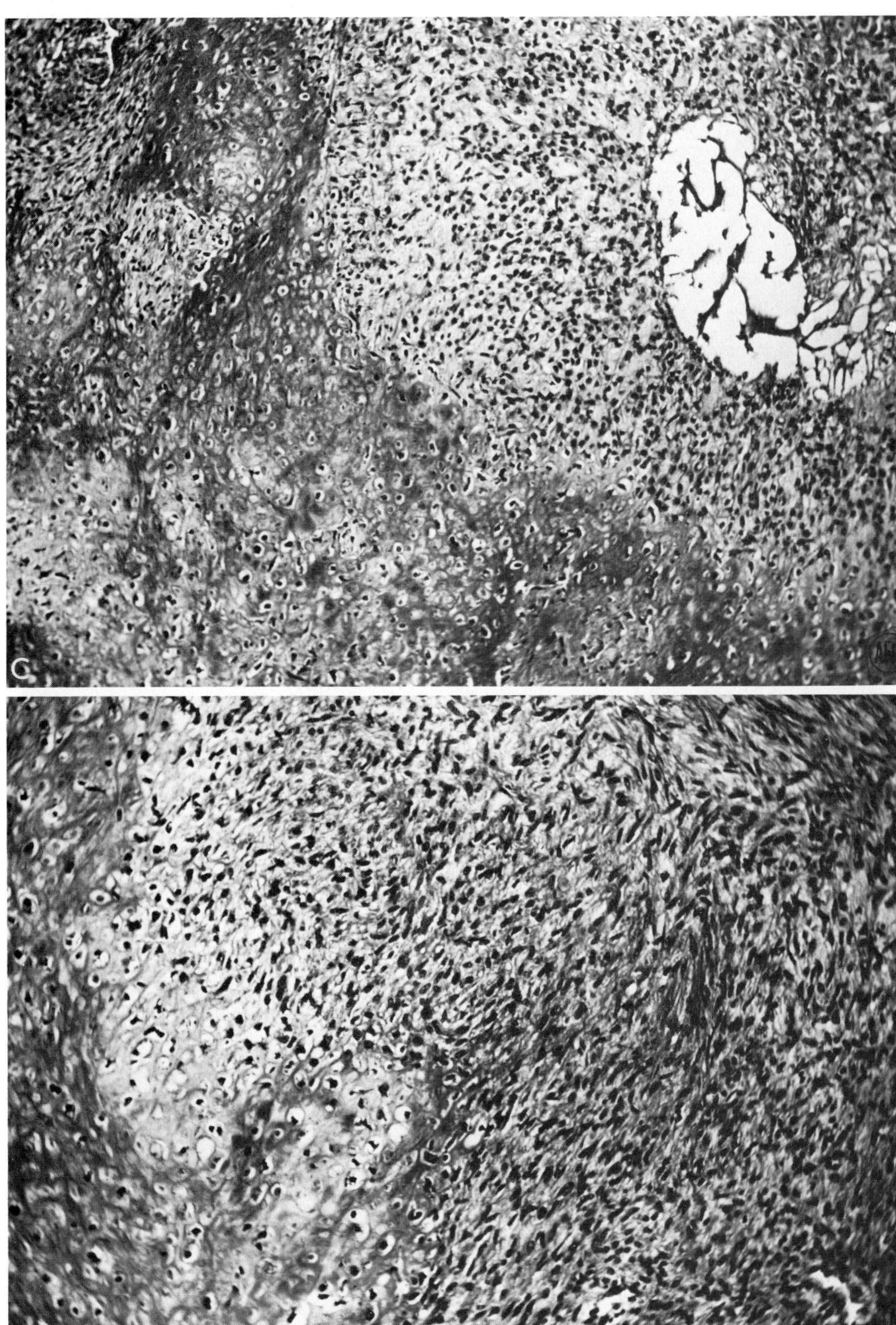

Figure 9–379 *Continued.*

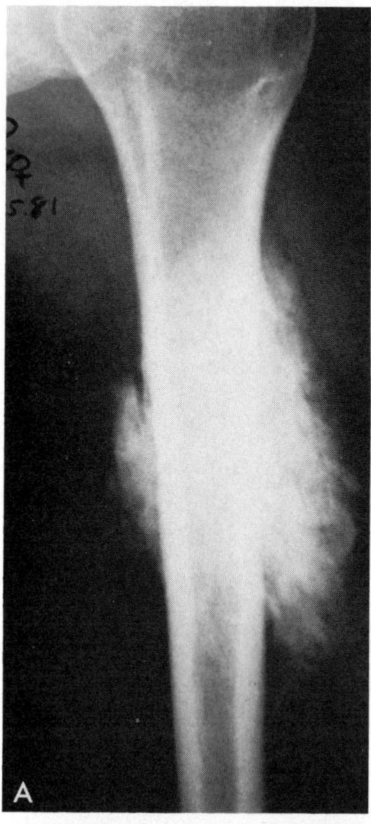

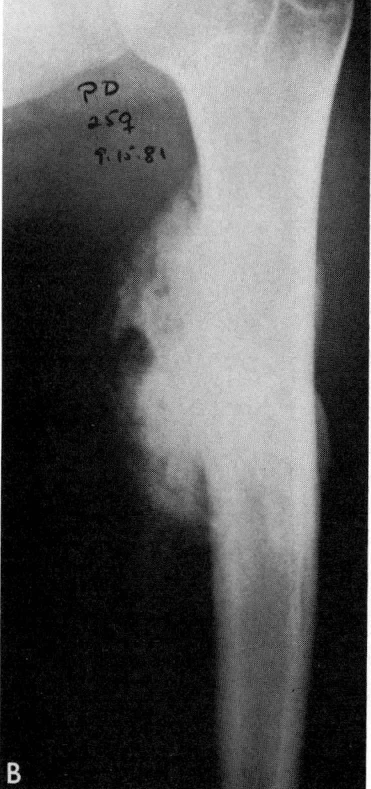

Figure 9–380. Parosteal sarcoma. Radiographs of the proximal humerus of a 25-year-old female who felt an asymptomatic mass in her arm while showering. Note the heavy ossification with preservation of the normal cortex throughout the lesion. There is a soft-tissue cap over the ossified portion.

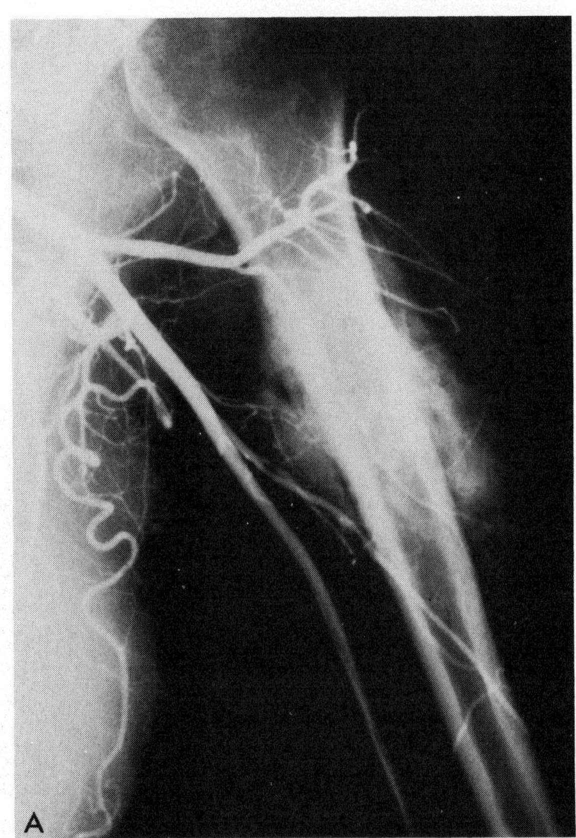

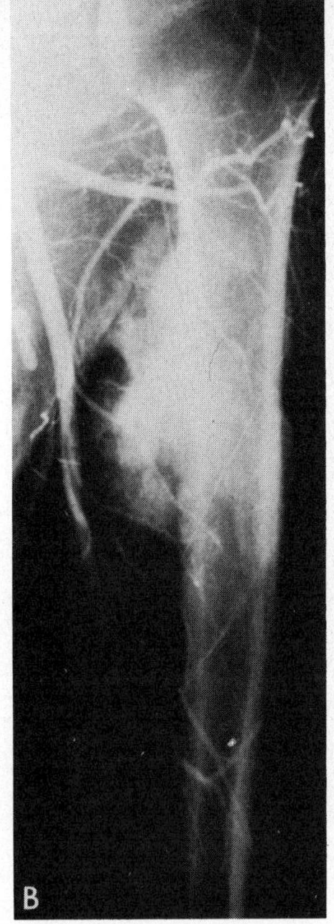

Figure 9–381. Parosteal sarcoma. Arteriograms of the lesion indicate relative avascularity, especially in the soft tissue component on the surface, which is almost devoid of vessels.

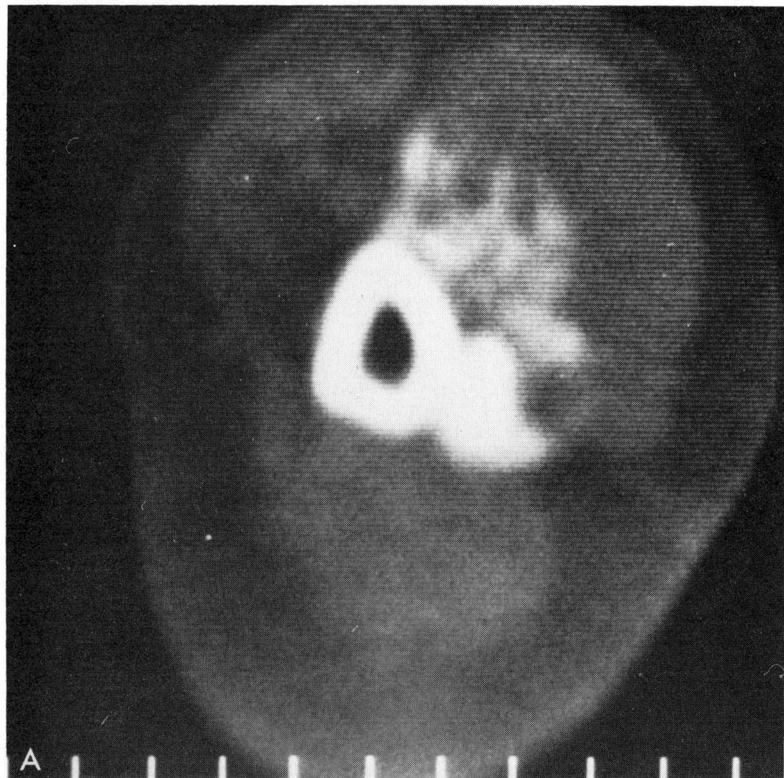

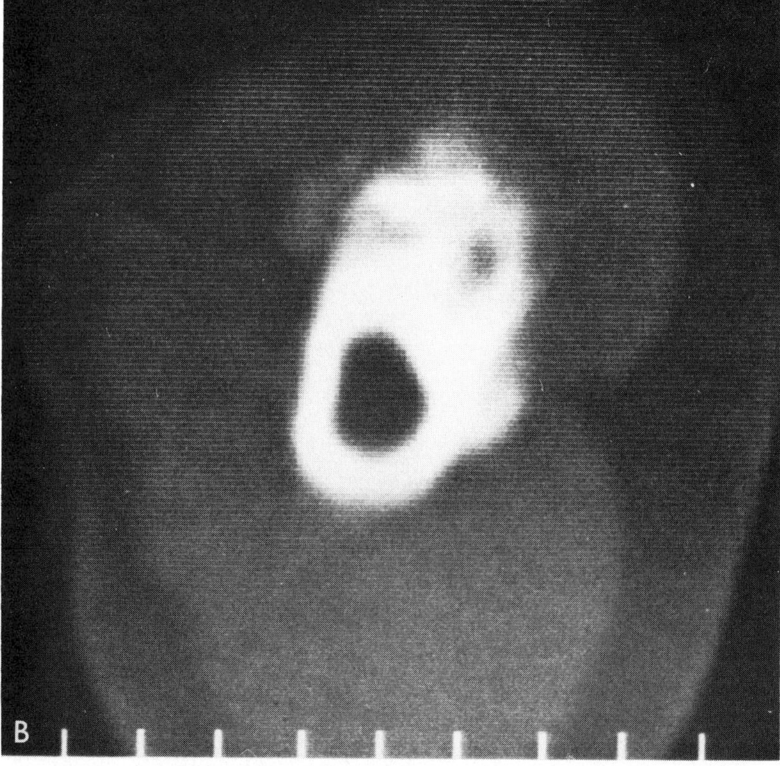

Figure 9–382. Parosteal sarcoma. CT scans through the proximal humerus illustrated in Figures 9–380 and 9–381. The lesion is entirely on the surface of the cortex, with no intramedullary involvement.

Illustration continued on following page

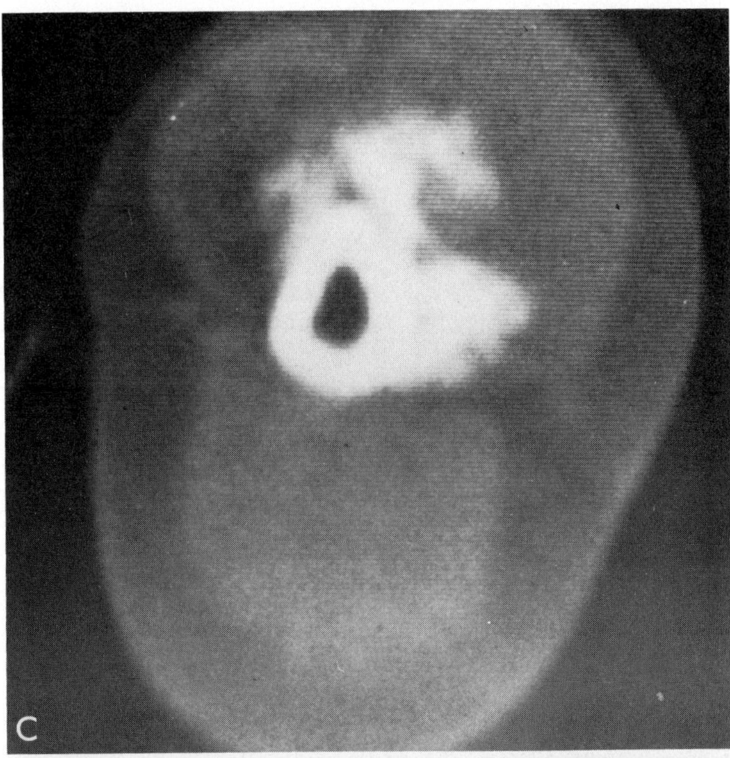

Figure 9–382 *Continued.*

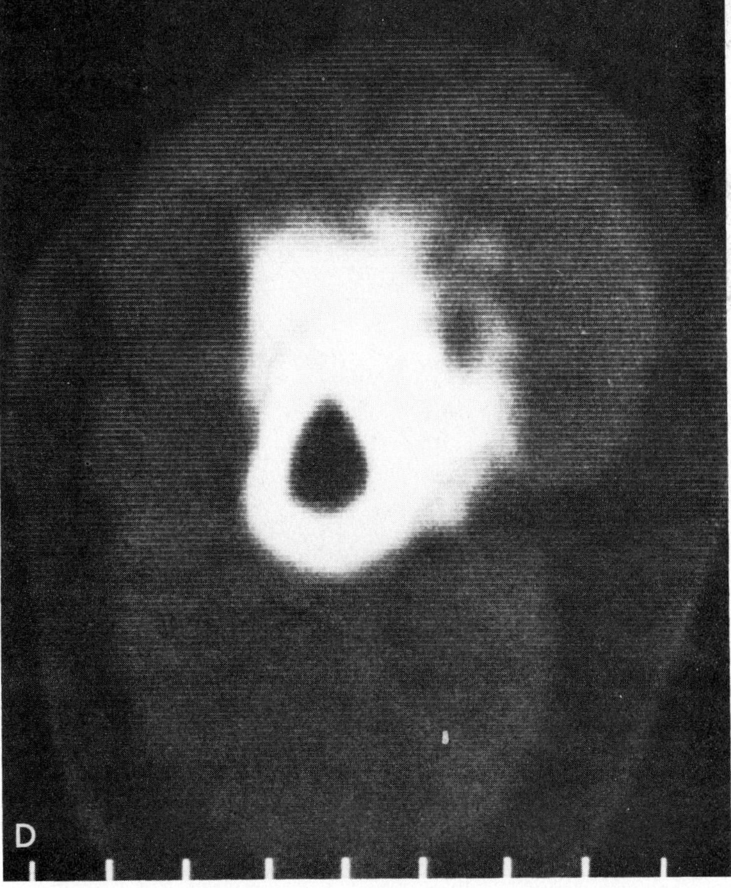

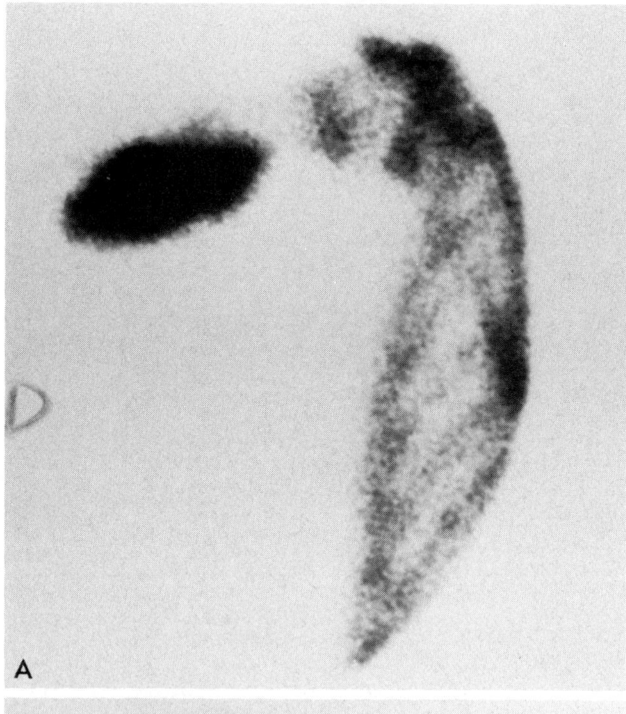

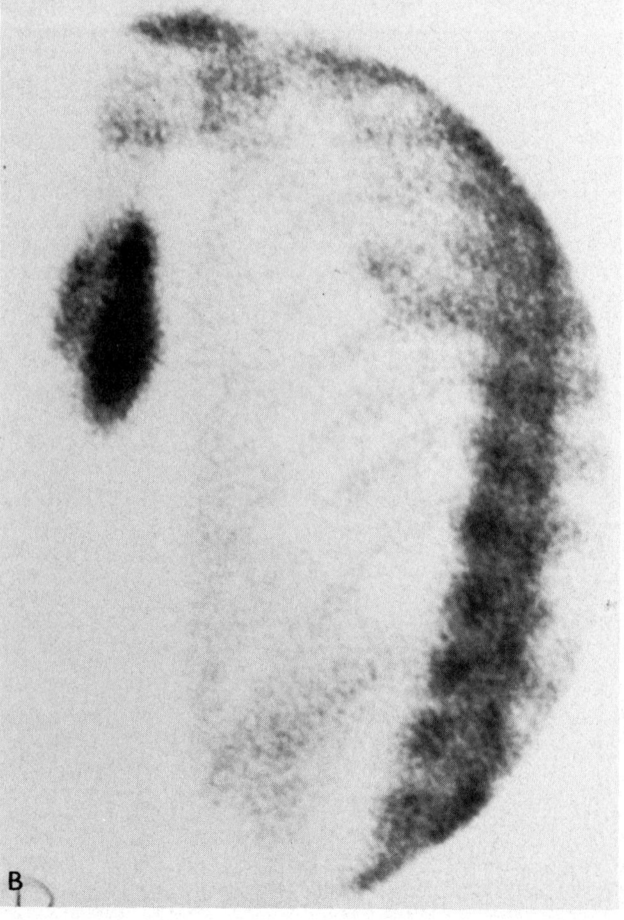

Figure 9–383. Parosteal sarcoma. Bone scans of the lesion shown in Figures 9–380 to 9–382. Note the heavy uptake of the radioisotope. *B* shows a clear zone in the center of the lesion, which represents the humeral shaft.

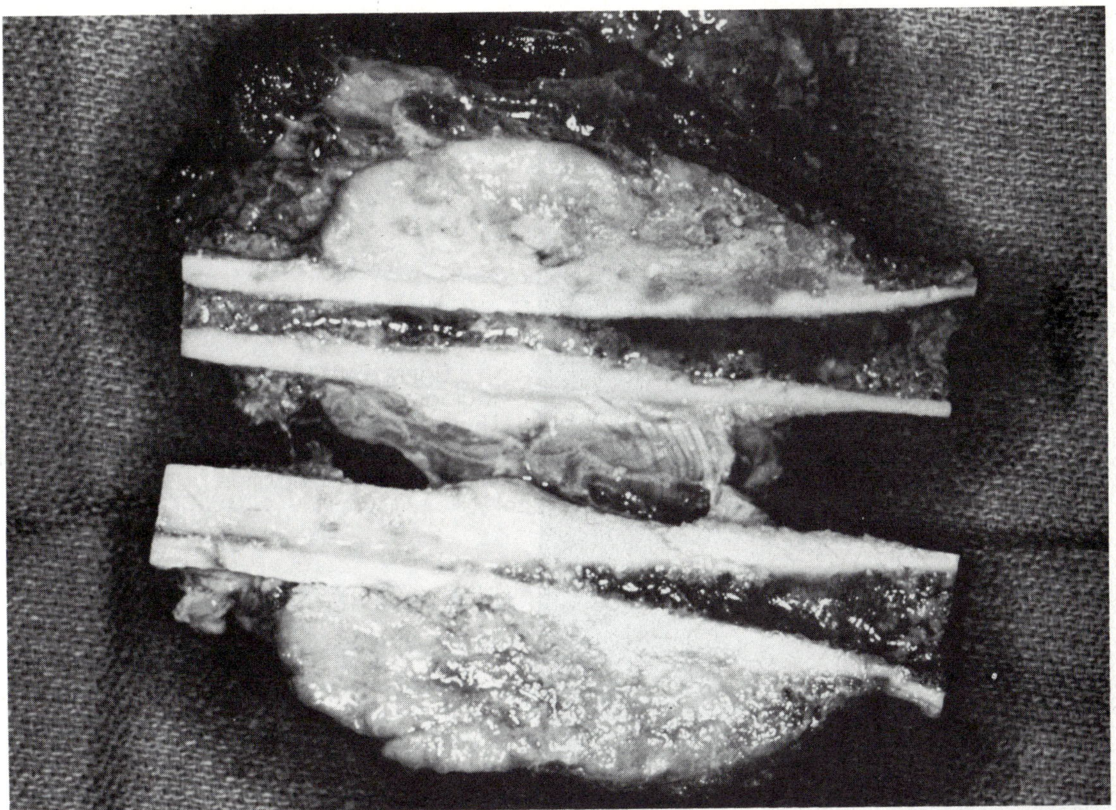

Figure 9–384. Parosteal sarcoma. Gross photograph of the cut surface of the resected humerus illustrated in Figures 9–380 to 9–383. The medullary cavity is completely free of tumor. Wide excision rather than amputation is often curative.

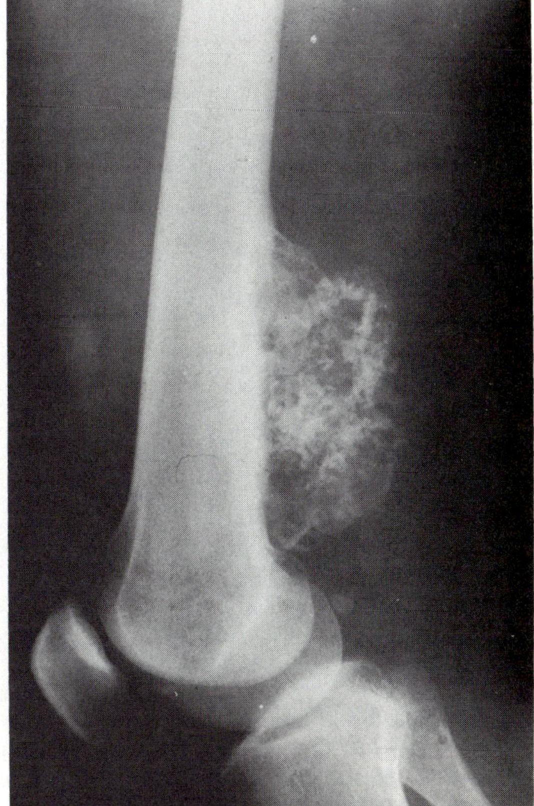

Figure 9–385. Parosteal sarcoma. Lateral radiograph of the distal femur with a large parosteal sarcoma projecting into the popliteal space. An attempt was made to remove this tumor by cutting through it, but a large portion was left behind with the underlying cortex intact.

Table 9–1. ANOMALIES AND NEOPLASMS: SUMMARY

The distinction between anomaly, benign neoplasm, and malignant neoplasm is often unclear, especially since most anomalies of bone exhibit varying tendencies for malignant transformation.

Benign Anomaly or Tumor	Malignant Counterpart

CARTILAGINOUS

Enchondroma
Benign cartilage tumor located within the medullary cavity of bone. Disseminated disease may be present: Ollier's disease or Maffucci's syndrome, the latter when associated with hemangiomas.

Radiology: Sharply circumscribed lytic defect, with flocculent matrix calcification.
Histology: Masses of cartilage, uniform cellular component, large lacunae with chondrocytes.

Chondrosarcoma
May be primary or may arise secondarily from pre-existing benign enchondroma.

Radiology: Markedly varied, but aggressive pattern demonstrated by moth-eaten or permeative destruction at the margins. Matrix calcification may or may not be present, and there may be radiographic evidence of a pre-existing enchondroma.
Histology: The tumor may exhibit marked variability, and generous biopsy is therefore necessary. The most subtle changes are alterations in the size of the chondrocyte and the filling of the lacunar space with a larger than normal number of chondrocytes per unit volume; myxoid change, spindling of chondrocytes, and, ultimately clear-cut malignant tumor occur. Various subtypes are indentifiable (e.g., clear cell chondrosarcoma, mesenchymal chondrosarcoma), but these are rare. Grading of tumor is related to prognosis.

Osteochondroma
Perichondrial proliferation with transformation to bone; may be single or multiple.
Radiology: Cartilage lesion on bony stalk. The lesion points away from the growth plate. Axial skeleton osteochondromas may reach enormous size.
Histology: Cartilage cap with transformation to bone. The transformation should mimic a growth plate.

Chondromyxoid Fibroma
Radiology: Metaphyseal, eccentric, sharply circumscribed, isolated lesion. Appearance identical with that of nonossifying fibroma of bone.
Histology: A myxoid ground substance is present, and there are numerous spindled cells with collagen formation, accompanied by giant cells. The lesion must be differentiated from a myxoid chondrosarcoma, which is usually more pleomorphic and has foci of clear-cut cartilage.

Chondroblastoma (Codman's Tumor)
Radiology: Epiphyseal location, sharply circumscribed lytic defect, occasional stippled calcification.
Histology: Foci of cartilage, extremely cellular, with numerous giant cells that may predominate, and "chicken-wire" calcification.

Isolated cases described in literature.

Miscellaneous
Bizarre lesions of cartilage that do not easily fit into established entities (not uncommon).

FIBROUS

Fibrous Dysplasia
Replacement of normal bony structure by a metaphyseal fibrous proliferation accompanied by poorly formed bone; occasional association with cartilage. May involve single bone (monostotic) or numerous bones (polyostotic). The lesions are unpredictable, and although they may remain arrested, destruction of cortical bone may lead to fracture. In disseminated disease, there is a tendency to skeletal deformity, and marked facial deformity may arise when skull bones are involved.

Isolated cases described in literature.

Table 9–1. ANOMALIES AND NEOPLASMS: SUMMARY (*Continued*)

Benign Anomaly or Tumor	Malignant Counterpart

FIBROUS (*Continued*)

Radiology: Defect usually involves full thickness of bone. It is lytic at first but may have a "ground-glass" appearance in older lesions.
Histology: Replacement of normal marrow by fibrous connective tissue that can vary in cellularity. Direct formation of bony trabeculae from the fibrous tissue. There are usually no identifiable osteoblasts, and only occasional osteoclasts are seen. Foci of cartilage may be present.

Nonossifying Fibroma (Fibroxanthoma)
Radiology: Metaphyseal, sharply circumscribed, eccentric.
Histology: Whorled fibrous pattern, cartwheel formation, numerous xanthoma cells, and little if any pleomorphism or mitotic activity. In older lesions, there may be calcification and secondary bone formation.

Fibrosarcoma
Radiology: Poorly defined lesion usually found in the metaphysis, with either moth-eaten or permeative destruction. Tendency to infarct fragments of bone. Periosteal reaction depends on rate of tumor growth.
Histology: Malignant fibroblasts, characterized by variation in cell size and shape. There is no direct osteoid formation by tumor cells, although the tumor may have foci of calcification that ultimately ossify.

Desmoplastic Fibroma
Histology: Dense, relatively acellular fibrous connective tissue simulating scar tissue. Focal calcification may be present.

Desmoplastic Fibrosarcoma
Histology: Same as that of desmoplastic fibroma, with increased pleomorphism. It is extremely difficult to differentiate a desmoplastic fibroma from its sarcomatous counterpart.

Fibrous Histiocytoma
Radiology: Circumscribed.
Histology: Fibrous stroma, xanthomatous, with round cell and spindled component.

Malignant Fibrous Histiocytoma
Radiology: Evidence of a pre-existing cyst or an infarct in large number of cases.
Histology: Histiocytic proliferation, fibrous stroma, giant cell and cellular proliferation.

Unicameral Bone Cyst
Radiology: Usually metaphyseal involving full thickness of bone, sometimes with expansion of cortex.
Histology: Cyst lining consists of single layered mesothelium with underlying connective tissue. Reactive bone formation, occasional neoplastic bone formation, or dense fibrous connective tissue.

Sarcoma Arising in Cyst Wall
Spindle cell tumor with evidence of pre-existing cyst. Rare.

Aneurysmal Bone Cyst
Always secondary to other primary processes.

Not described.

Cortical Fibrous Dysplasia (Ossifying Fibroma)
Radiology: Lesion arises in cortex and expands cortical margin internally and externally.
Histology: Similar to fibrous dysplasia, but fibrous connective tissues is intracortical. As opposed to fibrous dysplasia, this lesion has a prominent osteoblastic seam around each of the bony trabeculae.

Adamantinoma of Long Bone
Similar in location to cortical fibrous dysplasia but shows more aggressive growth pattern. Always exhibits a prominent intracortical component.
Histology: Biphasic tumor, including a fibrous and a more glandular type of epithelial component.

Table continued on following page

Benign Anomaly or Tumor	Malignant Counterpart

OSTEOID

Osteoid Osteoma
Radiology: Sharply localized, small nidus, excessive reaction; may be inflammatory or vascular process. May be in any bone. Diameter of nidus should not exceed 1 cm.
Histology: Bone formation without connective tissue, excessive vascularity, and uniform osteoblasts.

Osteoblastoma
Radiology: Sharply circumscribed, osteoid-forming, not necessarily calcified. Common in vertebrae.
Histology: Osteoblasts, with minimal pleomorphism, occasional extensive calcified osteoid formation, and clearly defined advancing margin.

Osteosarcoma
a. With extensive bone formation
b. With little bone
Radiology: Rapid growth pattern with periosteal reaction. Codman's triangle. Bone formation evident.
Histology: Neoplastic osteoid formed directly by the tumor. The presence or absence of this osteoid may vary, and there may be prominent vascular components or extensive sclerotic components, but there appears little difference in prognosis, regardless of histologic type.

Parosteal Osteosarcoma (Periosteal Osteosarcoma)
Formation of neoplastic osteoid by periosteal tumor, usually well differentiated, simulating a fibrous tumor. Must be distinguished from benign reactive process but usually exhibits poorly defined advancing margin.

OSTEOCLASTIC

Giant Cell Tumor of Bone
Radiology: Metaphyseal and epiphyseal after closure of growth plate; bubbly, expansile, usually sharp demarcation.
Histology: Numerous osteoclasts; also many stromal cells, which are similar to the osteoclasts. Occasional minute osteoid formation. The degree of pleomorphism varies, but predictibility of malignancy does not correlate well with histologic appearance.

Malignant Giant Cell Tumor
Histology: Pleomorphism, fibrous stroma, and increase in number of mitotic figures should alert observer to possibility of malignant tumor.

MARROW

NONE.

Ewing's Sarcoma
Radiology: Permeative destruction with periosteal reaction; no matrix formation.
Histology: Monomorphous round cell tumor, small nuclei, little if any cytoplasm, occasional positive glycogen stain.

Primary Lymphoma of Bone
Radiology: Permeative destruction. Tendency for minimal periosteal reaction.
Histology: Monomorphous infiltrate replacing marrow, but cells larger than those in Ewing's sarcoma, with more prominent cytoplasmic components.

Multiple Myeloma
Radiology: Punched-out lesions; no reactive bone formation. Sometimes, simple osteoporosis, pathologic fractures.
Histology: Replacement of marrow cavity by clusters or sheets of plasma cells. No reactive bone formation.

CITED REFERENCES

Arata, M. A., Peterson, H. A., and Dahlin, D. C.: Pathologic fractures through nonossifying fibromas—review of the Mayo Clinic experience. J. Bone Joint Surg. *63A*:980, 1981.

Biesecker, J. L., Marcove, R. C., Huvos, A. G., and Mike, V.: Aneurysmal bone cysts—a clinico-pathologic study of 66 cases. Cancer *26*:615, 1970.

Bogumill, G. P., Schultz, M. A., and Johnson, L. C.: Giant cell tumor, a metaphyseal lesion. J. Bone Joint Surg. *54A*:1558, 1972.

Boston, H. C., Dahlin, D. C., Ivins, J. C., and Cupps, R. E.: Malignant lymphoma (so-called reticulum cell sarcoma) of bone. Cancer *34*:1131, 1974.

Capanna, R., Dal Monte, A., Gitelis, S., and Campanacci, M.: The natural history of unicameral bone cyst after steroid injection. Clin. Orthop. *166*:204, 1982.

Case Records of the Massachusetts General Hospital (Case 7-1980). N. Engl. J. Med. *302*:456, 1980.

Case Records of the Massachusetts General Hospital (Case 40-1980). N. Engl. J. Med. *303*:866, 1980.

Dahlin, D. C.: Problems in the interpretation of results of treatment for osteosarcoma. Editorial. Mayo Clin. Proc. *54*:621, 1979.

Dahlin, D. C., and Salvador, A. H.: Chondrosarcomas of bones of the hands and feet—a study of 30 cases. Cancer *34*:755, 1974.

Dahlin, D. C., Unni, K. K., and Matsuno, T.: Malignant (fibrous) histiocytoma of bone—fact or fancy? Cancer *39*:1508, 1977.

Enneking, W. F., and Kagan, A.: "Skip" metastases in osteosarcoma. Cancer *36*:2192, 1975.

Hartman, K. S.: Histiocytosis X: a review of 114 cases with oral involvement. Oral Surg. *49*:38, 1980.

Huvos, A. G., and Higinbotham, N. L.: Primary fibrosarcoma of bone—a clinicopathologic study of 130 patients. Cancer *35*:837, 1975.

Huvos, A. G., Rosen, G., Bretsky, S. S., and Butler, A.: Telangiectatic osteogenic sarcoma: a clinicopathologic study of 124 patients. Cancer *49*:1679, 1982.

Johnson, L. C.: A general theory of bone tumors. Bull. N.Y. Acad. Med. *29*:164, 1953.

Johnson, L. C., Vetter H., and Putschar, W. G. J.: Sarcomas arising in bone cysts. Virchows Arch. Pathol. Anat. *335*:428, 1962.

Kyle, R. A.: Multiple myeloma—review of 869 cases. Mayo Clin. Proc. *50*:29, 1975.

Landon, G. C., Johnson, K. A., and Dahlin, D. C.: Subungual exostoses. J. Bone Joint Surg. *62A*:256, 1979.

Le Charpentier, Y., Forest, M., Postel, M., Tomeno, B., and Abelanet, R.: Clear-cell chondrosarcoma, a report of five cases including ultrastructural study. Cancer *44*:622, 1979.

Levy, W. M., Miller, A. S., Bonakdarpour, A., and Aegerter, E.: Aneurysmal bone cyst secondary to the other osseous lesions—report of 57 cases. Am. J. Clin. Pathol. *63*:1, 1975.

Lichtenstein, L., and Bernstein, D.: Unusual benign and malignant chondroid tumors of bone. Cancer *12*:1142, 1959.

Lieberman, P. H., Jones, C. R., Dargeon, H. W. K., and Begg, C. F.: A reappraisal of EG, HSC and LS syndrome. Medicine Baltimore *48*:357, 1969.

Mahoney, J. P., Spanier, S. S., and Morris, J. L.: Multifocal osteosarcoma—a case report with review of the literature. Cancer *44*:1897, 1979.

Mankin, H. J., Lange, T. A., and Spanier, S. S.: The hazards of biopsy in patients with malignant primary bone and soft tissue tumors. J. Bone Joint Surg. *64A*:1121, 1982.

Marcove, R. C., Weis, L. D., Vaghaiwalla, M. R., Pearson R., and Huvos, A. G.: Cryosurgery in the treatment of giant cell tumors of bone. Cancer *41*:957, 1978.

Markel, S. F.: Ossifying fibroma of long bone—its distinction from fibrous dysplasia and its association with adamantinoma of long bone. Am. J. Clin. Pathol. *69*:91, 1978.

Maurer, H. M.: Current concepts of cancer therapy. N. Engl. J. Med. *299*:1347, 1978.

McCarthy, E. F., and Dorfman, H. D.: Chondrosarcoma of bone with dedifferentiation: a study of eighteen cases. Hum. Pathol. *13*:36, 1982.

McCarthy, E. F., Matsuno, T., and Dorfman, H. D.: Malignant fibrous histiocytoma of bone—a study of 35 cases. Hum. Pathol. *10*:57, 1979.

Mickelson, M. R., and Bonfiglio, M.: Eosinophilic granuloma and its variations. Orthop. Clin. North Am. *8*:933, 1977.

Mirra, J. M., Kendrick, R. A., and Kendrick, R. E.: Pseudomalignant osteoblastoma versus arrested osteosarcoma—a case report. Cancer *37*:2005, 1976.

Revell, P. A., and Scholtz, C. L.: Aggressive osteoblastoma. J. Pathol. *127*:195, 1979.

Rodriguez, A. R., Lutcher, C. L., and Coleman, F. W.: Osteosclerotic myeloma. J.A.M.A. *236*:1872, 1976.

Rogers, J. S., II, Spahr, J., Judge, D. M., Varano, L. A., and Eyster, M. E.: IgE myeloma with osteoblastic lesions. Blood *49*:295, 1977.

Rosen, G., Marcove, R. C., Caparros, B., Nirenberg, A., Kosloff, C., and Huvos, A. G.: Primary osteogenic sarcoma—the rationale for preoperative chemotherapy and delayed surgery. Cancer *43*:2163, 1979.

Ruth, C. K., Lefkoe, R. T., and Schwamm, H. A.: Fibrous dysplasia in an elderly patient—a case report. Contemp. Orthop. *5*:61, 1982.

Salvador, A. H., Beabout, J. W., and Dahlin, D. C.: Mesenchymal chondrosarcoma: observations on 30 new cases. Cancer *28*:605, 1971.

Schlumberger, H. G.: Fibrous dysplasia of single bones (monostotic fibrous dysplasia). Milit. Surg. *99*:504, 1946.

Scranton, P. E., Jr., DeCicco, F. A., Totten, R. S., and Yunis, E. J.: Prognostic factors in osteosarcoma—a review of 20 years experience at the University of Pittsburgh Health Center Hospitals. Cancer 36:2179, 1975.

Simon, M. A.: Biopsy of musculoskeletal tumors. J. Bone Joint Surg. 64A:1253, 1982.

Spanier, S. S., Enneking, W. F., and Enriquez, P.: Primary malignant fibrous histiocytoma of bone. Cancer 36:2084, 1975.

Taylor, W. F., Ivins, J. C., Dahlin, D. C., Edmonson, J. H., and Pritchard, D. J.: Trends and variability in survival from osteosarcoma. Mayo Clin. Proc. 53:695, 1978.

Unni, K. K., and Dahlin, D. C.: Premalignant tumors and conditions of bone. Am. J. Surg. Pathol. 3:47, 1979.

Unni, K. K., Dahlin, D. C., Beabout, J. W., and Ivins, J. C.: Adamantinomas of long bones. Cancer 34:1796, 1974.

Unni, K. K., Dahlin, D. C., and Beabout, J. W.: Periosteal osteogenic sarcoma. Cancer 37:2476, 1976.

Unni, K. K., Dahlin, D. C., Beabout, J. W., and Ivins, J. C.: Parosteal osteogenic sarcoma. Cancer 37:2644 1976.

Unni, K. K., Dahlin, D. C., McLeod, R. A., and Pritchard, D. J.: Intraosseous well-differentiated osteosarcoma. Cancer 40:1337, 1977.

Weiss, S. W., and Dorfman, H. D.: Adamantinoma of long bone. Hum. Pathol. 8:141, 1977.

Wirman, J. A., Crissman, J. D., and Aron, B. F.: Metastatic chondroblastoma—report of an unusual case treated with radiotherapy. Cancer 44:87, 1979.

GENERAL REFERENCES

Aegerter, E., and Kirkpatrick, J. A., Jr.: Orthopedic Diseases. 4th ed. Philadelphia, W. B. Saunders Company, 1975.

Dahlin, D. C.: Bone Tumors, General Aspects and Data on 6,221 Cases. 3rd ed. Springfield, Ill., Charles C Thomas, 1978.

Greenfield, G. B.: Radiology of Bone Diseases. 3rd ed. Philadelphia, J. B. Lippincott Co., 1975.

Huvos, A. G.: Bone Tumors: Diagnosis, Treatment, Prognosis. Philadelphia, W. B. Saunders Company, 1979.

Jaffe, H. L.: Tumors and Tumorous Conditions of the Bones and Joints. Philadelphia, Lea & Febiger, 1958.

Jaffe, H. L.: Metabolic, Degenerative and Inflammatory Diseases of Bones and Joints. Philadelphia, Lea and Febiger, 1972.

Lichtenstein, L.: Bone Tumors. 4th ed. St. Louis, C. V. Mosby Co., 1972.

Lodwick, G. S.: The bones and joints. In Hodes, P. J. (Ed.): Atlas of Tumor Radiology. Chicago, Year Book Medical Publishers, Inc., 1971.

Madewell, J. E., Ragsdale, B. D., and Sweet, D. E.: Radiologic and pathologic analysis of solitary bone lesions. Part I: Internal margins. Radiol. Clin. North Am. 19:715, 1981.

Mirra, J.: Bone Tumors, Diagnosis and Treatment. Philadelphia, J. B. Lippincott Co., 1980.

Ragsdale, B. C., Madewell, J. E., and Sweet, D. E.: Radiologic and pathologic analysis of solitary bone lesions. Part II: Periosteal reactions. Radiol. Clin. North Am. 19:749, 1981.

Sehajowicz, F.: Tumors and Tumorlike Lesions of Bones and Joints. New York, Springer-Verlag, 1981.

Spjut, H. J., Dorfman, H. D., Fechner, R. E., and Ackerman, L. V.: Tumors of bone and cartilage. In Atlas of Tumors Pathology, second series, fasc. 5. Washington, D. C., Armed Forces Institute of Pathology, 1971.

Spjut, H. J., Fechner, R. E., and Ackerman, L. V.: Tumors of bone and cartilage (supplement). In Atlas of Tumor Pathology, second series, fasc. 5. Washington, D. C., Armed Forces Institute of Pathology, 1981.

Sweet, D. E., Madewell, J. E., and Ragsdale, B. D.: Radiologic and pathologic analysis of solitary bone lesions. Part III: Matrix patterns. Radiol. Clin. North Am. 19:785, 1981.

Unni, K. K.: Classification of bone tumours. Can. J. Surg. 20:504, 1977.

10

SYNOVIAL AND SELECTED SOFT-TISSUE LESIONS

The synovium is the cellular mesothelial layer that lines joint spaces, bursae, and tendon sheaths. Loose, fibrous connective tissue surrounds the synovial membrane and contains small blood vessels and lymphatics, some fat cells, fibroblasts, and tissue macrophages. More compact fibrous connective tissue is found near articular ligaments and tendons. Adipose tissue may predominate, depending on the anatomic location of the synovium. The inner lining consists of several layers of synovial cells without

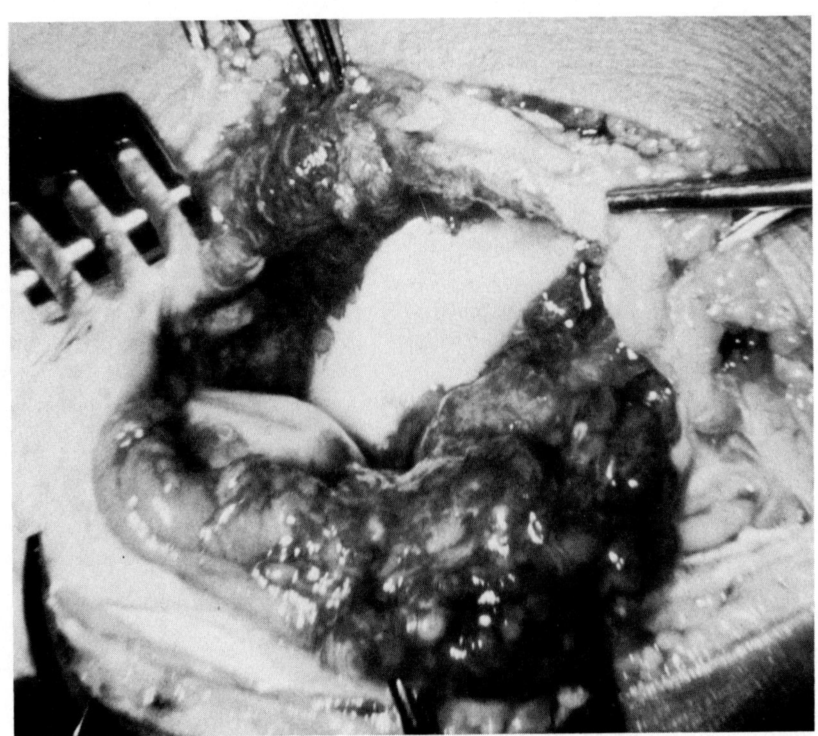

Figure 10–1. Pigmented villonodular synovitis. Surgical exposure of knee joint in 20-year-old male showing extensive involvement of the synovium. The articular cartilage is normal. The entire synovial lining is shaggy, showing numerous hypertrophic villi, and it is heavily pigmented with hemosiderin.

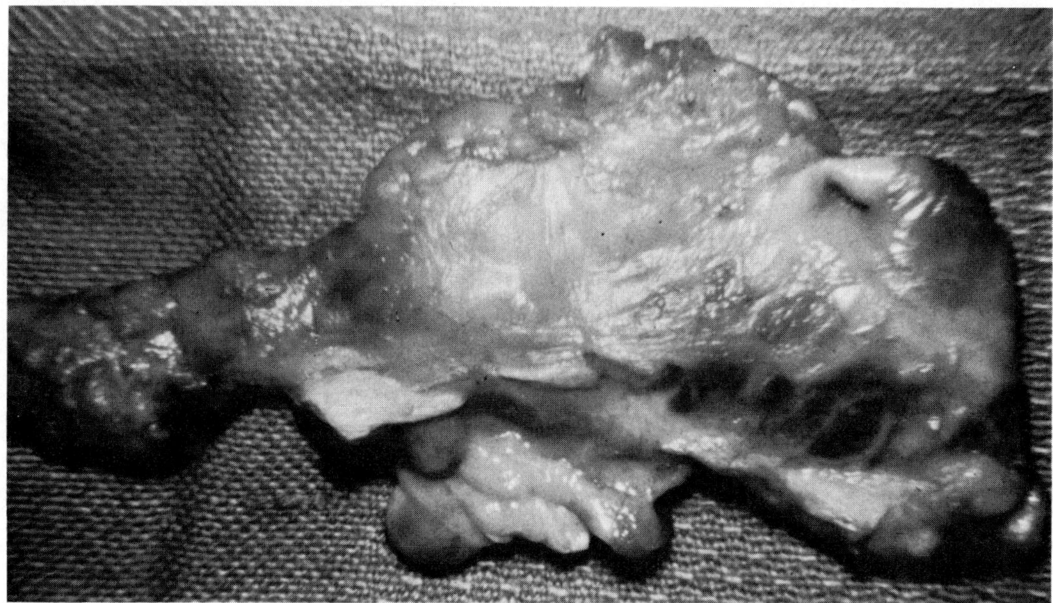

Figure 10–2. Pigmented villonodular synovitis. Gross specimen of a Baker's cyst taken from the knee illustrated in Figure 10–1. The cyst had been present for 4 years.

identifiable basement membrane. Type A cells, responsible for phagocytosis, are most numerous and resemble macrophages; type B cells are less numerous and may be intermediate cells or responsible for hyaluronic acid secretion.

Synovium heals after injury in the same manner that other soft tissue of mesenchymal origin does. There is capillary budding, fibroblastic proliferation, and cellular infiltration, and, depending on the etiologic agent, there may be acute, chronic, or

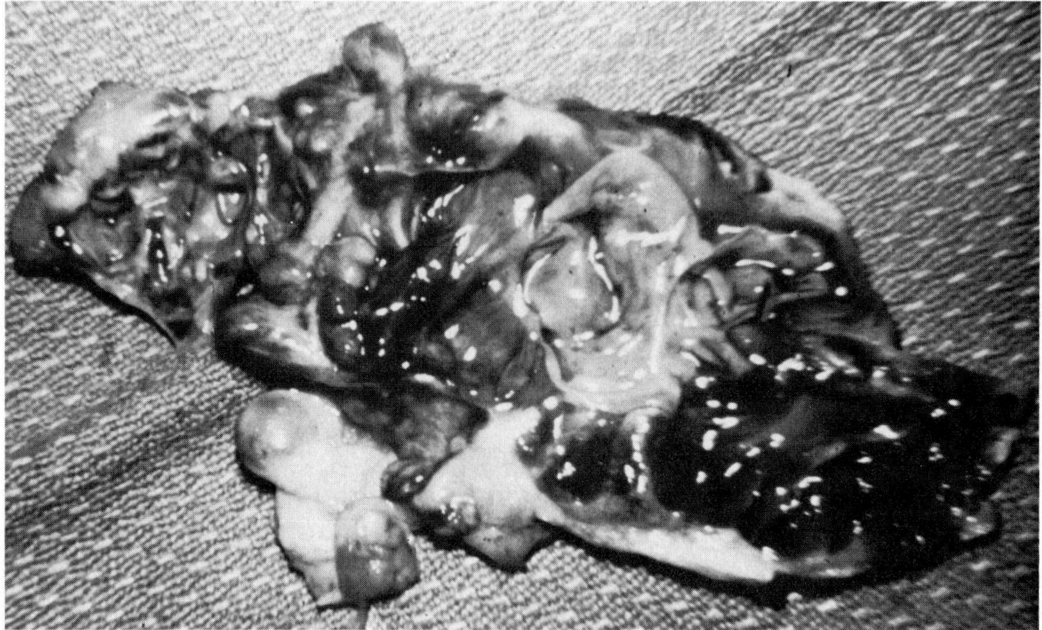

Figure 10–3. Pigmented villonodular synovitis. The entire synovial lining of the Baker's cyst is involved in the same villonodular synovitis process as the knee joint itself.

granulomatous inflammatory response. Synovial hypertrophy may result from trauma of any type, including relatively minor trauma. Tendons are often compressed in tendon sheaths with compact fibrous tissue about the mesothelial lining, which produces clinical entities such as "trigger finger" or de Quervain's disease. Hypertrophic villi develop as a response to stress (e.g., the mechanical changes of osteoarthritis). Such hypertrophied villi are also seen in infectious arthritis and collagen disease. Median nerve compression as a result of such hypertrophy of villous structure results in carpal tunnel syndrome.

PIGMENTED VILLONODULAR SYNOVITIS

Pigmented villonodular synovitis is thought to be a vascular anomaly that involves the entire synovial surface of one of the large joints. It is an extremely rare disease, usually involving the knee joint, but may be seen in any synovial lining and even in bursal linings. The term "pigmented" refers to the *grossly* apparent hemosiderin deposits in the joint lining; the term "villonodular" refers to the shaggy hypertrophied villous structure of the entire synovium of the joint.

Pigmented villonodular synovitis may show extreme variability in the mesenchymal proliferation of the synovium. Mistaken diagnosis of malignancy can be made. The lesion erodes the adjacent bone surfaces.

The histologic features consist of synovial villi that are composed of loose connective tissue and that contain numerous thin-walled blood vessels. Numerous hemosiderin-laden macrophages are present. Occasional multinucleated cells are also seen.

The differential diagnosis between pigmented villonodular synovitis and a giant cell tumor of tendon sheath (nodular synovitis) is based on the location, extent, and angiomatous component of the lesion rather than on histologic appearance.

Text continued on page 594

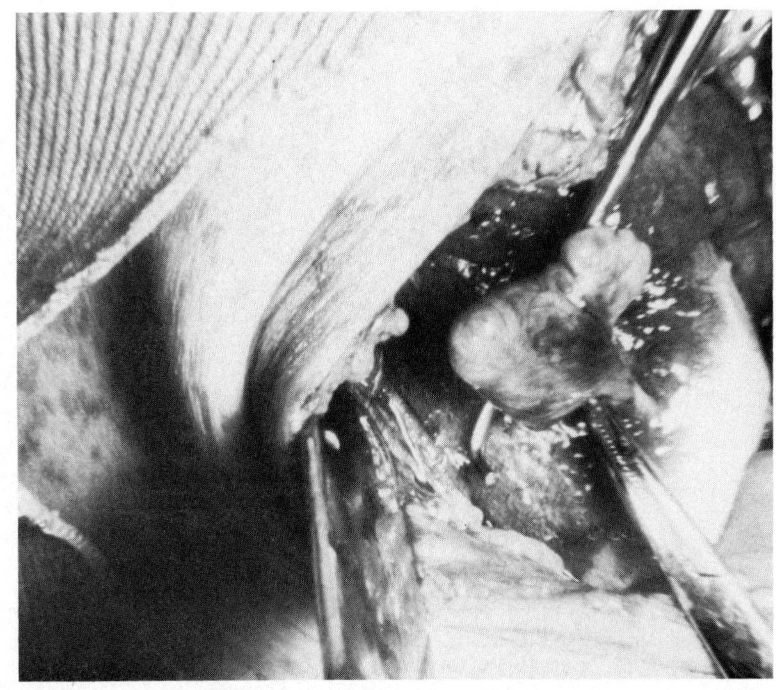

Figure 10–4. Nodular synovitis (giant cell tumor of tendon sheath) (compare with Fig. 10–1). A patient with a circumscribed nodule in the synovium of the knee. Although there are microscopic hemosiderin deposits in the synovium, the grossly visible pigmentation and hypertrophy of the lining that one would see in pigmented villonodular synovitis are not present. Nodular synovitis is a sharply localized tumor; pigmented villonodular synovitis is a diffuse lesion involving the synovial surface of the entire joint.

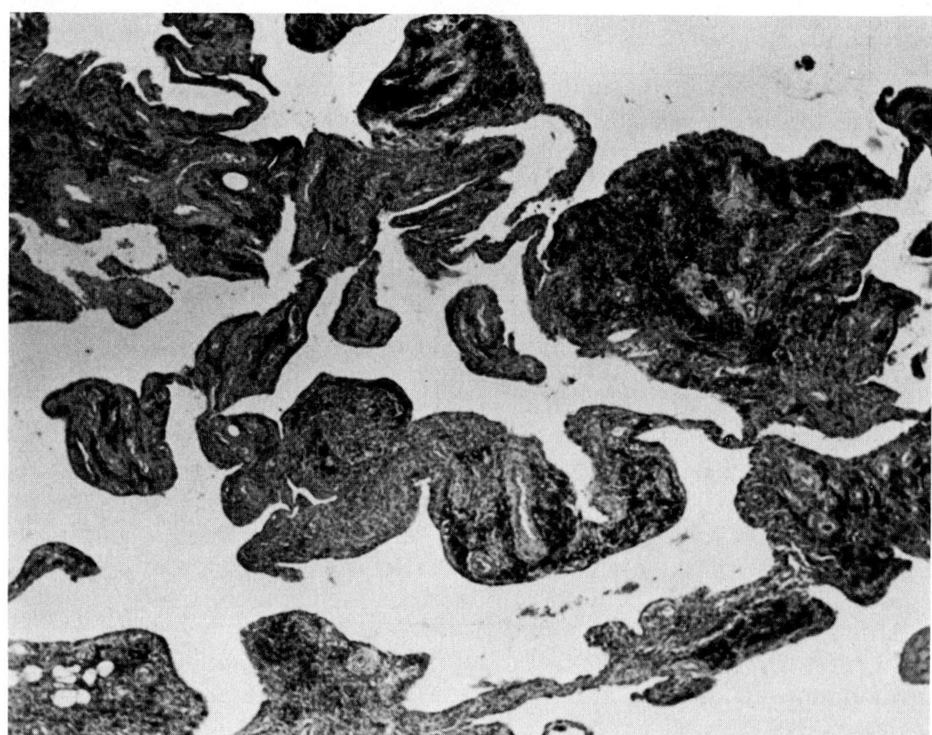

Figure 10–5. Histologic appearance of pigmented villonodular synovitis. The villous surface demonstrates extensive hypertrophy and numerous projections, some relatively nodular. All these projections have extensive hemosiderin deposits that are responsible for the readily identifiable pigmentation in the gross specimen.

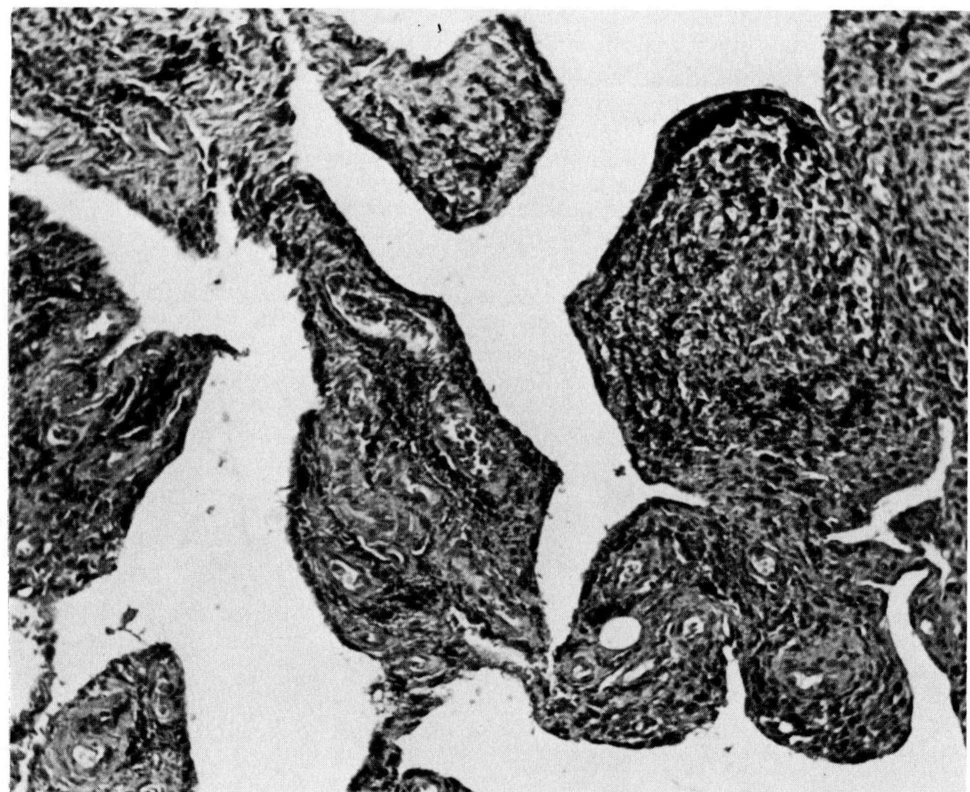

Figure 10–6. Pigmented villonodular synovitis. Higher-power view of a field similar to that illustrated in Figure 10–5. Note the nodular characteristics of the villi, many of which coalesce at their tips, leaving enclosed synovial spaces. There are numerous giant cells, histiocytes, and hemosiderin deposits throughout the tissue.

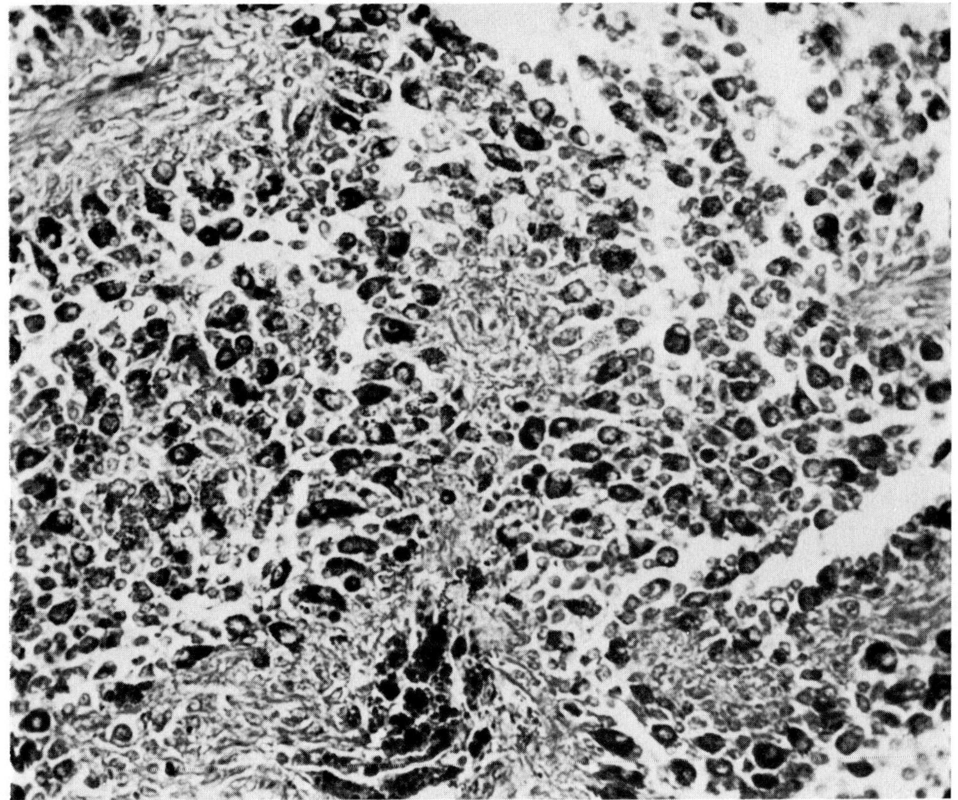

Figure 10–7. Pigmented villonodular synovitis. Higher-power view of a field similar to that shown in Figures 10–5 and 10–6. Note the extensive hemosiderin deposits in the hypertrophic villi. There are scattered giant cells throughout the lesion. Most of the hemosiderin is contained within histiocytes.

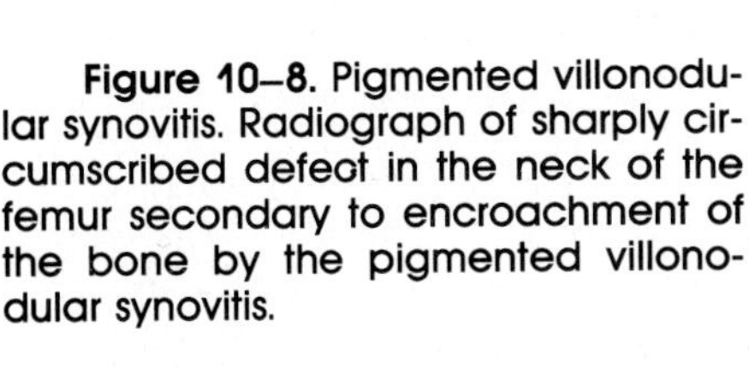

Figure 10–8. Pigmented villonodular synovitis. Radiograph of sharply circumscribed defect in the neck of the femur secondary to encroachment of the bone by the pigmented villonodular synovitis.

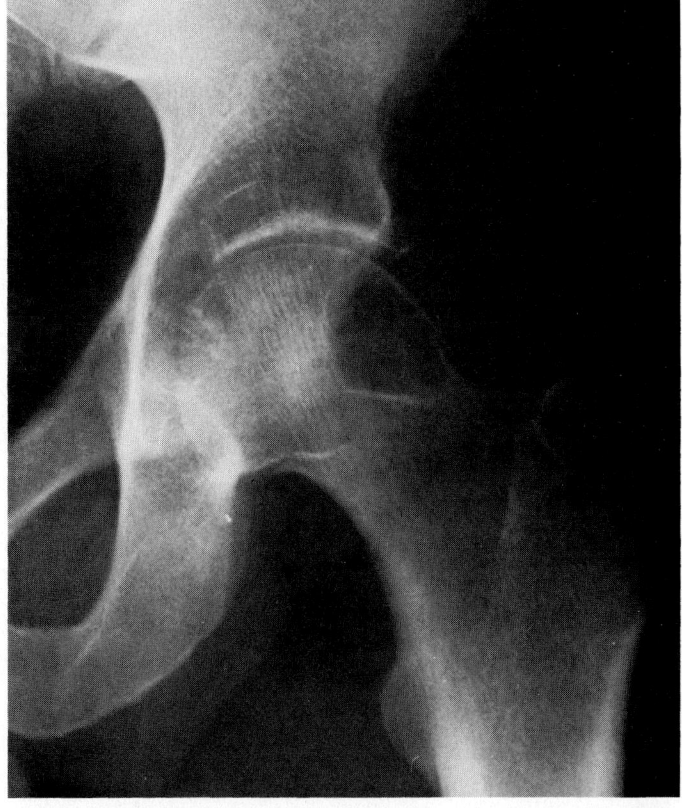

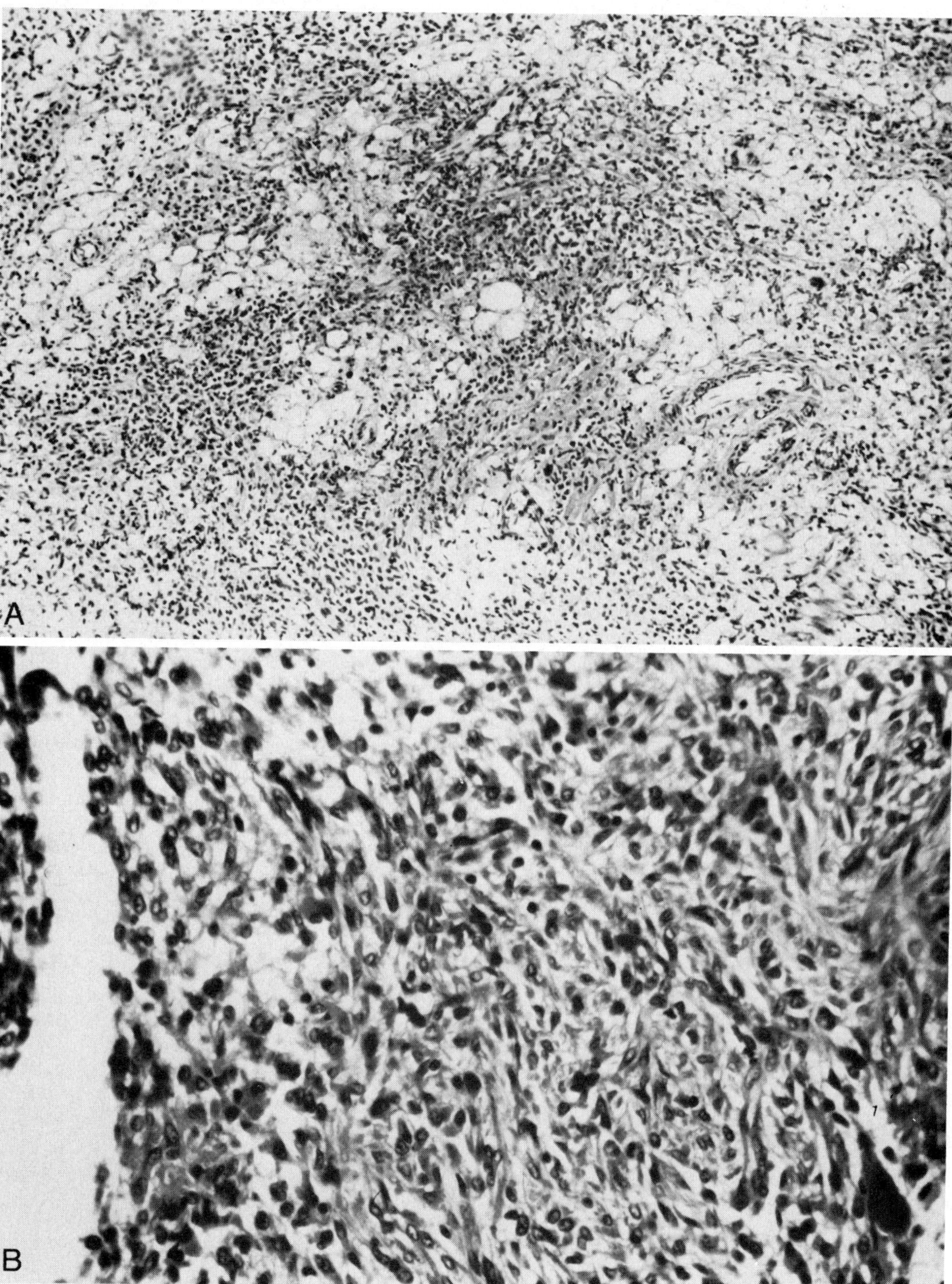

Figure 10–9. Histologic features of the lesion illustrated in Figure 10–8. Note the extensive vascularity (*C* and *D*), with numerous dilated vascular channels evident within the synovium. This vascularity is a regular feature of pigmented villonodular synovitis and is less pronounced in giant cell tumor of tendon sheath. Areas of fibrosis (*B*), hemosiderin deposition (*C*), giant cells (*B* and *C*), and xanthomatous deposits (*A*) are present. These histologic features are common to both pigmented villonodular synovitis and giant cell tumor of tendon sheath.

Illustration continued on opposite page

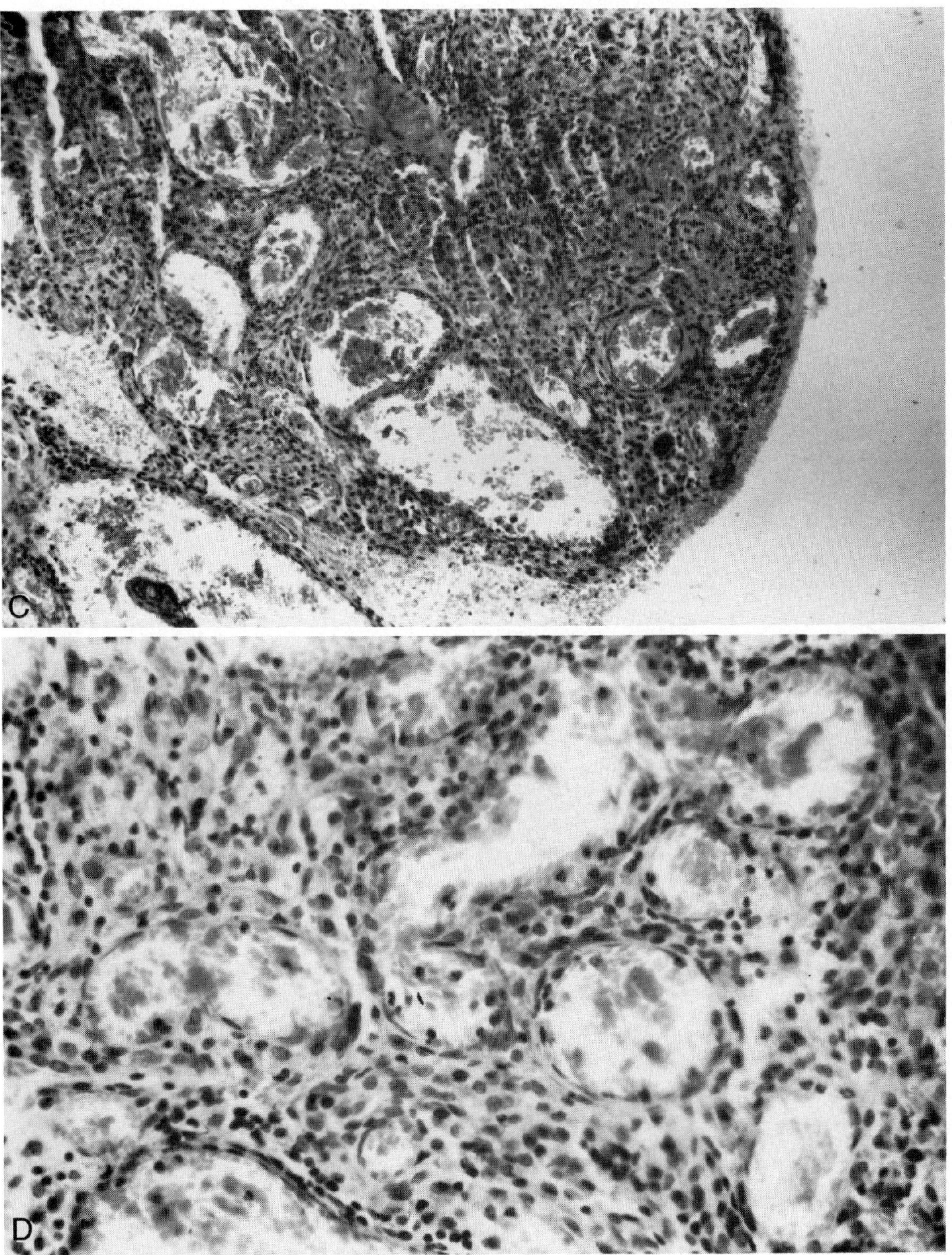

Figure 10–9 *Continued.*

GIANT CELL TUMOR OF TENDON SHEATH (NODULAR SYNOVITIS)

The giant cell tumor of tendon sheath (nodular synovitis) is a sharply localized lesion that is usually found in the synovial or tendinous spaces of the hands and feet, and it is a fairly common lesion in orthopaedic practice. These tumors are sharply localized and nodular, and they do not involve the entire synovial surface of the joint. The cut surface exhibits a characteristic yellow appearance that is due to the numerous xanthoma cells in the lesion. In the presence of focal hemorrhage, localized hemosiderin deposits may be observed, giving the lesion a yellowish-brown appearance.

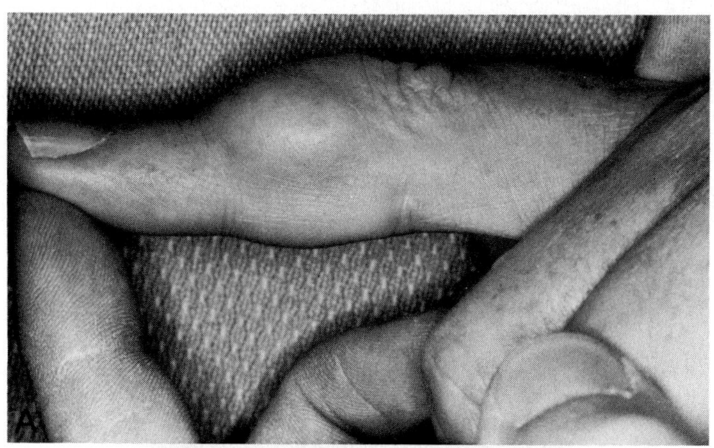

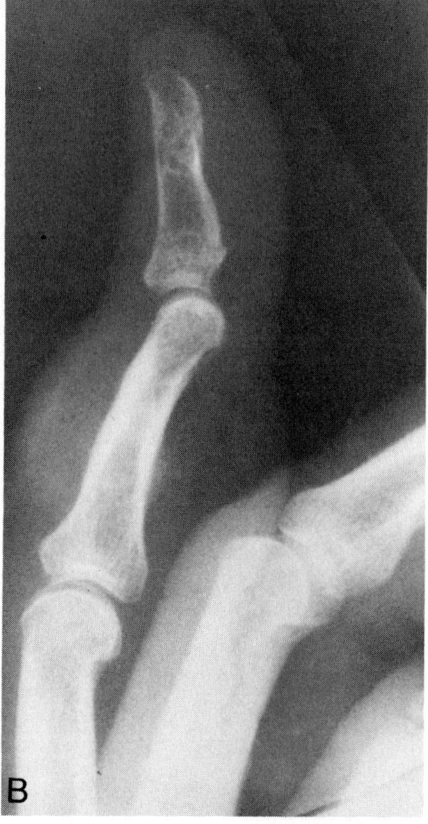

Figure 10–10. Giant cell tumor of tendon sheath. Clinical photograph (*A*) and lateral radiograph (*B*) of the finger showing a moderately extensive giant cell tumor of tendon sheath. The lesion has infiltrated around the side of the finger, and presents on both the dorsal and volar aspects. There is a soft-tissue density on the radiograph but no evidence of calcification. There is no erosion of bone, but there is a suggestion of periosteal elevation on the ventral aspect of the middle phalanx.

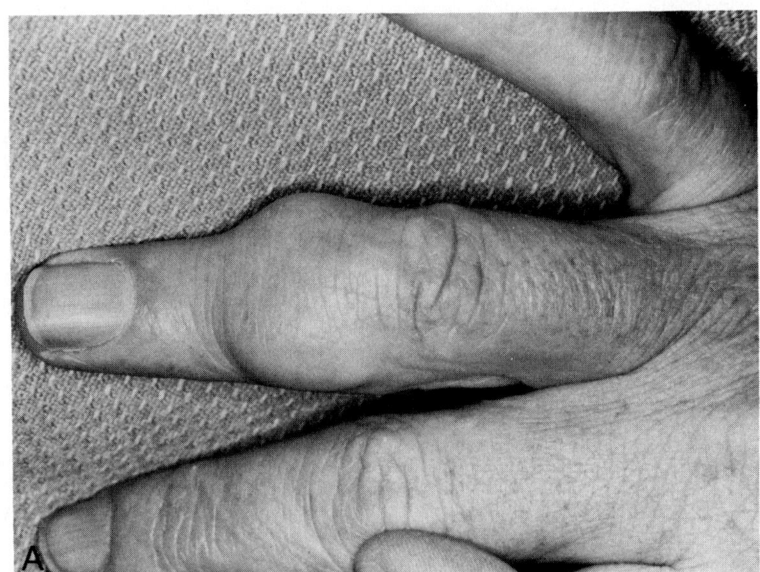

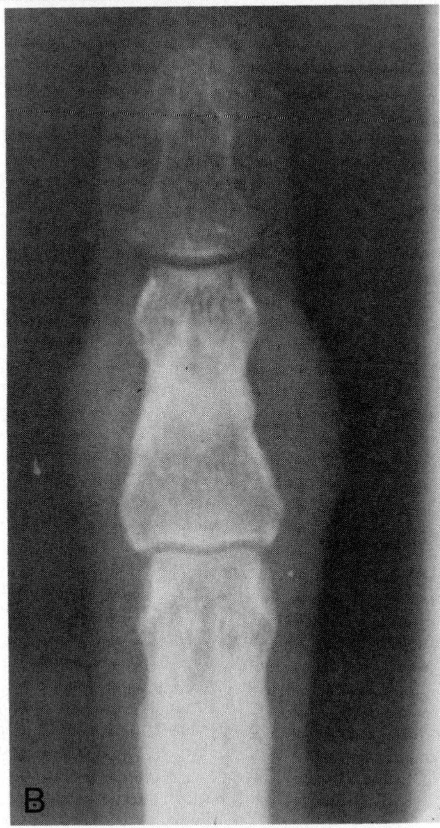

Figure 10–11. Giant cell tumor of tendon sheath. Posterior view (*A*) and radiograph (*B*) of the lesion shown in Figure 10–10. Most of the lesion has soft-tissue density, with a more radiolucent fat-density strip adjacent to the bone.

The histologic features of both pigmented villonodular synovitis and giant cell tumor of tendon sheath are very similar. Xanthoma cells, macrophages, giant cells in variable quantities, and proliferation of synovial lining cells are seen in both lesions. Both lesions are richly vascular. The preponderance of foam cells in the giant cell tumor of tendon sheath tends to offer clues as to the true nature of the lesion. It should be emphasized that pigmented villonodular synovitis is a lesion involving the entire synovial surface of a given joint, whereas giant cell tumor of tendon sheath is a sharply localized lesion, so differential diagnosis of the two should be easy.

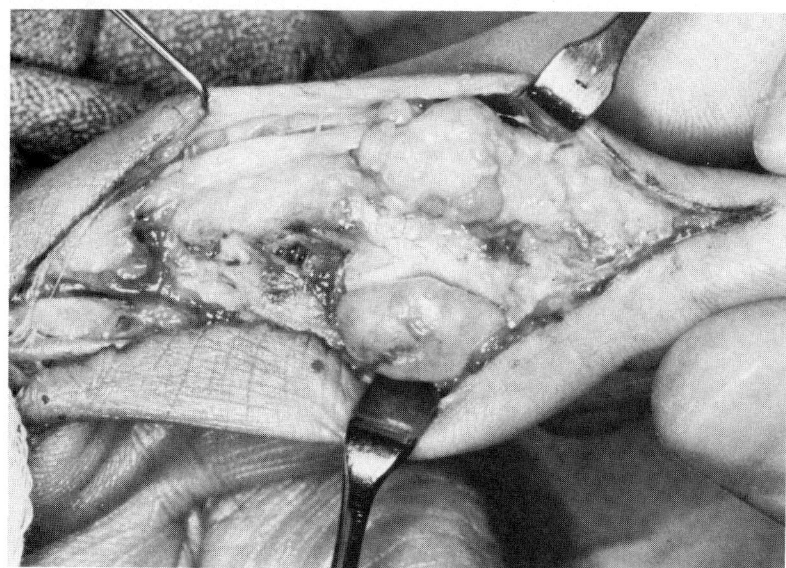

Figure 10–12. Giant cell tumor of tendon sheath. Surgical view of the lesion shown in Figures 10–10 and 10–11 illustrates the characteristic infiltration and dissection between the tendinous, vascular, and nervous structure of the digit. Because giant cell tumors of tendon sheath are slow-growing, painless lesions, the patient may postpone seeking treatment. When the patient finally does seek medical attention, there may be extensive infiltration that makes surgical removal more difficult and recurrences more common.

The giant cell tumor, with its rich vascular bed and proximity to bone, is commonly associated with erosions. It carries its own blood supply into the bone, and is easily "shelled-out," after which there are no remnants. Even with intraosseous involvement, most of the lesion remains on the surface. Multiple bones may be involved.

Text continued on page 606

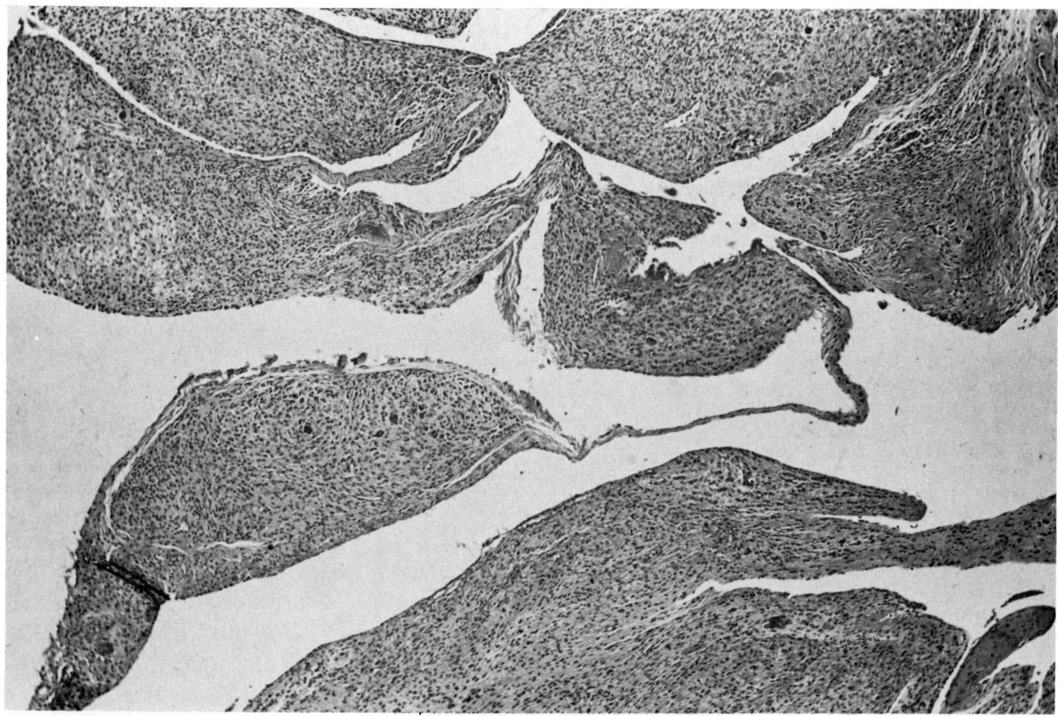

Figure 10–13. Low-power view of histologic specimen of giant cell tumor of tendon sheath. There are numerous villous structures, the majority thickened owing to increased cellularity. There is no significant edema, as one would see in an inflammatory process.

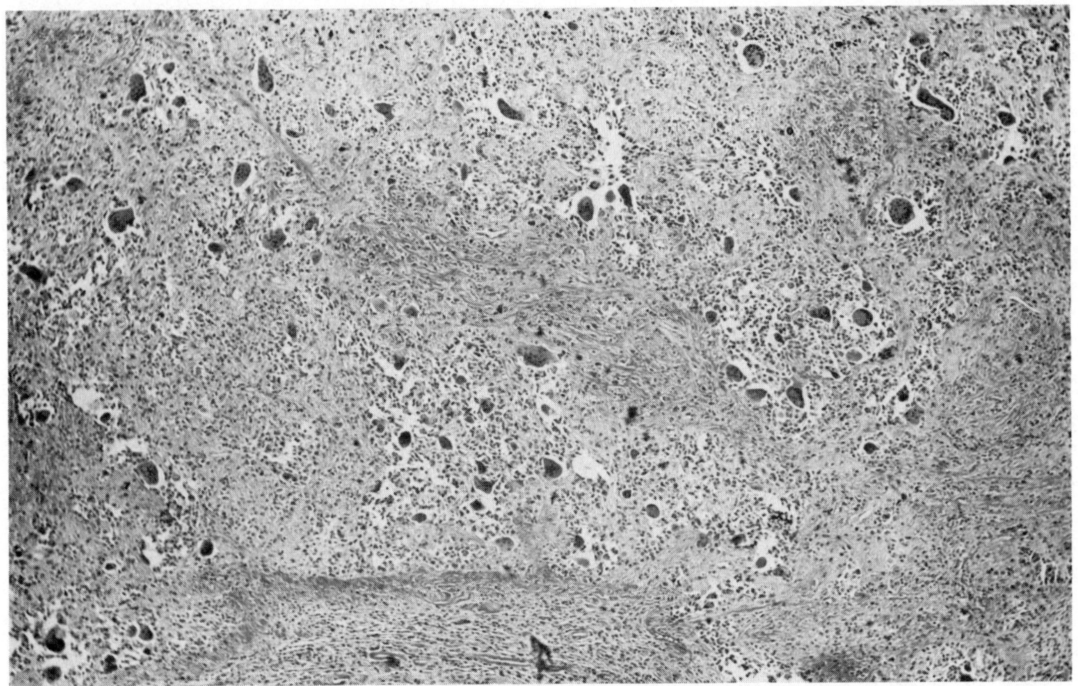

Figure 10–14. Giant cell tumor of tendon sheath. Low-power view of a typical nodule with numerous histiocytes. Giant cells are usually present and give the lesion its name. Fibrosis is always present and usually consists of strands of collagen coursing through the lesion, providing some coherence.

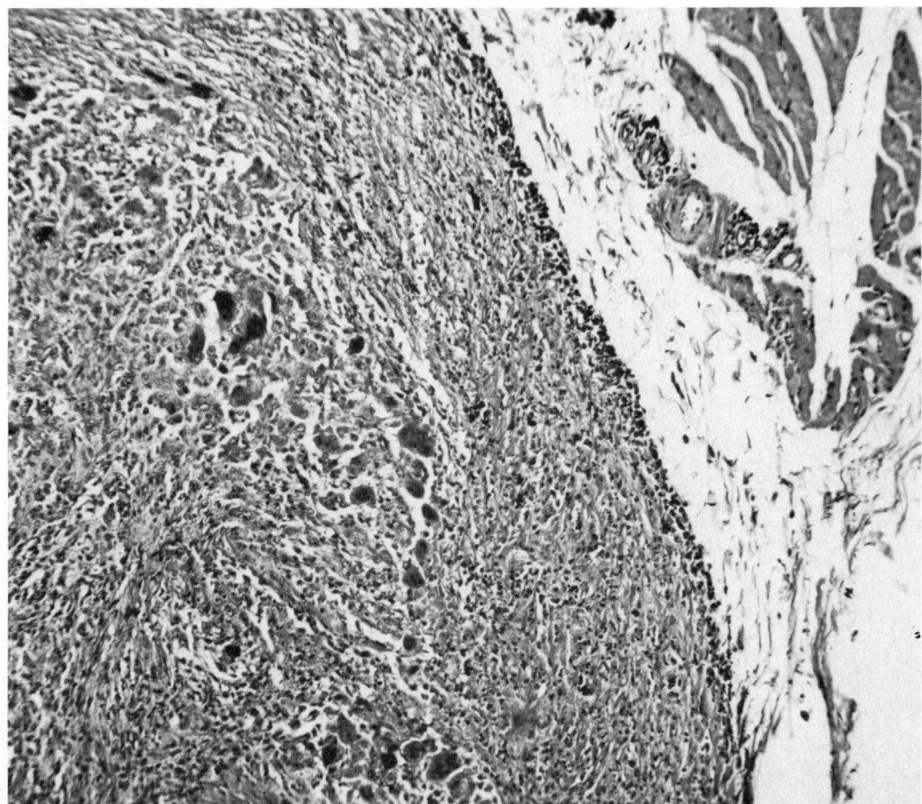

Figure 10–15. Giant cell tumor of tendon sheath. Higher-power view of the edge of a nodule. The numerous histiocytes, along with giant cells, constitute the basic cellular population of the lesion. The nodule grows by centrifugal expansion and not infiltration into the surrounding tissues. It tends to push aside the muscles, tendons, and vessels as it expands. The tumor is always surrounded by a pseudocapsule of compressed fibrous tissue.

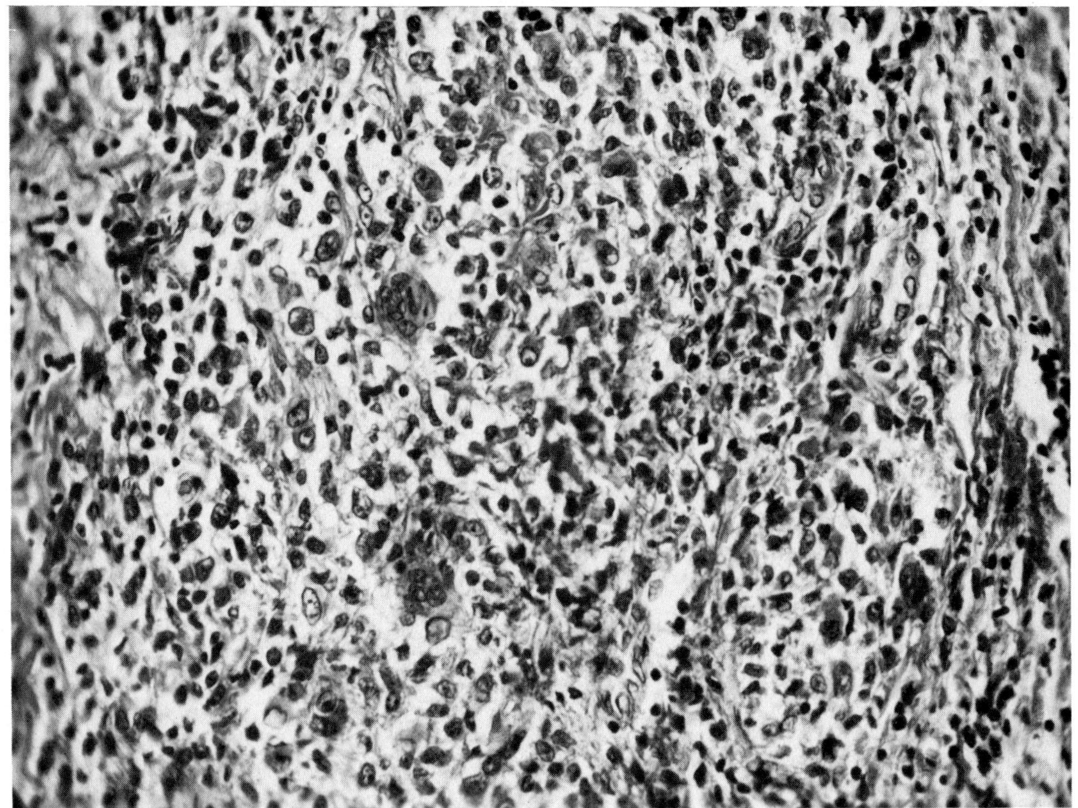

Figure 10–16. Giant cell tumor of tendon sheath. Higher-power view of a nodule with typical giant cells and stromal cells, mainly histiocytes, with a scattering of fibroblasts. Inflammation is not a prominent feature.

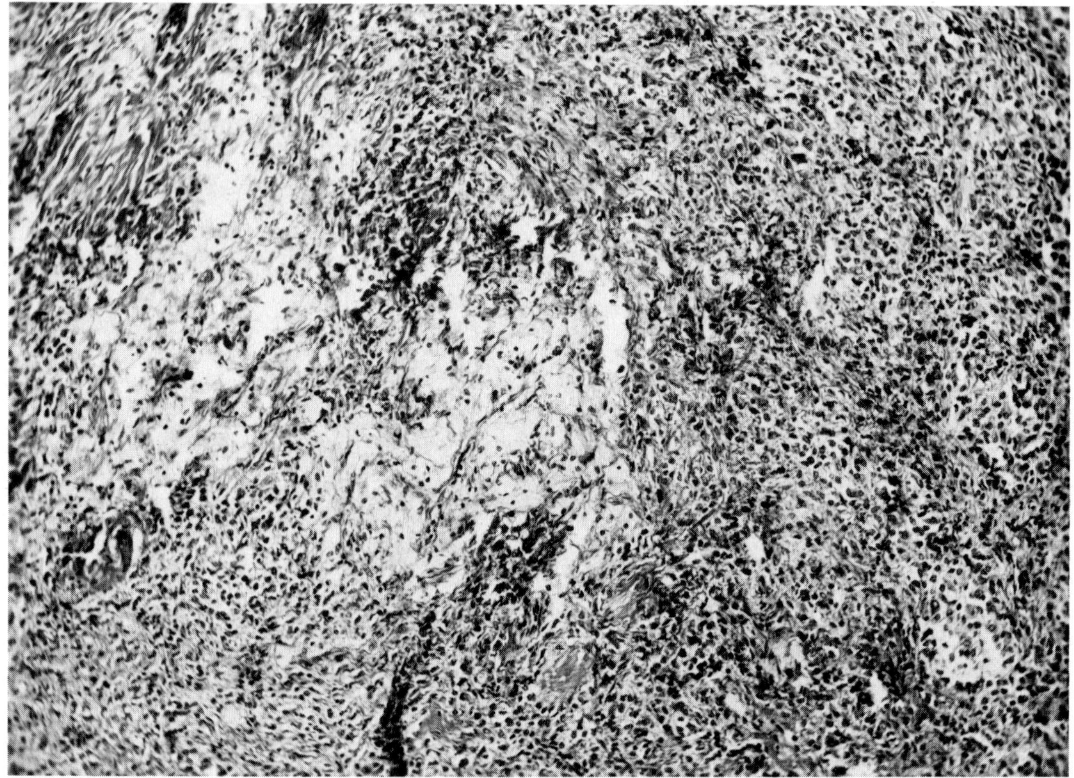

Figure 10–17. Giant cell tumor of tendon sheath with a field of xanthoma cells. Such cells are present in almost all lesions and are responsible for the yellow color seen on gross examination.

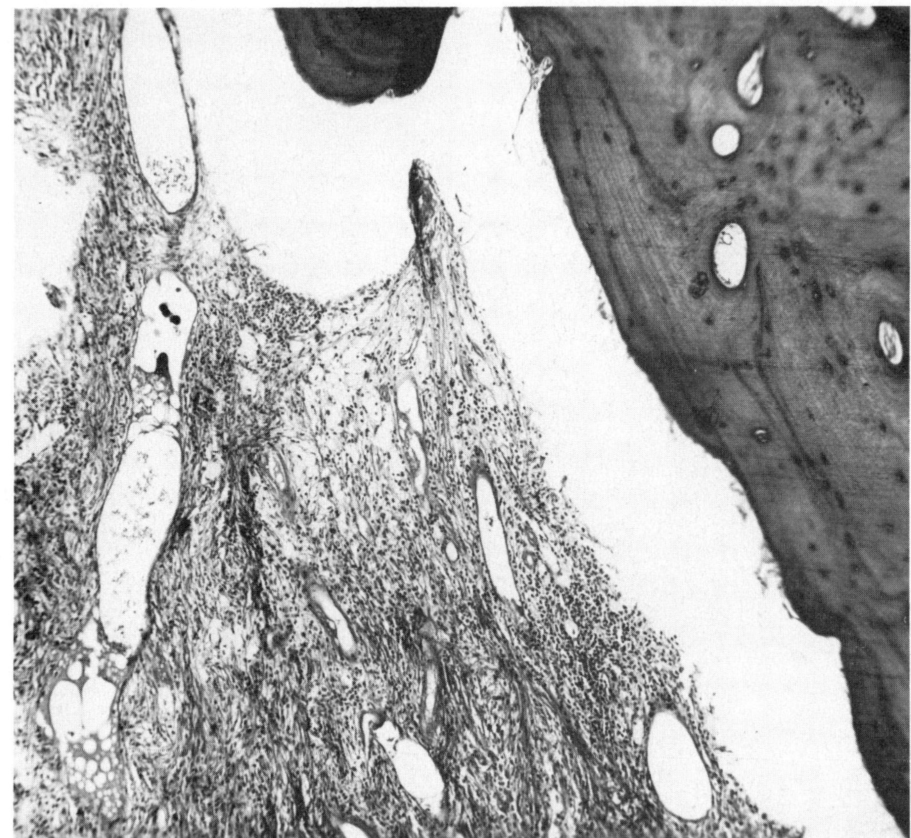

Figure 10–18. Low-power view of a giant cell tumor of tendon sheath invading bone. Even at this magnification one can recognize the areas of xanthoma cells. Numerous dilated vessels dispersed throughout the lesion are common.

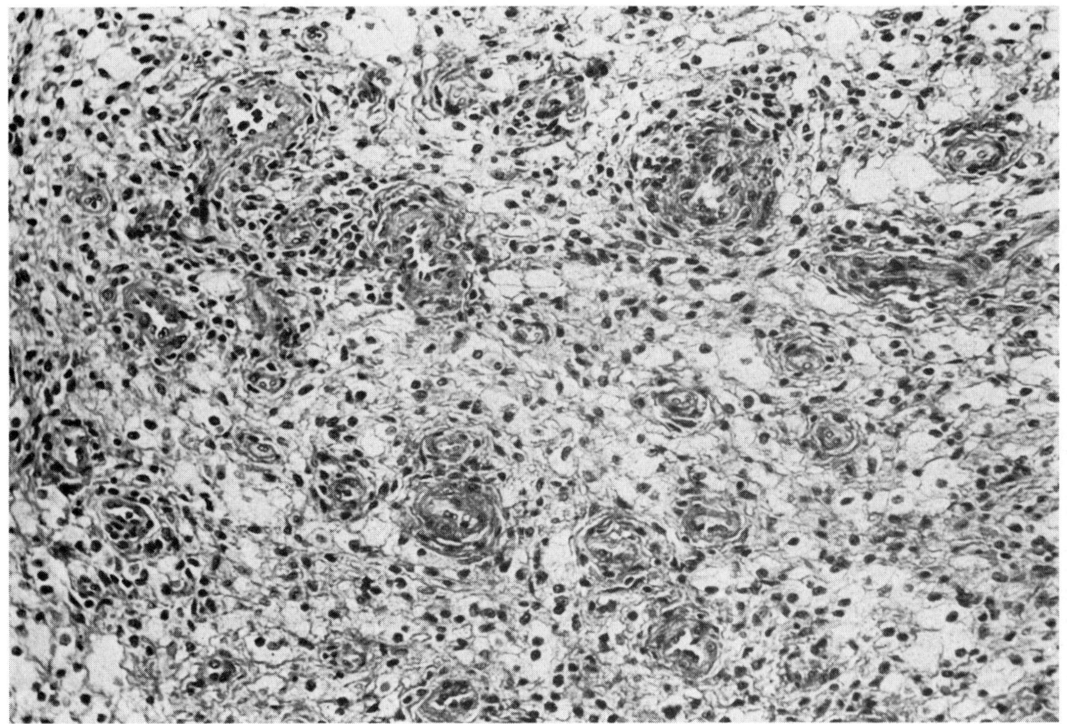

Figure 10–19. Giant cell tumor of tendon sheath. Higher-power view of a nodule containing large numbers of xanthoma cells and numerous vessels. When directly involving the bone surface, the active hyperemia will result in bone resorption.

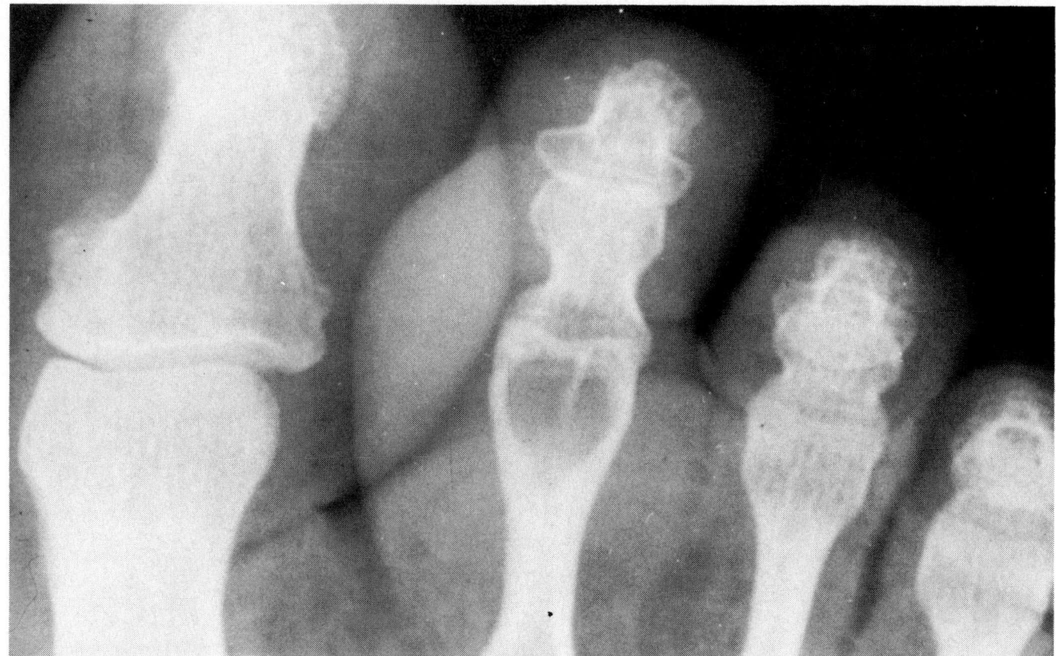

Figure 10–20. Anteroposterior radiograph of the foot with a giant cell tumor of tendon sheath invading the proximal phalanx of the second toe. There is a large soft-tissue mass without mineralization, and there is erosion of the distal end of the proximal phalanx.

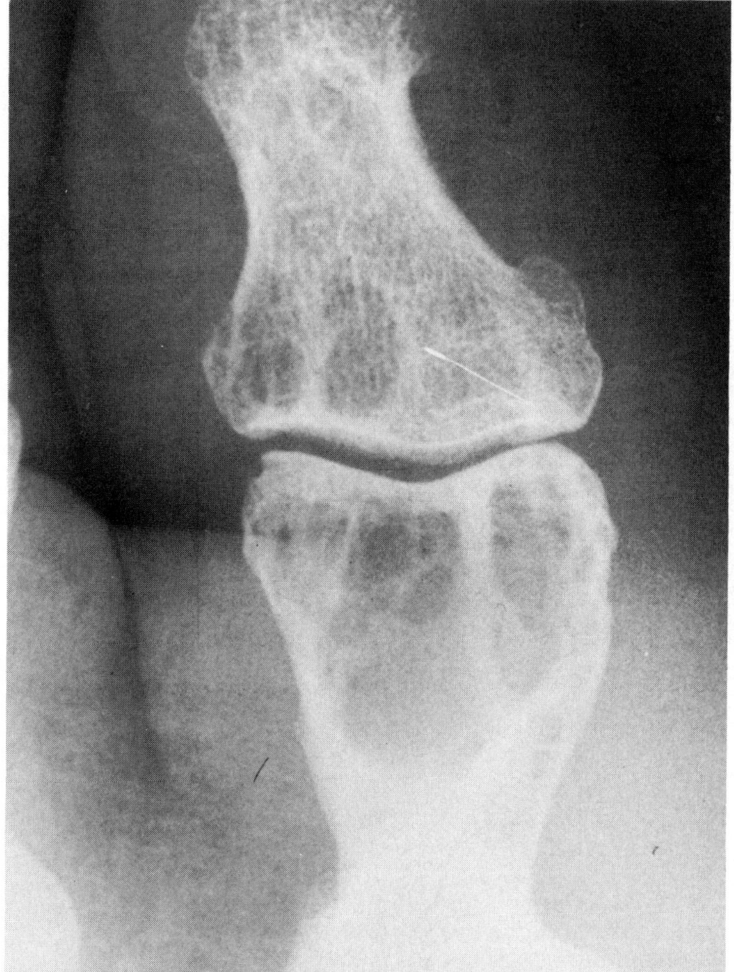

Figure 10–21. Radiograph of the great toe containing a giant cell tumor of tendon sheath. There is osseous invasion on both sides of the joint, with large lytic defects present in the contiguous bones.

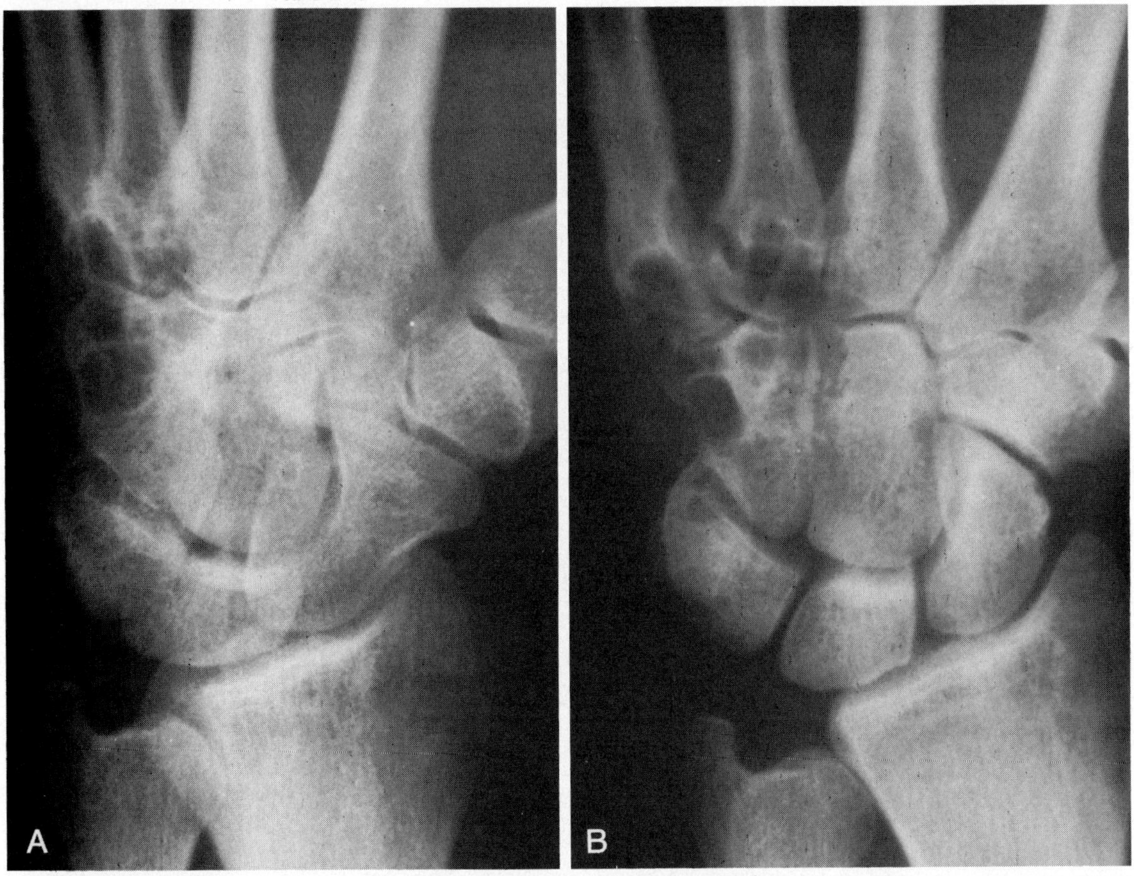

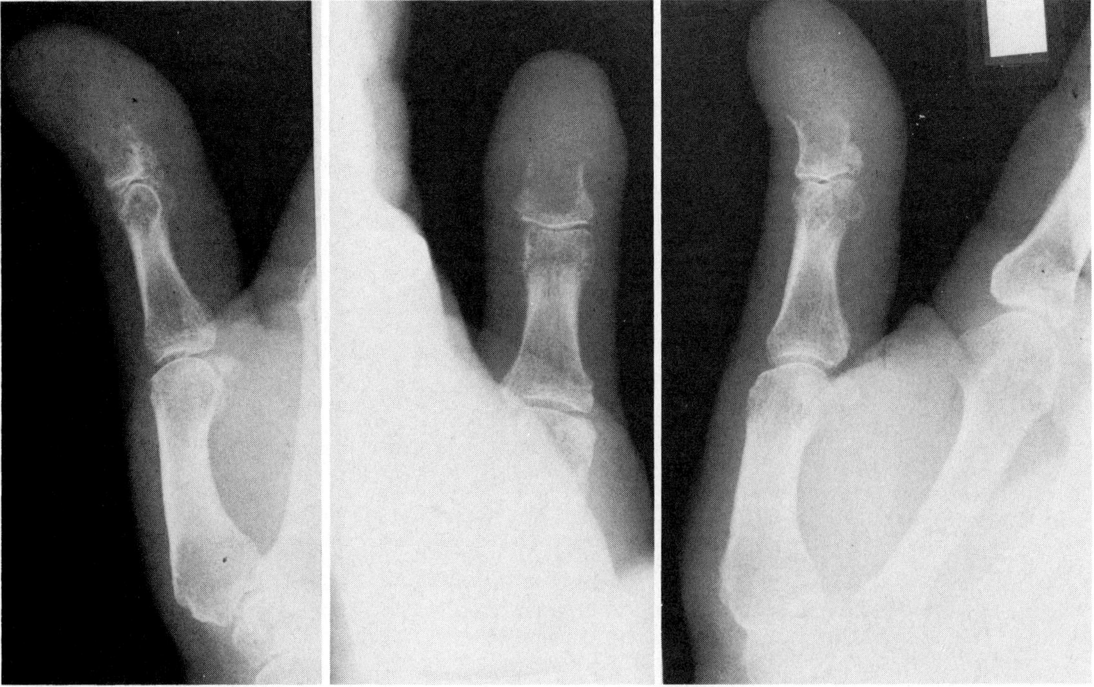

Figure 10–22. Giant cell tumor of tendon sheath. Radiographs of the wrist of a patient with giant cell tumor of tendon sheath on the ulnar aspect of the hand. It invades the bases of the fourth and fifth metacarpals as well as the hamate, and possibly the triquetrum. Such invasion of several bones around a joint should make one suspect nodular synovitis; tuberculosis, or angiomatous lesions.

Figure 10–23. Radiographs of the thumb of a patient with a giant cell tumor of tendon sheath destroying the terminal phalanx.

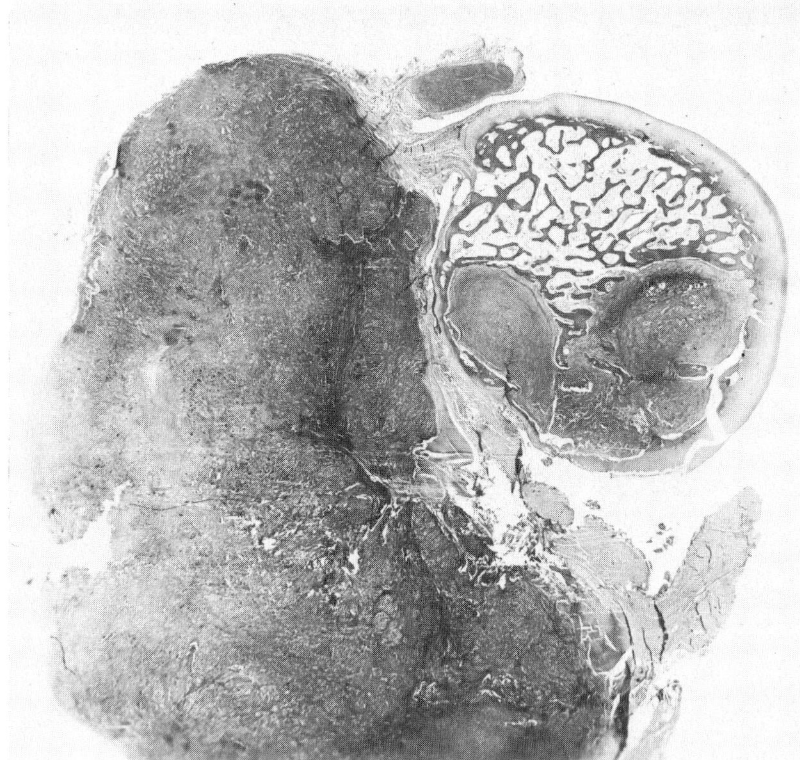

Figure 10–24. Macrosection of a large giant cell tumor of tendon sheath with osseous invasion. The bulk of the lesion is outside the bone, but there has been direct extension into the bone with destruction. Reactive bone formation with sclerosis around the lesion indicates a slow-growing process.

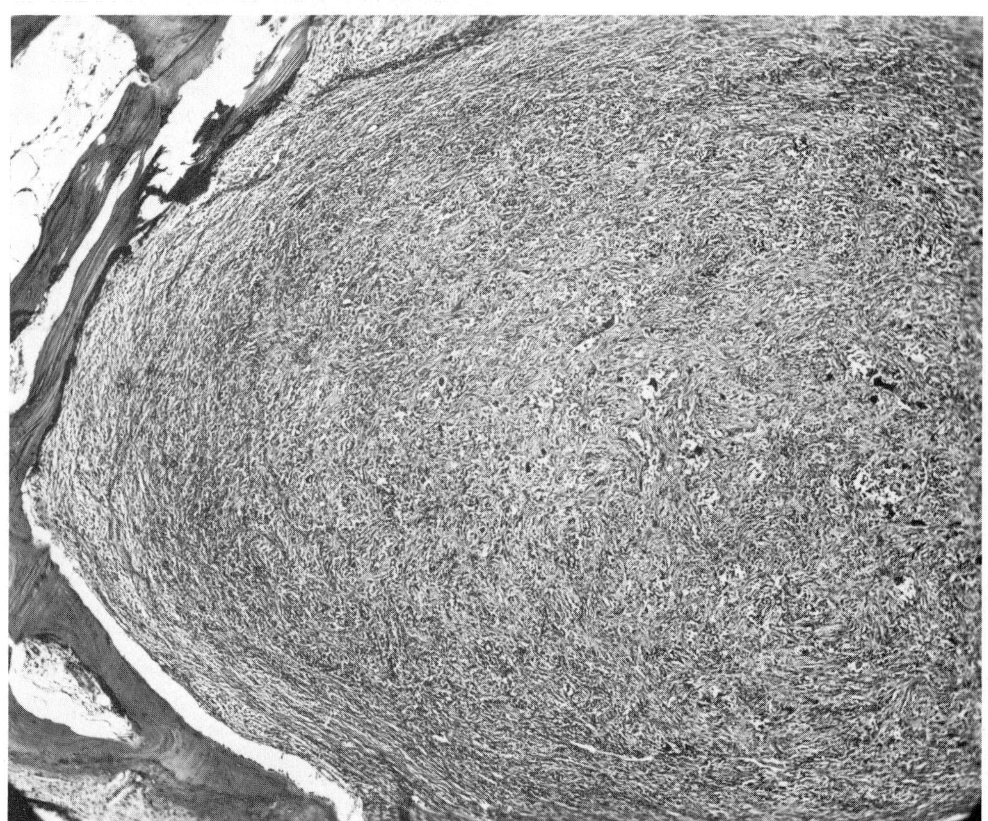

Figure 10–25. Giant cell tumor of tendon sheath. Histologic appearance of a nodule in the bone. Note that the invasion is by expansion and not infiltration between the trabeculae. Usually, the vascularity of the lesion causes osteoclastic removal of bone, but it does not infiltrate widely through the marrow spaces. The lesion carries its blood supply into the bone and is not nourished by the medullary blood supply. This facilitates complete removal by curettage.

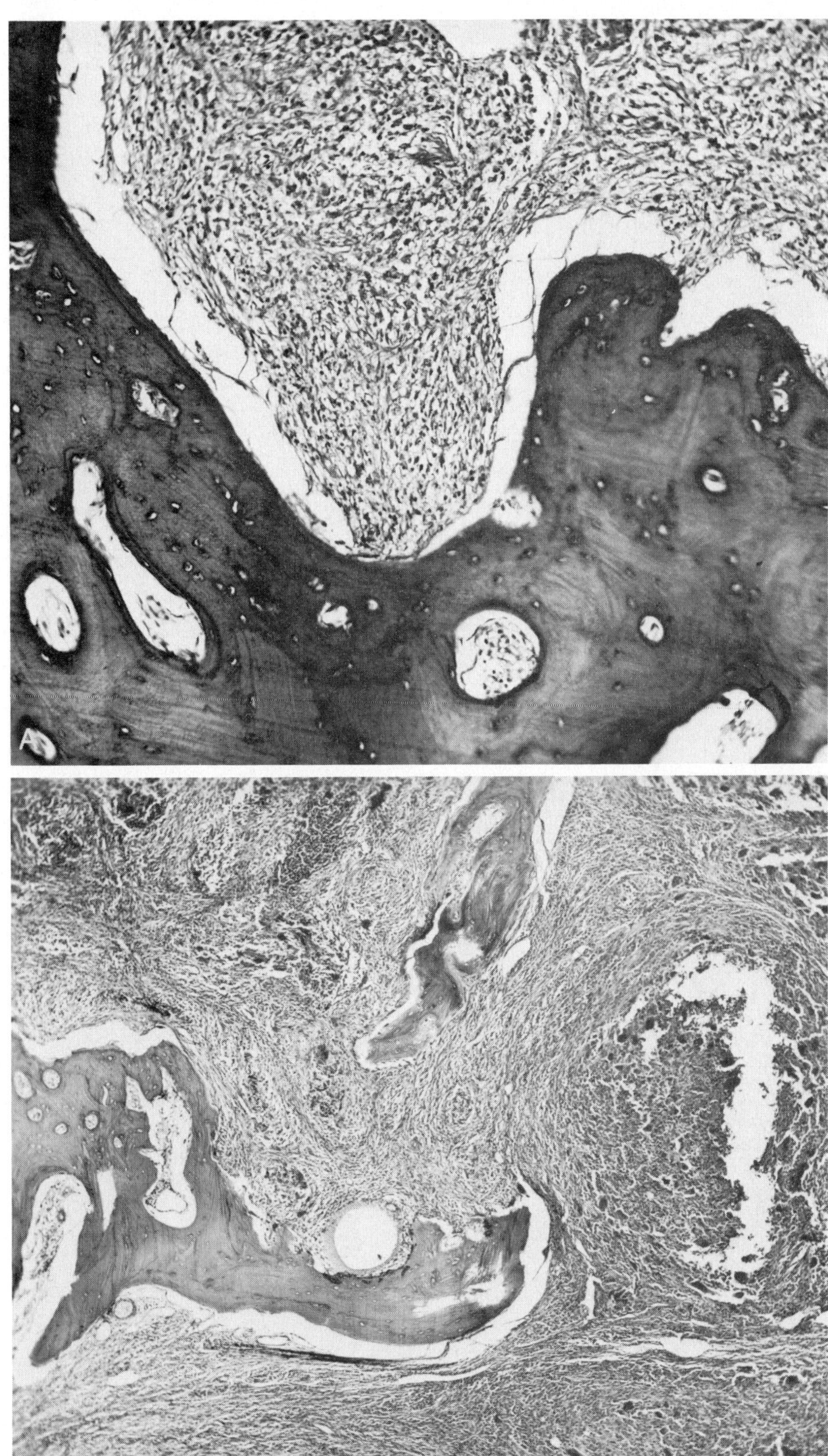

Figure 10–26. Giant cell tumor of tendon sheath. Histologic views of lesions in the bone demonstrating removal of cortical bone (*A*) and extension into the medullary spaces. In *B*, fragments of remaining cortical bone are surrounded by the nodules of the lesion. Such fragments are left in the interlocular spaces of the tumor and do not represent invasion between the pre-existing cancellous trabeculae.

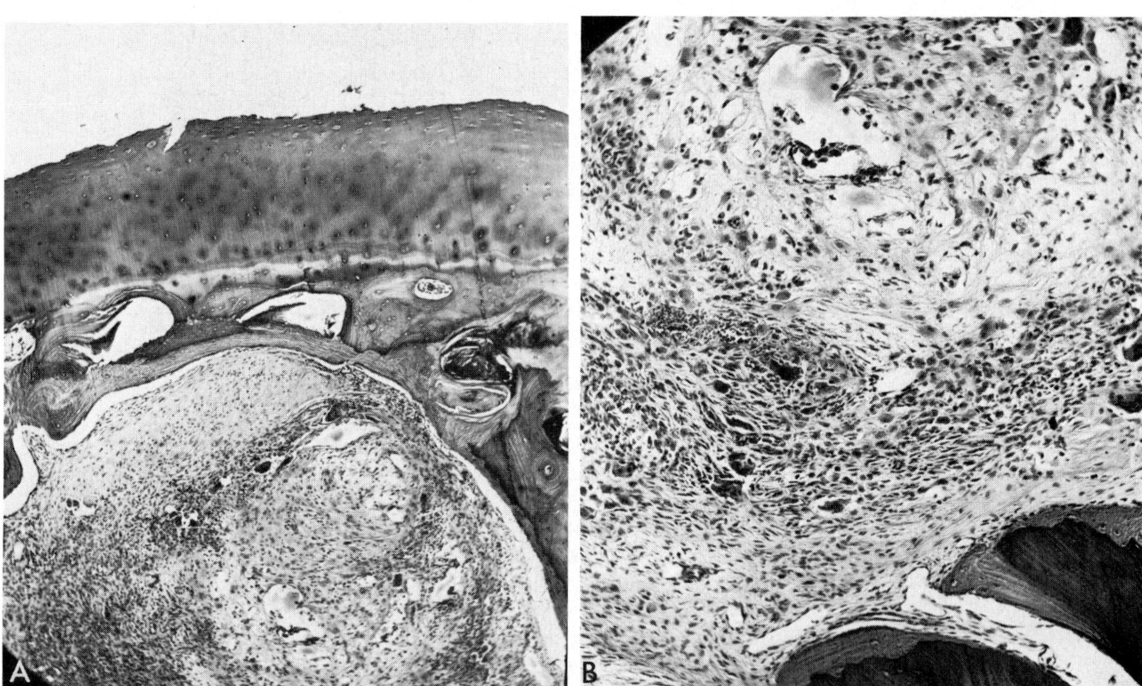

Figure 10–27. Giant cell tumor of tendon sheath. Histologic views of a lesion in bone demonstrating expansion into the subchondral spaces. This lesion has a small focus of cartilage metaplasia.

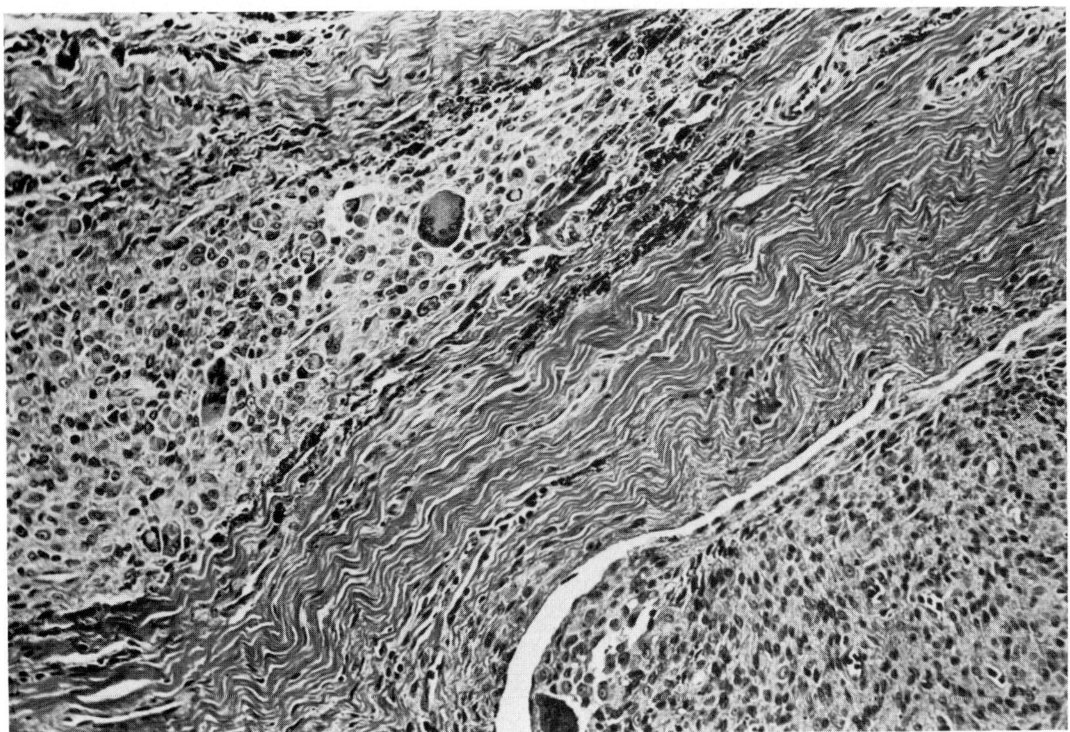

Figure 10–28. Giant cell tumor of tendon sheath. Hemosiderin deposits in giant cell tumors of tendon sheath are common because the lesions often occur in the digits, which are frequently exposed to trauma. Bleeding into the tissue imparts the brownish coloration to the gross appearance of the lesion.

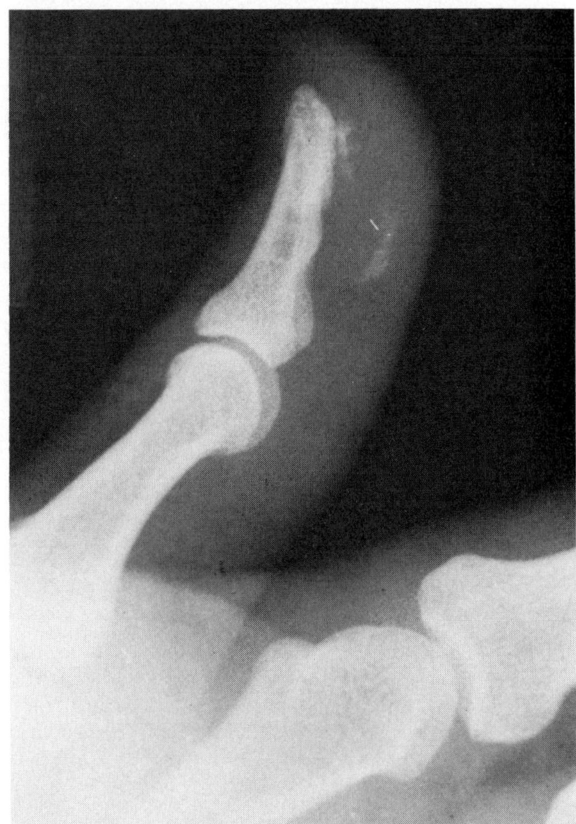

Figure 10–29. Calcification in a giant cell tumor of tendon sheath. The calcification is probably a result of trauma, although it may be a product of cartilage metaplasia.

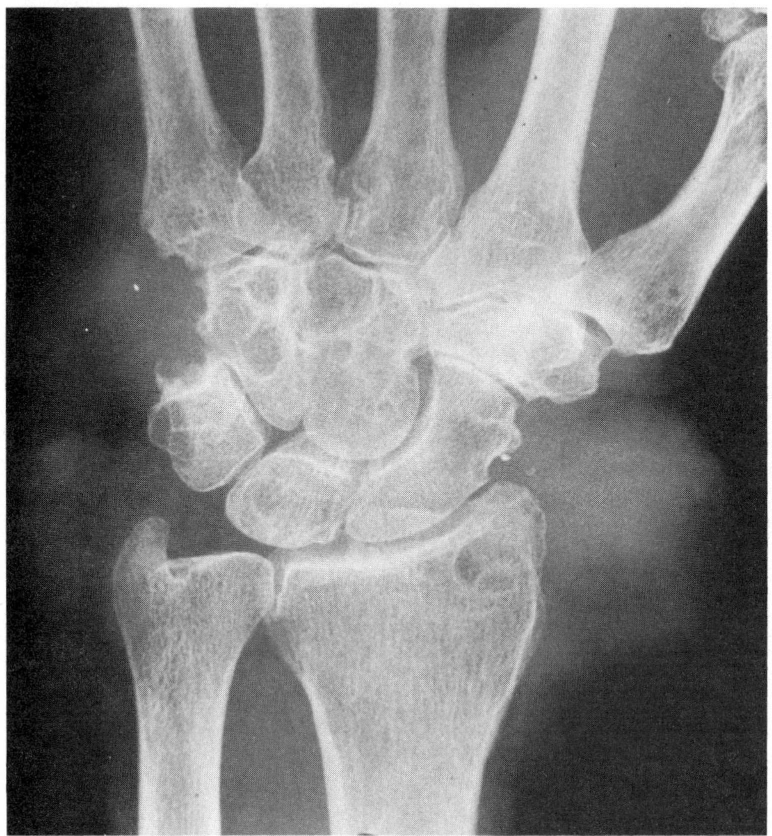

Figure 10–30. Synovial chondromatosis. Anteroposterior radiograph of the wrist of an 80-year-old man with large masses of unmineralized cartilage in the wrist joint. The soft-tissue density exhibits the lobulations characteristic of cartilage, even though there is no calcification. Sharply circumscribed defects in multiple bones associated with a soft-tissue mass are consistent with a benign soft-tissue tumor.

SYNOVIAL CHONDROMATOSIS

Synovium is capable of metaplasia into cartilage. The factors leading to this metaplasia are unknown. In true synovial chondromatosis, synovium undergoes metaplasia, and large cartilage masses are formed. These exhibit a greater degree of pleomorphism, mitotic activity, and increased cellularity when compared with benign intraosseous neoplastic cartilage. Identification of the synovial membrane that covers these cartilage masses should confirm that the lesion is synovial. Traumatic joint bodies are simply fragments of cartilage sheared off the articular surface that may continue to survive because they are nourished by joint fluid and do not require a blood supply. When such loose bodies secondarily attach to the synovium, they may be difficult to distinguish from the metaplastic process. Either variety may utilize the blood supply from the synovial attachment and eventually ossify in the center of the nodule.

Synovial chondromatosis rarely undergoes malignant transformation (Goldman, Unni). The moderate pleomorphism of cartilage should not be confused with malignant transformation.

Text continued on page 614

Figure 10–33. Synovial chondromatosis. Nodular focus of cartilage contained entirely within the synovium. The synovial membrane completely surrounds the nodule, indicating continuing attachment to the synovium itself. There are clearly defined cartilage cells and matrix without significant pleomorphism.

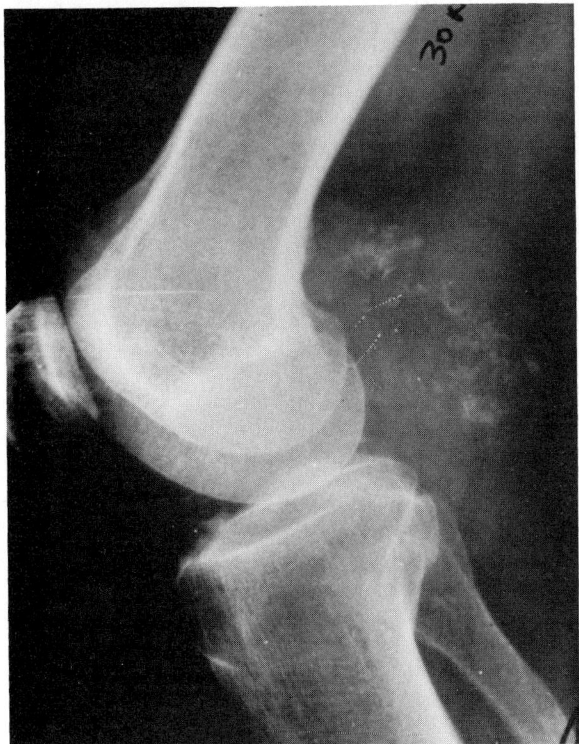

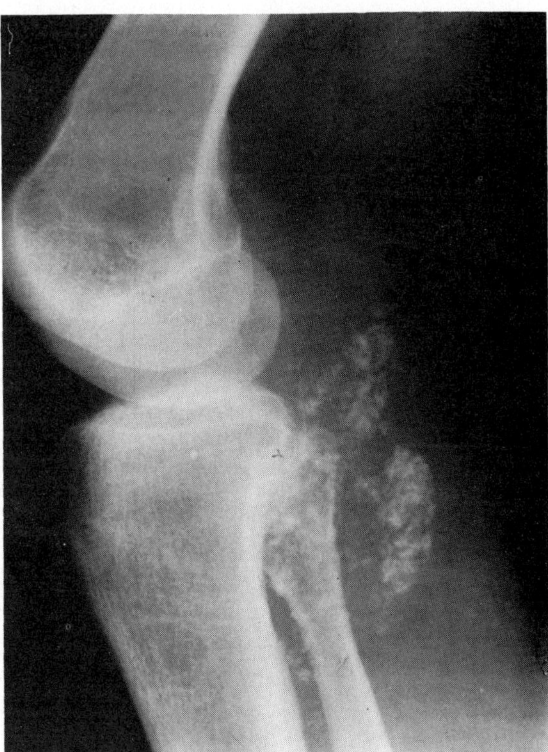

Figure 10–31

Figure 10–32

Figure 10–31. Synovial chondromatosis. Lateral radiograph of the knee showing numerous nodules of cartilage in the posterior compartments of the joint. The flocculent lobular characteristics of cartilage are readily demonstrated. The extent of calcification in these lesions can vary considerably.

Figure 10–32. Synovial chondromatosis. Lateral radiograph of the knee with characteristic large, irregular, flocculent lobules of calcified cartilage. Differential diagnosis includes osteochondritis dissecans and periosteal chondroma originating on the tibia.

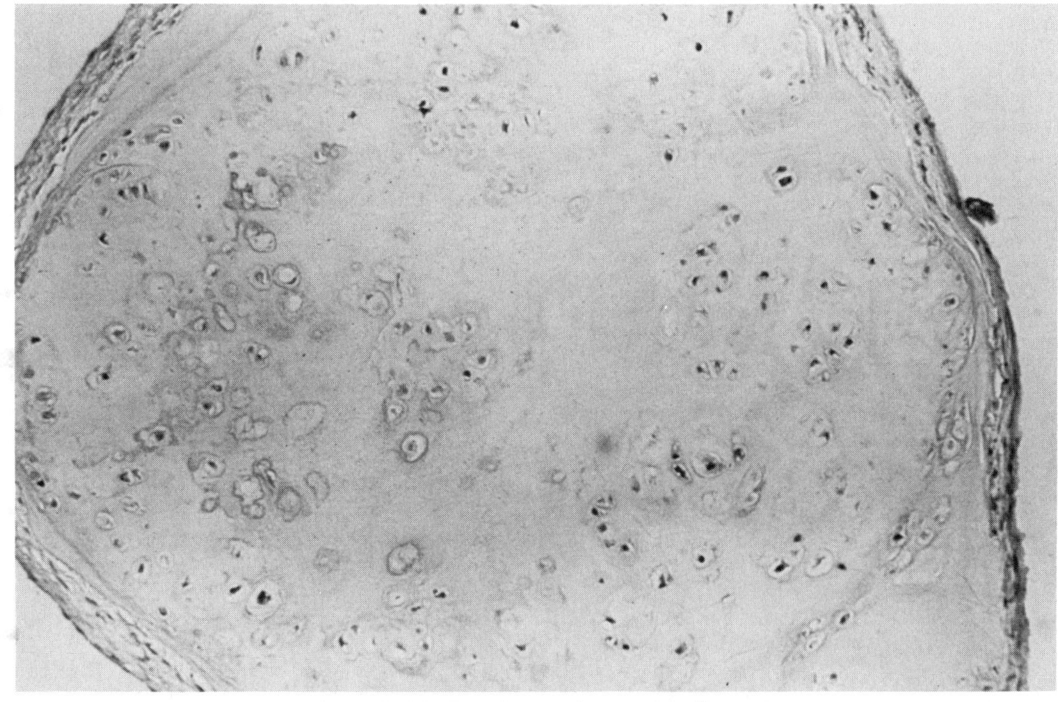

Figure 10–33. *See legend on opposite page*

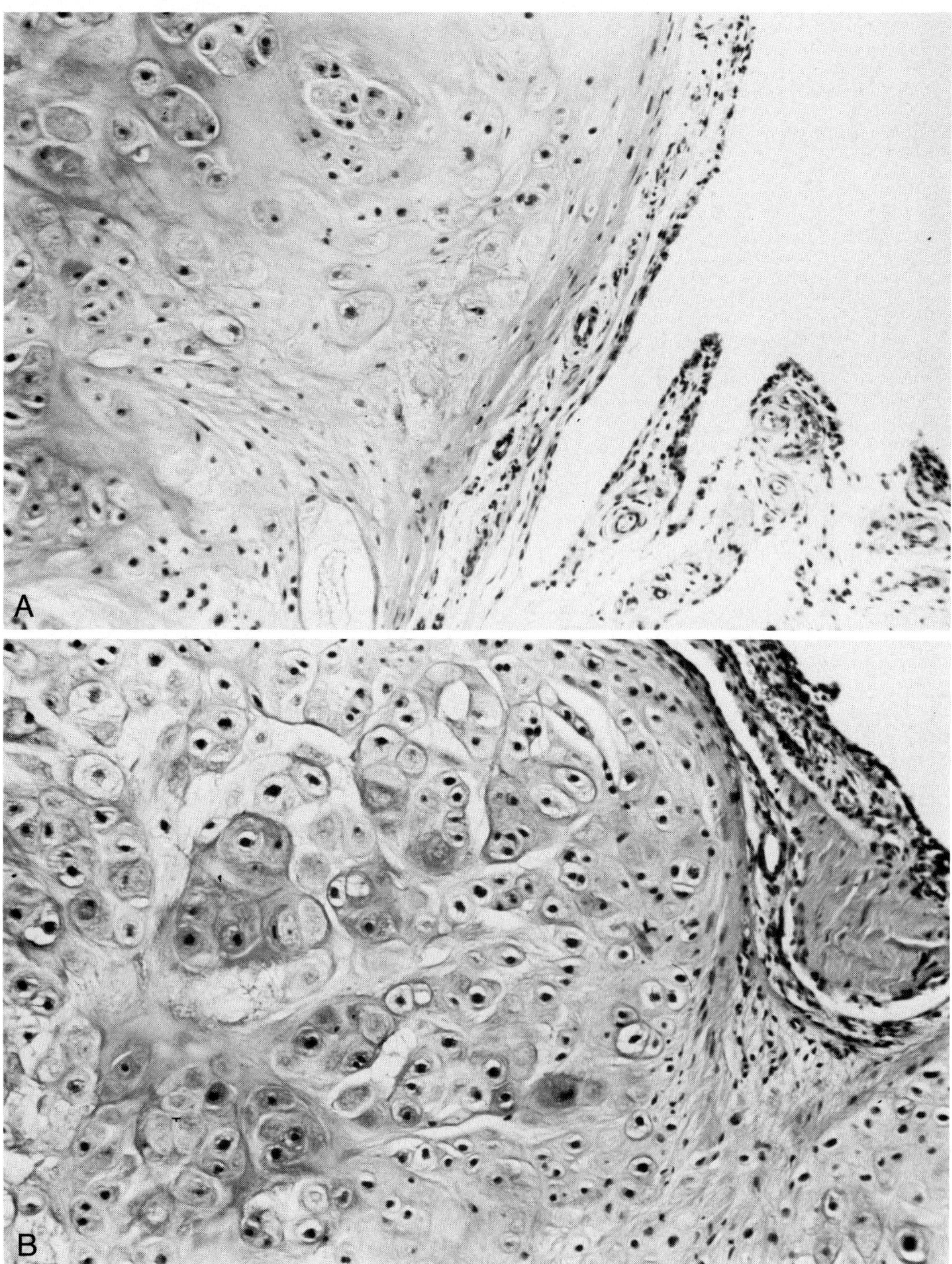

Figure 10–34. Synovial chondromatosis. A well-defined focus of cartilage metaplasia in the synovial membrane. Occasionally, the cartilage may exhibit significant pleomorphism, but these lesions rarely metastasize. The nodules may be free in the joint or may be retained by a stalk of synovium. The blood supply carried by the stalk can lead to further maturation with enchondral ossification.

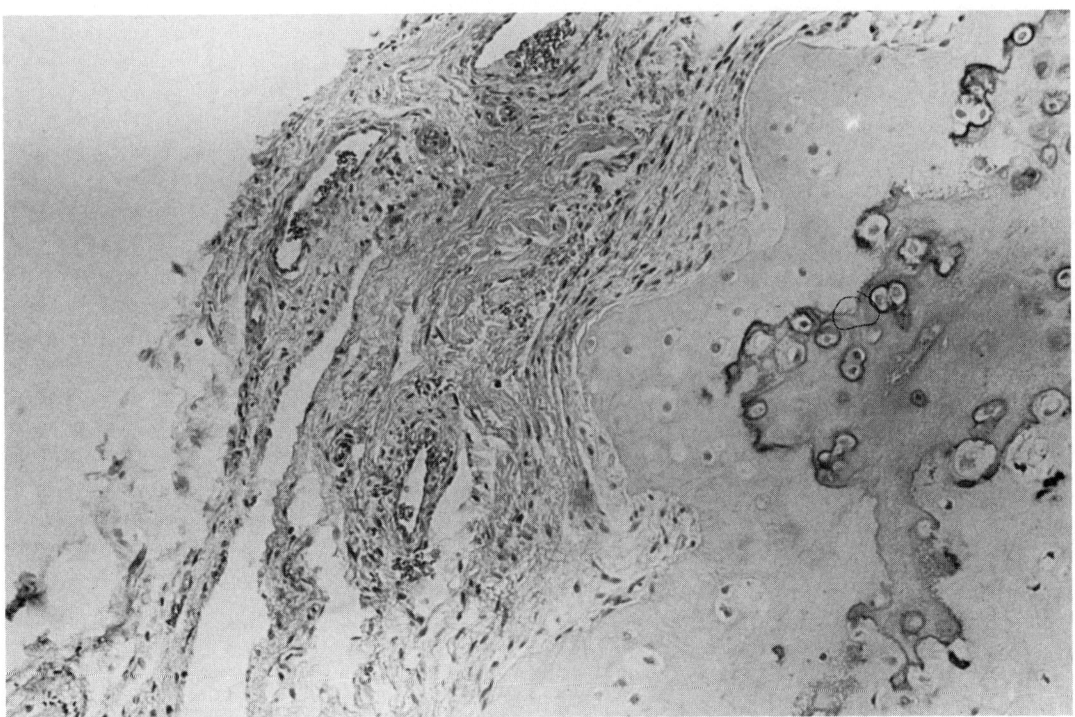

Figure 10–35. Synovial chondromatosis. Focus of cartilage covered by synovial membrane. The cartilage is undergoing characteristic maturation, demonstrating calcification of the matrix. Irregularity of cartilage formation and maturation produces the calcification seen radiographically.

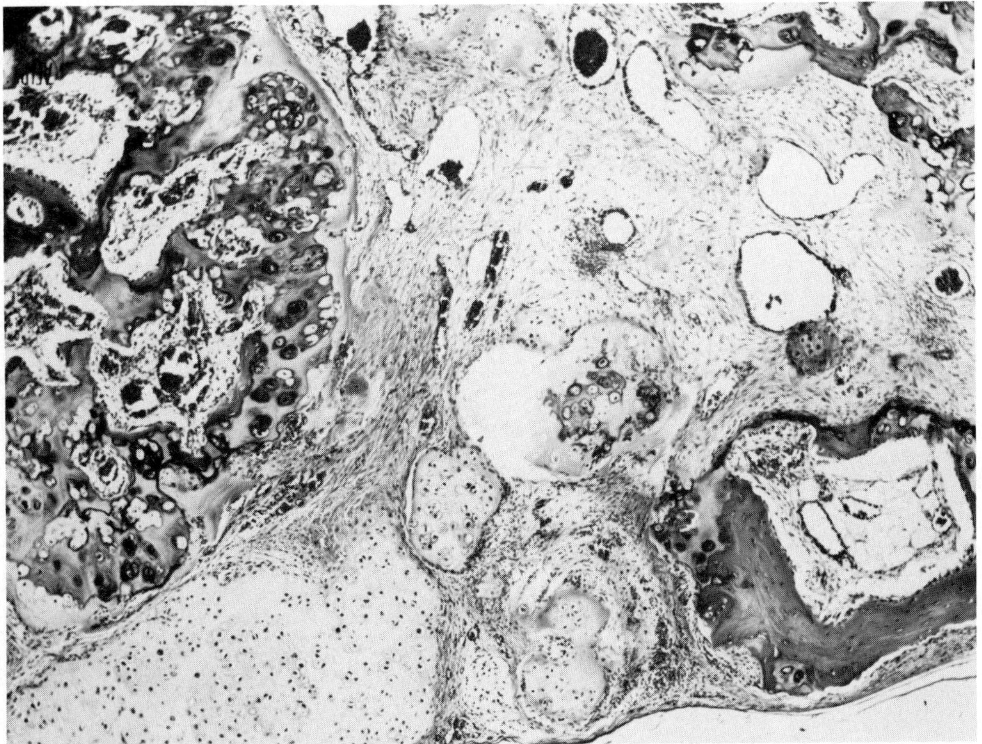

Figure 10–36. Synovial chondromatosis. Metaplastic cartilage focus undergoing further maturation, with replacement of calcified cartilage and production of bone. Calcification can occur without a blood supply, but ossification cannot. The presence of viable bone proves that this nodule is attached to the synovium.

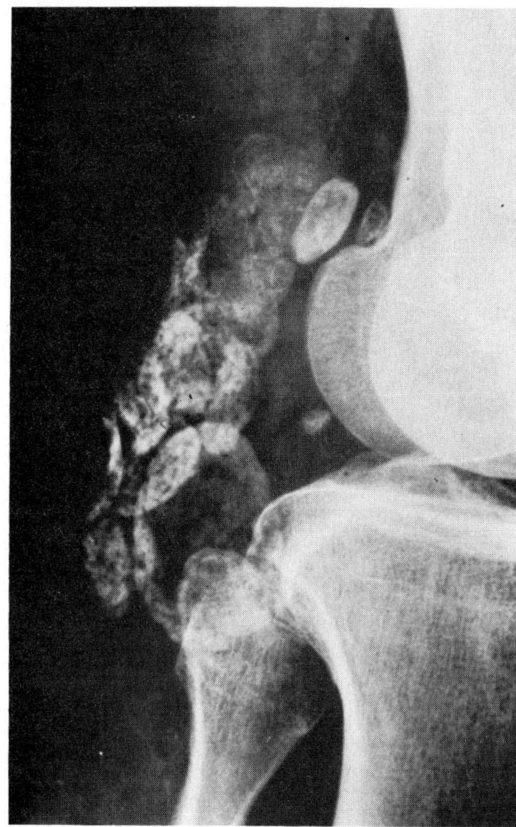

Figure 10–37. Synovial chondromatosis. Lateral radiograph of the knee showing large numbers of partially calcified and ossified nodular foci of cartilage.

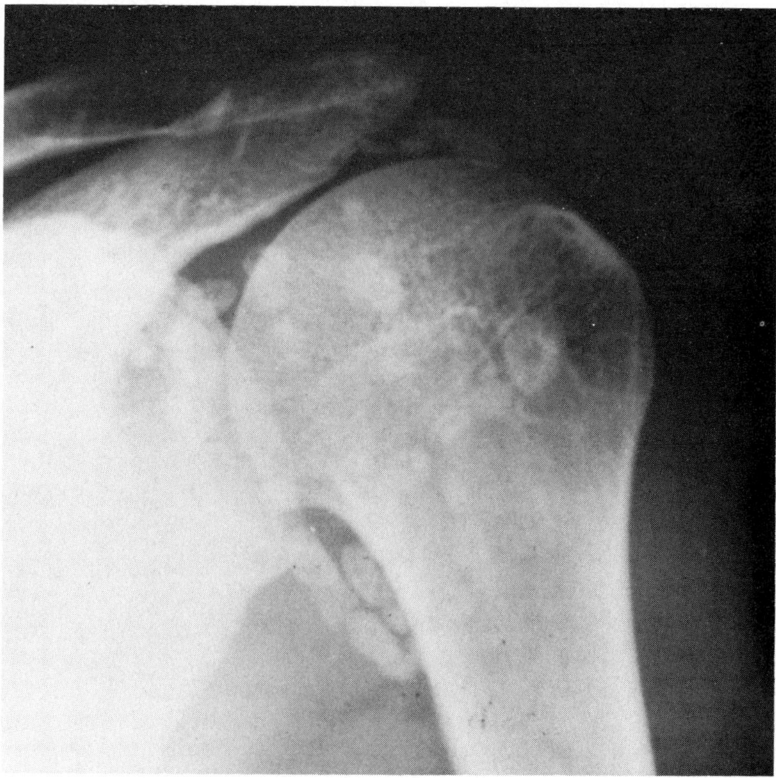

Figure 10–38. Synovial chondromatosis. Anteroposterior radiograph of a lesion demonstrating numerous ossified nodules in a shoulder joint.

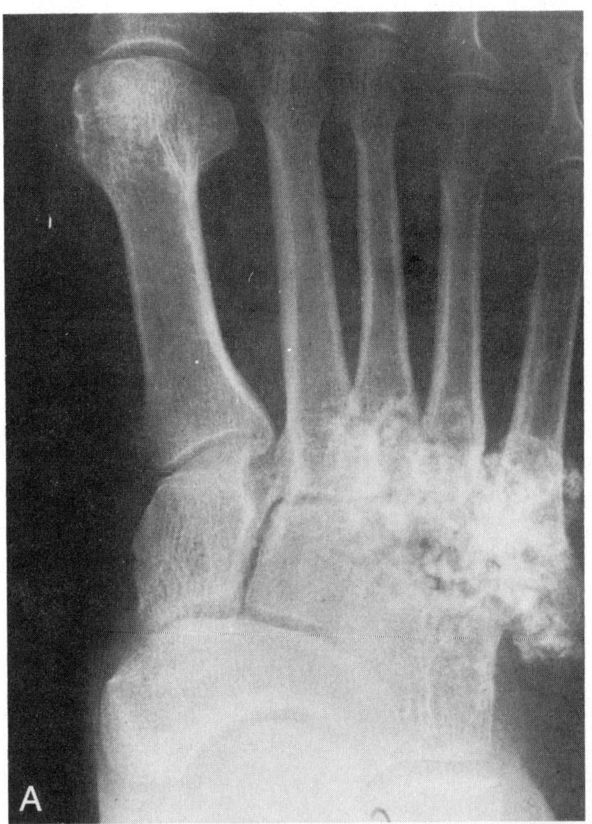

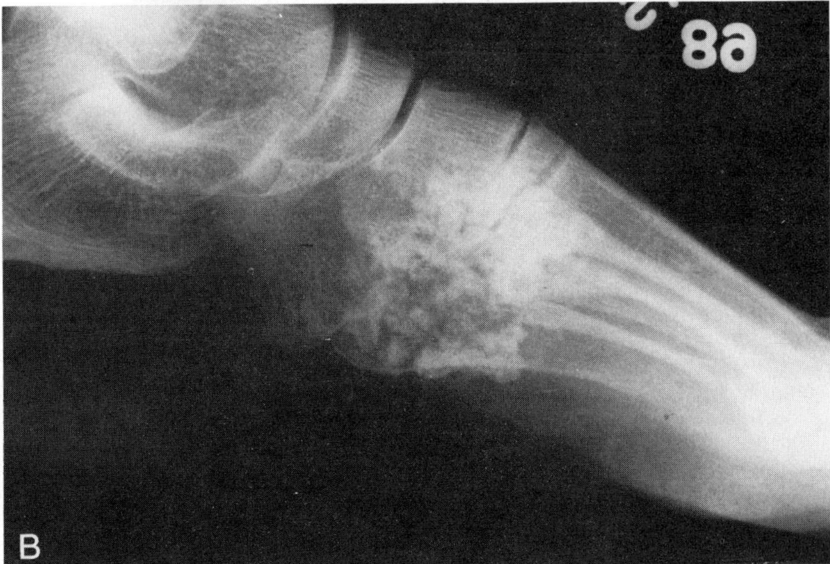

Figure 10–39. Synovial chondromatosis. Anteroposterior (*A*) and lateral (*B*) radiographs of a foot with extensive synovial chondromatosis at the base of the third, fourth, and fifth metatarsals. The nodules interfere with the function and nutrition of the joint and can actually cause erosions and deformity of the joint that lead to degenerative arthritis. Since the nodules frequently occur on a stalk, they can be trapped between the joint surfaces and cause symptoms of catching and locking.

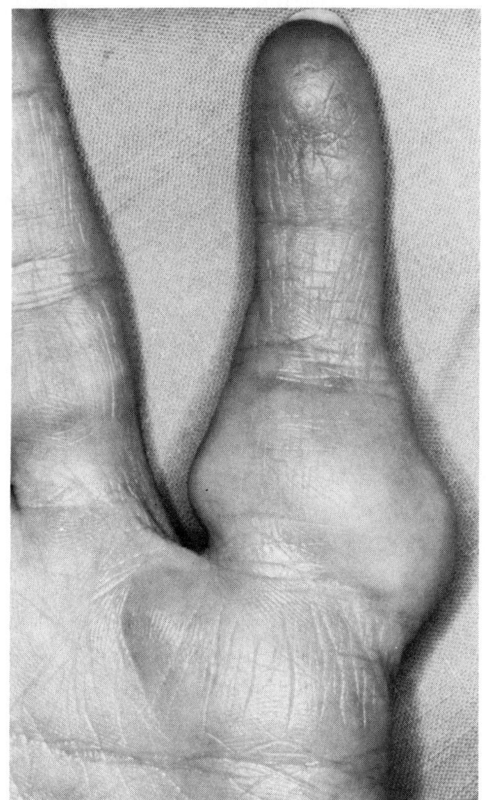

Figure 10–40. Synovial chondromatosis. Photograph of the hand of a 47-year-old female in whom a slowly enlarging mass in the little finger had been apparent for 8 years.

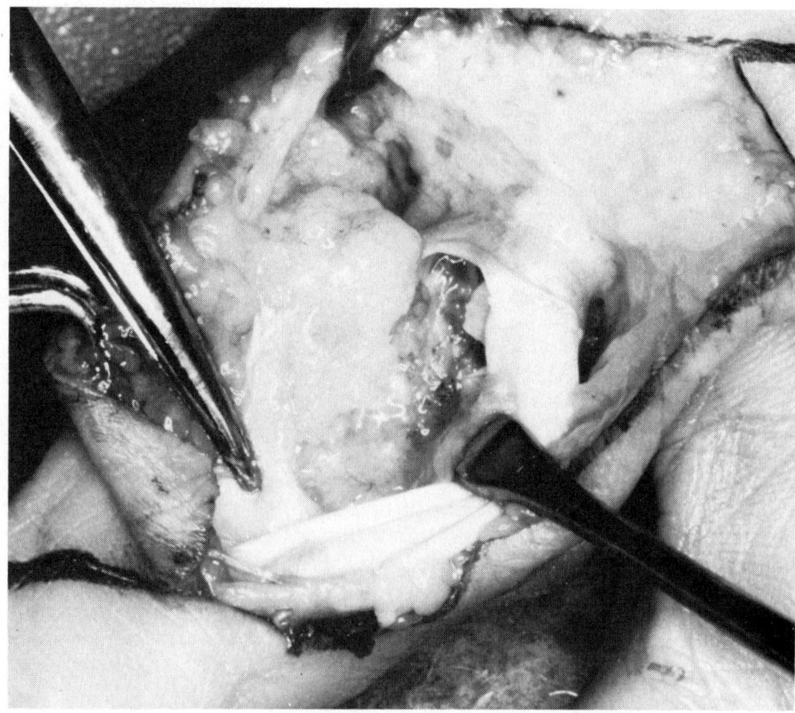

Figure 10–41. Synovial chondromatosis. Surgical exposure of the mass shown in Figure 10–39 reveals typical lobular cartilage. A blue, glistening surface is very characteristic. The prolonged presence of the lesion has allowed it to infiltrate extensively around the flexor and extensor tendons. Its origin from the joint is demonstrated by its presence beneath the volar plate and inside the joint capsule.

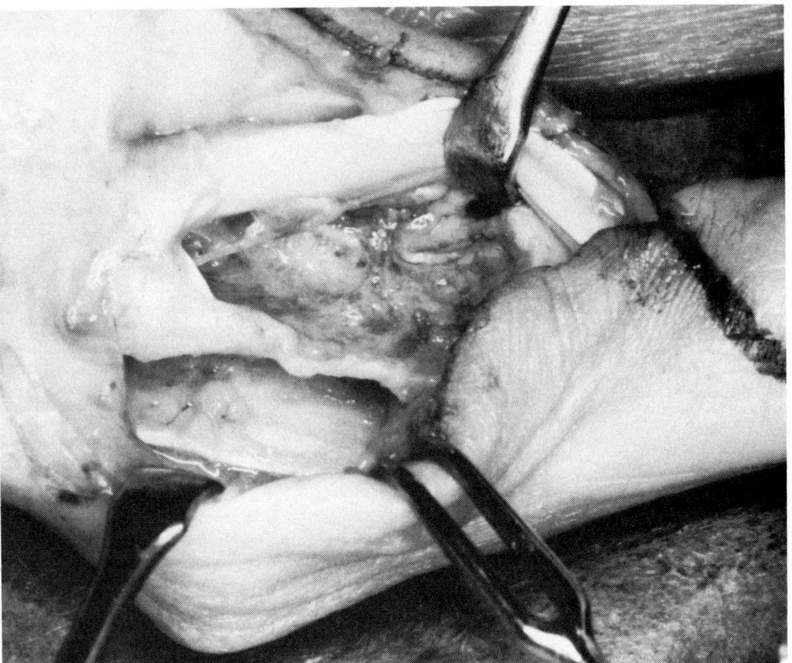

Figure 10–42. Synovial chondromatosis. Clinical photograph after removal of the cartilage. There has been extensive erosion of the phalanx on its dorsal and palmar surfaces over the long-term course of the lesion.

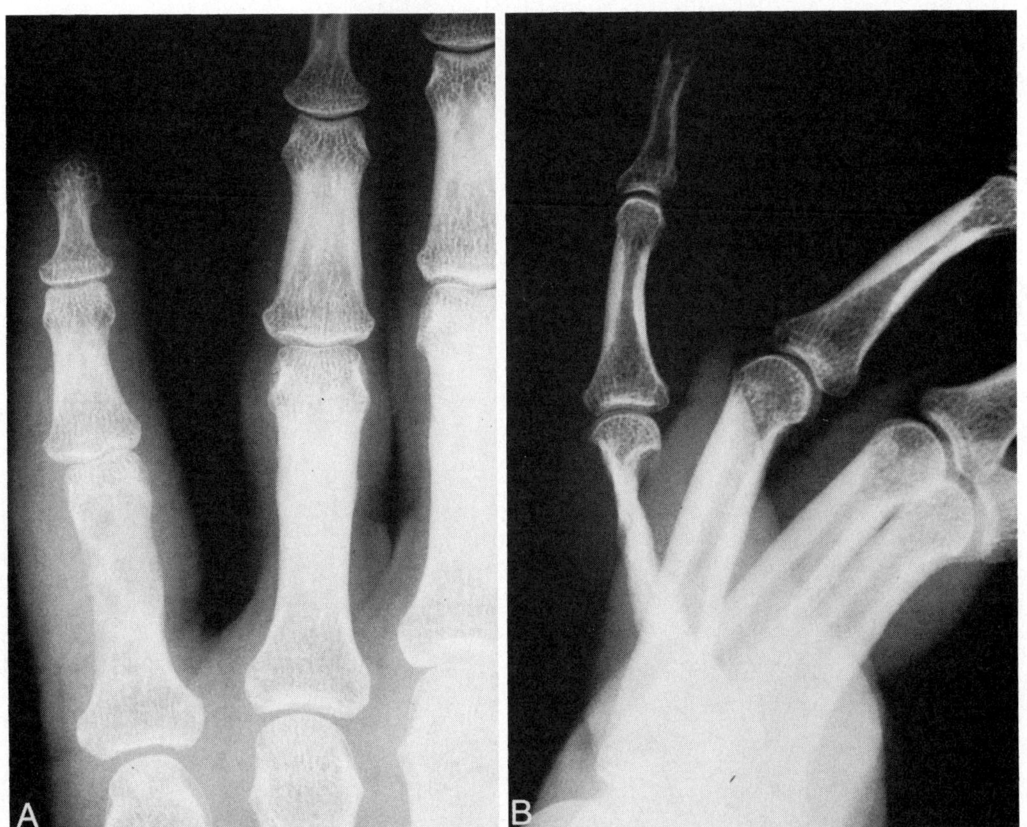

Figure 10–43. Synovial chondromatosis. Anteroposterior (*A*) and lateral (*B*) radiographs of the finger illustrated in Figures 10–40 to 10–42 following surgical removal of the lesion. No bone has been removed surgically, but a large portion of it has been eroded owing to the pressure exerted by the lesion.

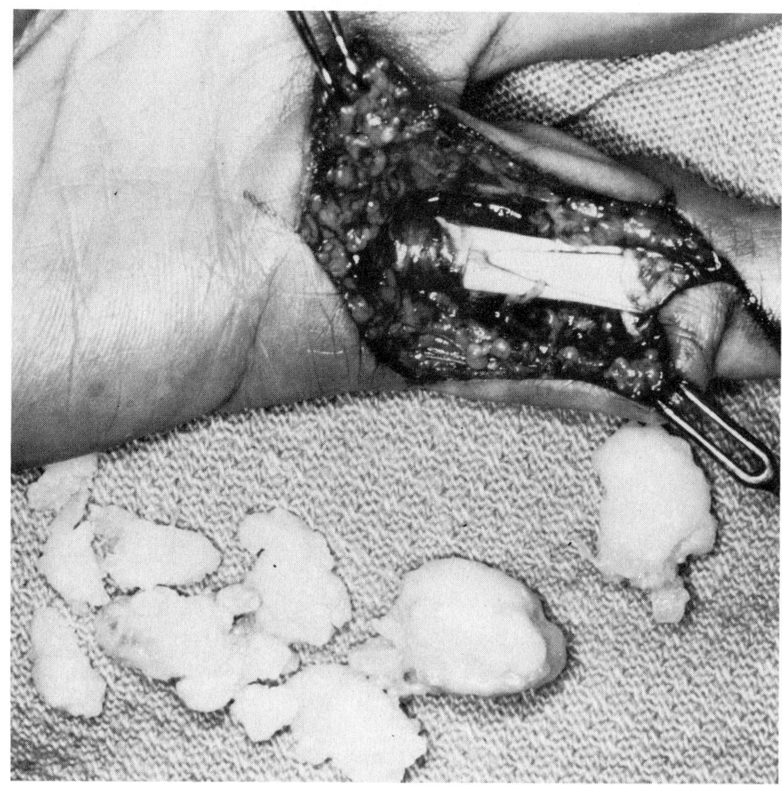

Figure 10–44. Synovial chondromatosis. Clinical photograph of the material resected from the tendon sheath, the joint, and the remainder of the finger shown in the preceding four figures. Note the large volume of tissue, which interfered with normal bone remodeling.

GANGLION

The ganglion, or ganglionic cyst, is a thinned-walled, fluid-filled sac. It appears to arise through a process of herniation of synovial lining of joint or tendon sheath through a defect in the fibrous capsule. Such a defect may result from trauma or

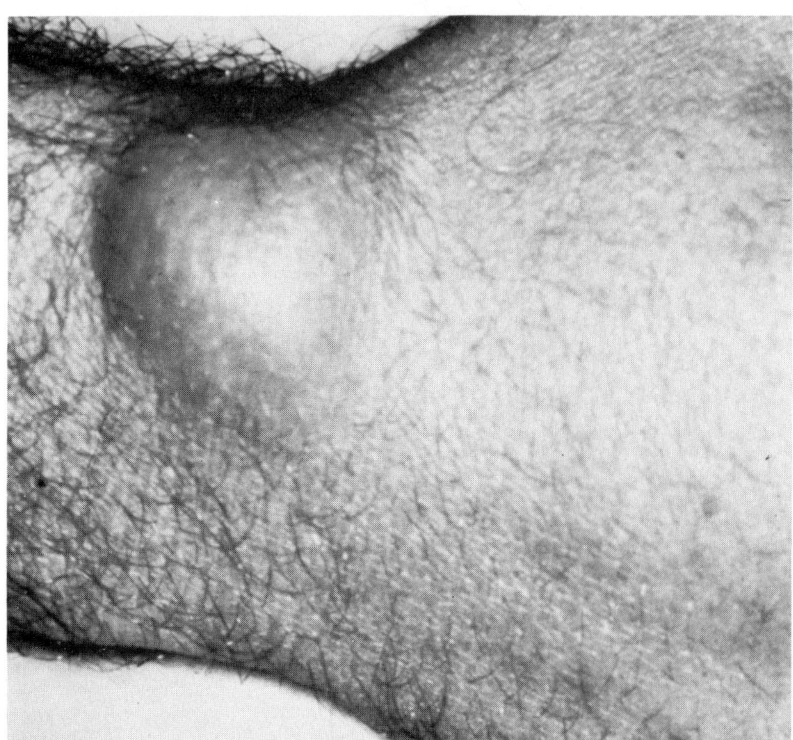

Figure 10–45. Ganglion. Clinical photograph of the hand and wrist of a 31-year-old male with a soft-tissue swelling over the dorsal radial aspect of the wrist. This figure represents the most characteristic location and appearance of a ganglion.

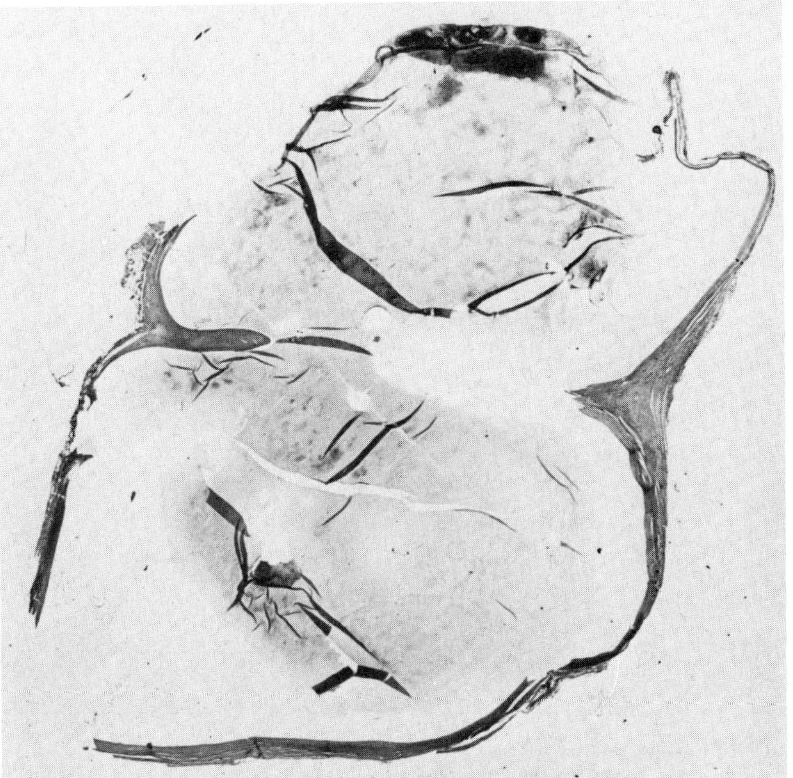

Figure 10–46. Section of an entire ganglion. Note the thin, partially septated wall. Such septation is common, but rarely does the ganglion have more than one cavity.

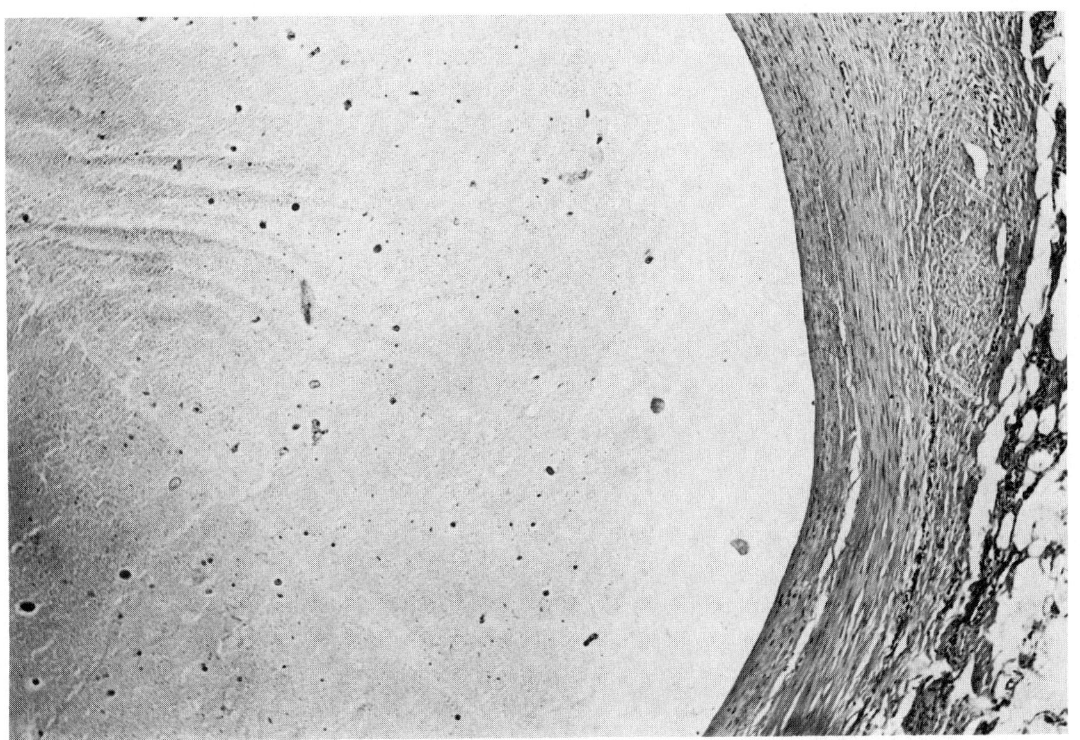

Figure 10–47. Fibrous wall of a typical ganglion. The early cyst has a much thinner wall, but with the passage of time the wall becomes thicker owing to the addition of new fibrous tissue. Initially, the wall is merely compacted subcutaneous tissue, pushed aside by the expanding cyst.

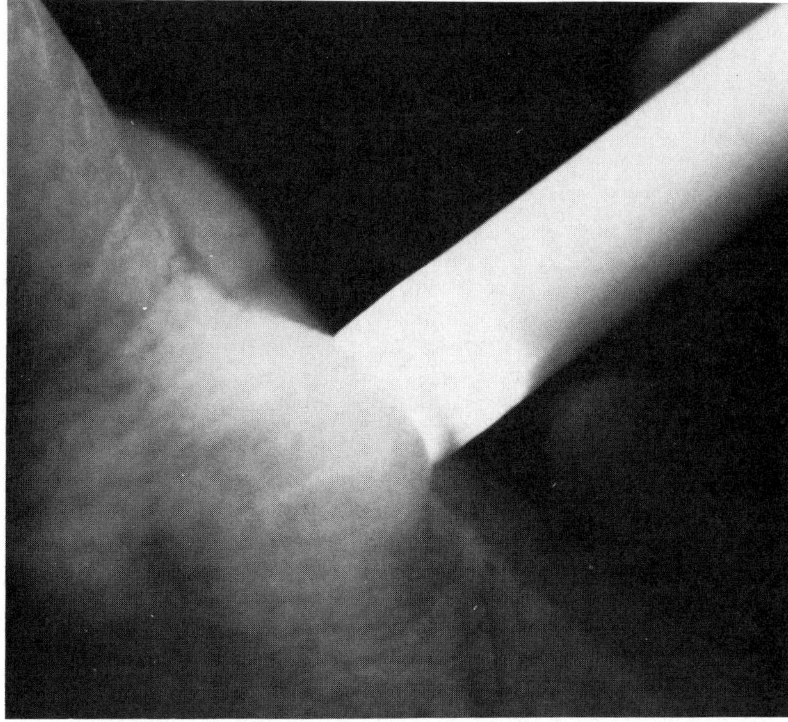

Figure 10–48. Ganglion. Since the lesion consists of a thin-walled, fluid-filled sac, a reliable test for a cyst is transillumination. Solid lesions will not transmit the light.

degenerative changes in the fibrous joint capsule. Approximately 50 per cent of ganglia connect with the underlying joint through a stalk that functions as a one-way valve, passing fluid from the joint to the cyst. Most stalks ultimately close by fibrosis.

Gross examination reveals a fibrous capsule, a smooth lining surface, and a cavity filled with a clear, white, somewhat mucoid fluid that is very similar to normal joint fluid. Ganglionic cysts show a central cavity but contain numerous smaller slitlike spaces lined by a similar synovial membrane. Retention of one of these smaller slits may account for the recurrence of previously partially excised lesions.

Text continued on page 622

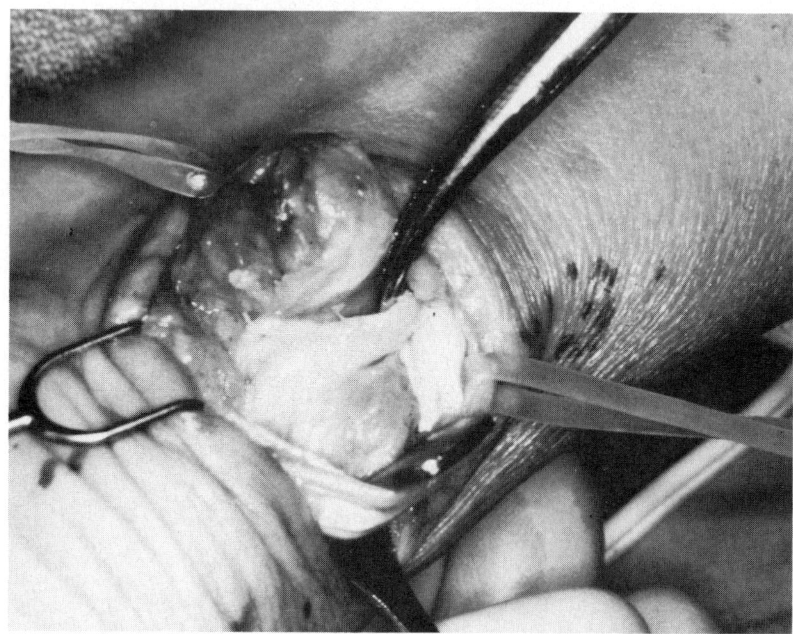

Figure 10–49. Ventral wrist ganglion. These commonly create problems for the surgeon because of their location beneath the radial artery. As the ganglion enlarges, it pushes in the path of least resistance and may appear on either side of the artery.

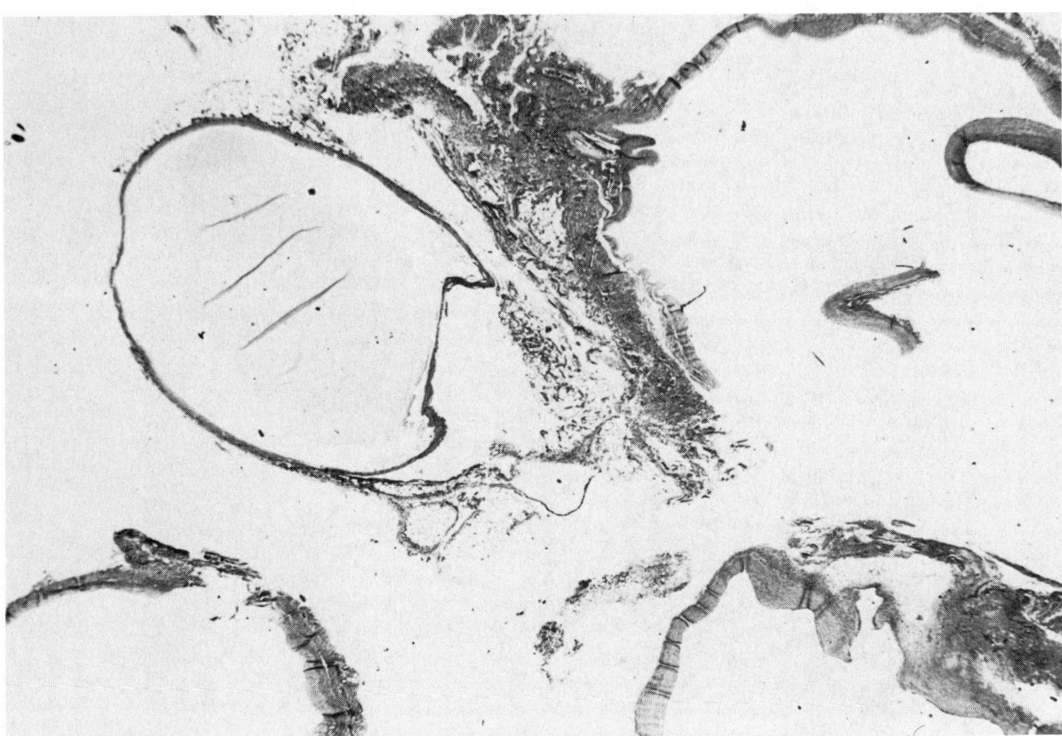

Figure 10–50. Histologic section of a ganglion that appears to have multiple cavities. The wall is of varying thickness, and the cavities are of different sizes. There is an irregular mix of fibrous and myxoid tissue in the septa between the loculations of the cyst.

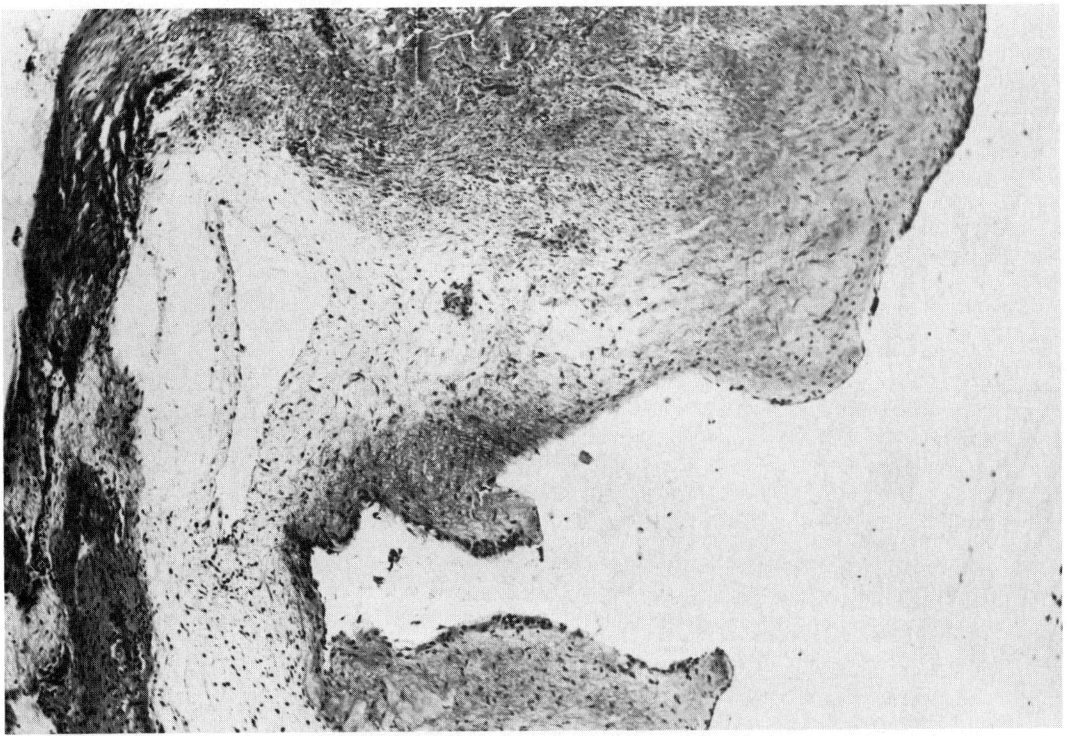

Figure 10–51. Ganglion. Higher-power view of· the cyst wall illustrated in the preceding figure demonstrates myxoid degeneration of the capsule wall, with formation of small daughter cysts. These usually reside in the fibrous capsule of the joint, from which the larger ganglion originates. If surgical excision involves tying the stalk rather than resecting this capsule, recurrences can arise from such daughter cysts.

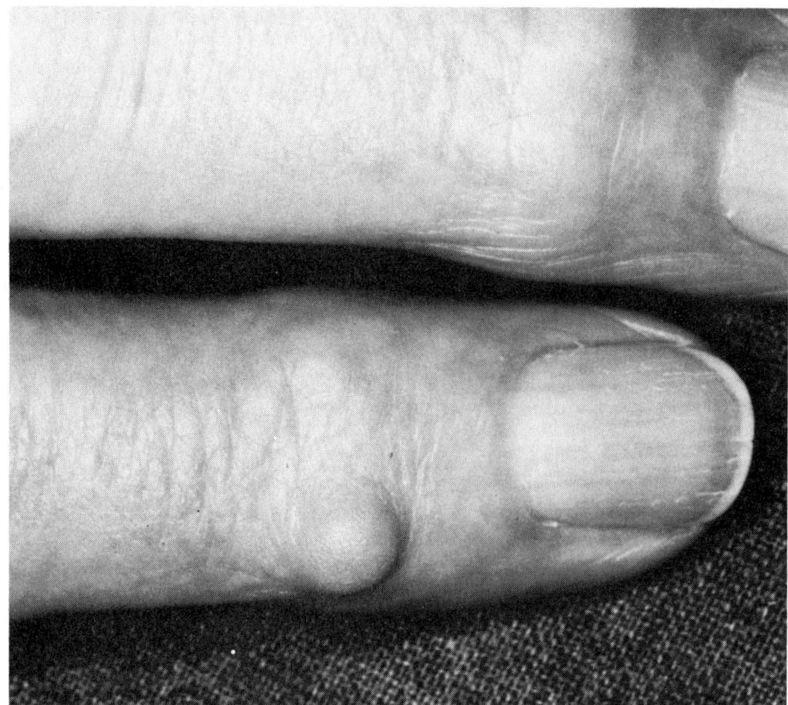

Figure 10–52. Mucous cyst. Clinical photograph of the fingers of a 74-year-old woman with a nodule overlying the distal interphalangeal joint. This has many of the characteristics of a ganglion, but is better known as a "mucous cyst."

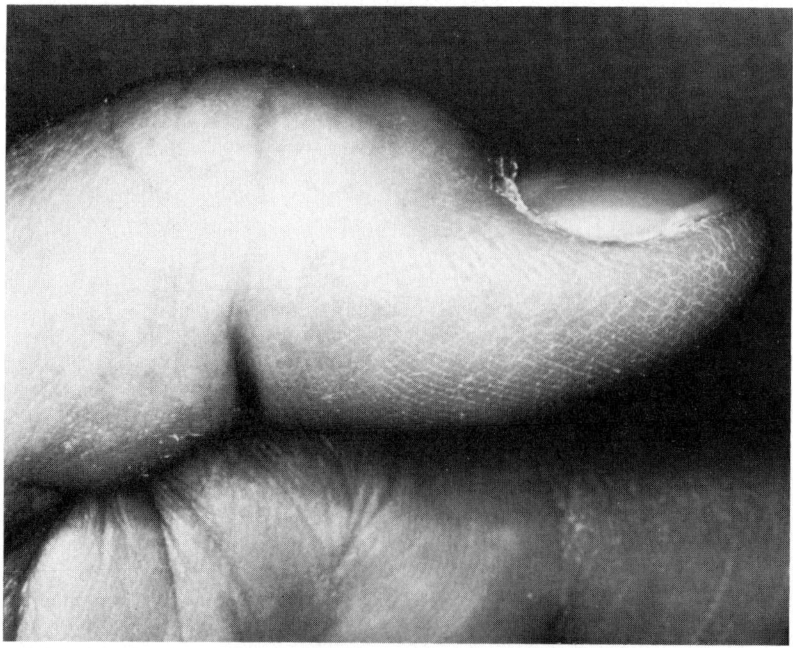

Figure 10–53. Mucous cyst. Lateral photograph of the thumb of a 59-year-old man with a cystic enlargement over the dorsum of the interphalangeal joint. This lesion is similar to that seen in Figure 10–52.

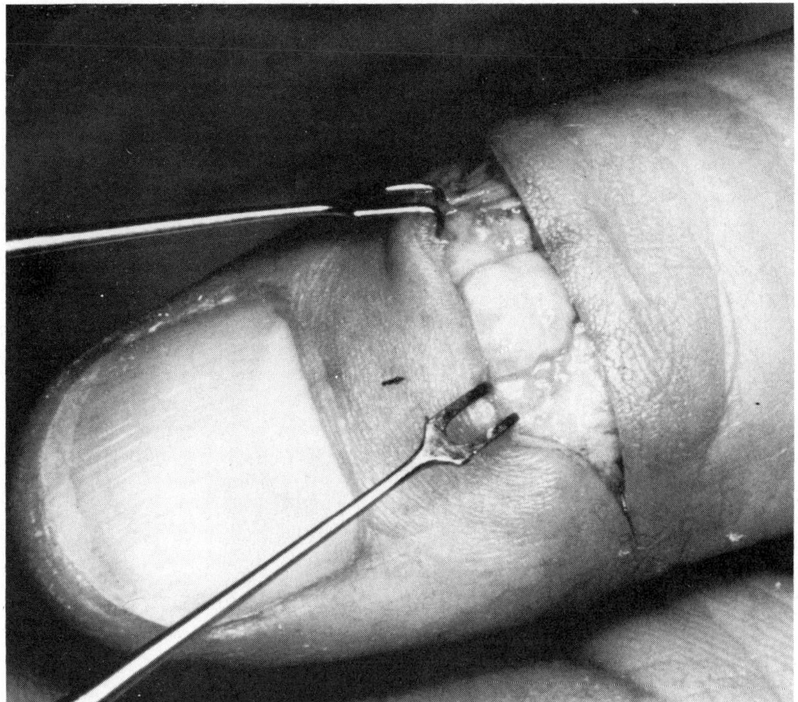

Figure 10–54. Mucous cyst. Surgical exposure of the lesion shown in Figure 10–53. Note the small cyst beside the extensor tendon bulging outward from the distal interphalangeal joint. Injection studies demonstrate communication with the joint.

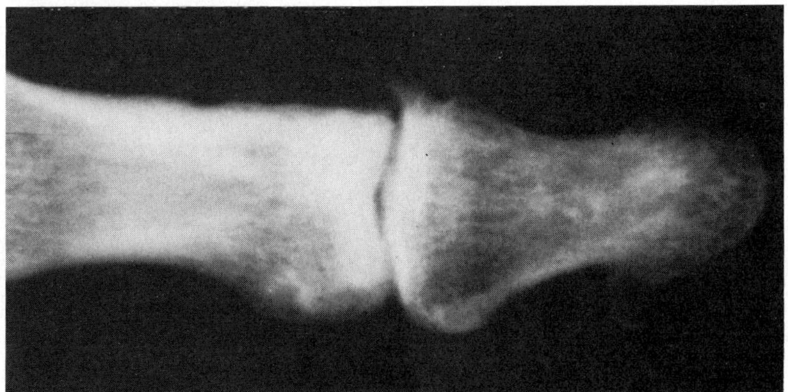

Figure 10–55. Mucous cyst. Radiograph of the interphalangeal joint shown in Figures 10–53 and 10–54. Classically, these cysts arise in degenerated joints characterized by thinning of the joint space, sclerosis of the bone ends, and osteophyte formation at the edge.

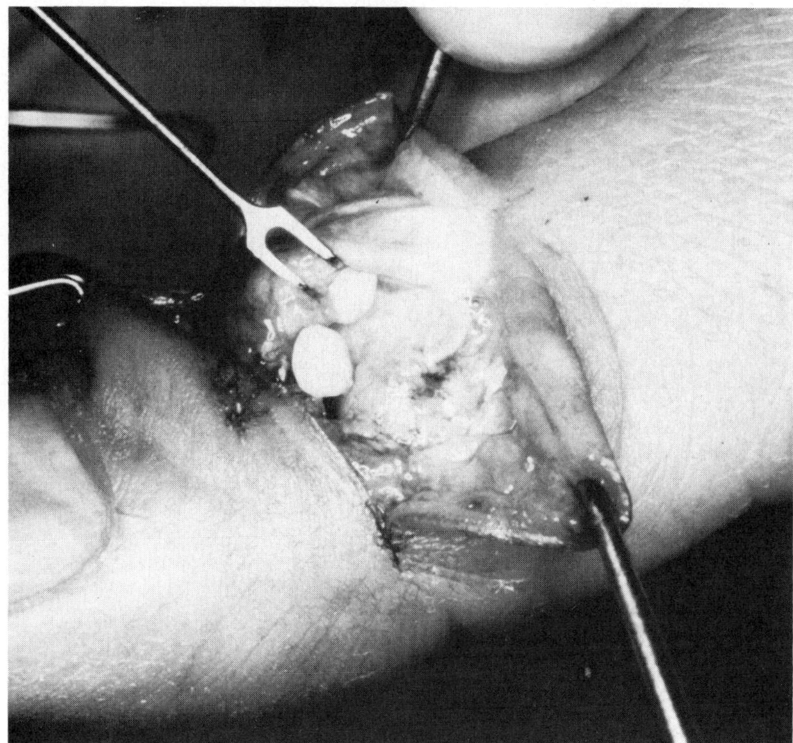

Figure 10–56. Mucous cyst. Surgical exposure of the interphalangeal joint shown in the preceding three figures. Note the several loose, extruding bodies, which are characteristic of degenerative arthritis.

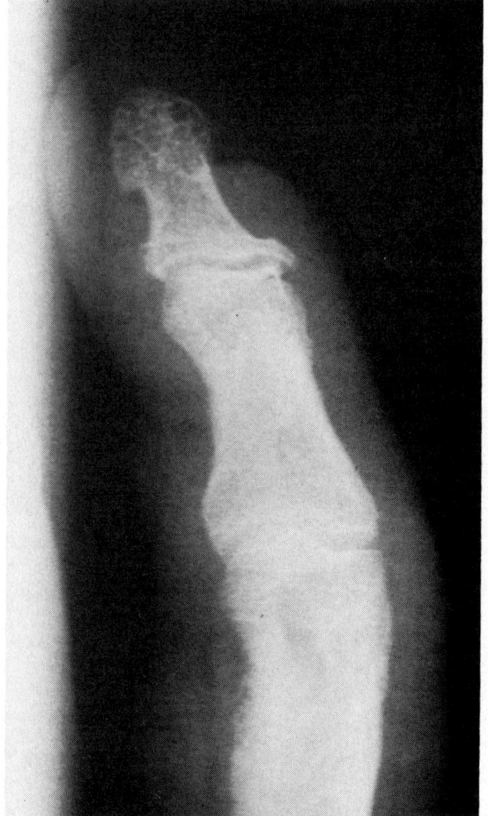

Figure 10–57. Mucous cyst. Oblique radiograph of a finger showing a large osteophyte projecting from the distal phalanx. Such osteophytes have been demonstrated to be the cause of such cysts. It may require oblique radiographs to demonstrate the osteophyte, but if looked for, they are found in the vast majority of cases.

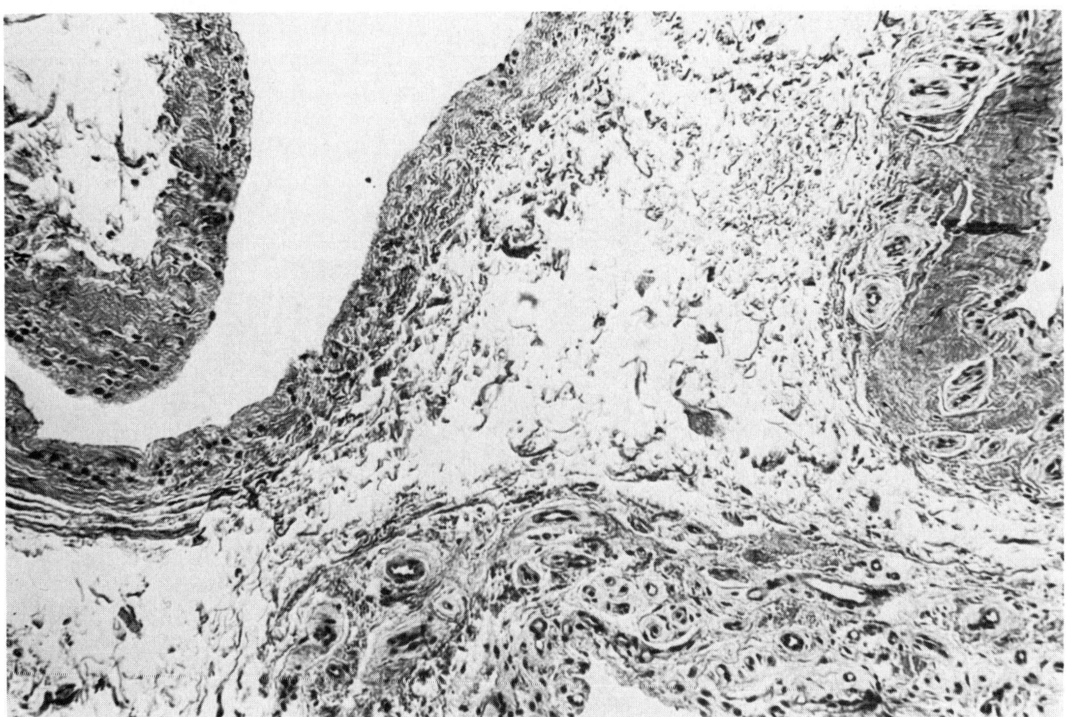

Figure 10–58. Microscopic section of the wall of a mucous cyst showing the lining of the cyst cavity and the myxoid degeneration of the tissue outside the lining.

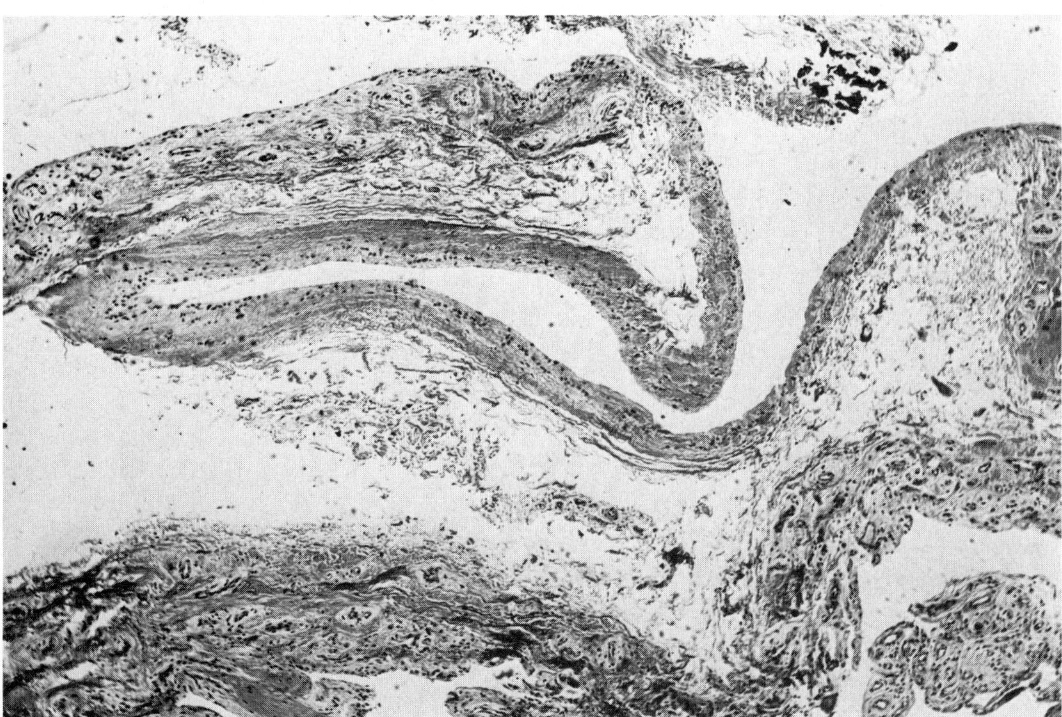

Figure 10–59. Lower-power view of the wall of a mucous cyst demonstrating marked myxoid changes in the tissues. Since the space between the skin surface and the bone is so small, marked thinning of the skin is common. Patients frequently self-treat these by puncturing them with a needle, and secondary infection is common.

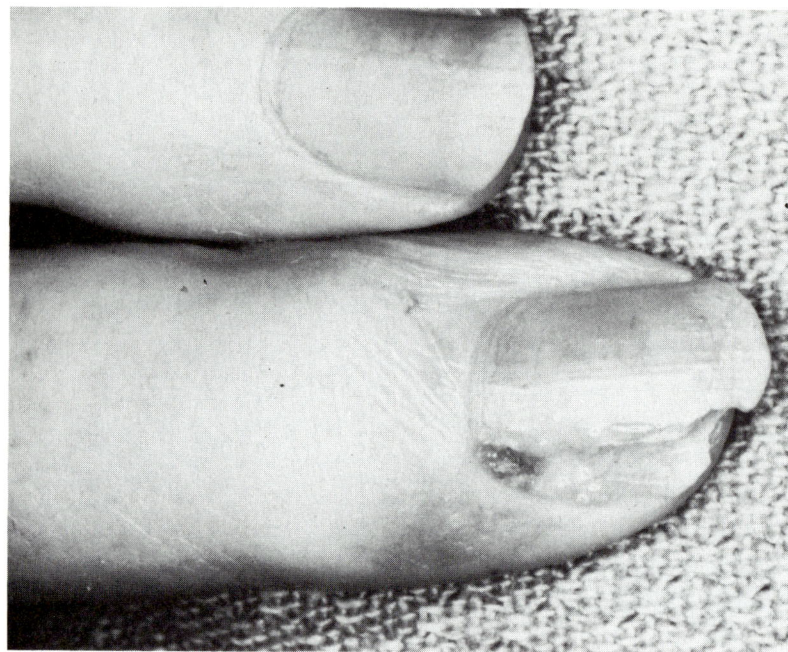

Figure 10–60. Mucous cyst. Since such lesions arise in the distal interphalangeal joint and are at the level of the germinal matrix of the finger nail, grooving of the nail is very common.

BURSITIS

Bursa is simply synovial membrane that undergoes the same pathologic transformations that may involve the synovial tissue. Thus, pigmented villonodular bursitis, nodular bursitis, and inflammatory bursitis are identical with their synovial counterparts. Indeed, there is no histologic method of differentiating synovial inflammatory disease from bursal inflammatory disease.

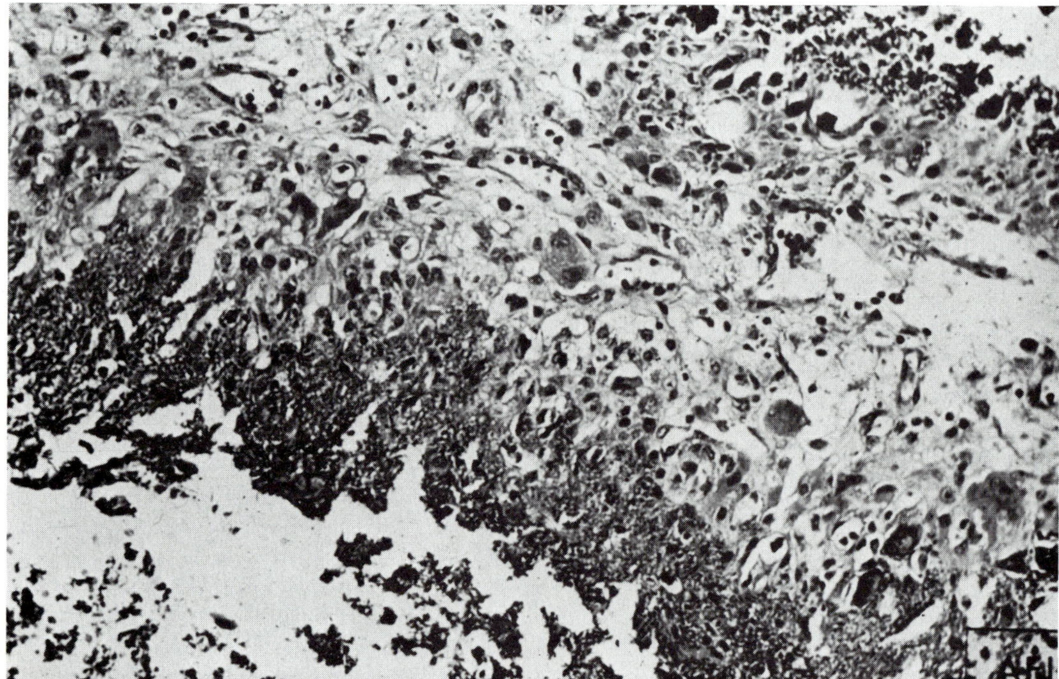

Figure 10–61. Section through the lining of a bursa demonstrating chronic inflammatory changes consistent with chronic bursitis. There is marked edema and fibrosis throughout the tissue, with increased vascularity and numerous inflammatory cells, including occasional giant cells.

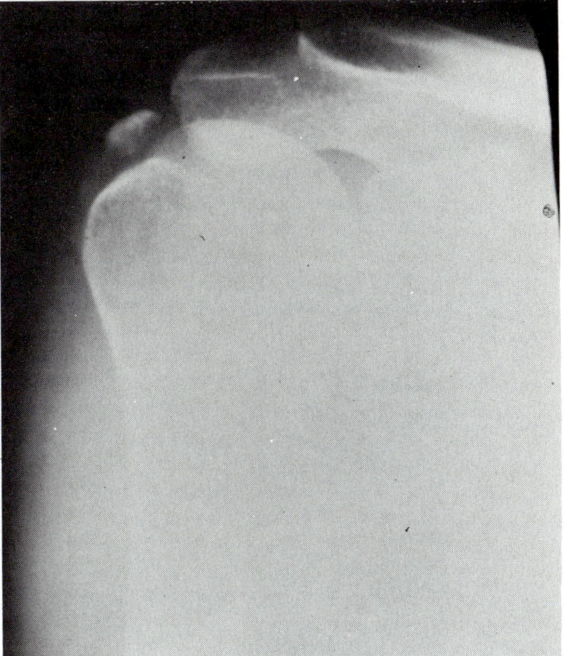

Figure 10–62. Bursitis with calcific tendonitis. Anteroposterior radiograph of a shoulder demonstrating calcification overlying the lateral aspect of the humeral head. Such calcification may be present in the supraspinatus tendon as a result of degeneration and dystrophic calcification, or it may burst out and become free within the subdeltoid and subacromial bursae.

Calcification of bursal tissue may occur secondary to repeated trauma. Thus, calcific bursitis is characterized by proliferation of bursal tissue and secondary amorphous calcification. Calcific bursitis may be secondary to adjacent tendon degeneration (e.g., supraspinatus syndrome).

Text continued on page 630

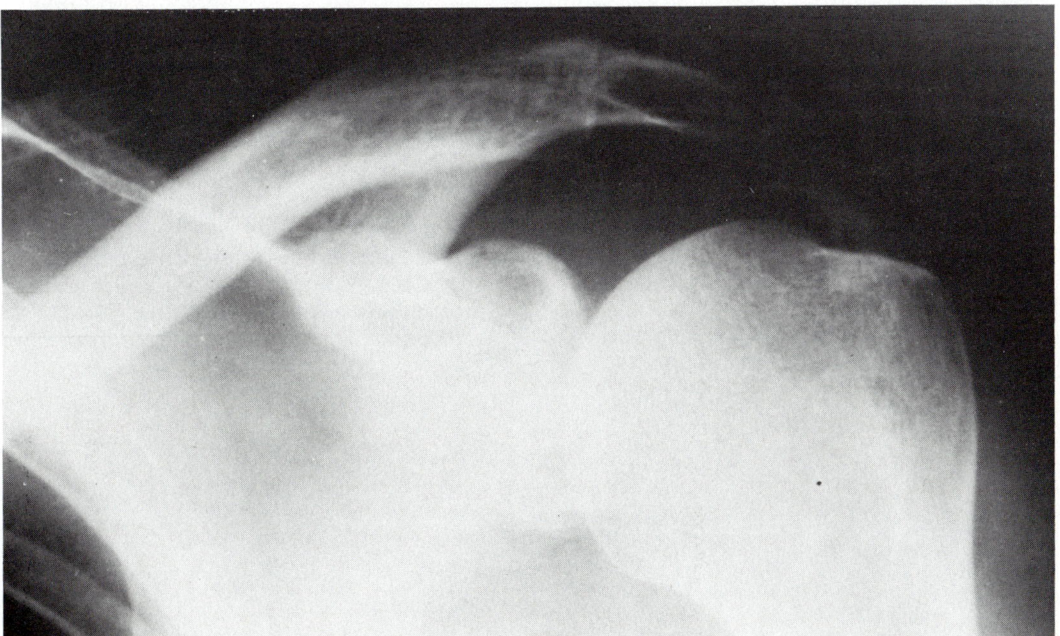

Figure 10–63. Anteroposterior radiograph of a shoulder showing calcification in the region of the greater tuberosity of the humerus. This deposit is more amorphous and less clear cut than that seen in the preceding figure. Frequently in this stage, the material is of a milky, semiliquid consistency and can be aspirated with a needle.

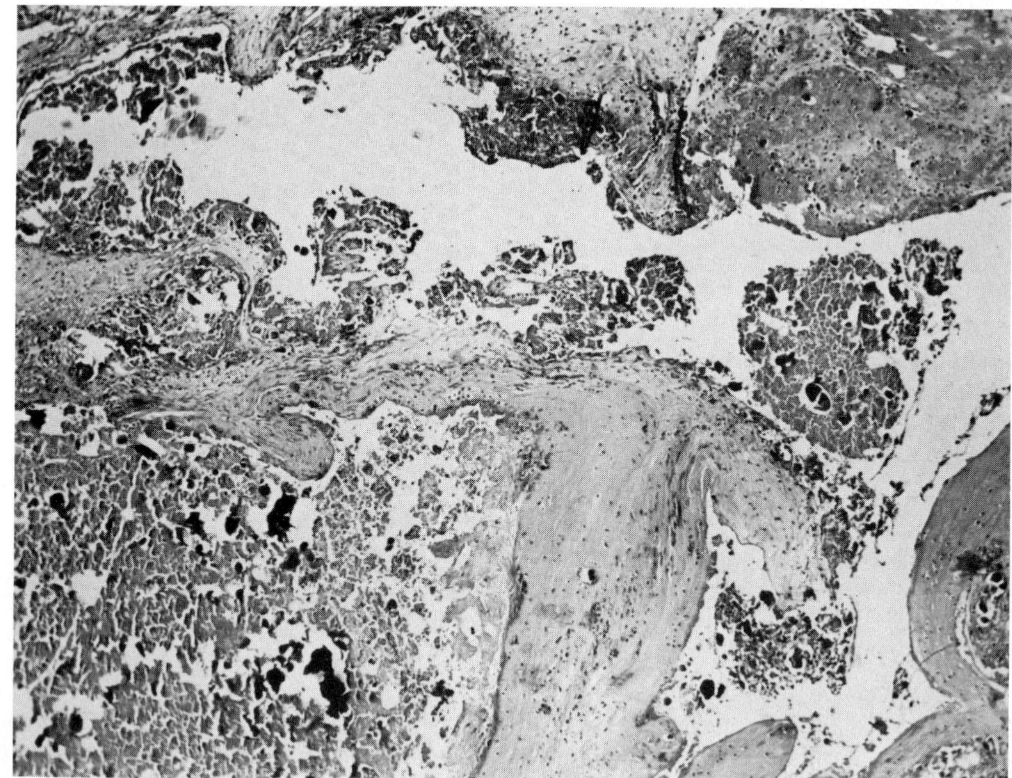

Figure 10–64. Histologic appearance of a section of calcific bursitis. Dense collagenized tissue is present as a centrally located band and may be a remnant of a disrupted tendon. There is a moderate amount of cellular debris, with amorphous calcium deposits. The bursal cavity is lined by irregular, hypertrophied villi, with increased thickness of lining cells. There are numerous inflammatory cells throughout.

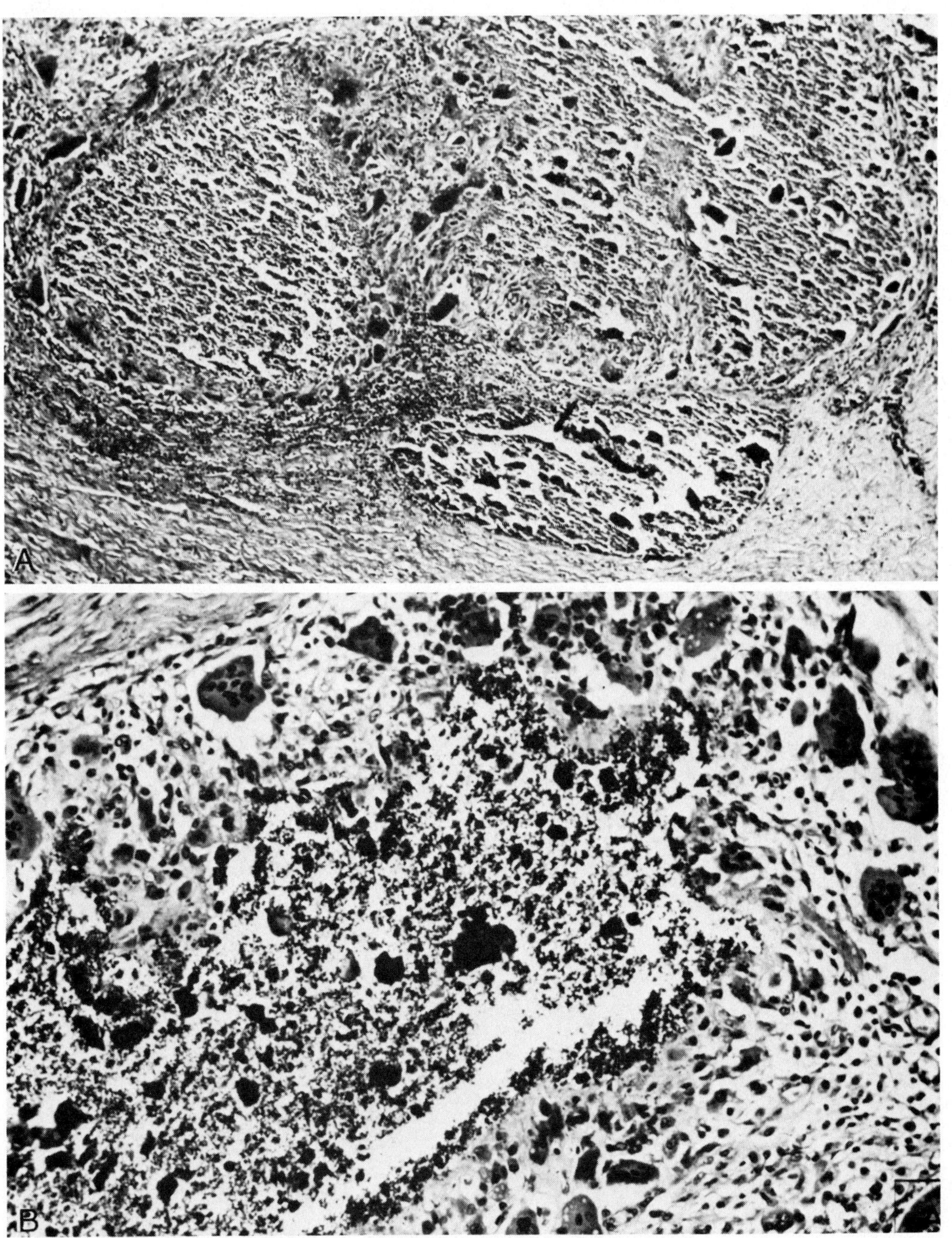

Figure 10–65. Bursitis. Sections through a degenerated tendon demonstrating chronic inflammatory cells and disorganized fibrosis, in addition to numerous calcium deposits that may be too small to be radiographically visible.

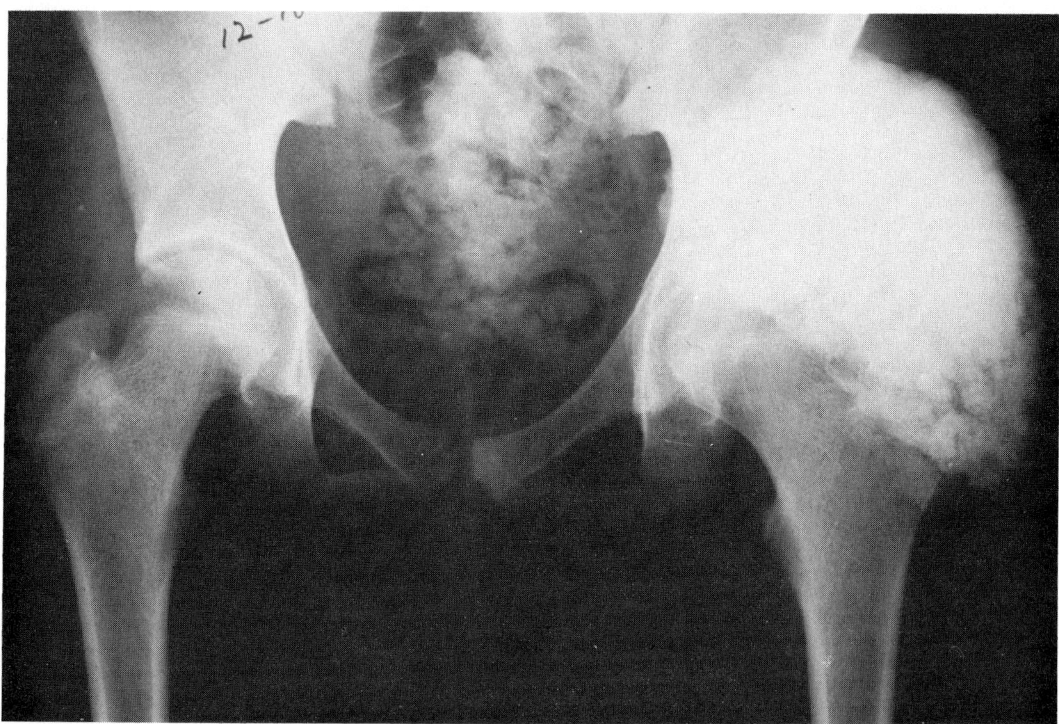

Figure 10–66. Bursitis. Tumoral calcinosis. Anteroposterior radiograph demonstrating large masses of calcium deposits around the proximal shaft and trochanters of the femur. These deposits are usually amorphous, crystalline deposits in the soft tissues about the joint, and with the associated fibrosis they can create painless, tumor-like masses that are quite frightening in appearance.

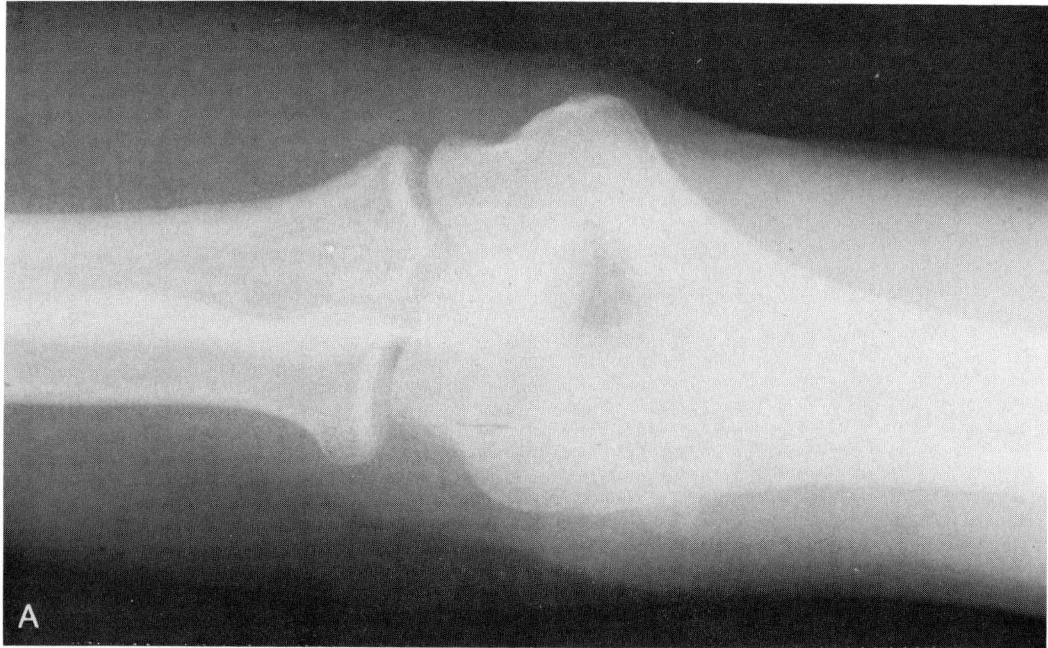

Figure 10–67. Bursitis. Tumoral calcinosis. Anteroposterior *(A)* and lateral *(B)* radiographs of the elbow showing a deposit in the triceps muscle, similar to that shown in Figure 10–66.

Illustration continued on opposite page

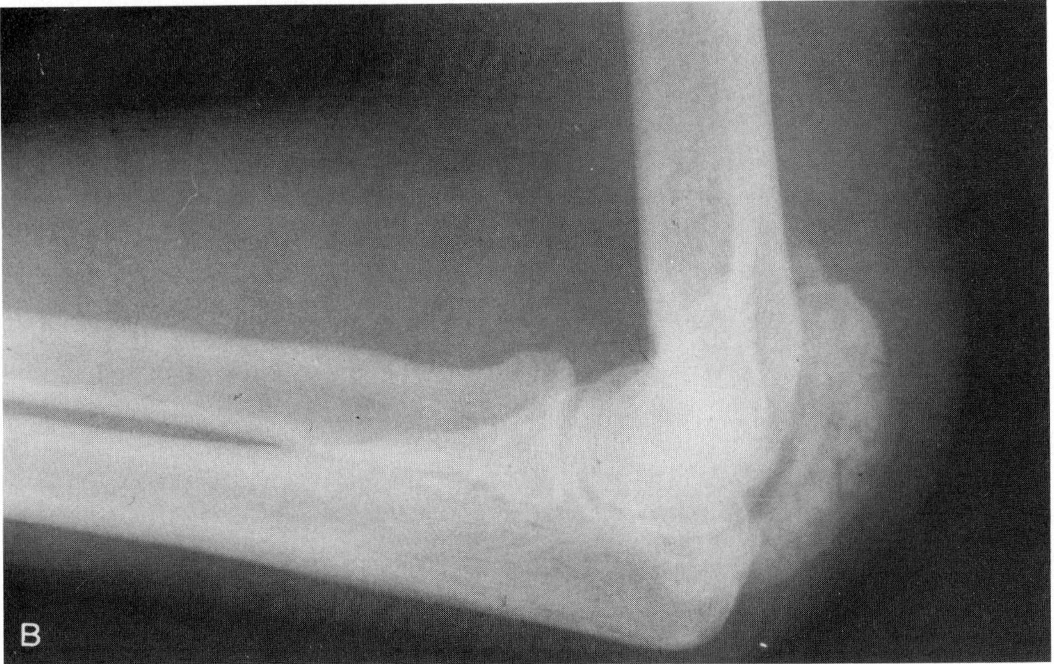

Figure 10–67 *Continued.*

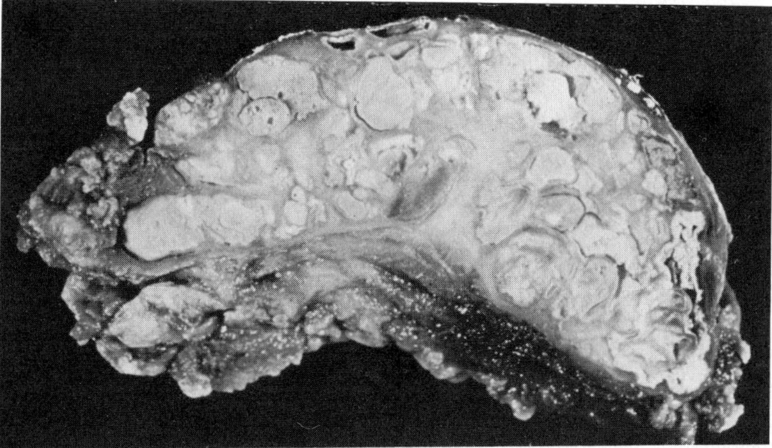

Figure 10–68. Bursitis. Excised specimen from the triceps muscle. These lesions are fairly well encapsulated and delineated, and they are relatively easy to resect surgically. If they are completely resected, they do not recur. They may have the clinical appearance of a myositis ossificans, although the calcification is usually more widespread throughout bursitis than in myositis ossificans, in which bone is formed primarily at the periphery of the lesion.

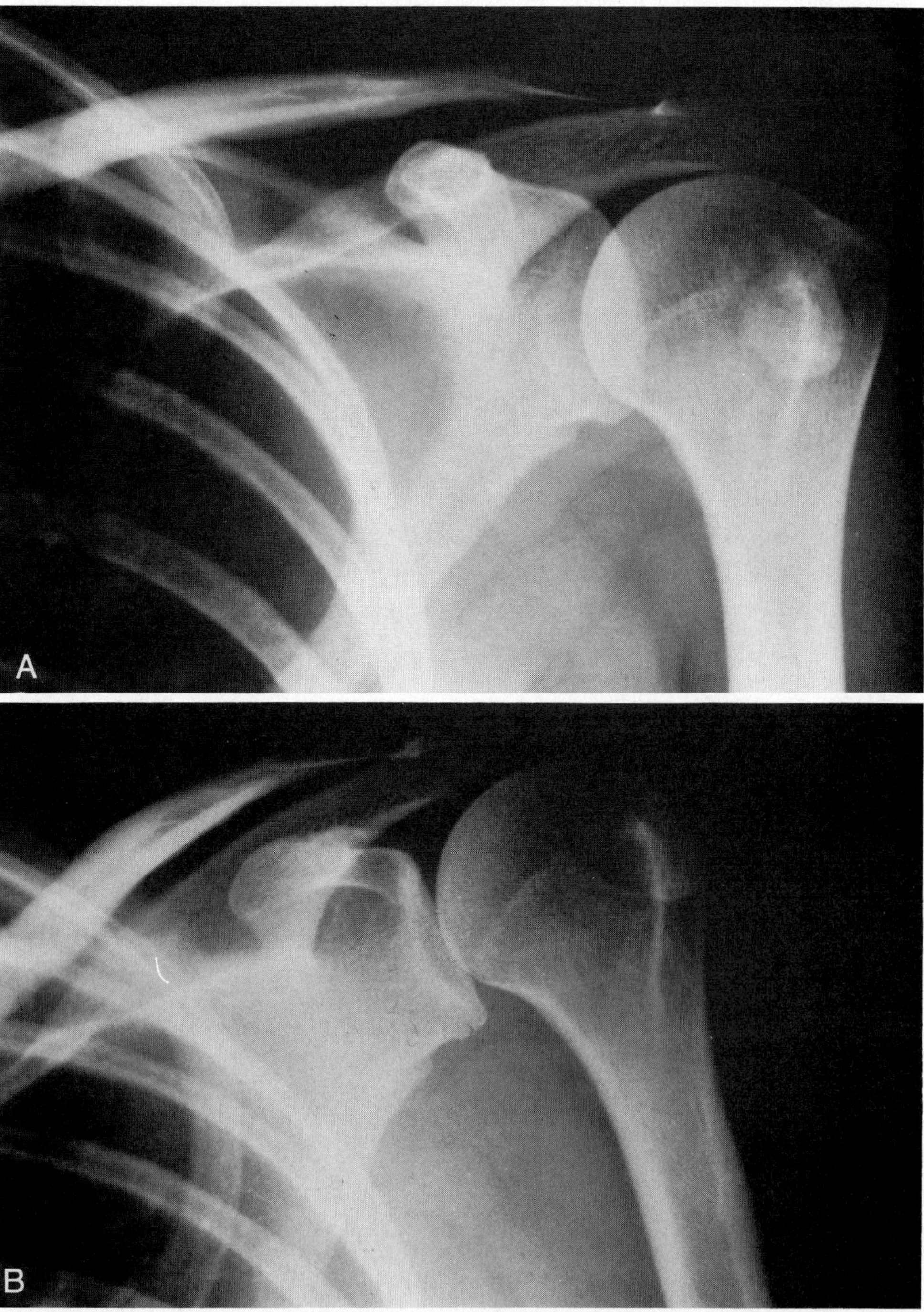

Figure 10–69. Bursitis. Proper positioning of the patient for radiographic demonstration of the calcified bursitis is necessary to avoid misinterpretation of the lesion. Note that only one of the four films *(D)* clearly demonstrates the extraosseous nature of the calcification process. The change in position of the lesion with different views alerts the physician to the extraosseous location.

Illustration continued on opposite page

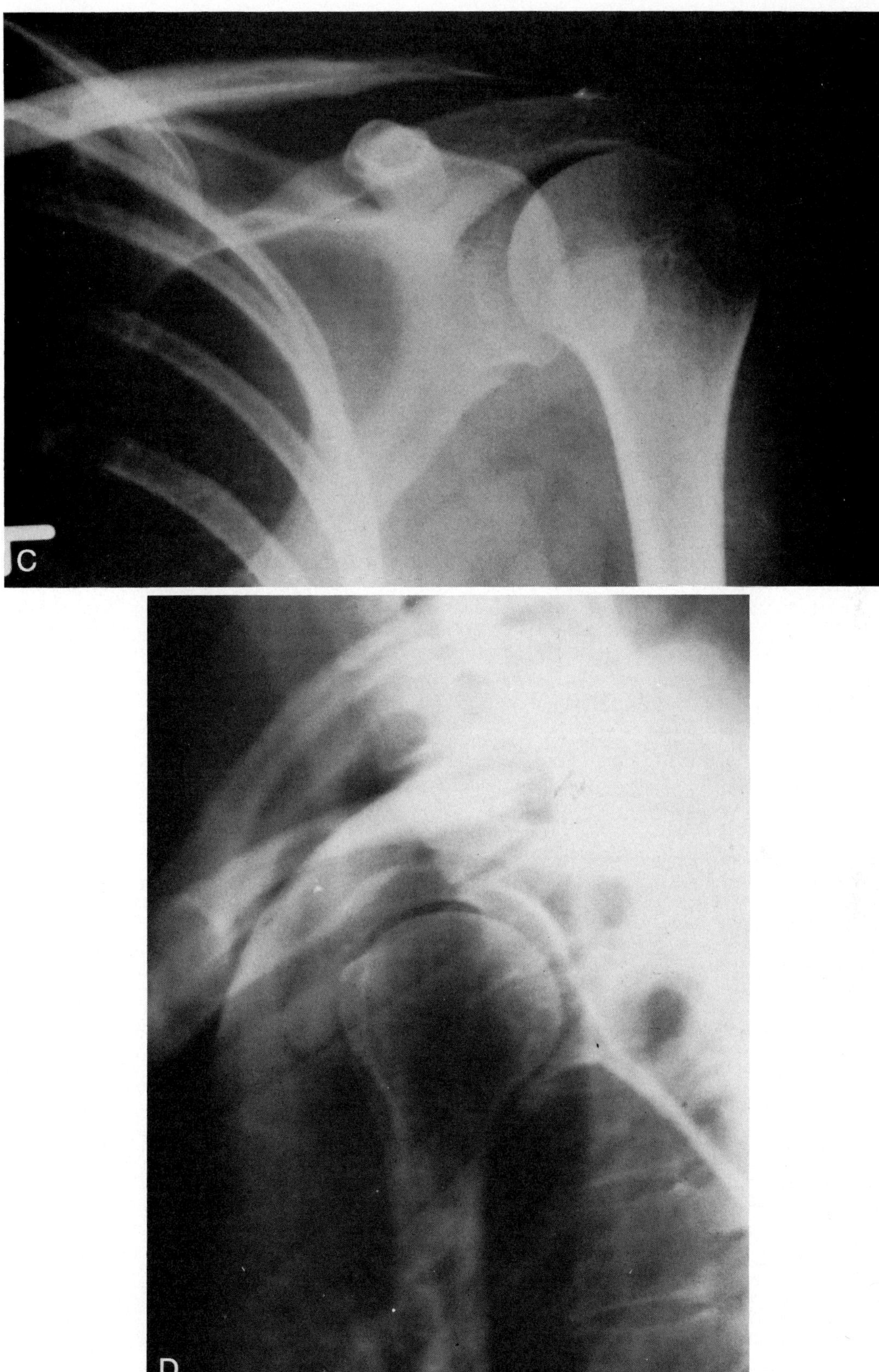

Figure 10–69 *Continued.*

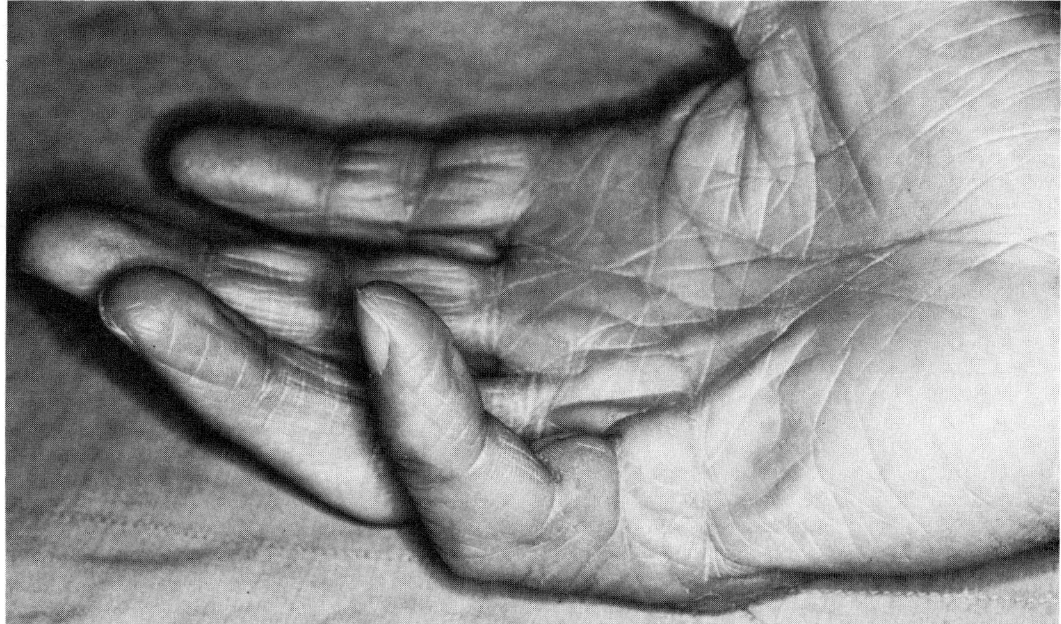

Figure 10–70. Clinical photograph of the hand of a patient with Dupuytren's contracture. The involvement of the palmar aponeurosis results in a combination of nodules and bands, with limitation of extension of the ring and little finger. The bands usually begin at the proximal palm and extend out toward the finger. Over a period of time, the contraction of these bands results in limitation of finger extension, although there is usually no limitation of flexion.

DUPUYTREN'S CONTRACTURE

Dupuytren's contracture is one of a series of fibromatoses that involve the palmar fascia of the hands and plantar fascia of the feet. It is a congenital inherited defect that results in characteristic bilateral contractures of the fingers. Histologically, it is

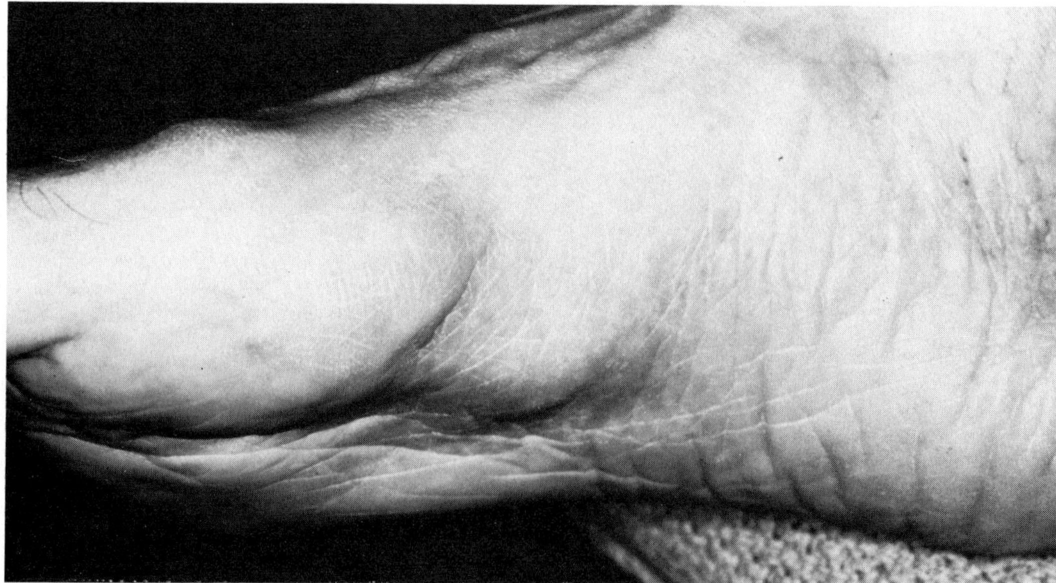

Figure 10–71. Clinical photograph of the foot of a 66-year-old man with Dupuytren's contracture. There are large nodules in the plantar fascia of the foot. Unlike nodules in the hand, these seldom cause contractures in the foot.

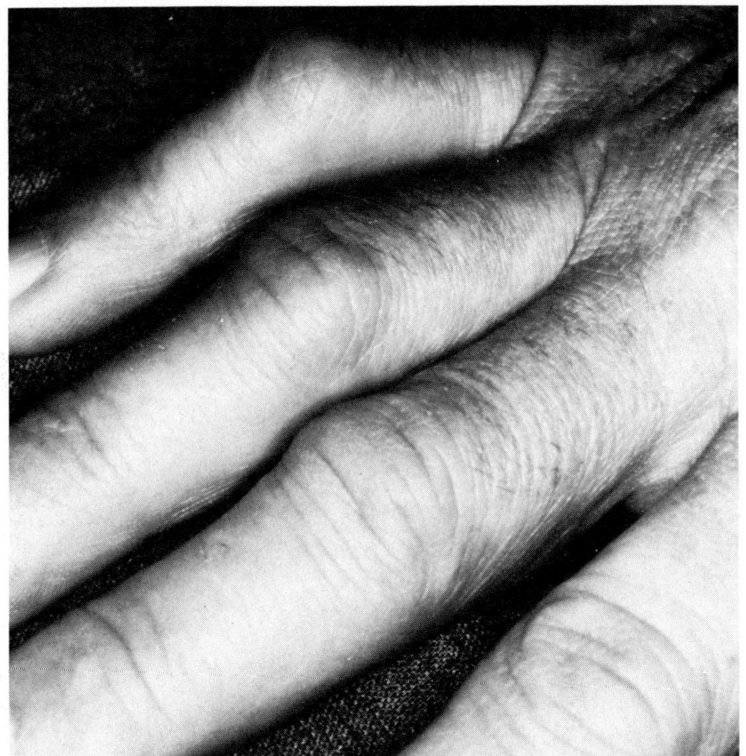

Figure 10–72. Dorsal view of the fingers of a 54-year-old patient with Dupuytren's contracture. Knuckle pads over the dorsal proximal interphalangeal joint are common in the disease. Histologically, they have the same appearance as the nodules in the palm; however, they do not cause extension contractures.

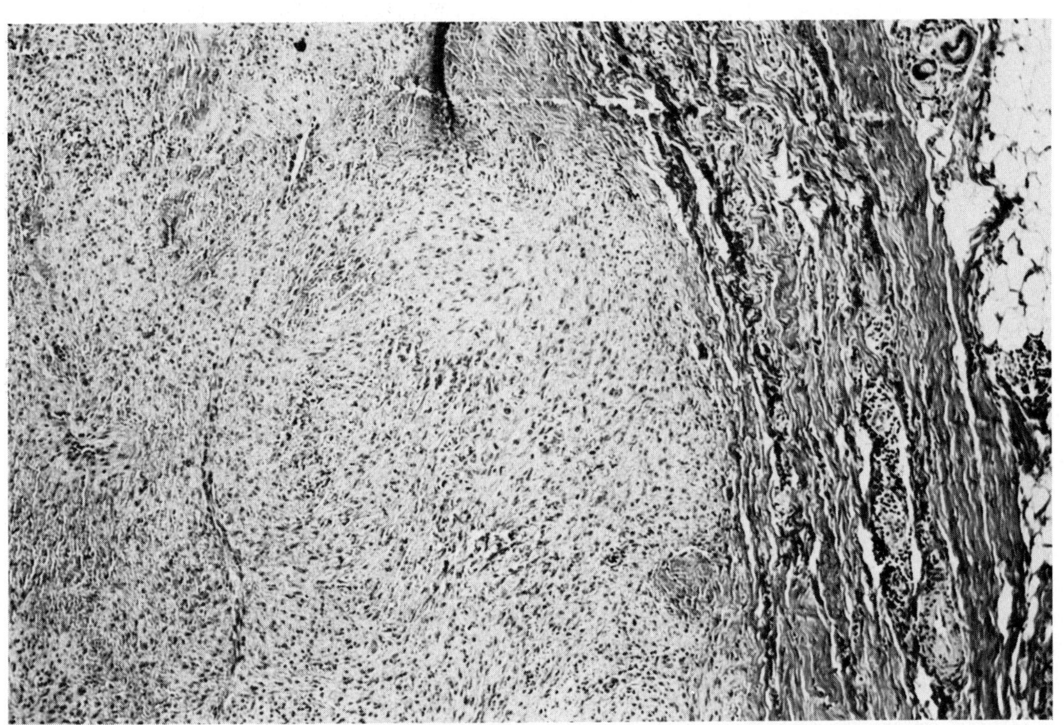

Figure 10–73. Low-power histologic appearance of an early Dupuytren's nodule from the palmar aponeurosis. The lesion is clearly demarcated from the subcutaneous fat. The immature lesions are quite cellular, without much collagen production.

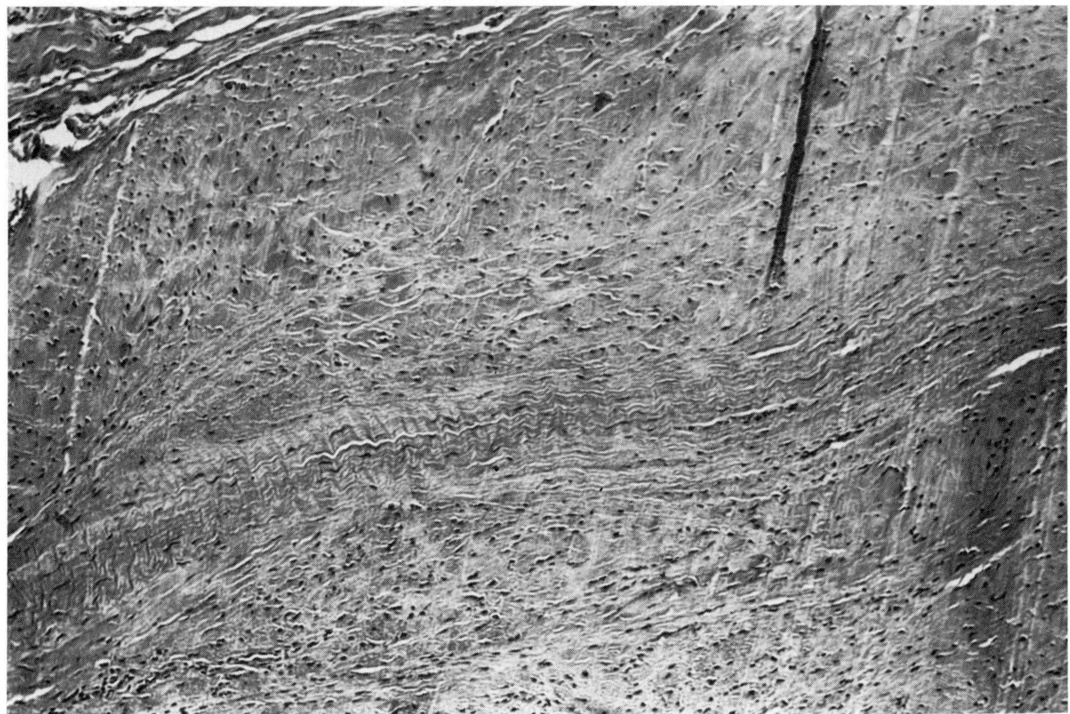

Figure 10–74. Histologic appearance of a mature nodule of Dupuytren's disease. Compared with Figure 10–73, this illustration demonstrates less cellularity, and unlike the previous figure, it shows extensive collagen fiber production.

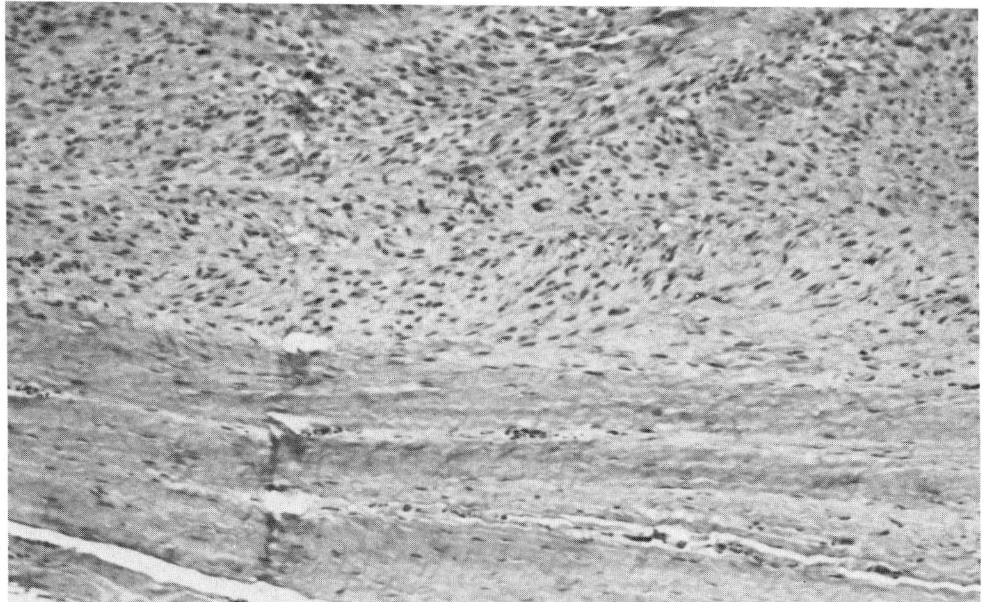

Figure 10–75. Dupuytren's contracture. Histology of a junction of a nodule with a cord. There is a heavy collagen production at the edge of the nodule. Some cellularity remains in the center of the lesion. Inflammatory cells and hemosiderin deposits are not prominent.

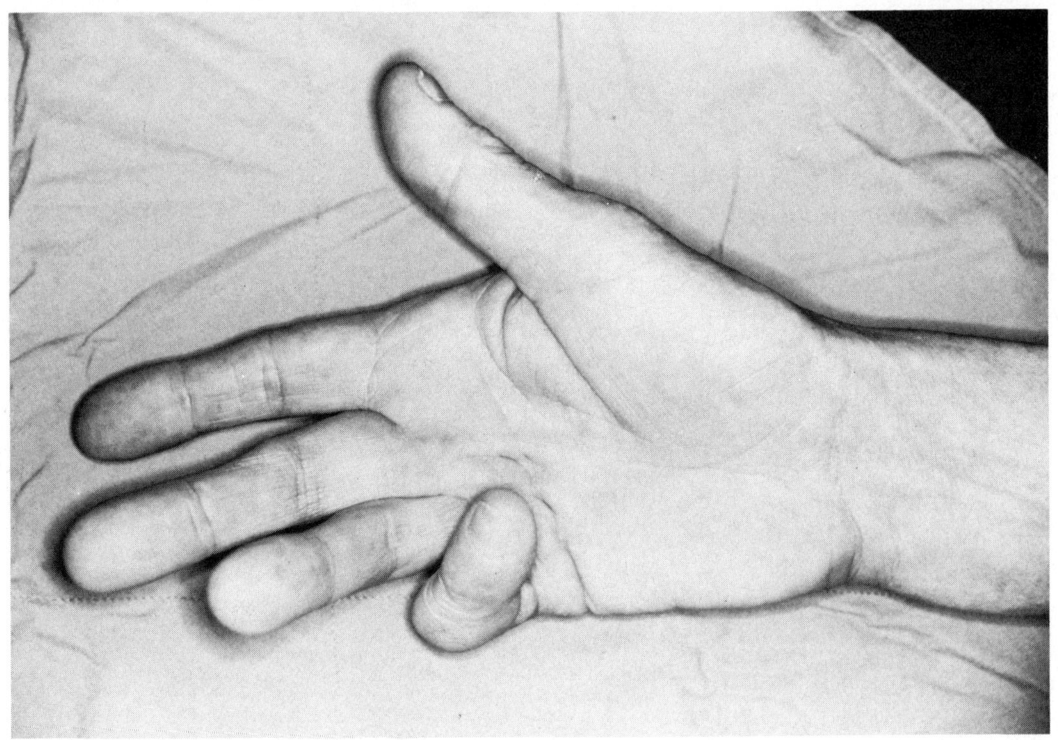

Figure 10–76. Clinical photograph of the hand of a 57-year-old man with Dupuytren's disease. The bands extend out to the middle, ring, and little fingers. Commonly, the abductor digiti minimi is extensively involved and causes rotation of the little finger along with its flexion contracture.

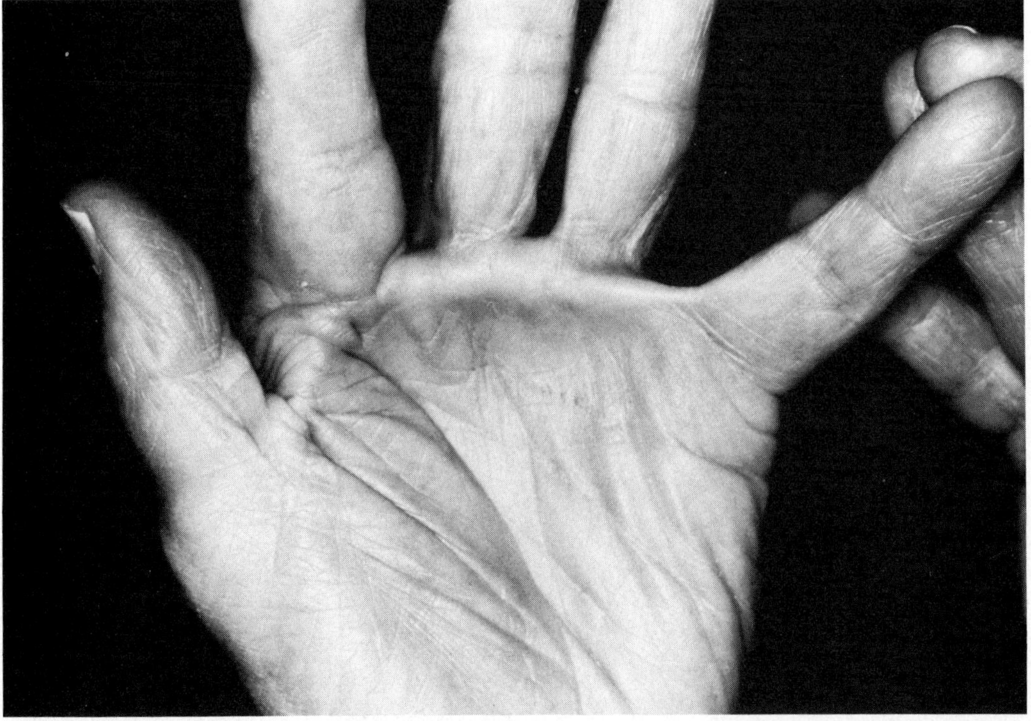

Figure 10–77. Dupuytren's contracture. In this hand, the natatory ligament is extensively involved, with limited separation of the fingers and the thumb. The longitudinal bands are much less prominent, although the other hand had extensive metacarpophalangeal and proximal interphalangeal contractures. The disease is usually bilateral, although clinical manifestation in the two hands may be quite different.

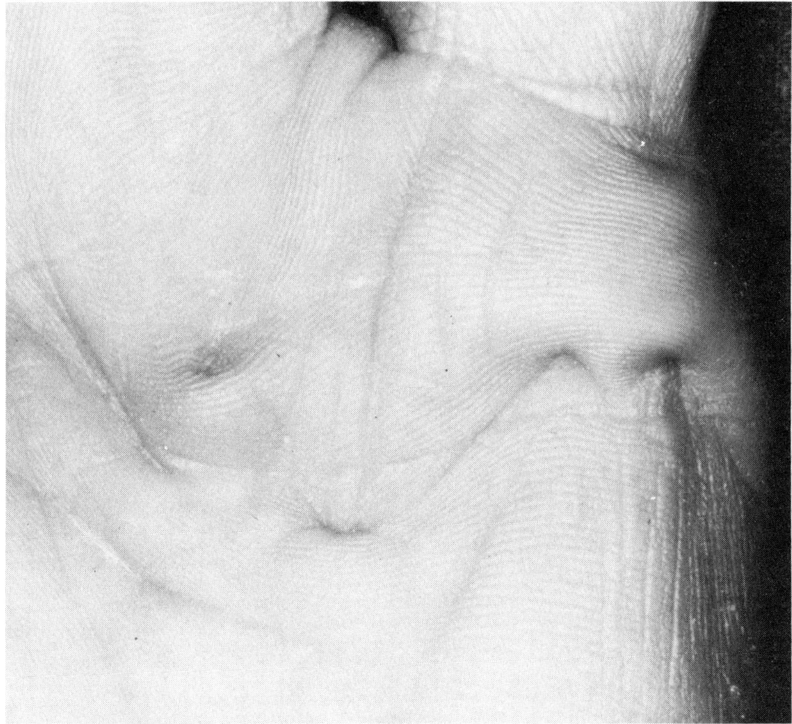

Figure 10–78. Nodules of Dupuytren's disease causing dimpling, or pits, in the skin surface. These are due to involvement of the septa between the skin and the palmar aponeurosis, which normally hold the skin in place during gripping activities.

characterized by areas of bland, relatively acellular connective tissue that alternate with nodules of cellular proliferation. The lesion is histologically similar to torticollis, extra-abdominal desmoid, and fibromatosis in numerous other locations within the skeletal musculature. Plantar fibromatosis, although histologically similar to palmar lesions, seldom results in contractures of the foot. All fibromatoses, regardless of site, have no metastatic potential, although their propensity to infiltrate into the adjacent tissue is well known. Dupuytren's contracture has limited potential for extension into adjacent soft tissue and tends to remain localized.

Text continued on page 642

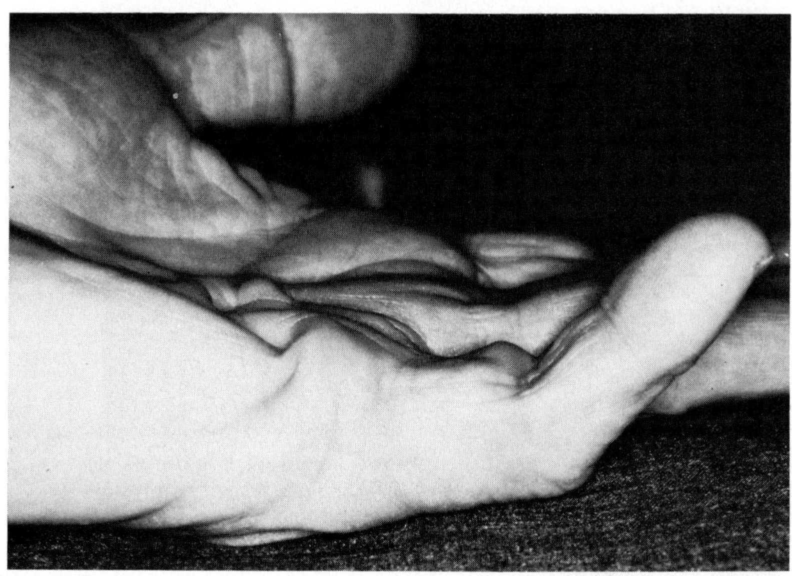

Figure 10–79. Dupuytren's contracture. Lateral photograph of the little finger showing marked dimpling that occurs when the patient attempts to extend. Nodules extending into the proximal phalanx of the finger cause contracture of the proximal joint.

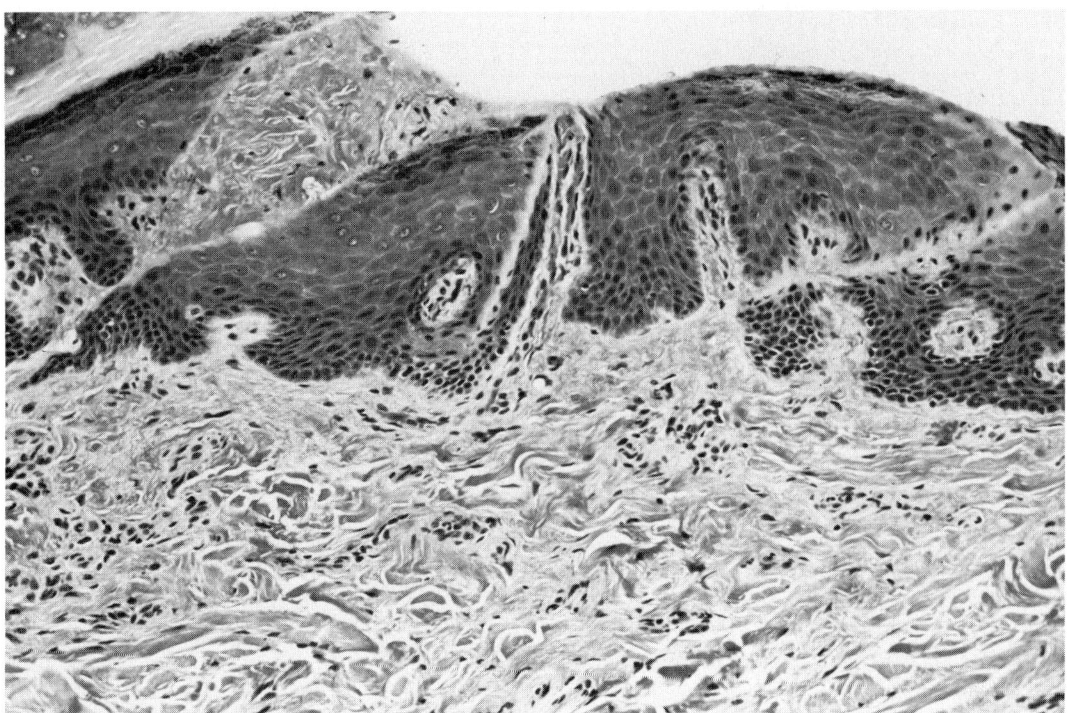

Figure 10–80. Dupuytren's contracture. Histologic appearance of skin demonstrating extensive involvement of the deep layers by the collagenized nodule. Note extension of collagenized tissue into the epidermis.

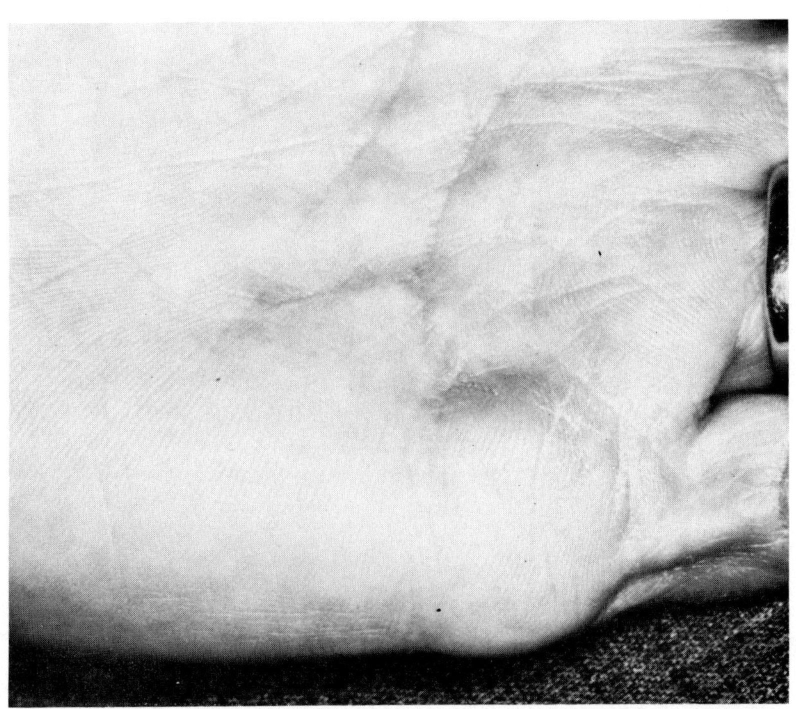

Figure 10–81. Clinical photograph of the hand of a 54-year-old man with different stages of active Dupuytren's disease. The cord extending to the long finger has been present for a number of years, the cord in the little finger has been present for 18 months, but the nodule overlying the metacarpophalangeal joint has been present for only 4 to 6 months, and during this time the patient experienced progressive contracture of the joint.

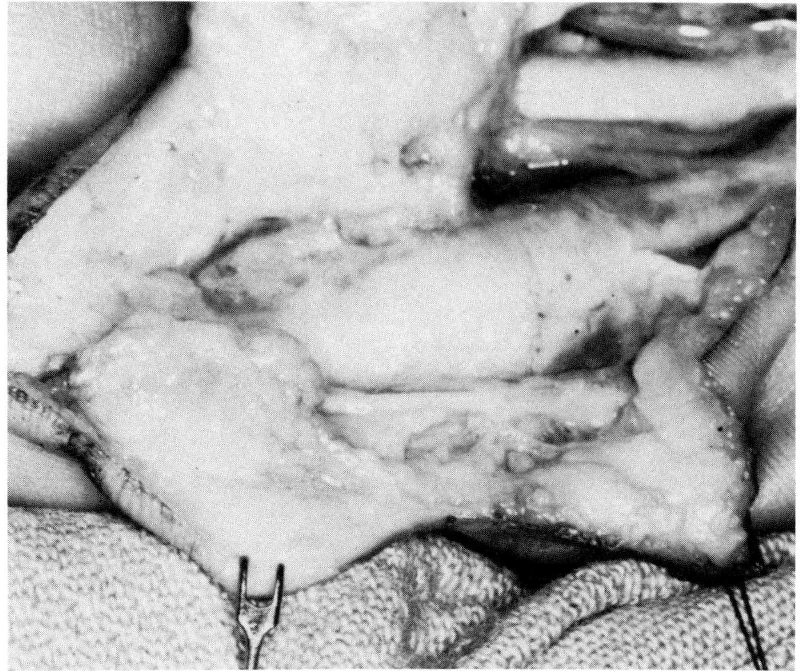

Figure 10–82. Dupuytren's contracture. Surgical exposure of the nodules evident in the previous figure. There is a large nodule in the tendon and insertion of the abductor digiti minimi. Extending distally from this is a cord that has been present for approximately 18 months.

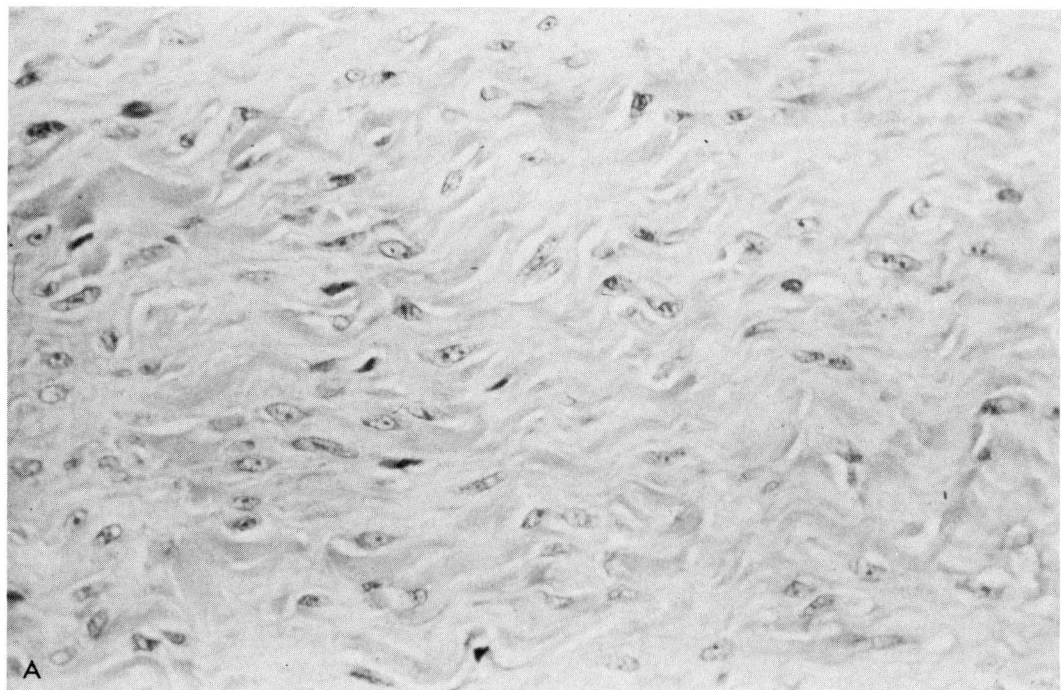

Figure 10–83. Dupuytren's contracture. These are sections taken from the 4- to 6-month-old nodule in the abductor digiti minimi of the hand shown in Figures 10–81 and 10–82. In *A*, there is moderate cellularity, with loose strands of collagen between the cells.

Illustration continued on opposite page

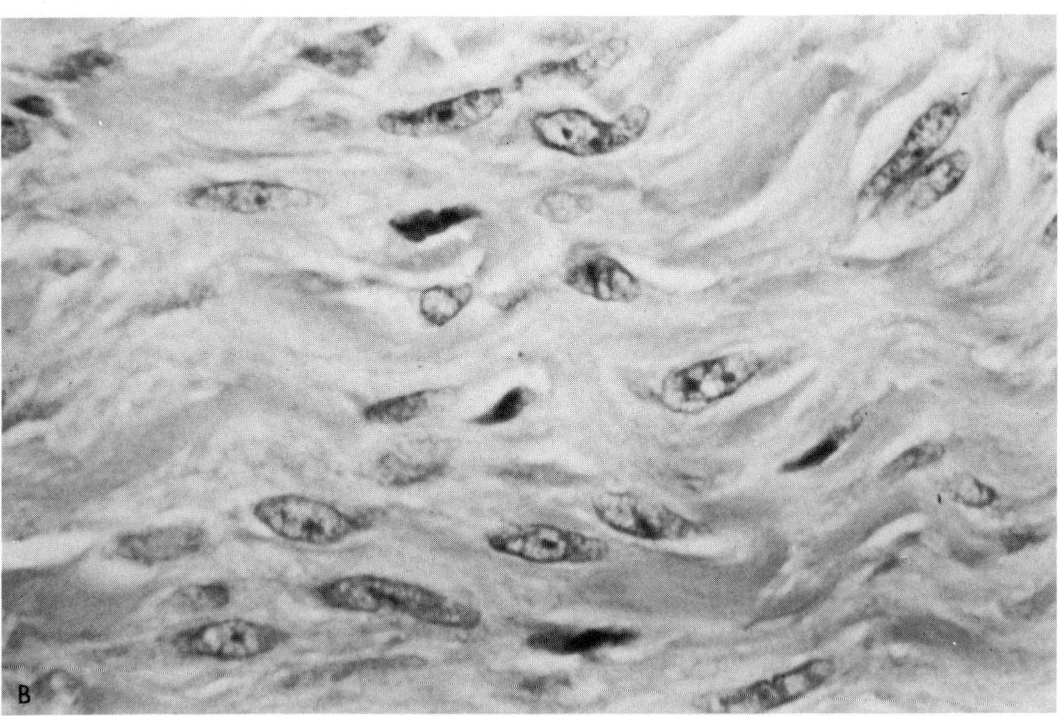

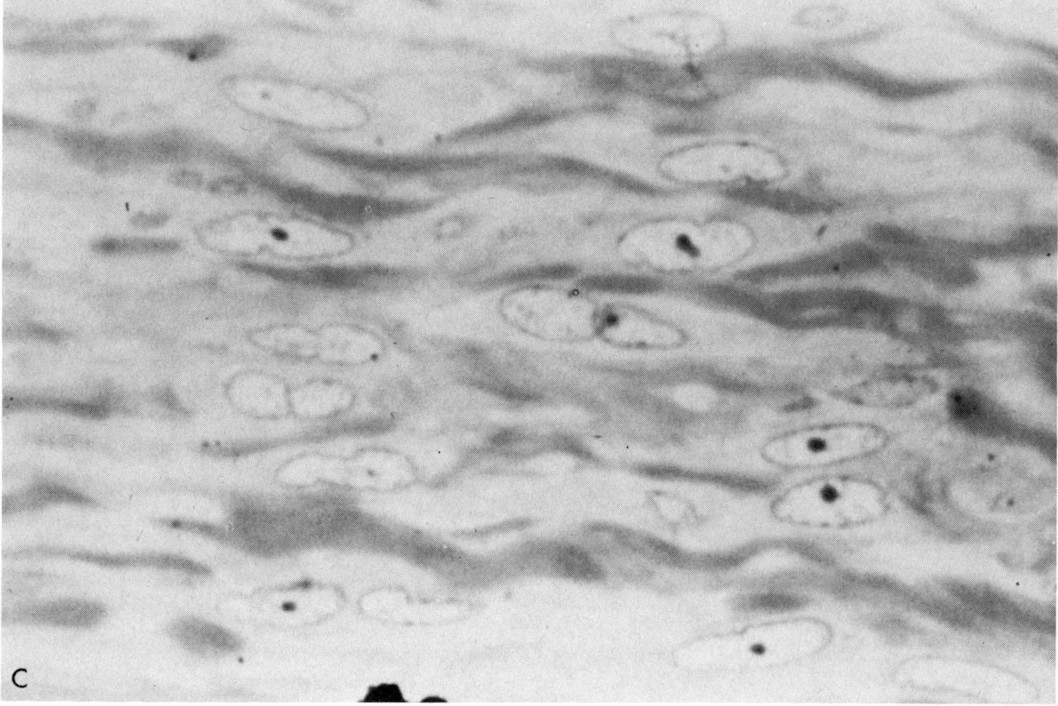

Figure 10–83 *(Continued)*. In *B*, the cell nuclei are quite distinct, with peripheral chromatin and a prominent nucleolus. Many of the nuclei are somewhat plump, although overall they are elongated, and there are numerous indentations along the nuclear surfaces. Collagen fibers are between the cells. In *C*, an ultrathin section from this nodule is depicted to show better nuclear detail. The peripheral chromatin and prominent nucleolus are characteristic of myofibroblasts because the cytoplasm contains fibers consistent with smooth muscle cells as well as a large amount of rough-surfaced endoplasmic reticulum, typical of pure fibroblasts. It is thought by some that this combination of contractile elements and collagen production leads to the progressive contracture.

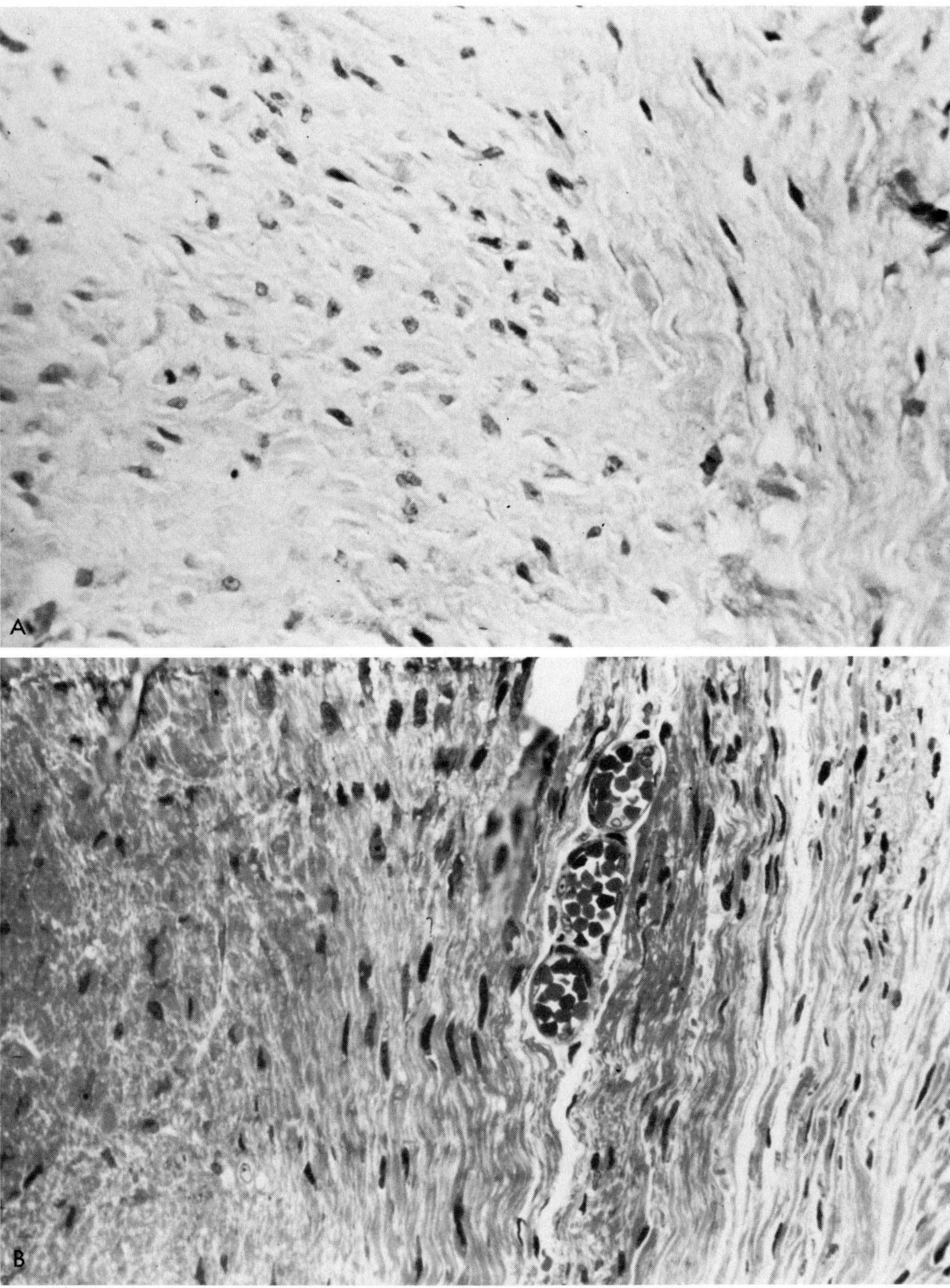

Figure 10–84. Dupuytren's contracture. Histologic sections from the 18-month-old nodular cord in the little finger of the hand shown in Figures 10–81 and 10–82. Note that there is much less cellularity here than in Figure 10–83. Also, the nuclei of the cells are more characteristic of normal fibroblasts, and the collagen is much better organized. The nuclei are elongated and lie between the collagen bundles. There is no significant indentation of the nuclei, and electromyography would not show the contractile elements in the cytoplasm.

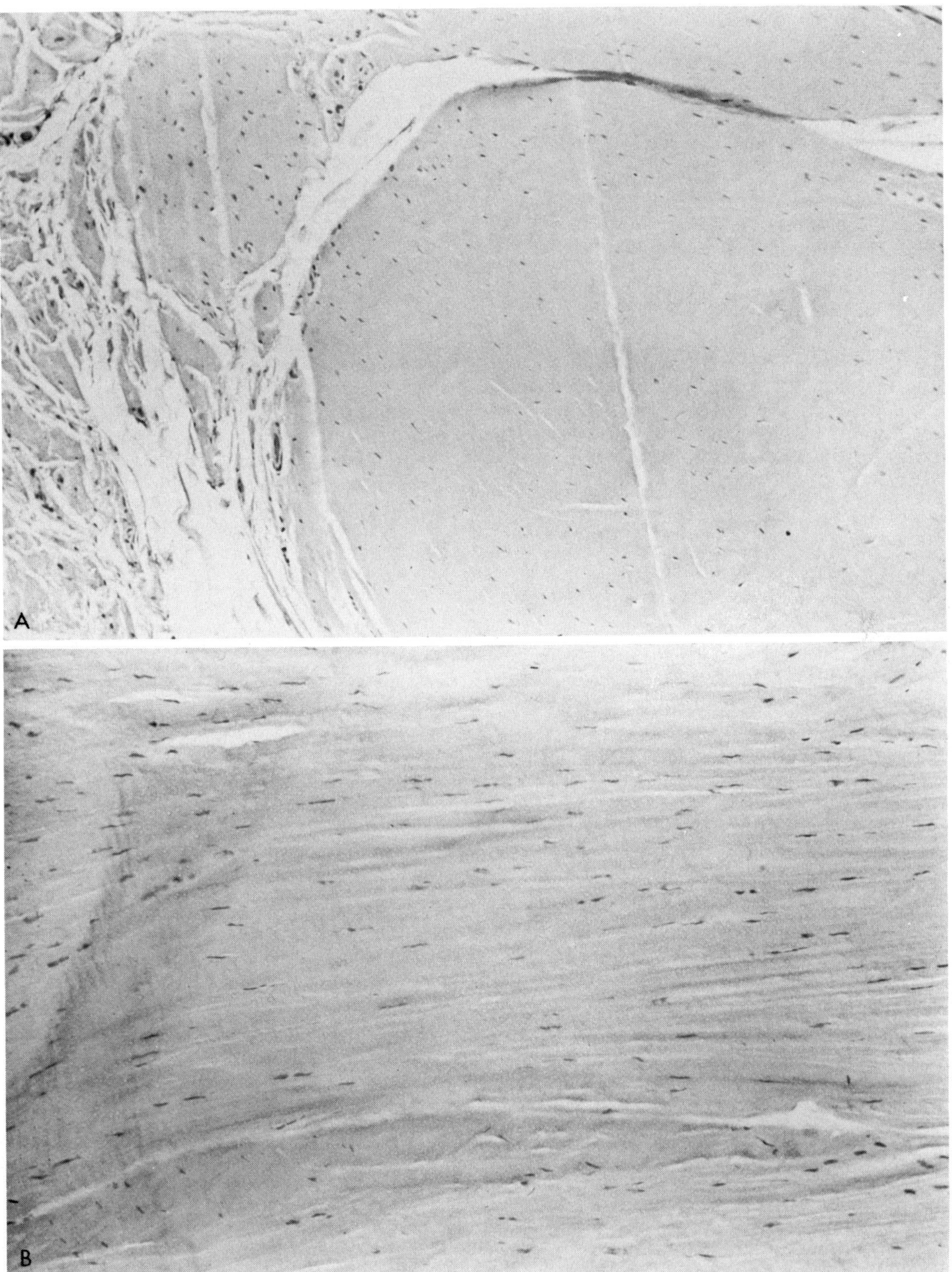

Figure 10–85. Dupuytren's contracture. Cross section *(A)* and longitudinal section *(B)* from the 12-year-old cord leading to the long finger of the hand illustrated in Figures 10–81 and 10–82. Here the cellularity is very sparse, and the collagen production and organization is very mature, almost tendon-like in consistency. This histologic picture is characteristic of the late cord. There are no contractile elements present.

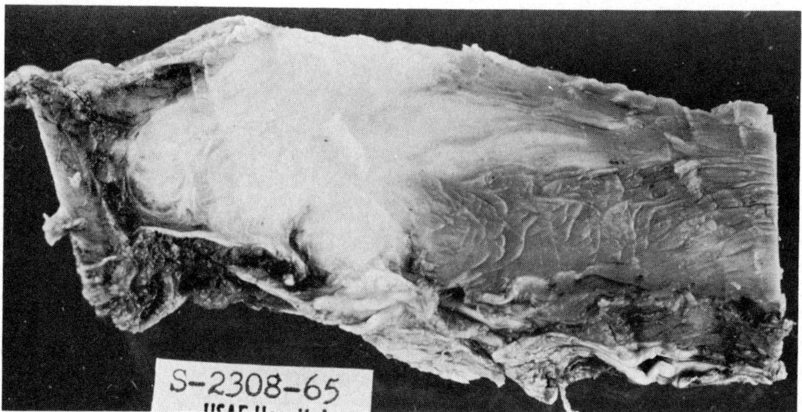

Figure 10–86. Fibromatosis (extra-abdominal desmoid). Fibromatosis involving the skeletal musculature of the extremities is locally aggressive. Note the insidious penetration of the deltoid muscle. There is danger that the surgeon will underestimate the degree of infiltration and perform an incomplete excision. The risk of subsequent recurrence is therefore high.

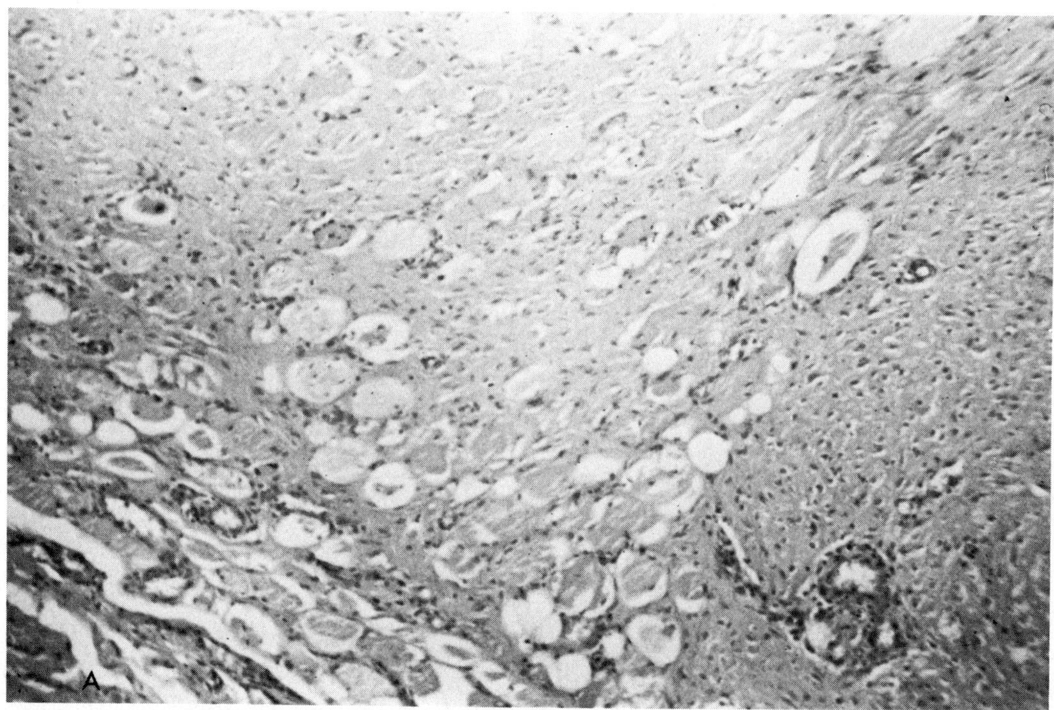

Figure 10–87. Histologic appearance of extra-abdominal desmoid illustrated in Figure 10–86. Infiltration of benign-appearing, heavily collagenized tissue into and around individual muscle fibers ultimately leads to atrophy of the fibers. This pattern of infiltration extends deeply into the muscle fibers and is responsible for the high recurrence rate.

Illustration continued on opposite page

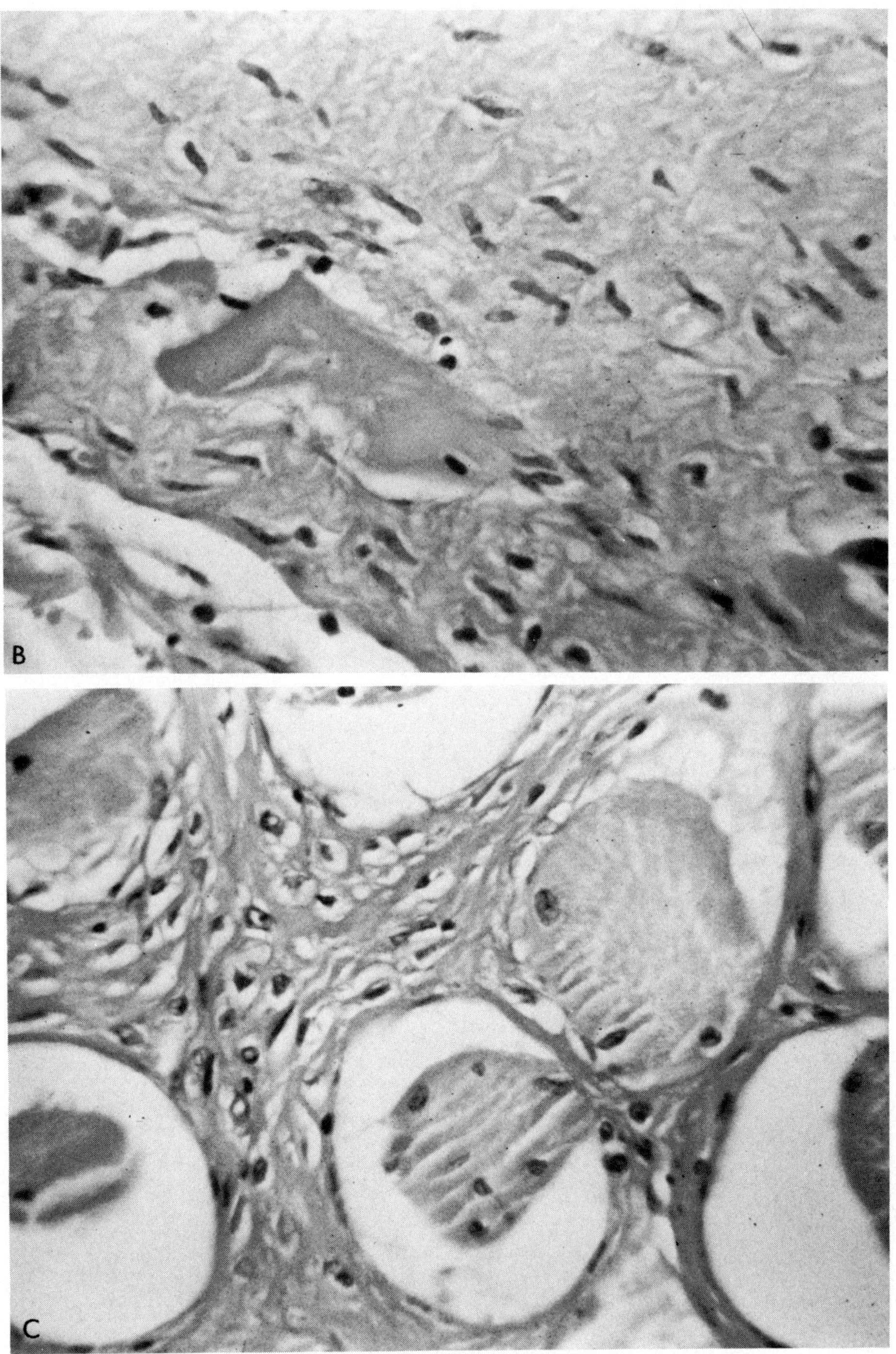

Figure 10–87 *Continued.*

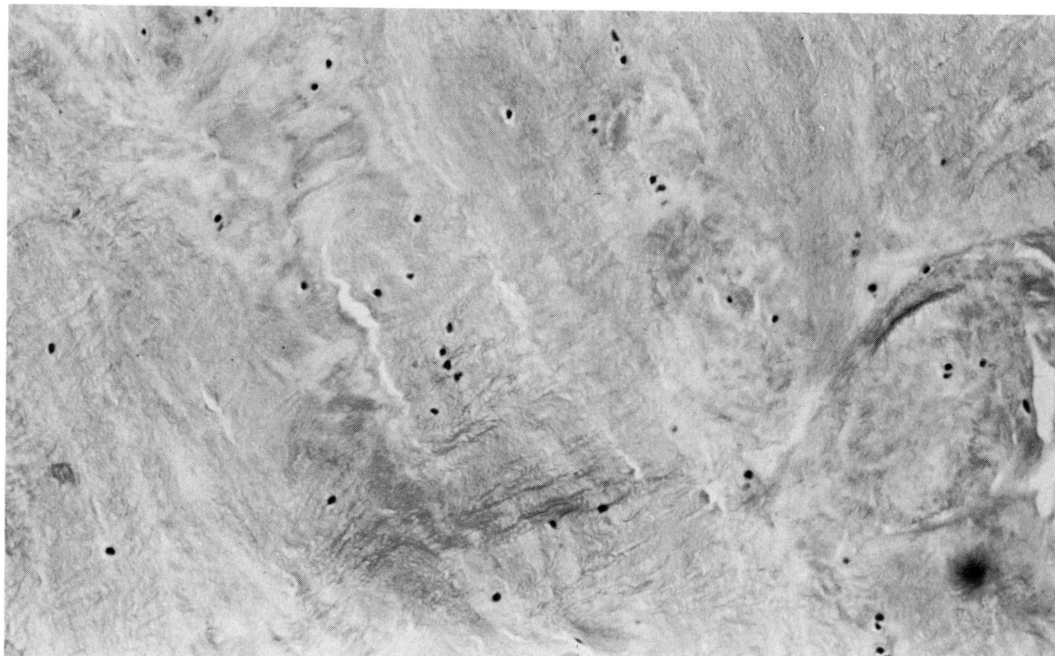

Figure 10–88. Meniscus. Heavily collagenized connective tissue characteristic of a normal meniscus.

MENISCAL INJURY

Under normal circumstances, the meniscus is composed of relatively acellular collagen bundles without clefts and demonstrates no chondroid metaplasia. Injury to the meniscus can be acute or cumulative. In the case of acute injury, no morphologic

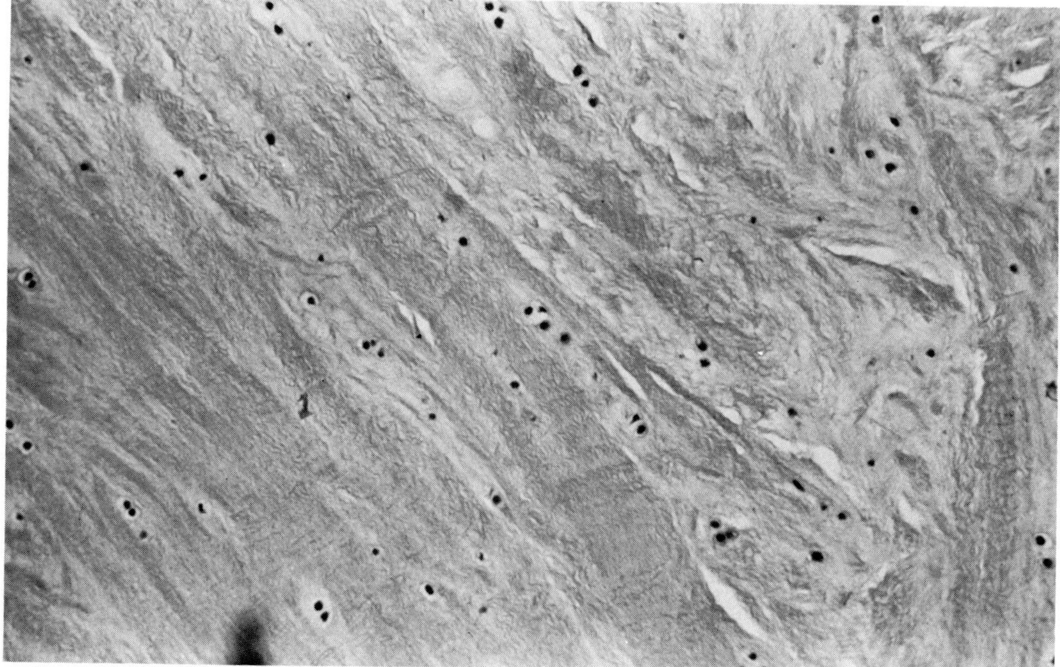

Figure 10–89. Fibrillary change in mild meniscal injury.

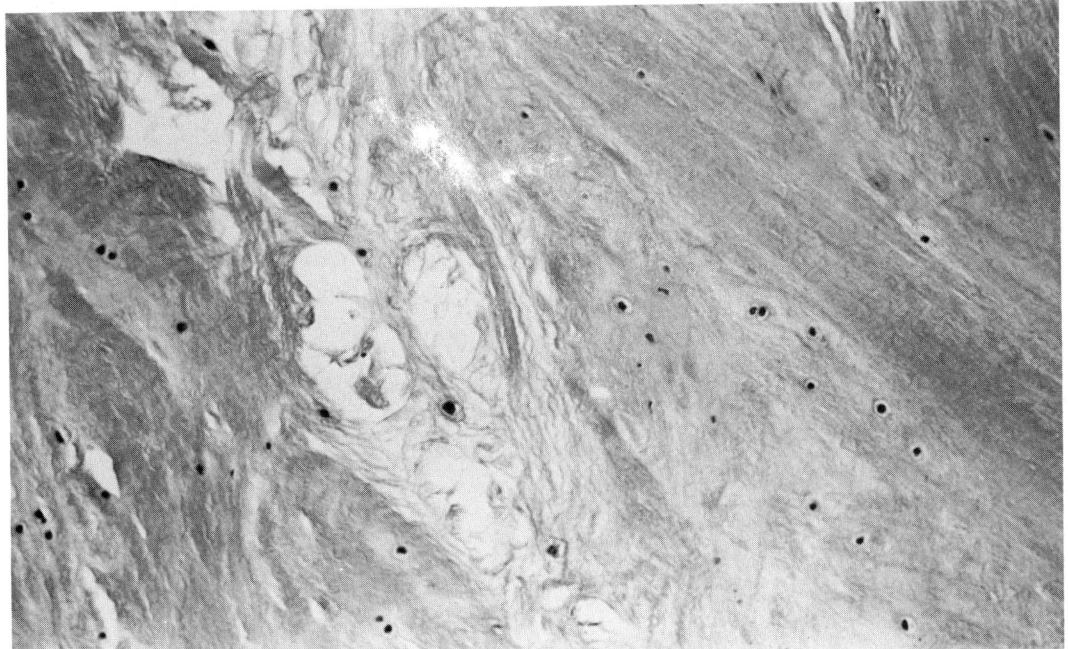

Figure 10–90. Early cyst formation in meniscal injury.

evidence of antecedent degeneration is noted. In those instances in which the injury is repetitive, degenerative changes are identified. These consist of cyst formation within the collagen bundles, chondroid metaplasia, and cleft formation. In severe injuries, cystic degeneration of the meniscus is identified.

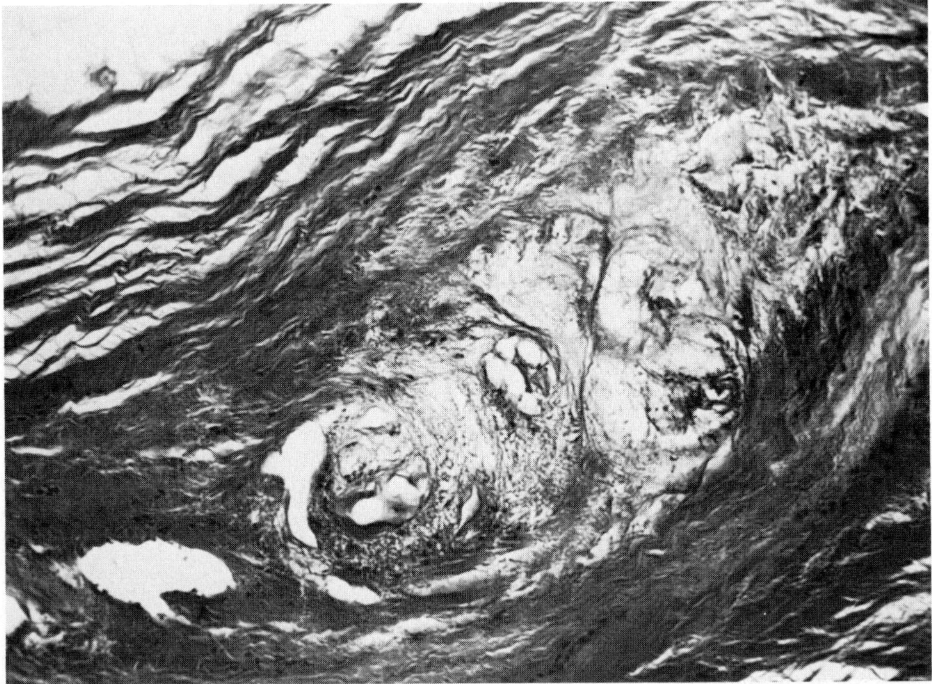

Figure 10–91. Severe myxoid degeneration of collagen leading to extensive cyst formation in meniscal injury.

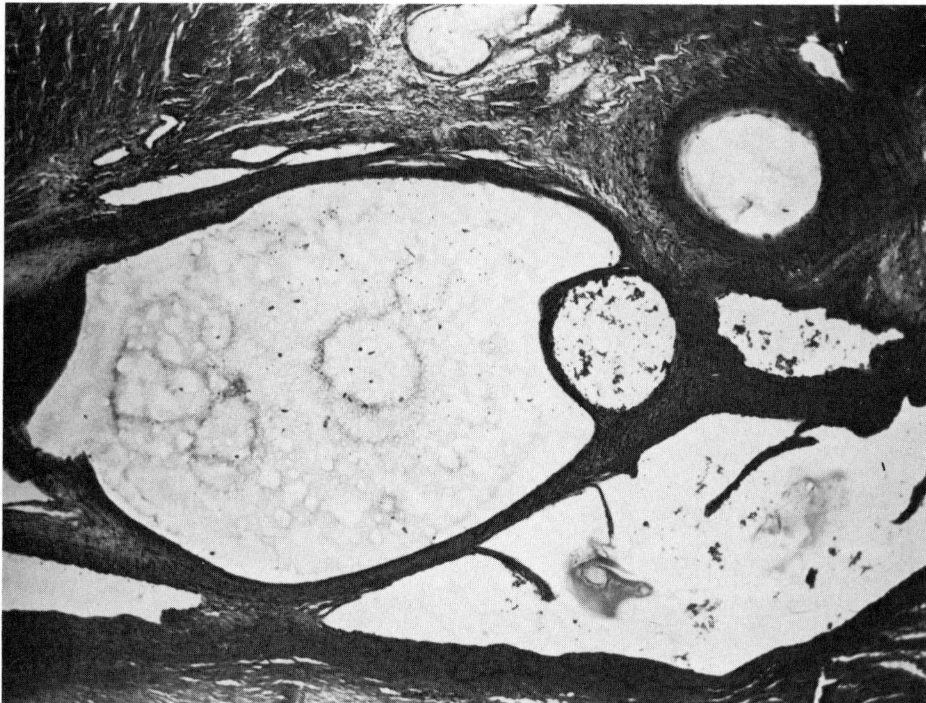

Figure 10–92. Advanced cyst formation a meniscal injury. The changes seen in Figure 10–91 represent a spectrum of traumatic injury and tissue reaction to the injury. Foci of cartilaginous metaplasia may be found in all injured menisci.

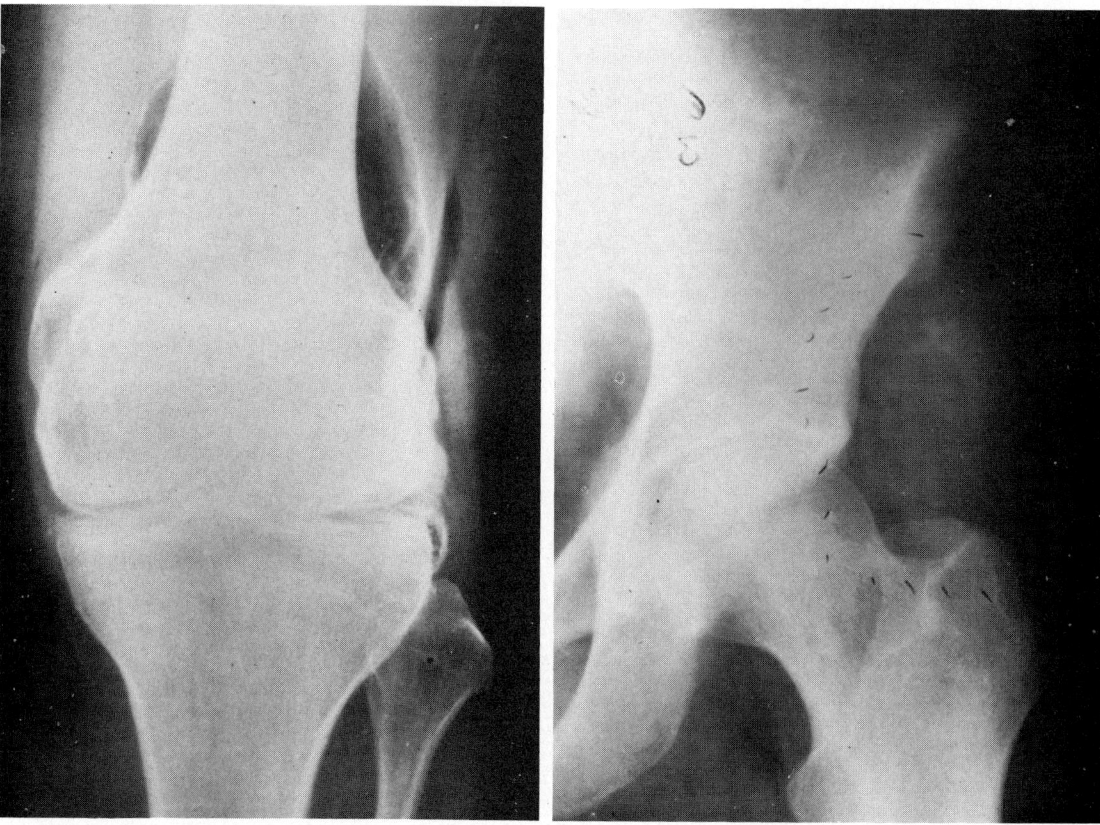

Figure 10–93

Figure 10–94

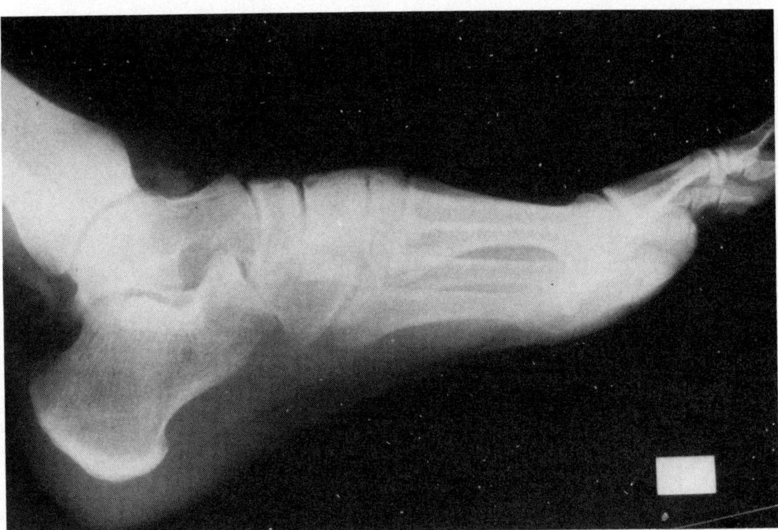

Figure 10–95. Synovial sarcoma. Radiograph of soft-tissue mass above the talus demonstrating hazy calcification. Calcification is not an invariable feature of synovial sarcoma, but it is present in more than 50 per cent of all tumors.

SYNOVIAL SARCOMA

Synovial sarcoma is a fairly common soft-tissue neoplasm that occurs in the para-articular regions. The lesion presents clinically as a soft-tissue mass, usually in proximity to the joint. It is uncommon for synovial sarcoma to be within the joint cavity. In a large number of cases it presents numerous small or spotty radiopacities caused by focal calcification within the lesion. This soft-tissue calcification suggests the diagnosis of synovial sarcoma. The more aggressive tumors secondarily involve bone.

One diagnoses the lesion by observing the characteristic spindle cell tumor. In most instances, a biphasic pattern is noted, with a spindle cell and a distinct epithelioid component. Careful observation and thorough sampling of the tumor usually disclose both cell types, although the spindle cell type may predominate.

The lesion has a history of dismal prognosis, even though long intervals between primary lesion and recurrence are documented. In recent years, the prognosis has improved somewhat, but the lesion is still associated with a 50 per cent mortality rate in most studies. Aggressive therapy is required when the lesion first presents itself.

Figure 10–93. Synovial sarcoma. Double-contrast arthrogram of a knee shows a partially calcified, poorly defined soft-tissue mass adjacent to the lateral condyle of the femur.

Figure 10–94. Synovial sarcoma. Radiograph of large soft-tissue mass with hazy, irregular calcification. The lack of maturation and zoning within the mass should cause the physician to suspect synovial sarcoma rather than myositis ossificans.

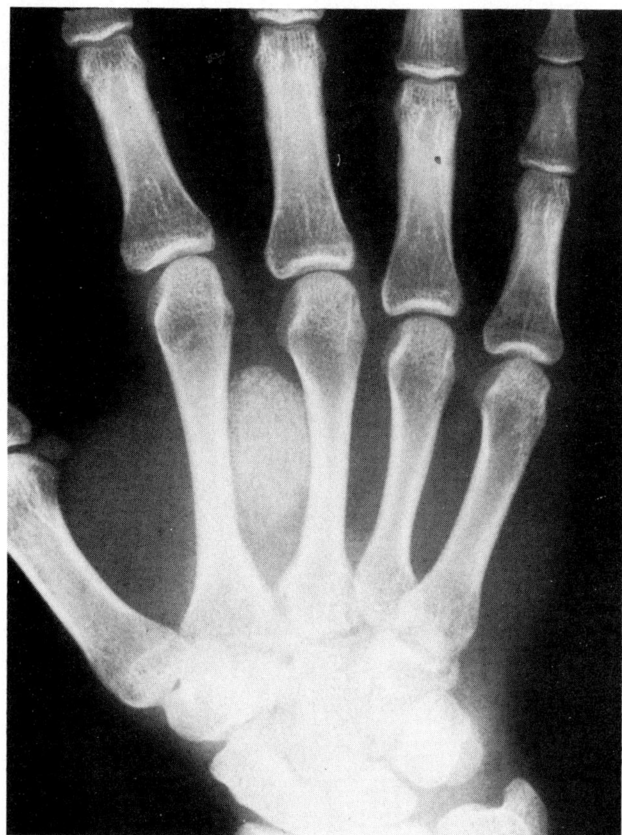

Figure 10–96. Synovial sarcoma. Radiograph of soft-tissue mass demonstrating extensive calcification adjacent to the second metacarpal. Despite this more intense calcification, neither zoning nor peripheral maturation is evident.

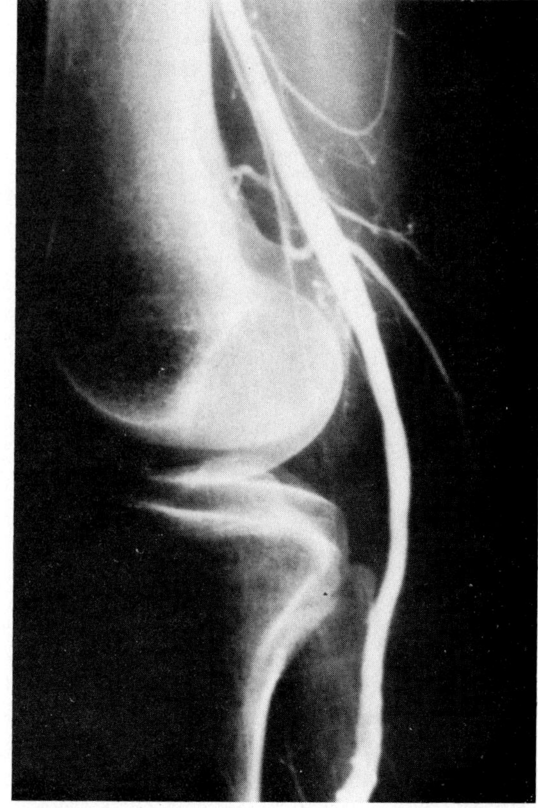

Figure 10–97. Lateral arteriogram of patient with popliteal synovial sarcoma. The tumor has no discernible calcification, but the extent of the lesion is detectable by the displacement of the popliteal artery.

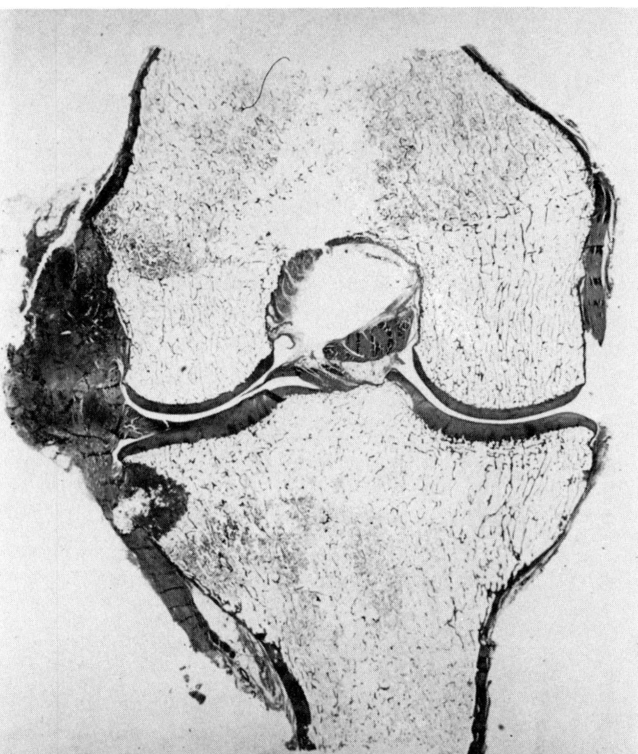

Figure 10–98. Macrospecimen of synovial sarcoma in soft tissue adjacent to the knee joint. Note the extension of the tumor into the tibia and femur.

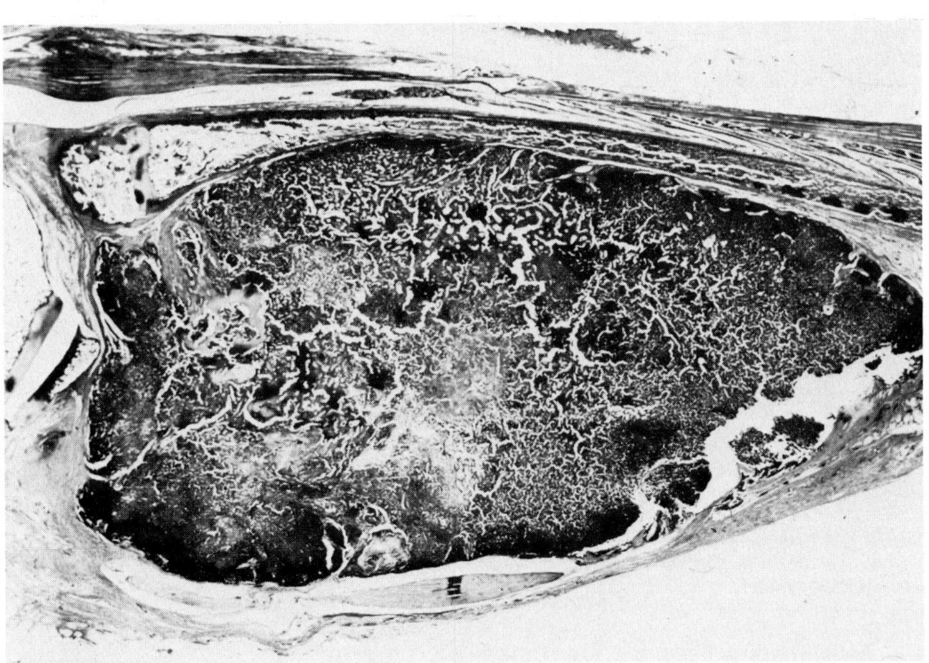

Figure 10–99. Synovial sarcoma. Macrospecimen of large circumscribed tumor in the soft tissue adjacent to the fibula. Despite apparent encapsulation, the tumor infiltrates into adjacent soft tissue. Simple excision of the nodule is almost invaribly followed by recurrence.

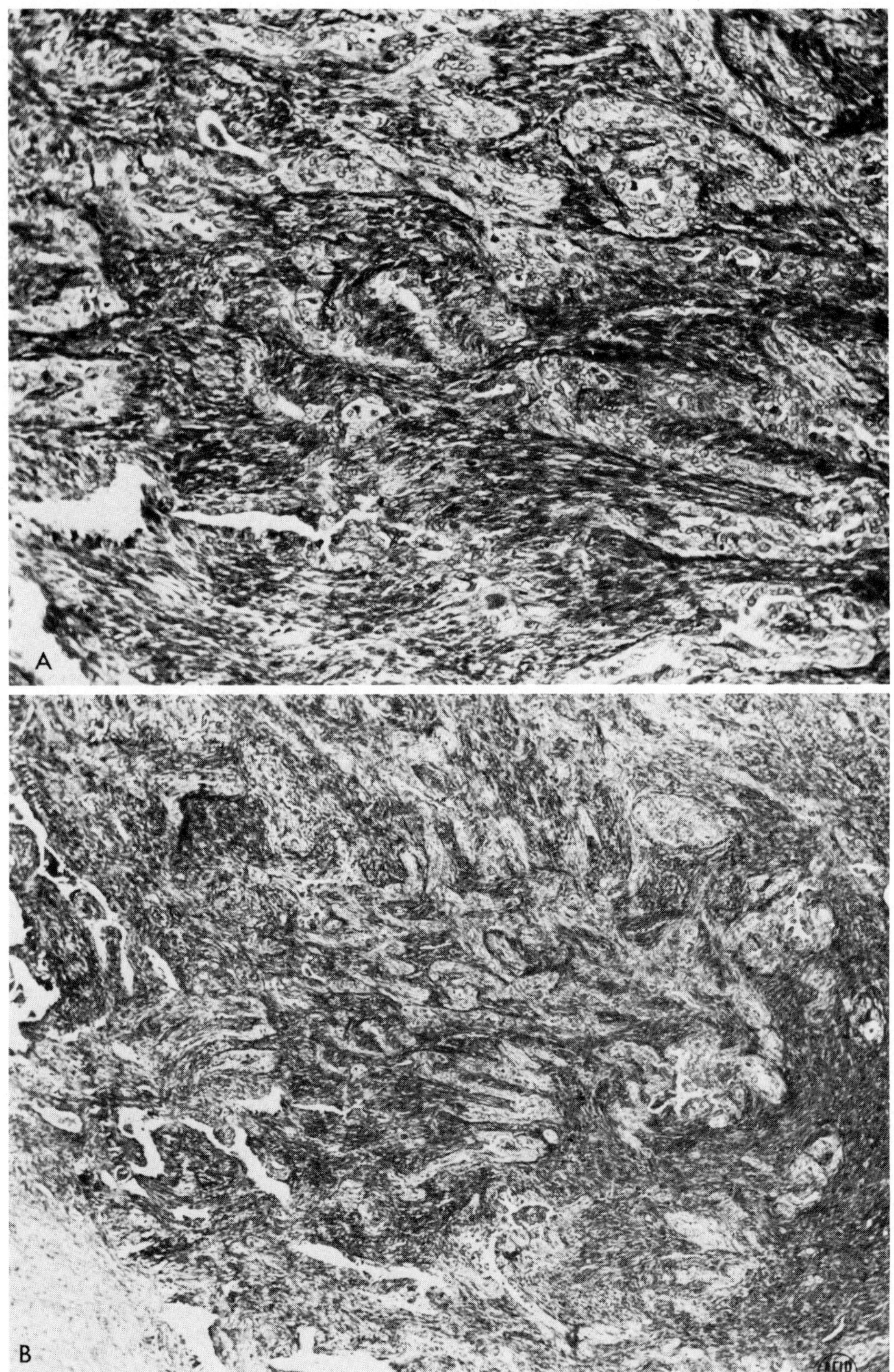

Figure 10–100. Biphasic pattern of synovial sarcoma is readily apparent in this illustration. A spindled, fibrosarcoma-like pattern is accompanied by clusters of tumor cells arranged in an epithelioid pattern.

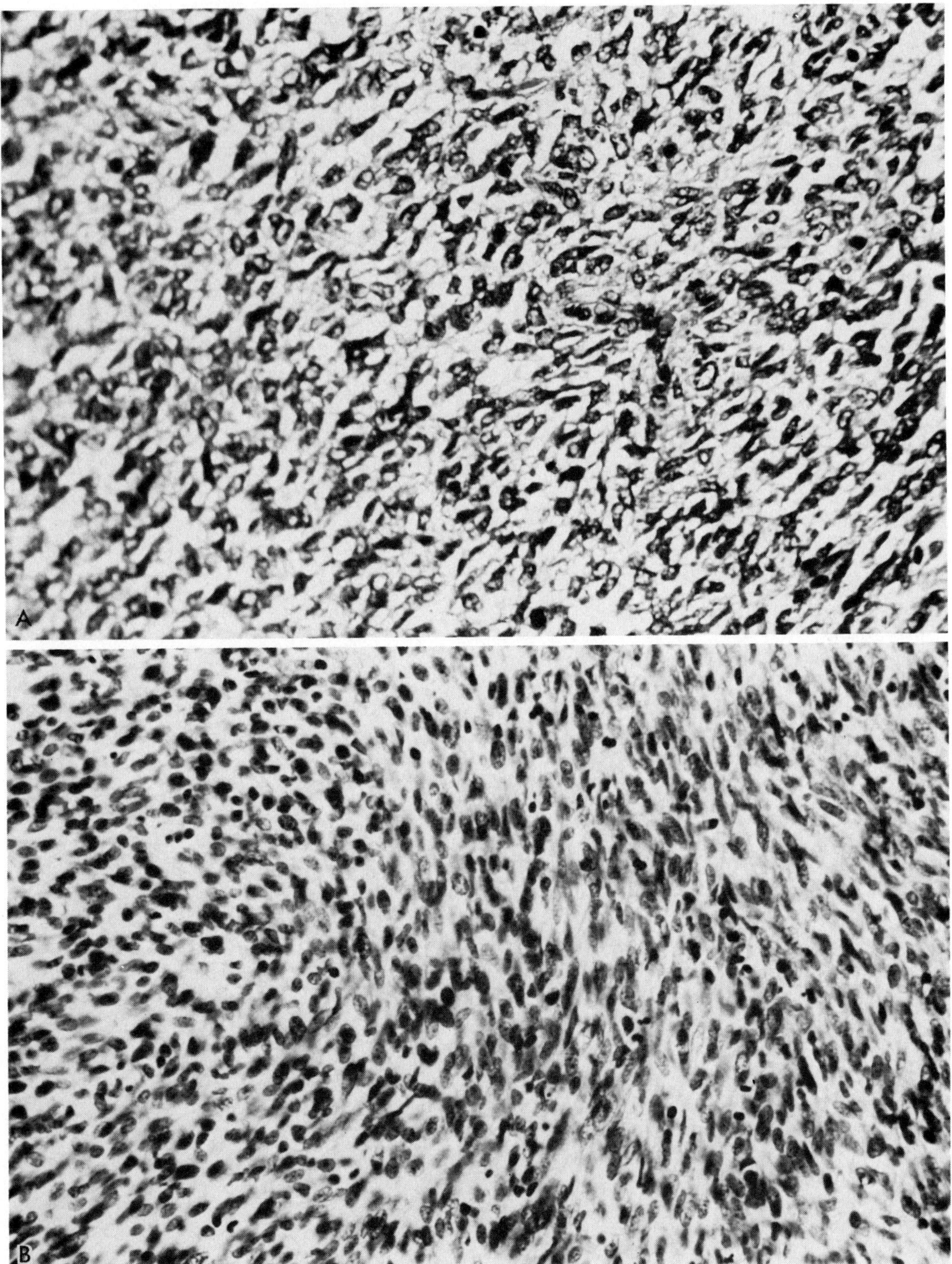

Figure 10–101. Higher magnification of the spindle-cell pattern in synovial sarcoma (compare with Figure 10–100). The tumor is highly cellular and moderately pleomorphic, but there is no discernible collagen formation.

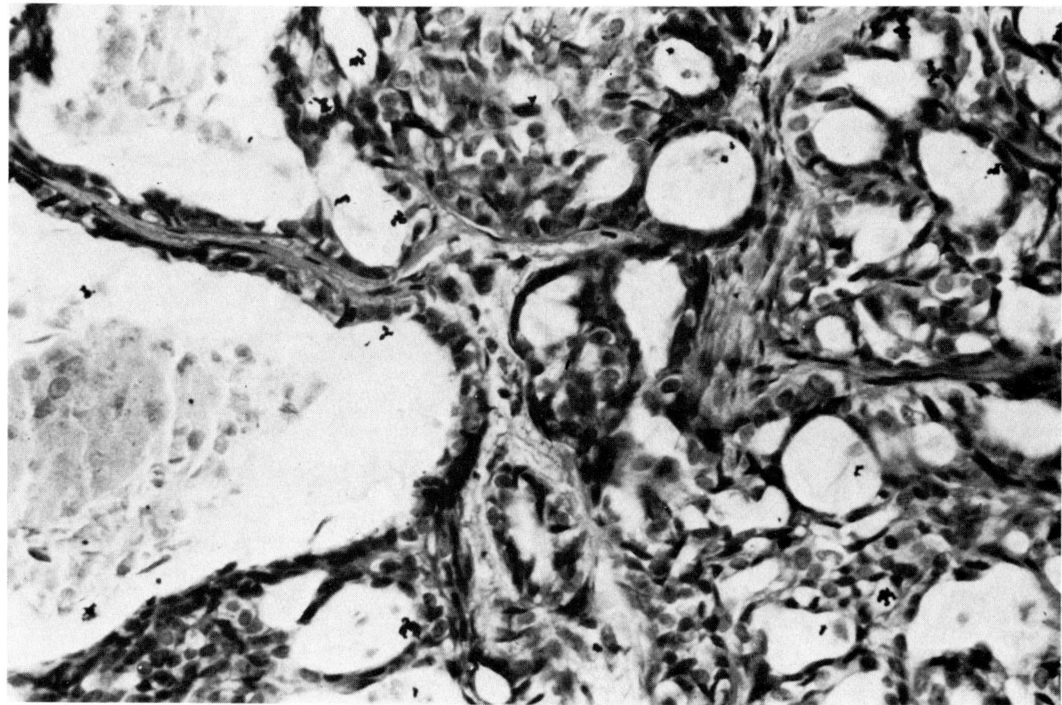

Figure 10–102. Higher magnification of epithelioid pattern in synovial sarcoma (compare with Figures 10–100 and 10–101). The pattern may be extensive and mimic an epithelial neoplasm. The secreted material is demonstrable with acid mucopolysaccharide stains (alcian blue).

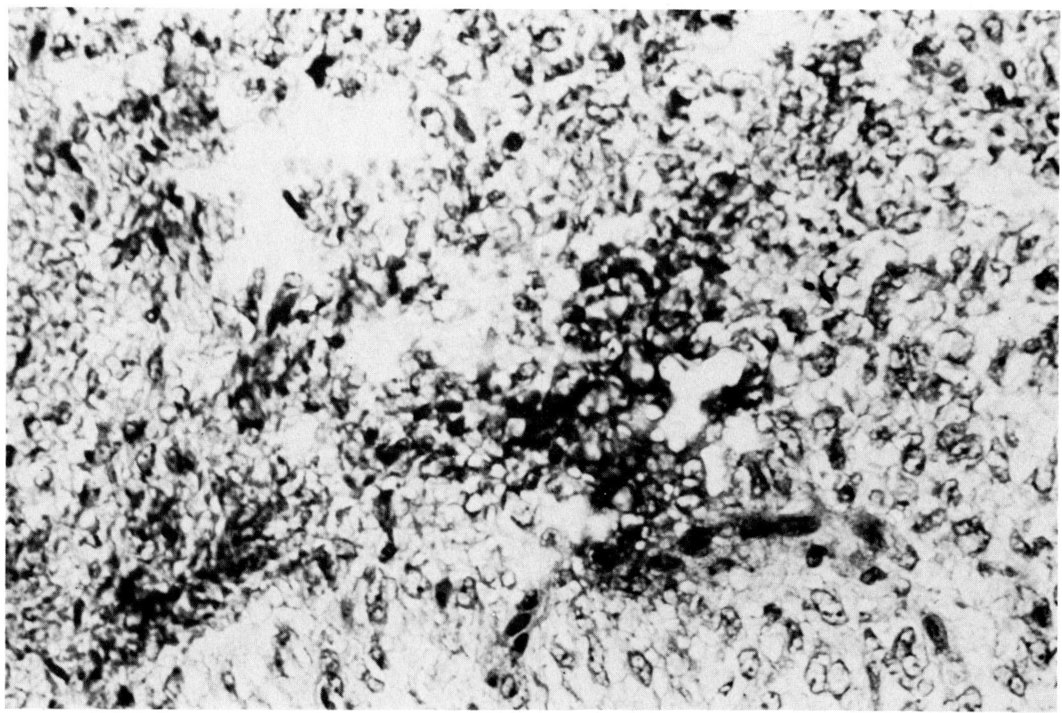

Figure 10–103. Focus of microscopic calcification in synovial sarcoma. Calcification, microscopic or grossly visible, is a common feature in synovial sarcoma.

GENERAL REFERENCE

Enzinger, F. M., and Weiss, S. W.: Soft Tissue Tumors. St. Louis, The C. V. Mosby Company, 1983.

CITED REFERENCES

Goldman, R. L., and Lichtenstein, L.: Synovial chondrosarcoma. Cancer 17:1233, 1964.
Unni, K. K., and Dahlin, D. C.: Premalignant tumors and conditions of bone. Am. J. Surg. Pathol. 3:47, 1979.

11

DIFFERENTIAL DIAGNOSIS OF BONE LESIONS

It has become an almost tiresome platitude that no bone biopsy should be performed without full exchange of data among clinician, radiologist, and pathologist prior to surgery. Despite this widely publicized admonition (Mankin, 1982; Simon, 1982), the pathologist often finds himself in the frozen-section area of the surgery suite confronted by an impatient surgeon, a fragment of tissue, no knowledge of clinical history or radiographic appearance, and the responsibility for attaching a diagnostic term to the disease process with its concurrent therapeutic implications. At other times, the pathologist is blessed with a "full" clinical history such as "lesion" or "tumor, left elbow" (with the insinuation that lesions of the left elbow are markedly different from those of the right). In most instances, the pathologist is not particularly well versed in differential diagnosis of the radiographic lesions, and the necessary effort to find the radiologist and discuss the differential with the surgeon often seems a logistically formidable task. Conversely, many clinicians are under the impression that the Deity converses with the pathologist directly from Mount Sinai, assuring absolute infallibility, or, in the event that communication is interrupted, that every nonossifying fibroma of bone has the letters "NOF" indelibly imprinted in hematoxylin and eosin on the slide the minute it emerges from the laboratory. Alas, there is no direct communication line to heaven; the subject is difficult; it is an art, not a science; despite logistical problems, full consultation is required to protect the patient from therapeutic misadventure. Disaster is avoided when all three specialists plan the approach together and assure themselves that the biopsy site is appropriate, that the biopsy diagnosis is consistent with the radiographic and clinical findings, and that the biologic potential of the process is correctly assessed prior to therapy.

The illustrations in this chapter are designed to demonstrate some of the problems in radiographic and histologic differential diagnosis. Fortunately, lesions that are problems to the pathologist can often be clarified with ease by the radiologist, and vice versa. But the two must talk with each other—and the clinician must ensure that they do so!

Introduction: Appropriate biopsy site.
Series 1: Fracture callus vs. osteosarcoma.
Series 2: Fracture callus vs. chondrosarcoma.
Series 3: Stress fracture vs. Looser's zone, tibia.
Series 4: Myositis ossificans vs. osteosarcoma, femur.
Series 5: Low-grade chondrosarcoma vs. myositis ossificans, femur.
Series 6: Osteoid osteoma, femur vs. osteomyelitis (focal osteitis), tibia vs. tertiary syphilis, radius and ulna.
Series 7: Osteoid osteoma, femur vs. osteomyelitis (focal osteitis), femur vs. diaphyseal dysplasia (Engelmann's disease), forearm.
Series 8: Osteomyelitis (focal osteitis), femur vs. adamantinoma vs. tertiary syphilis, tibia.
Series 9: Osteomyelitis (focal osteitis), humerus vs. eosinophilic granuloma, femur.
Series 10: Osteomyelitis vs. Ewing's sarcoma, humerus.
Series 11: Bone infarct vs. enchondroma, humerus.
Series 12: Bone infarct, tibia vs. chondrosarcoma, femur vs. osteosarcoma.
Series 13: Osteopetrosis vs. scurvy vs. lead poisoning, wrist.
Series 14: Rickets vs. scurvy vs. congenital syphilis, knee.
Series 15: Idiopathic osteoporosis vs. multiple myeloma vs. iatrogenic hypercorticoidism, spine.
Series 16: Paget's disease (osteitis deformans) vs. fibrous dysplasia.
Series 17: Paget's disease (osteitis deformans) vs. cortical fibrous dysplasia (ossifying fibroma), tibia.
Series 18: Paget's disease (osteitis deformans) vs. bone infarct, hip.
Series 19: Myelofibrosis vs. hyperparathyroidism.
Series 20: Hyperparathyroidism vs. Paget's disease (osteitis deformans), skull.
Series 21: Enchondroma vs. fibrous dysplasia, humerus.
Series 22: Synovial chondromatosis vs. joint bodies.
Series 23: Septic arthritis vs. rheumatoid arthritis vs. osteoarthritis, knee.
Series 24: Septic arthritis vs. granulomatous arthritis vs. neuropathic arthritis (Charcot's arthropathy), hip.
Series 25: Gouty tophus vs. rheumatoid nodule.
Series 26: Tuberculosis vs. rheumatoid nodule.
Series 27: Angioma vs. histiocytosis vs. multiple myeloma vs. metastatic carcinoma, skull.
Series 28: Metastatic carcinoma vs. osteochondroma vs. parosteal osteosarcoma vs. myositis ossificans, femur.
Series 29: Nonossifying fibroma vs. fibrosarcoma, tibia.
Series 30: Nonossifying fibroma vs. fibrous dysplasia vs. fibrosarcoma.
Series 31: Chronic osteomyelitis vs. giant cell tumor of bone vs. nonossifying fibroma, tibia.
Series 32: Chondroblastoma vs. giant cell tumor of bone.
Series 33: Giant cell tumor of bone vs. brown tumor of hyperparathyroidism.
Series 34: Loose bodies (synovial chondromatosis) vs. neuropathic arthritis (Charcot's arthropathy) vs. synovial sarcoma, ankle.
Series 35: Chondromyxoid fibroma vs. chondrosarcoma.
Series 36: Chordoma vs. chondrosarcoma.
Series 37: Aggressive enchondroma vs. chondrosarcoma vs. eosinophilic granuloma, femur.
Series 38: Enchondroma, femur vs. chondrosarcoma, tibia.
Series 39: Chondrosarcoma vs. osteosarcoma, femur.
Series 40: Osteoblastoma vs. osteosarcoma.
Series 41: Osteoid osteoma vs. osteoblastoma.

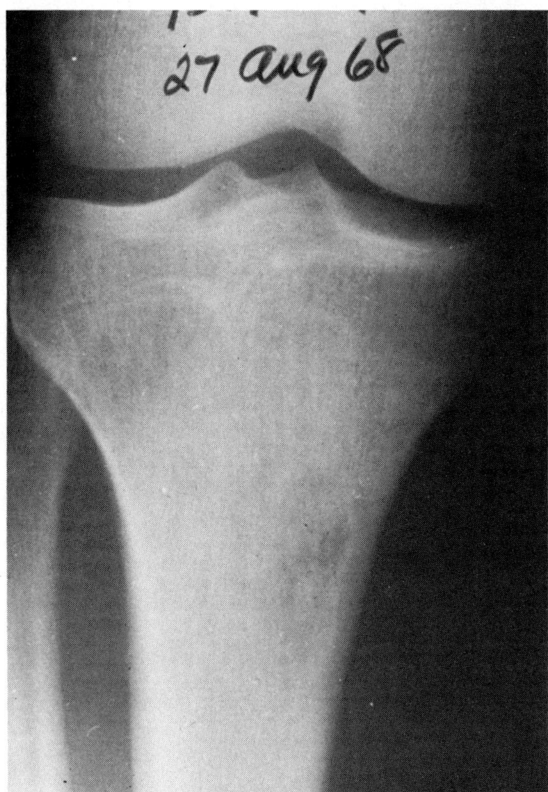

Figure 11–1. Radiograph exhibiting a poorly defined lytic process in the metaphysis of the tibia. There is no discernible periosteal reaction and minimal matrix calcification. The poorly defined margin is indicative of a fast-growing process, and the possibility that a neoplasm exists cannot be excluded.

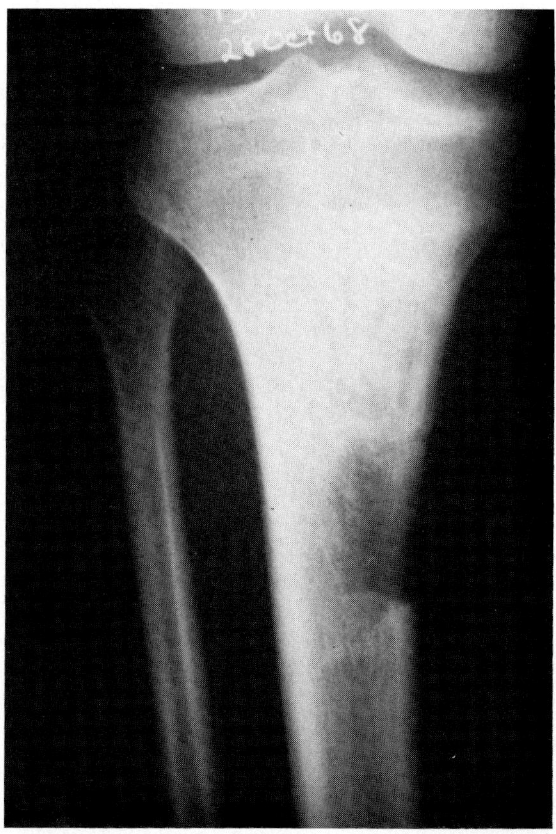

Figure 11–2. Radiograph of same tibia shown in Figure 11–1, 3 months later. Note the biopsy site in the lower metaphysis, below the lesion. The lesion has become increasingly sclerotic. It is still poorly defined but has grown towards the epiphysis. The matrix calcification is consistent with bone formation. There is no visible periosteal reaction.

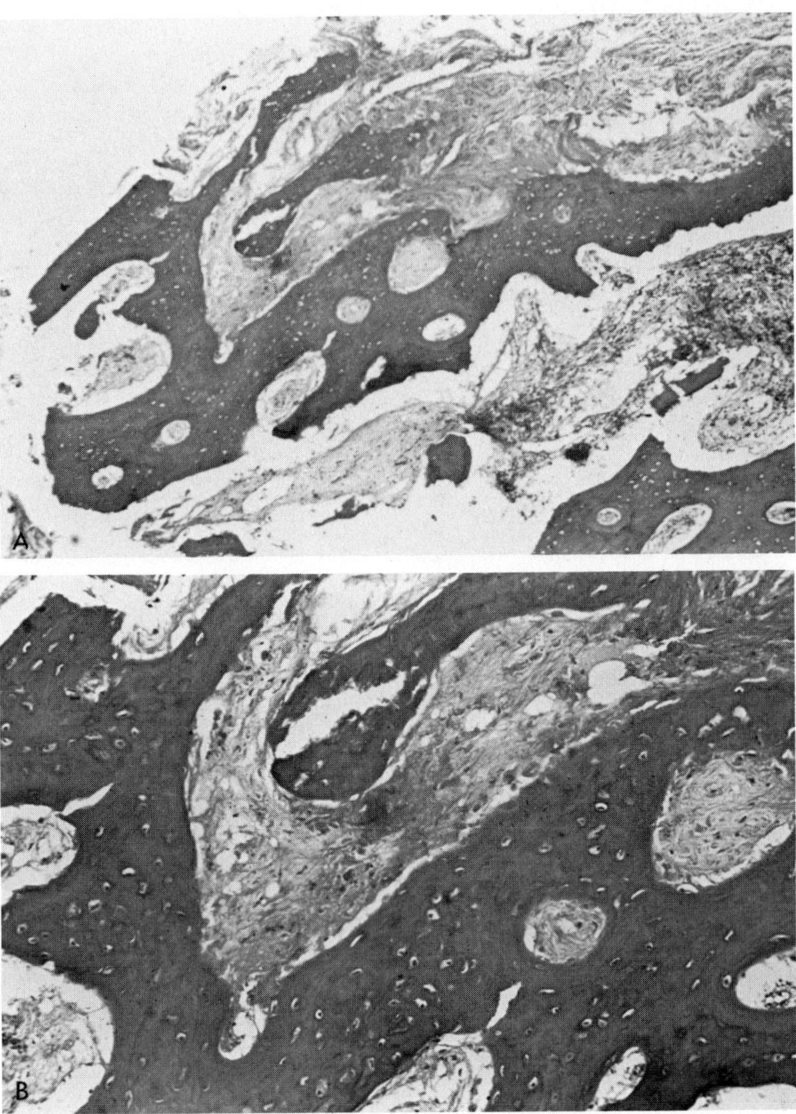

Figure 11–3. Histologic appearance of periosteal new bone formation, obtained at biopsy, and correctly diagnosed as reactive bone. Although the histologic diagnosis is correct on the basis of material available, the overall review of the case with the radiologist would have alerted the pathologist to the fact that the diagnosis of reactive bone is inconsistent with the radiographic appearance.

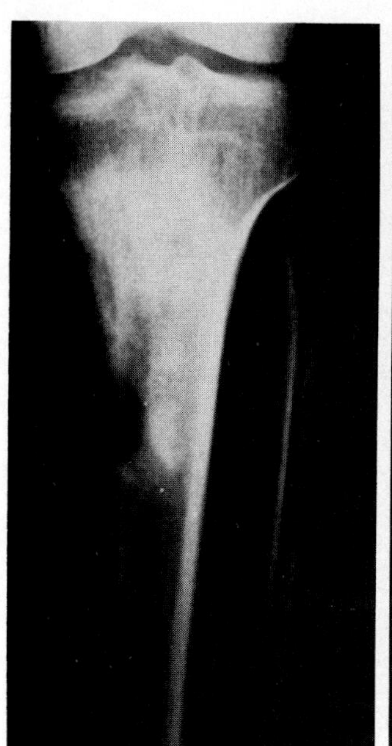
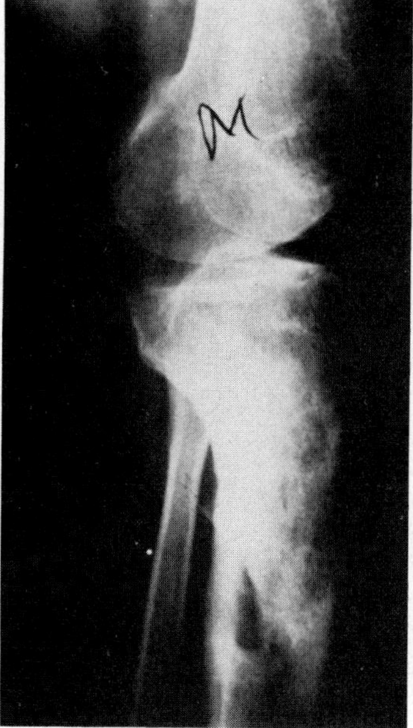

Figure 11–4

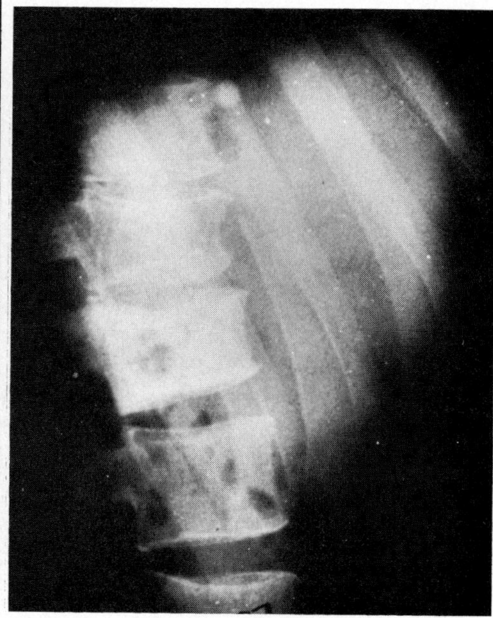

Figure 11–5

Figures 11–4, 11–5, 11–6. Radiographic appearance of lesion in tibia and vertebral body 2 years after previous biopsy. Radiograph exhibits extension of the lesion in the tibia and a sclerotic metastatic focus in the vertebral body; histologic examination of both the primary site in the tibia and the metastatic site in the vertebra reveals a virulent osteosarcoma.

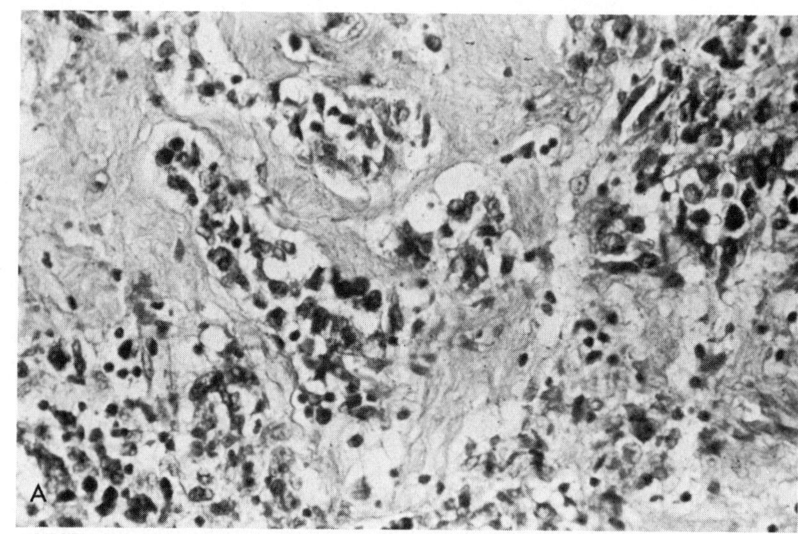

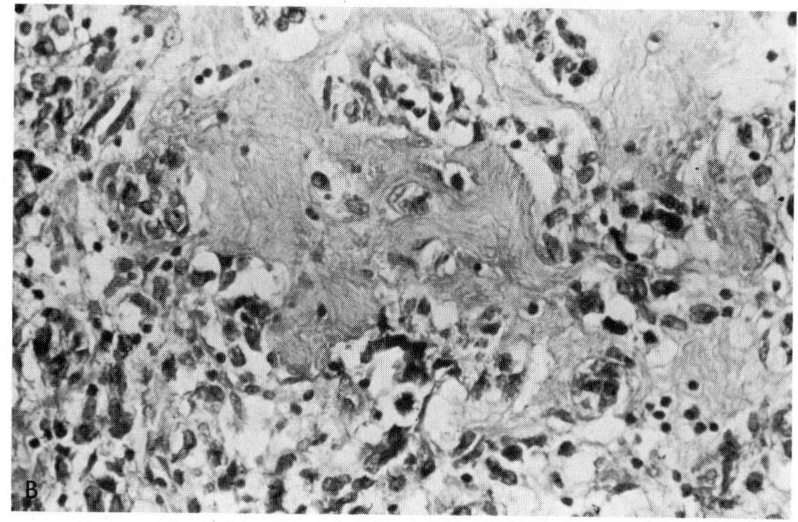

Figure 11–6

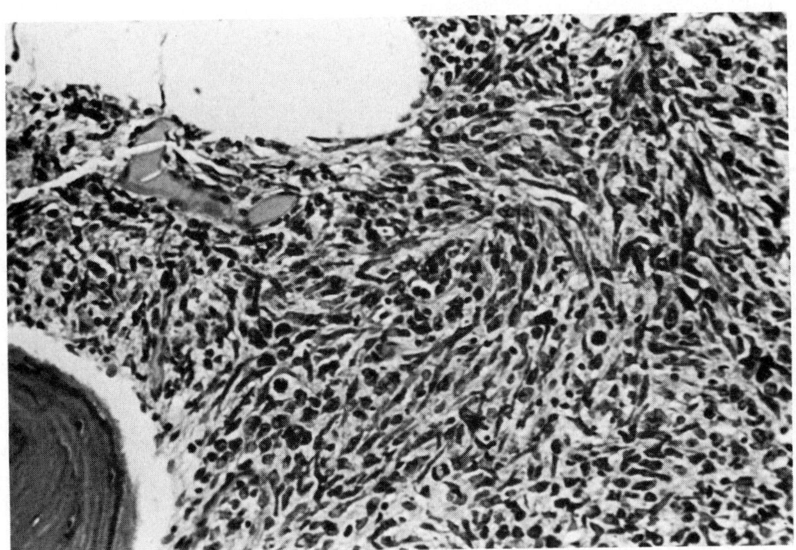

Figure 11–7

The history and radiographs usually establish the diagnosis unequivocally without difficulty. On rare occasions, pathologic fracture is the presenting syndrome of an underlying process, and biopsy, especially limited needle biopsy, may reveal only fragments of early callus. The pathologist must be aware of the radiographic appearance and biologic behavior of the entire lesion. Reactive bone at the margin of an osteosarcoma with pathologic fracture may be the correct histologic diagnosis of the specimen but totally inappropriate for the patient.

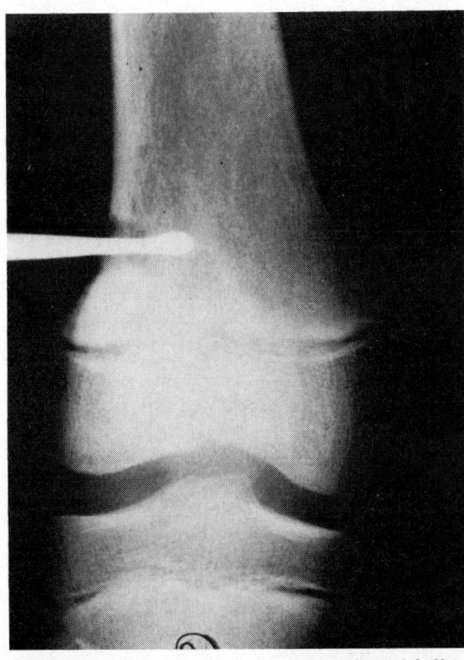

Figure 11–8. Eccentric, sharply circumscribed lytic lesion in metaphysis of the femur, showing neither matrix calcification nor periosteal reaction. Although the lesion has the radiographic appearance of a benign nonossifying fibroma, biopsy must confirm the radiographic appearance. Note the biopsy probe short of the lesion. Even if the biopsy is from the lesion itself, the approach from the lateral margin prevents adequate curettage and necessitates a second operative procedure.

It is absolutely imperative that the pathologist assure himself not only that the biopsy is from the correct site but also that he is involved in planning the site and extent of the biopsy as well as the appropriate therapy. If the expertise available to handle all aspects of the lesion is insufficient, the patient should be referred elsewhere.

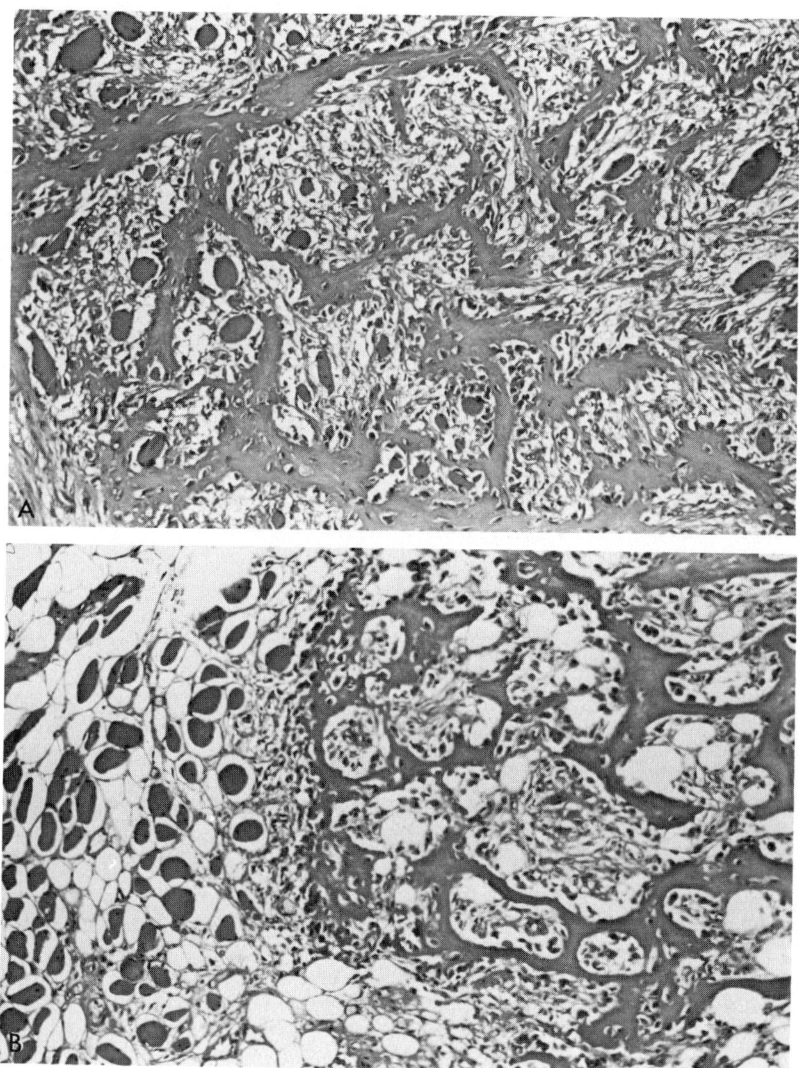

Figure 11–9. Fracture callus.

Illustration continued on page 660

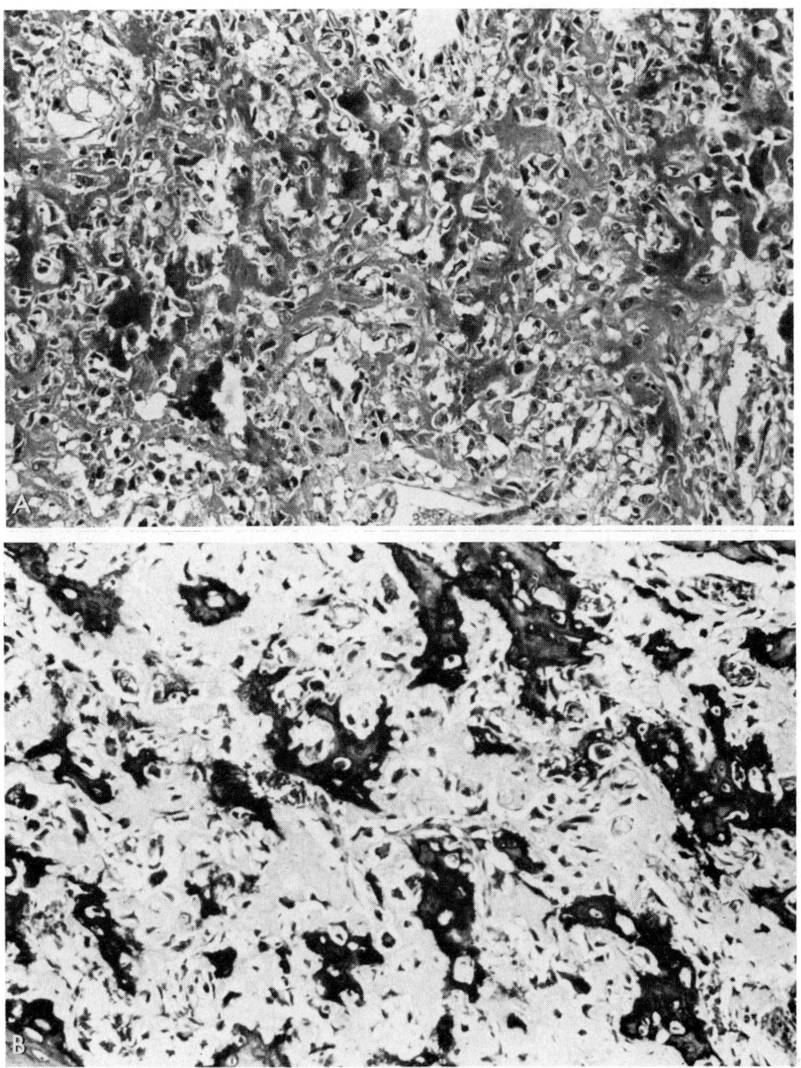

Figure 11–10. Osteosarcoma.

Illustration continued on page 661

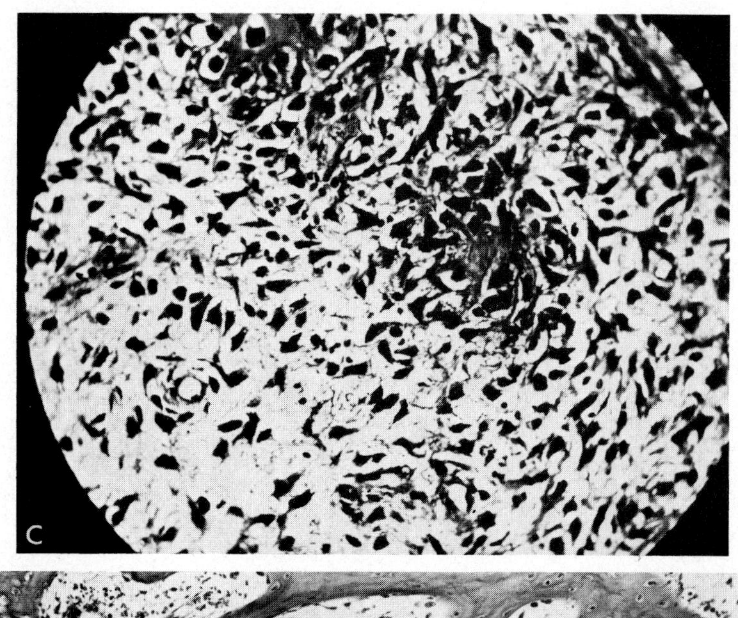

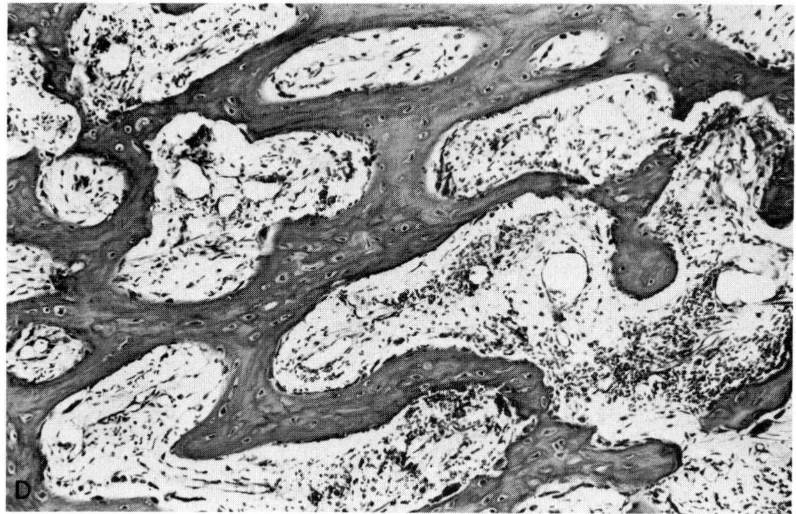

Figure 11–9 *Continued.* Fracture callus.

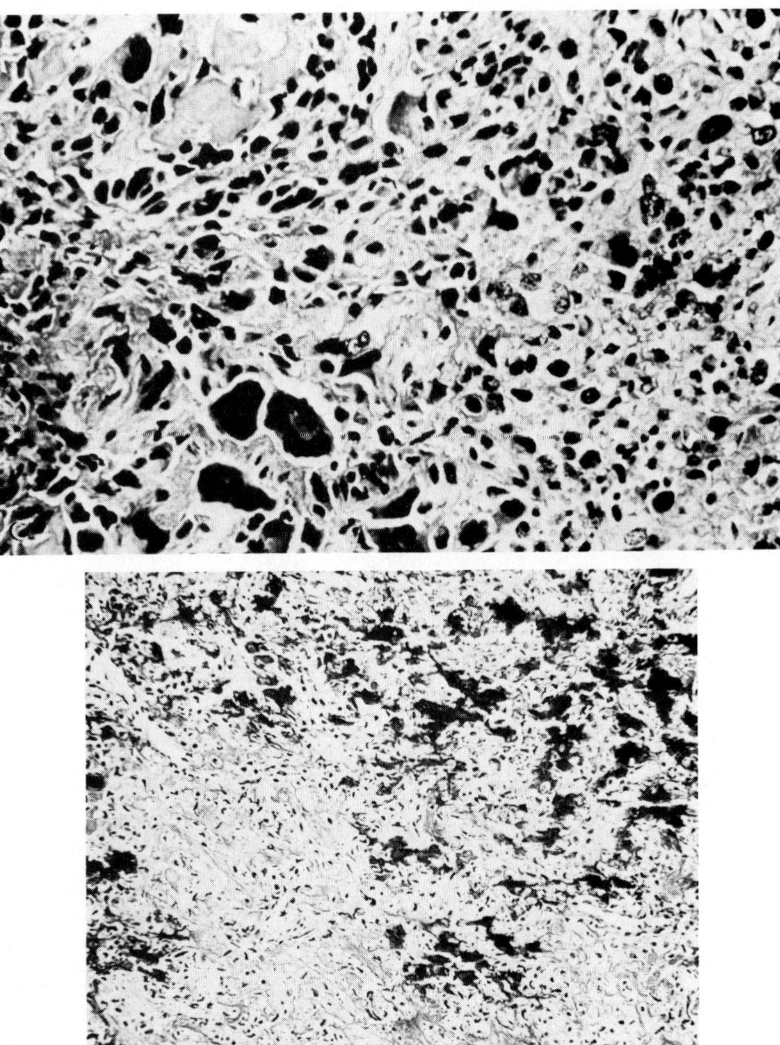

Figure 11–10 *Continued.* Osteosarcoma.

Series 1: Fracture callus vs. osteosarcoma. The callus contains well-delineated bony trabecula lined by uniform osteoblasts and cellular connective tissue between bone fragments. Note the bone formation in the midst of striated muscle. As the callus becomes more mature, the connective tissue between the newly formed trabecula also matures, becoming less cellular with numerous sinusoidal vessels.

The osteosarcoma exhibits irregular osteoid formation, accompanied by cellular stroma, with marked pleomorphism of the malignant osteoblasts. The bone is irregularly formed, with no evidence of a maturation pattern in either the bone or the connective tissue component between the neoplastic trabecula.

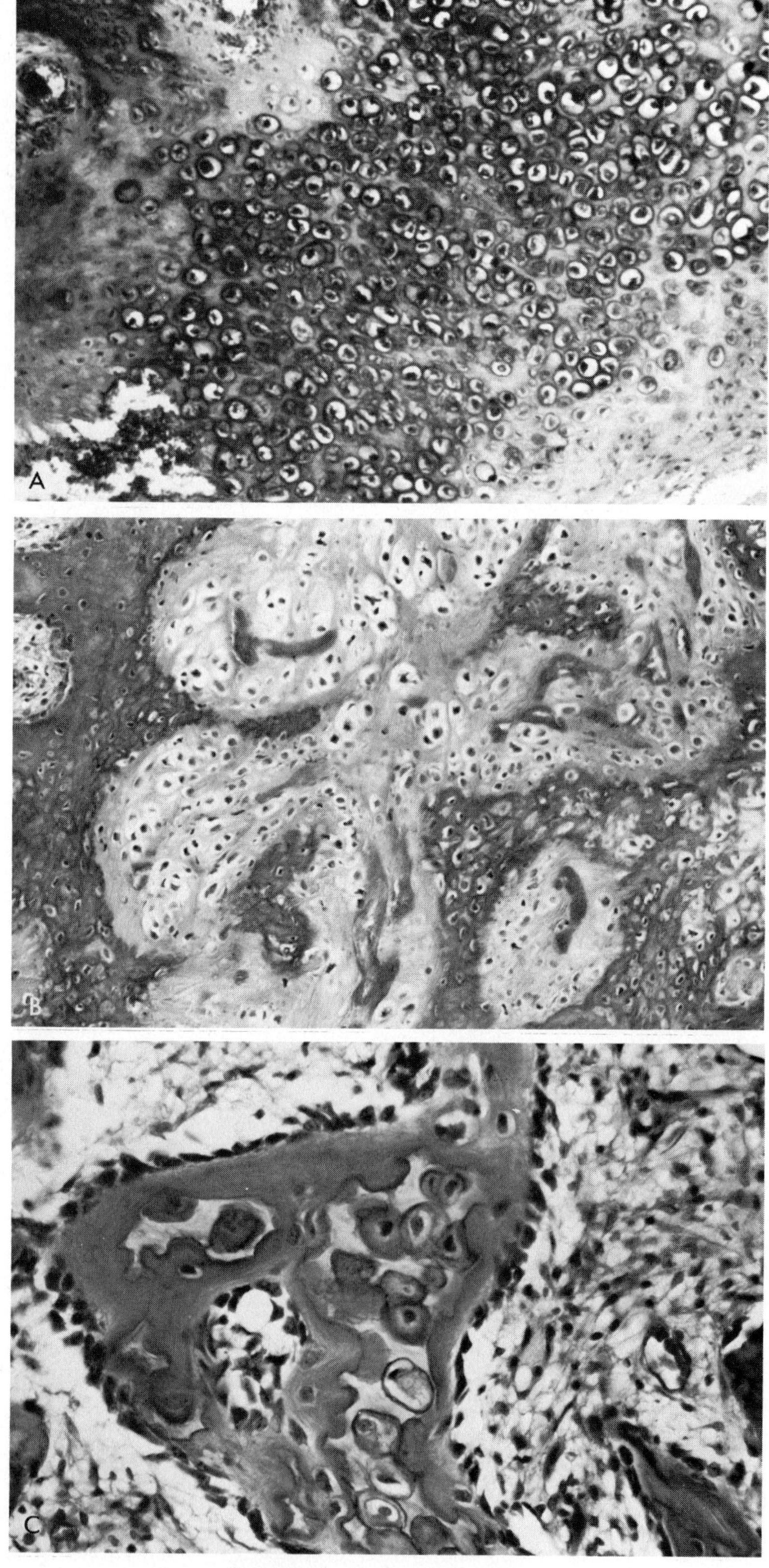

Figure 11–11. Fracture callus.

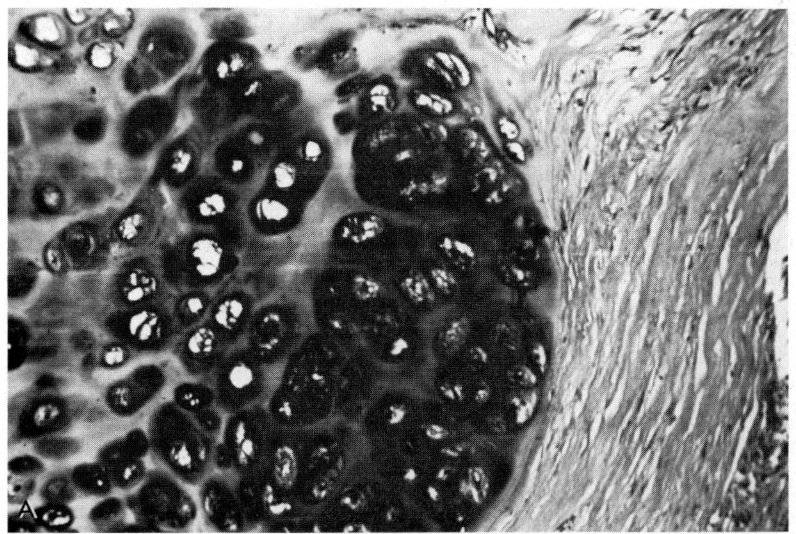

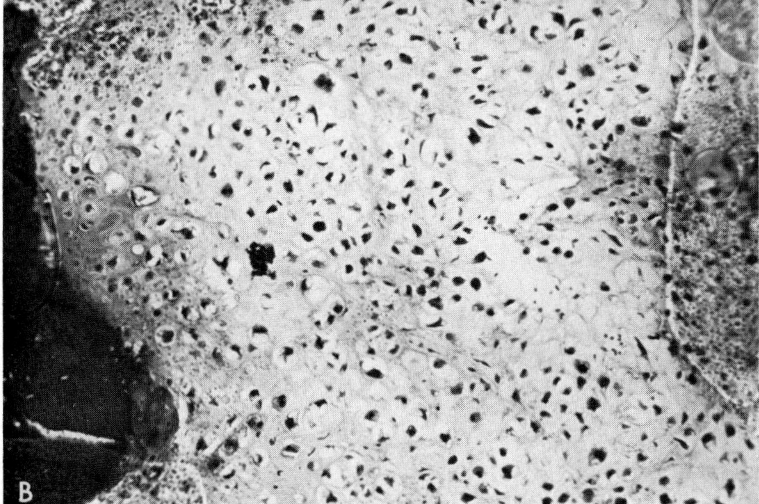

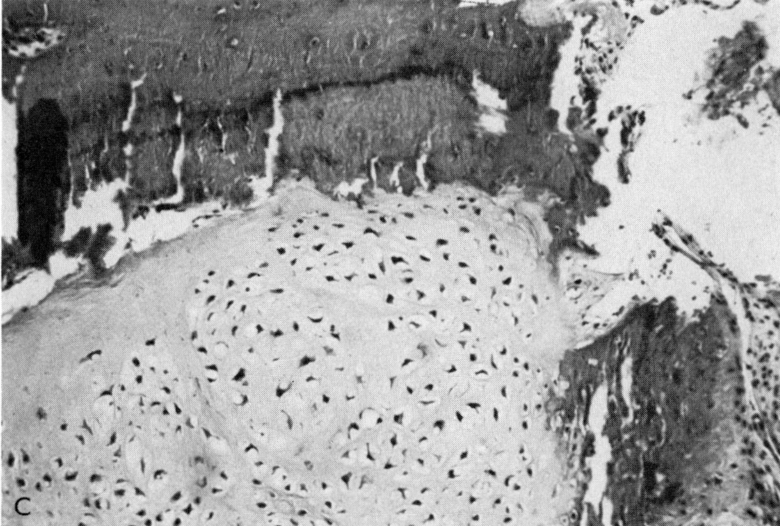

Figure 11–12. Chondrosarcoma.

Series 2: Fracture callus vs. chondrosarcoma. In a chondrosarcoma, the cartilage shows moderate to severe pleomorphism and hypercellularity, and it extends into the fibrous connective tissue. Calcification may be present. Note the sharp transition between neoplastic cartilage and normal residual trabecular bone or soft tissue.

In fracture callus, although the cartilage is quite cellular, the nuclear cytoplasmic ratio is maintained. Maturation and transition to bony trabecula may be noted even in the earliest callus. Note the incorporation of cellular cartilage within primitive trabecula lined by uniform osteoblasts, obviously benign.

The clinical and radiographic features that may lead to confusion between osteosarcoma and fracture callus apply equally to chondrosarcoma and callus. The extent of cartilage in callus depends on the vascular supply and immobilization of the fracture site (see Chapter 3, p. 76).

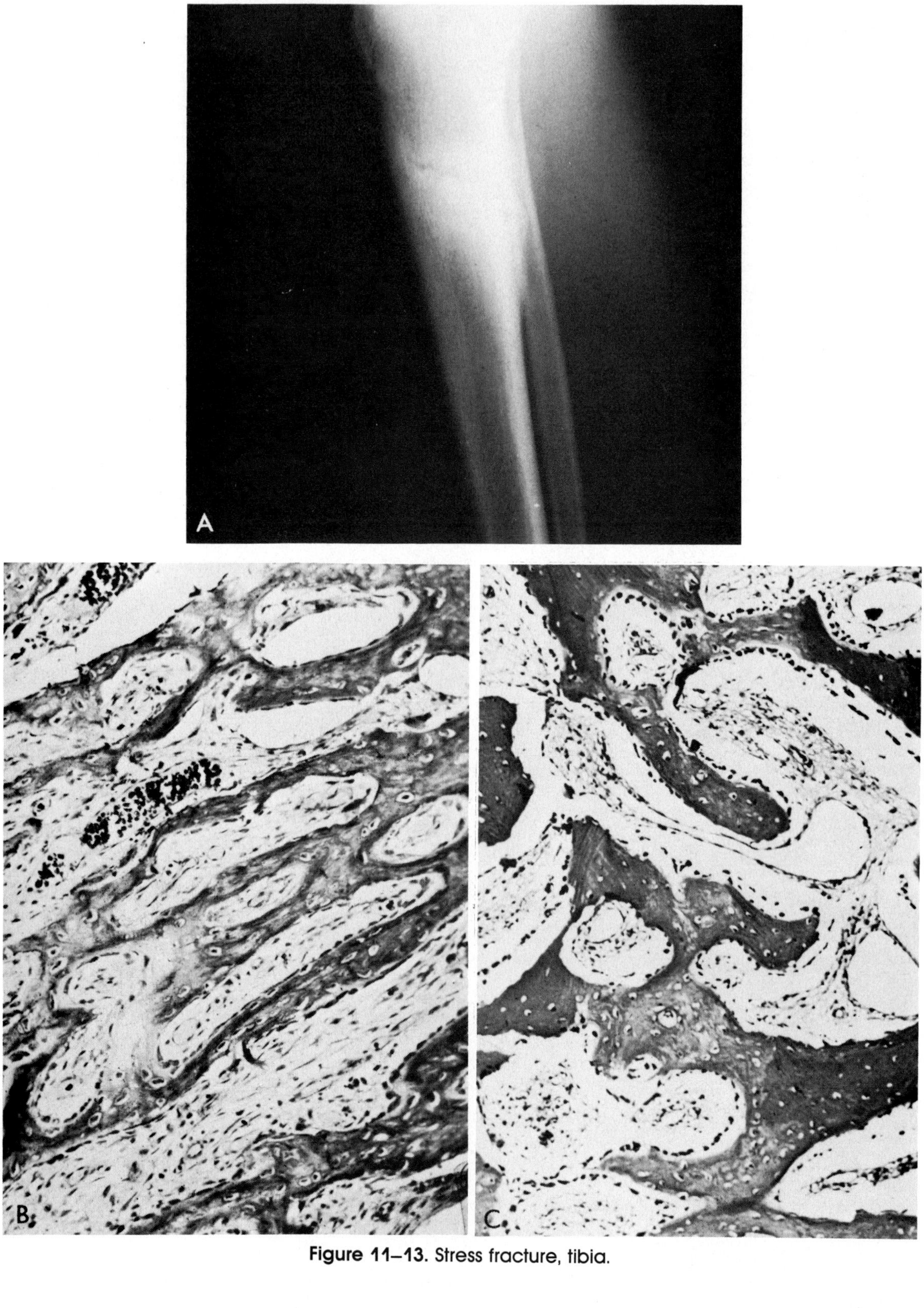

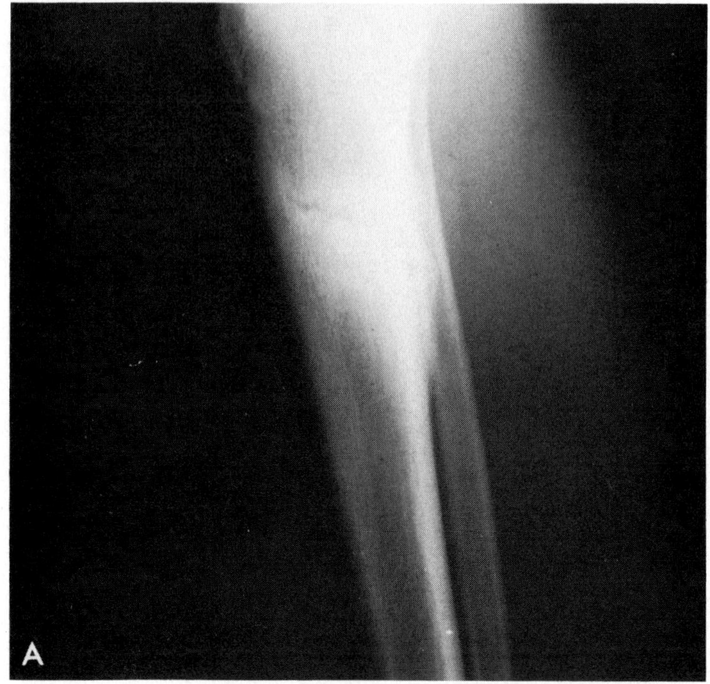

Figure 11–13. Stress fracture, tibia.

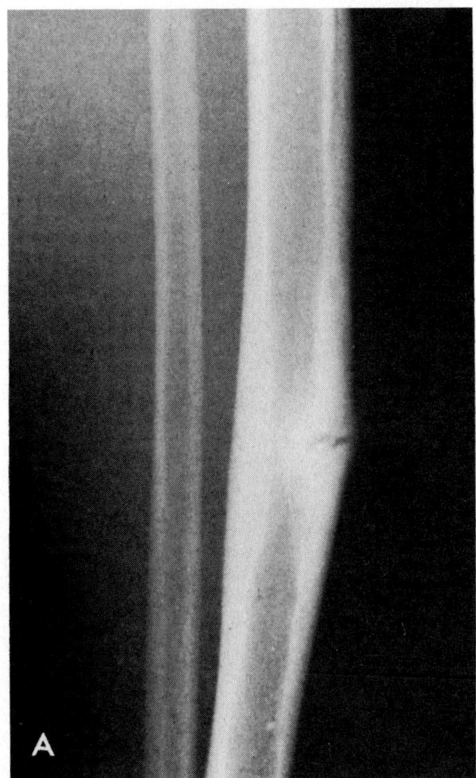

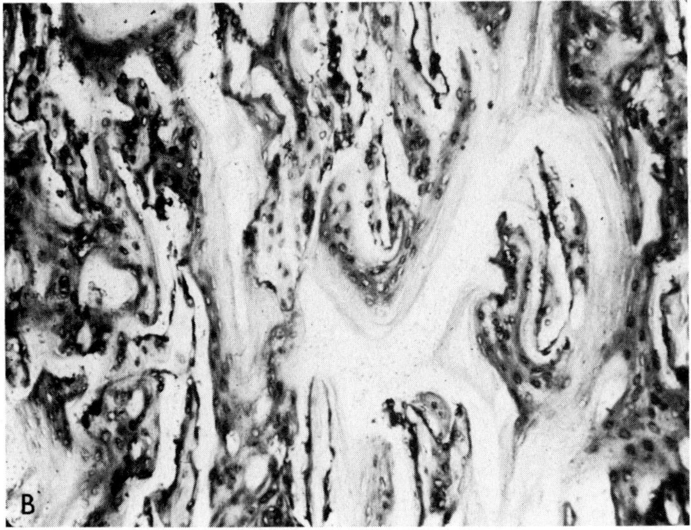

Figure 11–14. Looser's zone, tibia.

Series 3: Stress fracture vs. Looser's zone, tibia. Both processes represent localized zones of osteolysis in response to remodeling stimuli. In stress fracture, the resorptive tunneling of the cortex occurs in response to muscular stresses and elicits periosteal and endosteal repair, which may or may not be followed by the appearance of a fracture line.

The Looser's zone is initiated by similar stimuli in similar locations, but the repair attempt results in a fracture line filled with unmineralized osteomalacic material due to the underlying metabolic disease. Such osteomalacic seams may persist unchanged for a long time, whereas stress fractures heal promptly.

In stress reaction, the new periosteal bone is immature woven bone that is histologically normal.

Osteomalacia is characterized by large quantities of unmineralized osteoid. The osteoid seams are obviously enlarged, but undemineralized sections are required to prove the absence of calcium.

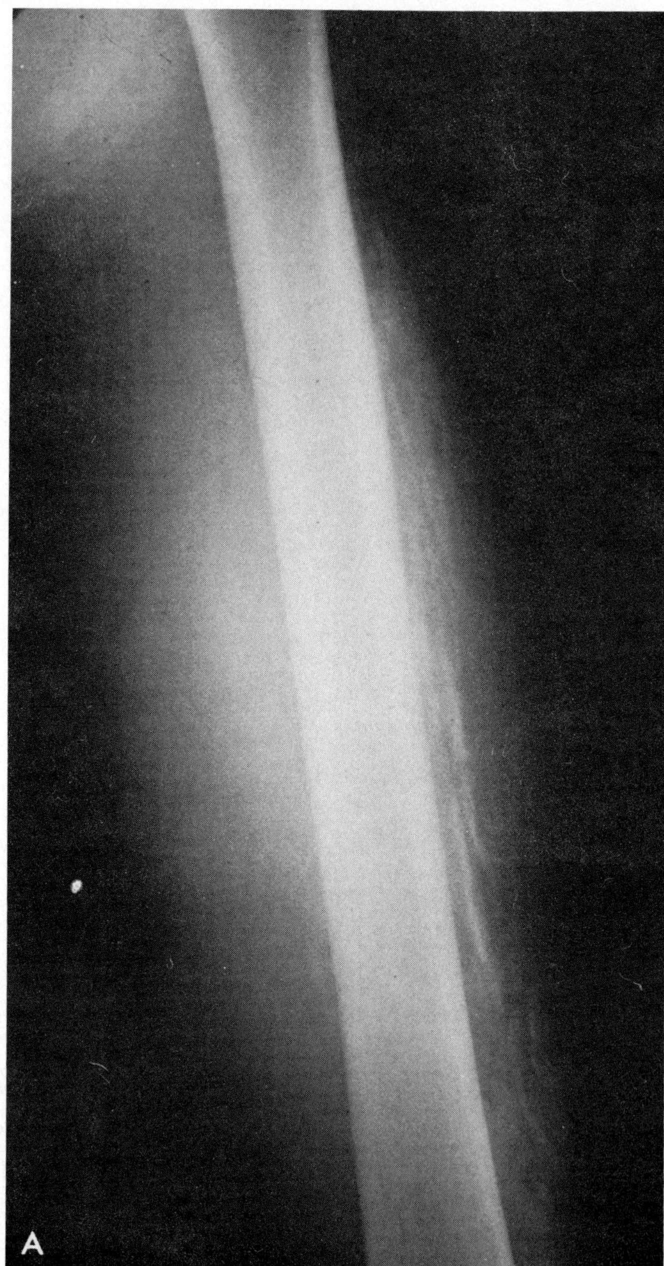

Figure 11–15. Myositis ossificans, femur.

Illustration continued on page 668

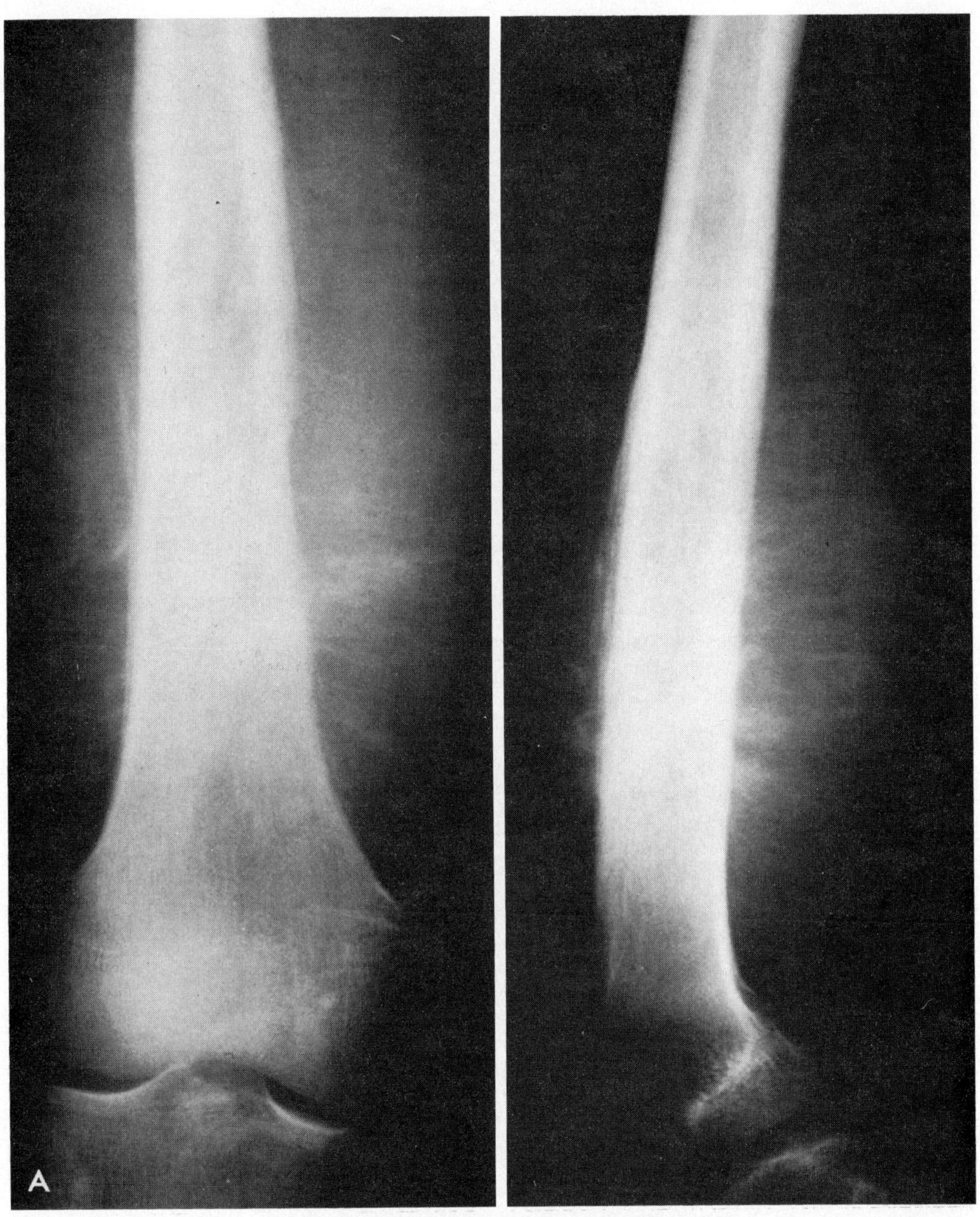

Figure 11–16. Osteosarcoma, femur.

Illustration continued on page 669

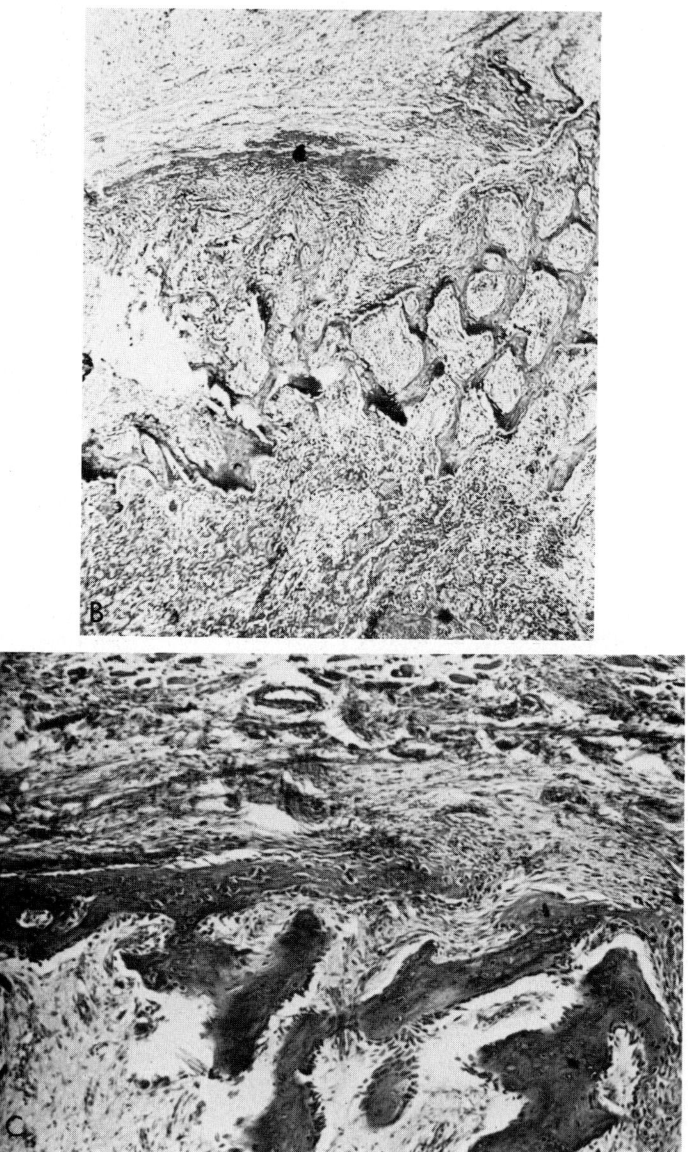

Figure 11–15 *Continued.* Myositis ossificans, femur.

Series 4: Myositis ossificans vs. osteosarcoma, femur. The soft-tissue swelling with veil-like ossification streamers near the surface of the femoral shaft raises the possibility of an aggressive, malignant lesion. Lack of bone change in the presence of an extensive lesion makes primary bone tumor unlikely and indicates that the lesion is in the muscle.

The intraosseous lesion, shown in anteroposterior and lateral views, has extensive "sunburst" bone production in the soft tissue; there is also a large soft-tissue mass with bone production in spiculated

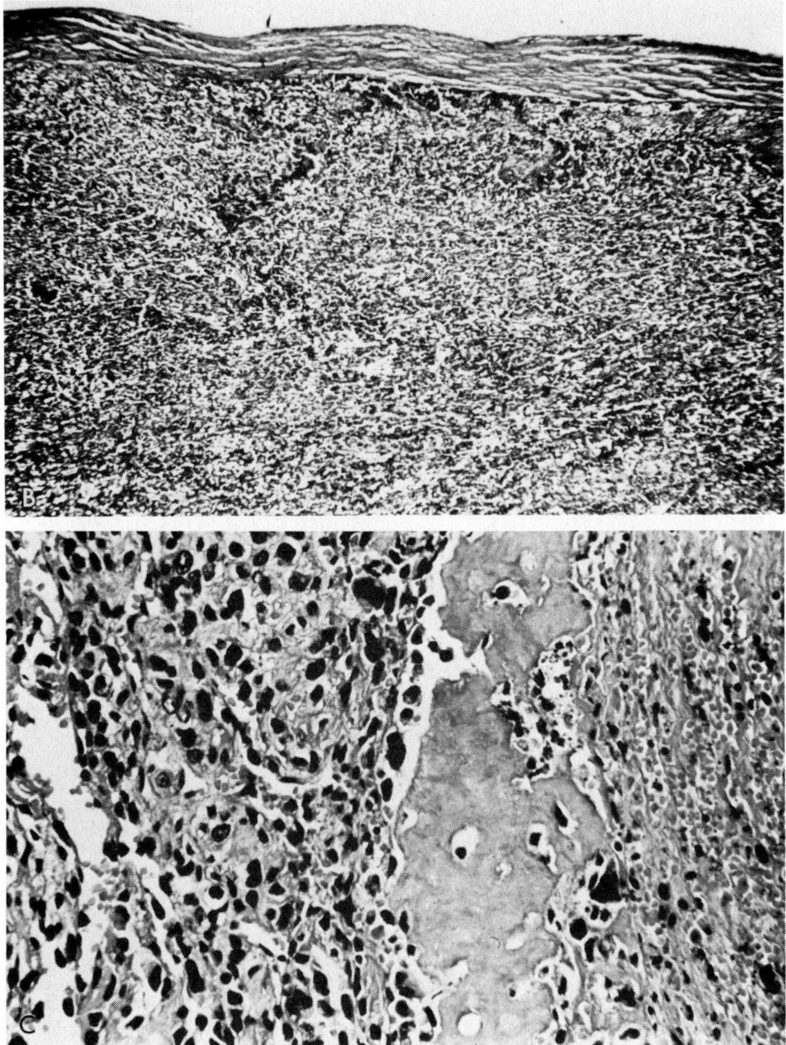

Figure 11–16 *Continued.* Osteosarcoma, femur.

streamers extending perpendicular to the cortex. The extensive changes of destruction and production inside the femur with a classic Codman's triangle and soft-tissue mass are consistent with osteosarcoma.

The histologic appearance of the osteosarcoma can be varied, quite cellular, or quite sclerotic. The advancing margin of the tumor is usually the least differentiated, and there is no relationship between tumor bone and the more cellular components of the sarcoma. Note the sharp demarcation of the myositis ossificans against the surrounding soft tissue, with the most mature elements visible at the periphery.

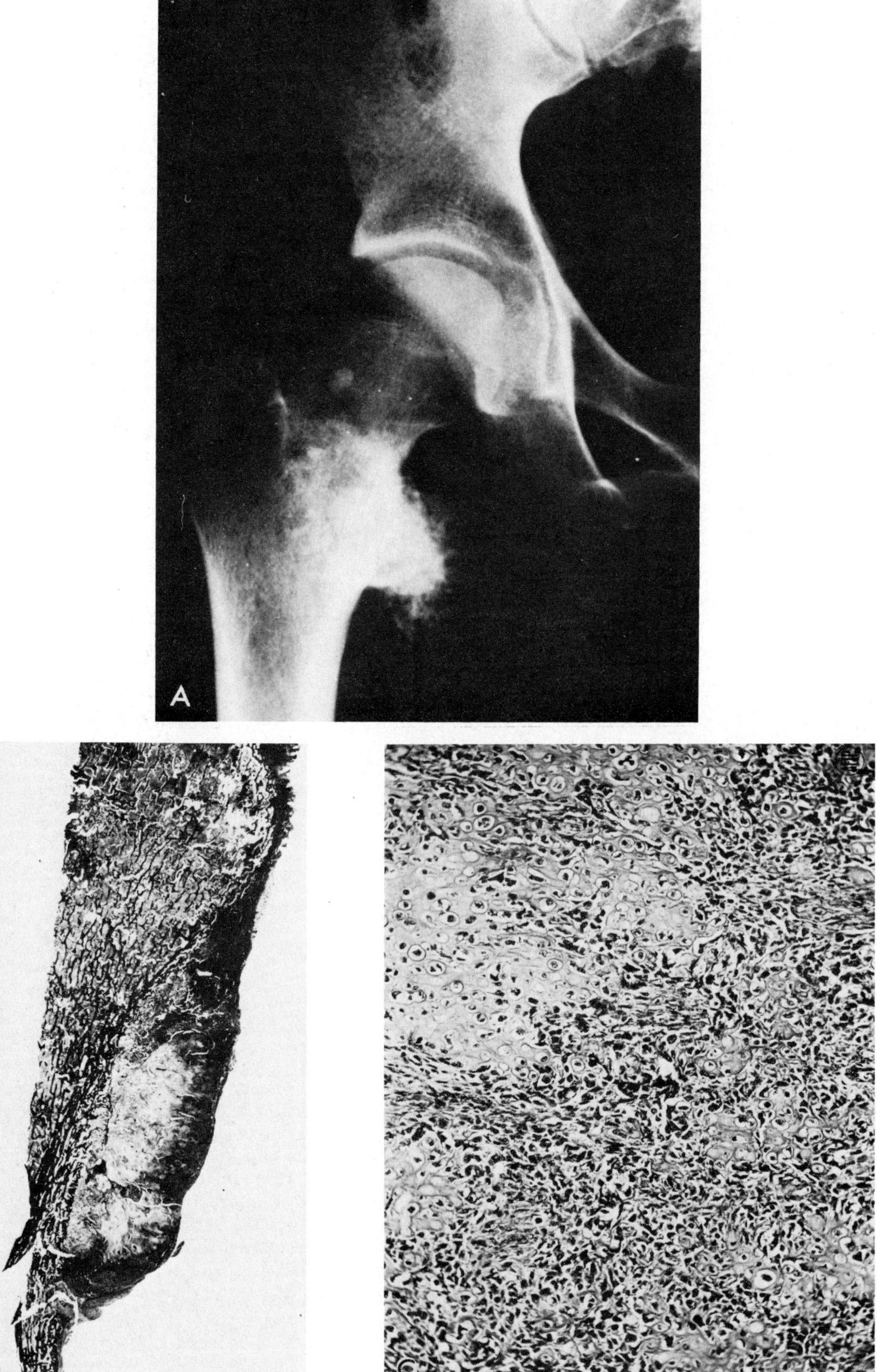

Figure 11–17. Low-grade chondrosarcoma, femur.

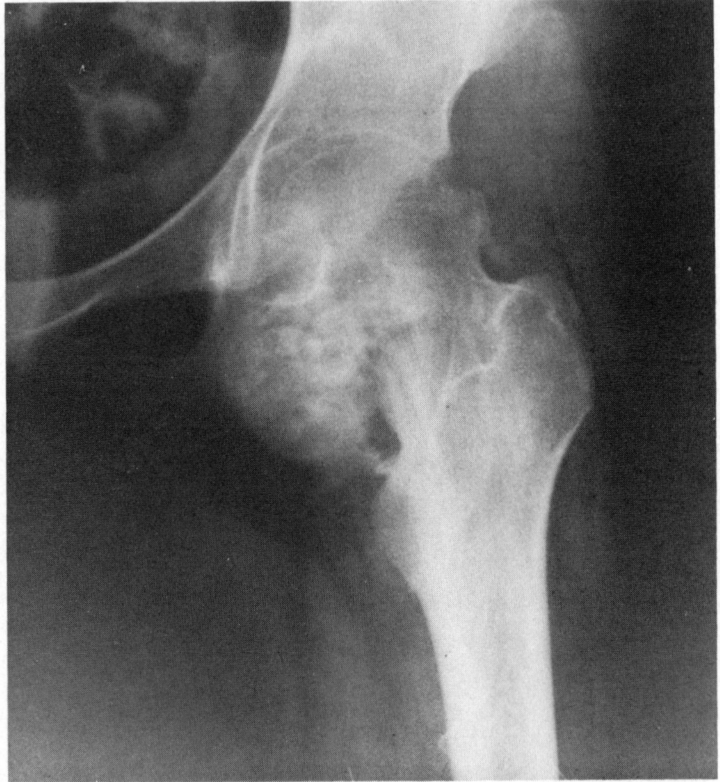

Figure 11–18. Myositis ossificans, femur.

Series 5: Low-grade chondrosarcoma vs. myositis ossificans, femur. The large lobulated exophytic growth with irregularly flocculent calcification suggests a cartilage lesion. The large size of the tumor and the extent of intramedullary involvement are consistent with malignant cartilage.

Myositis ossificans has a much smoother outline, without attachment to the femur. Several small pericapsular foci of bone formation in the soft tissues without significant change in the femur suggest a lesion arising in soft tissue, and the sharp margin of ossification indicates a benign process of mature myositis ossificans.

Chondrosarcoma may present with a small intraosseous focus and extensive involvement of adjacent soft tissue, mimicking a parosteal osteosarcoma or myositis ossificans. CT scans are necessary to exclude or document intramedullary involvement. Cartilage is usually not found in myositis ossificans unless it is secondarily fractured; the diagnosis of neoplastic versus reactive cartilage depends on the maintenance of normal cytologic criteria in benign entities and the transition to normal bone (see Series 2). Figure 11–17 exhibits the neoplastic, highly pleomorphic cartilage of the chondrosarcoma.

A careful history will usually document blunt trauma 1 to 2 months prior to the appearance of the myositis ossificans.

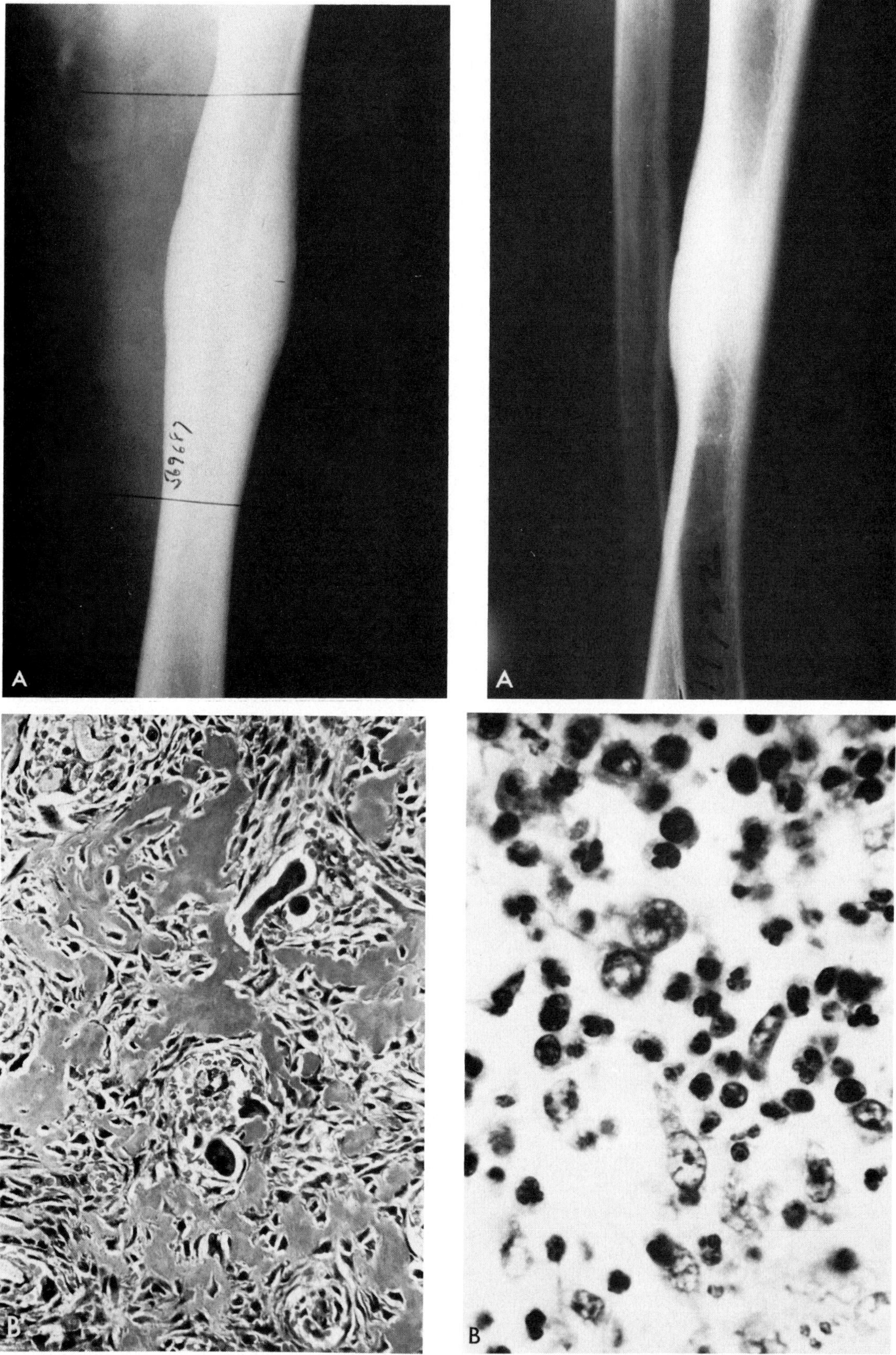

Figure 11–19. Osteoid osteoma, femur.

Figure 11–20. Osteomyelitis, tibia.

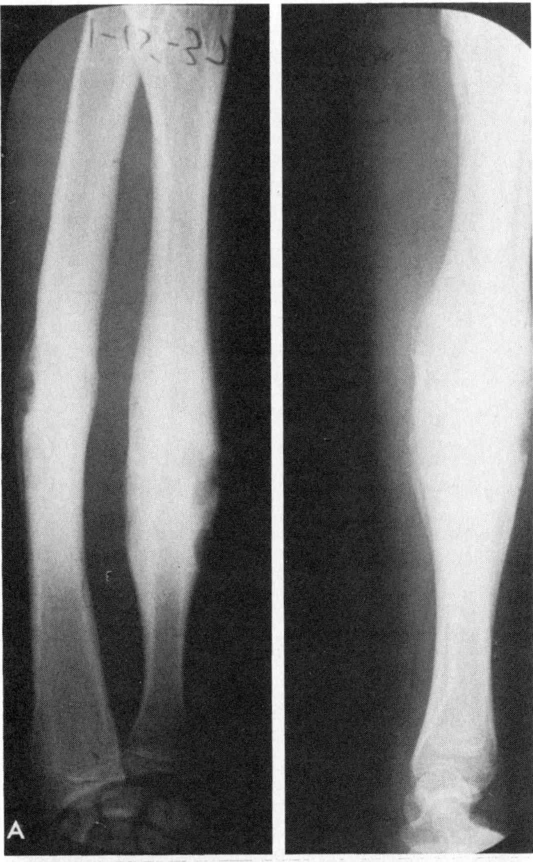

Series 6: Osteoid osteoma, femur vs. osteomyelitis (focal osteitis), tibia vs. tertiary syphilis, radius and ulna. Osteomyelitis in adults may be focal owing to penetrating injury. The subcutaneous tibia is often wounded by outside objects penetrating the skin and bone. Focal osteomyelitis in the tibial cortex causes a lytic focus (abscess) surrounded by dense reactive bone. This low-grade sclerotic process is similar to that elicited by an osteoid osteoma, which is usually a cortical lesion that is slow-growing and ultimately stationary, seldom exceeding 2 cm in diameter. The nidus may be hidden by the smooth outer surface of the dense homogeneous bone response, and tomograms may be required to demonstrate it. Biopsy and culture will confirm the diagnosis of osteomyelitis.

Luetic osteomyelitis in adults can cause diffuse hyperostosis secondary to periosteal thickening and endosteal bone production, and it can encroach upon the medullary cavity. The periosteal bone creates a large, dense, undulating contour, which may contain numerous radiolucent areas in the hyperostotic bone, representing gummas.

Syphilitic periostitis is characterized by a predominantly perivascular plasma cell infiltrate. Osteomyelitis with a small abscess cavity is characterized by an infiltrate of inflammatory cells with numerous polymorphonuclear leukocytes. The nidus of the osteoid osteoma is an extremely vascular osteoid-producing lesion without an inflammatory component.

Although the radiographic appearance of the three lesions is quite similar, the histologic appearance of each allows the trained observer to distinguish the three entities without difficulty.

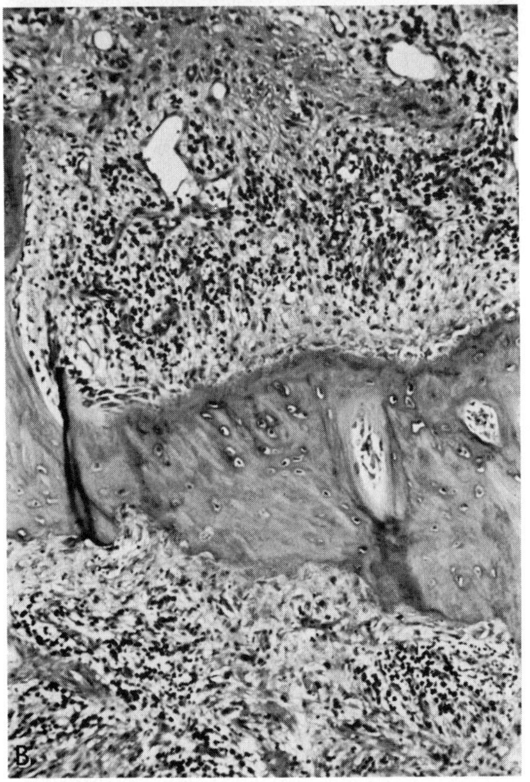

Figure 11–21. Tertiary syphilis, radius and ulna.

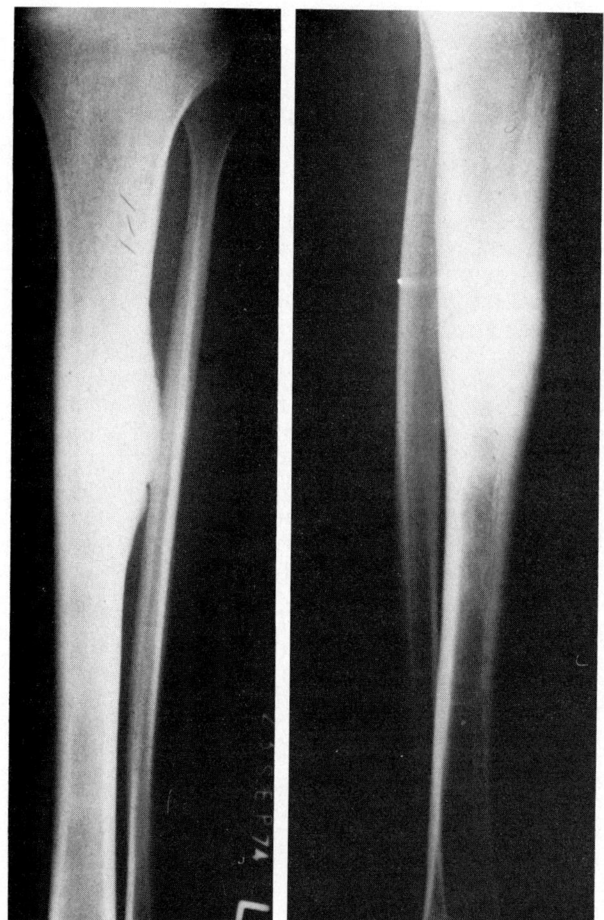

Figure 11–22. Osteoid osteoma, femur.

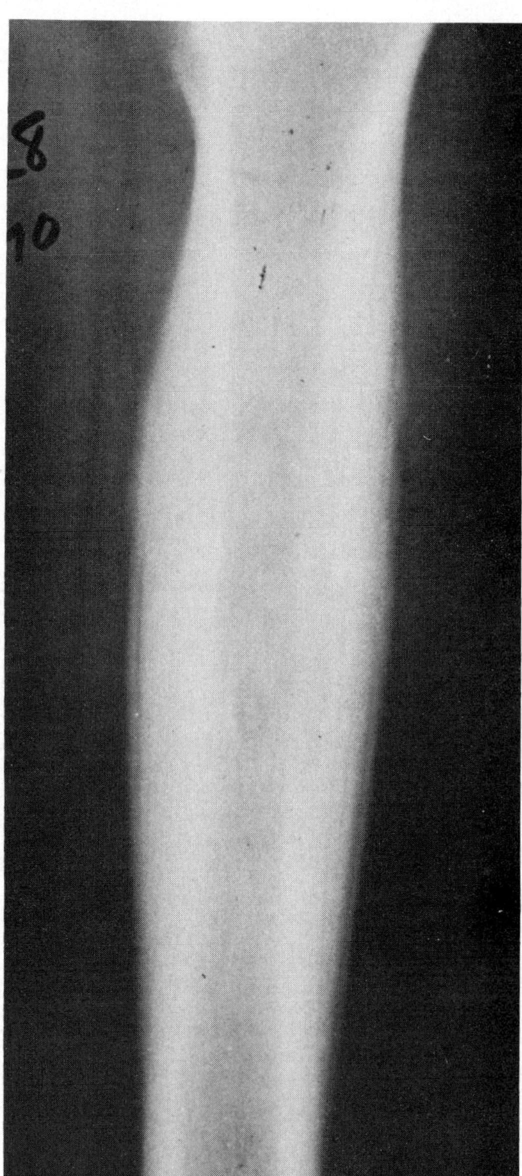

Figure 11–23. Osteomyelitis, femur.

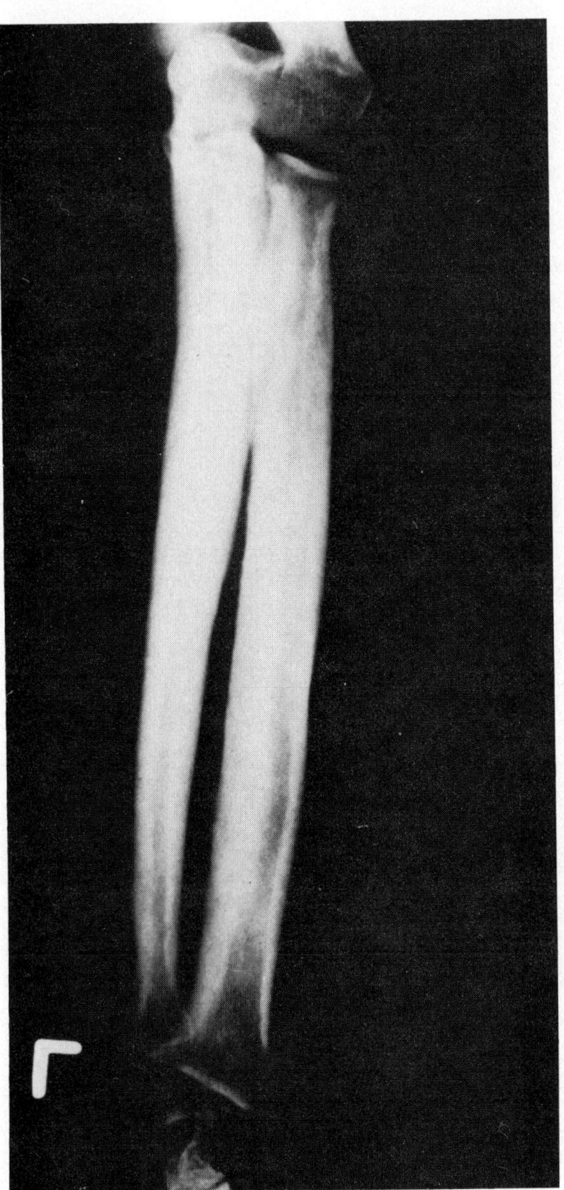

Figure 11–24. Diaphyseal dysplasia (Engelmann's disease).

Series 7: Osteoid osteoma, femur vs. osteomyelitis (focal osteitis), femur vs. diaphyseal dysplasia (Engelmann's disease), forearm. The reaction in all three lesions is predominantly cortical and diaphyseal with expansion of bone diameter. Osteoid osteoma causes marked, typically homogeneous rather than layered thickening of cortex on the endosteal and periosteal surfaces around a limited area of the diaphysis. A radiolucency may be evident inside the thickened cortex, particularly on tomograms. Osteomyelitis involves a longer segment of the diaphysis, with cortical resorption and several layers of periosteal new bone. Filling of the spaces between laminae of periosteal reaction is evidence of a slower rate of response and is more commonly seen in osteomyelitis than in a tumor. Engelmann's disease is an uncommon syndrome of unknown etiology in which the long bones demonstrate cortical thickening of the entire diaphysis with a normal epiphysis and metaphysis.

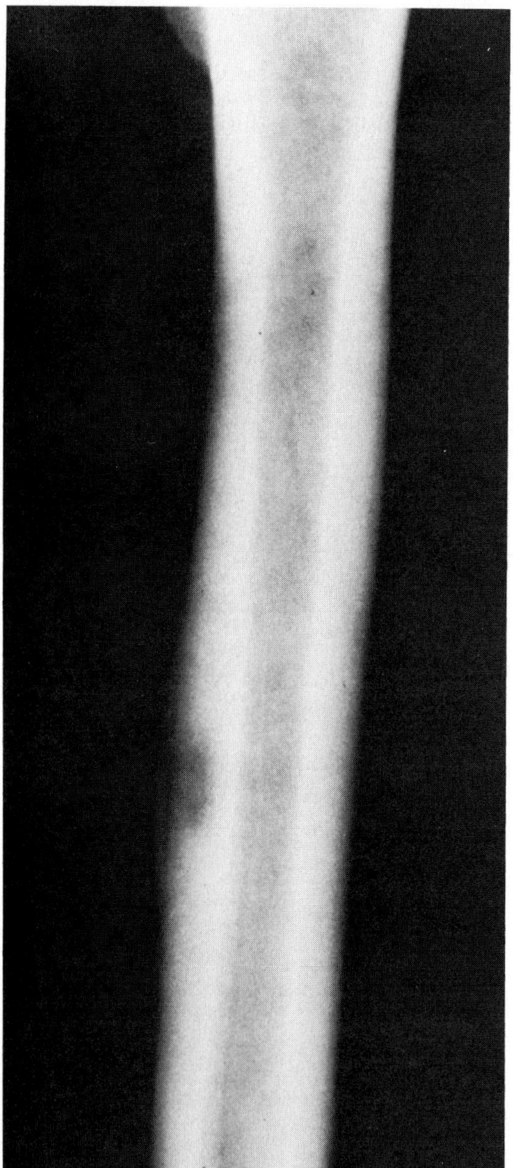

Figure 11–25. Focal osteitis, femur.

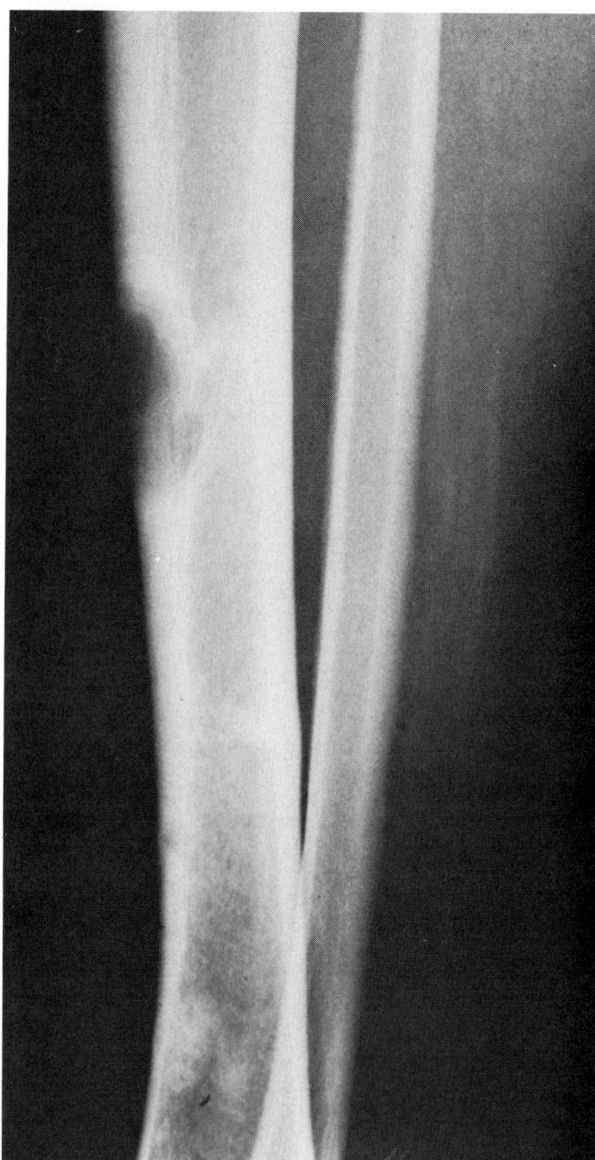

Figure 11–26. Adamantinoma, long bone.

Series 8: Osteomyelitis (focal osteitis), femur vs. adamantinoma of long bone vs. tertiary syphilis, tibia. The osteomyelitis is a localized cortical defect with thickening of the cortex and a thin layer of periosteal reaction indicating an active process. No intramedullary extension is evident, and no sequestrum is seen.

Adamantinoma of long bone is a neoplastic lesion of varying aggressiveness most commonly seen in the anterior tibial cortex. It is a cystic multilocular lesion with geographic destruction of the mid tibia, and the irregular radiolucency is combined with reactive thickening of the cortex without periosteal lamination, indicating a slow process. Multiple foci in the same bone are common. True intramedullary extension is uncommon unless the lesion is very aggressive or very large.

Syphilitic osteitis and periostitis produce multiple irregular radiolucencies (gummas) in a densely thickened cortex with an undulating surface and no acute periosteal lamination. Many bones are often involved.

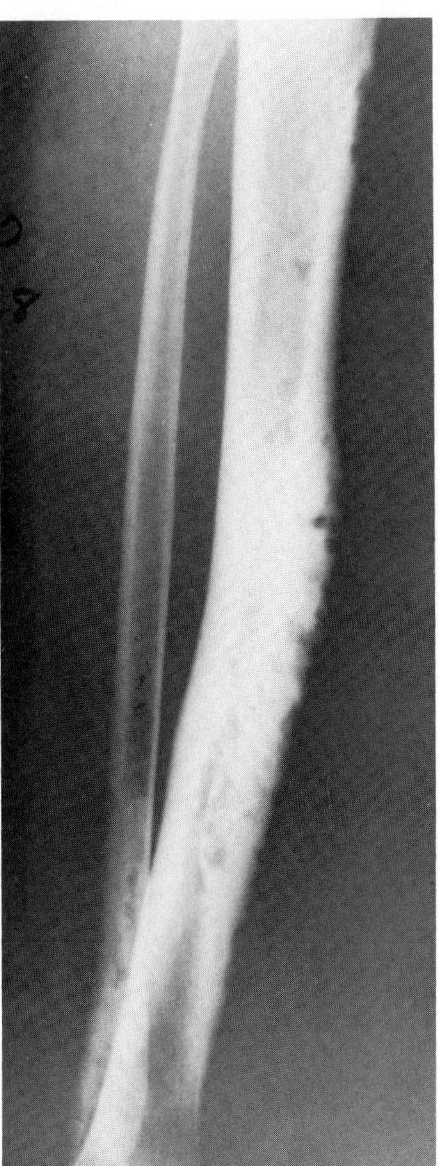

Figure 11–27. Tertiary syphilis, tibia.

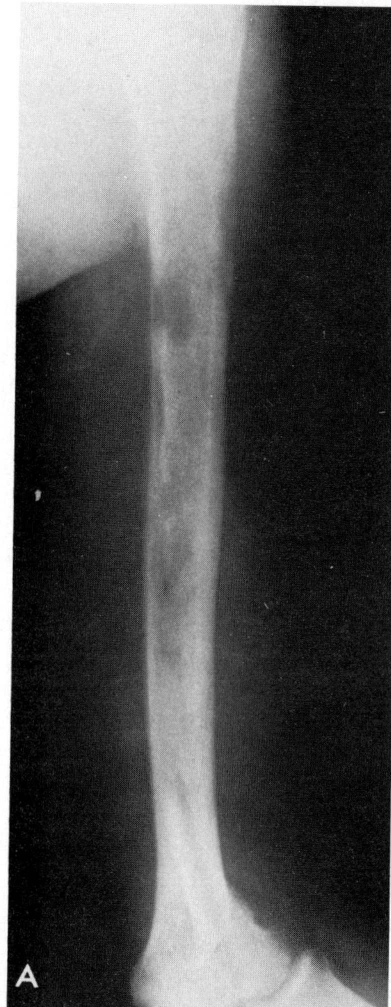
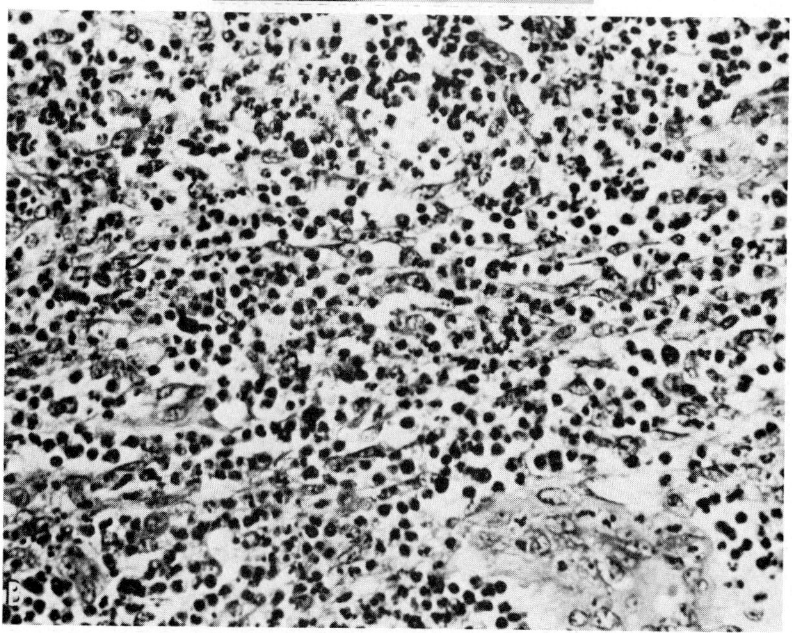

Figure 11–28. Osteomyelitis, humerus.

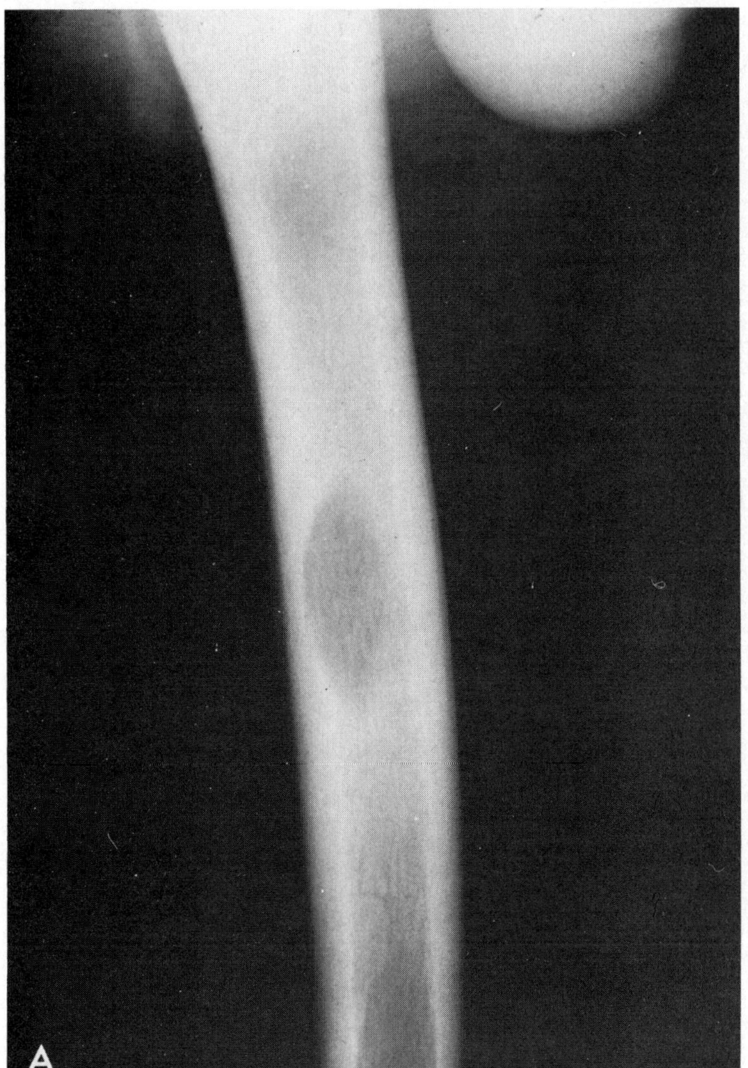

Series 9: Osteomyelitis (focal osteitis), humerus vs. eosinophilic granuloma, femur. The radiographic changes of osteomyelitis consist of moth-eaten and permeative patterns of osteolysis extending almost the entire length of the humeral diaphysis, with periosteal new bone formation visible proximally. There are cortical irregularities but no clear-cut sequestrum. There is no obvious soft-tissue swelling or mass. Bone destruction predominates over bone production. The histologic picture is characterized by a polymorphous inflammatory infiltrate consisting of granulocytes, lymphocytes, histiocytes, plasma cells, and thin strands of fibrin.

The eosinophilic granuloma shows an oval to round osteolytic diaphyseal focus with endosteal erosion and a sharply defined geographic margin. The trabecular reinforcement creates a sclerotic shell about the lesion. There is no matrix mineralization. The minimal early cortical expansion is produced by periosteal new bone that forms on the outer surface of the cortex adjacent to the endosteal erosion. Osseous reinforcement of the well-defined geographic margin is an indication that the process is benign and growing slowly, allowing the body to respond by "walling off" the irritative focus. The eosinophilic granuloma is characterized by an infiltrate of histiocytes, accompanied by a variable number of eosinophiles. Neutrophiles are not common and do not form a numerically significant component of the eosinophilic granuloma. In both osteomyelitis and eosinophilic granuloma, the normal fatty marrow is replaced by the infiltrate.

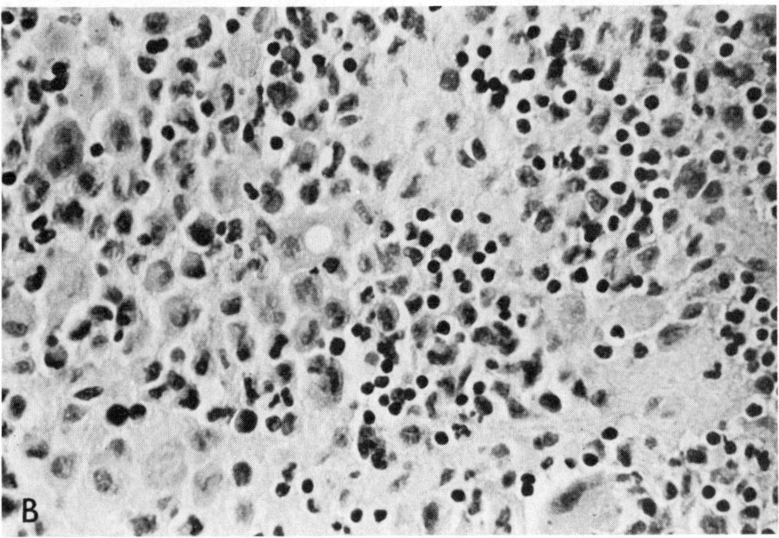

Figure 11–29. Eosinophilic granuloma, femur.

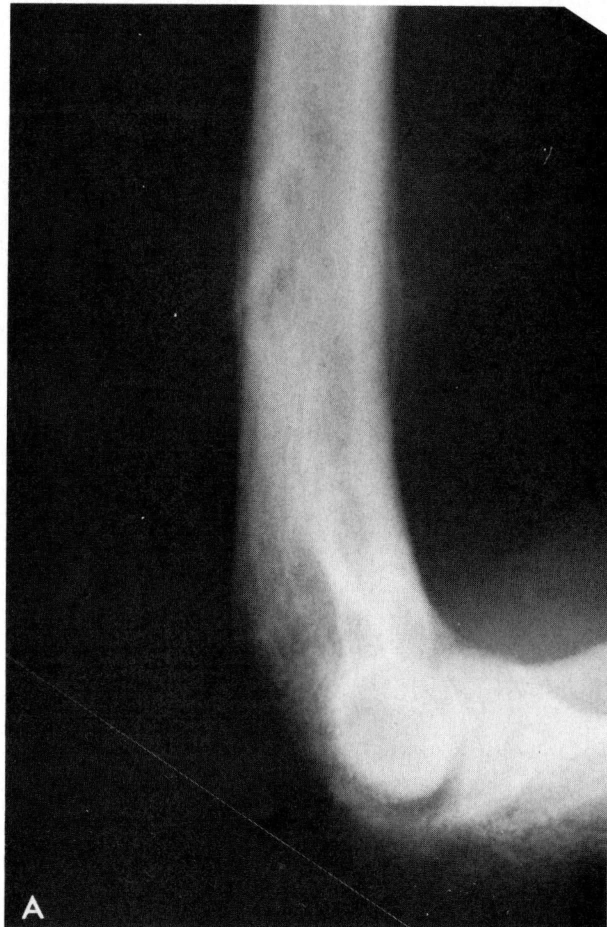

Figure 11–30. Osteomyelitis, humerus

Illustration continued on page 682

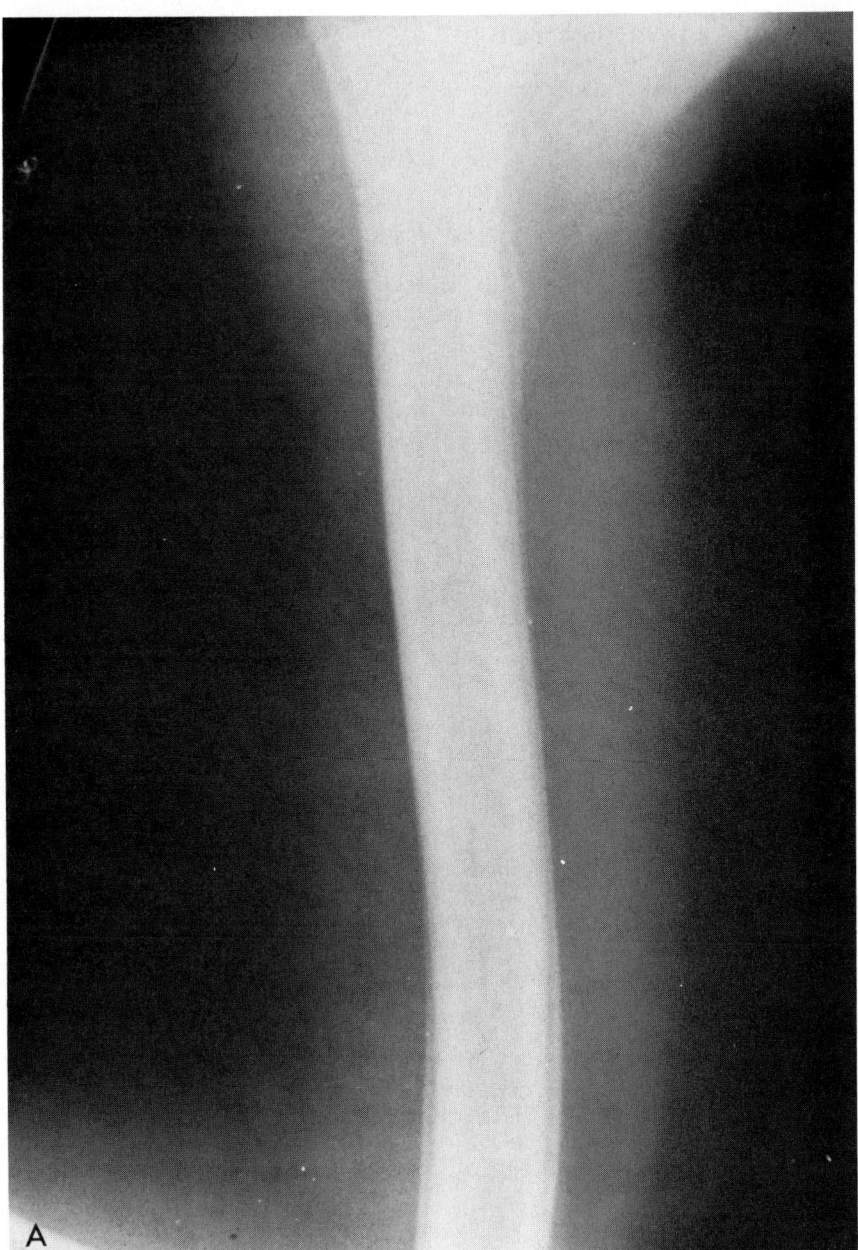

Figure 11–31. Ewing's sarcoma, humerus.

Illustration continued on page 683

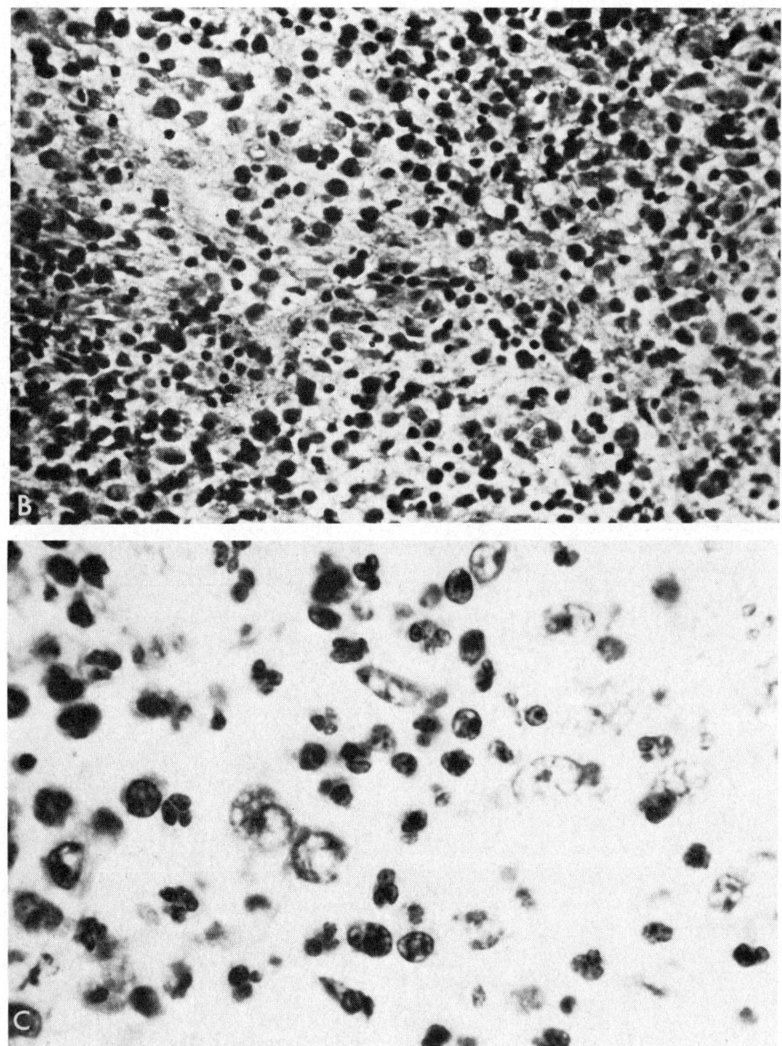

Figure 11–30 *Continued.* Osteomyelitis, humerus.

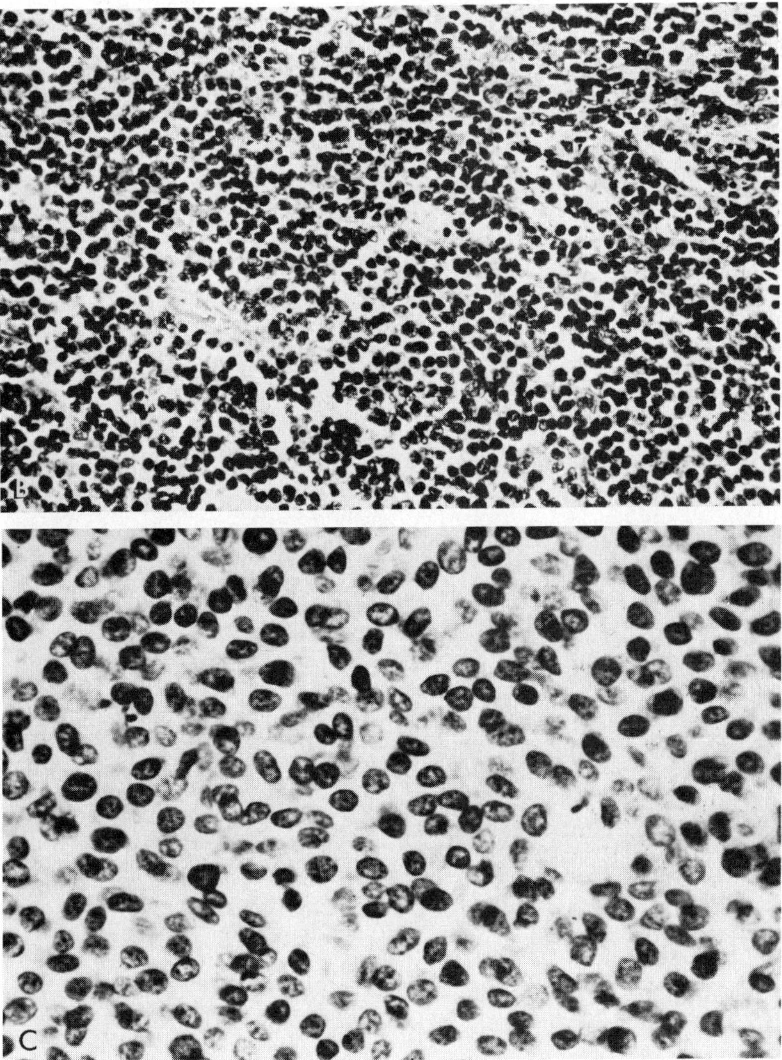

Figure 11–31 *Continued.* Ewing's sarcoma, humerus.

Series 10: Osteomyelitis vs. Ewing's sarcoma, humerus. Both lesions exhibit an ominous radiographic pattern of permeative destruction of medullary and cortical bone extending over a long segment of the humerus. Multiple layers of periosteal new bone ("onion skin") indicate intermittent activity. Spiculation of periosteal reaction ("sunburst" or "hair-on-end") as well as soft-tissue swelling can be seen with either process. Localization of the process to the metaphysis and thicker laminae of periosteal new bone are more common in osteomyelitis, whereas diaphyseal localization, especially full-length, favors Ewing's sarcoma. Clinical course of fever and chills with elevated sedimentation rate and white count can be seen in either process. The diagnosis cannot be ascertained on clinical or radiographic grounds alone but must be made on the basis of biopsy and culture. ("Biopsy every culture, culture every biopsy.") Ewing's sarcoma consists of a sheetlike infiltrate of uniform, small, oval to round cells with no discernible cytoplasm. Pseudorosettes may be identified. In contrast, osteomyelitis exhibits a polymorphous inflammatory infiltrate.

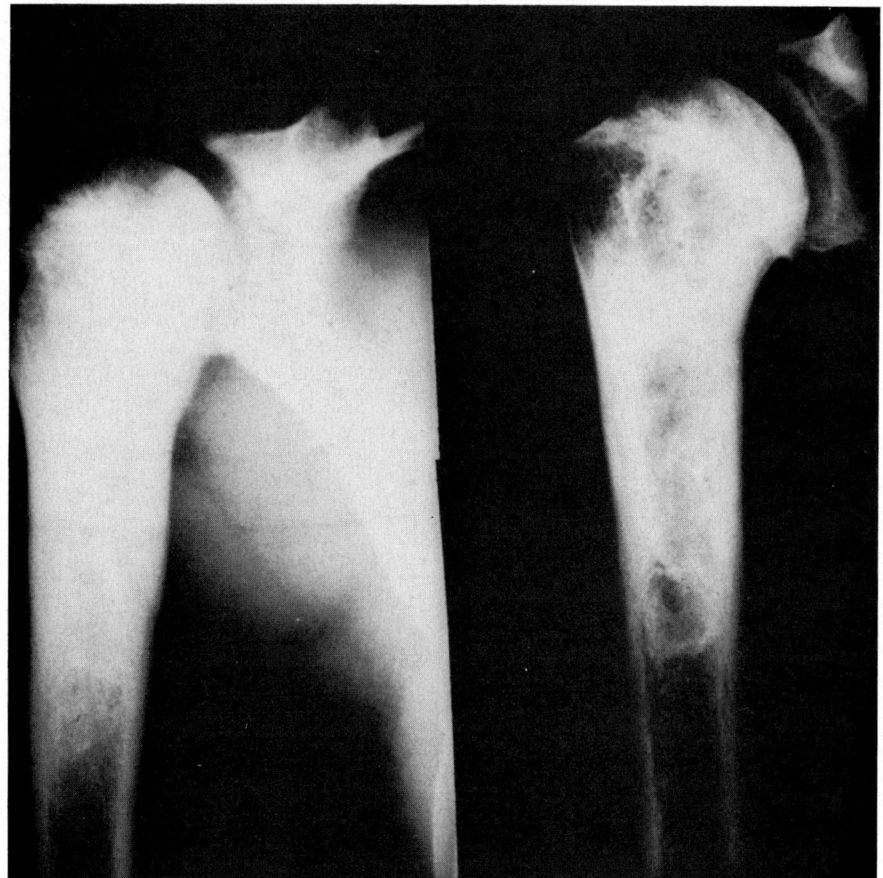

Figure 11–32. Infarct, humerus.

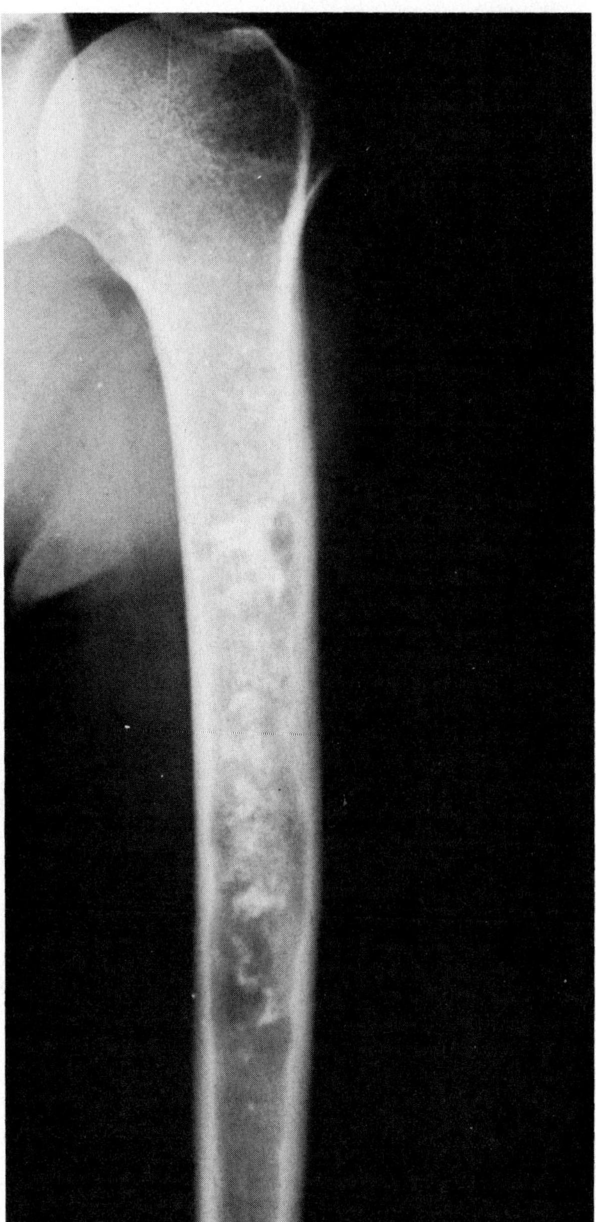

Figure 11–33. Enchondroma, humerus.

Series 11: Bone infarct, tibia vs. enchondroma, humerus. Infarct causes total necrosis of trabecular bone and marrow elements, mostly fat, commonly in the bone ends. Since the central area of the infarct is totally dead, the repair processes are seen around the periphery and consist of saponification (not usually evident on radiographs because the amount of calcium is minimal) and bony margination. Tomograms may be required to demonstrate the shell-like calcification and/or ossification of fat and ischemic bone.

Cartilage lesions are more often in the metaphysis or diaphysis. They show flocculent calcification in the shape of balls and rings, reflecting the normal process of enchondral ossification. Endosteal scalloping may be present in enchondroma, but bony expansion is uncommon in either lesion, except in smaller bones of hands and feet. Either lesion can involve many bones.

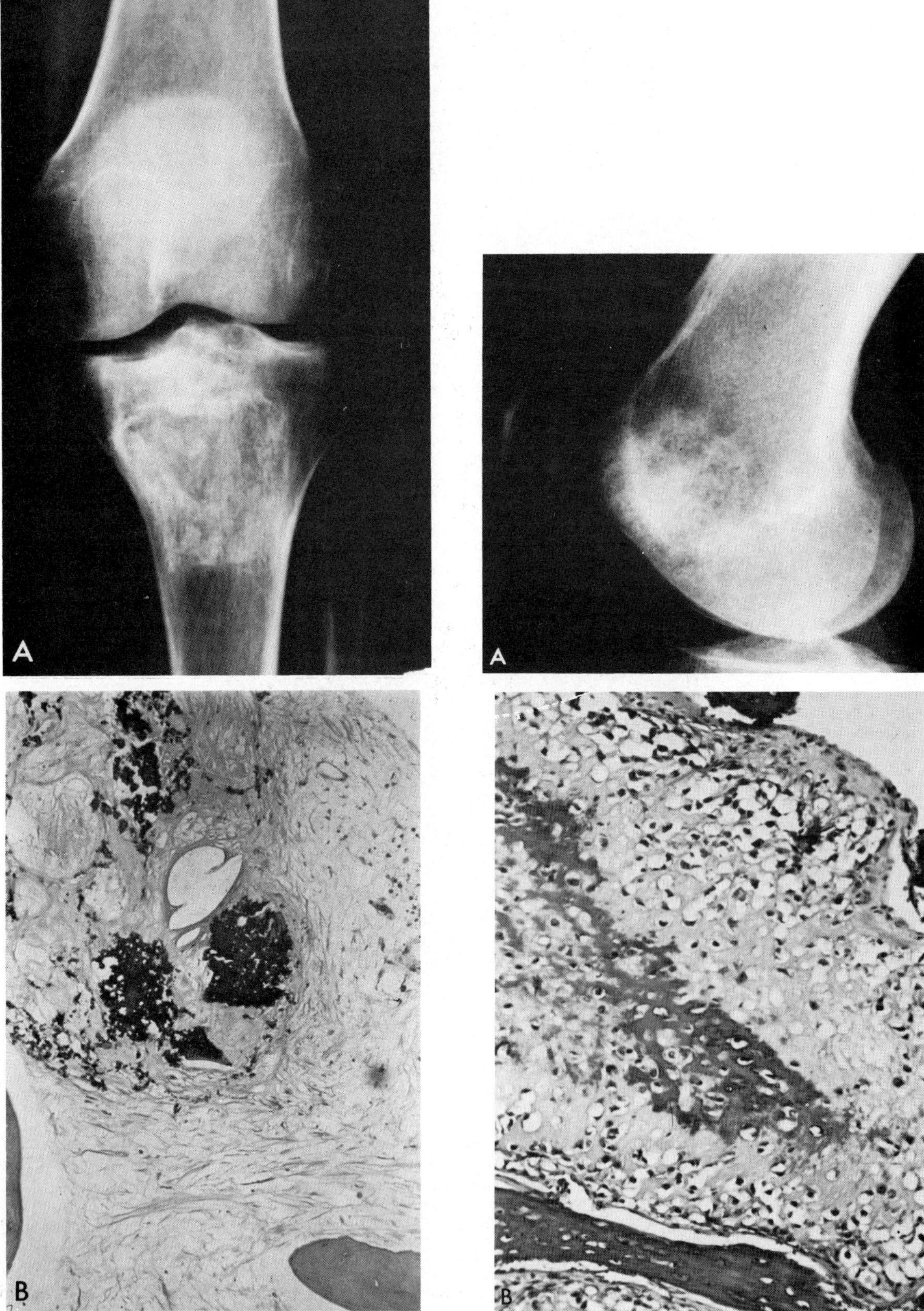

Figure 11-34. Bone infarct, tibia.

Figure 11-35. Chondrosarcoma, femur.

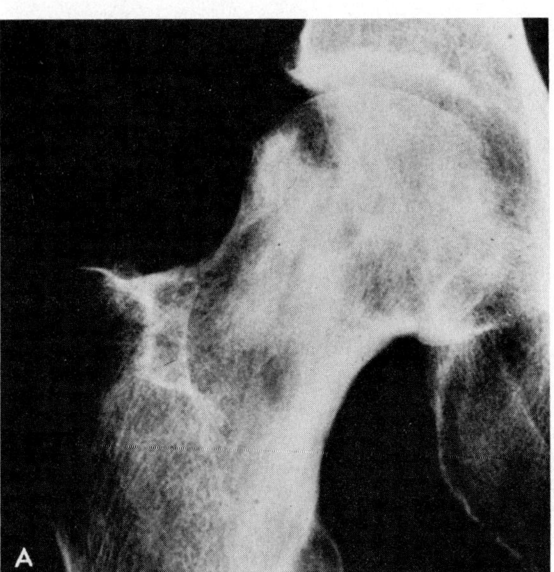

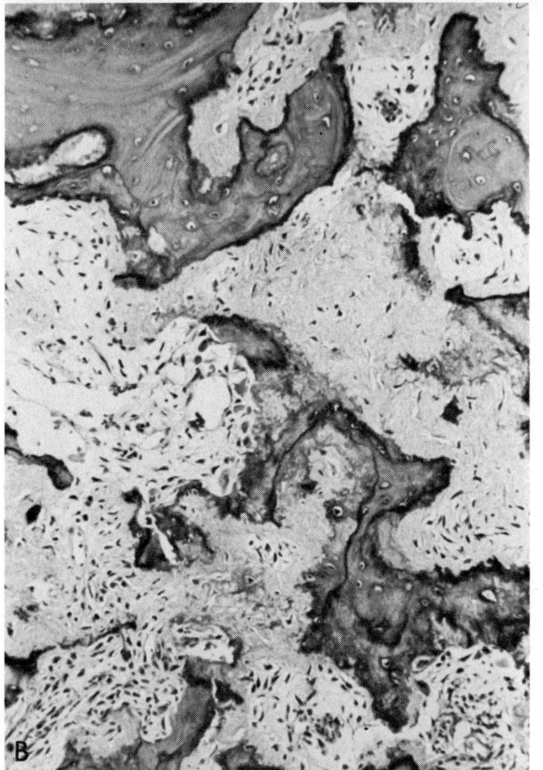

Figure 11–36. Osteosarcoma, femur.

Series 12: Bone infarct, tibia vs. chondrosarcoma, femur vs. osteosarcoma, femur. The juxta-articular tibial infarct occupies most of the proximal end of the bone with an irregular, distinct geographic margin that consists of a heavily mineralized shell. Some of the shell is poor quality ischemic bone in the reactive fibrous zone of the infarct. Weakening of subchondral support has resulted in fracture of the weight-bearing surface of the tibia.

The distal femoral lesion shows flocculent calcification without bone margination or bony matrix. A large predominantly osteolytic lesion with indistinct borders fading into the trabecular bone of the metaphysis are worrisome indicators of malignant change. The presence of pain supports the diagnosis of sarcoma. The flocculent calcification indicates chondrosarcoma; linear calcification would be indicative of osteosarcoma.

The calcification or saponification of necrotic fat in a bone infarct is characterized by dark blue discoloration of the fat without a significant cellular component. This is the poor quality ischemic bone. Osteosarcoma or chondrosarcoma may exhibit similar foci of calcification, but a cellular component is always present, and the cellularity is markedly pleomorphic.

Note the pleomorphic cartilage adjacent to normal trabecular bone with central calcification in the chondrosarcoma, as opposed to neoplastic osteoid formation on the surface of trabecular bone in osteosarcoma.

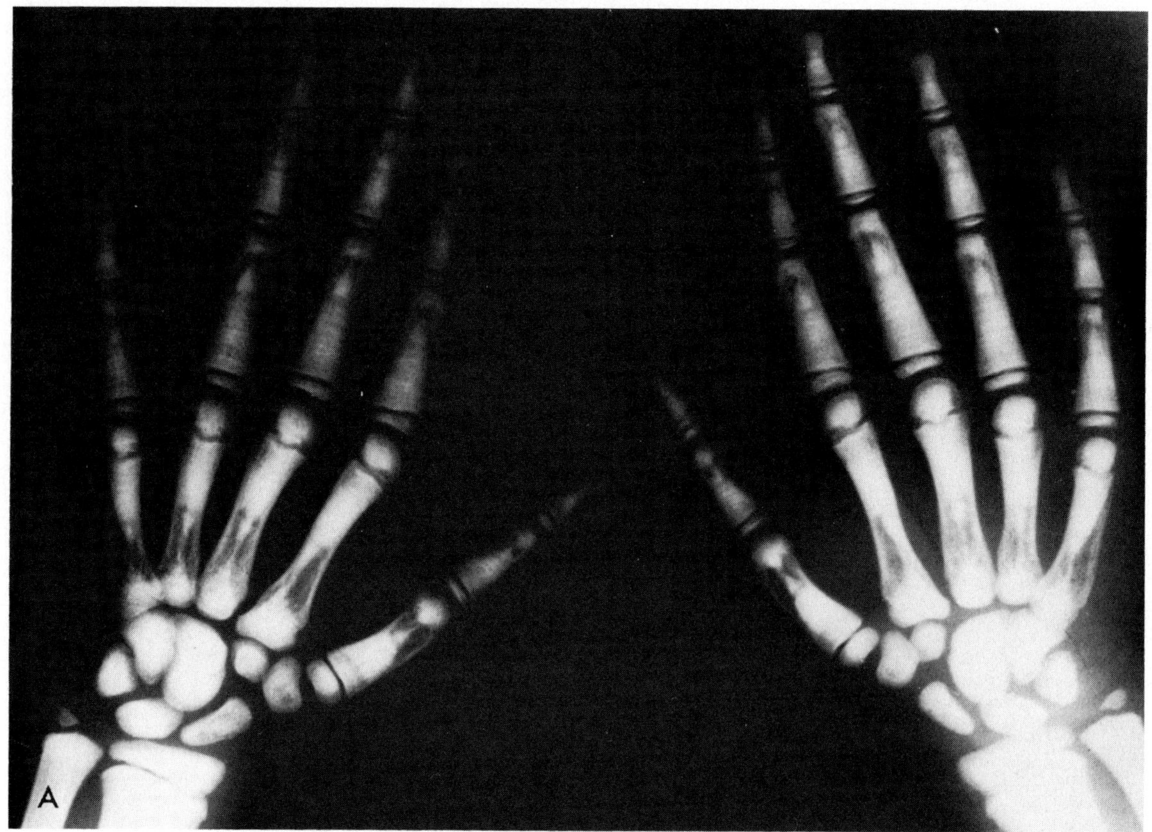

Figure 11–37. Osteopetrosis, wrist.

Illustration continued on page 690

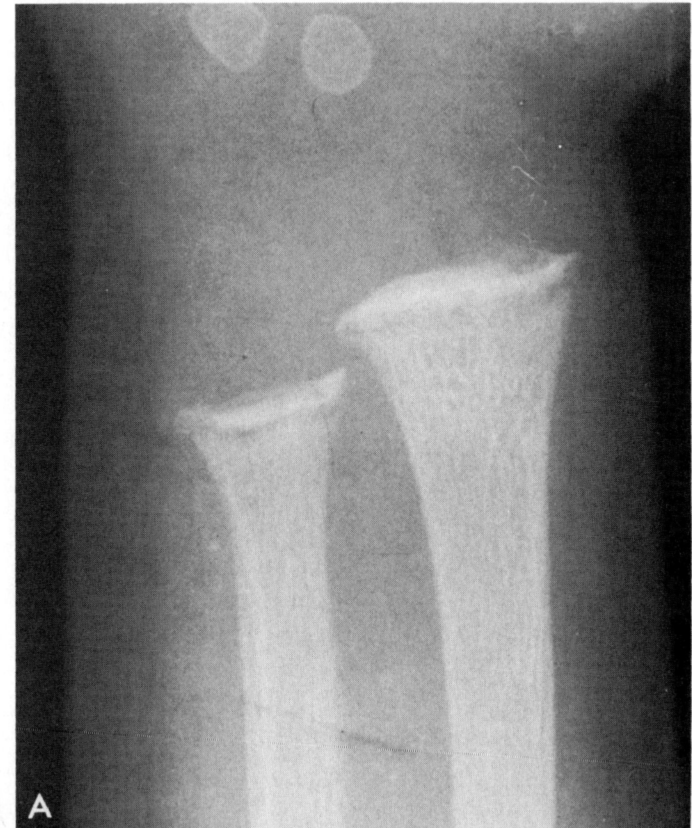

Figure 11–38. Scurvy, wrist.
Illustration continued on page 690

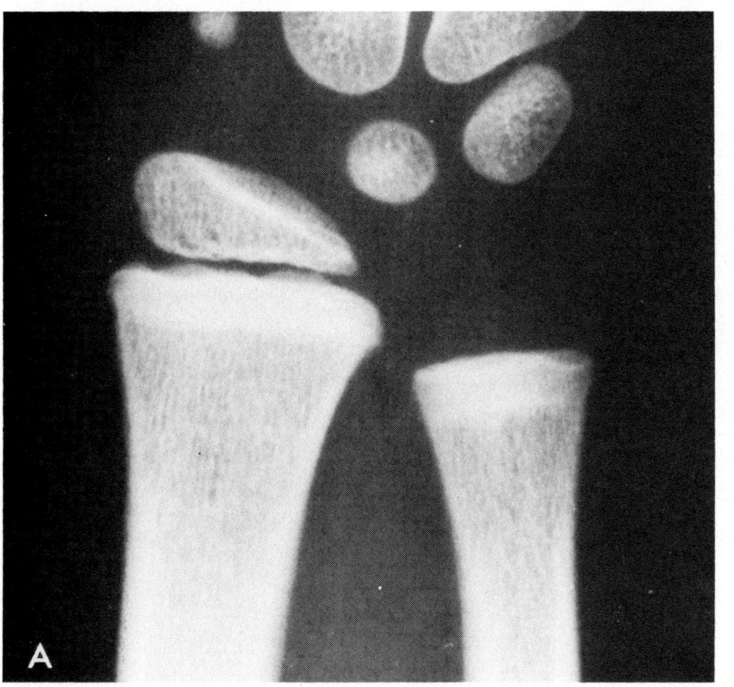

Figure 11–39. Lead poisoning, wrist.
Illustration continued on page 691

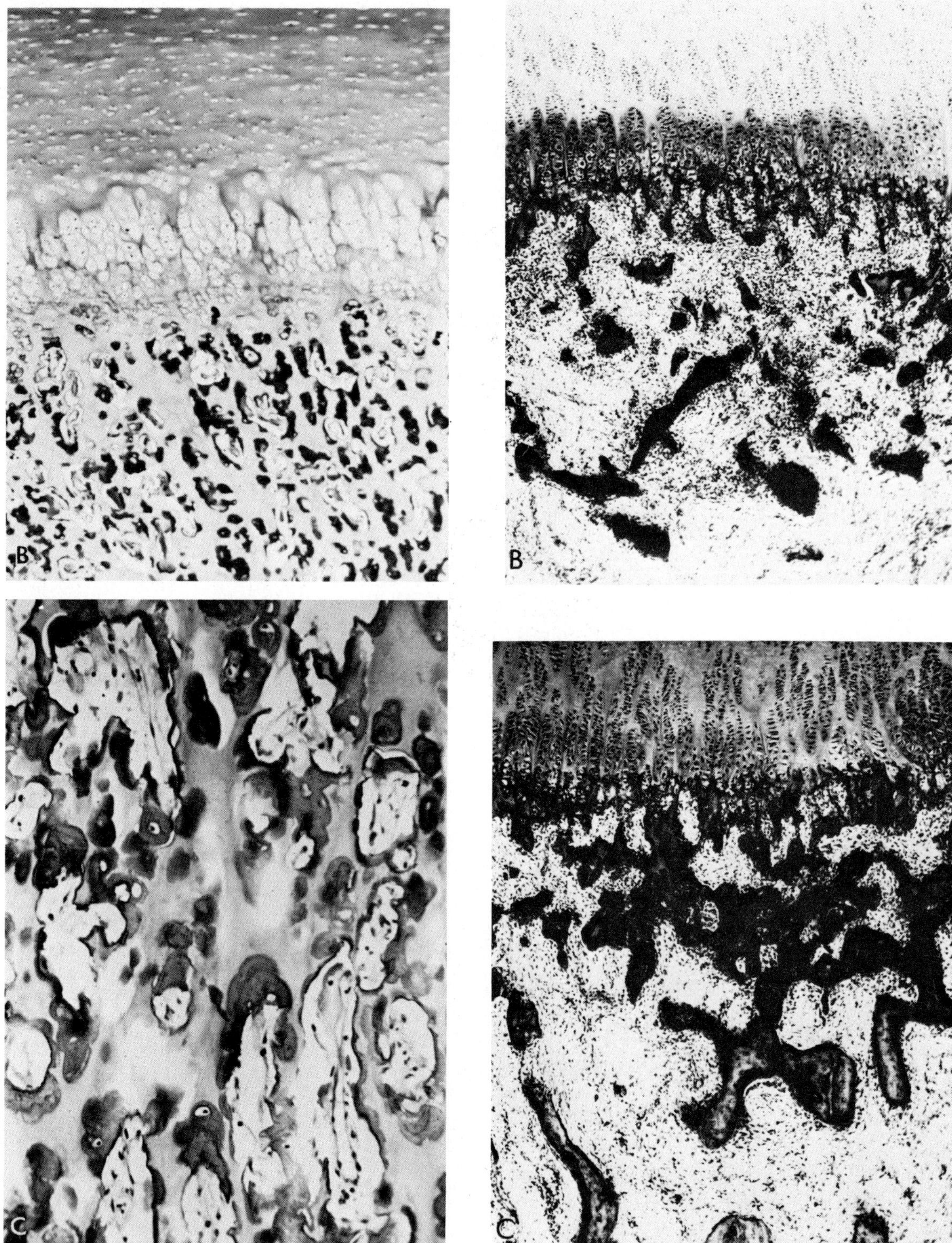

Figure 11–37 *Continued.* Osteopetrosis, wrist.

Figure 11–38 *Continued.* Scurvy, wrist.

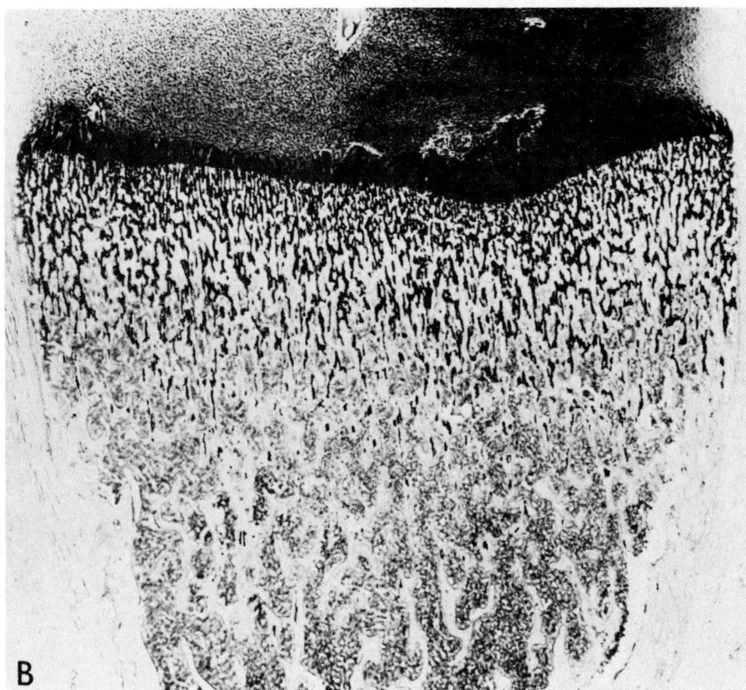

Figure 11–39 *Continued.* Lead poisoning, wrist.

Series 13: Osteopetrosis vs. scurvy vs. lead poisoning, wrist. Lead poisoning produces thick transverse radiodense lines on the metaphyseal side of the physis. Increased density is not due to lead salts, which are present in only minute quantities, but to persistence of calcified cartilage cores in primary trabecula due to inhibition of osteoclasts, resulting in interference with remodeling of both trabecula and the "cut-back zone" (see thorotrast toxicity, Chapter 2, Fig. 2–47).

Scurvy also has a dense zone of calcified cartilage in the metaphysis that is due to failure of functional osteoblasts to appear and produce bony trabecula. The zone of provisional calcification stands out clearly from the normally growing cartilage on one side and the failure of bone production on the other. Cortical bone production is depressed, producing osteoporosis where new bone should be formed. The bone formed before the deficiency of Vitamin C began is entirely normal.

In osteopetrosis, there is a decreased rate of bone and cartilage resorption, related to defective osteoclasts. Radiographs show transverse and longitudinal radiodensities or widespread osteosclerosis, which can present as "bone within a bone." Interference with remodeling results in widened metaphyses and diaphyses. Bones preformed in cartilage show the greatest abnormality, but the cranial vault can also be thickened.

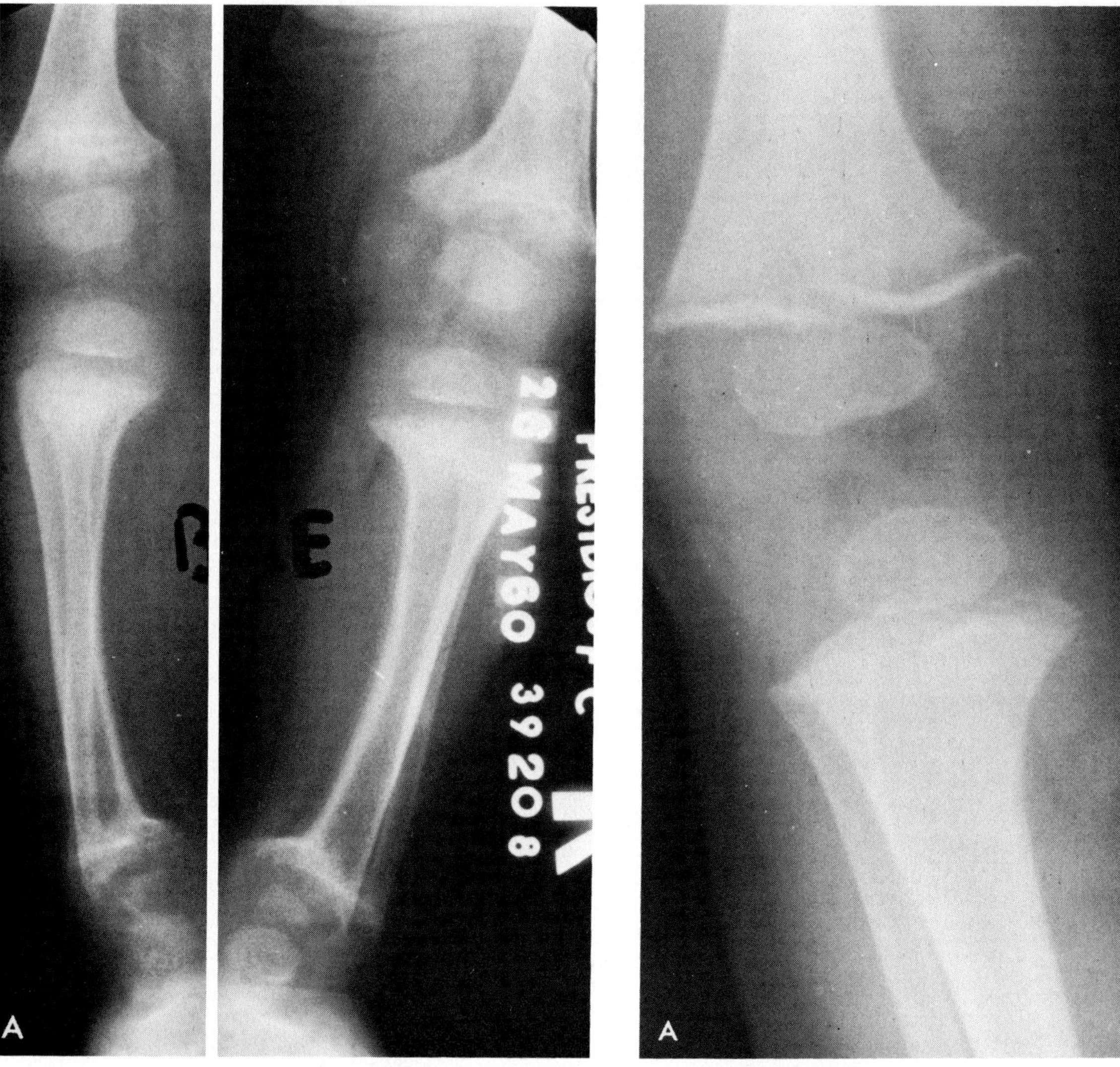

Figure 11–40. Rickets, knee.

Figure 11–41. Scurvy, knee.

Illustrations continued on page 694

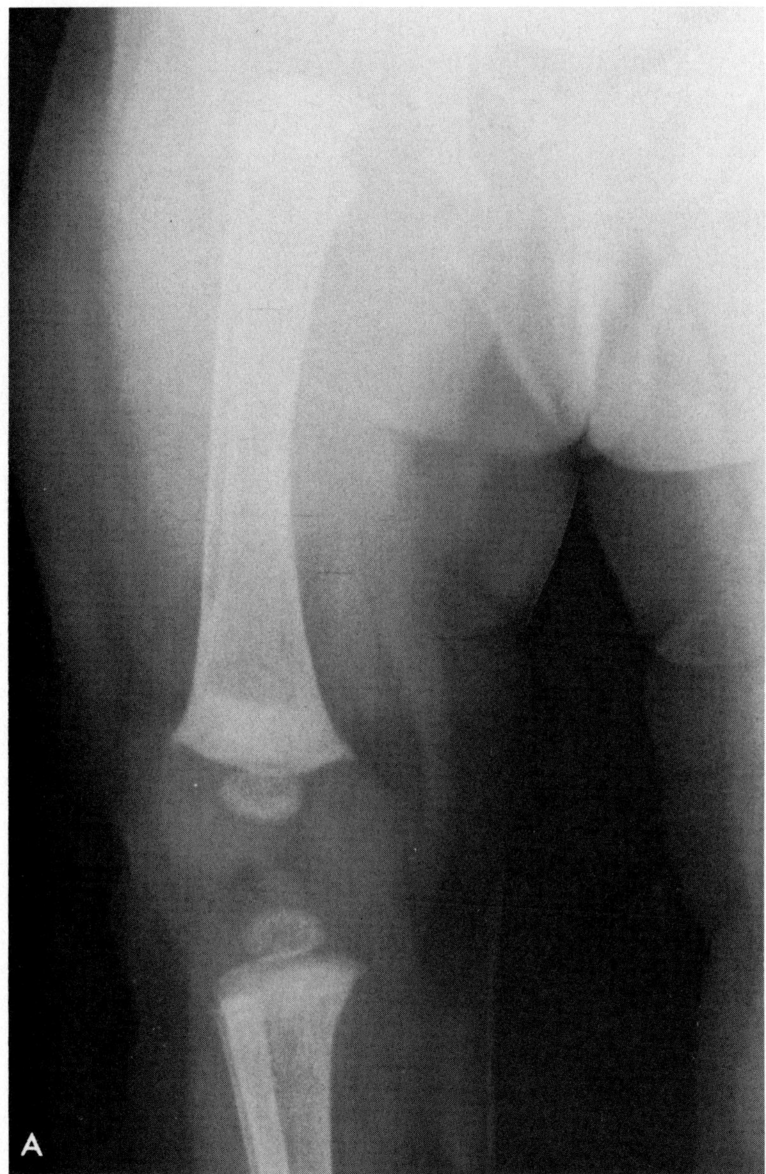

Figure 11–42. Congenital syphilis, knee.

Illustration continued on page 695

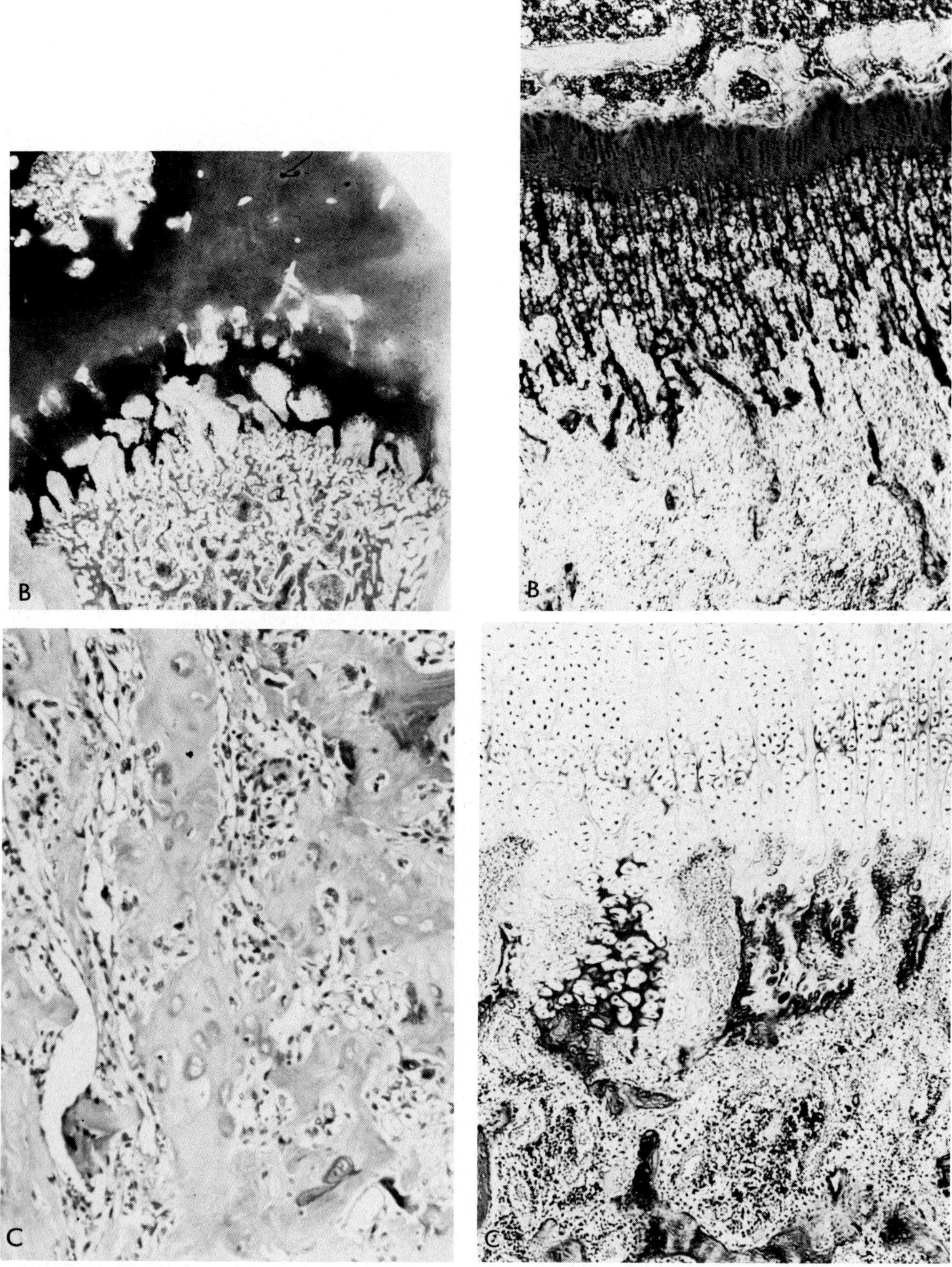

Figure 11–40 *Continued.* Rickets, knee.

Figure 11–41 *Continued.* Scurvy, knee.

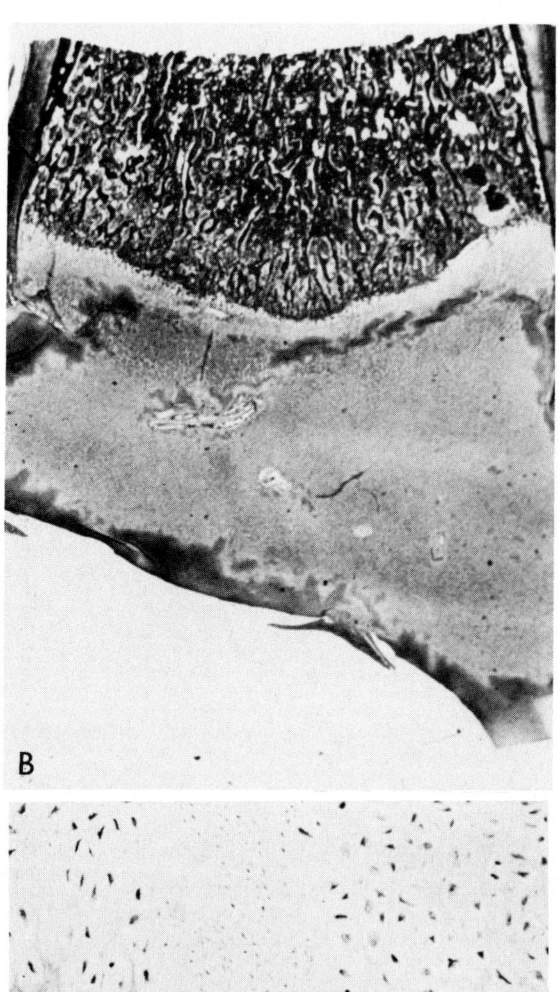

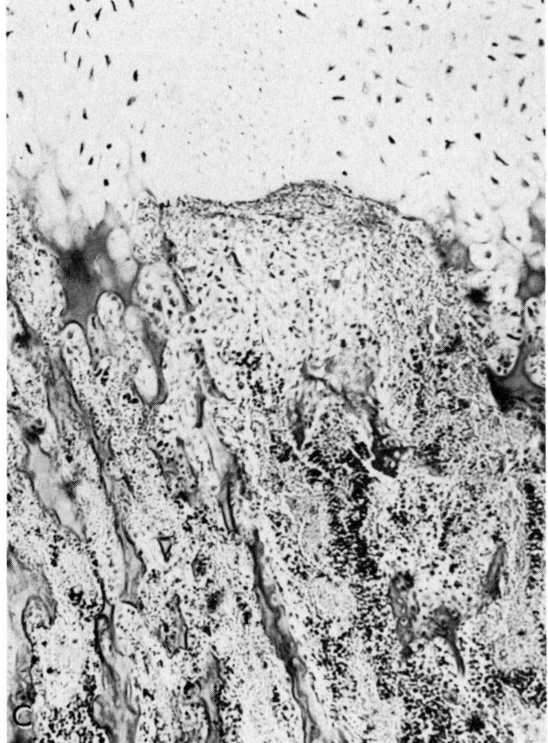

Figure 11–42 *Continued.* Congenital syphilis, knee.

Series 14: Rickets vs. scurvy vs. congenital syphilis, knee. Increased width of the physis, irregular mineralization of metaphysis, and flared bone ends with cupping of metaphysis are all characteristics of rickets. The changes consist of irregular prolongation of a hypertrophic cartilage zone without orderly maturation and results in gross deformities due to muscular stress on the elongated nonmineralized physis. Trabecular bone exhibits osteomalacia secondary to deposition of unmineralized osteoid.

In scurvy, the dense zone of provisional calcification stands out owing to lucency on both sides. The cortex is osteoporotic, but any bone present is normal. The physis is not elongated, since cartilage maturation is completed, and mineralization of the cartilage occurs in the normal zone.

In congenital syphilis, osteochondritic granulation tissue in the metaphysis prevents bone production, yielding an irregular radiographic lucent zone, similar to that seen in scurvy. The syphilitic granulations are quickly replaced when appropriate therapy is instituted. With subsequent growth, all stigmata of congenital syphilis in the metaphysis disappear. Diaphyseal changes occur early and consist of periosteal new bone production, which is evident prior to treatment. In scurvy, the periosteal new bone will not become radiographically visible until therapy is instituted.

Scurvy is often associated with rickets. Note the combination of defects in Figure 11–41, consisting of an elongated calcified cartilage base (scurvy) and foci of irregular incomplete cartilage maturation without calcification (rickets).

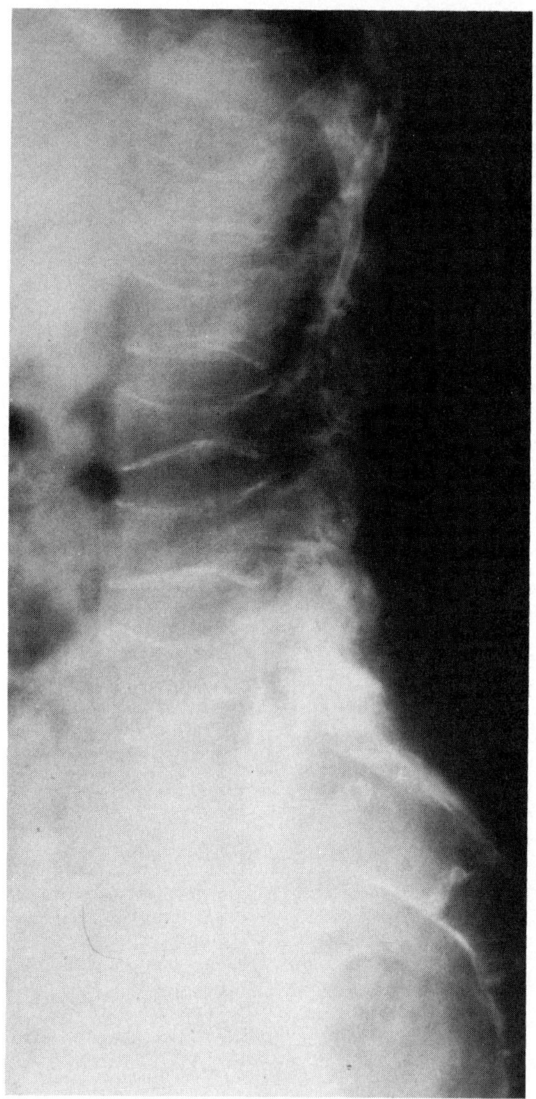

Figure 11–43. Idiopathic osteoporosis, spine.

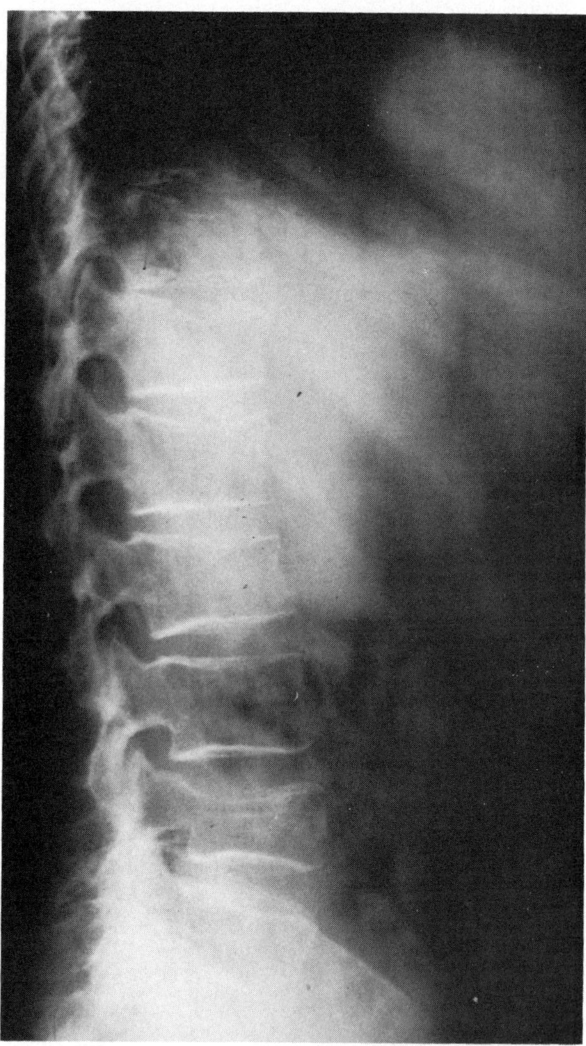

Figure 11–44. Multiple myeloma, spine.

Series 15: Idiopathic osteoporosis vs. multiple myeloma vs. iatrogenic hypercorticoidism, spine. All three entities are associated with marked loss of skeletal matrix and mineral and illustrate radiographic osteopenia. Secondary changes include wedging due to fractures with minimal trauma and cupping of vertebral end-plates as a result of regressive remodeling over time. Discrete lesions may be seen in myeloma, but severe osteopenia may be the only radiographic sign. Exogenous corticosteroid excess is radiographically indistinguishable from true Cushing's syndrome or postmenopausal osteoporosis. Differential diagnosis of these three entities is based on clinical history and laboratory findings.

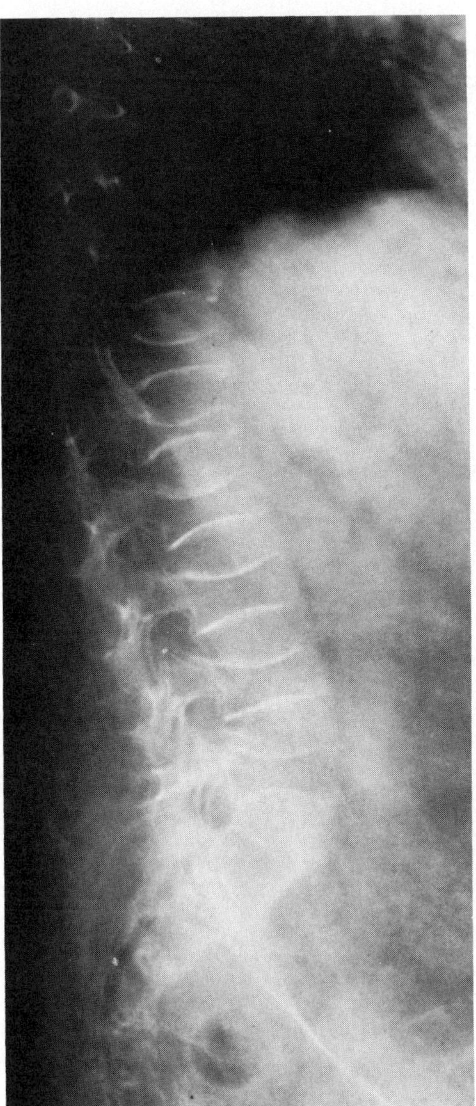

Figure 11–45. Iatrogenic hypercorticoidism, spine.

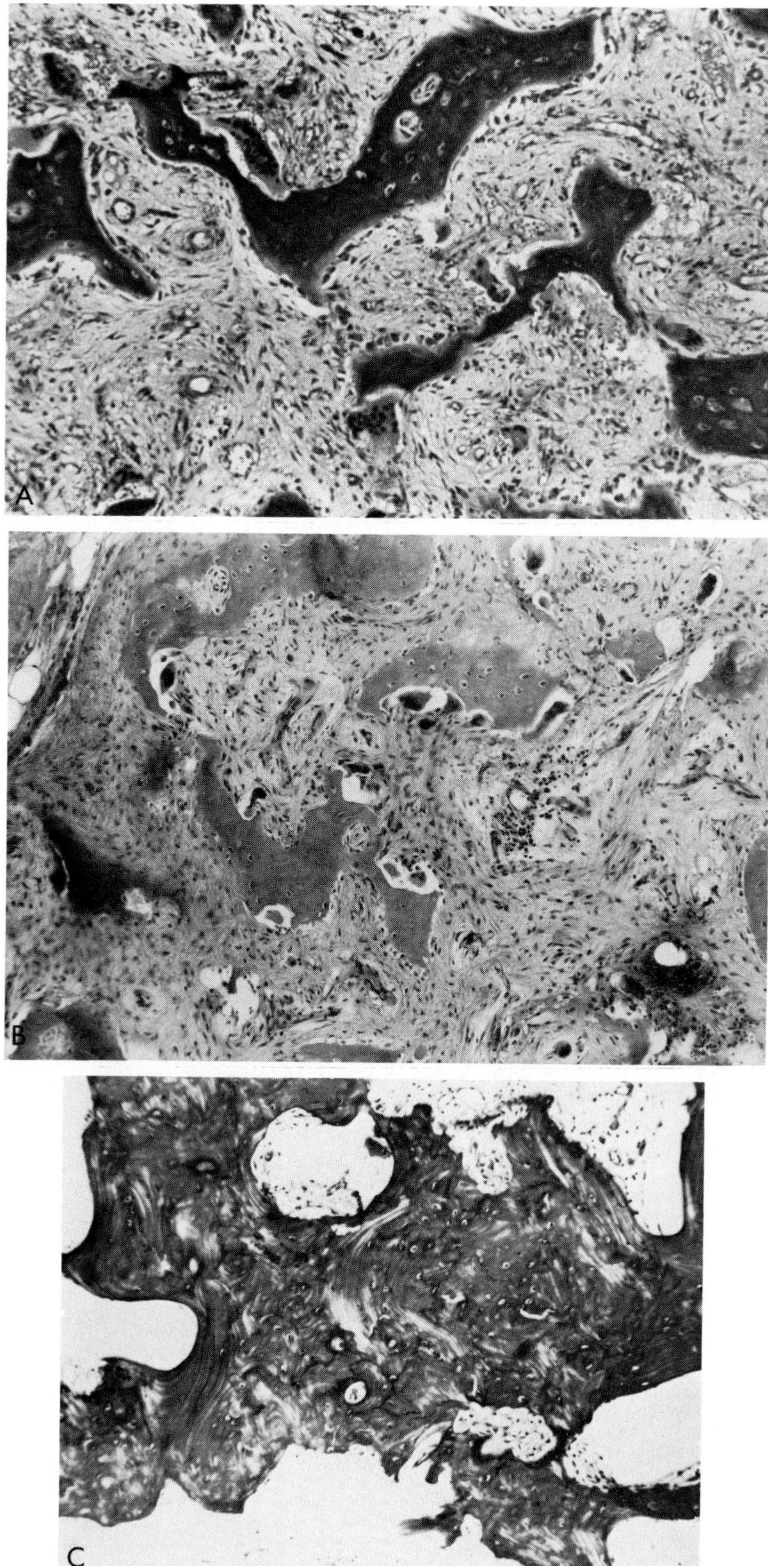

Figure 11–46. Osteitis deformans (Paget's disease).

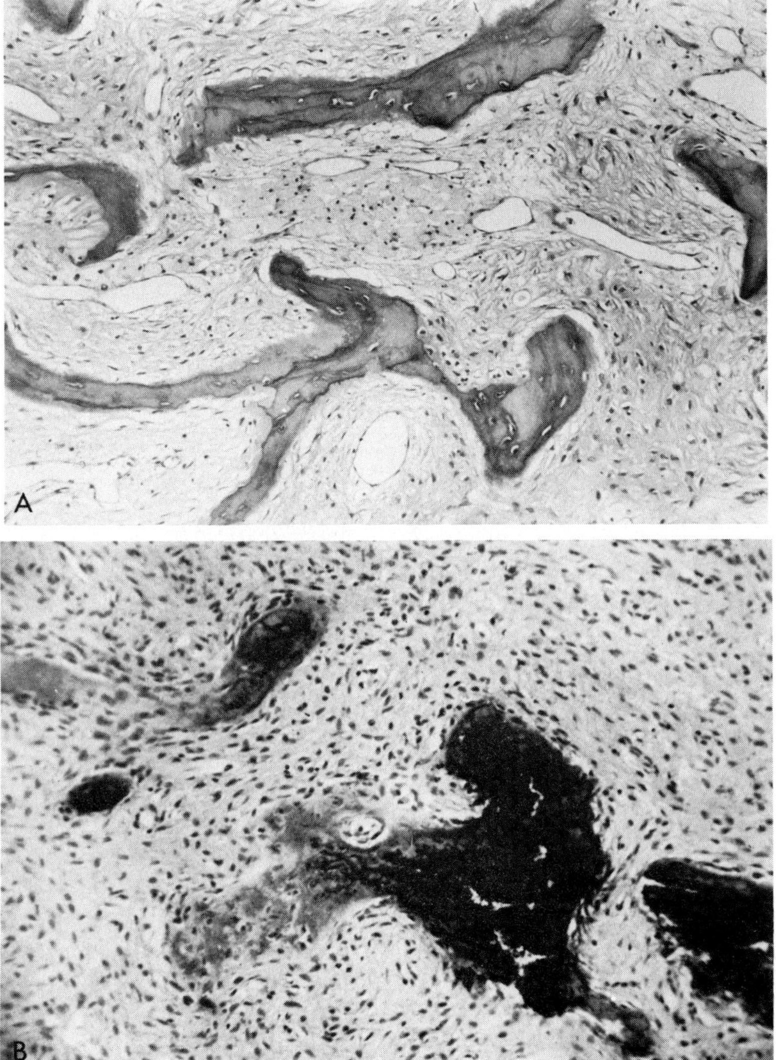

Figure 11–47. Fibrous dysplasia.

Series 16: Paget's disease (osteitis deformans) vs. fibrous dysplasia. The early lytic phase of Paget's disease is characterized by bone trabecula lined by osteoblasts accompanied by numerous osteoclasts. The stroma is fibrous and contains occasional inflammatory cells. The classic mosaic of Paget's disease is a later manifestation, associated with sclerosis.

Fibrous dysplasia is characterized by similar trabecula of bone, but the osteoblasts are generally absent, and giant cells, although they may be present in focal areas, are not a prominent feature.

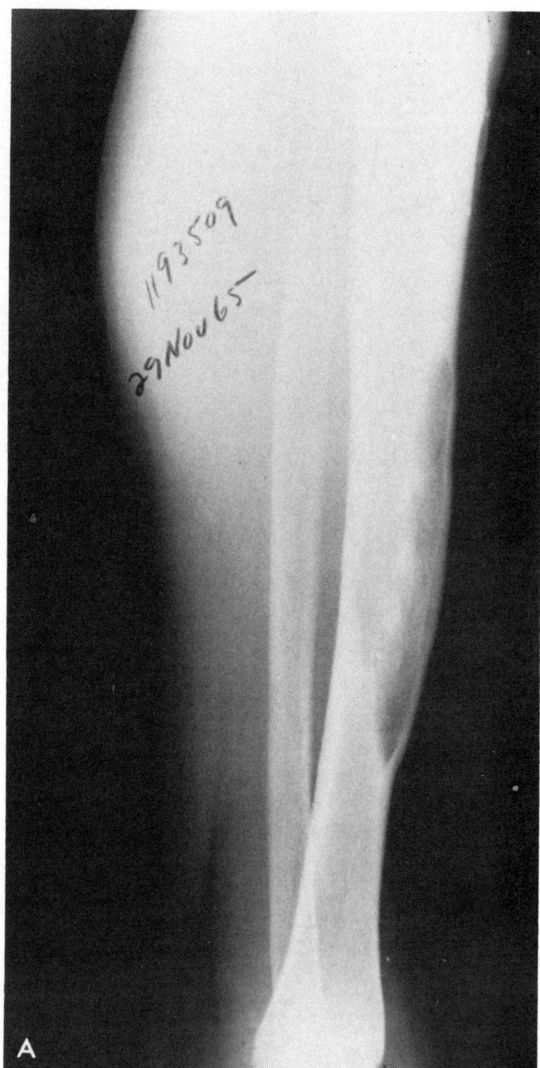

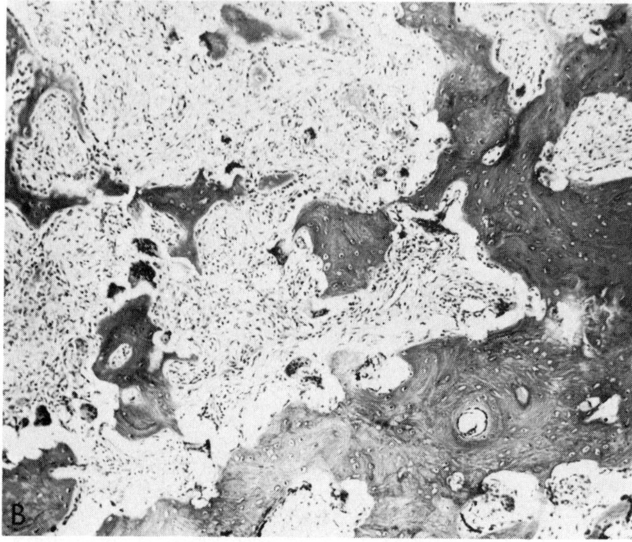

Figure 11–48. Osteitis deformans (Paget's disease), tibia.

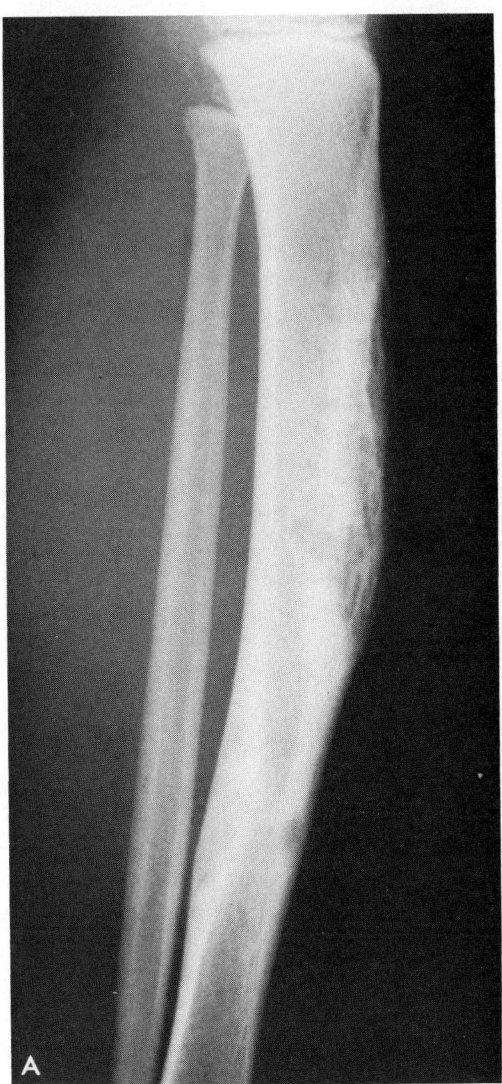

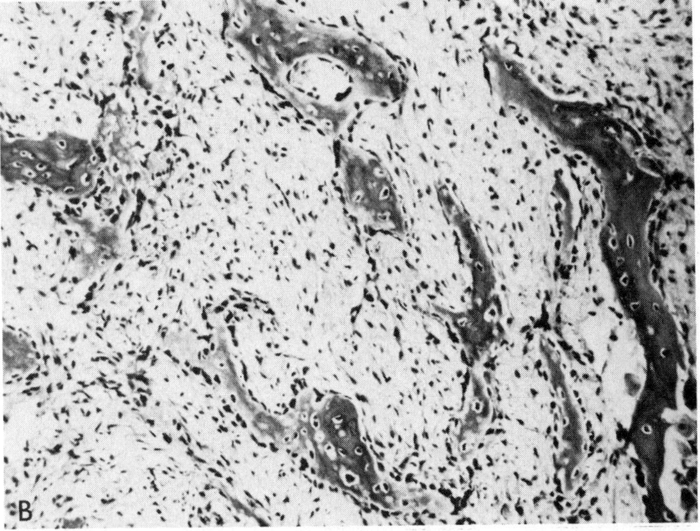

Figure 11–49. Cortical fibrous dysplasia (ossifying fibroma), tibia.

Series 17: Paget's disease (osteitis deformans) vs. cortical fibrous dysplasia (ossifying fibroma), tibia. Cortical fibrous dysplasia is a clearly defined, well-circumscribed, round or oval lesion entirely contained within the tibial cortex and always covered by a rim of bone. The matrix is usually radiolucent compared with the cortical surroundings, although it does contain varying numbers of bone spicules. The cortex is expanded and dense.

In Paget's disease, the initial phase is a wave of osteolysis in the cortex, with periosteal and endosteal reinforcement causing expansion. The unusually sharp margination has been likened to a "blade of grass" or "palette knife" and is due to the outline of the lytic process by cortical bone. Waves of repair will appear as irregular densities within the lytic zone of resorption.

The histologic evidence of cortical fibrous dysplasia consists of well-formed trabecula of bone surrounded by a rim of osteoblasts set in a fibrous connective tissue stroma. Paget's disease exhibits haphazard osteoclastic and osteoblastic activity and lacks the discrete spicule formation of cortical fibrous dysplasia.

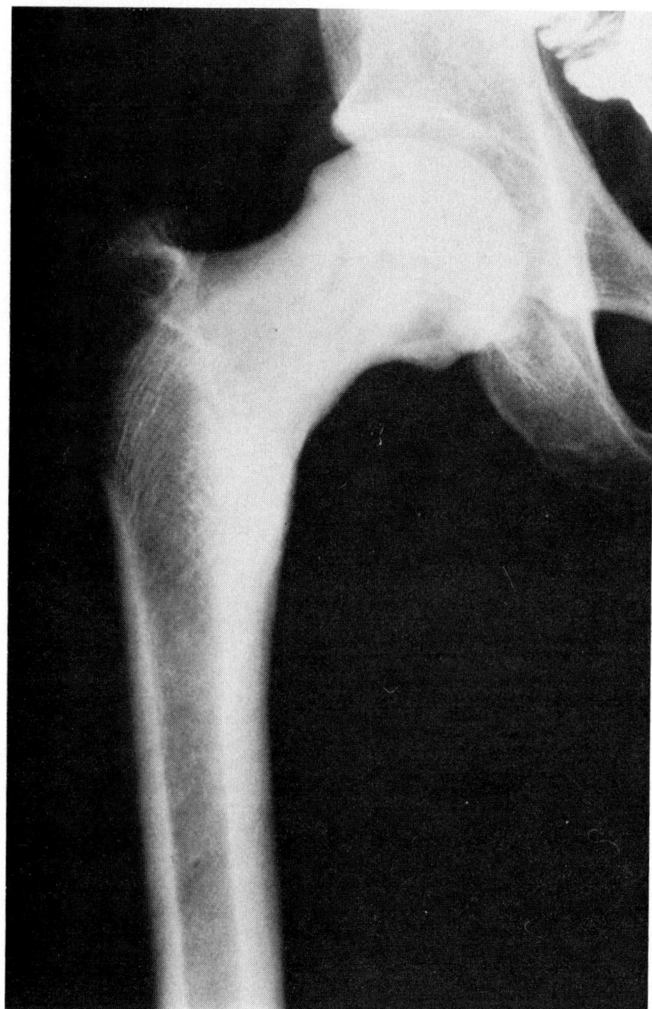

Figure 11–50. Osteitis deformans (Paget's disease), hip.

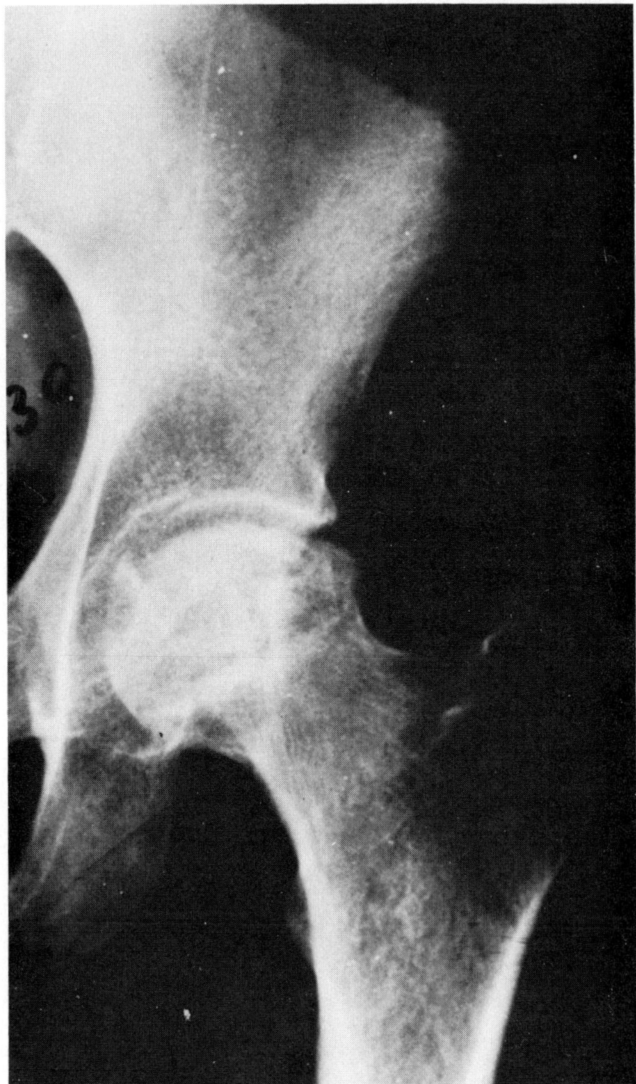

Figure 11–51. Aseptic necrosis, hip.

Series 18: Paget's disease (osteitis deformans) vs. bone infarct, hip. Paget's disease is initiated by an osteolytic phase followed by abnormal bone production. The bones become deformed by the eccentricity of this remodeling process. Increased bone production in the femoral head and neck results in radiographic density of the cortex and trabecular bone with some augmentation in lines of stress. This density extends below the level of the lesser trochanter. The histologic evidence of Paget's disease consists of massive osteoclastic activity and replacement of bone by nonspecific fibrous connective tissue. There is associated osteoblastic activity that ultimately leads to dense sclerotic bone with the classic mosaic pattern.

Infarct of the femoral head causes weakened bone, particularly during the revascularization phase, with impaction fractures and deformity. Areas of decreased density mixed with increased density are characteristic radiographic features of aseptic necrosis and indicate the healing phase ("creeping substitution"). Joint narrowing and degenerative joint disease are common in both entities when involving weight-bearing areas. The histologic evidence of aseptic necrosis consists of infarcted bone, ischemic bone, and osteoclastic removal of infarcted fragments at the line of "creeping substitution."

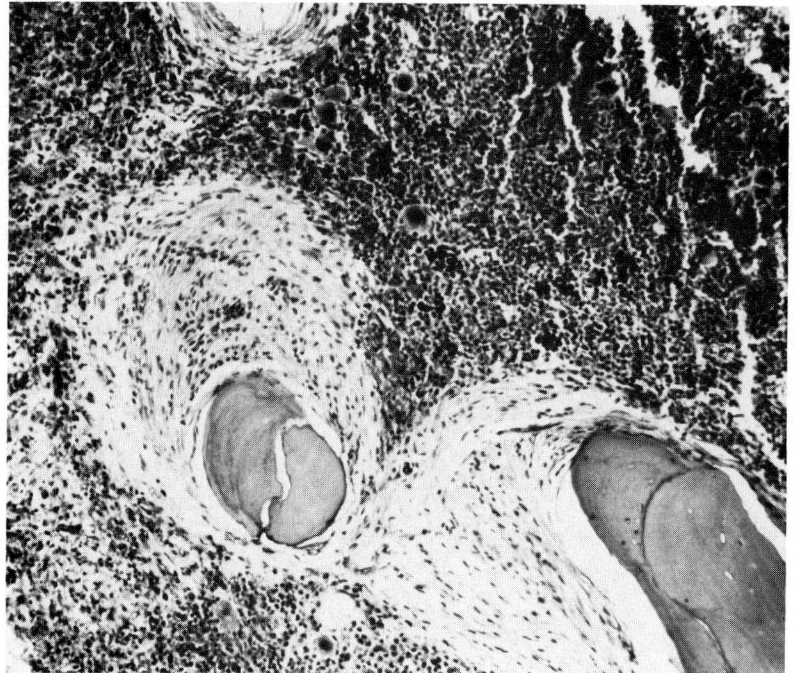

Figure 11–52. Myelofibrosis.

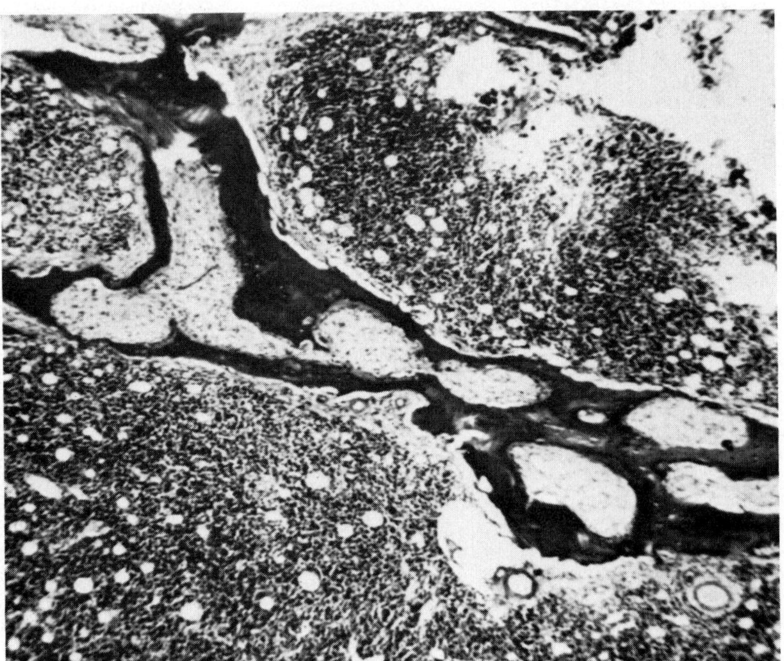

Figure 11–53. Hyperparathyroidism.

Series 19: Myelofibrosis vs. hyperparathyroidism. In myelofibrosis the fibrous connective tissue replaces the bone marrow but is on the outside of the trabeculum, and there is transition from fibrous connective tissue to bone. Note the appositional bone growth. In hyperparathyroidism, the mesenchymal connective tissue replaces bone, hollowing out the trabeculum, resulting in a net loss of bone.

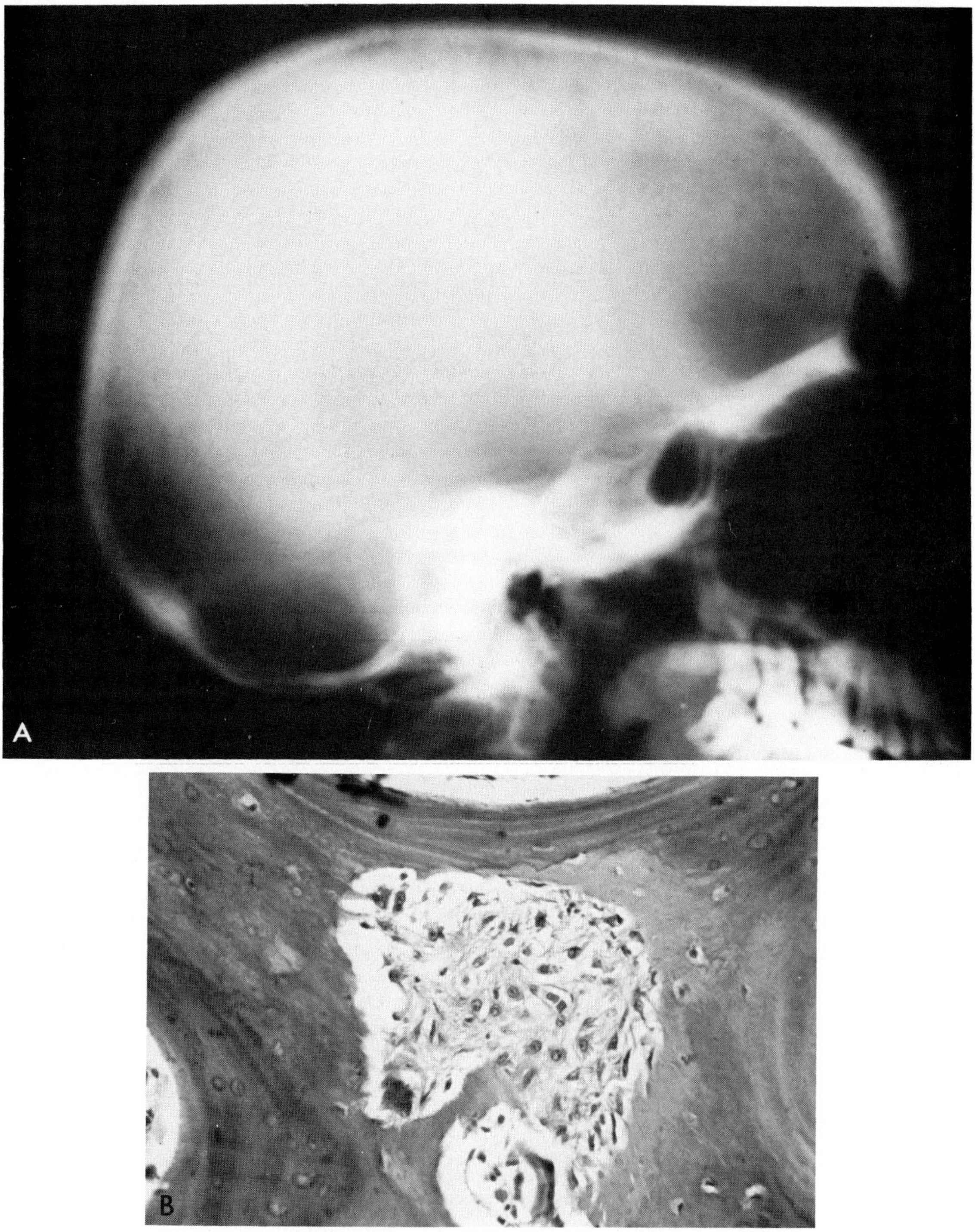

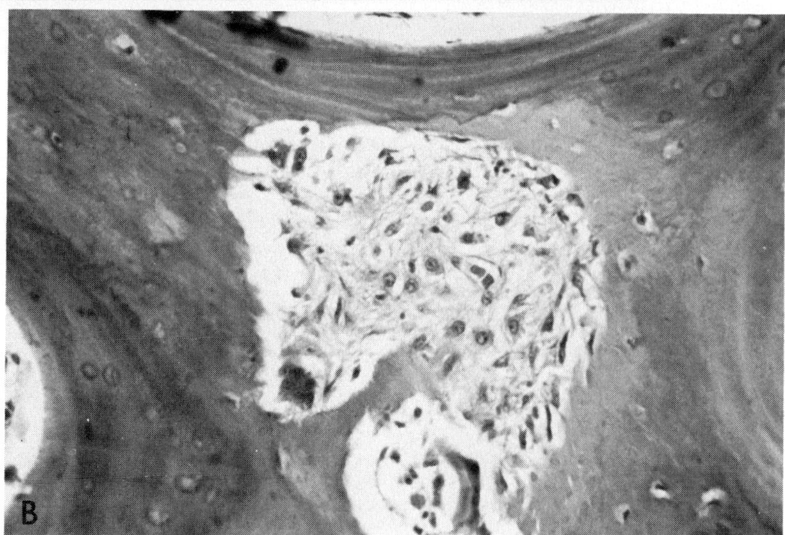

Figure 11–54. Hyperparathyroidism, skull.

Series 20: Hyperparathyroidism vs. Paget's disease (osteitis deformans), skull. Both entities are characterized by accelerated bone resorption and production in varying ratios. Hyperparathyroidism tends to be more diffuse, involving all trabecular and cortical surfaces and producing a fine "salt and pepper" appearance. The calvarium may become quite sclerotic.

In Paget's disease, the osteolysis is more irregular and tends to involve larger areas with adjacent uninvolved bone. Bone replacement is also more irregular, yielding larger "cotton-wool" patches.

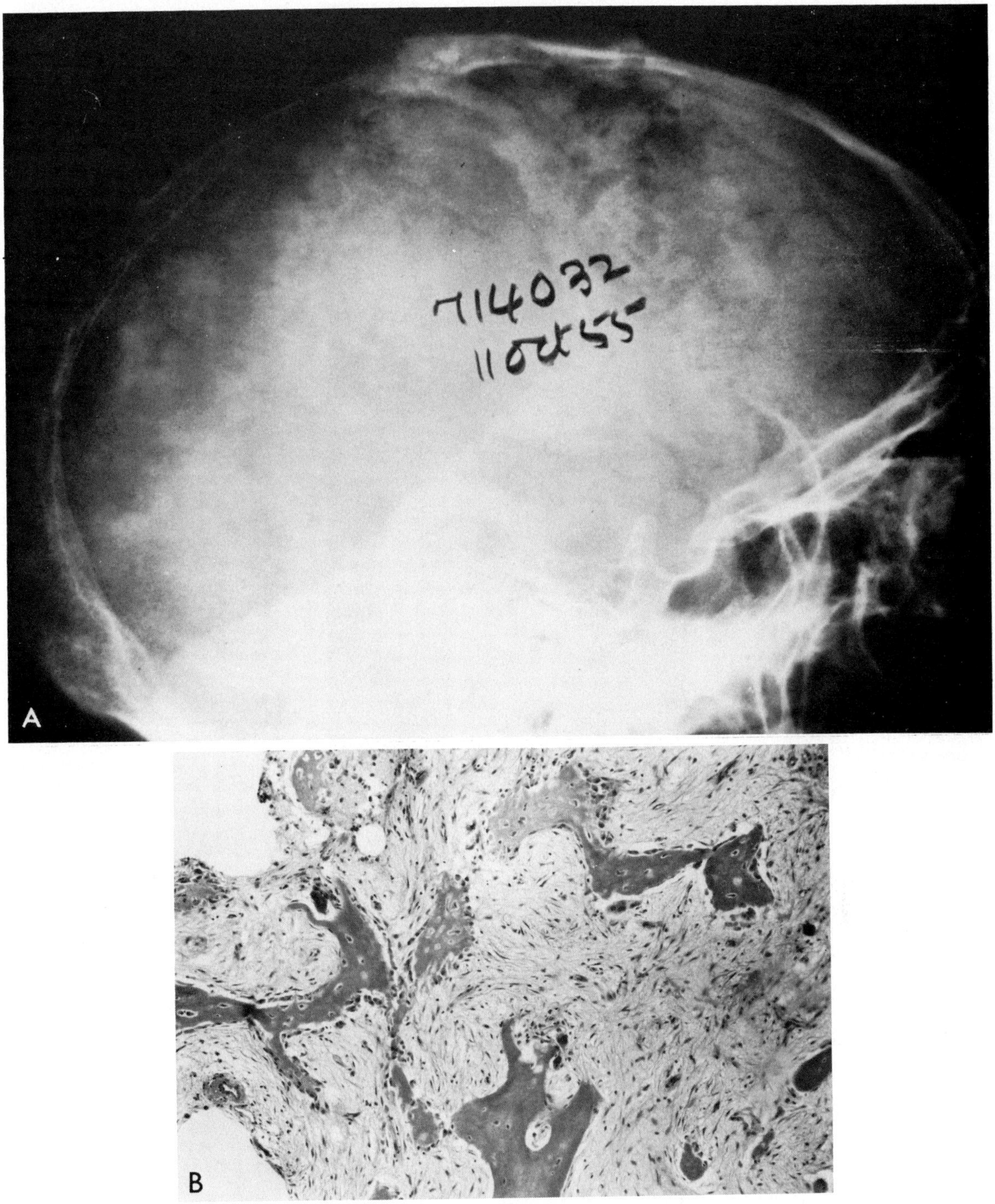

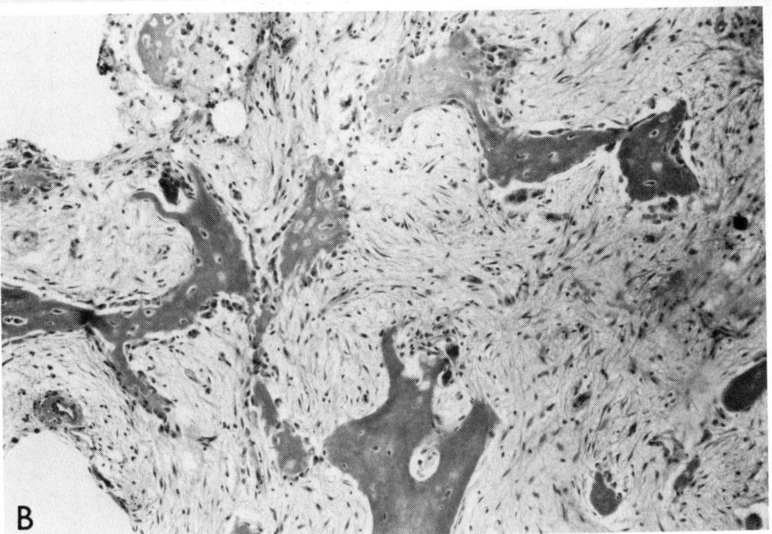

Figure 11–55. Osteitis deformans (Paget's disease), skull.

In hyperparathyroidism, the fibrous replacement of bone consists of hollowing out of trabecula; there may be some osteoblastic activity to reinforce trabecula in lines of stress. In Paget's disease, there is haphazard osteoblastic and osteoclastic activity, with fibrous replacement of cortical and spongiotic bone.

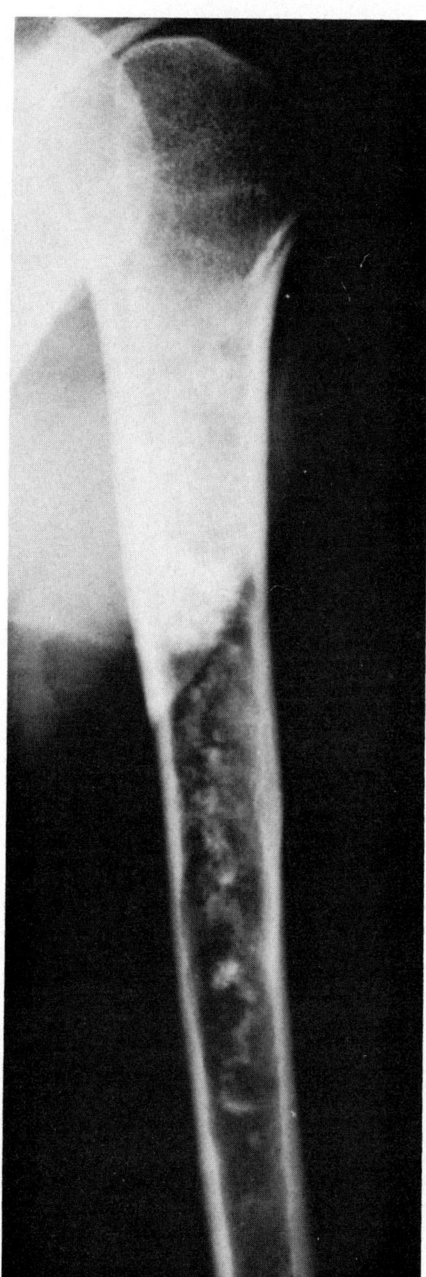

Figure 11–56. Enchondroma, humerus.

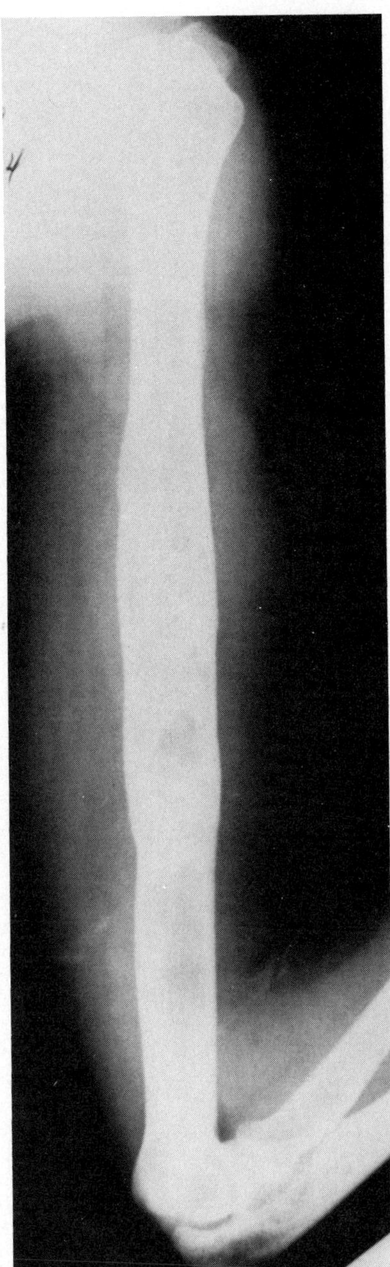

Figure 11–57. Fibrous dysplasia, humerus.

Series 21: Enchondroma vs. fibrous dysplasia, humerus. Elongated, irregularly convoluted and calcified intramedullary lesion with rings and balls of calcified cartilage is typical of enchondroma, as is the lack of change in the contour of host bone.

Fibrous dysplasia is usually elongated and has an irregular contour with frequent expansion of bone and no discrete mineralization of the matrix. Radiographic "ground glass" density results from large numbers of small ossified spicules in fibrous dysplastic matrix. Lack of periosteal reaction in either lesion indicates slow-growing or static condition.

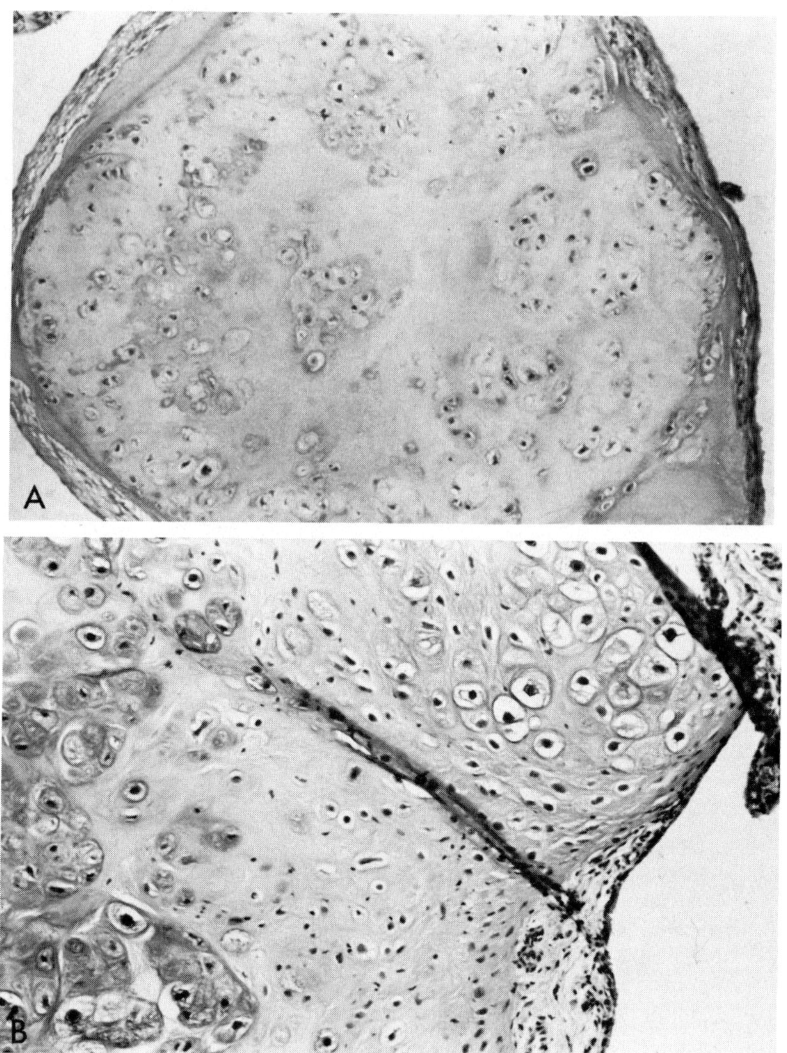

Figure 11–58. Synovial chondromatosis.

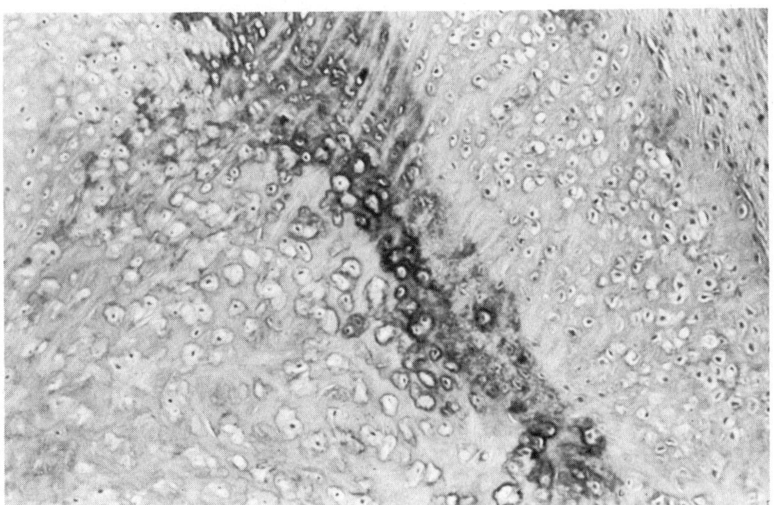

Figure 11–59. Joint body.

Series 22: Synovial chondromatosis vs. joint bodies. The loose body consists of cartilage desquamated into the synovial cavity, where cartilage continues to proliferate, nourished by synovial fluid. Focal areas of calcification may be present within the cartilage. Bone, if present, is infarcted. In contrast, synovial chondromatosis is always surrounded by a thin layer of edematous connective tissue and a synovial lining. The cartilage is a result of metaplasia of the synovial tissue and may be moderately pleomorphic. Viable bone may be present. The radiographic appearance of both lesions is identical, consisting of foci of calcification within the joint space.

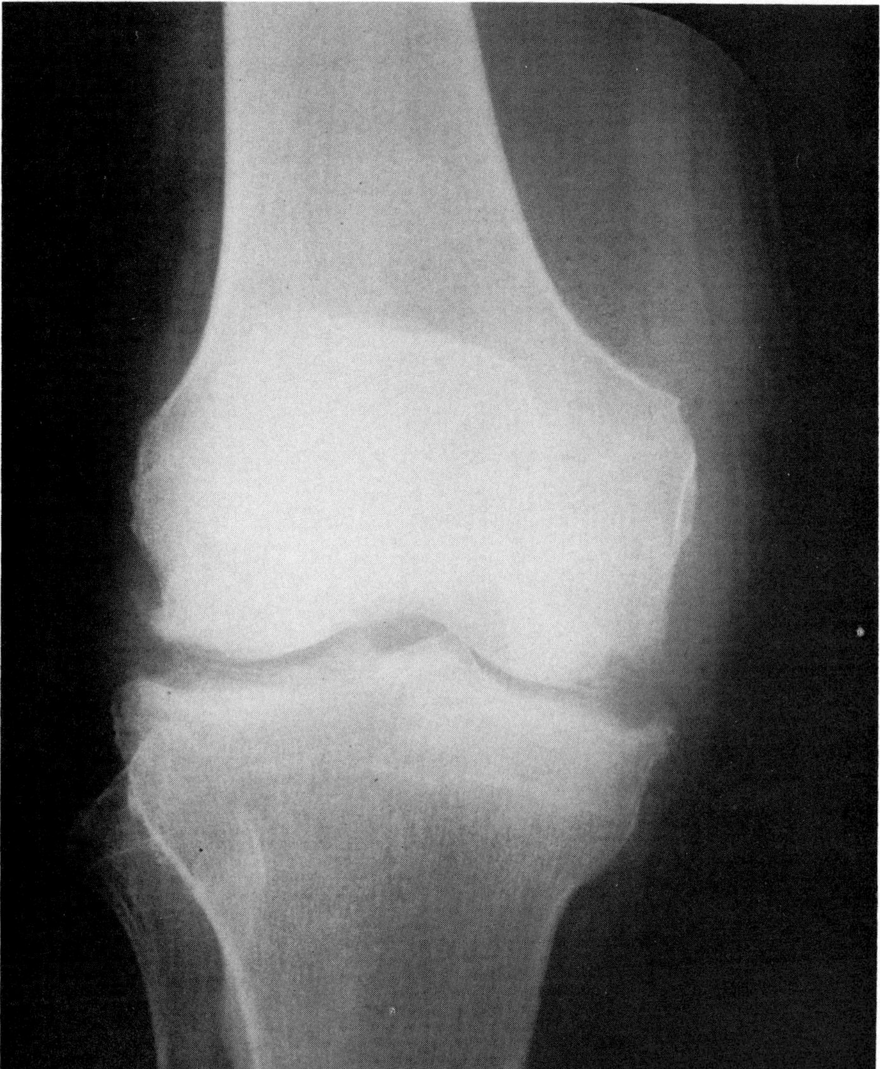

Figure 11–60. Septic arthritis, knee.

Series 23: Septic arthritis vs. rheumatoid arthritis vs. osteoarthritis, knee. Septic arthritis is characterized by destruction of cartilage due to enzymes in the inflammatory cells. Loss of cartilage thickness is seen radiographically as decrease in distance between bone ends. Invasion and destruction of adjacent bone cause irregularities in the bone ends, and osteomyelitis may be seen in either bone participating in the joint. The process may occur at any age and may be superimposed on pre existing degenerative arthritis. Rheumatoid arthritis also demonstrates thinned joint space due to destruction of cartilage by inflammatory cell enzymes. The process is usually slower, and para-articular osteoporosis is more evident, particularly in the hands and feet. Degenerative osteoarthritis is the end stage of either preceding entity, but it may also occur as primary disease. Histologic evidence of pannus formation is consistent with rheumatoid arthritis; degenerative arthritis simply exhibits fraying and destruction of cartilage. The weight-bearing surfaces in all three conditions are more involved than the margins, and the thinning of the joint space and the sharpening or "lipping" of joint margins due to osteophyte formation, subchondral erosions, or "cysts" are late manifestations in all three conditions.

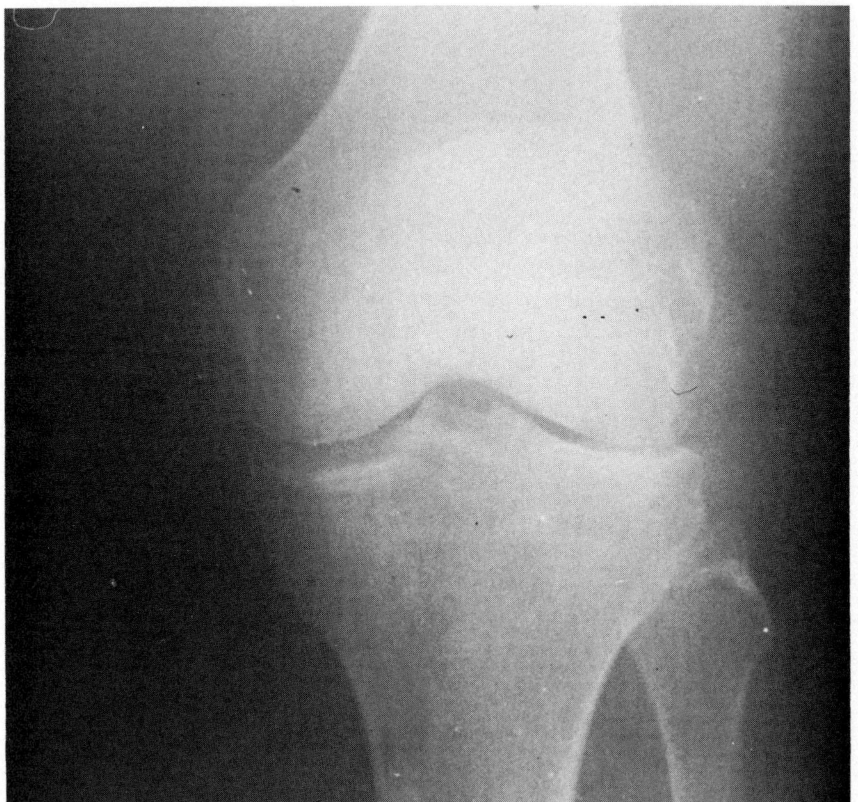

Figure 11–61. Rheumatoid arthritis, knee.

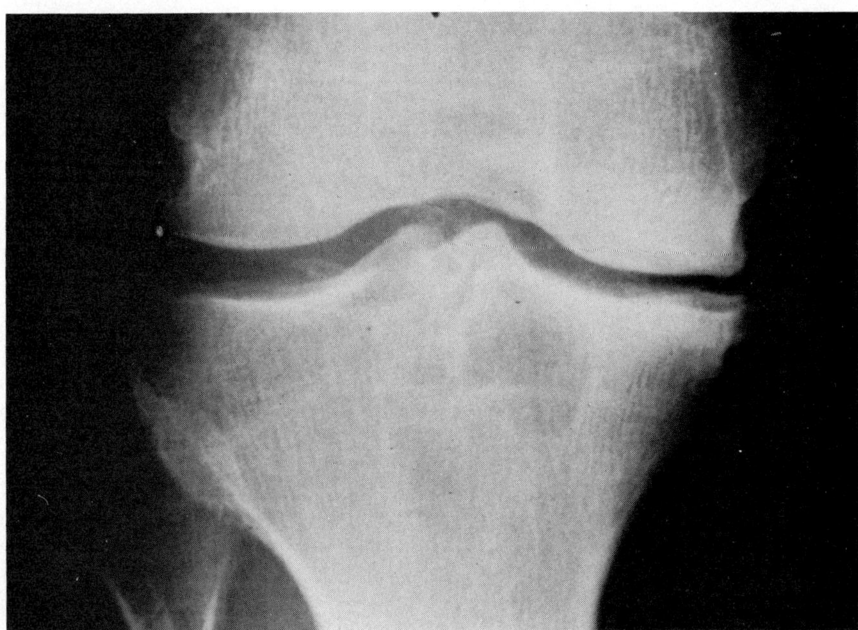

Figure 11–62. Osteoarthritis, knee.

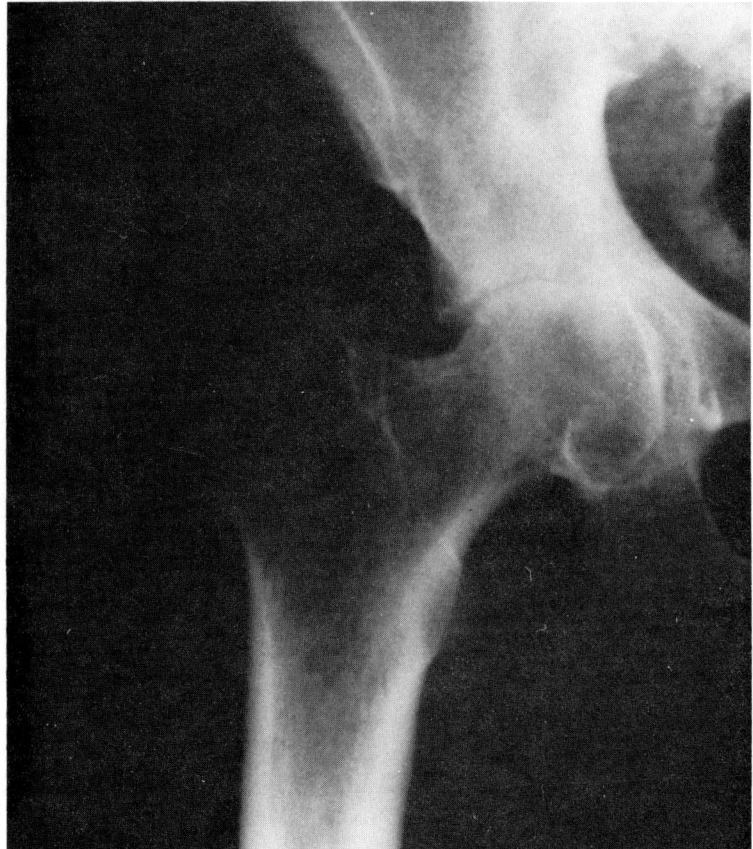

Figure 11–63. Septic arthritis, hip.

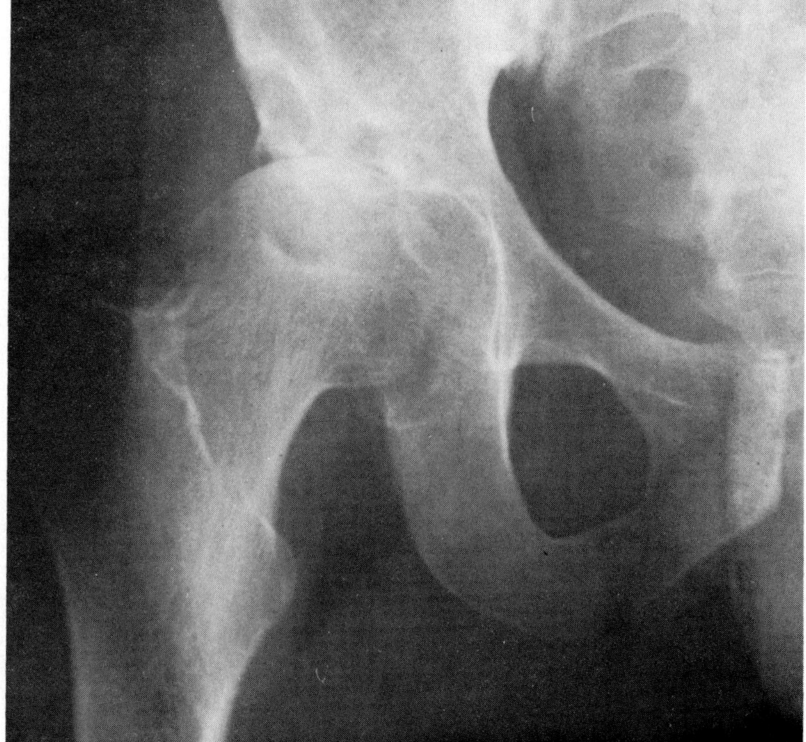

Figure 11–64. Granulomatous arthritis, hip.

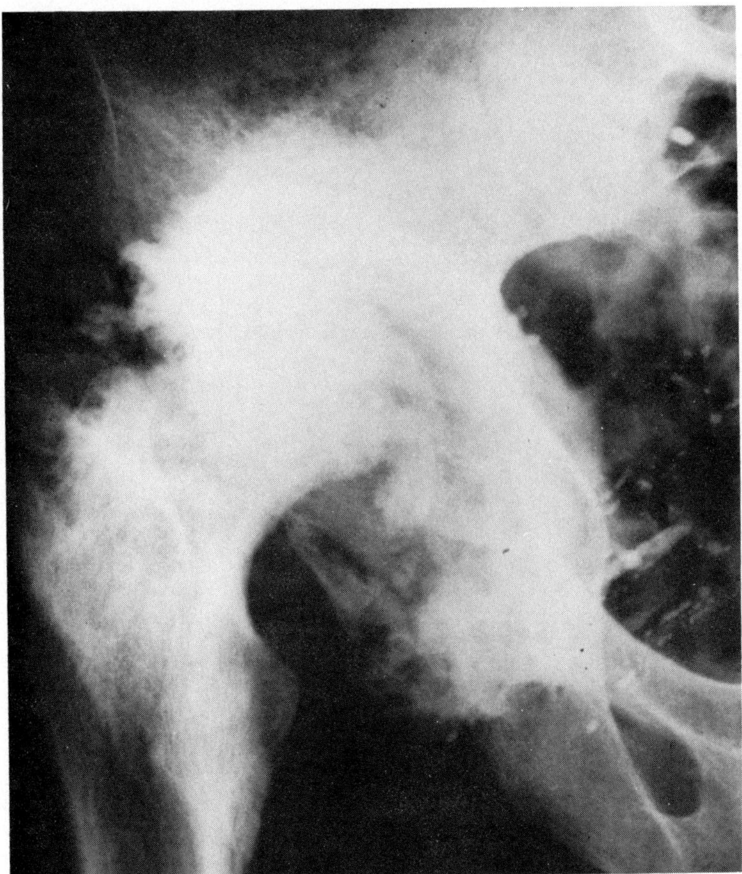

Figure 11–65. Neuropathic arthritis, hip.

Series 24: Septic arthritis vs. granulomatous arthritis vs. neuropathic arthritis (Charcot's arthropathy), hip. Septic arthritis causes uniform thinning of joint space by enzymatic destruction of articular cartilage, whereas tuberculous arthritis causes destruction by pannus formation from synovium with erosive destruction most marked at margins of the joint. In tuberculosis, the weight-bearing surface is spared until late in the disease. Neuropathic joints present as massive osteolysis with bone fragmentation and migration of fragments into recesses of the distended joints. Attempts at osseous repair produce osteophytes and sclerosis. Destruction and repair continue fairly rapidly until the architectural features of the joint are no longer recognizable. Massive destruction may occur in a few weeks. Any of the aforementioned processes can cause enough bone destruction to result in subluxation or dislocation of joints. The histologic features of tuberculosis are those of a caseating granulomatous process, usually involving the synovium and adjacent bone structures. Charcot's neuropathic arthritis will result in shards and fragments of cartilage phagocytosed by synovium, with a foreign body type granulomatous reaction but no caseation.

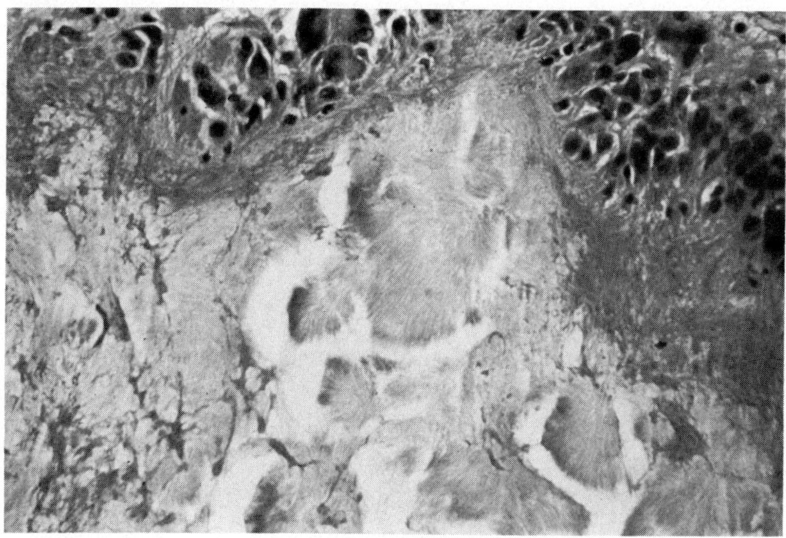

Figure 11–66. Gouty tophus.

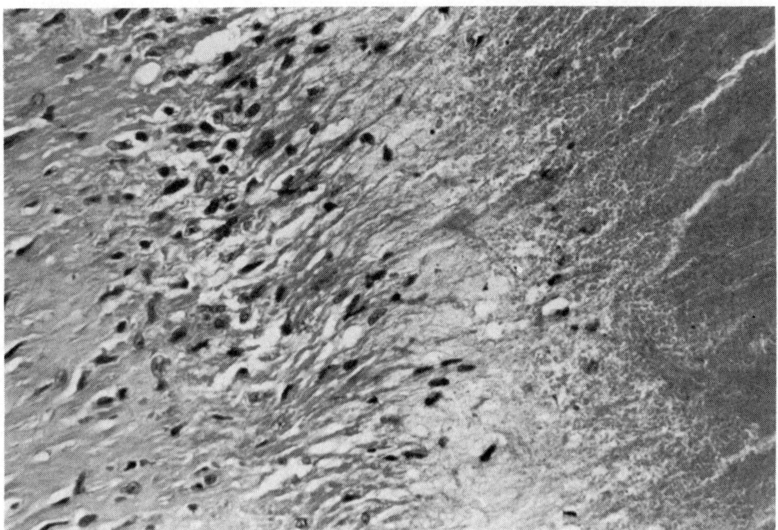

Figure 11–67. Rheumatoid nodule.

Series 25: Gouty tophus vs. rheumatoid nodule. The rheumatoid nodule consists of a central area of necrosis surrounded by giant cells and histiocytes, arranged in a stellate pattern. In gout, the needlelike crystal structure of the uric acid is identifiable, even in the formalin-fixed tissue. Giant cells are similar to those found in the rheumatoid nodule, and the histiocytes orient at right angles to the central area of crystalline deposition.

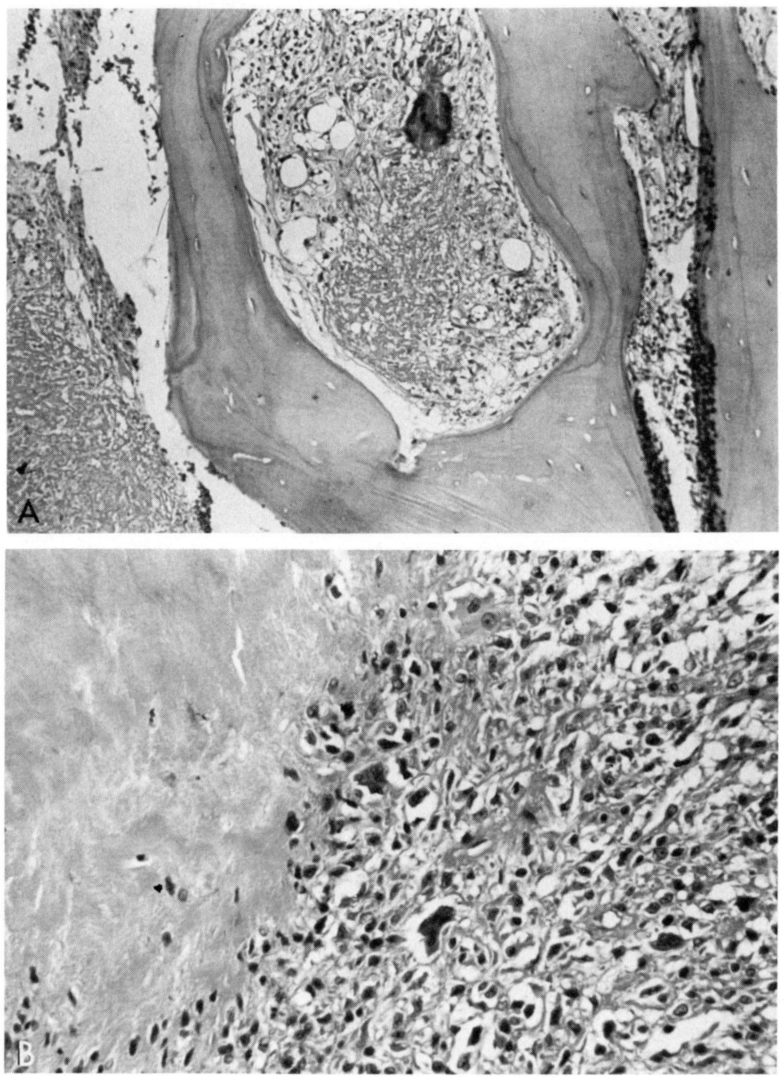

Figure 11–68. Tuberculosis.

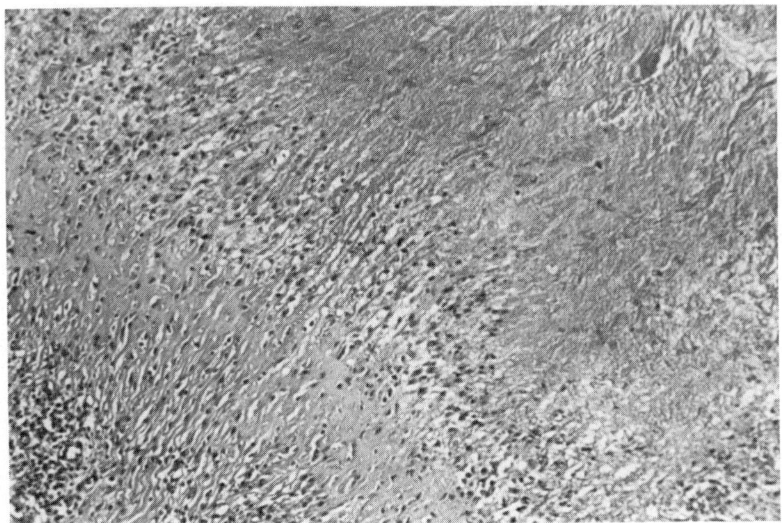

Figure 11–69. Rheumatoid nodule.

Series 26: Tuberculosis vs. rheumatoid nodule. The caseating granuloma of tuberculosis may be similar to the rheumatoid nodule. A
granulomatous process is characterized by the presence of epithelioid
cells and Langhans' giant cells. The stellate pattern usually associated
with the rheumatoid nodule is absent in tuberculosis.

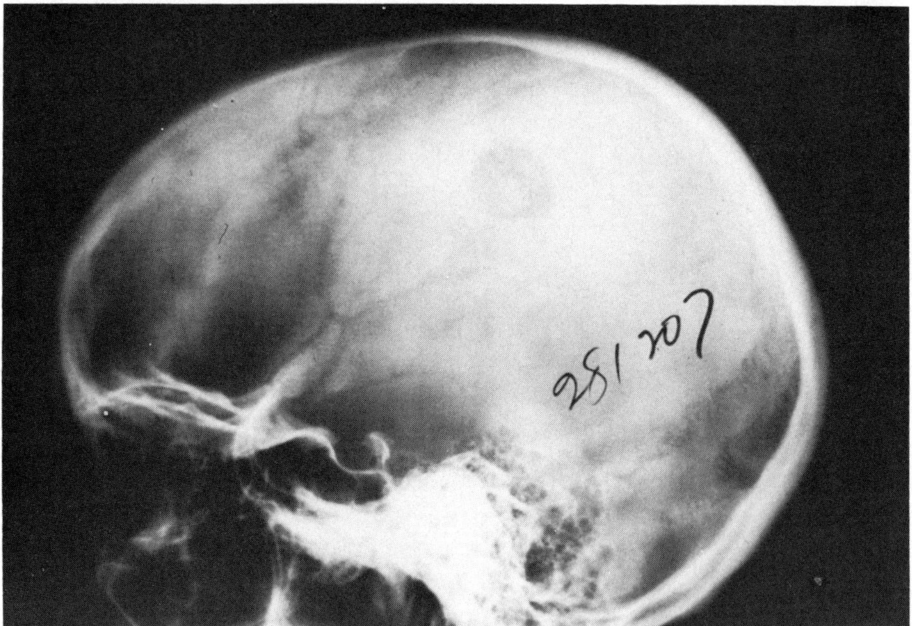

Figure 11–70. Hemangioma, skull.

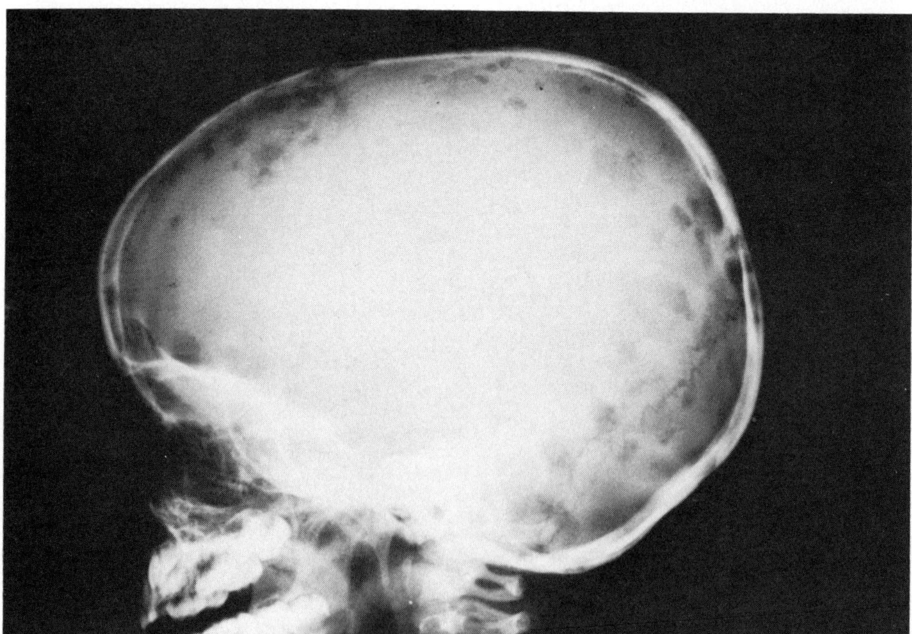

Figure 11–71. Histiocytosis, skull.

Series 27: Hemangioma vs. histiocytosis vs. multiple myeloma vs. metastatic carcinoma, skull. The hemangioma is a benign hamartoma that often presents as a solitary rounded lesion of the skull with streamers of bone in its matrix and surrounding trabecular reinforcement (sclerosis). The well-defined lesion with surrounding sclerosis is of variable size and may have beveled edges.

The presence of multiple lesions, particularly in a child, suggests histiocytosis, although metastases could present in a child as well as in adults. The lesions classically have minimal reaction around them.

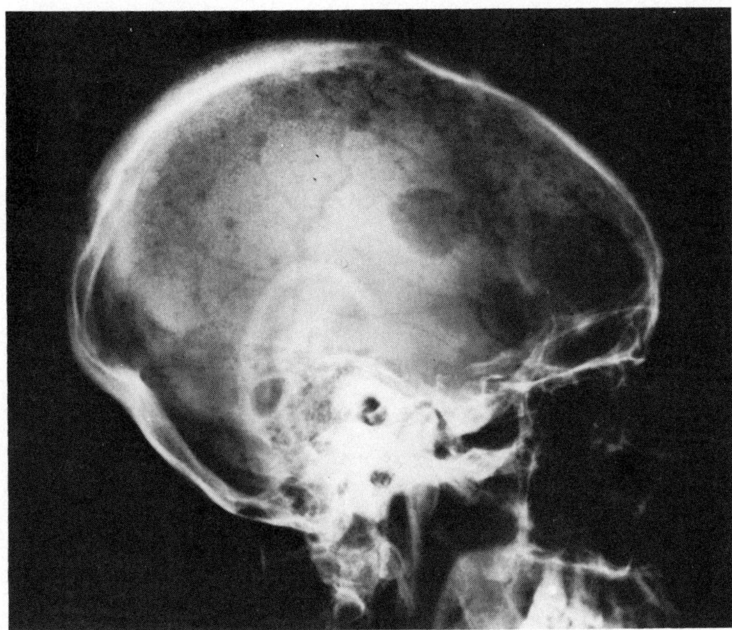

Figure 11–72. Multiple myeloma, skull.

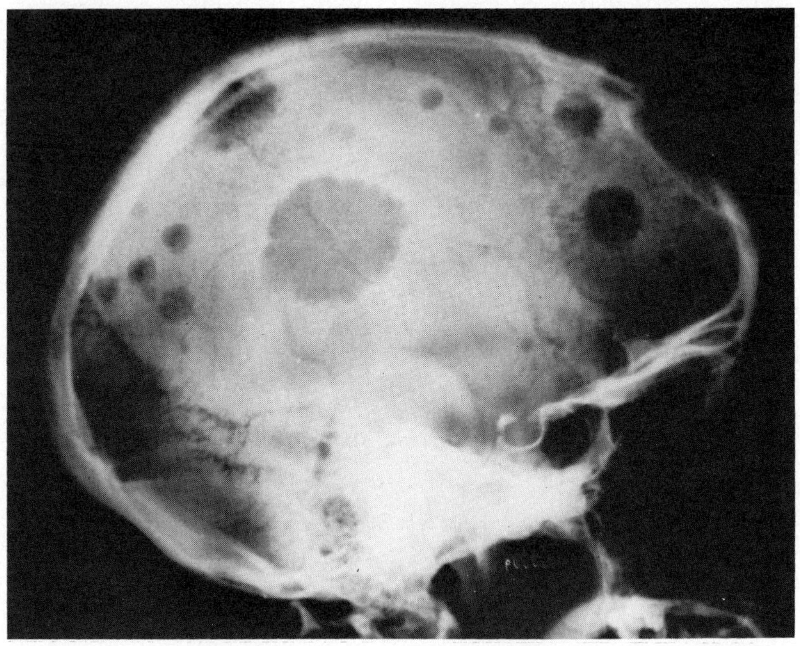

Figure 11–73. Metastatic carcinoma, skull.

Multiple myeloma frequently presents with multiple lesions in the calvarium. These are usually sharply marginated with no significant bony response.

Metastases will often present an identical radiographic picture, and the differential diagnosis must be based on a clinical history. Metastases may be lytic, blastic, or mixed.

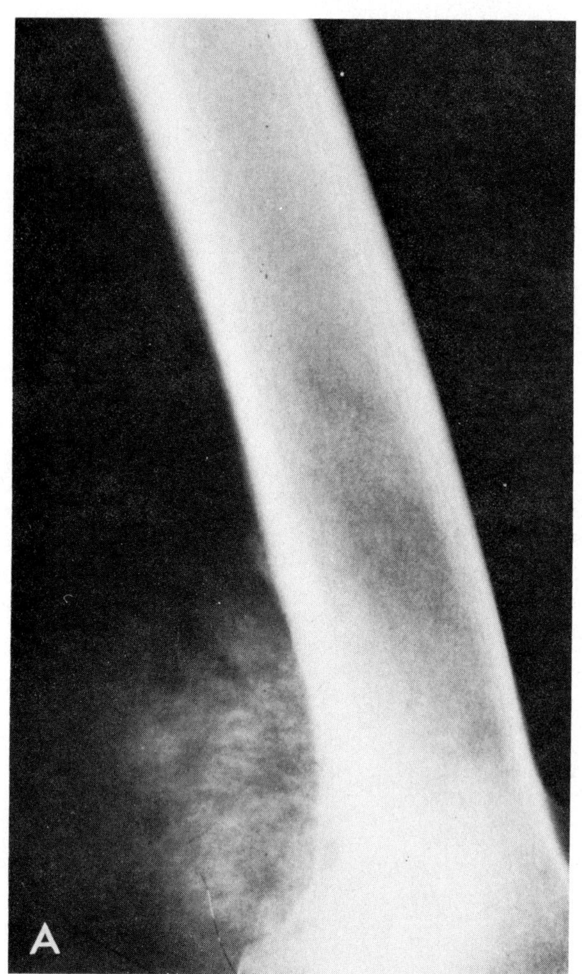

Figure 11–74. Metastatic carcinoma, femur.

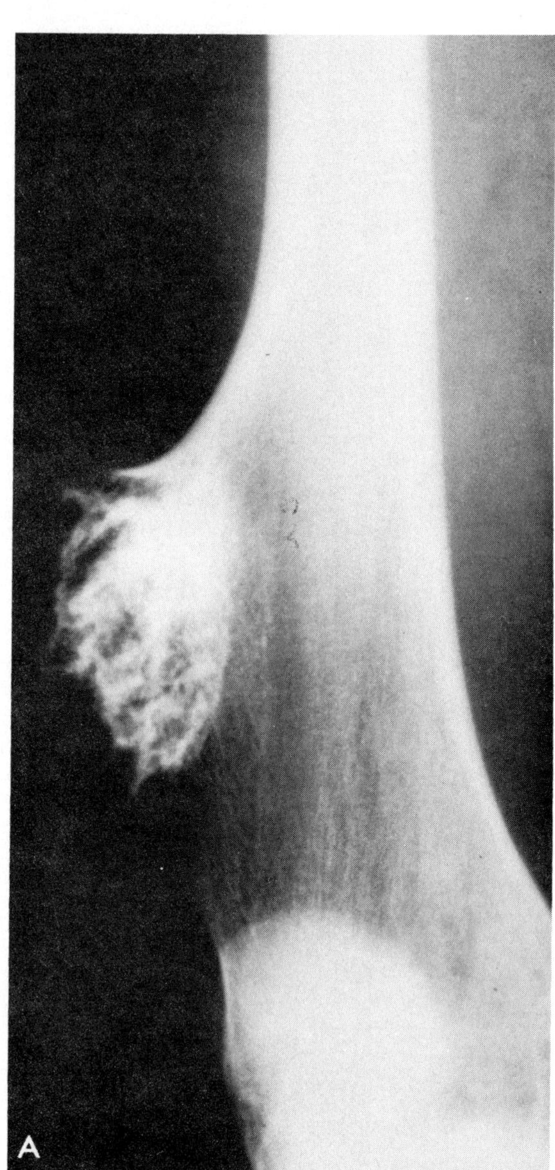

Figure 11–75. Osteochondroma, femur.

Illustrations continued on page 724

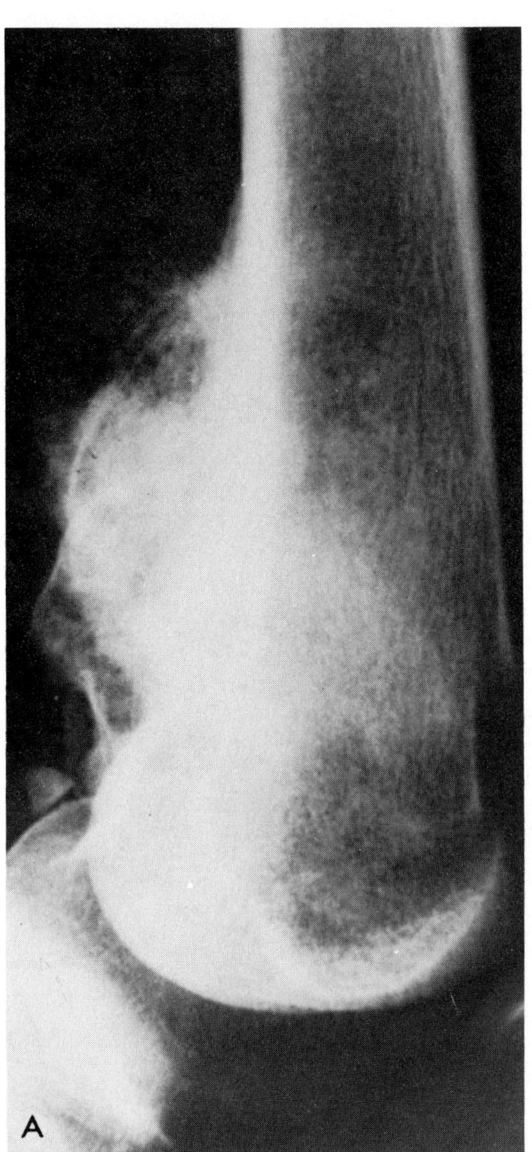

Figure 11–76. Parosteal sarcoma, femur.

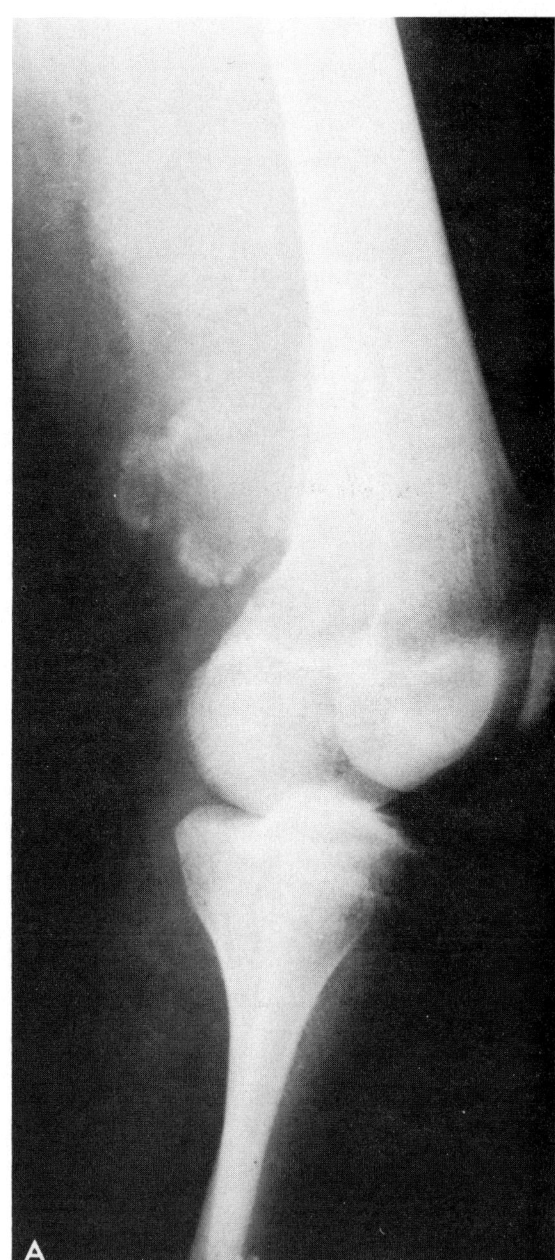

Figure 11–77. Myositis ossificans, femur.

Illustrations continued on page 725

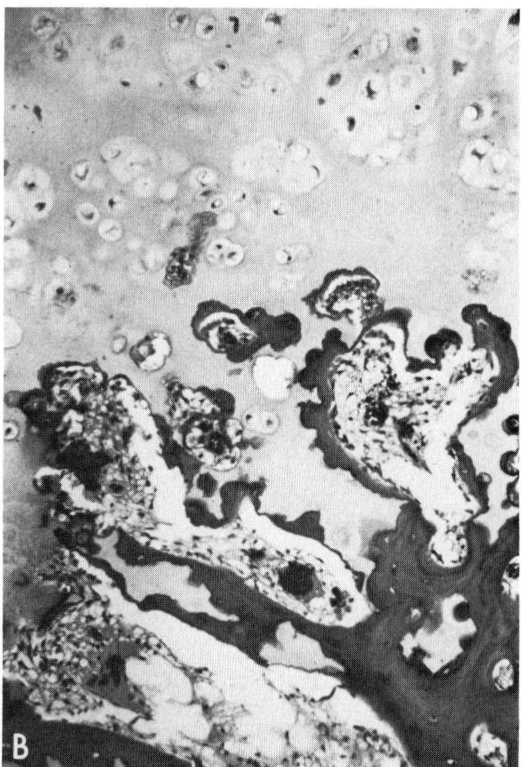

Figure 11–75 *Continued.* Osteochondroma, femur.

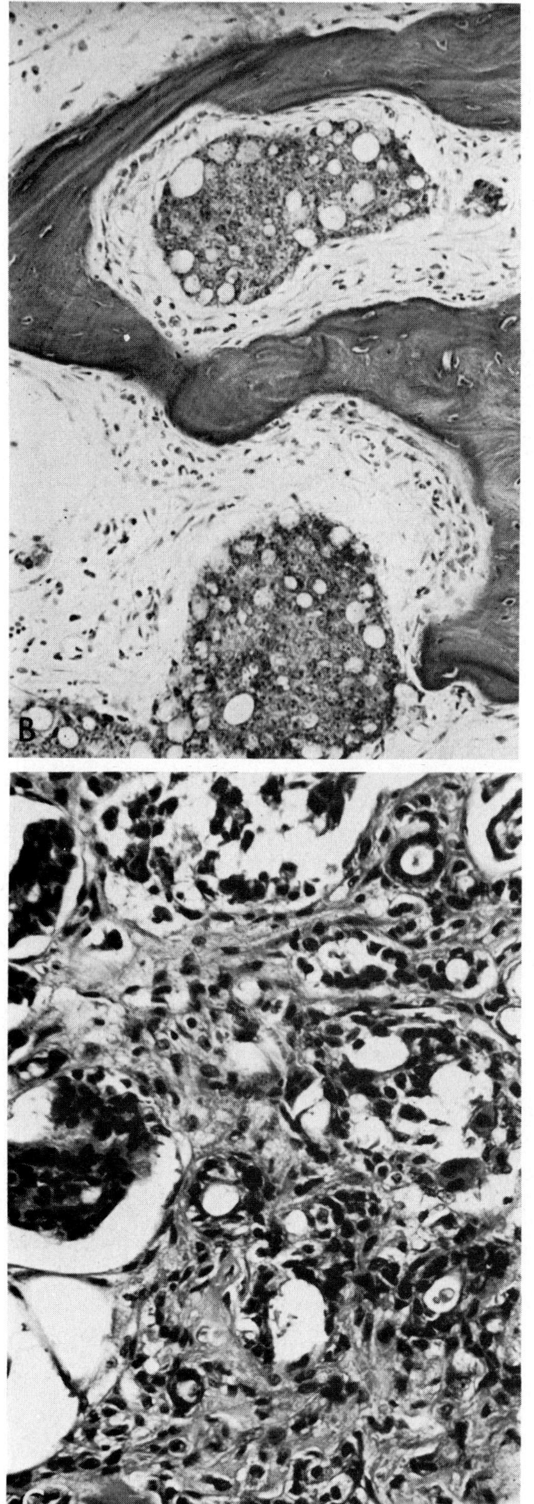

Figure 11–74 *Continued.* Metastatic carcinoma, femur.

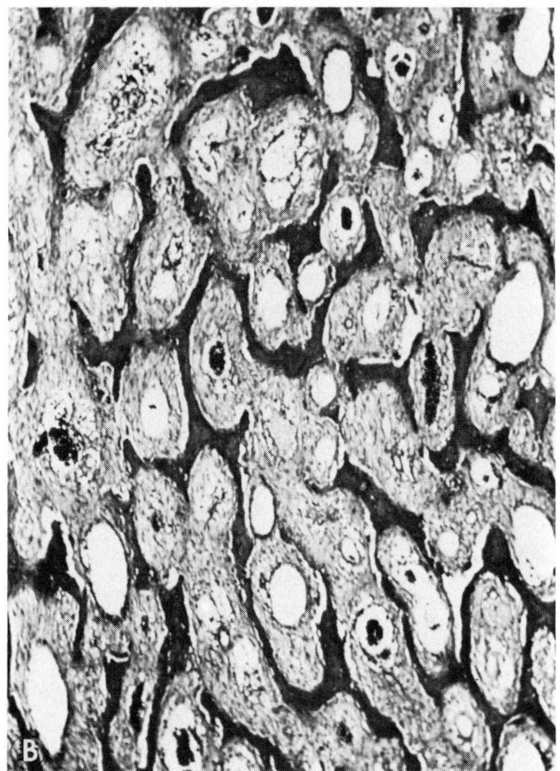

Figure 11–76 *Continued.* Parosteal sarcoma, femur.

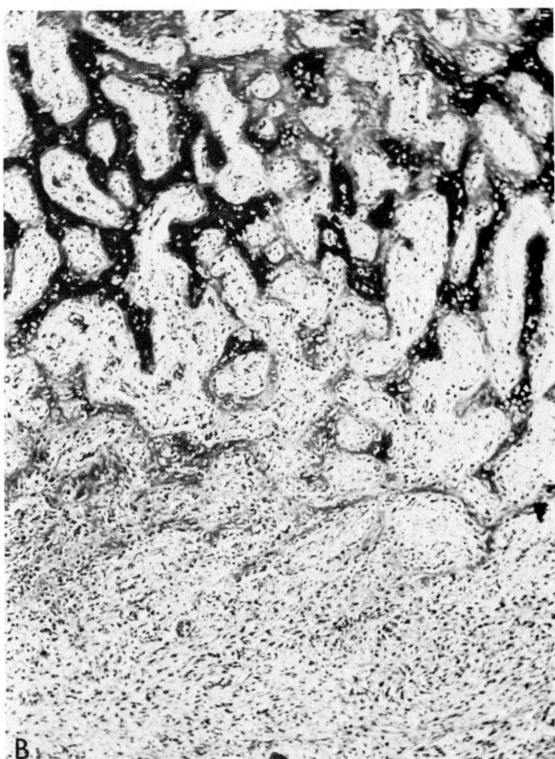

Figure 11–77 *Continued.* Myositis ossificans, femur.

Series 28: Metastatic carcinoma vs. osteochondroma vs. parosteal osteosarcoma vs. myositis ossificans, femur. The typical osteochondroma has a stalk of variable width that is sessile or pedunculated. The cortex of the stalk and spongiosa of the neoplasm are continuous with cortex and spongiosa of host bone. The cartilage cap may vary considerably in thickness, shape, and contour as well as radiographic density; none of these changes is diagnostic of aggressiveness or malignancy.

Parosteal (juxtacortical) sarcoma typically has broad attachment to underlying cortex, but the cortices are not continuous with the host bone cortex. A thin radiolucent cleavage plane is frequently seen between the tumor and the host bone. The medullary cavity of the neoplasm is filled with fibrous and well-differentiated osteoid rather than the normal marrow contained in an osteochondroma.

Metastatic carcinoma in bone and periarticular areas is the most common tumor of bone and can produce radiographic changes that can mimic any primary bone lesion. It must be constantly considered in the differential diagnosis at any age. The illustrations exhibit a glandular neoplasm replacing portions of the marrow. Higher magnification reveals an obviously glandular pattern.

Myositis ossificans is a soft tissue mass with peripheral calcification or ossification, irregular contour, hazy outline, and a central zone of relative radiolucency. It can occur in many locales but is most commonly seen in areas with large muscle mass or about joints.

The histologic evidence of an osteochondroma consists of a cartilage cap, transformation to bone similar to enchondral ossification, and the formation of marrow-containing spaces in the neoplastic bone. The parosteal osteosarcoma exhibits a fibrous stroma but no normal marrow elements within the neoplastic bone. Myositis ossificans exhibits reactive bone formation, with the most mature bone at the periphery of the lesion; parosteal osteosarcoma, however, exhibits the least differentiated portion at the periphery, even though the entire process may consist of relatively well-differentiated bony spicules. Metastatic carcinoma is usually easily identified, often with needle biopsy; however, metastatic carcinoma, especially renal cell carcinoma, may assume a pseudofibrous pattern when metastasizing to bone.

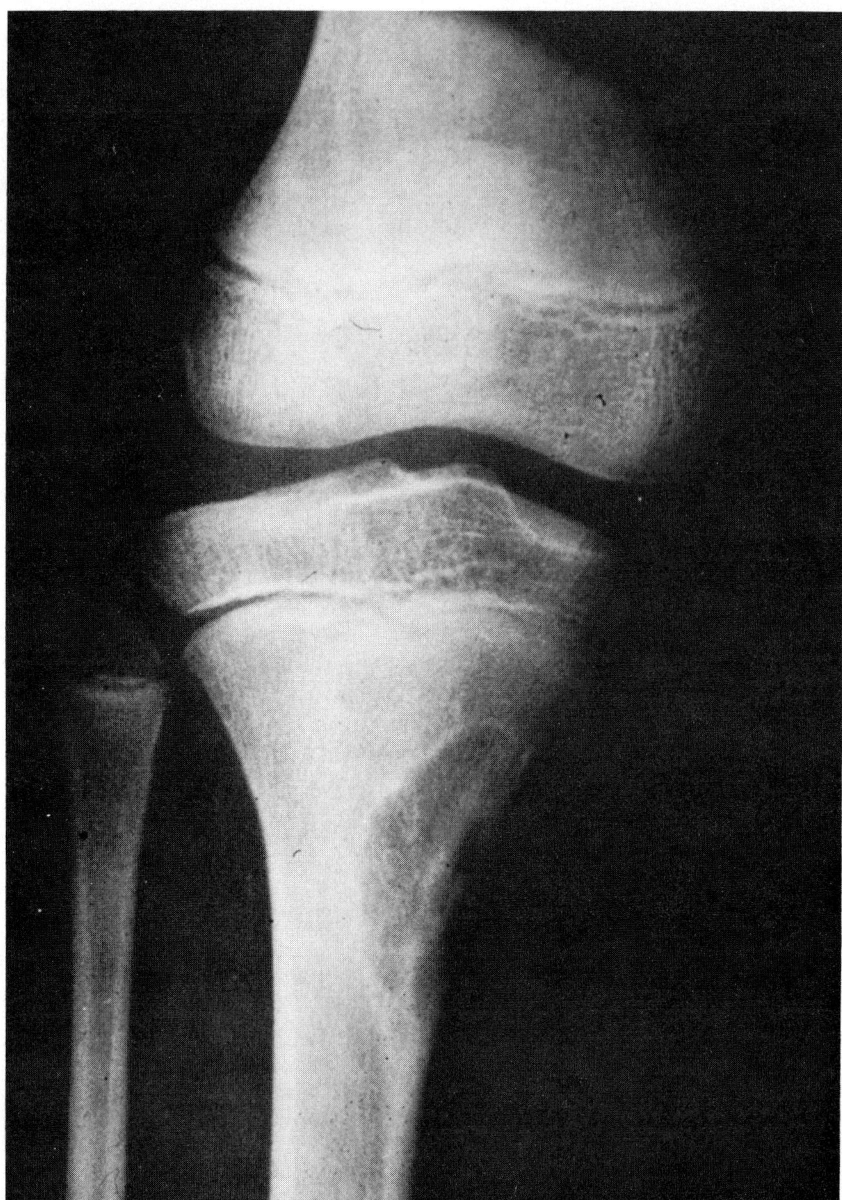

Figure 11–78. Nonossifying fibroma, tibia.

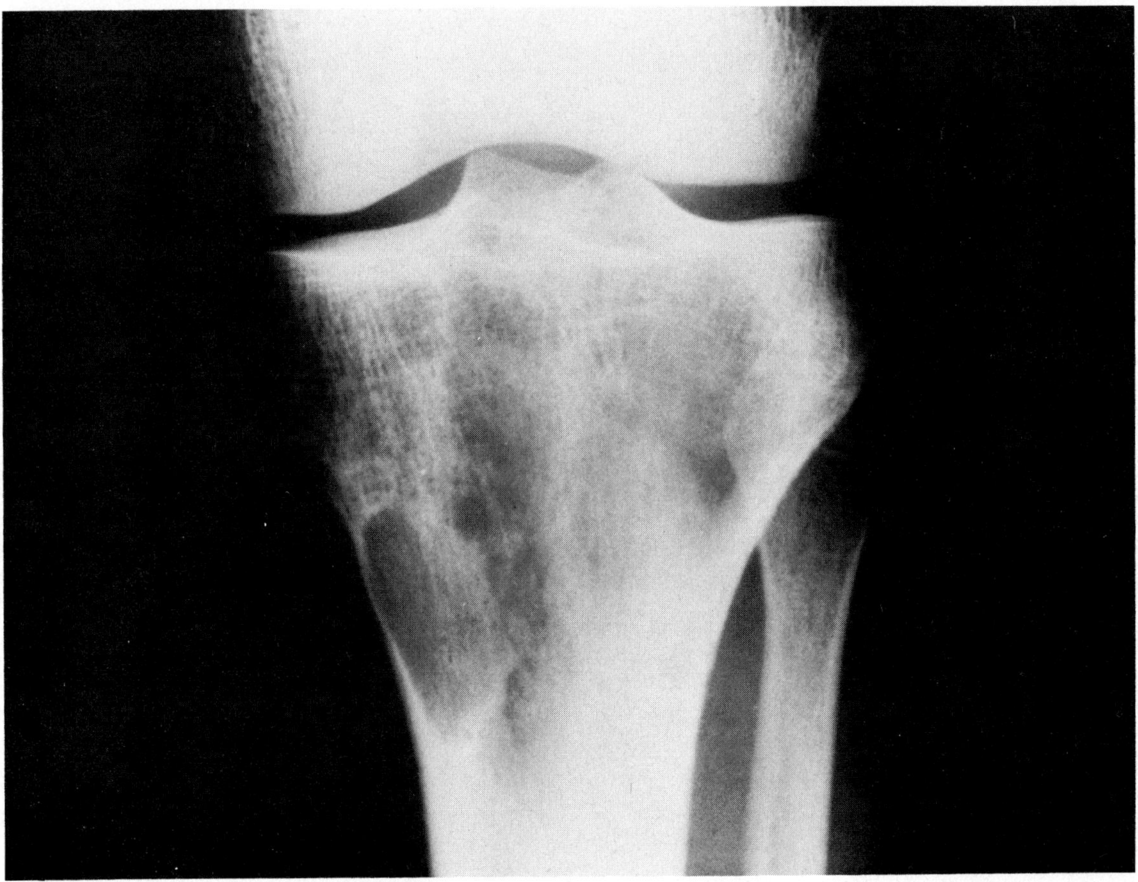

Figure 11–79. Fibrosarcoma, tibia.

Series 29: Nonossifying fibroma vs. fibrosarcoma, tibia. Eccentric, sharply marginated lucent lesion with sclerotic rim in the metaphyseal-diaphyseal junction of an adolescent is a classic picture of nonossifying fibroma.

The large, irregular radiolucent lesion in the adult tibia extending in irregular shape from the subchondral area well into the diaphysis indicates a more aggressive lesion. It is still contained inside the bone, and there is no periosteal reaction. The presence of a sclerotic, marginated portion near the cortex of the metaphyseal-diaphyseal junction raises the possibility that this fibrosarcoma arose in a nonossifying fibroma.

The initial biopsy from this lesion may well exhibit elements of a benign tumor. The pathologist must insist on biopsy from the area of permeative destruction.

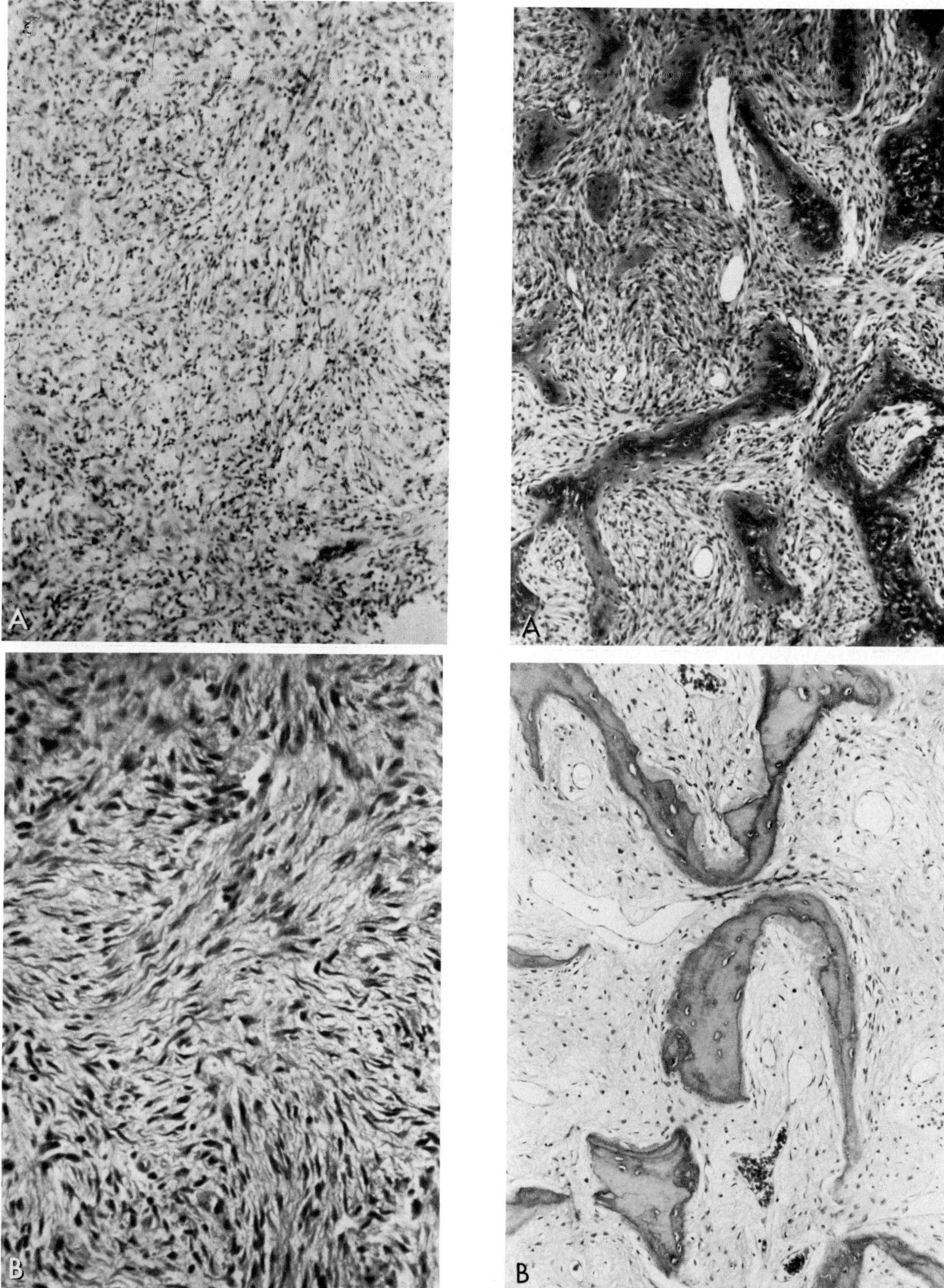

Figure 11–80. Nonossifying fibroma.

Figure 11–81. Fibrous dysplasia.

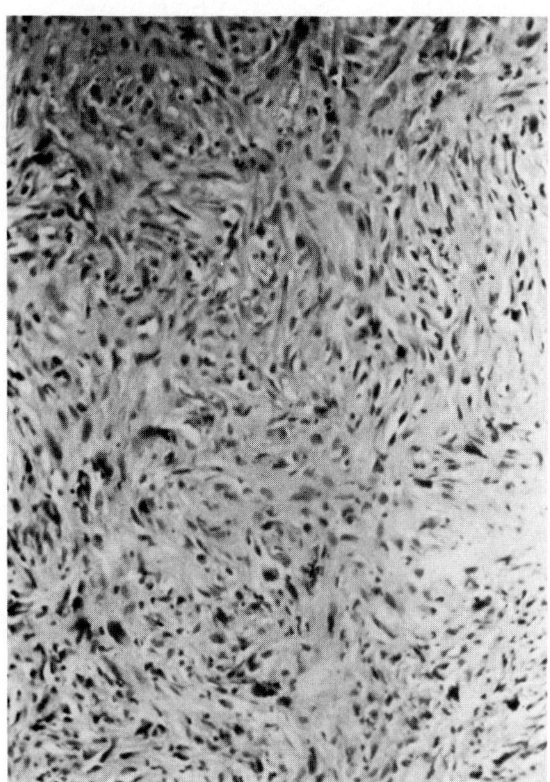

Figure 11–82. Fibrosarcoma.

Series 30: Nonossifying fibroma vs. fibrous dysplasia vs. fibrosarcoma. Cellular fibrous dysplasia exhibits transition from connective tissue to bone, but there is no significant pleomorphism. In older lesions the bone is more sclerotic, and the connective tissue is less cellular.

The fibrosarcoma is a pleomorphic collagen-producing tumor without identifiable osteoid or chondroid matrix production.

The nonossifying fibroma exhibits numerous fibroblasts with slender spindled cells and a "cartwheel" pattern, no significant pleomorphism or mitotic activity. Xanthomatous cells are usually present, and giant cells may be present in varying numbers. Calcification and ossification may occur, especially in older lesions.

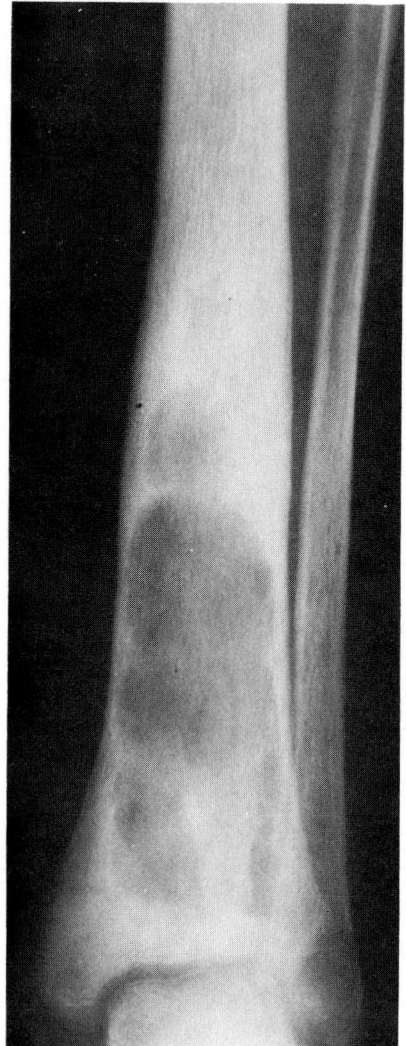

Figure 11–83. Chronic osteomyelitis, tibia.

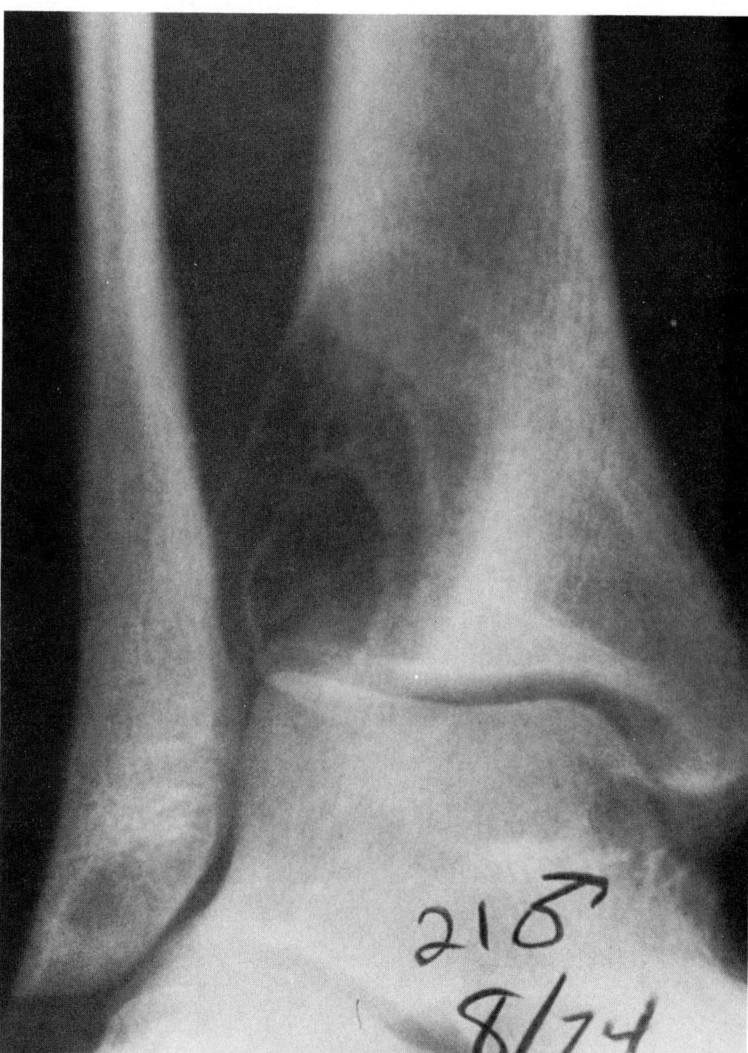

Figure 11–84. Giant cell tumor, tibia.

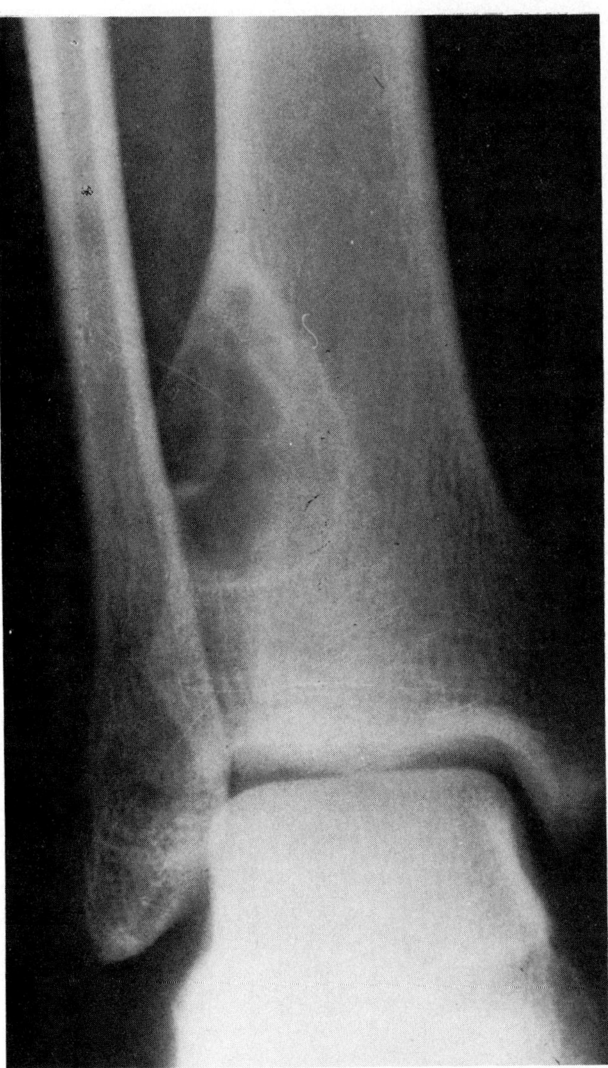

Figure 11–85. Nonossifying fibroma, tibia.

Series 31: Chronic osteomyelitis vs. giant cell tumor of bone vs. nonossifying fibroma, tibia. Organisms with low virulence (e.g., *Staphylococcus epidermidis*) can produce destructive lesions in bone, resulting in large cystic cavities that contain few organisms, but they do not elicit much cortical bony or periosteal reaction. Early antibiotic therapy can attenuate the response.

Giant cell tumor is located in the metaphyseal-epiphyseal region and is eccentrically placed in the bone. The matrix has no mineral production, and reaction of the host bone may be minimal because of slow growth of the tumor or because growth is too rapid to allow the periosteum to maintain an outer shell. The double-ring density is due to cortical resorption of anterior and posterior regions that overlap on the AP radiograph.

Nonossifying fibroma is also usually eccentric in the metaphyseal-diaphyseal zone. It can cause bone "expansion" by periosteal new bone keeping pace with endosteal surface resorption or by failure to remodel in the "cutback zone." This indicates a slow-growing, expansile process. There is no calcification in early lesions, but older lesions heal by ossifying from the diaphyseal end.

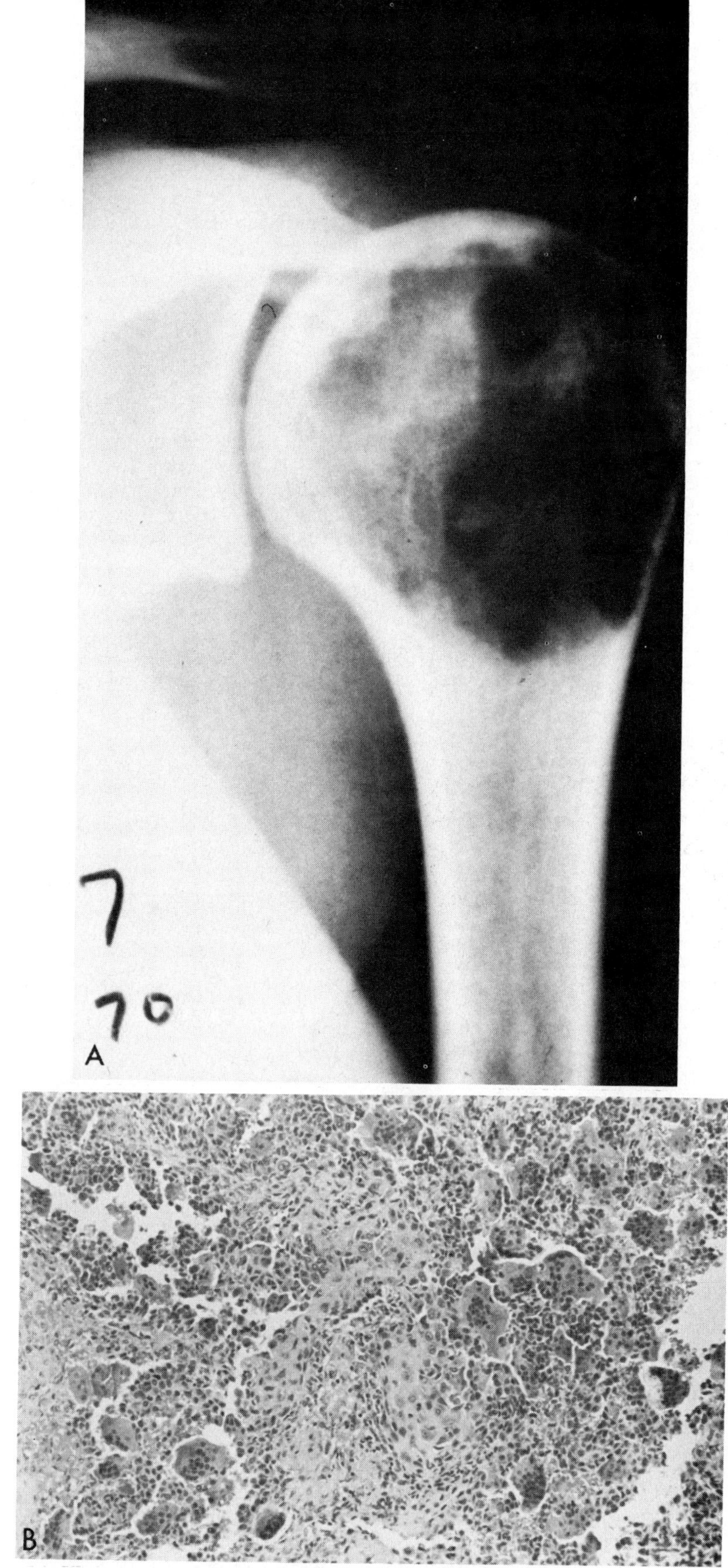

Figure 11–86. Chondroblastoma.

Series 32: Chondroblastoma vs. giant cell tumor of bone. The chondroblastoma is a sharply circumscribed defect in the epiphysis of a bone. Note that the center of the lesion is *above* the growth plate. When the growth plate has fused, the lesion will extend into the metaphysis.

The giant cell tumor of bone is a metaphyseal lesion, with its geographic center *below* the growth plate and extending into the epiphysis after the growth plate has fused.

The chondroblastoma, although it contains numerous giant cells that may predominate in the histologic picture, is always characterized by foci of cartilaginous differentiation. These foci are absent in a giant cell tumor of bone.

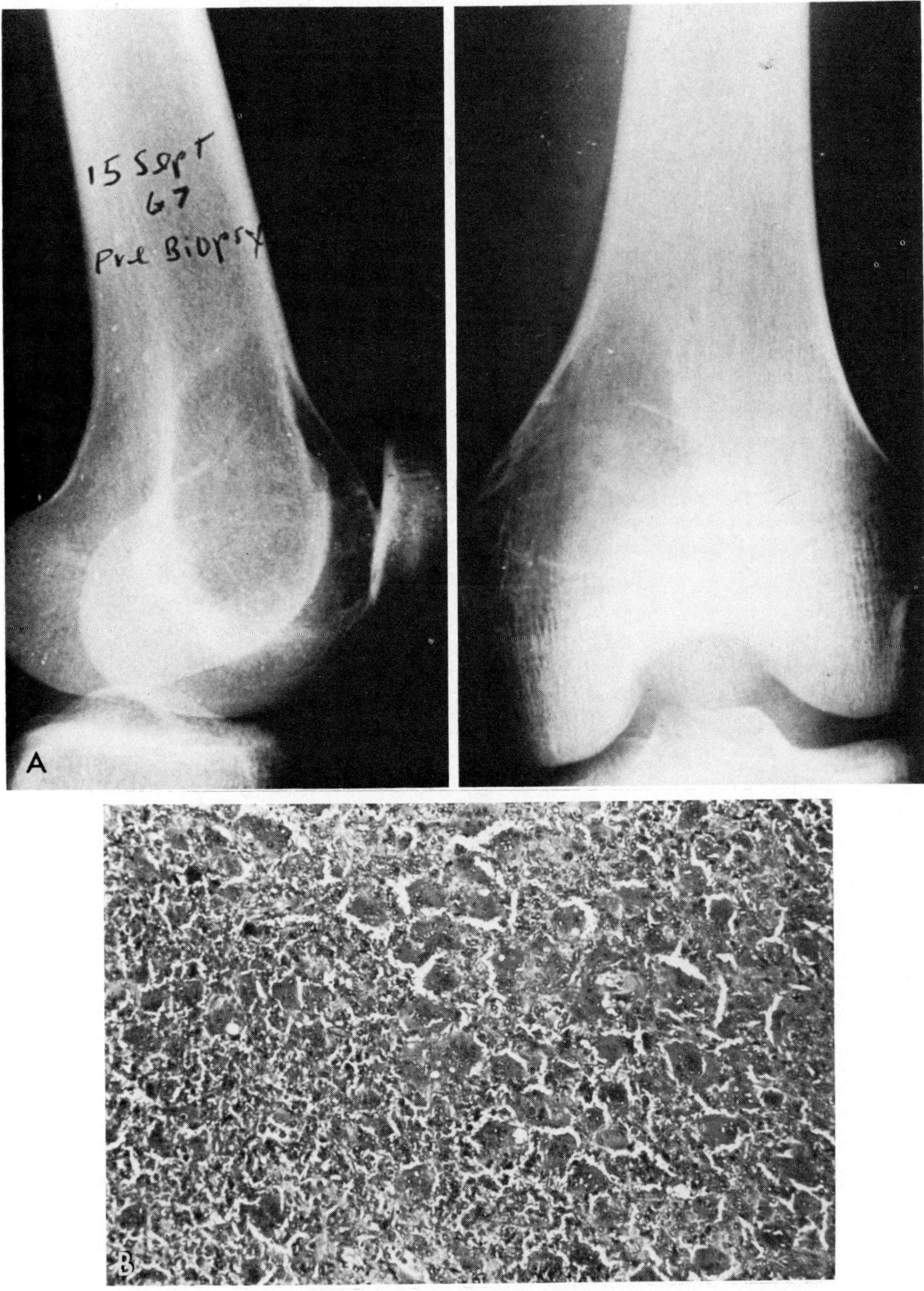

Figure 11–87. Giant cell tumor.

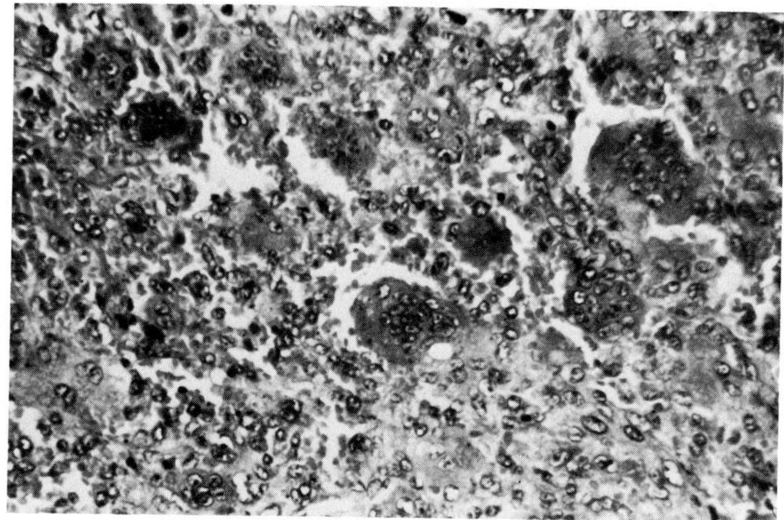

Figure 11–88. Giant cell tumor of bone.

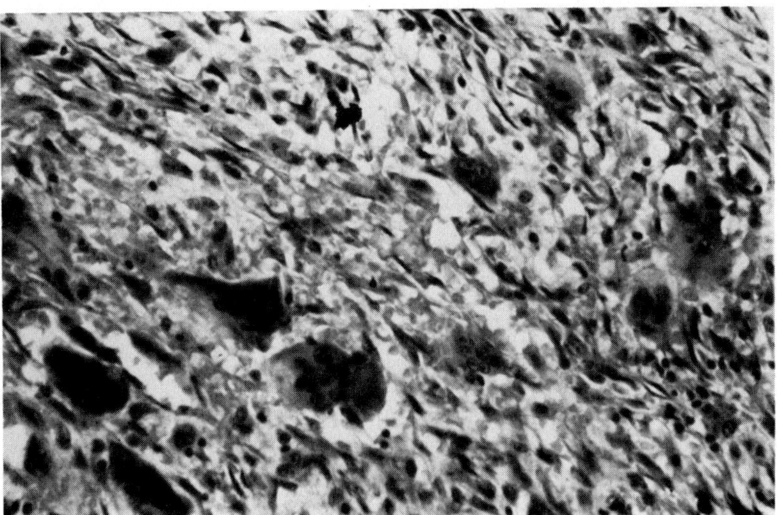

Figure 11–89. Brown tumor of hyperparathyroidism.

Series 33: Giant cell tumor of bone vs. brown tumor of hyperparathyroidism. The giant cell tumor of bone consists of osteoclasts; osteoclast and stromal cell nuclei are identical. The brown tumor of hyperparathyroidism is characterized by osteoclasts in a spindled mesenchymal stroma.

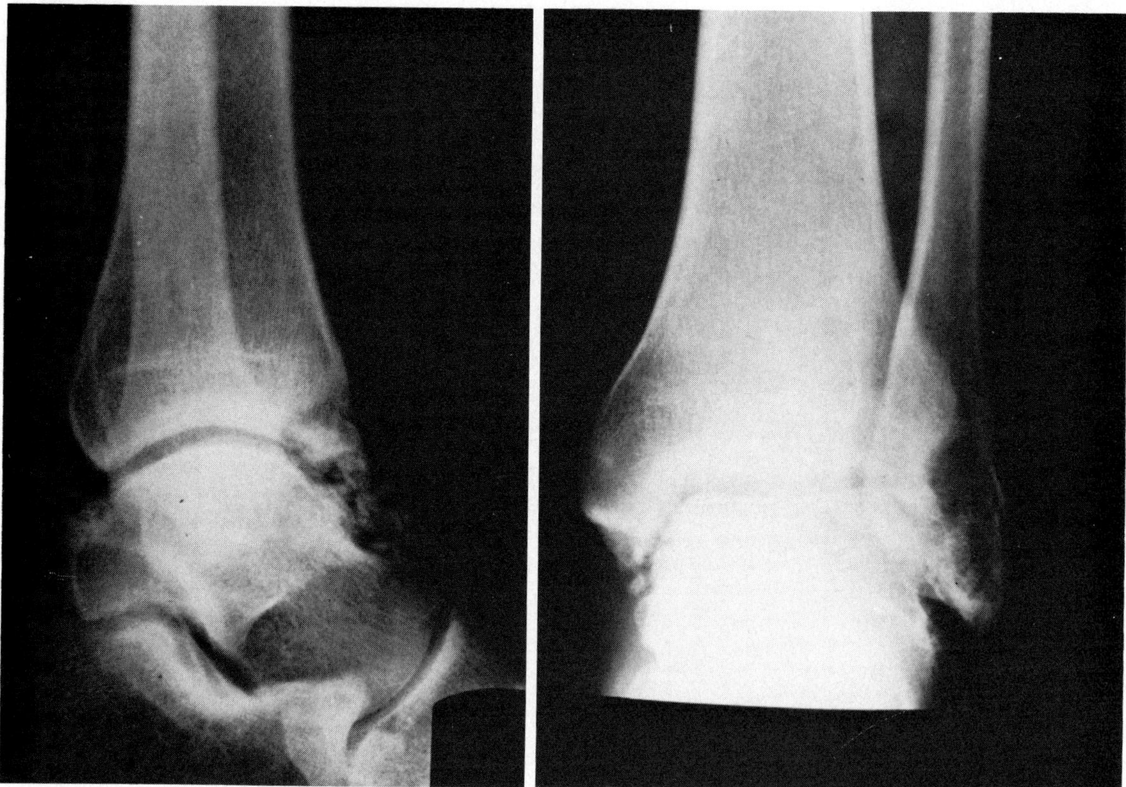

Figure 11–90. Loose joints (synovial chondromatosis).

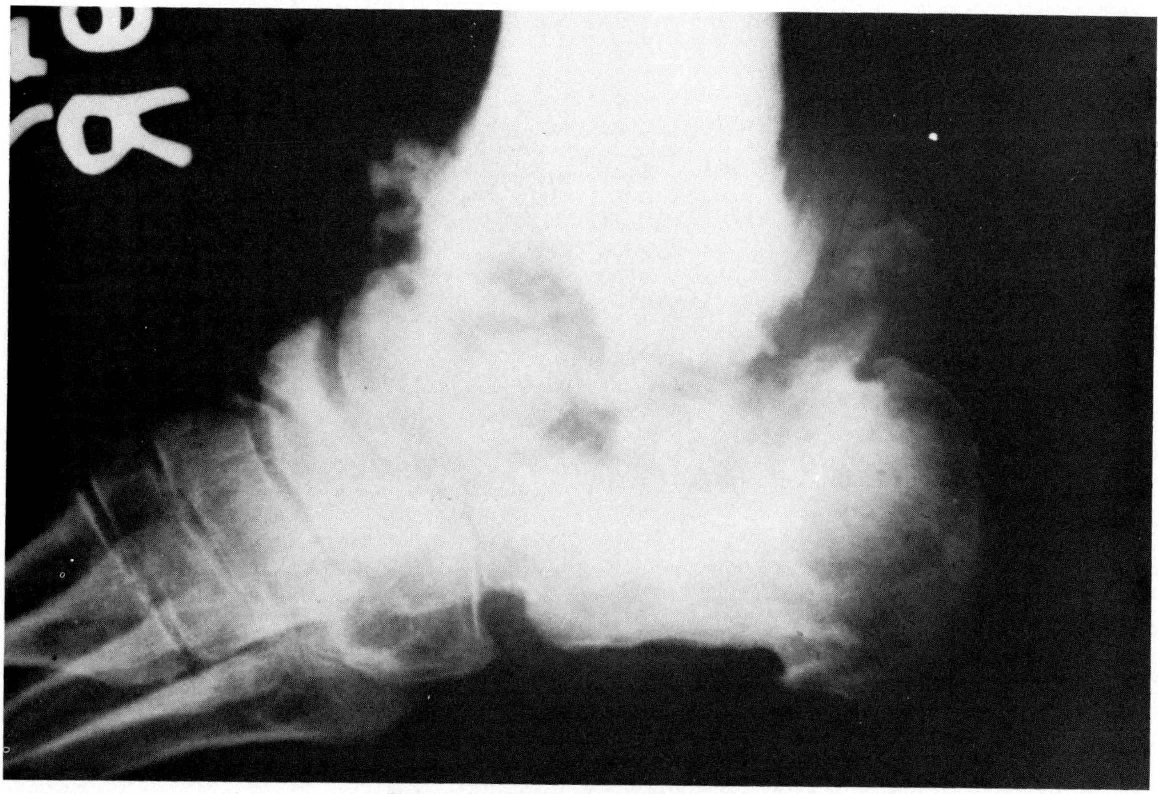

Figure 11–91. Neuropathy, ankle.

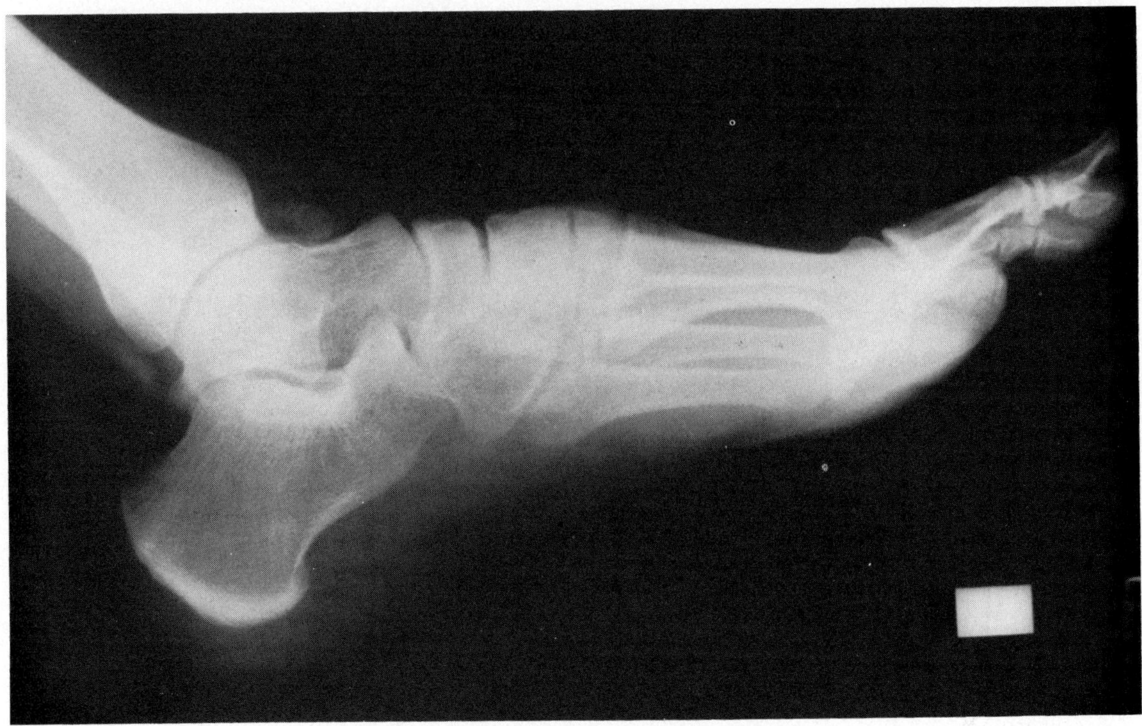

Figure 11–92. Synovial sarcoma, ankle.

Series 34: Loose joints (synovial chondromatosis) vs. neuropathic arthritis (Charcot's arthropathy) vs. synovial sarcoma, ankle. Loose bodies or synovial chondromatosis will exhibit multiple irregularly calcified and ossified nodules in the synovial cavity. Some are connected to the synovium by a stalk, others are embedded, and still others are loose in the joint. There may be associated irregularity at adjacent joint margins that is due to either interference with normal growth mechanisms or articular fragmentation (osteochondritis dissecans). The process may also be due to metaplasia within the synovium.

Neuropathic ankle joints are now more common in patients with diabetes or meningomyelocele than in patients with syphilis. Extensive destruction and fragmentation of adjacent bone ends and repair attempts produce multiple fragments of bone throughout the joint and gross distortion of the ankle.

Synovial sarcoma usually presents near but not within a joint. Approximately one half of all patients demonstrate soft-tissue calcification. Note calcification in soft tissue above the talus. The adjacent joint is usually normal.

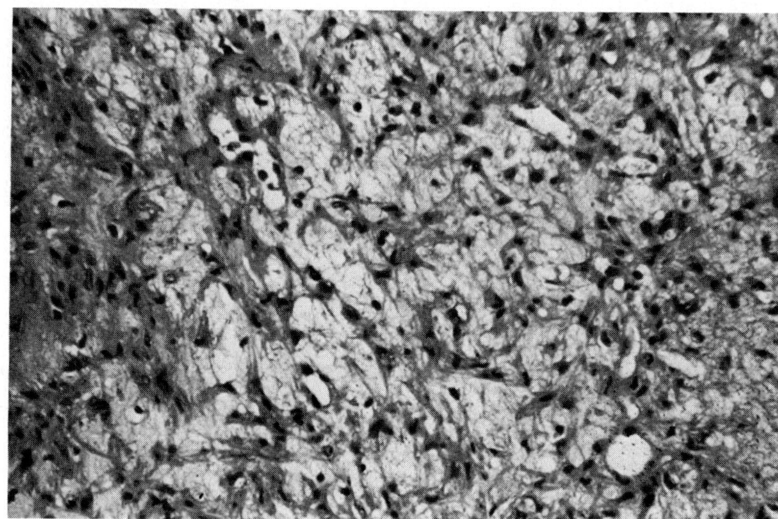

Figure 11–93. Chondromyxoid fibroma.

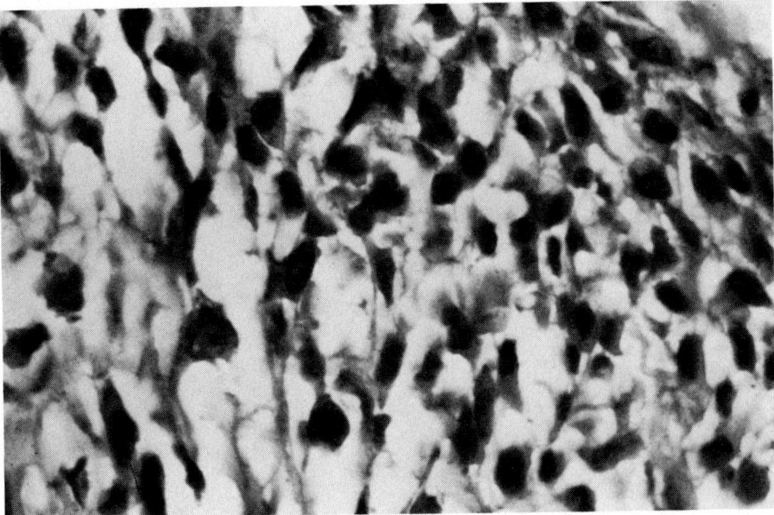

Figure 11–94. Chondrosarcoma.

Series 35: Chondromyxoid fibroma vs. chondrosarcoma. The chondromyxoid fibroma is composed of spindled fibroblasts set in a chondroid stroma. The cells are fairly uniform without significant pleomorphism or mitotic activity. The poorly differentiated chondrosarcoma consists of markedly pleomorphic spindled chondrocytes within a chondroid matrix.

Although the histologic appearance may be similar, radiographs offer clear-cut differentiation. The chondromyxoid fibroma is a lytic, sharply circumscribed defect, eccentrically located in metaphysis or diaphysis, without radiographic calcification. The radiographic appearance of chondrosarcoma may be quite variable, but the malignant process is reflected in indistinct margins, permeative or moth-eaten destruction, periosteal reaction, or evidence of matrix calcification.

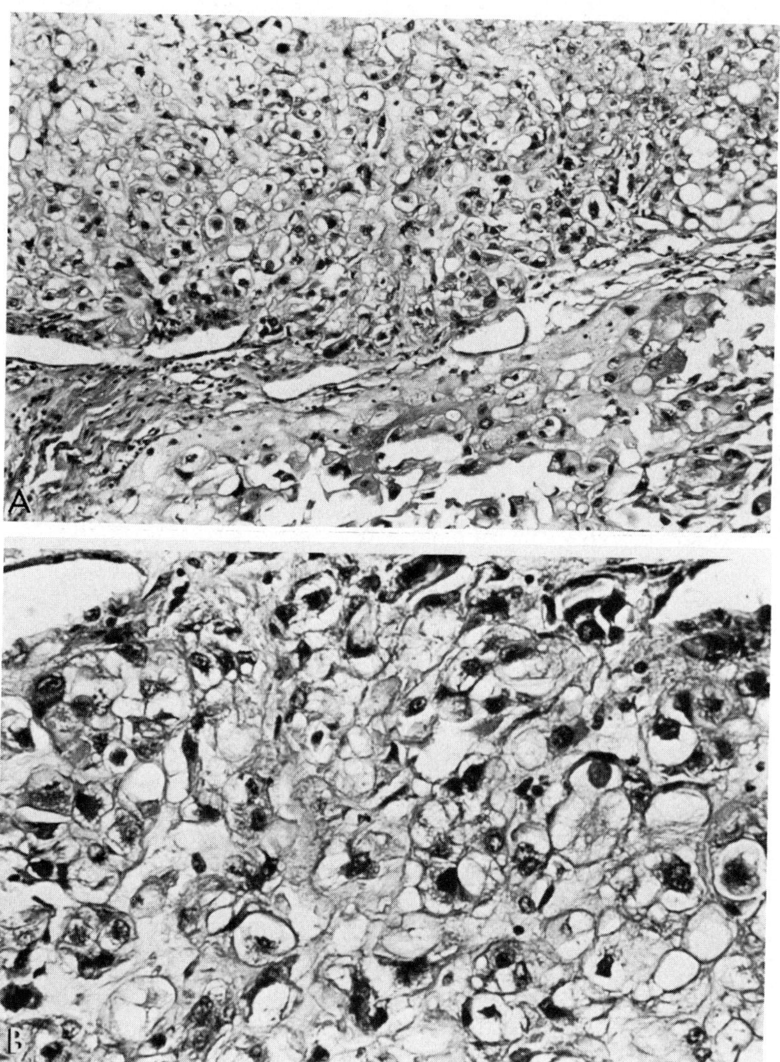

Figure 11–95. Chordoma.

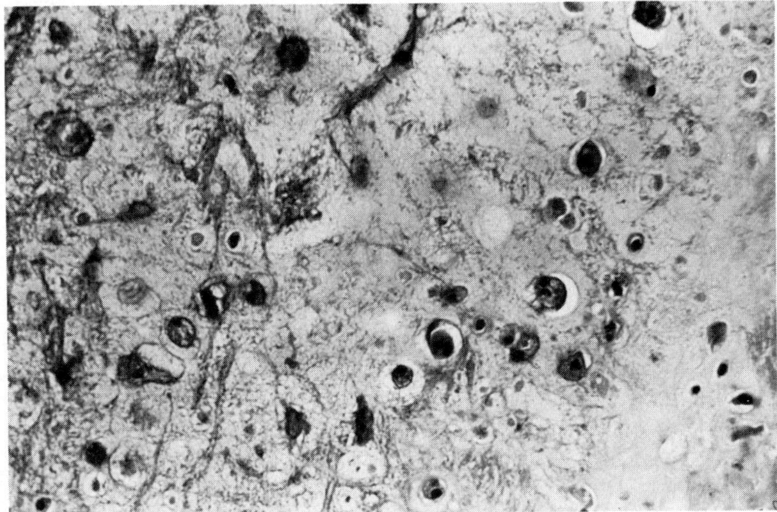

Figure 11–96. Chondrosarcoma.

Series 36: Chordoma vs. chondrosarcoma. The classic chordoma is characterized by the presence of numerous physaliferous cells, distinguished by central nuclei and bubbly, vacuolated cytoplasm. Chondrosarcomas, especially the more undifferentiated forms, consist of large nuclei filling the lacunar space. The matrix is chondroid, and although bubbly lacunae may be present, there are always foci in which the cartilage pattern is clearly identifiable.

Radiographs of the chordoma may demonstrate involvement of adjacent vertebral bodies, whereas vertebral chondrosarcoma tends to remain confined to a single bone.

There are occasional tumors that may contain features of both chondrosarcoma and chordoma: the "chondroid chordoma," usually originating in the base of the skull. The histogenesis of these lesions remains an issue requiring further clarification.

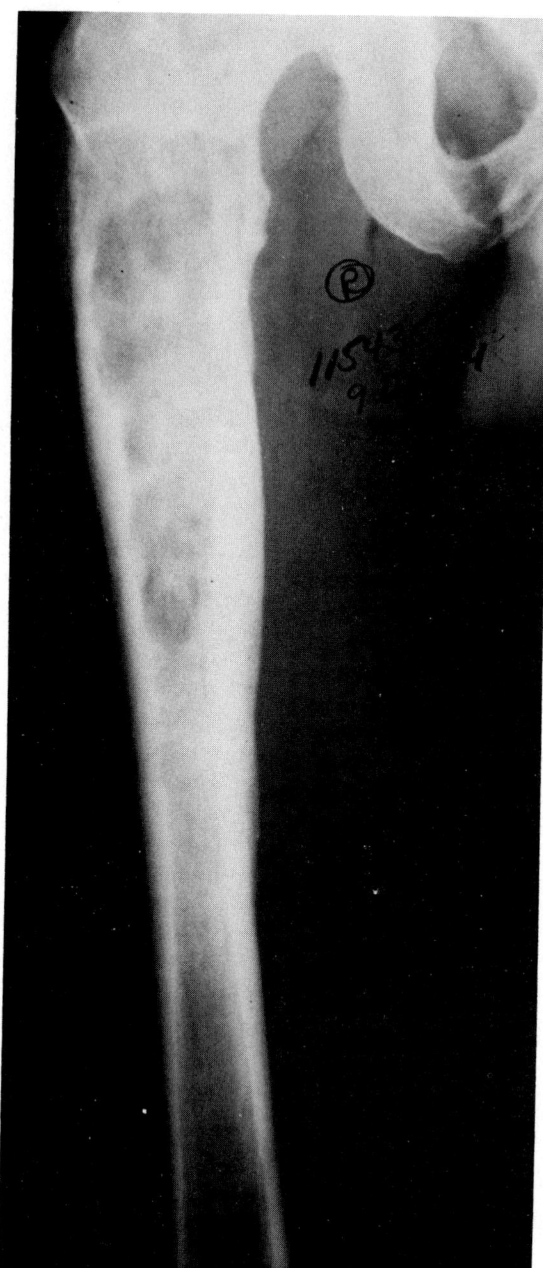

Figure 11–97. Aggressive enchondroma, femur.

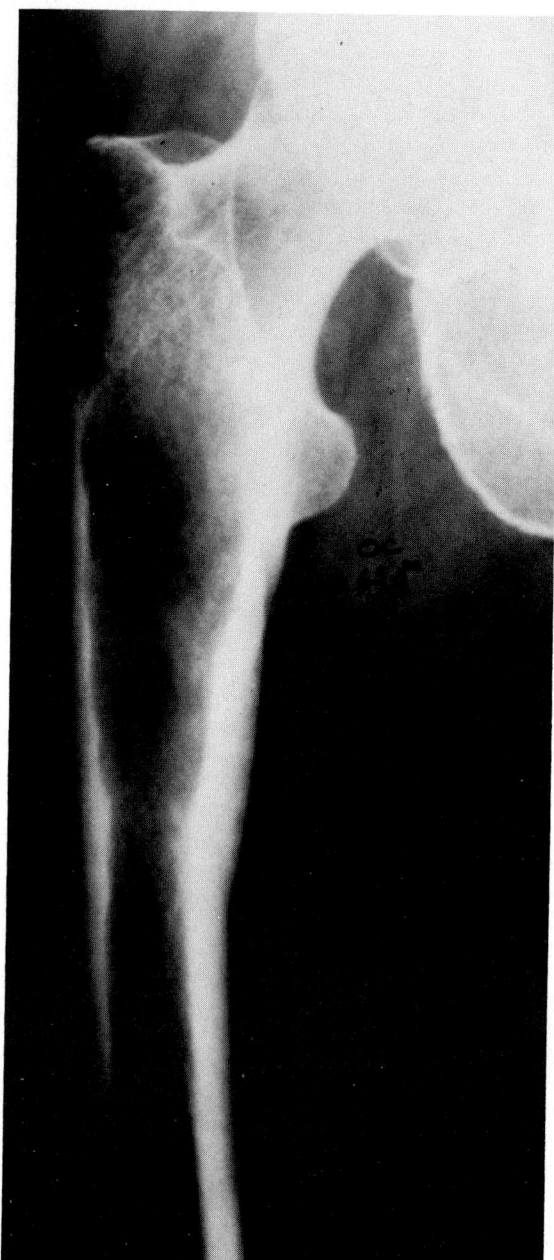

Figure 11–98. Chondrosarcoma, femur.

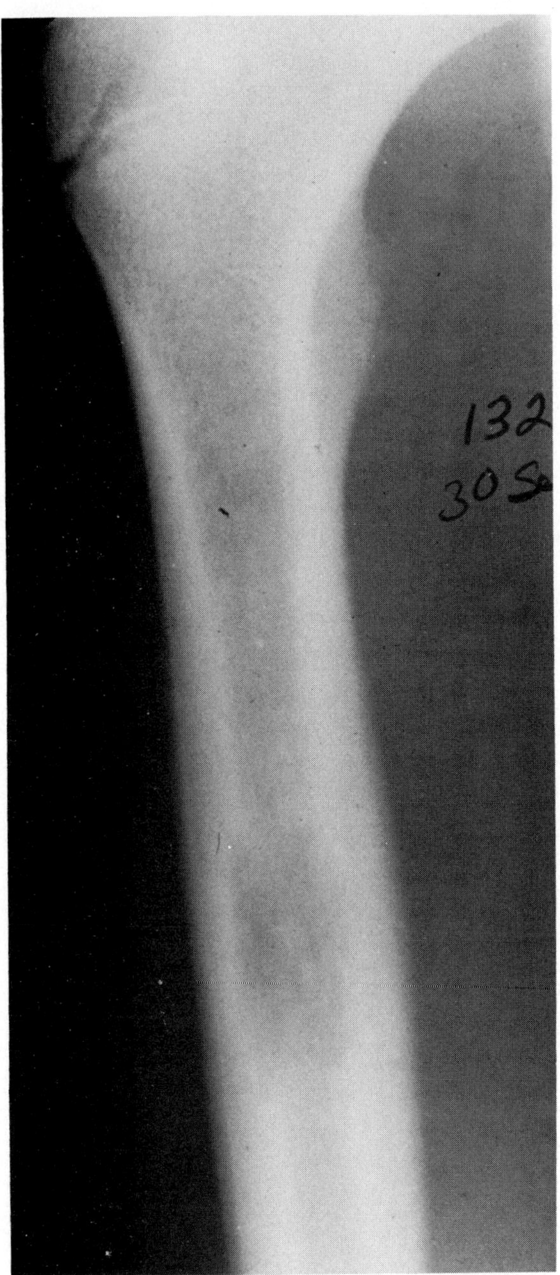

Figure 11–99. Eosinophilic granuloma, femur.

Series 37: Aggressive enchondroma vs. chondrosarcoma vs. eosinophilic granuloma, femur. The large expansile lesion with flocculent calcified matrix and rounded lobular surfaces causing endosteal scalloping are signs of a cartilage lesion. Cortical thickening and erosions indicate periosteal reaction and a relatively aggressive growth pattern. The histology, however, is benign.

The chondrosarcoma has fewer radiographic features that suggest malignant diagnosis, but the clinical symptoms of increasing pain and the histology indicate the malignant diagnosis. The water density and lack of calcification is consistent with the gross and histologic finding of predominant myxoid matrix.

The eosinophilic granuloma presents as an oval, lytic, intramedullary defect with endosteal resorption of cortex and periosteal stimulation to cause localized expansion and cortical thickening. These changes are consistent with the low-grade reactivity of an eosinophilic granuloma.

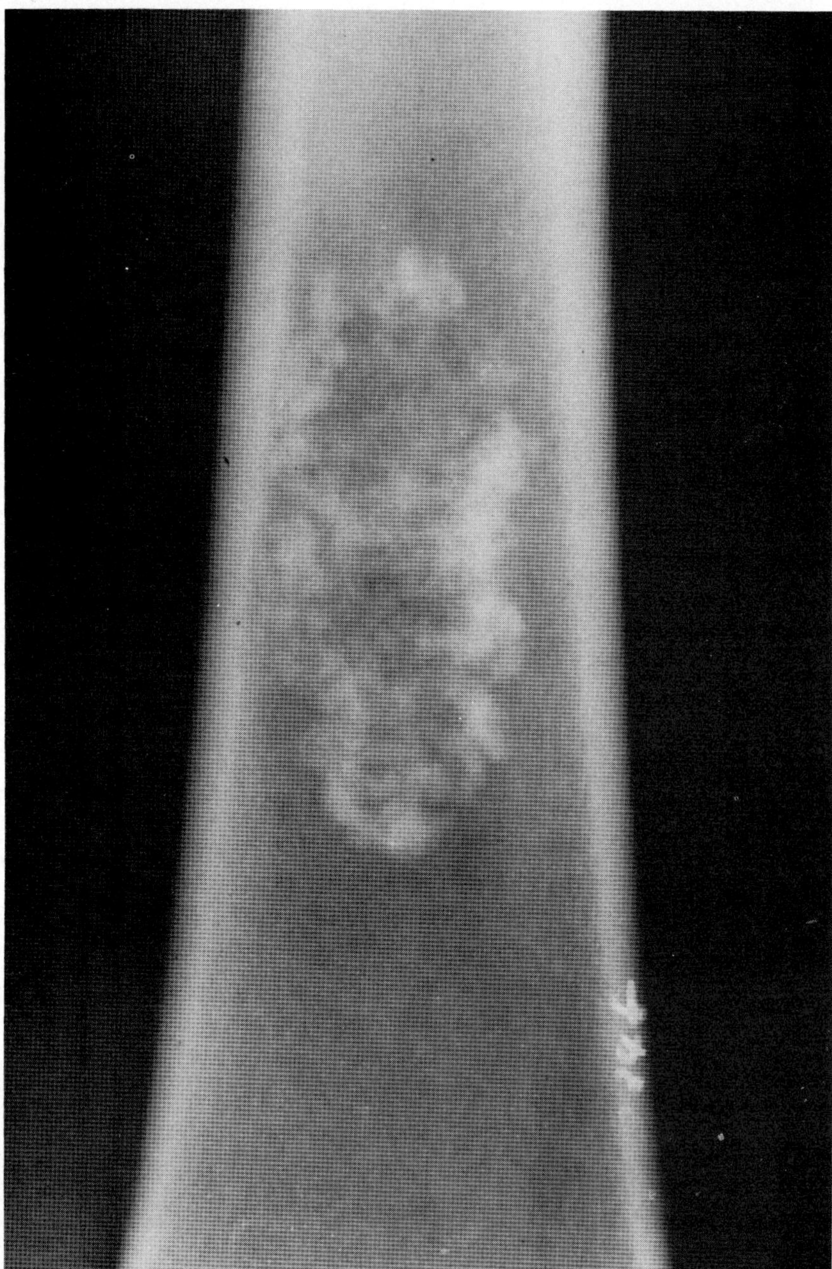

Figure 11–100. Enchondroma, femur.

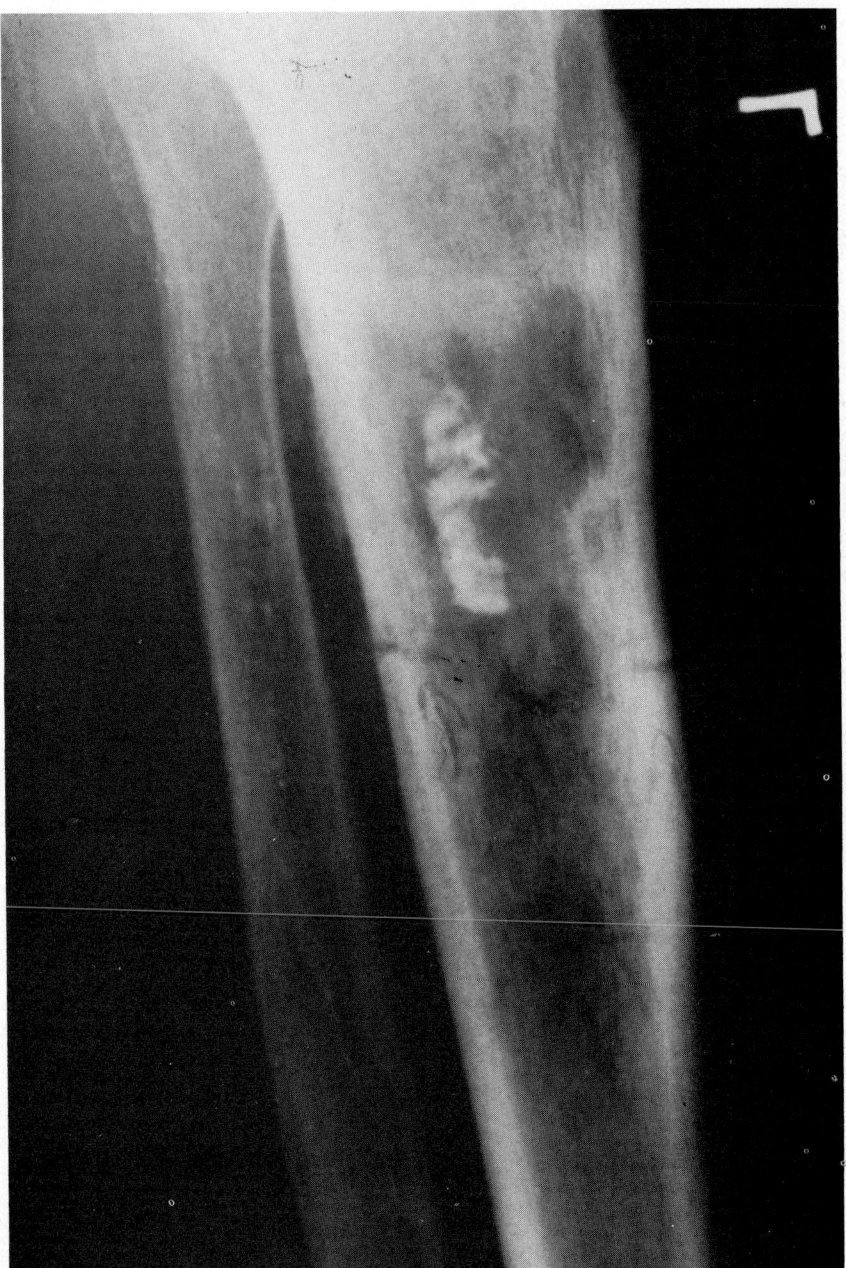

Figure 11–101. Chondrosarcoma, tibia.

Series 38: Enchondroma, femur vs. chondrosarcoma, tibia. The well-defined, clearly marginated lesion with flocculent calcification throughout the matrix proves the diagnosis of benign chondroma. Lack of response by bone around the lesion is consistent with a negative bone scan.

The tibial lesion has an irregular, densely calcified matrix within a larger, poorly defined radiolucent lesion. There is a pathologic fracture of undetermined age. Permeative resorption of the cortex, periosteal reactive new bone, and a fading, indistinct margin are consistent with chondrosarcoma arising in enchondroma.

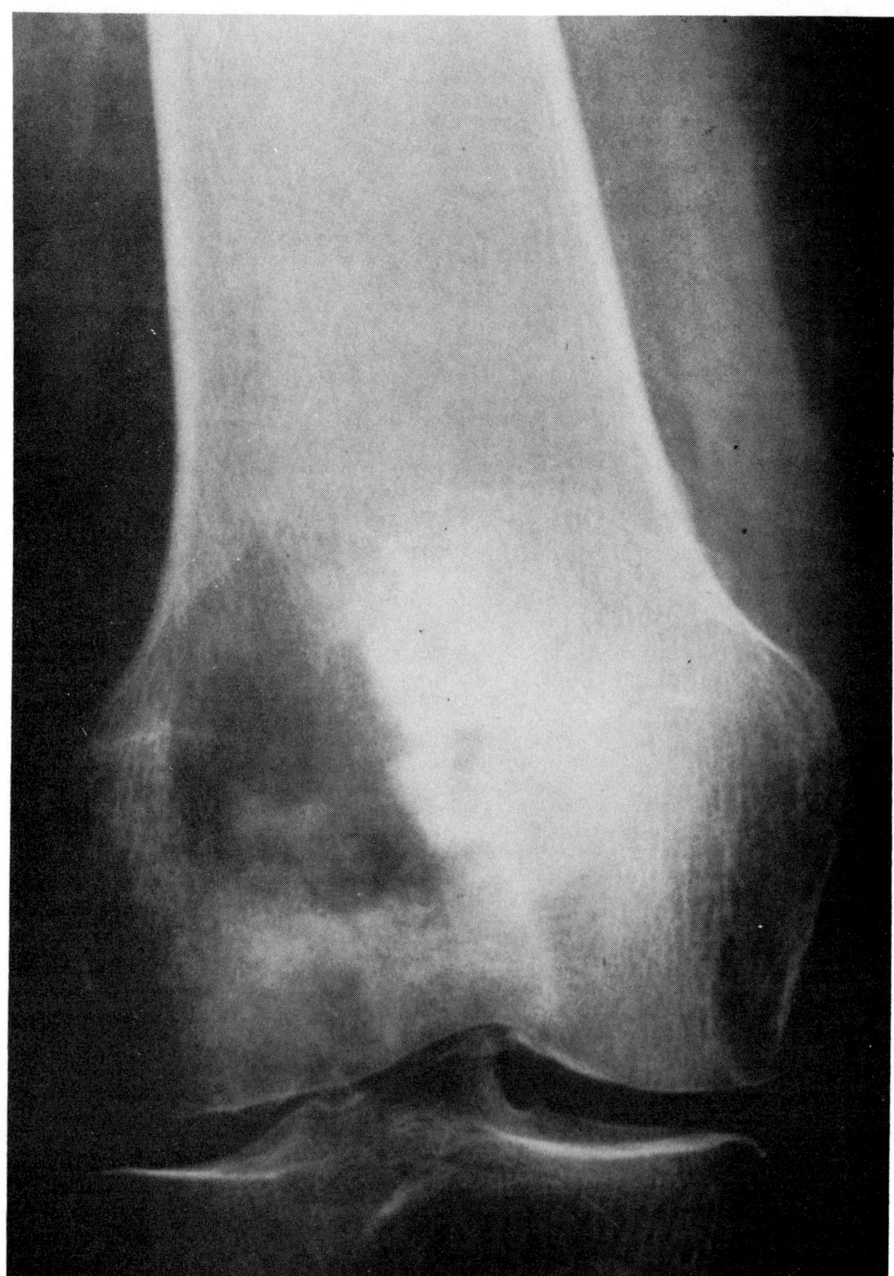

Figure 11–102. Chondrosarcoma, femur.

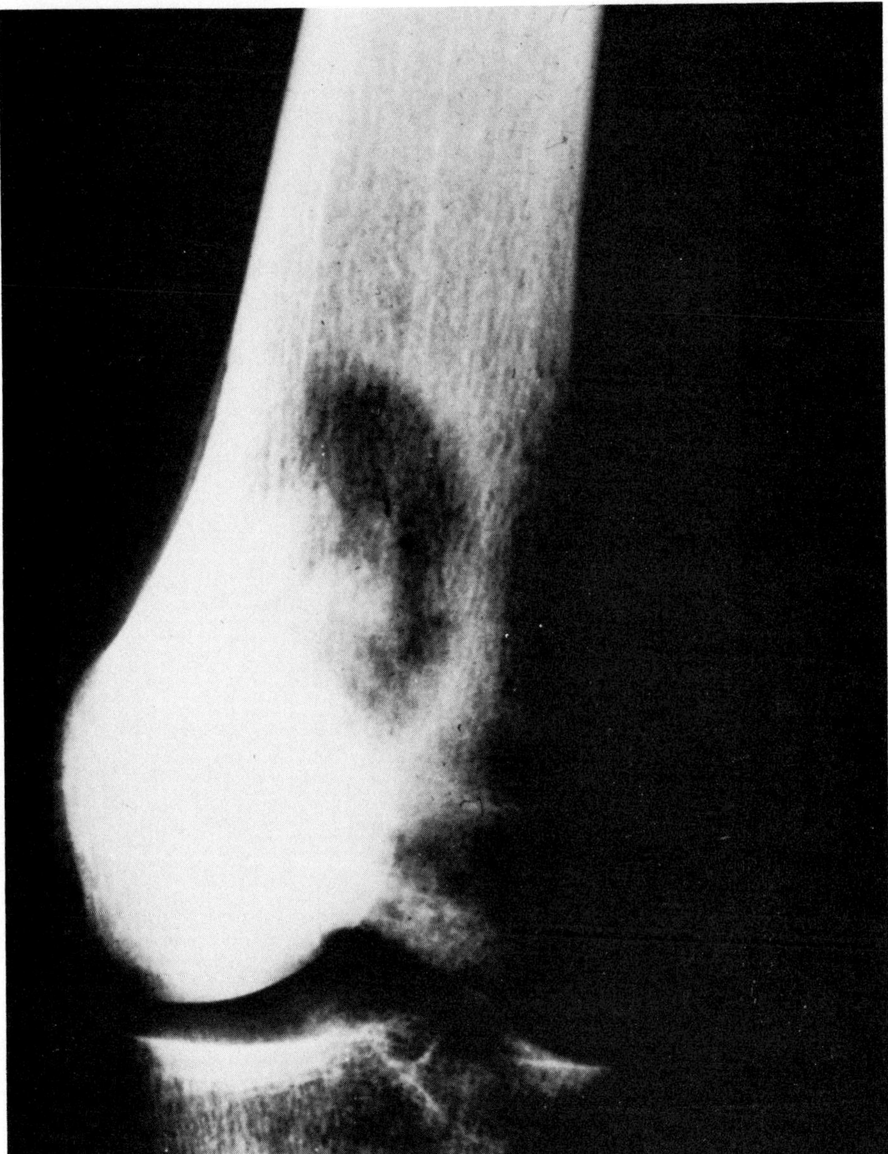

Figure 11–103. Osteosarcoma, femur.

Series 39: Chondrosarcoma vs. osteosarcoma, femur. Both lesions exhibit large osteolytic areas with poorly defined margins and extensive mineralized portions. The large size and destructive nature of the lesions with periosteal reaction are consistent with malignancy. The dense structureless matrix calcification suggests calcified cartilage, whereas the less dense mineral with pattern of trabecular reinforcement is more typical of bone.

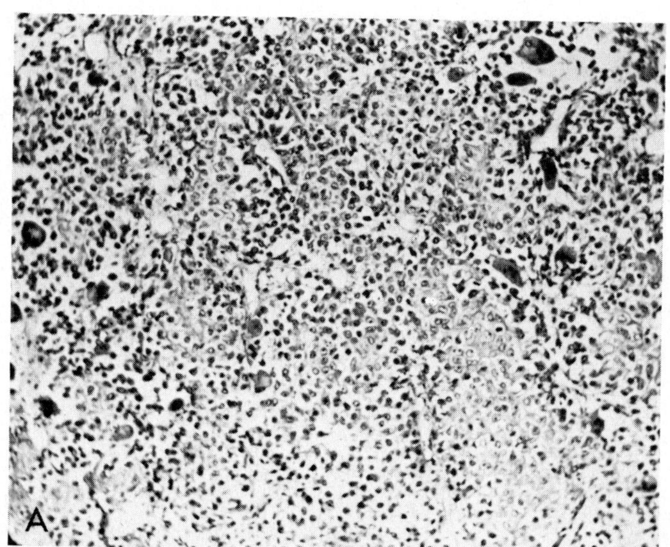

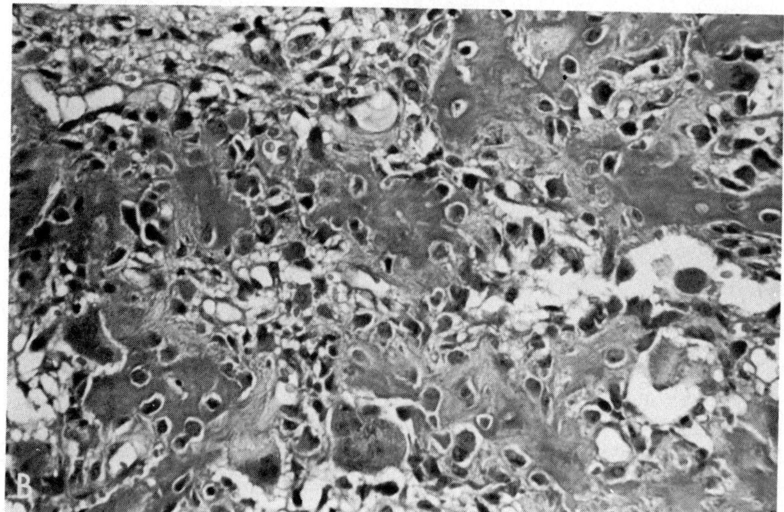

Figure 11–104. Osteoblastoma.

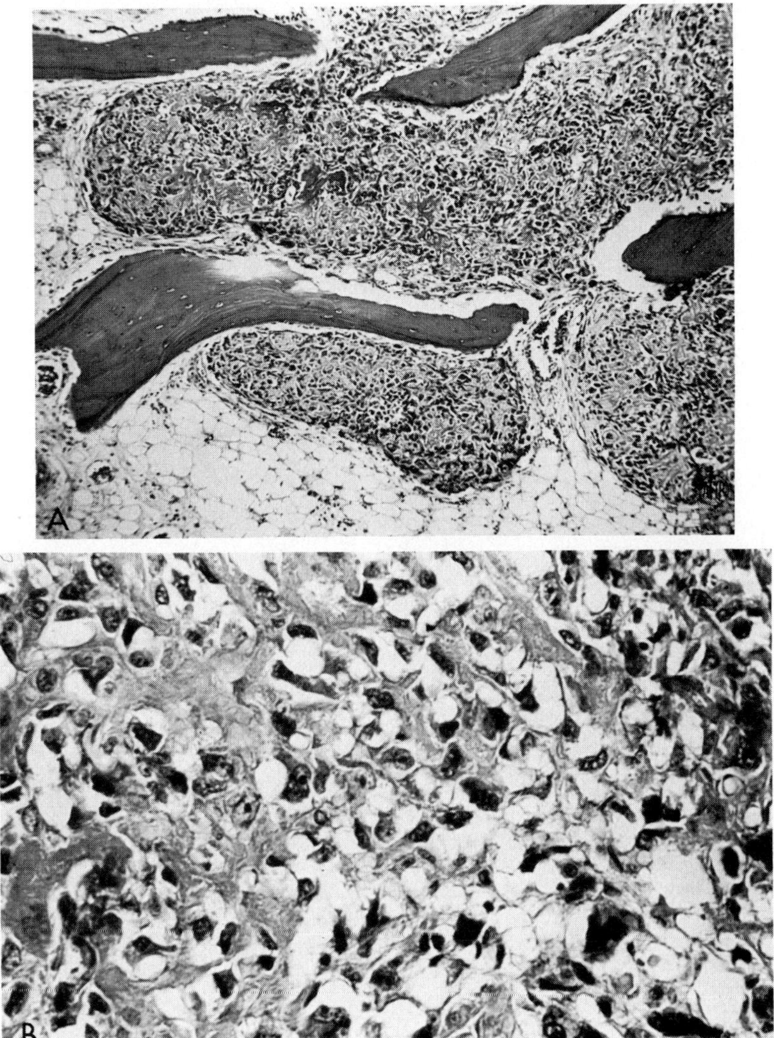

Figure 11–105. Osteosarcoma.

Series 40: Osteoblastoma vs. osteosarcoma. The osteosarcoma exhibits a fine, lacelike osteoid formation, with numerous, markedly pleomorphic osteoblasts. The osteoblastoma exhibits fairly uniform epithelioid osteoblasts forming osteoid. Neoplastic cartilage may be present in osteosarcoma, but not in osteoblastoma. The infiltrative growth pattern between trabecula of the marrow cavity indicates osteosarcoma.

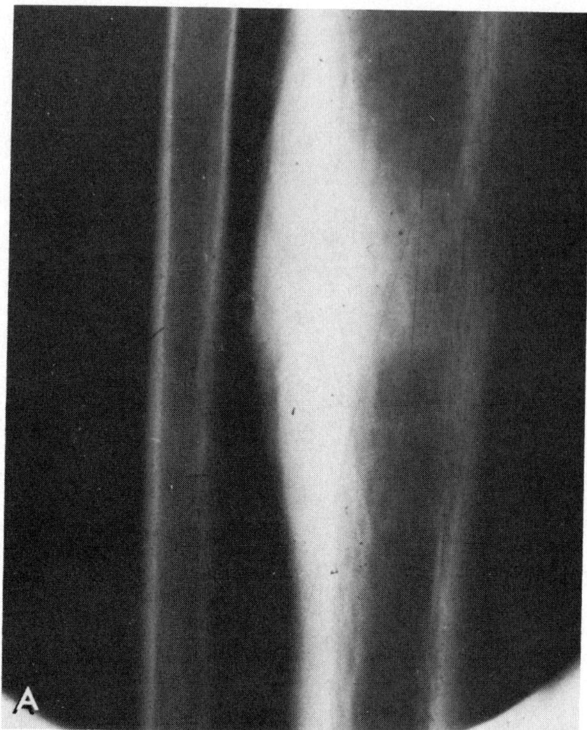

Figure 11–106. Osteoid osteoma.

Illustration continued on page 752

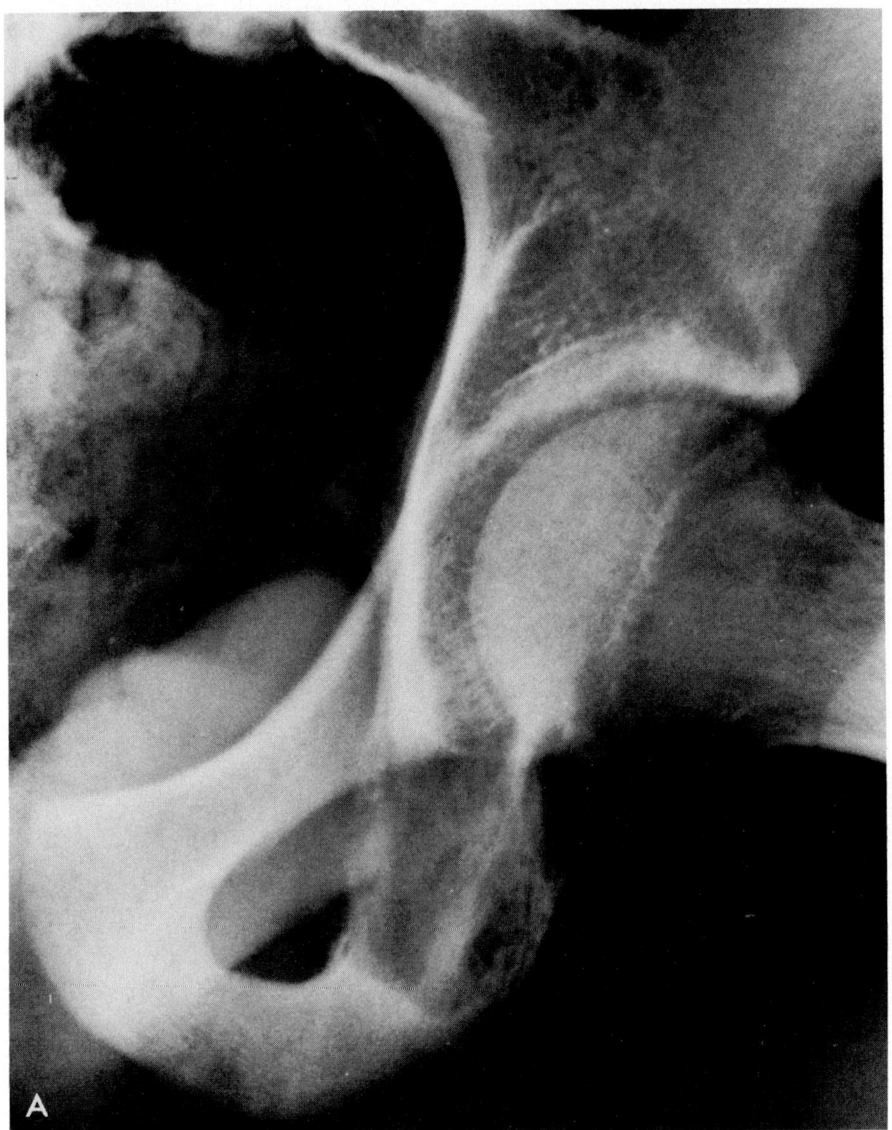

Figure 11–107. Osteoblastoma.

Illustration continued on page 753

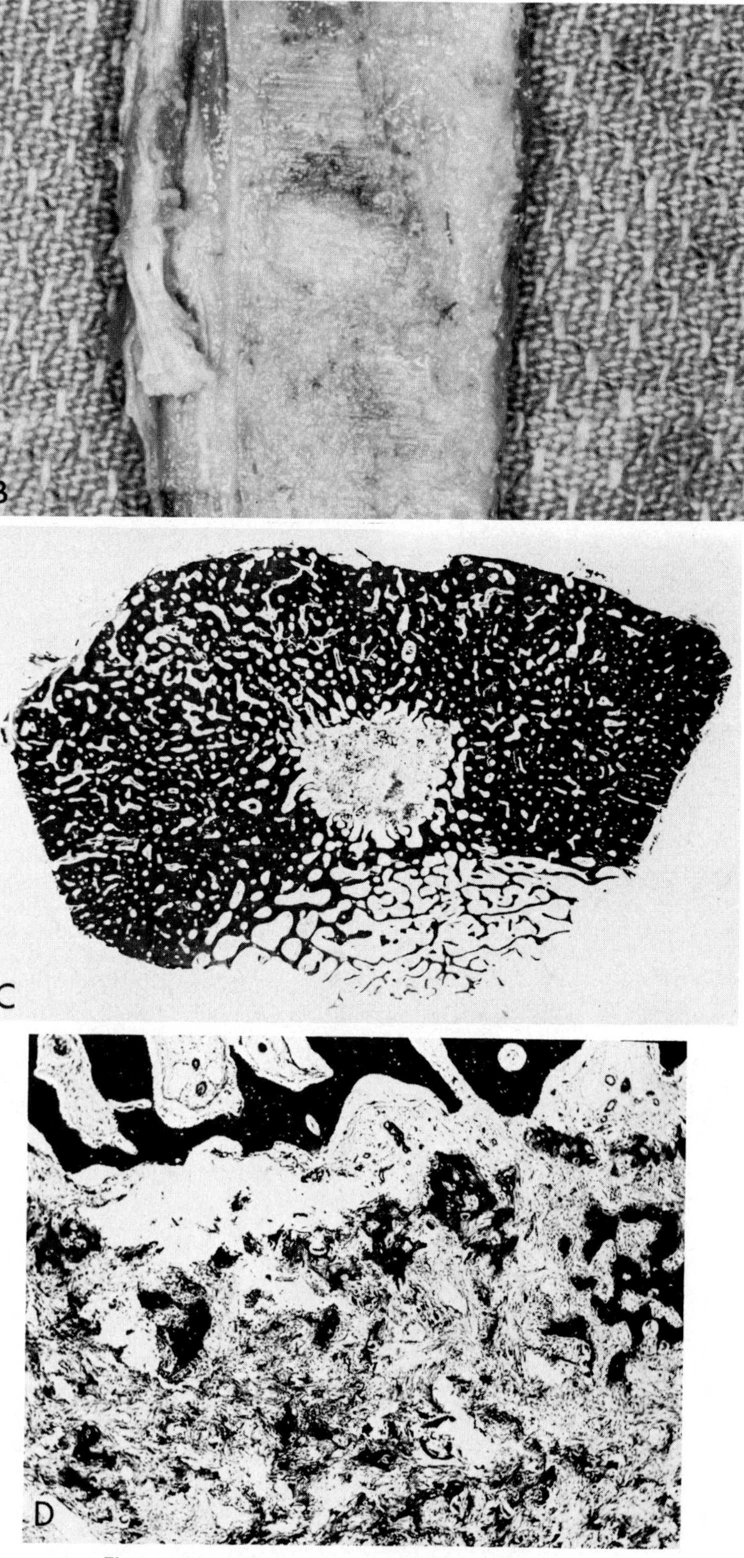

Figure 11–106 *Continued.* Osteoid osteoma.

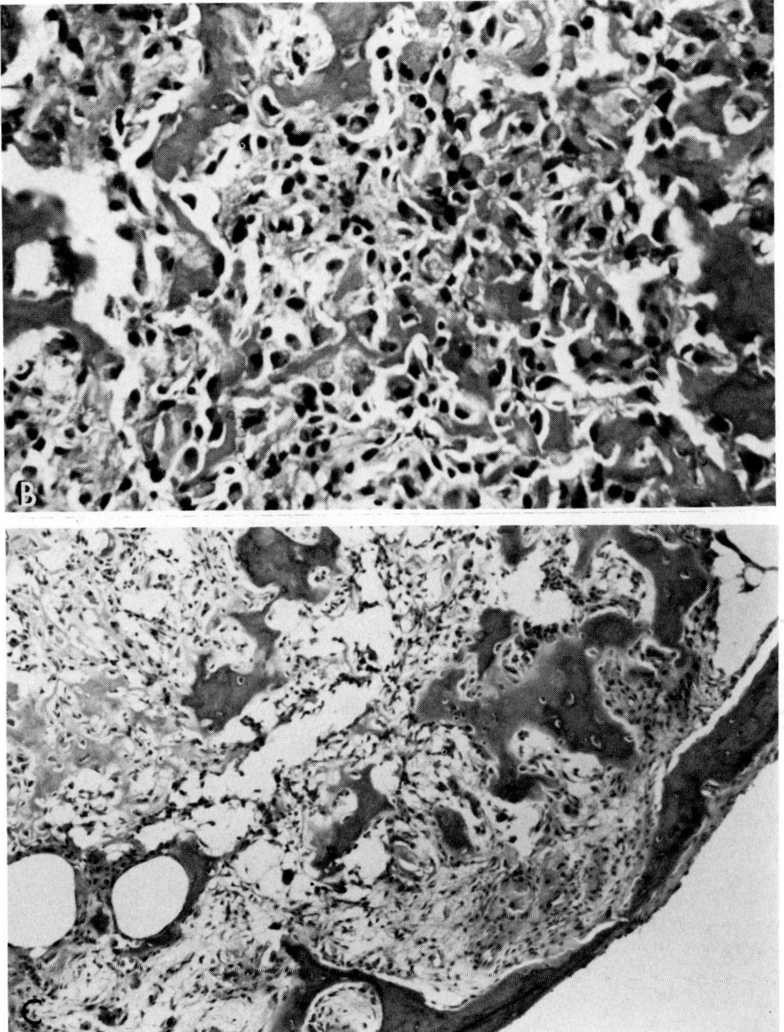

Figure 11–107 *Continued.* Osteoblastoma.

Series 41: Osteoid osteoma vs. osteoblastoma. The osteoid osteoma consists of a nidus with neoplastic osteoid formation surrounded by a dense sclerotic rim of bone with extensive reinforcement. In contrast, the osteoblastoma extends to the margin of the lesion without any rim of reinforced bone. Higher magnification of the osteoid osteoma reveals uniform osteoblasts with extensive cytoplasm, occasional multinucleated giant cells, and numerous vascular spaces. The osteoblastoma is similar, exhibiting numerous osteoblasts and well-formed osteoid. The nidus of an osteoid osteoma should not be larger than 1 cm in diameter.

CITED REFERENCES

Mankin, H. J., Lange, T. A., and Spanier, S. S.: The hazards of biopsy in patients with malignant primary bone and soft tissue tumors. J. Bone Joint Surg. 64A:1121, 1982.
Simon, M. A.: Biopsy of musculoskeletal tumors. J. Bone Joint Surg. 64A:1253, 1982.

CHAPTER ELEVEN
INDEX

Index